Handbuch der experimentellen Pharmakologie

Handbook of Experimental Pharmacology

Heffter-Heubner New Series

Vol. XXIII

Springer-Verlag Berlin Heidelberg GmbH 1968

Neurohypophysial Hormones and Similar Polypeptides

Contributors

W. Bargmann · P. J. Bentley · B. Berde · G. W. Bisset
R. A. Boissonnas · W. Doepfner · R. J. Fitzpatrick
M. Ginsburg · St. Guttmann · S. Jard · I. Krejčí · I. A. Mirsky · F. Morel
R. A. Munsick · J. Rudinger · K. Saameli · W. H. Sawyer
E. Stürmer · N. A. Thorn · H. Tuppy

Editor

B. Berde

With 150 Figures

Springer-Verlag Berlin Heidelberg GmbH 1968

ISBN 978-3-642-46129-3 ISBN 978-3-642-46127-9 (eBook)
DOI 10.1007/978-3-642-46127-9

Originally published by Springer-Verlag Berlin Heidelberg New York in 1968
Softcover reprint of the hardcover 1st edition 1968

Preface

> *"Science has but one language that of quantity, and but one argument, that of experiment."*
>
> E. H. Starling*

The pharmacology of the neurohypophysial hormones – and their physiology too, of course – has had the unbroken attention of a relatively wide circle of investigators for some ten years, and accordingly tremendous progress has been made. To summarise the present state of our knowledge, as is attempted in this volume, is hence a justified, if ambitious undertaking.

To what, it may be asked, are the great strides that have been made in this field to be attributed? Advances in polypeptide chemistry doubtless played a part by supplying the impetus to research in this area. Nevertheless, the breadth of our knowledge could not have been widened without specific, quantitative and accurate biological methods with which to exploit the opportunities offered by the chemists. On reading through the contributions to this volume, it will be readily apparent that the road to new findings was paved in most instances by reliable quantitative measurements. It may be surmised that further progress will be made by refinement and improvement of existing methods and more especially by the introduction of new ones.

A feature of work in this field over the last decade is that it has not been confined to problems of pharmacology and physiology in the narrow sense, but has been carried forward on a wide front extending from anatomy to biochemistry, from zoology to clinical medicine. This many-sidedness of the subject makes it possible to present a well-rounded picture; and it was my endeavour, when inviting the authors to contribute and deciding upon the topics to be covered in the various chapters, to illustrate this diversity of viewpoints. It need hardly be said that this meant forgoing any attempt to impose "unité de doctrine". However the approach adopted seems to me the more attractive, more logical one. In keeping with this policy the contributions of the different authors were to attuned to each other, but no one was required to sacrifice any important aspect of his subject in favour of another chapter. The contradictory views on this or that question are stimulating and not a source of annoyance. Overlapping has not occurred to any great extent, and where two authors have dealt with the same question, they have done so in such different ways that I consider it preferable to let both approaches to the subject stand on the grounds that "si duo faciunt idem, non est idem".

I should like to take this opportunity to express my warmest thanks to all those who have worked with me, as authors of the individual chapters, on the

---

* Lancet, **212**, 512 (1927)

production of this volume of the Handbook. If this joint enterprise has succeeded it is thanks to their competence, knowledge and application, for the editor's rôle is merely that of a coordinator.

My thanks are also due to Springer-Verlag, the publishers, who gave me every possible assistance in seeing this volume to completion. Dr. D. Maroske was kind enough to prepare the Subject Index.

And lastly I should like to voice my indebtedness to the Management of Sandoz Ltd., Basle, which allowed me to devote a not inconsiderable part of my time to the editing of this volume. I am also very grateful to a number of members of the staff of Sandoz Ltd.: to Mr. J.E. Smith, B. Sc., F.I. L., who translated some chapters and revised the language of others and to Miss Hannelore Straube and Miss Sonja Ebner for their valuable secreterial help.

Basle, January, 1968

B. Berde

Contents

Contributors

W. Bargmann, Anatomisches Institut der Universität Kiel, 2300 Kiel, Deutschland

P. J. Bentley, The Mount Sinai Graduate School of Biological Sciences of the City University of New York, New York, N.Y., U.S.A.

B. Berde, Medizinisch-Biologische Forschungslaboratorien, Sandoz A.G., 4000 Basel, Schweiz

G.W. Bisset, Medical Research Council, National Institute for Medical Research, Mill Hill, London, Great Britain

R. A. Boissonnas, Pharmazeutisch-Chemische Forschungslaboratorien, Sandoz A.G., 4000 Basel, Schweiz

W. Doepfner, Medizinisch-Biologische Forschungslaboratorien, Sandoz A.G., 4000 Basel, Schweiz

R. J. Fitzpatrick, Faculty of Veterinary Science, University of Liverpool, Liverpool, Great Britain

M. Ginsburg, Department of Pharmacology, Chelsea College of Science and Technology, University of London, London, Great Britain

St. Guttmann, Pharmazeutisch-Chemische Forschungslaboratorien, Sandoz A.G., 4000 Basel, Schweiz

S. Jard, Département de Biologie, Commissariat à l'Energie Atomique, C.E.N., Saclay, 91, France

I. Krejčí, Research Institute for Pharmacy and Biochemistry, Praha, ČSSR

I. A. Mirsky, Department of Clinical Science, University of Pittsburgh, Pittsburgh, Pa., 15213, U.S.A.

F. Morel, Département de Biologie, Commissariat à l'Energie Atomique, C.E.N., Saclay, 91, France

R.A. Munsick, Department of Obstetrics and Gynecology, School of Medicine, The University of New Mexico, Albuquerque, New Mexico, 87106, U.S.A.

J. Rudinger, Institute of Organic Chemistry and Biochemistry, Czechoslovak Academy of Science, Praha, ČSSR

K. Saameli, Medizinisch-Biologische Forschungslaboratorien, Sandoz A.G., 4000 Basel, Schweiz

W.H. Sawyer, Department of Pharmacology, College of Physicians and Surgeons of Columbia University, New York, N.Y., 10032, U.S.A.

E. Stürmer, Medizinisch-Biologische Forschungslaboratorien, Sandoz A.G., 4000 Basel, Schweiz

N.A. Thorn, Institute of Medical Physiology C, University of Copenhagen, København, Denmark

H. Tuppy, Institut für Biochemie, Universität Wien, 1090 Wien, Österreich

Neurohypophysis. Structure and Function

W. BARGMANN*

With 28 Figures

In the customary sense, the neurohypophysis is the posterior lobe (neural lobe) of the hypophysis (Fig. 1) situated together with the main substance of the adenohypophysis in the pituitary fossa of the sphenoid bone. Actually the posterior lobe is only a part of that portion of the hypothalamus which is to be defined as the neurohypophysis. For embryological and topographical reasons, one should consider the infundibulum of the third ventricle with the median eminence as the *pars proximalis*, and the posterior lobe as the *pars distalis of the neurohypophysis*. These two are connected by the infundibular stem (cf. DIEPEN, 1962). Like the distal portion of the neurohypophysis, the proximal part is attached to a part of the adenohypophysis, the pars infundibularis adenohypophyseos. The three parts of the neurohypophysis — infundibulum and median eminence, infundibular stem, and posterior lobe — have a similar structural pattern. Both the proximal and the distal neurohypophysis will be discussed in this introductory chapter, as the structure and function of the posterior lobe cannot be fully understood without taking into consideration the median eminence.

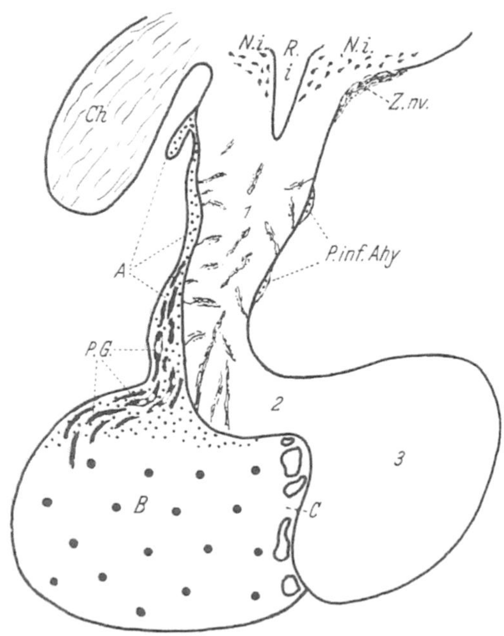

Fig. 1. Hypophysis of the adult human, sagittal section. A. Pars infundibularis adenohypophyseos. Note the terminal swelling just behind the chiasma and the slight development on the posterior surface of the infundibulum (1); Z.nv. Zona neurovasculosa of GREEN; 2 "lower stem"; 3 neural lobe; B. anterior lobe; C. Zona intermedia; P.G. Portal vessels; N.i. Nucleus infundibularis of the Tuber cinereum. From DIEPEN (1962)

It must be emphasized that the neurohypophysis does not have the character of an organ which can be isolated but rather embodies the terminal part of certain hypothalamic neuronal systems, i.e. of the nucleus supraopticus, paraventricularis and infundibularis. The quantitative development of these nuclei determines the size of the entire neurohypophysis.

Topography and morphology of the proximal as well as the distal neurohypophysis vary greatly according to the species; thus a detailed description of special peculiarities cannot be given. The experimenting research worker is referred to the literature reviewed by ROMEIS (1940), DIEPEN (1962) and GABE (1966). It goes

* Dedicated to Professor Dr. FRITZ HAHN (Freiburg/Br.) on his 60th birthday in friendship.

without saying that exact knowledge of morphological details is absolutely necessary for judging the results of experiments. This applies, for example, to the relationships between the neurohypophysis and the pars intermedia of the hypophysis (cf. p. 31).

Vascularization of the Hypophysis, Hypophysial Portal System

Since the proximal and distal neurohypophysis as well as the adenohypophysis have a close vascular relationship, information concerning the vascularization of the hypophysis and its portal system (Fig. 1 and 2) should be presented first.

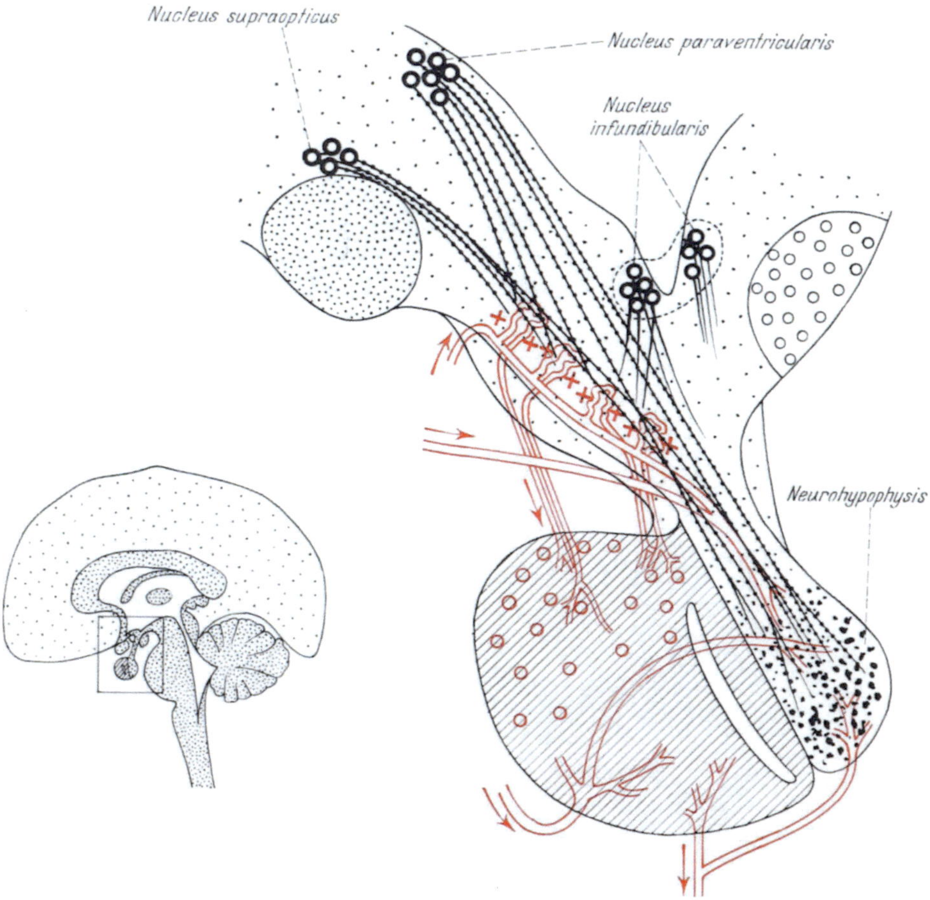

Fig. 2. Diagram of the hypothalamic-neurohypophysial neuronal systems and of the hypophysial portal system, represented in the human infundibulum and hypophysis. The arrows indicate the direction of flow, + = special vessels (capillary loops) in the median eminence. Sketch and drawing by Prof. Dr. J. VAN DE KAMER, Utrecht

Vascularization of the hypophysis in *mammals* is provided by the A. hypophysea superior from the Circulus arteriosus Willisi, whose rami, the Aa. infundibulares, supply the infundibular part of the adenohypophysis, and the A. hypophysea inferior which enters the organ at the posterior circumference of the distal neurohypophysis (neural lobe). The Aa. infundibulares form a capillary network on the external surface of the infundibulum, the "Mantelplexus" (ROMEIS, 1940), from which the so-called special capillary loops penetrate through the wall of the infundibulum (Fig. 3 and 4). The blood flows from these into the capillary system of the

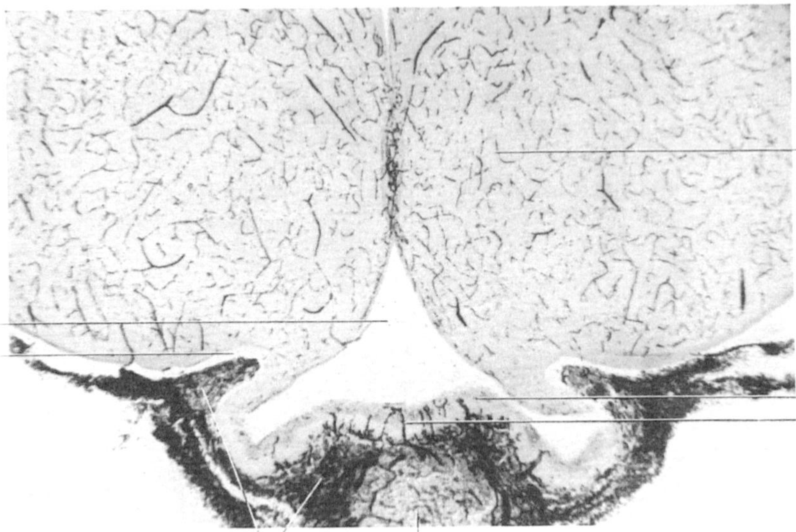

Fig. 3. Transverse section through the infundibulum of the cat, demonstrating the blood vessels, after SLONIMSKI-CUNGE (benzidine method, 22 × magnification).
Note the difference between the fine capillary network of the Tuber cinereum and the coarse loops of the infundibular special vessels. The latter are connected with the adenohypophysial capillary net or with the so-called portal vessels. Lateral portions of the infundibulum and dorsal wall of the infundibulum poorly vascularized. From NOWAKOWSKI (1951)

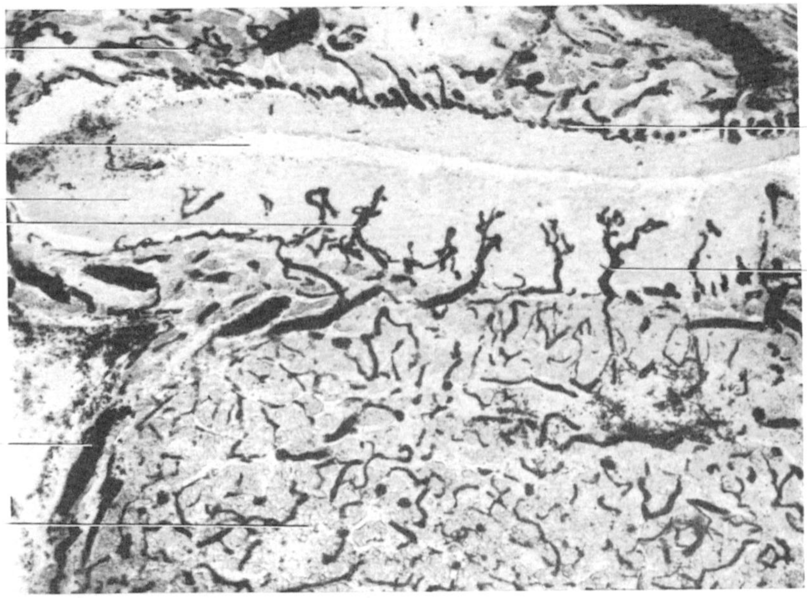

Fig. 4. Frontal section through the infundibulum of the cat (quite far caudally). Vessels demonstrated as in Fig. 3. Note the connections of the infundibular special vessels with the vascular network of the adenohypophysis. 60 × magnification. From NOWAKOWSKI (1951)

pars infundibularis of the adenohypophysis. Special capillary loops and the infundibular capillary net are the origin of wide portal vessels which direct the blood into the sinusoidal capillaries of the anterior lobe. In vivo observations have clarified the question often asked concerning the direction of flow, by showing that the blood flows from the infundibulum toward the anterior lobe. This observation does not exclude the possibility that there may be a reversal of flow within the anterior lobe (literature in DIEPEN, 1962). In some animals (rat, Guinea-pig, rabbit,

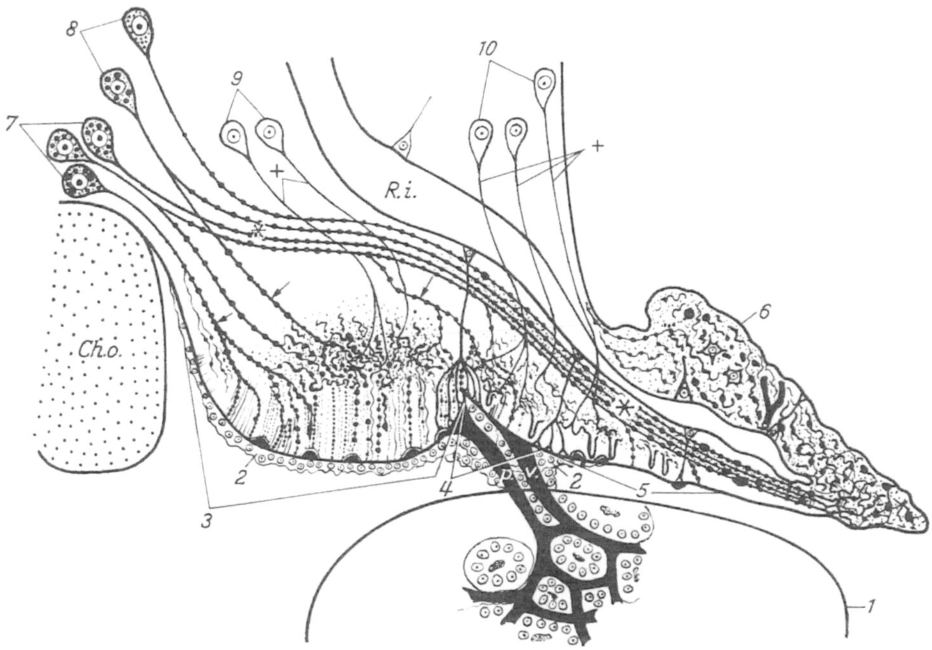

Fig. 5. Lateral sagittal section through the infundibulum and neural lobe of the white-crowned sparrow (*Zonotrichia leucophrys* Gambelii). In birds the infundibulum contains a rostral portion (3), within which in the Zona externa infundibuli as well gomoripositive neurosecretory fibers from the supraoptico-hypophysial system (+) are abundant. In addition, endings of the Tr. tubero-hypophyseus (+) are in the rostral portion: the majority of these endings, however, are located in the caudal portion (4). Many of these fibres form loops. 1 anterior lobe; 2 Pars infundibularis adenohypophyseos; 5 infundibular stem; 6 neural lobe; 7 and 8 Nucleus supraopticus and paraventricularis; 9 and 10 Nucleus infundibularis; R.i. Recessus infundibuli; Ch.o. Chiasma opticum; P.v. Portal vessels. Modified after OKSCHE (1961), from DIEPEN (1962)

cat, dog, *Macaca mulatta*; literature in DIEPEN, 1962) communications also exist between the "Mantelplexus" of the solid portion of the infundibulum and the capillary net within the posterior lobe. In the rat a communication of the plexus in the anterior and posterior lobes through the intermediate part has been observed (CLEMENTS and HARRISON, 1966). Apparently there are no sexual differences with regard to the development of the portal system (CLEMENTS and HARRISON, 1966, rat).

VITUMS, MIKAMI, OKSCHE, and FARNER (1964) give an accurate description of the vascularization of the median eminence and of the distal neurohypophysis in the *bird* (Fig. 5). The median eminence and the posterior lobe receive their blood supply from the A. infundibularis, an anterior ramus of the A. carotis interna. As Fig. 5 shows, the A. infundibularis divides into an anterior primary capillary plexus in the region of the median eminence. Portal vessels extend from here, which spread into the cephalic lobe of the adenohypophysis. Secondly the A. infundibularis forms a posterior primary capillary plexus in the posterior part of the median eminence. This posterior capillary plexus leads into a posterior group of portal vessels, which penetrate the caudal region of the adenohypophysis. Finally from the A. infundibularis an artery extends, which, on one hand, participates in forming the posterior primary capillary plexus in the caudal part of the median eminence, and on the other hand supplies the distal neurohypophysis (posterior lobe). The blood from the anterior and posterior lobes flows through the sinus cavernosus system and the Vv. caroticae to the V. jugularis. There is no communication between the venous capillaries of the posterior lobe and the sinusoids of the anterior

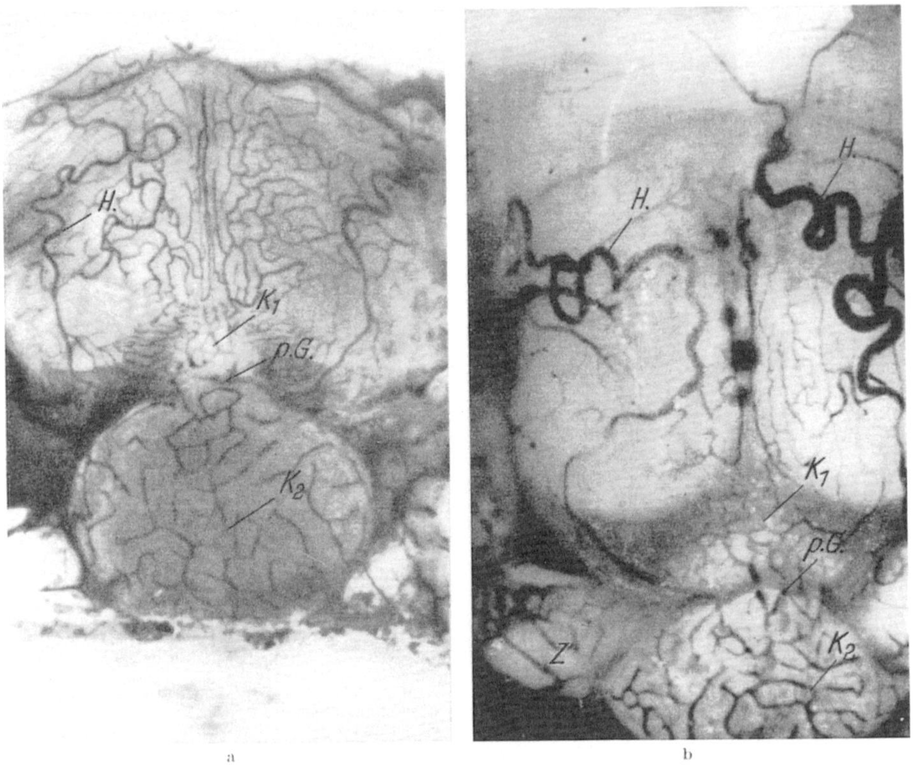

a b

Fig. 6a and b. Injection of the hypophysial vascular system of *Rana temporaria* with india ink-gelatine. Basal view of the hypothalamus and the anterior lobe of the hypophysis. Ca. 30× magnification. a: H. Hypophysial branch of the hypothalamic artery; K_1 primary capillary network over the median eminence; p.G. portal vessels; K_2 sinusoidal capillaries in the Pars distalis adenohypophyseos; Z intermediate lobe (visible only in b) b: Superscription as in Fig. 6. a. More pronounced vascular pattern than in Fig. 6. a. From W. MAUTNER (1964)

lobe. The distinct spatial separation of the anterior and posterior lobes in birds thus is manifested in angioarchitectonics as well. In addition the particular position of the median eminence in its relationships to the adenohypophysis becomes clearly apparent here (with regard to development of the hypophysial portal vessel system in birds, cf. VITUMS, ONO, OKSCHE, FARNER, and KING, 1966).

In vivo observations of *amphibians* (Anura) also have shown that the blood stream of the hypophysial portal system (Fig. 6) flows from the infundibulum to the distal part of the adenohypophysis (MAUTNER, 1964, literature and further methodological and morphological details).

A. Pars Proximalis Neurohypophyseos (Infundibulum, Median Eminence)

The infundibulum of *humans* and *mammals* is separated externally from the Tuber cinereum (Fig. 7) at the floor of the diencephalon by the sulcus hypothalamoinfundibularis or tubero-infundibularis. Its proximal part contains the Recessus infundibuli. In some species (hedgehog, cat) this extends into the posterior lobe, but as a rule it is restricted to the infundibulum. The compact portion of the infundibulum tapers off distally. The infundibular part of the adenohypophysis, the

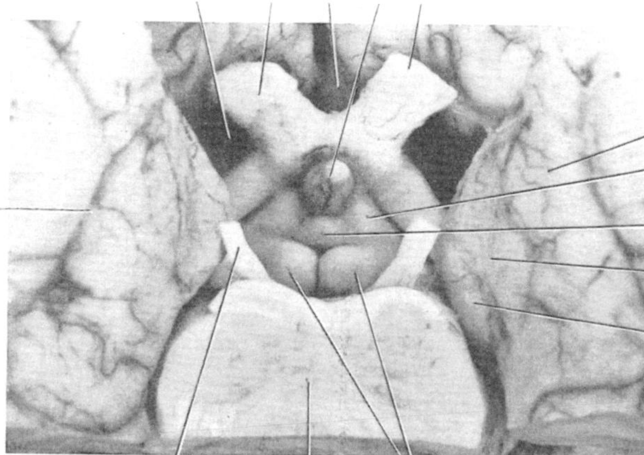

Fig. 7. Basal surface of the Tuber cinereum of the Human. Hy. st. Hypophysial stem; Em. lat. Eminentia lateralis; Em. p. inf. Eminentia postinfundibularis; subcall. Gyrus subcallosus; amb. Gyrus ambiens; semilun. Gyrus semilunaris; F. pal. neoc. Fissura palaeo-neocorticalis after SPATZ; perf. ant. Substantia perforata anterior; mam. Corpus mamillare; Unc. Uncus. From CHRIST (1951)

so-called "Trichterbelag", embraces the infundibulum (Fig. 1); in numerous animals, however, more or less large portions of the dorsal circumference of the infundibulum remain free of an adenohypophysial covering (cf. HANSTRÖM, 1952, 1953, and DIEPEN, 1962).

In *birds* a remarkably strong development of the proximal portion of the neurohypophysis has been observed; there are also corresponding characteristic angioarchitectonics (Fig. 5). Recently the median eminence of birds has attracted the particular interest of experimental morphologists (cf. p. 9).

1. *Light-Microscopy*

The proximal neurohypophysis has basically the same structure in the majority of *mammals* up to the lower primates. In the higher primates and in humans more complicated conditions are present. The architecture of the proximal neurohypophysis can be particularly clearly studied on the infundibulum of the cat (NOWAKOWSKI, 1951; Fig. 8). The wall of the infundibulum consists of two longitudinal zones, namely the *Zona interna* containing many cells, and a *Zona externa infundibuli* which, as a rule, contains a smaller number of cellular elements. The Zona externa fits closely against the infundibular portion of the adenohypophysis (contact zone). The Zona interna is traversed by the neurosecretory Tractus supraoptico-hypophyseus; this zone includes numerous glia cells (pituicytes). The Zona externa is also traversed by nerve fibers, but they are tiny and are free from neurosecretory material visible with the light-microscope. The fibers of the external zone probably originate from the nucleus infundibularis, perhaps also from the nucleus ventromedialis (DIEPEN, 1962). At the beginning of the infundibulum are situated cells of the nucleus infundibularis tuberis, which may be observed along the ventricle into the infundibular wall. The Zona externa disappears in the direction of the posterior lobe so that the Zona interna and the "nasal duplication zone" of the pars intermedia come into contact in a so-called infundibular stem. In humans an external zone of the infundibulum is only slightly developed or not at all. Here the

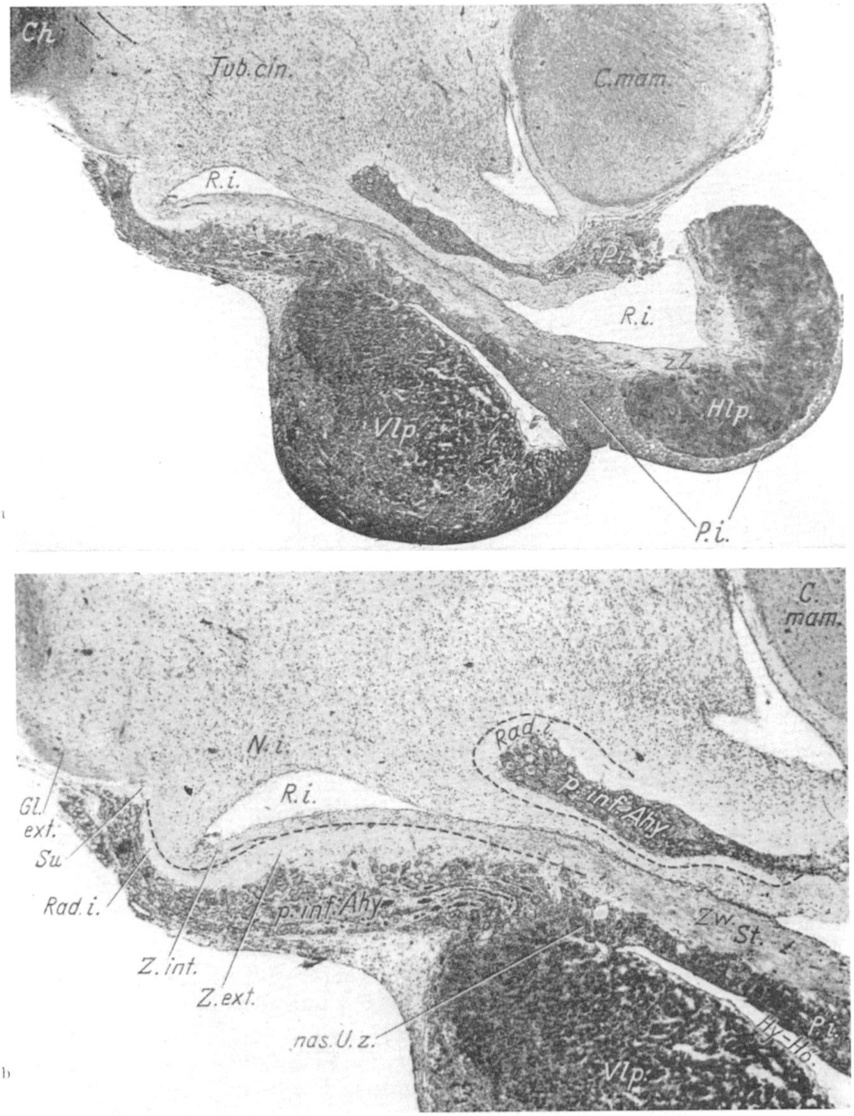

Fig. 8. a Sagittal section through the hypophysis of the cat (chromalum-hematoxylin-phloxin, 15 μ. b Enlarged section from the proximal hypophysis. The dotted line shows the border between the Zona interna and the Zona externa infundibuli. The Zona externa extends distally only as far as the Pars infundibularis (P. inf. Ahy.) spreads out on the adenohypophysial side. N.i. Nucl. infundibularis; Rad.i. Radix infundibuli; P.i. Pars intermedia of the hypophysis; Vl. anterior lobe; Hl. neural lobe; Hyhö. cavum hypophyseos; Ch. chiasma; C.mam. Corpus mamillare; R.i. Rec. infundibuli; Gl.ext. external layer of glial fibres; Su.i. Sulcus tubero-infundibularis; Zw.St. infundibular stem; z.Z. central zone of the neural lobe; nas.U.z. Nasal zone of duplication of Romeis. From Nowakowski (1951)

entire wall of the infundibulum is penetrated by the nerve fibers of the Tractus supraoptico-hypophyseus. This system is pierced by vessels which are surrounded by fine webs from the Tractus tubero-hypophyseus (pericapillary islands). Diepen (1962) discusses further details observed in the various species.

At the zone of contact mentioned above and in the infundibular stem numerous blood capillaries from the so-called "Mantelplexus" (see p. 2) force their way into the ventral wall of the infundibulum perpendicularly to the direction of the nerve fibers. These special infundibular vessels (Nowakowski, 1951; Spatz, 1951; cf. Diepen, 1962) form twisted capillary loops with an afferent and efferent limb; they are surrounded by a well-developed sheath of argyrophilic fibrils. Many of the loops are connected with the adenohypophysial vascular system, thus belonging to the portal system. In some mammals fibers rich in neurosecretory material have been observed on the surface of the capillary loops (Bargmann, 1953; Rothballer, 1953, etc., cf. literature in Diepen, 1962).

In *birds* the median eminence is developed into a storage organ rich in neurosecretory material (Oksche, Laws, Kamemoto, and Farner, 1959; Oksche, Wilson, and Farner, 1964, etc., Fig. 9b). Investigation by light-microscopy shows that the median eminence, for example of the zebra finch (*Taenopygia castanotis*), consists of a Zona interna with a stratum ependymale and stratum fibrosum as well as a Zona externa with a stratum reticulare and a stratum palisadicum (Oksche, Farner, Serventy, Wolff, and Nicholls, 1963). The stratum fibrosum contains contorted neurosecretory fibers from the Tractus supraoptico-hypophyseus and scattered tubero-hypophyseal fibers. The stratum reticulare is traversed by a network of nerve fibers from the same nuclei. The sometimes perpendicularly oriented nerve fibers coming from the stratum reticulare end in the stratum palisadicum; these fibers are rich in neurosecretory material, stainable with aldehyde-fuchsin (Kobayashi, Hirano, and Matsui, 1966; Bern, Nishioka, Mewaldt, and Farner, 1966, literature). A part of the nerve fibers reaches the capillaries of the portal vessels in the basal zone of the median eminence (for further histological data cf. Oksche et al., 1963). The significance of the glia in the median eminence is unclear (cf. Bern and Hishioka, 1965).

In the median eminence of the *anurans* numerous nerve fibers end at the capillaries of the portal system (Dawson, 1952). According to Dierickx and van den Abeele (1959) aldehyde-fuchsin-positive fibers from the nucleus praeopticus containing large amounts of neurosecretory material force their way into the Zona externa. Thus this region can be compared to the posterior lobe since these fibers enter into a close relationship with the blood capillaries (Mautner, 1964). Aldehyde-fuchsin-negative fibers come from the area periventricularis of the ventral portion of the Tuber cinereum (Dierickx, 1965).

2. Electron-Microscopy

Electron microscopical investigations reveal unmyelinated axons with granules of various types in the median eminence of *mammals* (rat, Kobayashi, 1964, a.o., hedgehog, Campbell and Holmes, 1966). Their distribution within the median eminence is not regular and differs from one species to another. According to Kobayashi (1964) and Matsui (1966) as well as Kobayashi, Oota, Uemura, and Hirano (1966, rat), one finds here 1. unmyelinated nerve fibres with large granules (90—160 mμ diameter) and vesicles like synaptic vesicles, 2. fibres with small granules (70—150 mμ diameter) as well as vesicles and 3. axons which contain only vesicles. Fibres with small granules are copious in the external zone, those with large elementary granules are scarce. The small electron dense elementary granules are thought to contain monoamines (Zambrano and de Robertis, 1967, dog), the large granules to carry neurohypophysial hormones or polypeptides related to them, and the vesicles to contain acetylcholine, possibly acetylcholine-esterase as well (Kobayashi, 1964). Kobayashi (1964) considers it possible that the vesicles in fibres with small granules contain acetylcholine-esterase and monoaminoxidase (cf. Matsui and Kobayashi, 1965). Monroe (1967) points out that small elementary granules (diameter less than 1000 Å) are characteristic for the tiny infundibular axons which end at the primary capillaries of the portal system (rat).

As Bern and Nishioka (1965) emphasize, there is similarity in the axons of the median eminence of *birds*. Typical neurosecretory elementary granules (average diameter 1700 Å), smaller granules (average diameter 1000 Å), supposedly adrenergic in type, and small vesicles of the type of synaptic vesicles occur. The authors regard the last as cholinergic vesicles. All of these particles can be present within one and the same axon.

3. *Functional Changes of the Median Eminence and their Significance*

In an impressive way, histological investigations of the median eminence of *birds* support the opinion that the median eminence is an organ comparable to the posterior lobe (Fig. 9) but reacting differently from the latter (cf. Assenmacher and Benoit, 1958; Benoit, 1964). As Oksche, Laws, Kamemoto, and Farner (1959) found, the median eminence of the North American white crowned sparrow (*Zonotrichia leucophrys*) can contain so much neurosecretory material that it resembles the posterior lobe. The amount of neurosecretory substance in the median eminence of this animal shows striking seasonal fluctuations (cf. Fig. 9). In early summer the median eminence contains very small amounts of neurosecretory substance. However, in autumn, when the birds are refractory to photoperiodic stimulation there are considerable accumulations of neurosecretion. The median eminence of birds which had been held since late-autumn or winter on short daily photoperiodes of 8 h, also in spring and early summer, has large accumulations of neurosecretory material. During June-August, with birds held since previous autumn on 8-h-days, the increase of the daily photoperiod to 20 h causes, in 20 days, a considerable increase in body weight and testicular weight (deposition of fat due to hyperphagia). At the same time there is a diminution of neurosecretory material in the median eminence. In the posterior lobe, on the other hand, the deposit of secretory material remains unchanged. Darkness effects a reaccumulation of the neurosecretory substance in the median eminence. The median eminence of male and female castrates contains more neurosecretory material in the early summer than does that of control animals. In contrast to the median eminence, the distal neurohypophysis clearly reacts to osmotic stress with a depletion of its stainable neurosecretory material (cf. also Oksche, Wilson, and Farner, 1964, *Coturnix japonica*, Oksche, Mautner, and Farner, 1964). Studies on the zebra finch (*Taenogypia castanotis*), made by Farner, Oksche, and Lorenzen (1962) as well as by Oksche, Farner et al. (1963) show that the sexual activity of not every species is photoperiodically determined, and that their median eminence and gonads correspondingly do not react to a lengthening of the photoperiod.

The findings of Oksche, Farner et al. as well as those of Dierickx (1965) which have been mentioned only in part, are in agreement with the concept that the median eminence is the site where hypothalamic hormones enter the hypophysial portal system and in this way reach the cells of the anterior lobe. This concept is also valid for the median eminence in *mammals*. G.W. Harris (1965, lit.) and coworkers have gathered extensive experimental evidence for such neurohormonal control of the anterior lobe. The substrate of this control consists of neurosecretory nerve endings on the infundibular capillary loops (Bargmann, 1953; Barry and Cotte, 1961, etc.) as well as unmyelinated thin fibres with elementary granules of the type of the monoamine granules (Monroe, 1967; Hök-

FELT, 1967). According to electron-microscopical investigations made by BRADBURY and HARRIS (1964, quoted from HARRIS, 1965), the same alterations occur

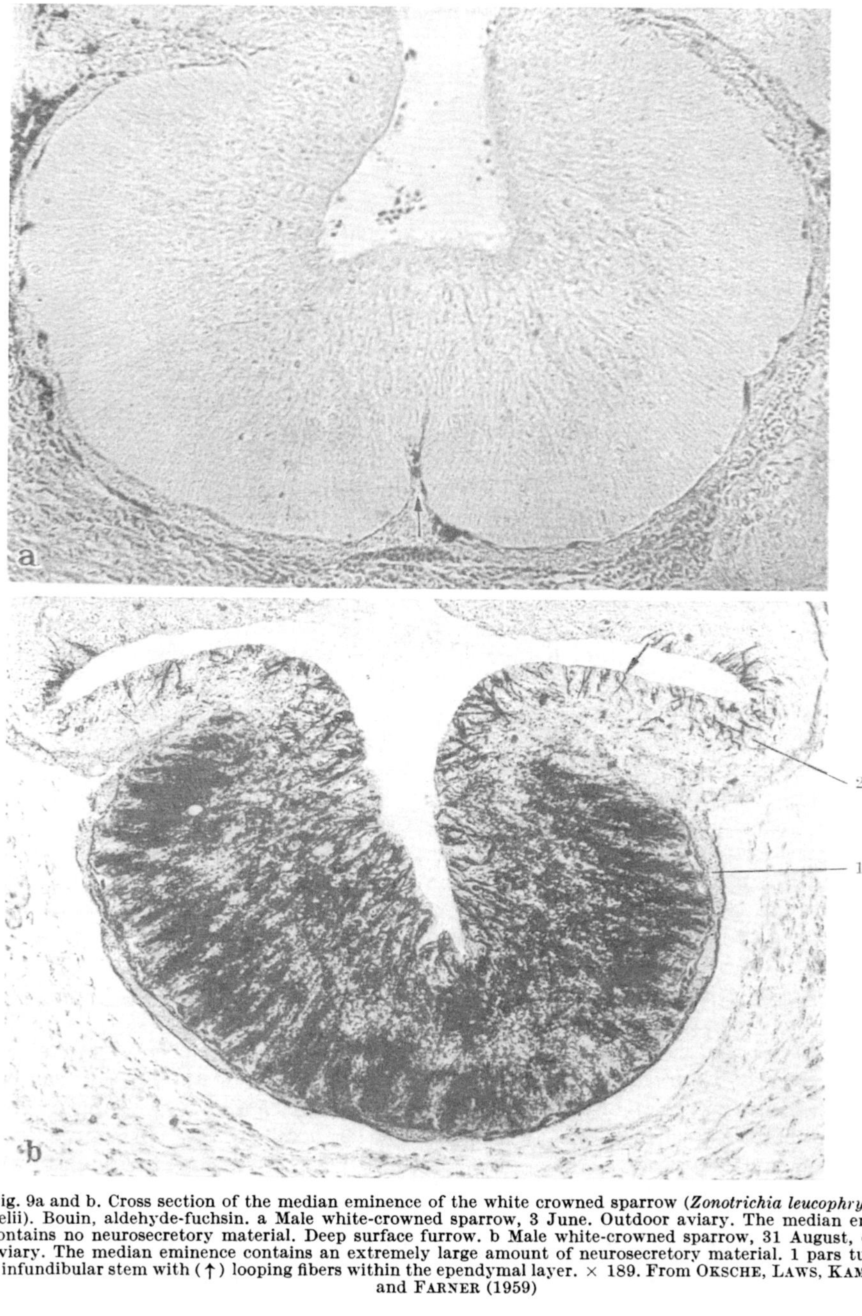

Fig. 9a and b. Cross section of the median eminence of the white crowned sparrow (*Zonotrichia leucophrys* Gambelii). Bouin, aldehyde-fuchsin. a Male white-crowned sparrow, 3 June. Outdoor aviary. The median eminence contains no neurosecretory material. Deep surface furrow. b Male white-crowned sparrow, 31 August, outdoor aviary. The median eminence contains an extremely large amount of neurosecretory material. 1 pars tuberalis, 2 infundibular stem with (↑) looping fibers within the ependymal layer. × 189. From OKSCHE, LAWS, KAMEMOTO, and FARNER (1959)

in the nerve endings at the portal vessels in rabbit's post coitum, i.e. with reflectory release of luteinizing hormones, which are observed after stimulation at the nerve endings in the posterior lobe and in the medulla of the adrenal gland.

Streefkerk (1967) is of the opinion that the infundibular catecholamines do not play an important role as releasing factors in the regulation of the adenohypophysis, since the amount of fluorescent material in the median eminence of the rat is not visibly changed under the conditions of stress and dehydration.

Findings obtained from investigation of *anura* as well support the opinion that substances are released in the median eminence which induce the cells of the adenohypophysis to release hormones. In the aldehyde-fuchsin-negative fibres in the median eminence of *Rana temporaria*, Dierickx (1964, 1965, lit.) describes the axons of a gonadotropic center in the Tuber cinereum, which is responsible for the seasonal cyclic development of the ovaries, eggs and oviducts and the development of the thumb pads in the males. This conclusion is based on the following experiment: total interruption of the nervous pathway to the median eminence and hypophysis without disturbance of the blood supply to the hypophysis causes absence of the seasonal cyclic development of eggs, ovaries and oviducts. Incomplete interruption of this nervous pathway results in correspondingly inadequate development of the gonads. According to Rodriguez (1966) the median eminence of the toad *Bufo arenarum* Hensel is also the site of release of substances stimulating the epithelial cells of the anterior lobe.

The interpretation of the structural pattern of the median eminence with regard to neurohormonal influence of the anterior lobe can proceed from the following working hypothesis: the neurosecretory fibres at the capillaries of the median eminence release the same hormones which are also released in the posterior lobe, namely vasopressin and oxytocin or their equivalents in lower vertebrates. It is conceivable that these substances reach and influence the cells of the anterior lobe via the blood stream. However, it has been shown that substances can be extracted from the median eminence which effect a release of hormones in the anterior lobe, the so-called releasing factors (RF, cf. Guillemin, 1964), but which are not identical with the octapeptides of the posterior lobe. These are polypeptides whose molecular weight belongs to the same order of magnitude as that of the polypeptides of the posterior lobe. One can distinguish between releasing factors which effect a release of ACTH, LH, and other hormones of the anterior lobe. In all probability the RF are contained completely or partially, in the neurosecretory material within the median eminence which can be traced by means of light-microscopy. There is question concerning the meaning of the diencephalic fibres with small elementary granules which are visible in the median eminence under the electron-microscope, further, of the axons which mainly contain small vesicles of the type of the synaptic vesicles (Oota and Kobayashi, 1962, 1963; Oota, 1963). If the information of Kobayashi (1964) is correct, whereby the median eminence of the frog, turtle, and bird contains neurohypophysial hormones, with a higher ratio of vasopressin to oxytocin than is indicated for the posterior lobe, one must wonder whether releasing factors and neurohypophysial hormones, both produced in the hypothalamus, are released in the median eminence simultaneously. Oota and Kobayashi (1962, 1963) as well as Oota (1963) consider it possible that a release of a cholinergic substance from the synaptic vesicles of nonsecretory fibers causes the release of neurohormones in the capillaries.

B. Pars Distalis Neurohypophyseos (Posterior Lobe, Neural Lobe)

As Fig. 10 and 11 show, the distal neurohypophysis, the posterior lobe, can have the shape of a cup-like thickening of the wall of the infundibulum (e.g. cyclostomes) or of a bulging formation. Against the posterior lobe lies the pars intermedia closely attached like a cap. In other cases there is a pocket-shaped posterior lobe which surrounds the lumen of the infundibulum (e.g. in turtles). In primates

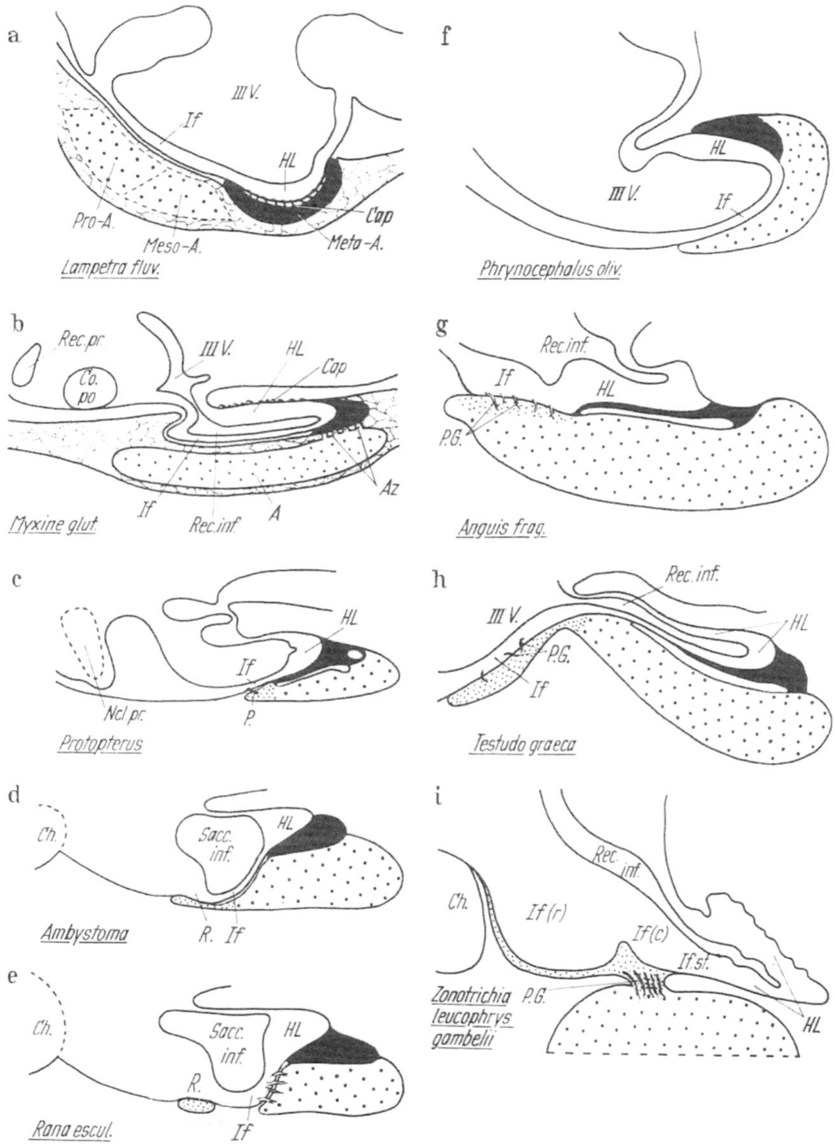

Fig. 10 a—i. Diagram of median sagittal sections through the hypophysis of various vertebrates. Anterior lobe indicated by large dots, Pars infundibularis by small dots, Pars intermedia black. Hl. neural lobe; If. infundibulum. a *Lampetra fluviatilis*. Pro-A. Pro-Adenohypophysis; Meso-A. Meso-Adenohypophysis; Meta-A. Meta-Adenohypophysis; Cap. capillaries between neural lobe and Meta-Adenohypophysis. b. *Myxine glutinosa*. A. Adenohypophysis; Az. "Auflockerungszone"; Cap. capillaries on the surface of the neural lobe; Rec.inf. Recessus infundibuli; Co.po. Commissura postoptica; Rec.pr. Recessus praeopticus. c *Protopterus*. P. portal vessels. The hypophysis of the lungfishes is much more similar to that of the tetrapods (cf. d, e) than to the hypophysis of the teleostean fishes. d *Ambystoma*. Note the Pars infundibularis of the adenohypophysis of the mammals which extends far rostrally (the neighbouring region of the infundibulum corresponds to the Radix infundibuli, R.). e *Rana esculenta*. The rostral portion of the Pars infundibularis hypophyseos is not connected with the anterior lobe here. The infundibulum is thicker compared to that of the Urodeles. f *Phrynocephalus Olivieri* (Lacertilia). Noticeably weak development of the proximal as well as distal portion of the neurohypophysis ("Sphenodontypus", Wingstrand). g *Anguis fragilis*. Infundibulum overlaps the anterior pole of the posterior lobe closely. h *Testudo graeca*. i white-crowned sparrow (*Zonotrichia leucophrys* Gambelii). If(r) rostral portion of the infundibulum (Zona externa with gomoripositive nerve endings); If(c) caudal portion of the infundibulum; If.st. infundibular stem; P.G. portal vessels. The median eminence is lacking. From Diepen (1962)

one finds compact neural lobes whose nasal convexity is always covered by a layer of intermediate lobe tissue, while the lower and posterior periphery of the organ is covered with a pars intermedia, in some cases more (*Callithrix*), in others less

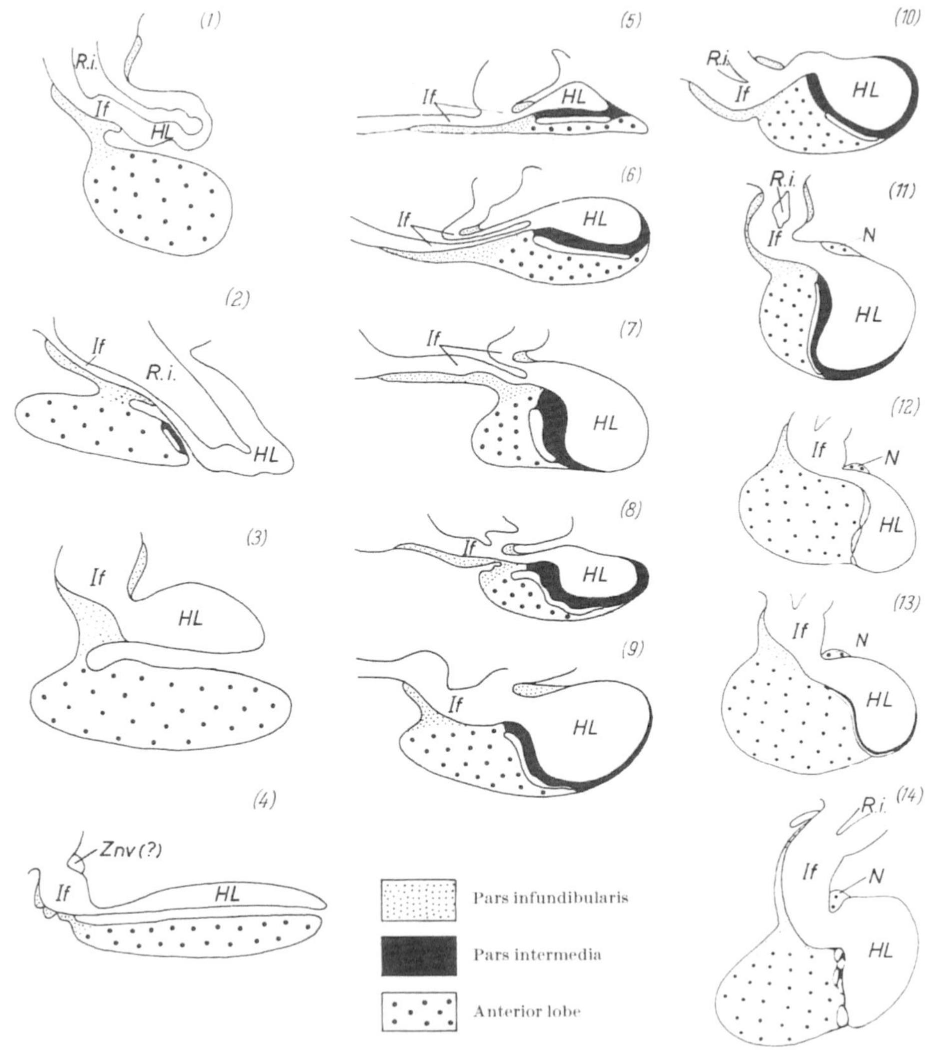

Fig. 11. Schematic median sagittal sections through the hypophysis of various animals. 1—4 Types in which the Pars intermedia is lacking: 1 Bird hypophysis, *Garrulus glandarius*; 2 *Tachyglossus setosus* (Monotremata, rudimentary Pars intermedia); 3 Whale hypophysis (*Tursiops*); 4 Indian elephant, Znv. Zona neurovasculosa; 5—14 Hypophyses from the series insectivores — *Tupaia glis* — primates; 5 *Sorex*; 6 *Erinaceus europaeus*; 7 *Galemys pyrenaicus*; 8 *Tupaia glis*; 9 *Nycticebus coucang* (Prosimiae); 10 *Callithrix jacchus* (*Hapale*); 11 *Macaca mulatta*; 12 and 13 chimpanzee and orangutan; 14 *homo sapiens*. Note the reduced Pars intermedia rich in cysts — "Zona intermedia" — in the Summoprimates (12 and 14). N. neck hypophysis (belongs cytologically to the anterior lobe). From DIEPEN (1962)

(*Macaca mulatta*), sometimes not at all (chimpanzee, humans, Fig. 11). There is no contact with an intermediate lobe in birds, whales (HOLZMANN, 1960) and in elephants. Here one finds a septum of connective tissue between the distal neurohypophysis and the adenohypophysis (cf. ROMEIS, 1942; DIEPEN, 1962).

In fish there are particularly complicated conditions. In the Selacians as well as in a number of the Teleostean fishes, combs and strands of tissue from the posterior lobe penetrate deeply into the adenohypophysis; the strands break up into individual fibres and in many cases are joined with the epithelial cells of the meta-adenohypophysis; the latter is considered to be the homologue of the pars intermedia (cf. p. 31). Removal of the pars intermedia can thus mean the removal of tissue from the neurohypophysis in some species, and obtaining extracts from the intermediate tissue can sometimes mean extraction at the same time of hormones which are contained in the processes of the posterior lobe tissue within the pars intermedia. That similar conditions are also to be considered in some mammals as well, is mentioned on p. 33.

The isolated posterior lobe of the adult human is generally comparable to a berry about the size of a pea, with a stem; in addition to round shapes, there are also club-shaped flattened posterior lobes. The surface of the neural lobe is humpy, particularly on the side facing outward, and often stands out in pronounced ridges. Thus individual variations in the shape of the posterior lobe occur, as can be seen in the investigations of Romeis (1940) on isolated human hypophyses; this also applies to animal hypophyses.

There are relatively few data concerning the *weight of the posterior lobe.*

Rasmussen (1928, 1934; cf. Romeis, 1940) gives the following average values as the *absolute weight* of the posterior lobe of the *human* hypophysis: in the *male* 117.3 mg (anterior lobe 387.6 mg, Zona intermedia-parenchyma 3.1 mg, Zona intermedia-colloid 3.3. mg), in the *female* (non-pregnant) 109.3 mg (anterior lobe 500 mg, Zona intermedia-parenchyma 3.5 mg, Zona intermedia-colloid 3.7 mg), in the *pregnant female* 103.8 mg (anterior lobe 598.3 mg, Zona intermedia-parenchyma 2.4 mg, Zona intermedia-colloid 3.7 mg). In the *male* in contrast to the reduction of weight of the anterior lobe which sets in during the fourth or fifth decade of life, the posterior lobe gains weight somewhat with advanced age. In the *female* a very slight increase in the weight of the posterior lobe occurs, while the weight of the anterior lobe remains the same.

The *relative weight* of the portions of the organ in the human male and female (average values) with relation to the entire organ are: posterior lobe 23.10% male, 17.99% female; anterior lobe 74.80% male, 80.49% female; Zona intermedia-parenchyma 0.85% male, 0.65% female; Zona intermedia-colloid 1.20% male, 0.95% female.

According to Hammar (1933; cf. Romeis, 1940) the following values are valid for the *rabbit*: posterior lobe 14.1—19.0%, anterior lobe 66.2—73.5% and intermediate lobe 10.0 to 15.1% of the weight of the entire organ.

The pars intermedia is strongly developed in a number of animals which live under conditions of extreme aridity — among them certain rodents. In these cases one must count on a considerable shift of the weight relationships between anterior, intermediate and posterior lobes in these animals. In addition the weight of the posterior lobe, the site of release of vasopressin-adiuretin, is probably quite various in animals with differences in habitat. Apparently there are no systematic quantitative investigations available on this topic.

1. Light-Microscopy

As conventional slides show (Fig. 12), the posterior lobe of the *mammals* consists of a dense felt-work of very thin unmyelinated nerve fibers, in which glia cells (pituicytes) and blood capillaries are embedded (Fig. 13), the latter accompanied by argyrophilic fibrils. Nerve cells do not belong to the regular components of the posterior lobe; ganglionic cells are to be observed in the neurohypophysis in a number of *fishes* (Bargmann, 1953; Fujita, 1963) and of the *ox* (Stutinsky, 1948). In *humans* and in some *mammals* strands and nests of epithelial intermedia cells often extend into the neurohypophysis ("invasion" of basophils, Fig. 14).

Under low magnification irregular, more dense and lighter areas within the posterior lobe are to be seen, the "Verdichtungszonen" and "Zwischenstreifen" (Romeis, 1940, Fig. 13). A particular lobulation is characteristic for the neurohypophysis of the opossum (*Didelphys virginiana*, BODIAN, 1951; BARGMANN, 1955; Fig. 15).

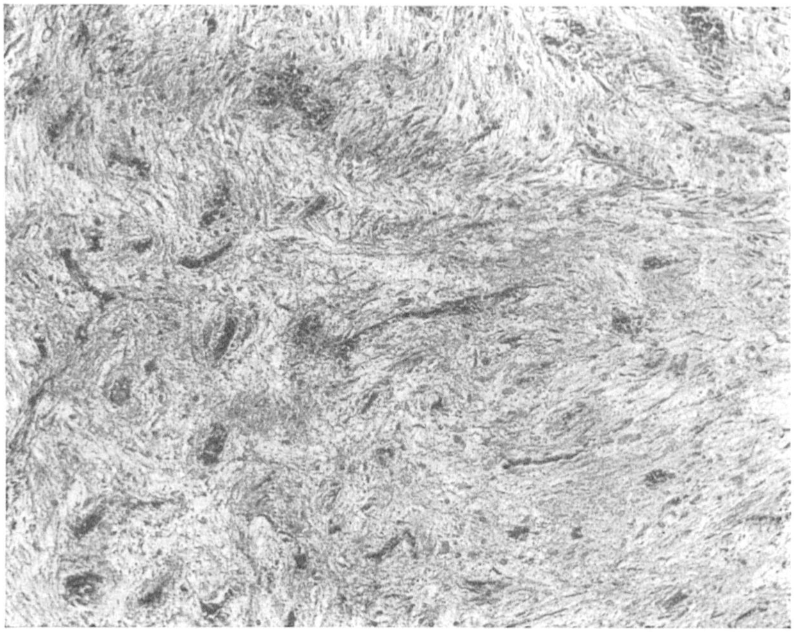

Fig. 12. Neural lobe of the hypophysis of an adult human (Susafixation, thickness of the slide 8 μ, Azan stain). 130× magnification. From BARGMANN (1954)

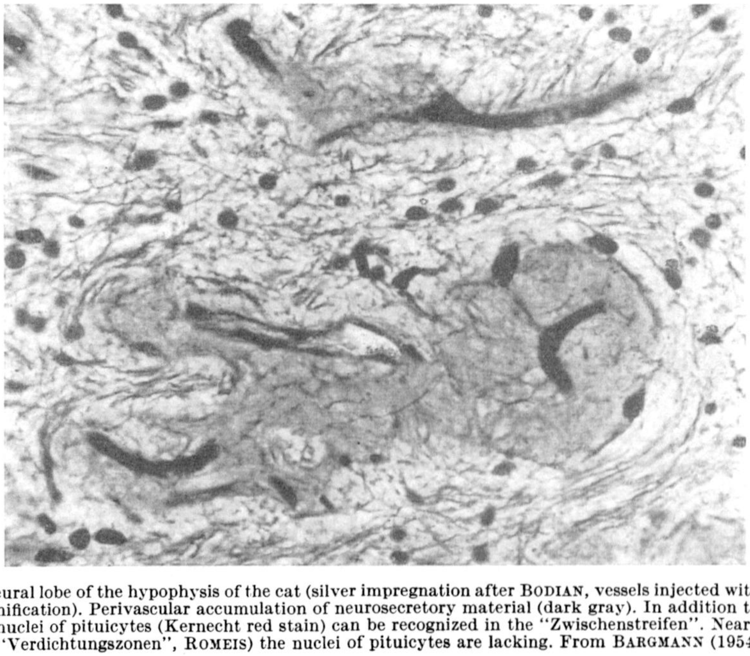

Fig. 13. Neural lobe of the hypophysis of the cat (silver impregnation after BODIAN, vessels injected with india ink, 310× magnification). Perivascular accumulation of neurosecretory material (dark gray). In addition to the nerve fibres, the nuclei of pituicytes (Kernecht red stain) can be recognized in the "Zwischenstreifen". Near the vessels ("Verdichtungszonen", ROMEIS) the nuclei of pituicytes are lacking. From BARGMANN (1954)

a) *Nerve Fibers.* The abundance of unmyelinated nerve fibers in the neurohypophysis and their relation to the blood capillaries is revealed only with silver impregnations. One can observe that the fine nerve fibres in the "Zwischenstreifen"

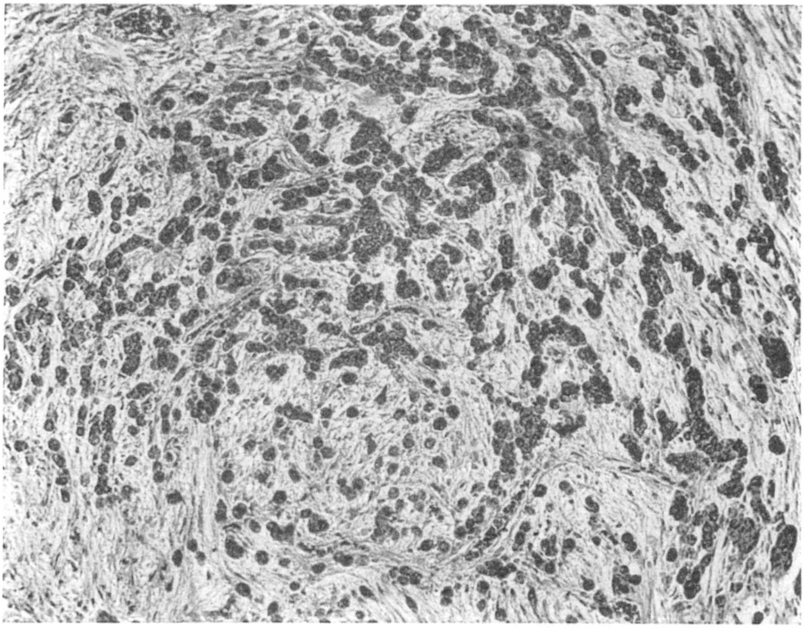

Fig. 14. Neural lobe of the hypophysis of an adult male with invasion of basophiles. (Susafixation, 8 μ, Azan stain) 130 × magnification. From BARGMANN (1954)

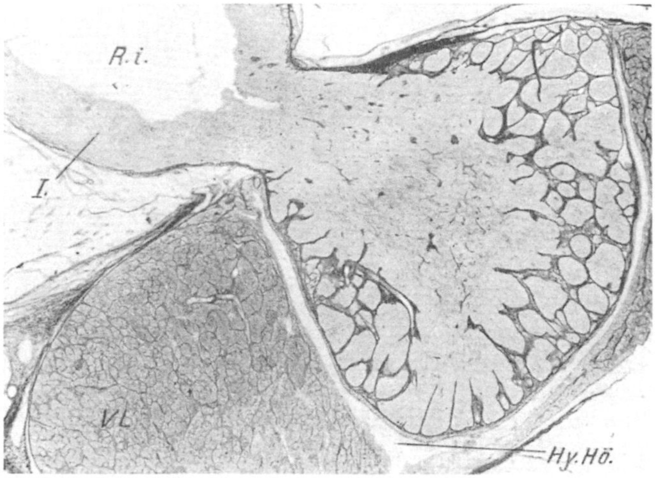

Fig. 15. Hypophysis of the opossum (*Didelphys virginiana*). Impregnation of the argyrophile connective tissue after PERDRAU, 15 μ. 21 × magnification. Lobulation of the peripheral parts of the neural lobe. R. i. Recessus infundibuli; Vl. anterior lobe; HyHö. Cavum hypophyseos. I. infundibulum. From DIEPEN (1962)

are for the most part parallelized and loosely distributed, while in the "Verdichtungszonen" they are quite tangled, often surrounding the twisted blood capillaries in a circular manner. In the "Zwischenstreifen" they accompany the more or less straight capillaries predominantly in longitudinal direction. The centers of the "Verdichtungszonen" in which the blood capillaries are situated remain light in nerve impregnations. GREVING (1925) called these areas "islands". Myelinated nerve fibers occur only occasionally in the posterior lobe (e.g. in the Guinea-pig).

The origin of the neurohypophysial nerve fibers has been revealed to a great extent in connection with investigations of the hypothalamic neurosecretion (E. and B. SCHARRER, 1954; BARGMANN, 1949, 1954), after it became possible to stain selectively the perikarya of the Nucleus supraopticus and paraventricularis and their unmyelinated processes as a *neurosecretory pathway* (BARGMANN, 1949). This "via neurosecretoria" joins the hypothalamic nuclei with the neurohypophysis. After staining with chromalum-haematoxylin (BARGMANN), with aldehyde-fuchsin (GABE) or alzian blue (SLOPER) the terminals of the pathway in the

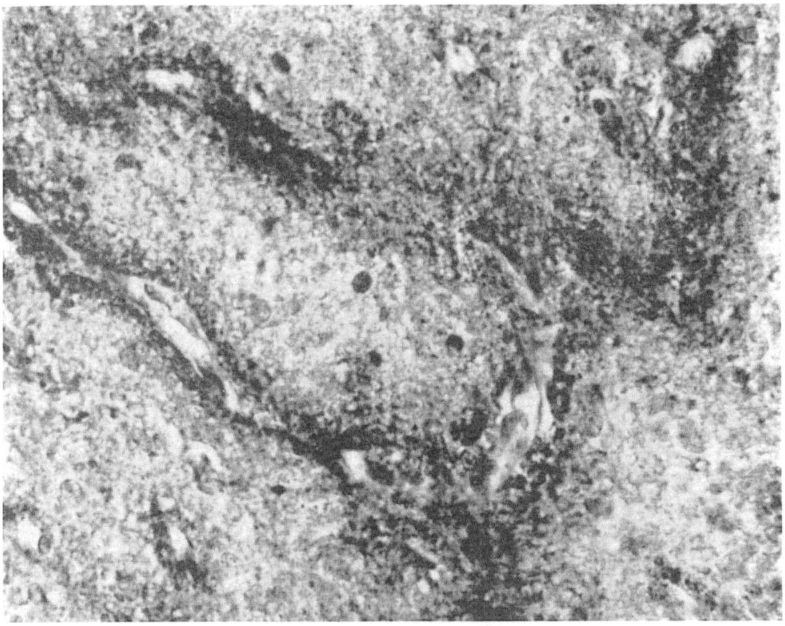

Fig. 16. Neural lobe of a cat. Perivascular accumulation of neurosecretory material. Stained with chromalum-hematoxylin-phloxin, 480× magnification

neurohypophysis appear as a felt-work which contains neurosecretory material. Thickenings of the nerve fibres, called *Herring bodies*, are filled with neurosecretory material. The pericapillary "Verdichtungszonen" are particularly rich in neurosecretory substance (Fig. 16). In addition neurosecretory material is accumulated in the immediate vicinity of the blood capillaries which are located on the borderline between the posterior lobe and the Pars intermedia. In the lobulated neurohypophysis of the opossum, the marginal regions of the lobules ("palisadic zone") are particularly rich in stainable neurosecretory material (BODIAN, 1951; BARGMANN, 1955).

The significance of the diencephalic neurosecretory system was clarified by combination of experimental morphological (cf. p. 23) and pharmacological studies. Since the investigations by HILD and ZETLER (1951, 1952, 1953) it is known that the entire neurosecretory pathway, i.e. the secretory nuclei in the hypothalamus, the unmyelinated fiber tract to the neurohypophysis and its terminals in the posterior lobe, contain the hormones vasopressin and oxytocin. These hormones are released into the blood stream at the endings of the secretory nerve cells in the neurohypophysis (cf. p. 26). Since the hormones are produced in the perikarya of the secretory hypothalamic neurons, they should be designated as hypothalamic hormones and not as posterior lobe hormones (Bargmann, 1954). The fact that these hormones are octapeptides leads Bargmann, Lindner, and Andres (1967) to propose that in analogy to cholinergic and aminergic neurons these nerve cells which synthesize these hormones should be termed *peptidergic neurons*.

Findings obtained by means of isolation of nerve endings from the bovine posterior pituitary (subcellular fractions) support the hypothesis "that a given neurosecretory cell synthesizes, stores and secretes only one of the peptide hormones" vasopressin and oxytocin (Bindler, Labella, and Sanwal, 1967).

It has not been clarified satisfactorily whether besides the central nerve fibres mentioned above the Plexus caroticus penetrates into the distal neurohypophysis (Romeis, 1940).

b) *Pituicytes.* Bucy (1930, 1932) described glia cells provided with processes within the posterior lobe of cattle, the pituicytes. Romeis (1940) succeeded in demonstrating at least four various types of these elements and their transitional stages in the human posterior lobe. Romeis speaks on one hand of *reticulocytes*, forming a three-dimensional network, cells which are rich in cytoplasm, and further of *micropituicytes*, small isolated elements presenting a ragged appearance. The *fibropituicytes* also occur isolated and are noticeable because of their size and the length of their thin processes. The *adenopituicytes*, which are sometimes isolated and sometimes in groups, resemble glandular cells; the cytoplasm of these glial elements is often vacuolized. All pituicytes, primarily the fibropituicytes, can contain granules of lipofuscin, particularly in advanced age. The occurrence of extremely tiny granules and vacuoles in the cytoplasm of the pituicytes causes Romeis to assume a secretory activity of all types of these cells. Since up till now there has been no systematic investigation concerning the morphology of the pituicytes of other species, the question is open whether the findings of Romeis are valid only for the posterior lobe of humans. Stutinsky (1957, lit.) described different types of pituicytes of mammals.

The relationships of the pituicytes to the terminals of the unmyelinated nerve fibres in the posterior lobe have been elucidated to a certain degree electron-microscopically (cf. p. 19). *Mitoses* of the pituicytes have been observed by many investigators. According to Ortmann (1951, lit.; also Diepen, 1962, lit.) they are numerous enough to mention only when the amount of neurosecretory material has been considerably reduced following stress of the diencephalic neurosecretory system. Ortmann (1951) considers the individual fluctuation scale of the number of mitoses (rat) to be considerable.

c) *Epithelial Cells in the Posterior Lobe.* In the posterior lobe of the human hypophysis there are often webs and strands of basophilic epithelial cells which originate in the Pars intermedia (Romeis, 1940, Fig. 14). Such an invasion of basophils is observed primarily in older individuals. According to Hanström (1948, 1950, 1952, 1953, literature in Diepen, 1962) this invasion also occurs to a greater or lesser extent in mammals, including anthropomorphs. As Bargmann and Knoop (1960) emphasize, nerve fibres with swellings containing neurosecretory material accumulate on the surface of the basophilic epithelial cells. These findings have led to the misinterpretation that the immigrated cells of the intermediate lobe are transformed into colloid.

d) *Connective Tissue and Blood Capillaries in the Posterior Lobe.* The surface of the posterior lobe is covered with a capsule of *connective tissue* which consists of collagen and elastic fibres. At the border with the intermediate lobe, only a thin, usually interrupted zone of connective tissue is developed. *Argyrophilic fibrils* predominante in the interior of the posterior lobe (Fig. 17); these fibrils accompany the blood vessels in the form of irregular networks. Argyrophilic fibrils extending from the perivascular sheath permeate the intercapillary tissue of the posterior lobe. Romeis (1940) observed quantitative regional differences in the development

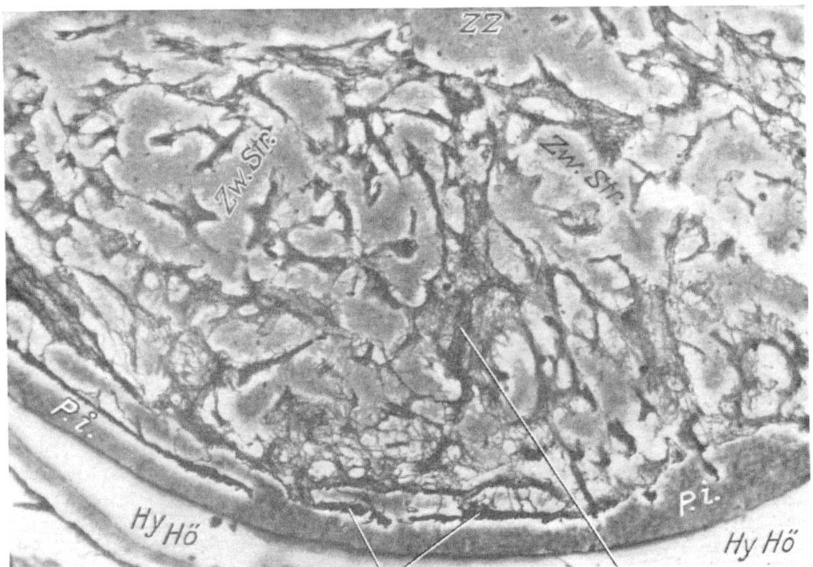

Fig. 17. Neural lobe of the cat (sagittal section) (impregnation after Perdrau). The figure shows the abundance of argyrophile fibers surrounding the blood vessels. Z.Z. central zone; Zw.Str. "Zwischenstreifen" (Romeis); Verd.Z. perivascular zones (Romeis); Intermed. Plex. plexus of blood vessels in the marginal zone of the neural lobe; HyHö. Cavum hypophyseos; P.i. Pars intermedia. 25× magnification. From Nowakowski (1951)

of the argyrophilic net. For example, many perivascular argyrophilic fibres are particularly to be found in the upper quarter and on the dorsal side of the posterior lobe. In the lobulated posterior lobe of *Didelphys virginiana* each lobule is sheathed by a network of argyrophilic fibrils (Diepen, 1962, Fig. 15).

Many *mast cells* occur in the neurohypophysis of the opossum (Bodian, 1963).

2. *Electron-Microscopy*

As is to be expected on the basis of light-microscopical observations, many tiny unmyelinated nerve fibres which lie close together appear on electron-micrographs of the posterior lobe (Fig. 18). There is no intercellular space in the sense of light-microscopy. Individual fibres are sometimes deeply embedded into the cytoplasm of the pituicytes (Fig. 19). Occasionally it has been observed that the glia cells of the posterior lobe are wrapped around the axons (Legait and Legait, 1958; Bargmann and Knoop, 1960). *Synapses* between neurosecretory fibres and pituicytes are to be discerned under the electron-microscope, as pointed out by Knowles and Vollrath (1965, 1966, eel) and Wittkowsi (1967, Guinea-pig). The cytoplasm of the pituicytes, which shows no signs of secretory activity, is permeated by numerous filaments (Barer and Lederis, 1966, rabbit). Often it contains in-

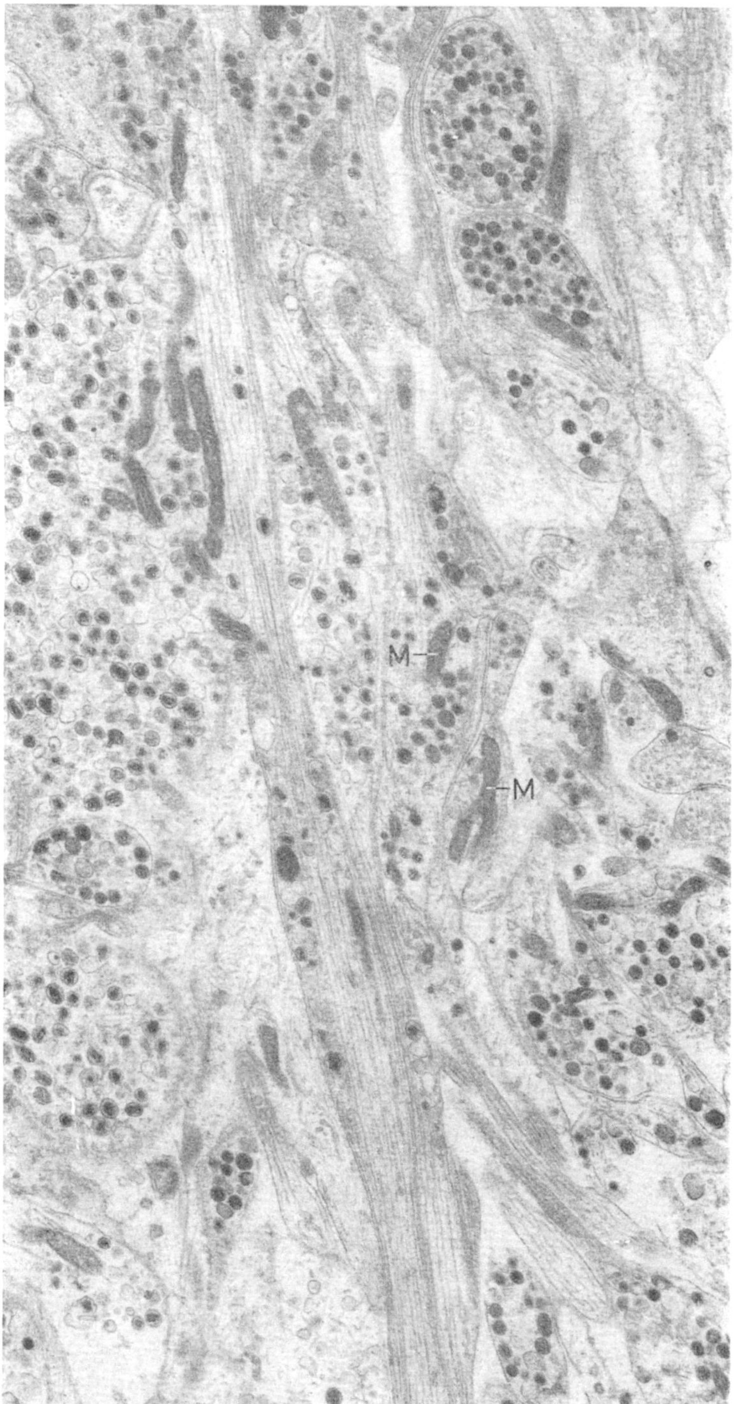

Fig. 18. Neural lobe of the hypophysis of the cat. Nerve fibers cut horizontally and longitudinally can be recognized which contain elementary granules of the neurosecretory material. M = Mitochondrion. Electron micrograph, 17,500× magnification

clusions of lipids and pigment granules (cf. p. 18). Different types of pituicytes are described by FUJITA and HARTMANN (1961, rabbit, astrocytes, microglia).

Apart from the conventional neurofilaments, neurotubules and mitochondria with cristae (PALAY, 1955; BARGMANN, KNOOP, and THIEL, 1957, etc.), there are distributed within the neuroplasm of the axons in the posterior lobe the so-called *elementary granules* i.e. spheroidal or ovoid particles having diameters of 800 to 3000 Å, depending upon species (Fig. 18). These elementary granules are separated from the neuroplasm by a membrane and enclose an electron-dense substance.

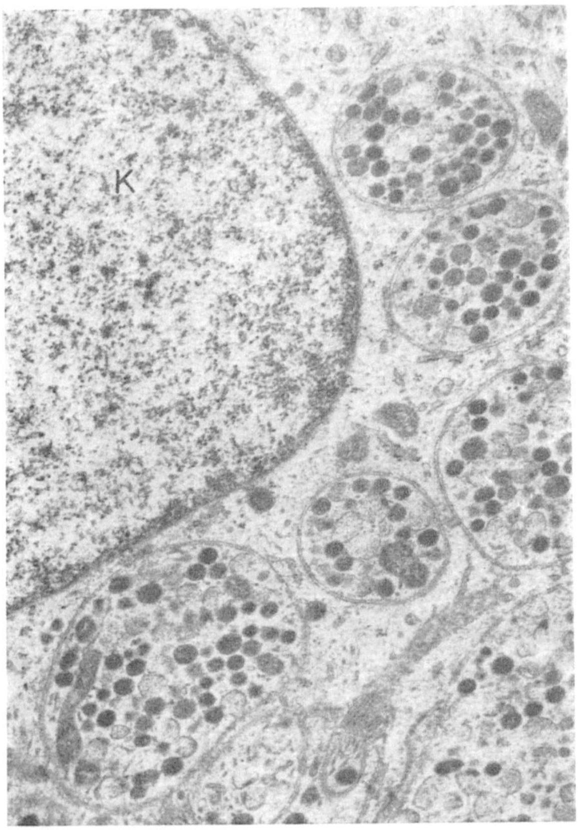

Fig. 19. Pituicyte in the neural lobe of the cat, in whose cytoplasm neurosecretory nerve fibers are embedded. K = nucleus of the pituicyte. Electron micrograph, 15,000 × magnification. From BARGMANN, Histologie und mikroskopische Anatomie des Menschen, 6. Aufl., G. Thieme-Verlag Stuttgart, 1967

Electron-Microscopically empty or only partly filled vesicles are to be considered as granules which have released their contents (see below). *Synaptic vesicles* occur in addition to the granules in the axonal endings which approach the basement membranes of the posterior lobe capillaries or which reach the perivascular spaces (see below). Circumscribed thickenings of the nerve fibers, which can be rich in elementary granules and mitochondria, correspond to the Herring bodies already mentioned. In *Tropidonotus natrix* BARGMANN, KNOOP, and THIEL (1957) found swellings of the nerve fibres filled with closely packed elementary granules which apparently coalesced into a compact mass. Even the myelinated nerve fibres of the posterior lobe, which occur occasionally in some animals (e.g. rabbits), can be provided with elementary granules (BARER and LEDERIS, 1966).

The elementary granules are without a doubt *the submicroscopic equivalent of the neurosecretory material* which can be made visible in light-microscopy by selective staining. With excessive demand on the water metabolism, e.g. in thirst, the

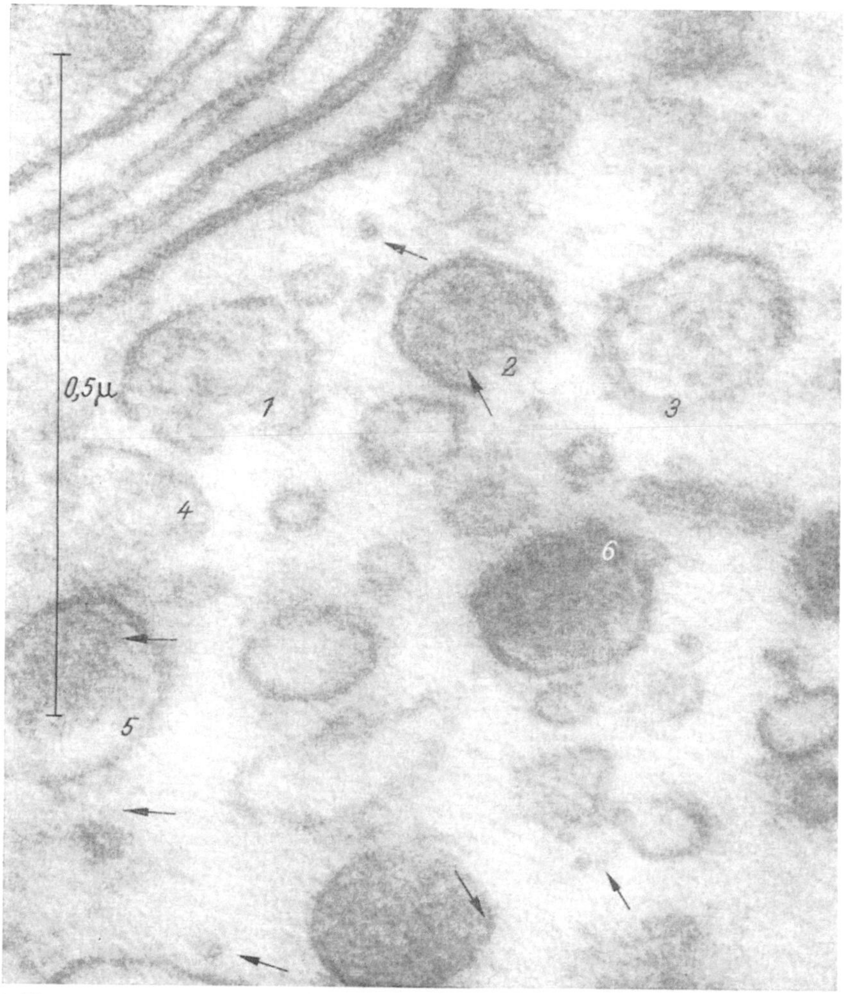

Fig. 20. Human neurohypophysis. Internal structure of the elementary granule content. In granules 1—7 vesicular structures can be seen; similar and larger microvesicles are discernible outside the elementary granules (arrows). 176,000 × magnification. Elmiscope I; uranyl acetate stain. From LEDERIS (1965)

posterior lobe loses neurosecretory material. This process corresponds to a transformation of the elementary granules into "empty" vesicles (Fig. 24 and 25). Further, it has become evident that the elementary granules which are produced in the secretory nuclei of the hypothalamus (Nucleus supraopticus and paraventricularis) and which are transported into the posterior lobe by means of axonal flow (HILD, 1954; FLAMENT-DURAND, 1966), contain octapeptide hormones (vasopressin, oxytocin, mesotocin, isotocin, etc., LEDERIS, 1962). According to BINDLER and coworkers (1967) the individual nerve terminals filled with elementary granules store only *one* of the hypothalamic octapeptides, vasopressin *or* oxytocin (cf. p. 18, bovine posterior pituitary). LEDERIS (1965) assumes that the microvesicles observed in the interior of the granules (see also BODIAN, 1963, opossum, Fig. 20) could be macromolecular aggregates of hormone and neurophysin, the inert carrier substance (protein) of the posterior lobe hormone (ACHER, 1958, 1960).

As more recent investigations show, the population of granules in the neurosecretory diencephalic system is not uniform. According to HOLMES (1964) fibres occur in the neural lobe of the hedgehog, which contain granules of differing nature. HOLMES not only found spheroidal elementary granules of the type just described, but also ovoid particles with hexagonal, crystalloid inclusions (diameter up to 5000 Å) and finally small granules with an electron-dense core, which correspond to catecholamine granules in size and shape (cf. HÖKFELT and others, 1967). According to CAMPBELL and HOLMES (1966) the fibres, which have probably monoamine granules, in the hedgehog are situated primarily in the superior region of the infundibular stem.

The sites of production of the crystalloid particles as well are the Nucleus supraopticus and paraventricularis. The functional significance of the granules with crystalloid inclusions is still unknown. There is likewise no clear idea concerning the nature of the irregularly shaped, electron-dense, often granulated particles and lamellated structures which have been observed in some axons. Some of them may possibly be lysosomes. In other species, however (e.g. rodents, primates) the crystalloid particles were not found (HOLMES, 1964). But even here a mixed population of inclusions is present: in addition to large and small *vesicles*, 1. large and 2. small electron-dense *granules* occur in the nerve endings. The dimorphism of the neurosecretory granules is especially evident in *fish*, in which neurohypophysial fibres penetrate into the Pars distalis (adenohypophysis, e.g. eel). KNOWLES and VOLLRATH (1966) described large A-granules (diameter 1000—1400 Å) and small B-granules (diameter 500—700 Å). It is not yet known what effect the corresponding neurosecretory A- and B-fibres have on the various cells of the adenohypophysis (cf. also BARGMANN, 1966, lit., and p. 32).

The *blood capillaries* of the posterior lobe are distinguished by an endothelium which is provided with so-called pores ("fenestrated endothelium"). These pores are closed by a diaphragm (BARGMANN and KNOOP, 1960; MONROE and SCOTT, 1966; BARER and LEDERIS, 1966; cf. DIEPEN, 1962). The pericapillary space is sometimes wide, sometimes narrow, and contains fibrocytes (LEDERIS, 1965, humans; BARER and LEDERIS, 1966, rabbit). In addition it is bridged by processes of pituicytes whose pedicles lie adjacent to the surface of the basement membrane. In some places the pericapillary space is extended in channels which are lined with basement membranes (BARER and LEDERIS, 1966).

The paraventricular and supraoptic nuclei and their axons are provided with aminergic and cholinergic synapses (FALCK, 1964; BARGMANN, 1966, lit.). These endings belong presumably to the fibre systems originating in the brain stem (ROTHBALLER, 1966) that regulate the release of hypothalamic neurons as demonstrated by electrophysiological experiments.

C. Functional Changes of the Posterior Lobe

The amount of neurosecretory material in the posterior lobe in all vertebrates fluctuates according to the status of the water metabolism. In addition it changes with parturition (STUTINSKY, 1953), lactation, with the annual sexual cycle in some animals, with the influence of drugs, and with various types of nonspecific stress.

Thirst. In amphibians which have been kept in a dry environment for a few days, in thirsting birds and mammals, or in animals to which salt was administered in the drinking water, there is a considerable diminution of neurosecretory material in the neural lobe (Fig. 21). This diminution can be recognized on slides stained with chromalum-haematoxyline (KRATZSCH, 1951; ORTMANN, 1951; EICHNER, 1954; and others). The depletion of the posterior lobe corresponds to a release of antidiuretic active vasopressin.

Lactation. The ultrastructure of the posterior lobe tissue in mammals was investigated in the lactating rat (MONROE and SCOTT, 1966), in which a diminution of the amount of stainable neurosecretory material had already been described (STUTINSKY, 1953; MALANDRA, 1956; and others, cf. GABE, 1966, lit.). In lactating

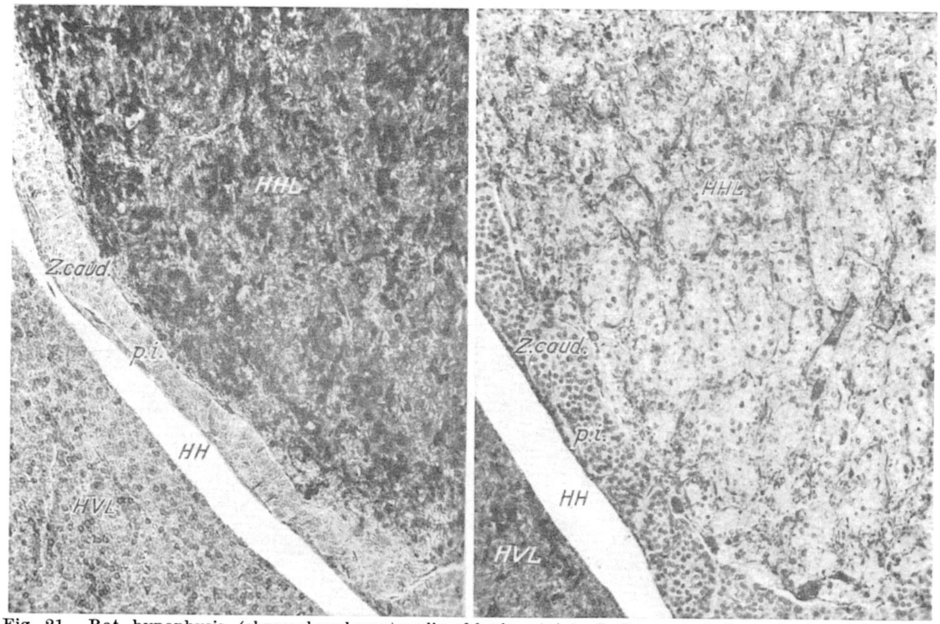

Fig. 21. Rat hypophysis (chromalum-hematoxylin-phloxin stain). Left: normal hypophysis; right: after 7 days without water. HHL. neural lobe of the hypophysis; HVL. anterior lobe of the hypophysis; Z.caud.p.i. Caudal zone of the intermediate lobe; HH. Cavum hypophyseos. Ca. 100 × magnification. From ENGELHARDT (1962)

animals the number of elementary granules with an electron-dense core is greatly reduced, while the number of electron-microscopically empty vesicles is considerably increased (MONROE and SCOTT, 1966). The structural changes in the posterior lobe observed during lactation are to be interpreted as the equivalent of a reflectory release of oxytocin, i.e. of the milk let-down factor, which causes the myoepithelial cells of the mammary gland to contract and thus contributes toward the release of milk (cf. BERDE, 1959). Already within 15 min after the suckling young animals have been separated from the mother, a considerable restoration takes place (MONROE and SCOTT, 1966). One hour later the elementary granules with electron-dense cores prevail again.

Hibernation. Investigations of the posterior lobe of a hibernating mammal (*Eliomys quercinus*, E. LEGAIT, H. LEGAIT, C. BURLET, and A. BURLET, 1966, literature on hibernation, also in DIEPEN, 1962) have revealed that the volume of the organ increases during hibernation and the amount of neurosecretory material increases at the same time. In this process there is enlargement and vacuolization of the pituicytes. When the animal awakens the posterior lobe decreases in size, the amount of neurosecretory material diminishes, and the pituicytes lose their vacuoles. The level of acid phosphatase and acetylcholine-esterase increases in the posterior lobe during hibernation and decreases considerably upon awakening. After

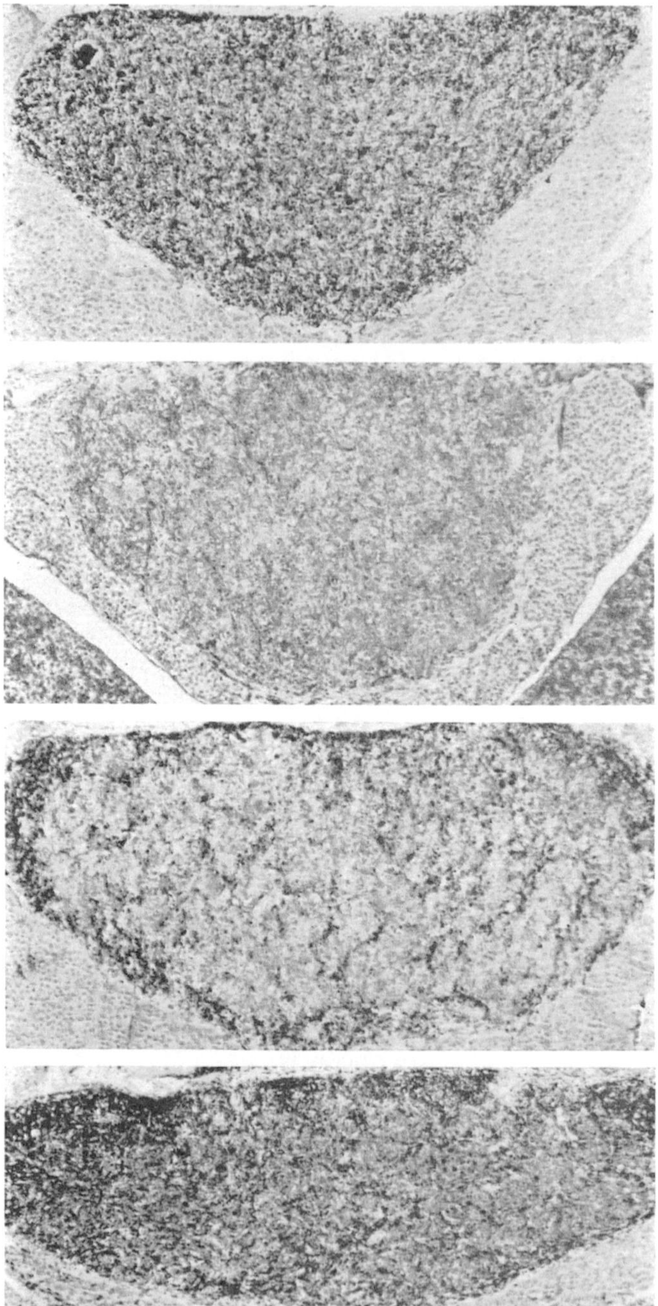

a

b

c

d

Fig. 22 a—d. a Neurohypophysis of a rat which was killed 30 min after an injection of 2 mg morphium sulfate. No diminution of neurosecretory material. Normal structure of the neural lobe. Frontal section. 6 μ thickness, chromalum-hematoxylin-phloxin stain after GOMORI, 85× magnification (Panphot, Leitz).
b Neurohypophysis of rat which was killed 3 days after the beginning of the experiment and which had received 2 mg morphium sulfate twice daily by injection. Definite diminution of neurosecretory material, which only remains distributed finely dispersed and diffuse in the neural lobe.
c Neurohypophysis of a rat which was killed 10 days after the beginning of the experiment and which had received 2 mg morphium sulfate twice daily by injection. Reaccumulation of neurosecretory material: particular perivascular accumulation of the secretory material, therefore strong concentration in the border regions of the neural lobe.
d Neurohypophysis of a rat which was killed 20 days after the beginning of the experiment and which had received 2 mg morphium sulfate twice daily by injection. Neural lobe especially rich in neurosecretory material. From RODECK and BRAUKMANN (1966)

hibernation has ended, the alkaliphosphatase activity increases into the wall of the capillary walls.

Drugs, Stress. After administration of various substances which have an antidiuretic effect, the quantity of neurosecretory material in the posterior lobe likewise sinks considerably. This applies for example to nicotinic acid and morphium sulfate (Rodeck and Braukmann, 1966; Fig. 22). A diminution in the amount of neurosecretory material has also been observed after administration of histamine (Fr. Hartmann, 1958) and pilocarpine (Fujita and Hartmann, 1961). Alloxan diabetes (rat) is combined with a reduction of the neurosecretory substance in the

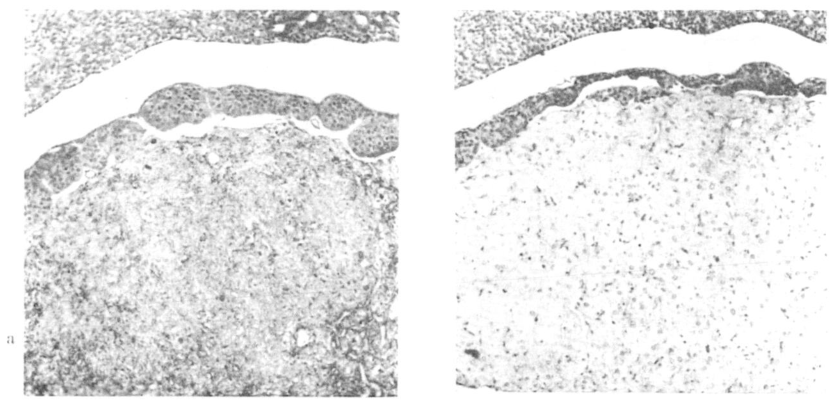

Fig. 23. a Frontal section through the neural lobe of a normal rat with accumulation of neurosecretory material. b Frontal section through the neural lobe emptied of neurosecretory material in an animal intoxicated with Alloxan. Chromalum-hematoxylin-phloxin stain. 74× magnification. From E. Kratzsch (1951/52)

neurohypophysis (Kratzsch, 1951; Fig. 23). In the nerve endings in the neurohypophysis of the opossum (*Didelphys virginiana*) Bodian (1963) found numerous empty vesicles after administering urea. The same phenomenon can be observed after anesthesia with ether, i.e. after a stimulus which effects hormonal release (Kivalo, 1966, Barer and Lederis, 1966, rabbit).

Non-specific factors like cold (Braukmann and Rodeck, 1966), hunger (Breuer, 1966) and pain (Rothballer, 1963; Streefkerk, 1967) cause a similar process.

The increase in number and size of secretory granules to be observed electronmicroscopically in the neurohypophysis (rabbit) after injection of adrenaline has been interpreted as an equivalent of a blockade of the hormone release (Fujita and Hartmann, 1961).

D. The Mechanism of Release

The question of what factors effect the release of hypothalamic hormones on the perivascular endings of the peptidergic neurons in the posterior lobe and how this release is performed belongs to the topics of neuroendocrinology, which are of particular interest (cf. Bargmann, 1966, 1967).

Verney (1947) has shown that an increase of the osmotic blood pressure is followed by a release of antidiuretic hormone in the posterior lobe, if the blood reaches the hypothalamic secretory nuclei. In addition, the intracarotid injection of hypertonic saline results in release of the oxytocic hormone (Anderson, 1951; Abrahams and Pickford, 1953) producing responses of the mammary gland and the uterus. It is not known whether the blood exerts an immediate influence upon the perikarya belonging to the Nucleus supraopticus and paraventricularis or whether the stimulation of the neurosecretory cells is caused by action of the

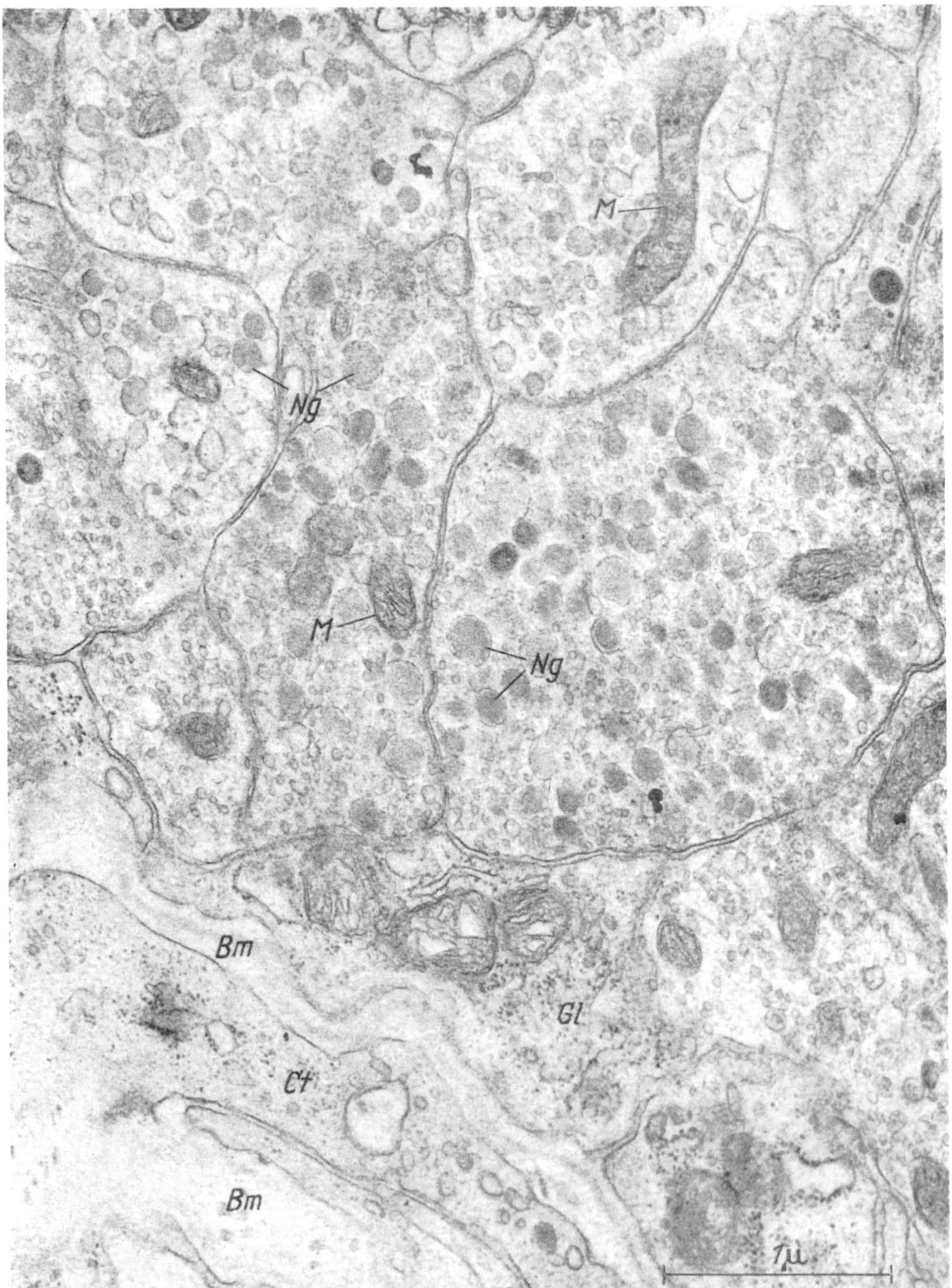

Fig. 24. Pars nervosa of the hypophysis from an "osmotic-control" bird (*Zonotrichia leucophrys* Gambelii). All axons contain small vesicles. Larger axons also contain neurosecretory granules (Ng). As in the median eminence a glial "cuff" (Gl) separates axons from basement-membrane region (Bm). Fibroblast process (Ct) within basement-membrane region. M, mitochondria; En, endothelium. From BERN, NISHIOKA, MEWALDT, and FARNER (1966)

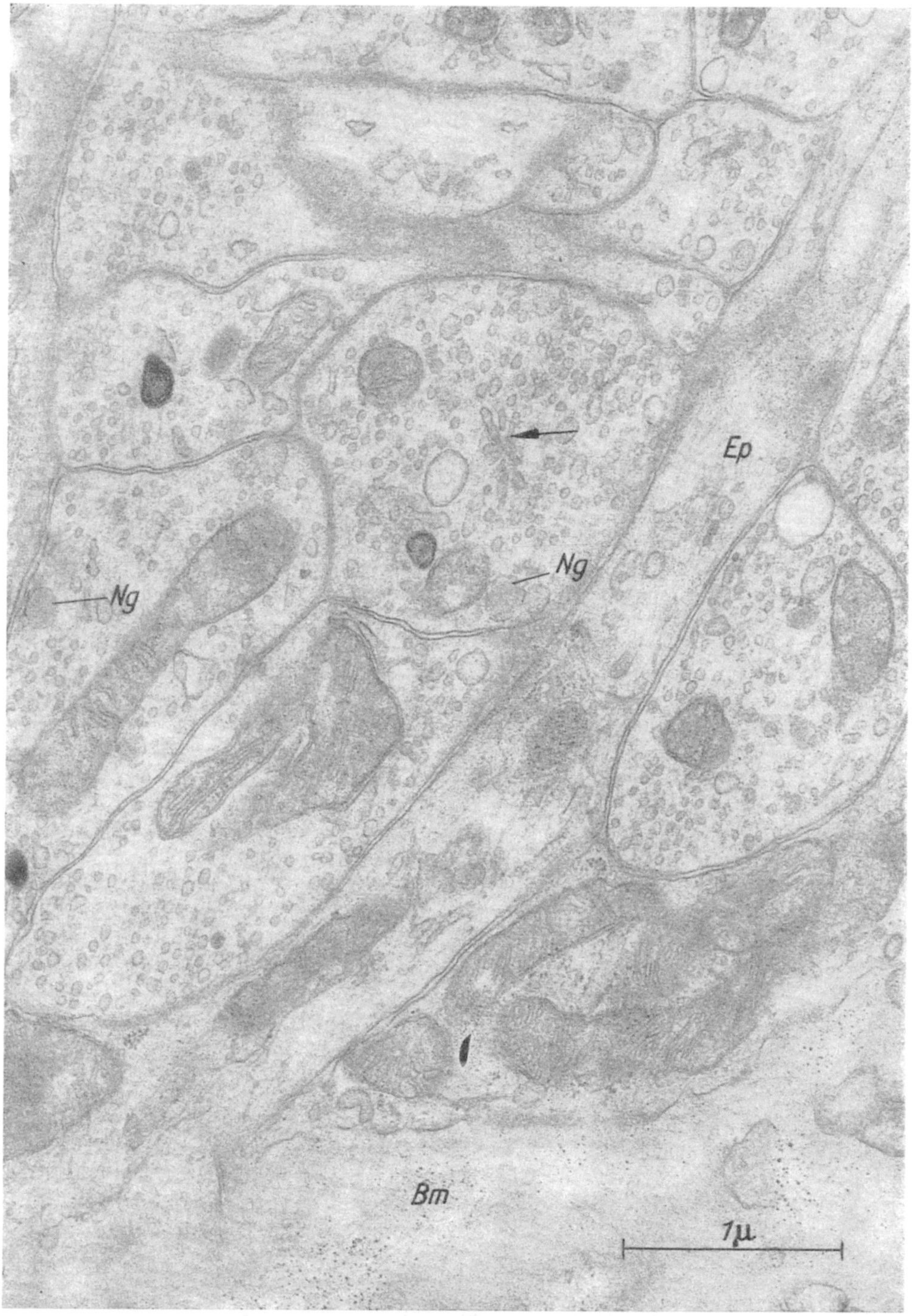

Fig. 25. Pars nervosa of a "chronic-osmotic" bird (*Zonotrichia leucophrys* Gambelii). The "chronic-osmotic" group was given graded dosages of NaCl up to 0.5 M interspersed with tap water for 8 days and killed. Axons contain many small vesicles, some of which appear elongated (arrow). Some neurosecretory granules (Ng) also present. Ependymal process (Ep) with "foot" on capillary basement-membrane region (Bm). From BERN, NISHIOKA, MEWALDT, and FARNER (1966)

synapses on these elements. Such synapses can be detected in great number by means of fluorescence-microscopy (FALCK, 1964) and electron-microscopy. In addition, synapses are to be found on the axons of neurosecretory fibres running to the posterior lobe (OOTA, 1963; OOTA and KOBAYASHI, 1963; BARGMANN and LINDNER, 1964, unpublished observations; BARGMANN, 1966). Most synapses are observed on the neurosecretory fibres in the median eminence (mice, birds, turtles, frogs, cf. p. 23). Typical synapses were also found on fibre swellings filled with secretory material in the neurohypophysis of the rat (BARGMANN, 1966).

Electrophysiological investigations (BENNETT and FOX, 1962; KOBAYASHI, 1964; BERN, 1962; BERN and YAGI, 1964), show that neurosecretory cells conduct impulses. It can be assumed as certain that secretory neurons whose endings for the most part reach the capillaries in the posterior lobe, also conduct impulses and that this impulse conduction is followed by the release of hormones (cf. M. PICKFORD, 1945). According to G.W. HARRIS electric stimulation of the neurosecretory centers provoques a release of neurohormones from the neurohypophysis. We do not yet know whether the axosomatic and axon-axonal synapses existing between nonsecretory neurons and secretory nerve cells are exclusively excitatory ones (cf. BARGMANN, 1966, lit.).

As already mentioned, the release of hormones from the nerve endings in the hypophysis corresponds to a transformation of the elementary granules into vesicles (Fig. 24 and 25). In addition to having elementary granules, the endings of the neurosecretory fibres also contain synaptic vesicles which are considered to be carriers of acetylcholine. Further, acetylcholine or a similar substance was found in the neurohypophysis of mammals (KOBAYASHI and OOTA, 1964; LEDERIS, 1966, 1967; DANIEL and LEDERIS, 1967, lit.). Acetylcholin injected intravenously or in the nucleus supraopticus (chloralosed dog) indices an inhibition of the rate of urine flow caused by the liberation of vasopressin into the circulation (M. PICKFORD, 1947). For these reasons the following hypothesis may be proposed (cf. also DE ROBERTIS, 1964): due to excitation of the neurosecretory cells acetylcholine is liberated from the synaptic vesicles. It causes an alteration in the membranes which envelop the elementary granules so that they become permeable for the peptide hormones in these granules. The hormones enter the surrounding axoplasm (cf. H.A. BERN, 1966). The plasmalemma of the axonal endings is possibly influenced by the acetylcholine in the same manner. After passing through the membrane of the elementary granules, the neuroplasm and the plasmalemma of the nerve endings, the hormones must penetrate the following barriers: basement membrane — perivascular space — basement membrane — endothelium (pinocytosis?). KOELLE and GEESEY (1961) are also of the opinion that a cholinergic mechanism plays a part in the release at the nerve terminals in the posterior lobe, since the authors found acetylcholine-esterase in the neurohypophysis of the cat. These findings were confirmed by KOBAYASHI and FARNER (birds, cf. KOBAYASHI and OOTA, 1964). Further investigations must prove the validity of this hypothesis. In this respect the role of calcium is to be considered (literature in H.A. BERN, 1966). An emptying of the elementary granules, i.e. the release of posterior lobe hormones occurs only when calcium is present (BIE and THORN, 1966). The presence of Ca^{2+} seems to diminish the binding of vasopressin and oxytocin to the carrier substance of these hormones (for lit. cf. DANIEL and LEDERIS, 1967), theoretically postulated by BARGMANN (1949) and proved by ACHER (1958) to be an inert protein (neurophysin).

Further, one must clarify the behaviour of the *carrier protein* (see p. 23). Up till now there have only been data by BARER and LEDERIS (1966), according to which the electronmicroscopical equivalent of this substance in the elementary granules could correspond to tiny vesicles (Fig. 20) inside these particles. Their fate during the course of release is not known. Likewise unclear is whether the elementary granules, emptied by the release of hormones, are again filled with electron-dense substance or whether they are fragmented and broken down.

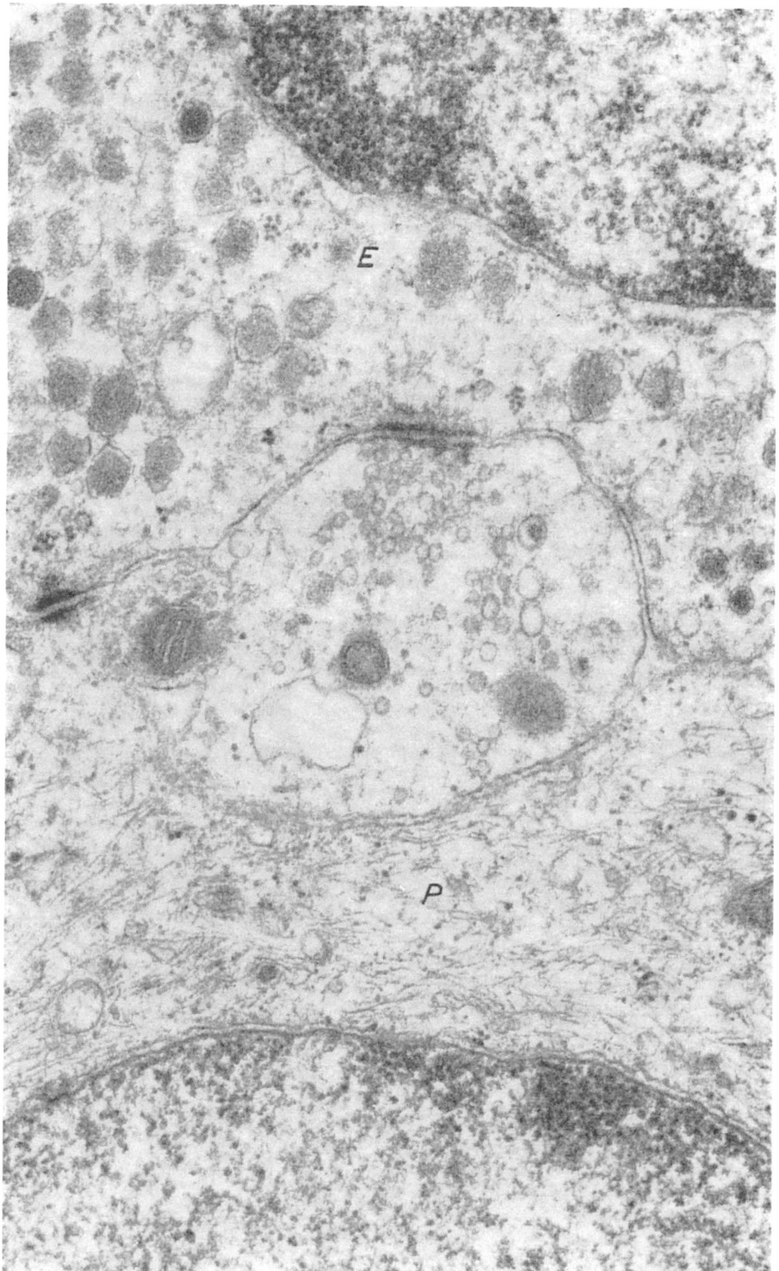

Fig. 26. Synapse on epithelial cell (E) of the Pars intermedia (cat). P. palisade cell, whose cytoplasm contains tiny filaments. Ca. 45,000× magnification. From BARGMANN, LINDNER, and ANDRES (1967)

E. Neurohypophysis and Pars Intermedia

In many species the neurohypophysis and Pars intermedia of the adenohypophysis are not sharply separated from each other. In a number of *Selacians* and *Teleosts*, *secretory nerve fibres* from the posterior lobe invade deeply into the intermediate lobe of the hypophysis (SCHARRER, 1952; BARGMANN, 1953). According

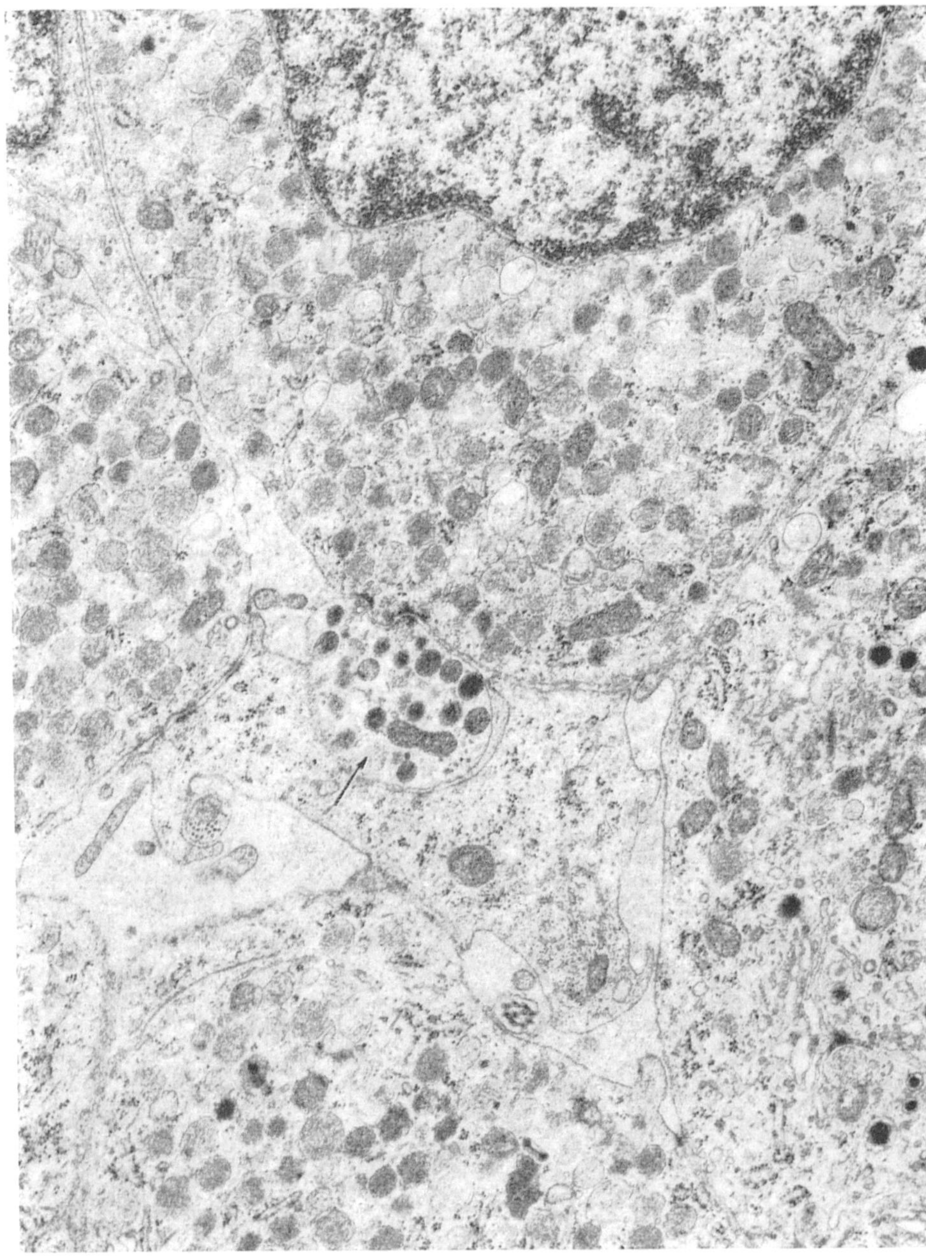

Fig. 27. Synapse (arrow) with neurosecretory elementary granules on the surface of an epithelial cell of the Pars intermedia (cat). 17,500× magnification. From BARGMANN, LINDNER, and ANDRES (1967)

to SMOLLER (1967) neurosecretory axons possibly regulating the secretion of intermedin enter the pars intermedia of the treefrog (*Hyla regilla*). Neurosecretory nerve fibres in the intermediate lobe of *mammals* have been demonstrated with chrom-alum-haematoxyline and silver impregnations; they are sometimes in close contact with follicles of the Pars intermedia (BARGMANN, 1949, 1966; EICHNER, 1954, etc.). *Adrenergic nerve fibres* probably of hypothalamic origin have been observed with fluorescence-microscopy in the pars intermedia of the pituitary in the toad

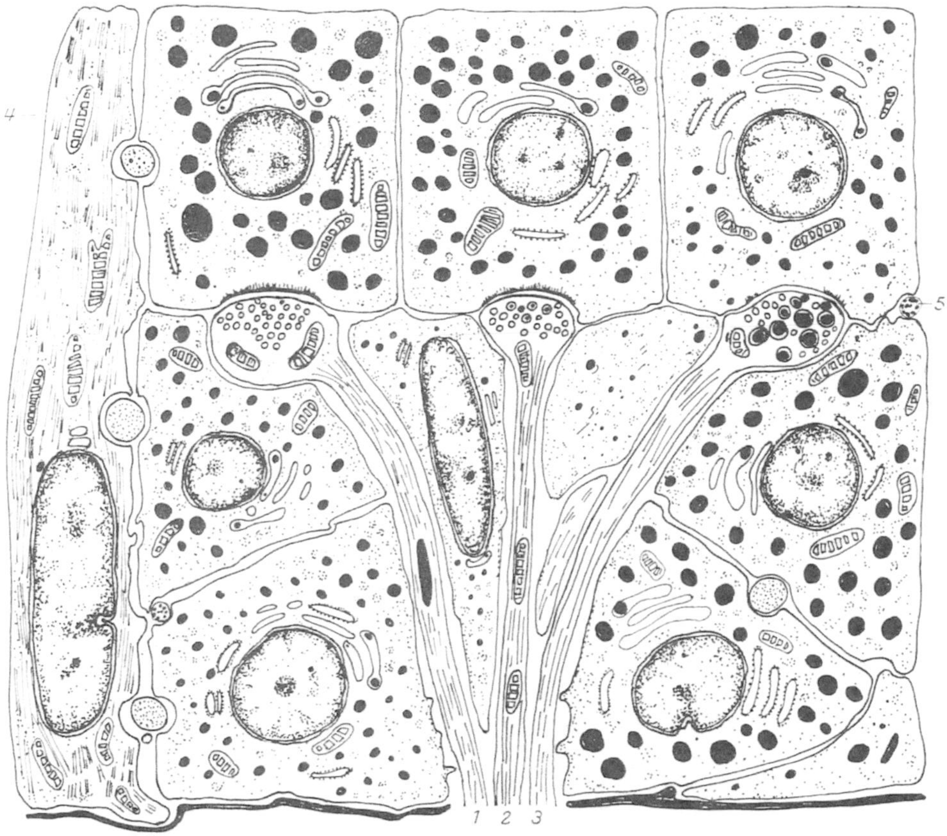

Fig. 28. Diagram of the innervation of the epithelial cells in the intermediate lobe of the hypophysis by means of cholinergic (1), adrenergic (2), and peptidergic (3) nerve fibers or synapses. 4 palisade cell; 5 cross section of a cilium. From BARGMANN, LINDNER, and ANDRES (1967)

(*Bufo arenarum*, ENEMAR, FALCK, and ITURRIZA, 1967). As shown by electron-microscopical investigations (LEGAIT and LEGAIT, 1957; BARGMANN and KNOOP, 1960) there is close contact between the *neurosecretory fibres* and the epithelial cells of the Pars intermedia in teleosts which resembles synapses. VOLLRATH (1967) proved direct contact between the neurosecretory fibres and the hormone-producing cells of the Pars intermedia and the anterior lobe in *Hippocampus cuda*. Partly it is a matter of contacts without synaptic vesicles and thickenings of the presynaptic membrane, partly of contacts with synaptic vesicles and thickenings of the membranes. In other species (e.g. *Tinca tinca*) the endings of the neurosecretory fibres are separated from the plasmalemma of the epithelial cells by a single or double basement membrane. Synapses between the nerve fibres from the posterior lobe and cells of the intermediate lobe in *mammals* (Fig. 26, 27 and 28) were shown by Bargmann, Lindner, and Andres (1967) in the intermediate lobe of the cat with the electron-microscope. These synapses are partly of the cholinergic, partly of the adrenergic type; in addition there are contacts between the neurosecretory fibres and the surface of the epithelial cells (peptidergic synapses, cf. p. 18). The question whether the so-called invasion of basophils (cf. p. 18) is a special case of this kind of contact relationship remains open.

The possibility of contacts or interdigitations between the neurohypophysis and the intermediate lobe must be taken into particular consideration by research workers who draw conclusions from the results of extraction experiments. Extracts from the Pars intermedia of teleosts (e.g. *Gadus morrhua*) and also of mammals (see above) may contain substances from the hypothalamic nerve fibres which are included within this part of the hypophysis.

F. Regeneration of the Neurohypophysis, Stalk Section

Some results of experiments reveal that after the hypophysial stem has been removed or destroyed, differentiation of an "Ersatzhinterlappen" (rat) may occur, if the interruption of the fibres leading from the hypothalamus to the posterior lobe is not followed by a retrograde degeneration of the Nuclei supraopticus and paraventricularis (Gaupp and Spatz, 1955; Stutinsky, Bonvallet, and Dell, 1949/50; Moll, 1957, etc., literature in Diepen, 1962; Dierickx, 1965).

The reaction of the neurosecretory tractus supraoptico-hypophyseus after *section* of the hypothalamic-hypophysial pathway (stalk section) is described by Hild (1951, anura), Hild and Zetler (1953, dog), Iturriza and Restelli (1967, toad) and others (for lit. cf. Diepen, 1962). After dissection of the hypophysial stalk neurosecretory material accumulates in the proximal stumps of the interrupted fibres. This finding speaks in favour of the theory that the hypothalamic neurosecretion is transported to the distal neurohypophysis (cf. Bargmann, 1966, lit.). In this connection the investigations by Sloper et al. (1960), Ficq and Flament-Durand (1963) are of peculiar importance demonstrating that radioactive substances are transported through axonal flow from the secretory nuclei towards the neurohypophysis.

G. Neurohypophysial Tissue Cultivated In Vitro

Tissue from the posterior lobe of mammals was cultivated *in vitro* by Geiling and Lewis (1935), Anderson and Haymaker (1935/36) and Hild (1935/54). After about a week the neurohypophysial axons had degenerated, the intraaxonal neurosecretory material is no longer demonstrable by staining (Hild, 1954). On the other hand the pituicytes became very prominent. The processes of these elements resembling protoplasmic astrocytes are in contact with each other. Like other glia cells, the transformed pituicytes make peculiar undulating movements which have been recorded on film. These cells penetrate more slowly into the periphery of the culture than the spindle-shaped cells growing out of the sparse connective tissue in the posterior lobe. Posterior lobe hormones which were transferred into the culture medium together with the tissue disappear in the course of a week, i.e. during the degeneration of the secretory nerve fibres. Neural lobe tissue taken from dehydrated animals and cultivated *in vitro* does not contain and produce neurohypophysial hormones.

Summary

As described in the foregoing chapters, hypothalamic nerve cells of various kinds participate in the structure of the proximal and distal neurohypophysis.

Among these elements the so-called *neurosecretory* cells assume a peculiar position: they are neurons whose endings reach the capillaries in the median eminence and in the neural lobe and to a small extent also the pituicytes in the neurohypophysis and the epithelial cells of the intermediate lobe. Up till now these cells were considered to be neurons which could not be classified in the conventional system of the nerve cells because they 1. produce secretions which are detectable by light-microscopy and which contain hormones, and 2. do not enter into a synaptic contact with other cells but release their specific products into the blood stream (glandular nerve cells, E. SCHARRER).

More recently doubt has been expressed (BARGMANN, LINDNER, and ANDRES, 1967) whether it is necessary to regard the neurosecretory cells as special neurons that are difficult to classify. It has been shown — contrary to previous concepts — that terminals of secretory nerve cells of lower vertebrates as well as of mammals have contacts with cells of the hypophysis (LEGAIT and LEGAIT, 1957; BARGMANN and KNOOP, 1960; KNOWLES, 1963; BARGMANN, 1965; VOLLRATH, 1967). According to BARGMANN, LINDNER, and ANDRES (1967, cat) and VOLLRATH (1967) the endings of neurosecretory fibres form *synapses* on the surface of the intermediate lobe cells. These synapses contain synaptic vesicles as well as neurosecretory elementary granules. Admittedly it is not known in what way and with what effect octapeptides released from the endings — in the manner of transmitter substances? — influence the epithelial cells of the intermediate lobe. In spite of this fact BARGMANN and co-workers consider it justifiable to describe those nerve cells that produce vasopressin, oxytocin and releasing factors as *peptidergic neurons*, of which some have *peptidergic synapses*, and in this way to classify them along with the previously known cholinergic, aminergic, etc. neurons.

In the *proximal neurohypophysis* (median eminence) there are nerve endings which contain smaller elementary granules, very probably monoamine granules (KOBAYASHI and co-workers, 1966; MONROE, 1967; HÖKFELT, 1967). Like the endings of the classic neurosecretory cells these terminals also enter into close relationships to the capillaries. Since the granules of these diencephalic cells containing monoamines are probably formed in the same manner as the elementary granules of the typical neurosecretory cells and the granules of peripheral adrenergic neurons (DAHLSTRÖM, 1966), namely in the perikaryon, and since granules of this type are transported distally and intra-axonally just like the neurosecretory elementary granules (DAHLSTRÖM, 1966) one must ask why the aminergic neurons should not also be listed as neurosecretory cells. One does not have to answer this question if one follows the proven principle of classifying the nerve cells according to their mode of activity and not merely according to their morphological behaviour.

The precise and by no means completed study of the neurohypophysis has thus resulted in the realization that we are dealing with 1. a complex of storage and release sites that is built up by neurons of the ventral, poorly myelinated hypothalamus (cf. BARGMANN and SCHARRER, 1951), and 2. with a system whose specific hormonal effects are brought about mainly by peptidergic neurons. The storage and release of polypeptides which are produced in hypothalamic centers are apparently the most important functions of the neurohypophysis. Conventional and aminergic diencephalic-neurohypophysial nerve fibres with synaptic vesicles and monoamine granules respectively possibly participate in the release of polypeptides. Further it is not yet clear what part is played by the perivascular hypothalamic neurons in the proximal neurohypophysis containing granules of the monoamine type. If some of these cells should release their products into the capillaries in the median eminence, a neurohumoral stimulation of the anterior lobe by aminergic cells, i.e. not only be peptidergic neurons seems conceivable (cf. FUXE,

1964). The function of the *glia cells* in the median eminence and in the posterior lobe of the neurohypophysis is still unknown.

References

Abrahams, V.C., and M. Pickford: Simultaneous observations on urine flow and uterine activity in the conscious bitch. J. Physiol. (Lond.) **12**, 56 (1953).

Acher, R.: Etat naturel des principes oxytocique et vasopressique de la neurohypophyse. II. Int. Symposium über Neurosekretion, Lund 1957, p. 71—78. Hrsg. von W. Bargmann, B. Hanström, B. u. E. Scharrer. Berlin-Göttingen-Heidelberg: Springer 1958.

— Biochemistry of the protein hormones. Ann. Rev. Biochem. **29**, 547—576 (1960).

Anderson, B.: Some observations on the neurohormonal regulation of milk-ejection. Acta physiol. scand. **23**, 1—7 (1951).

Anderson, E., and W. Haymaker: Elaboration of hormones by pituitary cells growing *in vitro*. Proc. Soc. exp. Biol. (N.Y.) **33**, 313—316 (1935).

Assenmacher, I., et J. Benoit: Quelques aspects du contrôle hypothalamique de la fonction gonadotrope de la préhypophyse. In: Pathophysiologia diencephalica, p. 401—426. Wien: Springer 1958.

Barer, R., and K. Lederis: Ultrastructure of the rabbit neurohypophysis with special reference to the release of hormones. Z. Zellforsch. **75**, 201—239 (1966).

Bargmann, W.: Über die neurosekretorische Verknüpfung von Hypothalamus und Neurohypophyse. Z. Zellforsch. **34**, 610—634 (1949).

— Über das Zwischenhirn-Hypophysensystem von Fischen. Z. Zellforsch. **38**, 275—298 (1953).

— Das Zwischenhirn-Hypophysensystem. Berlin-Göttingen-Heidelberg: Springer 1954.

— Weitere Untersuchungen am neurosekretorischen Zwischenhirn-Hypophysensystem. Z. Zellforsch. **42**, 247—272 (1955).

— Über Synapsen im endokrinen System. Nova Acta Leopoldina N.F. **30**, 199—206 (1965).

— Neurosecretion. Int. Rev. Cytol. **19**, 183—201 (1966).

— Über neuroendokrine Zwischenhirnsysteme. Freiburger Universitätsreden N.F. Heft 42. Freiburg/Br.: Hans Ferdinand Schulz 1967.

—, u. A. Knoop: Über die morphologischen Beziehungen des neurosekretorischen Zwischenhirnsystems zum Zwischenlappen der Hypophyse (licht- und elektronenmikroskopische Untersuchungen). Z. Zellforsch. **52**, 256—277 (1960).

— — u. A. Thiel: Elektronenmikroskopische Studie an der Neurohypophyse von Tropidonotus natrix. Z. Zellforsch. **47**, 114—126 (1957).

—, u. E. Lindner: Über den Feinbau des Nebennierenmarkes des Igels (*Erinaceus europaeus* L.). Z. Zellforsch. **64**, 868—912 (1964).

— — u. K.H. Andres: Über Synapsen an endokrinen Epithelzellen und die Definition sekretorischer Neurone. Untersuchungen am Zwischenlappen der Katzenhypophyse. Z. Zellforsch. **77**, 282—298 (1967).

—, and E. Scharrer: The site of origin of the hormones of the posterior pituitary. Amer. Scientist **39**, 255—259 (1951).

Barry, I., et G. Cotte: Etude préliminaire, au microscope électronique, de l'éminence médiane du cobaye. Z. Zellforsch. **53**, 714—724 (1961).

Bennett, M.V.L., and S. Fox: Electrophysiology of caudal neurosecretory cells in the skate and fluke. Gen. comp. Endocr. **2**, 77—96 (1962).

Benoit, J.: The structural components of the hypothalamo-hypophyseal pathway, with particular reference to photostimulation of the gonads in birds. Ann. N.Y. Acad. Sci. **117**, 23—34 (1964).

Berde, B.: Recent progress in oxytocin research. Springfield/Ill.: Charles C. Thomas 1959.

Bern, H.A.: The properties of neurosecretory cells. Gen. comp. Endocr. Suppl. **1**, 117—132 (1962).

— On the production of hormones by neurons and the rôle of neurosecretion in neuroendocrine mechanisms. Symp. Soc. exp. Biol. **20**, 325—344 (1966).

—, and R.S. Nishioka: Fine structure of the median eminence of some passerine birds. Proc. Zool. Soc. Calcutta **18**, 107—119 (1965).

— —, L.R. Mewaldt, and D.S. Farner: Photoperiodic and osmotic influences on the ultrastructure of the hypothalamic neurosecretory system of the white-crowned sparrow (*Zonotrichia leucophrys Gambelii*). Z. Zellforsch. **69**, 198—227 (1966).

—, and K. Yagi: Electrophysiology of neurosecretory systems. Excerpta Med. Int. Congress Ser. No. **83**, 577—583 (1964).

Bie, P., and N.A. Thorn: Studies of the possible release of antidiuretic hormone from hypothalamic tissue *in vitro*. Acta physiol. scand. **68** (suppl. 277), 26 (1966).

Bindler, E., Fr. S. Labella, and M. Sanwal: Isolated nerve endings (neurosecretosomes) from the posterior pituitary. Partial separation of Vasopressin and Oxytocin and the isolation of microvesicles. Cell Biol. **34**, 185—205 (1967).
Bodian, D.: Nerve endings, neurosecretory substance and lobular organization of the neurohypophysis. Bull. Johns Hopk. Hosp. **89**, 354—376 (1951).
— Cytological aspects of neurosecretion in opossum neurohypophysis. Bull. Johns Hopk. Hosp. **113**, 57—93 (1963).
Breuer, H. A.: Untersuchungen über die Auswirkung des Hungers auf die postnatale Entwicklung der Regulationszentren des Wasserhaushaltes. Z. Kinderheilk. **96**, 308—321 (1966).
Bucy, P. C.: The pars nervosa of the bovine hypophysis. J. comp. Neurol. **50**, 505—520 (1930).
Campbell, D. J., and R. L. Holmes: Further studies on the neurohypophysis of the hedgehog (*Erinaceus europaeus*). Z. Zellforsch. **75**, 35—46 (1966).
Clements, J. P., and T. P. Harrison: Variations in the distribution of the portal vessels of the rat's hypophysis cerebri. Communic. Anat. Soc. of Great Britain and Ireland 1966, 36 (Ref. No. 44).
Dahlström, Annica: The intraneuronal distribution of noradrenaline and the transport and life-span of amine storage granules in the sympathetic adrenergic neuron. A histochemical and biochemical study. Stockholm 1966.
Daniel, A. R., and K. Lederis: Release of neurohypophysial hormones *in vitro*. J. Physiol. (Lond.) **190**, 171—187 (1967).
Dawson, A. B.: Hypothalamo-hypophysial relationship in Rana pipiens demonstrated by Gomoris' chromalum-hematoxylin method. Anat. Rec. **112**, 443—444 (1952).
Diepen, R.: Der Hypothalamus. In: Handbuch der mikroskopischen Anatomie des Menschen, Bd. IV, S. 7. Hrsg. von W. Bargmann. Berlin-Göttingen-Heidelberg: Springer 1962.
Dierickx, K., and A. van den Abeele: On the relations between the hypothalamus and the anterior pituitary in Rana temporaria. Z. Zellforsch. **51**, 78—87 (1959).
— The nerve fibres controlling the gonadotropic activity of the hypophysis of Rana temporaria. Z. Zellforsch. **63**, 938—949 (1964).
— Regeneration of the neural lobe of the hypophysis after extirpation of the median eminence in Rana temporaria. Acta anat. (Basel) **60**, 181—186 (1965).
— The origin of the aldehyde-fuchsin-negative nerve fibres of the median eminence of the hypophysis: a gonadotropic centre. Z. Zellforsch. **66**, 504—518 (1965).
Eichner, D.: Zur Morphologie des neurosekretorischen hypothalamisch-hypophysären Systems beim Goldhamster (*Cricetus auratus*) unter normalen und experimentellen Bedingungen. Z. Zellforsch. **40**, 151—161 (1954).
Enemar, A., B. Falck, and F. C. Iturriza: Adrenergic nerves in the pars intermedia of the pituitary in the toad (*Bufo arenarum*). Z. Zellforsch. **77**, 325—330 (1967).
Falck, B.: Cellular localization of monoamines. Progr. Brain Res. 8, 28—44 (1964).
Farner, D. S., A. Oksche, and L. Lorenzen: Hypothalamic neurosecretion and the photoperiodic testicular response in the white-crowned sparrow (*Zonotrichia leucophrys gambelii*). In: Proc. 3rd Int. Symposium on Neurosecretion, Bristol 1961.
— The photoperiodic control of reproduction cycles in birds. Amer. Scientist **52**, 137—156 (1964).
Ficq, A., and J. Flament-Durand: Autoradiography in endocrine research. In: Techniques in endocrine research, pp. 73—85. Ed. by P. Eckstein and Fr. Knowles. New York: Academic Press 1963.
Fujita, H., and J. Fr. Hartmann: Electron microscopy of neurohypophysis in normal, adrenaline-treated and pilocarpine-treated rabbits. Z. Zellforsch. **54**, 734—763 (1961).
Fujita, T.: Über das Zwischenhirn-Hypophysensystem von Chimaera monstrosa. Z. Zellforsch. **60**, 147—162 (1963).
Fuxe, K.: Cellular localization of monoamines in the median eminence and the infundibular stem of some mammals. Z. Zellforsch. **61**, 710—724 (1964).
Gabe, M.: Neurosecretion. Oxford-London-Edinburgh-New York-Toronto-Paris-Braunschweig: Pergamon Press 1966.
Gaupp, V., u. H. Spatz: Hypophysenstieldurchtrennung und Geschlechtsreifung. Über Regenerationserscheinungen an der suprasellären Hypophyse. Acta neuroveg. (Wien) **12**, 285—328 (1955).
Geiling, E. M. M., and M. R. Lewis: Further information regarding the melanophore hormone of the hypophysis cerebri. Amer. J. Physiol. **113**, 534—537 (1935).
Greving, R.: Beitrag zur Innervation der Hypophyse. Klin. Wschr. **4**, 218 (1925).
Guillemin, R.: Hypothalamic-hypophysial interrelationships in the production of pituitary hormones *in vitro*. In: Hypothalamic-hypophysial interrelationships. Ed. by W. S. Fields. Springfield/Ill.: Charles C. Thomas 1956.
— Hypothalamic factors releasing pituitary hormones. Recent Progr. Hormone Res. **20**, 89—121 (1964).

HANSTRÖM, B.: The hypophysis in some South African insectivora, Carnivora, Hyracoidea, Proboscidea, Artiodactyla and Primates. Arkiv. Zool. **4**, 187—294 (1952).
— The neurohypophysis in the series of mammals. Z. Zellforsch. **39**, 241—259 (1953).
HARRIS, G.W.: Neural control of the Pituitary gland. Monographs of the Physiological Society. London: Edward Arnold (Publishers) Ltd. 1955.
— Entwicklung und heutiger Stand der Neuroendokrinologie. Dtsch. med. Wschr. **90**, 61—65 (1965).
HILD, W.: Experimentell-morphologische Untersuchungen über das Verhalten der „Neurosekretorischen Bahn" nach Hypophysenstieldurchtrennungen, Eingriffen in den Wasserhaushalt mit Belastung der Osmoregulation. Virchows Arch. path. Anat. **319**, 526—546 1951).
— Elaboration of so-called posterior lobe hormones in the hypothalamus. Biol. Bull. **105**, 360—361 (1953).
— Histological and endocrinological observations in tissue cultures of posterior pituitary of dog and rat. Tex. Rep. Biol. Med. **12**, 474—488 (1954).
— Das morphologische, kinetische und endokrinologische Verhalten von hypothalamischem und neurohypophysärem Gewebe *in vitro*. Z. Zellforsch. **40**, 257—312 (1954).
—, and G. ZETLER: Über das Vorkommen der Hypophysenhinterlappenhormone im Zwischenhirn. Arch. exp. Pathol. Pharmakol. **213**, 139—153 (1951).
— — Vergleichende Untersuchungen über das Vorkommen der Hypophysenhinterlappenhormone im Zwischenhirn einiger Säugetiere. Dtsch. Z. Nervenheilk. **167**, 205—214 (1952).
— — Über die Funktion des Neurosekrets im Zwischenhirn-Neurohypophysensystem als Trägersubstanz für Vasopressin, Adiuretin und Oxytocin. Z. ges. exp. Med. **120**, 236—243 (1953).
— — Experimenteller Beweis für die Entstehung der sog. Hypophysenhinterlappenwirkstoffe im Hypothalamus. Pflügers Arch. ges. Physiol. **257**, 169—201 (1953).
HÖKFELT, T.: The possible ultrastructural identification of tubero-infundibular dopamine-containing nerve endings in the median eminence of the rat. Brain Res. **5**, 121—123 (1967).
HOLMES, R.L.: Comparative observations on inclusions in nerve fibres of the mammalian neurohypophysis. Z. Zellforsch. **64**, 474—492 (1964).
— The fine structure of the infundibular process in the hedgehog. Z. Zellforsch. **61**, 894—912 (1964).
HOLZMANN, K.: Die neurosekretorische Verknüpfung von Hypothalamus und Hypophyse bei Balaenoptera borealis. Z. Zellforsch. **51**, 185—208 (1960).
ITURRIZA, F.C., and M.A. RESTELLI: Neurosecretion in the distal stump of the sectioned hypothalamic-hypophyseal tract in the toad. Z. Zellforsch. **81**, 297—302 (1967).
KIVALO, J.: Effect of some anesthetic agents on diuresis and hypothalamo-hypophysial neurosecretion in the rat. Ann. Med. exp. Fenn. **44** (Suppl. No. 5).
KNOWLES, FR.: Neuroendocrine correlations at the level of ultrastructure. Arch. Anat. Microscop. Morphol. Exper. **54**, 343—358 (1965).
—, and L. VOLLRATH: Synaptic contacts between neurosecretory fibres and pituicytes in the pituitary of the eel. Nature (Lond.) **206**, 1168—1169 (1965).
— — Neurosecretory innervation of the pituitary of the eels Anguilla and Conger. Proc. roy. Soc. **250**, 311—342 (1966).
— — Changes in the pituitary of the migrating european eel during its journey from rivers to the sea. Z. Zellforsch. **75**, 317—327 (1966).
KOBAYASHI, H.: Histochemical, electron-microscopic and pharmacologic studies on the median eminence. Excerpta Med. Int. Congr. Ser. No. 83, 570—576 (1964).
—, T. HIRANO, and T. MATSUI: Accumulation of aldehyde-fuchsin stainable material in the posterior median eminence following total hypophysectomy or adenohypophysectomy in the pigeon. J. Fac. Sci., Univ. Tokyo, Sec. IV, **11**, 1—9 (1966).
—, Y. OOTA, H. UEMURA, and T. HIRANO: Electron-microscopic and pharmacological studies on the rat median eminence. Z. Zellforsch. **71**, 387—404 (1966).
KRATZSCH, E.: Experimentell-morphologische Untersuchungen am Zwischenhirn-Hypophysensystem der Ratte bei Polyurie infolge Alloxanvergiftung. (Mit besonderer Berücksichtigung der Pituicyten.) Z. Zellforsch. **36**, 371—380 (1951).
LEDERIS, K.: Ultrastructure of the hypothalamo-neurohypophysial system in teleost fishes and isolation of hormone-containing granules from the neurohypophysis of the cod (*Gadus morrhua*). Z. Zellforsch. **58**, 192—213 (1962).
— An electron-microscopical study of the human neurohypophysis. Z. Zellforsch. **65**, 847—868 (1965).
— Acetylcholin in the mammalian neurohypophysis. J. Endocr. **37**, 24—25 (1966).
— Beziehung zwischen der Ultrastruktur der Neurohypophyse und der subcellulären Verteilung von biologisch aktiven Substanzen. Naunyn-Schmiedebergs Arch. Path. Pharmak. **257**, 83—93 (1967).

Legait, H., et E. Legait: Terminaisons neurosécrétoires au niveau de l'adénohypophyse chez quelques téléostéens. Etude au microscope électronique. C.R. Soc. Biol. (Paris) **151**, **1943** à 1946 (1957).

— — Recherches sur l'ultrastructure de l'hypophyse de quelques téléostéens. C.R. Soc. Biol. (Paris) **152**, 130—133 (1958).

— —, C. Burlet, et A. Burlet: Recherches histo-enzymologiques sur le système hypothalamo-neurohypophysaire du Lérot (*Eliomys quercinus* L.). Bull. Ass. Anat. 51. Réun. Marseille 1966.

Malandra, B.: Beobachtungen am neurosekretorischen Zwischenhirnsystem der normalen, trächtigen und laktierenden Ratte. Z. Zellforsch. **43**, 594—610 (1956).

Matsui, T.: Fine structure of the median eminence of the rat. J. Fac. Sci. Univ. Tokyo, Sec. IV, **11**, 71—96 (1966).

—, and H. Kobayashi: Histochemical demonstration of monoamine oxidase in the hypothalamo-hypophysial system of the tree sparrow and the rat. Z. Zellforsch. **68**, 172—182 (1965).

Mautner, W.: Das räumliche Bild des neurosekretorischen Zwischenhirnsystems und der portalen Hypophysengefäße von Rana temporaria und einigen anderen Anuren. Mit Lebendbeobachtungen am portalen Hypophysenkreislauf. Z. Zellforsch. **64**, 813—826 (1964).

Moll, J.: Regeneration of the supraoptico-hypophysial and paraventriculo-hypophysial tracts in the hypophysectomized rat. Z. Zellforsch. **46**, 686—709 (1957).

Monroe, Barbara G.: A comparative study on the ultrastructure of the median eminence, infundibular stem and neural lobe of the hypophysis of the rat. Z. Zellforsch. **76**, 405—432 (1967).

—, and D.E. Scott: Ultrastructural changes in the neural lobe of the hypophysis of the rat during lactation and suckling. J. Ultrastruct. Res. **14**, 497—517 (1966).

Nowakowski, H.: Infundibulum und Tuber cinereum der Katze. Dtsch. Z. Nervenheilk. **165**, 261—339 (1951).

Oksche, A., D.S. Farner, D.L. Serventy, F. Wolff, and C.A. Nicholls: The hypothalamohypophysial neurosecretory system of the Zebra finch (*Taeniopygia castanotis*). Z. Zellforsch. **58**, 846—914 (1963).

—, D.F. Laws, F.I. Kamemoto, and D.S. Farner: The hypothalamo-hypophysial neurosecretory system of the white-crowned sparrow (*Zonotrichia leucophrys Gambelii*). Z. Zellforsch. **51**, 1—42 (1959).

—, W.O. Wilson, and D.S. Farner: The hypothalamic neurosecretory system of *Coturnix coturnix japonica*. Z. Zellforsch. **61**, 688—709 (1964).

Oota, Y.: On the synaptic vesicles in the neurosecretory organs of the carp, bullfrog, pigeon and mouse. Annot. Zool. Jap. **36**, 167—172 (1963).

—, and H. Kobayashi: Fine structures of the median eminence and pars nervosa of the pigeon. Annot. Zool. Jap. **35**, 128—138 (1962).

— — Fine structure of the median eminence and the pars nervosa of the bullfrog (*Rana catesbeiana*). Z. Zellforsch. **60**, 667—687 (1963).

Ortmann, R.: Über experimentelle Veränderungen der Morphologie des Hypophysen-Zwischenhirnsystems und die Beziehung der sog. „Gomorisubstanz" zum Adiuretin. Z. Zellforsch. **36**, 92—140 (1951).

Pickford, M.: Control of the secretion of antidiuretic hormone from the pars nervosa of the pituitary gland. Physiol. Rev. **25**, 573—595 (1945).

— The action of acetylcholine in the supraoptic nucleus of the chloralosed dog. J. Physiol. (Lond.) **106**, 264—270 (1947).

Ranson, S.W., C. Fisher, and W.R. Ingram: The hypothalamico-hypophysial mechanism in diabetes insipidus. Res. Publ. Ass. nerv. ment. Dis. **17**, 410—432 (1938).

Rasmussen, A.T.: The weight of the principal components of the normal male adult human hypophysis cerebri. Amer. J. Anat. **42**, 1—27 (1928).

— The weight of the principal components of the normal hypophysis cerebri of the adult human female. Amer. J. Anat. **55**, 253—275 (1934).

Rinne, U.K.: Ultrastructure of the median eminence of the rat. Z. Zellforsch. **74**, 98—122 (1966).

de Robertis, E.: Histophysiology of synapses and neurosecretion. Oxford-London-Edinburgh-New York-Paris-Frankfurt: Pergamon Press 1964.

Rodeck, H., u. R. Braukmann: Zur Frage der Wirkung von Morphiumsulfat auf das neurosekretorische System. Z. Zellforsch. **75**, 517—526 (1966).

Rodriguez, E.M.: Differences between median eminence and neural lobe in amphibians. Z. Zellforsch. **74**, 308—316 (1966).

Romeis, B.: Die Hypophyse. In: Handbuch der mikroskopischen Anatomie des Menschen. Hrsg. von W. v. Möllendorff, Bd. VI, S. 3. Berlin: Springer 1940.

ROTHBALLER, A.B.: Changes in the rat neurohypophysis induced by painful stimuli with particular reference at neurosecretory material. Anat. Rec. **115**, 23—36 (1953).

— Pathways of secretion and regulation of posterior pituitary factors. Res. Publ. Ass. nerv. ment. Dis. **43**, 86—131 (1966).

SARRAT, R.: Modificaciones de la pars intermedia y posterior de la hipófisis producidas por el hambre y la sed. An. Anat. **16**, 59—98 (1967).

SCHARRER, E.: Das Hypophysen-Zwischenhirnsystem von Scyllium stellare. Z. Zellforsch. **37**, 196—204 (1952).

— Neurosecretion in the vertebrates: a survey. Publ. Staz. zool. Napoli **24** (Suppl.). Convegno sulla Neurosecrezione 1954, 18—20.

—, u. B. SCHARRER: Neurosekretion. In: Handbuch der mikroskopischen Anatomie des Menschen, Bd. VI, S. 5. Hrsg. von W. BARGMANN. Berlin-Göttingen-Heidelberg: Springer 1954.

SLOPER, J.C., D.J. ARNOTT, and B.C. KING: Sulphin metabolism in the pituitary and hypothalamus of the rat. A study of radioisotope-uptake after the injection of ^{35}S O-L-Cysteine, Methionine, and sodium sulphate. J. Endocr. **20**, 9—23 (1960).

SMOLLER, C.G.: Ultrastructural studies on the developing neurohypophysis of the Pacific treefrog (*Hyla regilla*). Gen. comp. Endocr. **7**, 44—73 (1966).

SPATZ, H.: Neues über die Verknüpfung von Hypophyse und Hypothalamus. Acta neuroveg. (Wien) **3**, 5—49 (1951).

STREEFKERK, J.G.: Functional changes in the morphological appearance of the hypothalamo-hypophyseal neurosecretory and cholaminergic neural system, and in the adenohypophysis of the rat. Acad. Proefschrift, 1—110. Drukkerij W.G. van Soest N.V., Amsterdam 1967.

STUTINSKY, F.: Sur l'existence de cellules ganglionnaires dans la neurohypophyse de Boeuf. C.R. Soc. Biol. (Paris) **142**, 63—65 (1948).

— La neurosécrétion au cours de la gestation et le post-partum chez la rate. Ann. Endocr. (Paris) **14**, 722—725 (1953).

— Recherches morphologiques sur le complexe hypothalamo-neurohypophysaire. Bull. Micr. appl. Mémoire Lors série No. 2. Paris 1957.

—, M. BONVALLET, and P. DELL: Les modifications hypophysaires au cours du diabète insipide expérimental chez le chien. I, II. Ann. Endocr. (Paris) **10**, 505 (1949); **11**, 1 (1950).

VERNEY, E.B.: The antidiuretic hormone and the factors which determine its release. Proc. roy. Soc. B **135**, 27—106 (1947).

VITUMS, A., SH.-I. MIKAMI, A. OKSCHE, and D.S. FARNER: Vascularization of the hypothalamo-hypophysial complex in the white-crowned sparrow (*Zonotrichia leucophrys Gambelii*). Z. Zellforsch. **64**, 541—569 (1964).

—, K. ONO, A. OKSCHE, D.S. FARNER, and J.R. KING: The development of the hypophysial portal system in the white-crowned sparrow (*Zonotrichia leucophrys Gambelii*). Z. Zellforsch. **73**, 335—366 (1966).

VOLLRATH, L.: Über die neurosekretorische Innervation der Adenohypophyse von Teleostiern, insbesondere von *Hippocampus cuda* und *Tinca tinca*. Z. Zellforsch. **78**, 234—260 (1967).

WITTKOWSKI, W.: Synaptische Strukturen und Elementargranula in der Neurohypophyse des Meerschweinchens. Z. Zellforsch. **82**, 434—458 (1967).

ZAMBRANO, D., and E. DE ROBERTIS: Ultrastructure of the hypothalamic neurosecretory system of the dog. Z. Zellforsch. **81**, 264—282 (1967).

Chemistry of the Neurohypophysial Hormones

R. A. BOISSONNAS and ST. GUTTMANN

With 21 Figures

Seven chemically related hormones have been detected up to now in the neurohypophyses of mammals, birds, amphibians and fish: oxytocin, vasopressin, lysine-vasopressin, vasotocin, mesotocin, isotocin and glumitocin. As can be seen from their chemical structure (Fig. 1), they all consist of a peptide chain of nine amino acid residues and are therefore, strictly speaking, nonapeptides. The two half cystine residues occupying the 1st and the 6th positions of the chain are linked together by their sulphur atoms, thus forming a ring of 20 atoms. As these two half cystine residues constitute together *one* cystine residue, some authors formerly designated these hormones as octapeptides, but this nomenclature is now considered illogical, for it is impossible to apply it in the case of more complicated peptides like insulin, which have nevertheless the same 20 atom ring.

These neurohypophysial hormones differ among themselves in the nature of the amino acid residues occupying positions 3, 4 and/or 8. In all these hormones the amino group of the first half cystine residue is free and the carboxyl groups are amidified by ammonia. As a result all of them, even those which do not contain basic amino acids, are bases which form salts with acids and migrate towards the cathode at neutral pH.

The flavianate (PIERCE et al., 1952) and the p-hydroxybenzene-p′-sulphonate (BODANSZKY and DU VIGNEAUD, 1959d) of oxytocin have occasionally been

Oxytocin

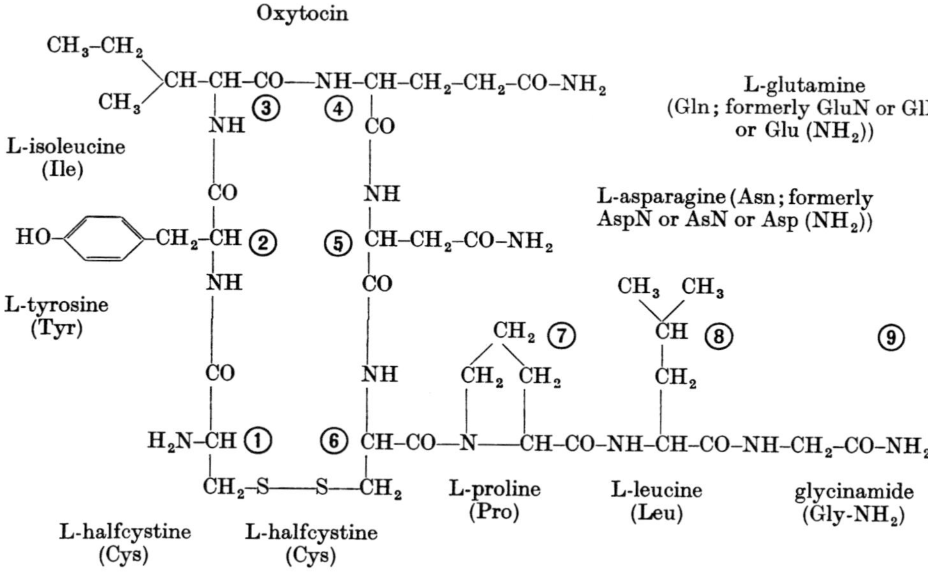

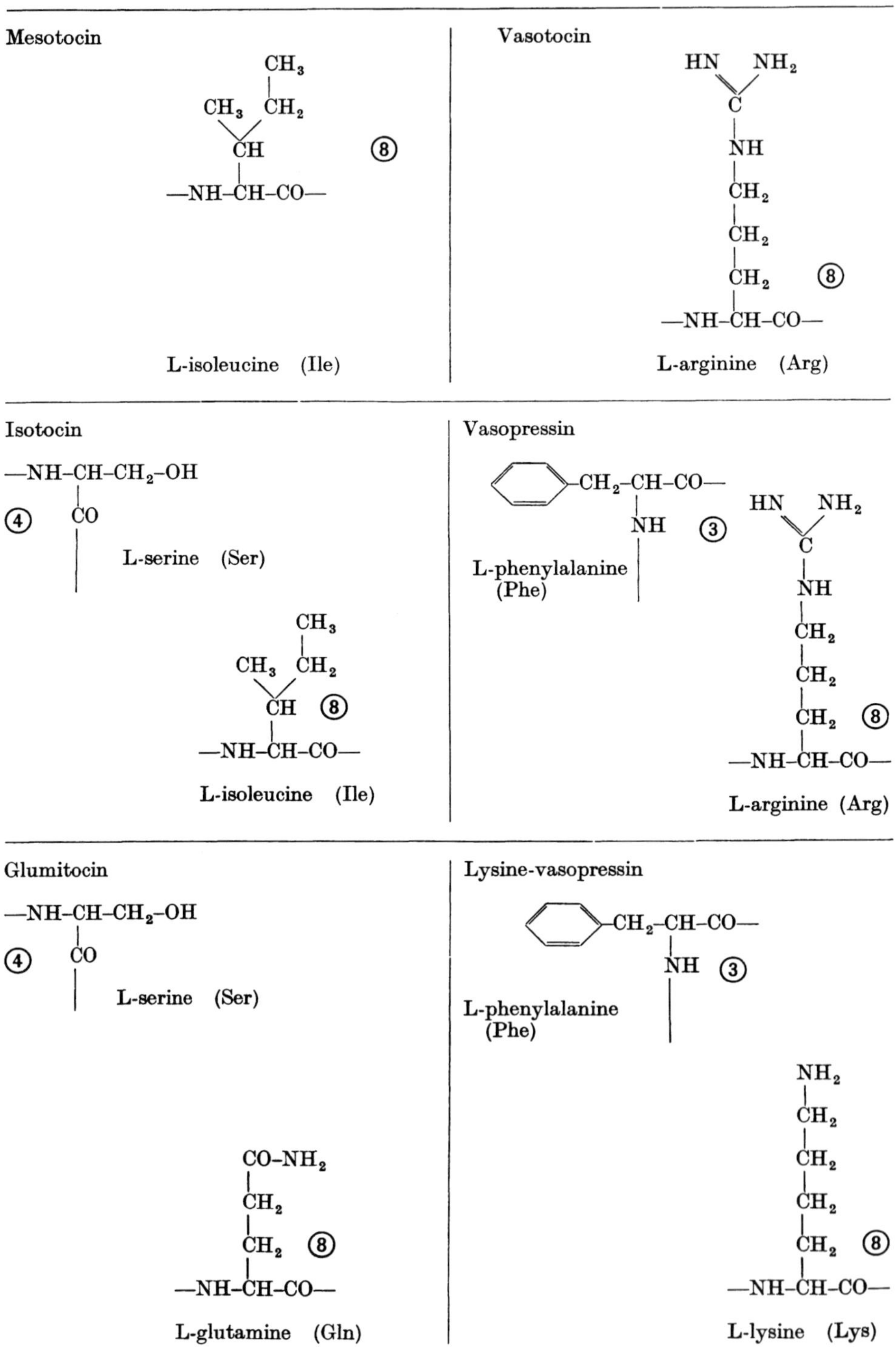

Fig. 1. Structure of the neurohypophysial hormones

obtained in crystalline form. The reactivity of the N-terminal amino group has been studied in more detail in oxytocin than for the other members of the family. Oxytocin can be acylated by acylating agents or reacted with isocyanates to the corresponding carbamates (SMYTH, 1965) and with acetone to a Schiff's base (YAMASHIRO et al., 1965).

The terminal amide group as well as the lateral amide group of the glutamine and asparagine residues are susceptible to hydrolysis, especially by aqueous acids the speed of hydrolysis increasing with temperature and hydrogen ion concentration. In alkaline medium the amide group of the asparagine residue is split with the formation of the corresponding imide, which can re-open, giving a β-peptide linkage. All these reactions yield products deprived of the original biological activities and largely account for the slow inactivation of the peptides which occurs on heating their aqueous solutions.

The phenolic hydroxyl group of the tyrosine residue can be acylated under special conditions, but, in most cases, this reaction has not been thoroughly investigated.

The disulphide bridge of these hormones is opened by reducing agents, two thiol groups being formed. When this reduction is effected by Raney nickel (TURNER et al., 1951) the thiol groups formed are replaced by hydrogen atoms, this introducing two alanine residues in place of the original half cystine residues.

Oxidation by performic acid also opens the ring, in this case by converting both half cystine residues to cysteic acid residues (cf. e. g. MUELLER et al., 1951). At alkaline pH this oxidation reaction may even occur, although slowly, merely in the presence of air.

In their normal, active, form these hormones have an intramolecular disulphide bridge. Besides this monomeric form they can also exist as polymers, in which the disulphide bridges are intermolecular (RESSLER, 1958; SCHALLY and GUILLEMIN, 1964 cf. also HEATON et al., 1956). These polymeric forms seem to be inactive or to possess only a low activity. It is difficult to decide whether such polymers possess low activity or are totally devoid of activity, for partial reconversion to the normal active monomeric form can occur during the assay procedure.

In the blood, as in most solutions used for pharmacological or medical purposes, these hormones are in a very dilute state, which strongly favours their monomeric, active form. Upon concentration the equilibrium shifts more and more towards the polymeric forms. This equilibrium establishes itself rapidly at neutral or slightly alkaline pH in presence of catalytic amounts of metallic ions and of compounds with thiol groups. On dilution, the equilibrium is reversed toward the prefential formation of the monomeric form. In moderately acid solution, the equilibrium establishes itself much more slowly, and the rate of formation of the inactive polymers on concentration is also retarded as is their reconversion into active monomers on dilution.

The behaviour in the dry state is analogous to their behaviour in highly concentrated solution. Only neutral salts with nonvolatile acids are stable. Acid salts bring on the hydrolysis of the amide groups by the included water. Salts with weak volatile acids, such as acetic acid, tend to lose their volatile acid component to give the free base, which by autocatalysis yields polymers.

It follows from these considerations that these hormones are best stored as dilute, slightly acidic aqueous solutions.

It must be kept in mind that the chemical formulae, as drawn in extended form in Fig. 1 for the sake of clarity, do not give an idea of the compactness of these molecules. The peptide chain is like the vertebral column of a coiled hedgehog and the characteristic side groups of the amino acid residues protrude outside like prickles. These hormones can therefore come in contact with other large molecules (e. g. receptors) only with their characteristic side groups. This explains why even very small changes in these side groups affect their biological properties so profoundly.

In the following paragraphs of this chapter the isolation, the determination of the structure and the synthesis of each of these hormones is briefly reviewed[1].

I. Oxytocin

A. Isolation

Since DUDLEY described the existence of an oxytocic and a pressor factor in the pituitary gland in 1919, a large number of workers have attempted to isolate them in pure state.

The first real purification of oxytocin was achieved by KAMM et al. (1928) who extracted acetonic hypophysial powder with hot dilute acetic acid. On saturating the obtained solution with salt both the oxytocic and pressor factors were precipitated. After extraction with glacial acetic acid, followed by fractional precipitation with acetone, ether and petrol ether, a dry material possessing 160 IU oxytocic and 6 IU pressoric activity per mg was obtained. With the aid of a slightly different procedure (STEHLE and FRASER, 1935) the activity of the material was raised to 250 IU oxytocic activity per mg.

Chromatographic purification on zeolite columns led to almost pure oxytocin (POTTS and GALLAGHTER, 1942, 1944). The oxytocin was finally obtained in an analytically pure state by LIVERMORE and DU VIGNEAUD (1949) after submitting the product purified by the Kamm procedure to two successive counter-current distributions. An activity of 865 IU/mg was given in the first reports, but this value was later corrected by the same authors (PIERCE et al., 1952), who found that despite extensive counter current distribution and several crystallisations of its flavianate, the product could not be purified above 490 IU/mg. The same degree of activity was also obtained for oxytocin purified by a slightly different procedure by French authors (MAIER-HUESER et al., 1953) and for oxytocin obtained by total synthesis.

For the purification of very small quantities, CONDLIFFE (1955) has proposed a purification by partition chromatography on Hyflo Supercel.

A recent and relatively simple method of purification uses a combination of ion-exchange chromatography and zone electrophoresis (PORATH, 1957). This should permit the preparation of pure oxytocin on a gramme scale. Another rapid method of purification employs ion exchange chromatography on CM-cellulose (SCHALLY et al., 1959).

A useful method for the isolation of very small quantities of oxytocin and of vasopressin is based on the properties of these hormones to associate with the protein neurophysin (ACHER et al., 1958b). The complex formed can be dissociated by treatement with trichloracetic acid. Human (LIGHT and DU VIGNEAUD, 1958), ox, hog (ACHER et al., 1958b), horse (ACHER et al., 1958a, 1959a), sheep (ACHER et al., 1959b) and whale oxytocin (ACHER et al., 1963) have been isolated by this procedure.

---

[1] The abbreviations used for the amino acid residues are indicated in Fig. 1 along with the chemical structures. The schemes of synthesis are written in the usual abbreviated manner, i. e. the chemical functions only of the peptide are given and its skeleton is represented by a heavy line crossing the thin lines corresponding to the amino acid residues it contains. The abbreviations used for the protecting groups are all summarized at the bottom of Fig. 2.

Gel filtration alone (LINDNER et al., 1959; PORATH and SCHALLY, 1962) or associated with partition chromatography (YAMASHIRO, 1964) has been used recently to prepare pure oxytocin.

B. Elucidation of the Structure of Oxytocin

The amino acid composition of oxytocin was established for the first time by PIERCE and DU VIGNEAUD (1950). After hydrolysis of the hormone in 5.8 N HCl for 20 hours at 110°, the resulting amino acids were separated by chromatography on a starch column and quantitatively measured by reacting them with ninhydrine. The following amino acid composition was found: leucine, isoleucine, tyrosine, proline, glutamic acid, aspartic acid, glycine and cystine in equimolar amounts as well as a little more than three equivalents of ammonia. This amino acid composition was later confirmed on the hydrolysate of pure hog and bovine oxytocins obtained via their crystalline flavianates (PIERCE et al., 1952).

The structure of oxytocin was elucidated independently and at about the same time by DU VIGNEAUD et al. (1953b) and by TUPPY (TUPPY, 1953; TUPPY and MICHL, 1953). DU VIGNEAUD deduced the sequence of the amino acids in oxytocin on the basis of the amino acid composition of the different peptides obtained after mild hydrolysis and of the results given by Edman's degradation of some of these fragments. Postulating that all the amino acids were most probably bound together by α-amide linkages and that the three moles of ammonia amidified the three carboxyl groups not taking part in peptide linkages, DU VIGNEAUD proposed the following structure for oxytocin:

$$\text{H–}\underline{\text{Cys–Tyr–Ile–Gln–Asn–Cys}}\text{–Pro–Leu–Gly–NH}_2$$

Working with oxidised oxytocin and applying slightly different techniques TUPPY (TUPPY, 1953; TUPPY and MICHL, 1953) arrived simultaneously and independently at the same structure, which, some months later, was confirmed by the brilliant total synthesis of DU VIGNEAUD et al. (1953a).

Oxytocin has been isolated and chemically characterised in the following species: hog and beef (DU VIGNEAUD et al., 1953b), horse (ACHER et al., 1958, 1959a), man (LIGHT and DU VIGNEAUD, 1958), domestic fowl (ACHER et al., 1960a), sheep (CHAUVET et al., 1960a) and whale (ACHER et al., 1963).

C. Action of Enzymes on Oxytocin

Oxytocin is relatively resistant to proteolytic enzymes. Carboxypeptidase and trypsin are, as expected, without effect, chymotrypsin and leucinaminopeptidase attack it only very slowly. Subtilisin liberates glycinamide from oxytocin, but not from its oxidised derivative (ACHER et al., 1959a, b).

Oxytocin is readily inactivated by the enzyme, named oxytocinase, which can be found in body fluids, especially in serum, and in tissue homogenates (see: TUPPY, 1960, 1961). Oxytocinase possesses amino-peptidase-like activity and splits oxytocin between Cys and Tyr. It is present in greater concentration in the serum of pregnant women, its concentration reaching a maximum just before term and then rapidly decreasing (MENDEZ-BAUER et al., 1961). Oxytocinase of serum origin has been purified and characterised (TUPPY and WINTERSBERGER, 1960). For its standardisation L-cystine-di-β-naphthylamide was used as substrate (TUPPY and NESWADBA, 1957). According to RYCHLIK (1964) the inactivation of oxytocin by tissue extracts proceeds in two steps: in the first step the disulphide bridge is opened by reduction and in the second an aminopeptidase-like enzyme, which is unable to attack the intact molecule, splits the N-terminal amino acid residues.

Recently two enzymes possessing oxytocin inactivating activity have been isolated from retroplacental serum (SJÖHOLM, 1964). They act by liberating cysteine and tyrosine from oxytocin.

D. Synthesis of Oxytocin

Having elucidated the structure of oxytocin, DU VIGNEAUD et al. (1953a, 1954a) confirmed it by synthesis (Fig. 2). They synthesised the sequences 3—5 and 6—9 and coupled them together in order to form the heptapeptide 3—9, which was in turn condensed with the dipeptide 1—2 to yield the protected nonapeptide

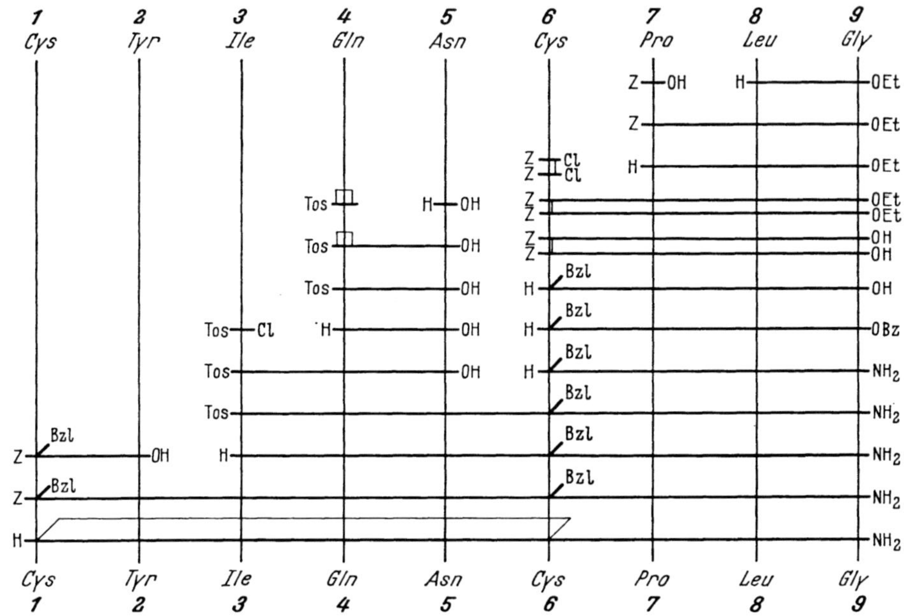

Fig. 2. Synthesis of oxytocin (DU VIGNEAUD et al., 1953a and 1954)

Abbreviations:

	Trt = trityl	Et = ethyl
	EC = ethylcarbamoyl	Me = methyl
Z = benzyloxycarbonyl	NO_2-Z = p-nitrobenzyloxycarbonyl	But = tert. butyl
Tos = p-toluenesulphonyl	Bz = benzoyl	NP = p-nitrophenyl
Boc = tert. butyloxycarbonyl	Bzl = benzyl	CP = 2, 4, 5-trichlorphenyl

1—9. All the protecting groups were removed by treatment with sodium in liquid ammonia and the thiol groups of the H-Cys(H)-Tyr-Ile-Gln-Asn-Cys(H)-Pro-Leu-Gly-NH_2 thus obtained were oxidised with air in order to form the disulphide bridge. As had been expected, this oxidation gave rise to several side products besides the desired cyclic nonapeptide. After purification by counter current distribution DU VIGNEAUD and his collaborators succeeded in obtaining pure synthetic oxytocin which proved to be identical in all respects with the natural hormone. A crystalline flavianate which was identical with the one formerly obtained with the natural hormone (PIERCE et al., 1952), was also produced.

The brilliant work of DU VIGNEAUD thus not only confirmed that the structure proposed by him for oxytocin was correct, but also showed for the first time that large biologically active peptides could be produced by synthesis. However, this first synthesis of oxytocin was rather long and complicated. Moreover it necessitated several treatments with sodium in liquid ammonia, which, as later work in peptide chemistry has shown, is not without detriment to peptide chains. For these reasons, du Vigneaud himself, as well as numerous other workers, have endeavoured to improve the synthesis of oxytocin.

In a first new approach (Boissonnas et al., 1955), the three tripeptides 1—3, 4—6 and 7—9 were synthesised by stepwise elongation from the C-terminal end (Fig. 3). The sequences 4—6 and 7—9 were then linked together, and the hexapeptide obtained, after removal of its N-terminal protecting group, was coupled

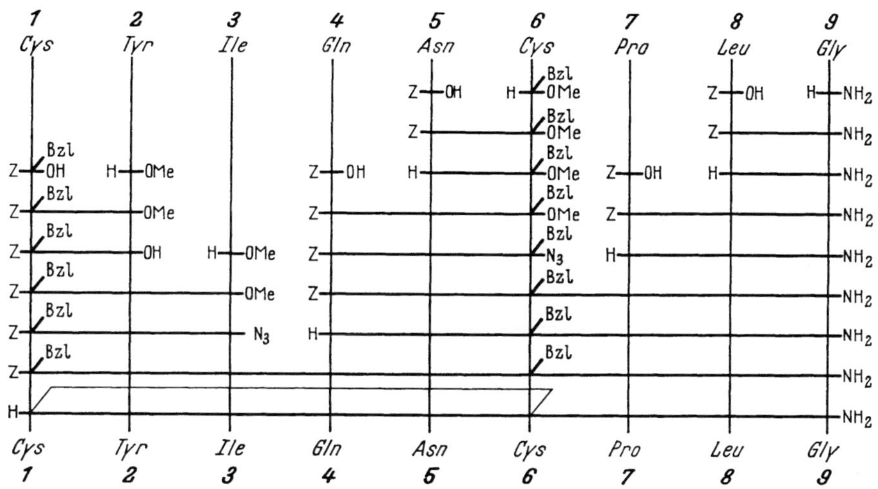

Fig. 3. Synthesis of oxytocin (Boissonnas et al., 1955)

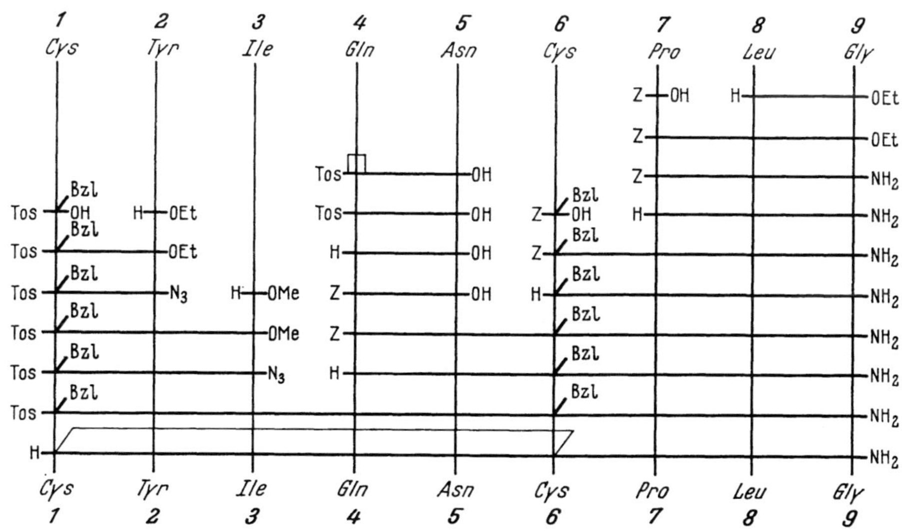

Fig. 4. Synthesis of oxytocin (Rudinger et al., 1956)

with the N-terminal tripeptide, yielding the same protected nonapeptide as formerly obtained by du Vigneaud. This improved scheme of synthesis, which led to the first industrial production of oxytocin requires a fewer number of steps and affords higher yields. It has the additional advantage that it avoids the danger of racemisation. In a third scheme of synthesis (RUDINGER et al., 1956) (Fig. 4), which is intermediate between the above two procedures, the nonapeptide is protected at its N-terminal end by a tosyl group.

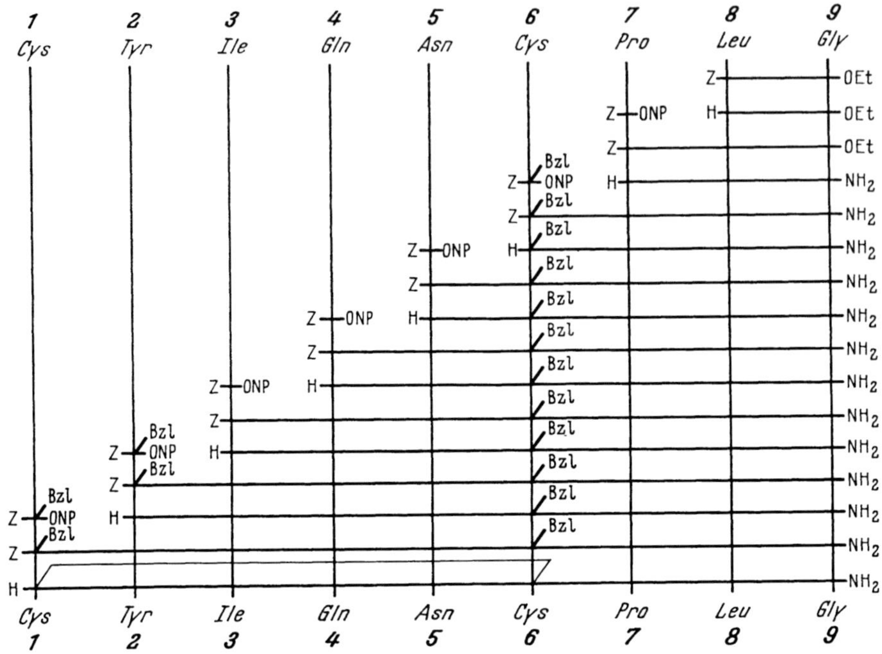

Fig. 5. Synthesis of oxytocin (BODANSZKY and DU VIGNEAUD, 1959b, c)

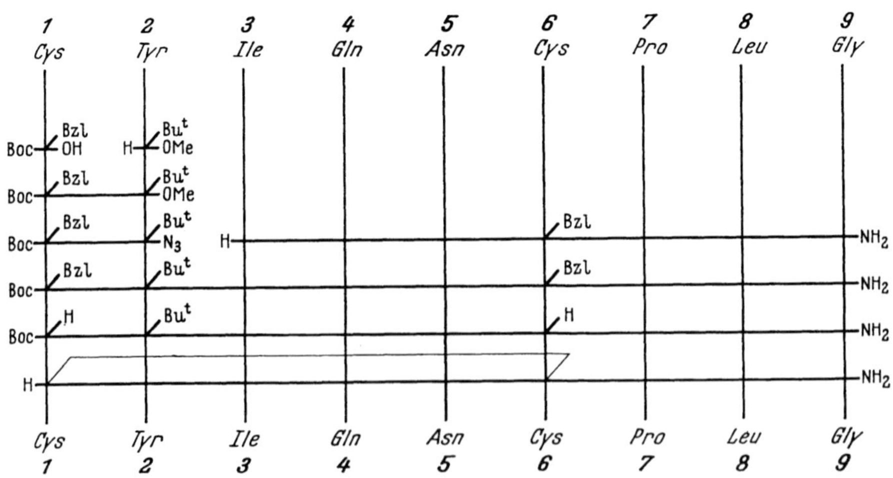

Fig. 6. Synthesis of oxytocin (STURM et al., 1964)

In each of these three syntheses the building of peptide bonds was achieved by activating the carboxyl groups in form of their chloride, azide or mixed anhydride. The introduction of dicyclohexyl-carbodiimide as reagent in peptide chemistry (SHEEHAN and HESS, 1955) and the use of p-nitrophenyl esters (BODANSZKY, 1955) led to other improved syntheses of oxytocin.

In a general study on the synthesis of oxytocin (BODANSZKY and DU VIGNEAUD, 1959a) the sequences 1—5 and 6—9 were linked together by several methods, including the dicyclohexylcarbodiimide method.

In a further approach to the synthesis of oxytocin (BEYERMAN et al., 1959) extensive use was made of dicyclohexylcarbodiimide for the synthesis of sequences 1—3 and 4—9. The condensation of the sequence 1—3 with the sequence 4—9 was performed with high yield in a rather unusual aqueous organic medium. Unfortunately no biological activities are given in this description.

The next synthesis of oxytocin (BODANSZKY and DU VIGNEAUD, 1959b, c) (Fig. 5) represented a new approach in peptide synthesis. The whole molecule of oxytocin was built up by adding the different amino acids one by one in form of their protected active esters. Thus the peptide chain grew stepwise from its

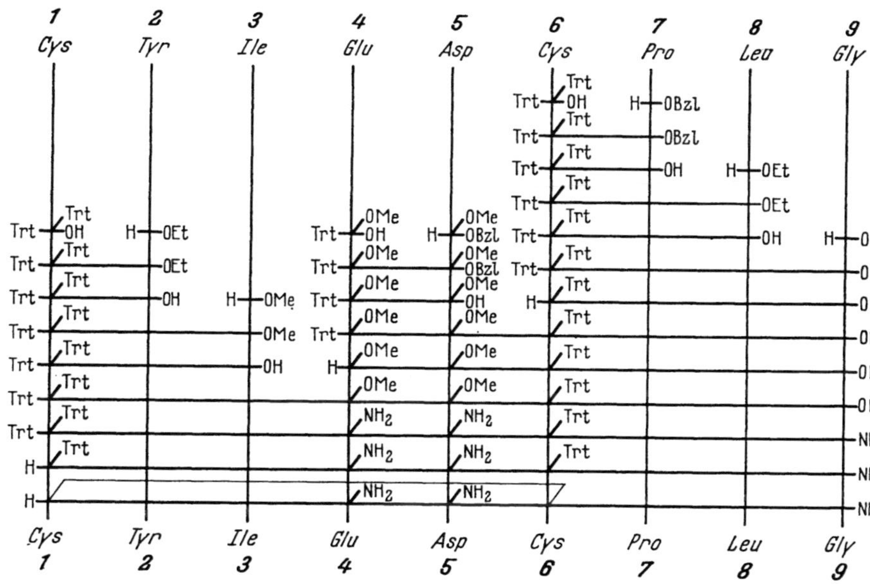

Fig. 7. Synthesis of oxytocin (VELLUZ et al., 1956)

C-terminal end towards its N-terminal end. Each step was performed with nearly quantitative yields by using a slight excess of activated amino acid at each step. By this method of synthesis the protected nonapeptide described earlier was obtained in a better overall yield in spite of the higher number of intermediary steps.

In all the syntheses described above, the thiol groups of the cysteine residues were protected by a benzyl group and the N-terminal amino group, by a benzyloxycarbonyl or a tosyl group. In the final step all protecting groups were removed together by treatment with sodium in liquid ammonia. In another synthesis (STURM et al., 1964) (Fig. 6) a tert.-butyloxycarbonyl group was used to protect the amino group of the N-terminal cysteine residue. The benzyl groups protecting the thiol groups were first split off with sodium in liquid ammonia. This treatment left the tert.-butyloxycarbonyl group intact. A sparingly soluble partially protected nonapeptide was thus obtained, which was easily purified before the oxidation step. After cleavage of the amino-protecting group by treatment with trifluoracetic acid or hydrochloric acid and conversion into the corresponding acetate, pure oxytocine acetate was isolated. This, after oxidation with air, yielded oxytocin in high yield.

A common feature of all these syntheses of oxytocin is the protection of the thiol groups of both cysteine residues with the aid of benzyl groups. The removal of these groups necessitates treatment with sodium in liquid ammonia, which, as mentioned above, may lead to undesired side reactions.

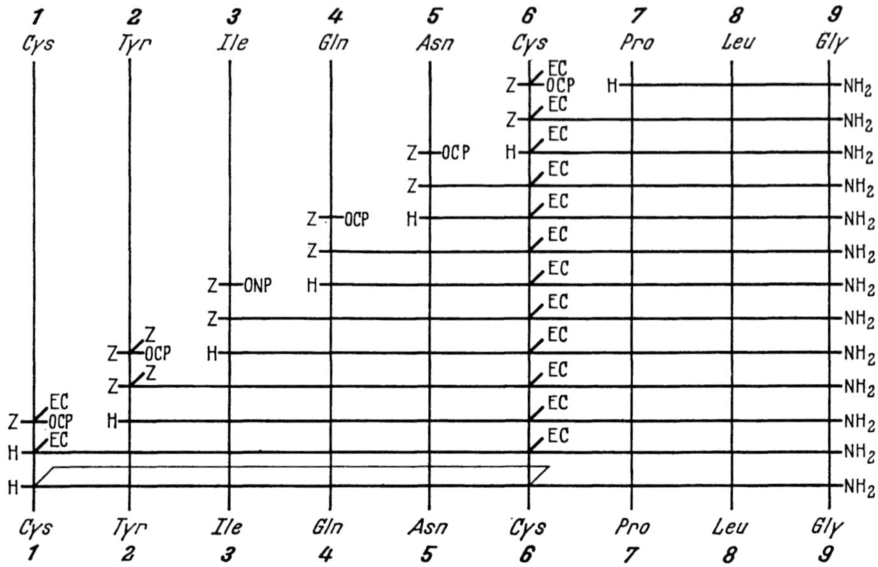

Fig. 8. Synthesis of oxytocin (GUTTMANN, 1963 and 1966)

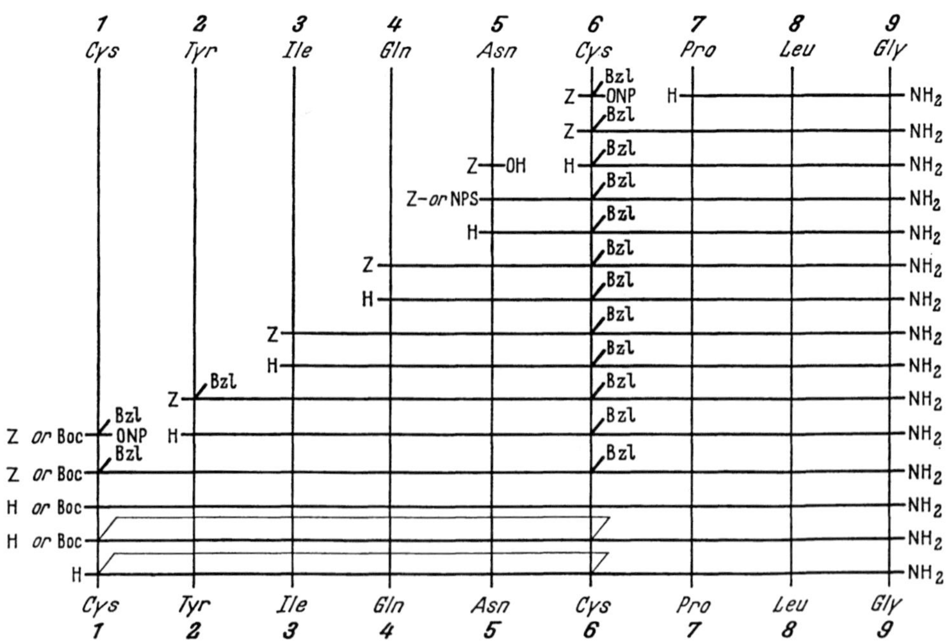

Fig. 9. Synthesis of oxytocin (PHOTAKI, 1966)

The following approaches represent attempts to avoid this shortcoming by using new thiol protecting groups which can be removed under mild conditions.

A first and very original approach (Velluz et al., 1956) used triphenylmethyl groups to protect the N-terminal amino group as well as the thiol groups (Fig. 7). The condensation steps were performed with the aid of dicyclohexylcarbodiimide, the yields at each step being over 70 %. Dangers of racemisation were not, however, excluded in this way of synthesis. In the final step the triphenylmethyl groups were removed by relatively mild treatment with aqueous 10 N hydrochloric acid in methylene chloride.

In a further approach along the same line (Guttmann, 1963, 1966) (Fig. 8), the ethylcarbamoyl group was used for the first time to protect the thiol group of both cysteine residues. The synthesis proceeded by stepwise elongation as in the scheme of Bodanszky and du Vigneaud (1959b, c), but 2, 4, 5-trichlorphenyl esters were employed to activate the carboxyl groups at each condensation step. At the end of the synthesis the thiol-protecting groups were removed with methanolic ammonia. The oxytocin thus obtained exhibited a biological activity of 510 ± 23 IU/mg.

The benzoyl group was also used to protect the thiol groups (Photaki, 1964, 1966) (Fig. 9). These S-benzoyl groups were removed at the end of the synthesis by mild treatment with sodium methylate, and ethylene iodide was employed for oxidation of the thiol groups to produce the S-S-bridge.

In the latest approach to the synthesis of oxytocin (Sakakibara et al., 1965) the thiol groups of the cysteines were protected with p-methoxybenzyl groups, which were removed in the last step with hot trifluoracetic acid or, still better, with anhydrous hydrofluoric acid.

E. Radioactive Oxytocin

Randomly tritium labelled oxytocin was obtained by exposure of oxytocin to tritium gas (du Vigneaud et al., 1962). By this procedure all the amino acids were labelled, glycine and tyrosine to a somewhat greater extent than the others. However the specific radioactivity obtained by this method did not exceed 12.4 microcuries/mg. Oxytocin, specifically tritium labelled in the leucyl residue situated at position 8, was prepared by the same authors (du Vigneaud et al., 1962) by incorporating labelled leucine into oxytocin by total synthesis. A radioactivity of 130 microcuries/mg was then obtained. Oxytocin labelled with tritium in the tyrosyl residue situated at position 2 has been obtained by iodination of oxytocin followed by catalytic reduction with tritium (Agishi and Dingman, 1965). Its specific radioactivity was 228 microcuries/mg.

Similarly labelled oxytocin was also obtained by total synthesis using tritium labelled tyrosine (Carlsson and Sjöholm, 1966). This material exhibited a specific radioactivity of 2900 microcuries/mg.

II. Vasopressins

The history of the vasopressins is closely related to that of oxytocin. Vasopressin (arginine-vasopressin) is present in the pituitary of all mammals hitherto investigated with the exception of the hog and some related mammals such as the peccary and hippopotamus, which possess lysine-vasopressin.

A. Isolation

The first really highly active vasopressin preparation was obtained by Stehle and Fraser (1935) by fractionated precipitation of pituitary extracts. A further purification by electrophoresis gave a product with an activity of 200 IU/mg (IRVING et al., 1941), but still contaminated with oxytocin. Shortly afterwards a vasopressin preparation with an activity of 450 IU/mg was obtained by adsorbing the contaminating oxytocin on zeolite (POTTS and GALLAGHER, 1942, 1944). Vasopressin in the high state of purity required for structural studies was first obtained by purification by counter-current distribution (TURNER et al., 1951). The same state of purity was also achieved by ionophoresis (ACHER and FROMAGEOT, 1955).

Vasopressin was also isolated via a protein complex (ACHER et al., 1958b). The complex of neurophysin with vasopressin and oxytocin was extracted from pituitary powder under very mild acidic conditions, salted out with sodium chloride and then freed from salts by dialysis. Treatment with 5% trichloroacetic acid liberated both peptidic hormones and precipitated the proteinic neurophysin. Vasopressin and oxytocin were adsorbed on Amberlite IRC-50 from the supernatant solution. Oxytocin and then vasopressin in that order were eluted with an ammonium acetate buffer. The vasopressin obtained by this method exhibited a very high purity, as evidenced by paper chromatography, paper electrophoresis and column chromatography. The same procedure was applied to isolate human (LIGHT and DU VIGNEAUD, 1958), bovine (ACHER et al., 1958b), equine (ACHER et al., 1958a), ovine (ACHER et al., 1959b), chicken (CHAUVET et al., 1960b) and whale (ACHER et al., 1963) vasopressins. It was also employed to isolate hog lysine-vasopressin (ACHER et al., 1958b) which had been formerly obtained by counter current distribution (POPENOE et al., 1952).

Partition chromatography on Hyflo-Super-Cel in the system sec-butanol/0.1% acetic acid has been applied for purification of very small quantities (3 mg) of pressor material of bovine and hog origin (CONDLIFFE, 1955). Hog lysine-vasopressin has also been obtained in a pure state by zone electrophoresis on cellulose (PORATH, 1957).

Ion exchange chromatography on carboxymethylcellulose yielded highly purified bovine vasopressin (380 IU/mg) and hog lysine-vasopressin (260 IU/mg) (WARD and GUILLEMIN, 1957; SCHALLY et al., 1959). This procedure permits the purification of large quantities of material, as does another ingenious method recently reported (SAFFRAN et al., 1962) in which pituitary powder is percolated in a continuously varying mixture of ethanol, water and acetic acid. The material thus obtained possessed a pressor activity of 60 IU/mg. Further purification by curtain electrophoresis yielded pure vasopressin (450 IU/mg).

B. Elucidation of the Structure of Vasopressin (Arginine-Vasopressin)

Total hydrolysis of highly purified vasopressin of bovine origin yielded phenylalanine, tyrosine, proline, glutamic acid, aspartic acid, glycine, arginine and cystine in approximately equimolar amounts, as well as three equivalents of ammonia (TURNER et al., 1951; ACHER and CHAUVET, 1953).

The method used to elucidate the structure of vasopressin (POPENOE and DU VIGNEAUD, 1953, 1954) was very similar to that used for oxytocin. Vasopressin was oxidised with performic acid and yielded the same amino acids as the intact material except that two equivalents of cysteic acid were found in place of cystine (POPENOE and DU VIGNEAUD, 1953). The oxidised vasopressin behaved as a single substance in counter-current distribution and in paper or ion exchange chromatography. Sanger's DNP method showed the N-terminal residue to be cysteic acid. Treatment with bromine water liberated $CySO_3H$-Tyr$(Br)_2$-OH and a single large peptide with phenylalanine in its N-terminal position. It was possible therefore to conclude that $CySO_3H$-Tyr-Phe was the N-terminal sequence of performic oxidised vasopressin. After partial acid hydrolysis eleven fractions were separated by ion exchange chromatography and their amino acid composition was determined.

From these findings the following partial sequence was established for oxidised vasopressin:

$$CySO_3H\text{–Tyr–Phe–Gln–Asn–}CySO_3H\text{–[Pro, Arg, Gly]–}NH_2$$

As digestion of vasopressin with trypsin liberated glycinamide (DU VIGNEAUD et al., 1953c), this showing that arginine immediately preceded glycine, only one position was possible for proline. The following structure was therefore proposed for vasopressin:

$$\underbrace{\text{Cys–Tyr–Phe–Gln–Asn–Cys}}\text{–Pro–Arg–Gly–}NH_2$$

The assumption that Gln and Asn were linked by α-peptidic linkages was confirmed later by the results obtained on digestion with papain (LAWER et al., 1954). The same conclusion was also arrived at using Edman's and Sanger's method to identify the N-terminal amino acid residue of the fragments obtained by partial hydrolysis (ACHER and CHAUVET, 1954).

C. Elucidation of the Structure of Lysine-Vasopressin

Total hydrolysis of highly purified vasopressin of hog origin yielded phenylalanine, tyrosine, glutamic acid, aspartic acid, proline, glycine, lysine and cystine in approximately equimolar ratio, as well as three equivalents of ammonia (POPENOE et al., 1952). Thus the amino acid contents of both vasopressine were identical, except for the basic amino acids, arginine and lysine.

The following structure was therefore proposed, merely on the grounds of analogy (DU VIGNEAUD et al., 1953c):

$$\underbrace{\text{Cys–Tyr–Phe–Gln–Asn–Cys}}\text{–Pro–Lys–Gly–}NH_2$$

This provisional structure was fully confirmed by total synthesis.

D. Synthesis of Vasopressin (Arginine-Vasopressin)

The first synthesis of vasopressin was achieved by DU VIGNEAUD's team in 1954 (DU VIGNEAUD et al., 1954b; cf. also KATSOYANNIS et al., 1957). As the arginyl residue in position 8 bears a reactive guanido group, this should be protected during the synthesis in order to avoid side reactions. DU VIGNEAUD's team partially resolved this problem by protonating this guanido group during the synthesis.

The protected nonapeptide was built up according to the scheme 5+(2+2) (Fig. 10). The two dipeptides 6—7 and 8—9 were prepared by the acid chloride method which is now rather hardly ever used in peptide chemistry. These two fragments were coupled together using tetraethylpyrophosphite as a condensing agent. The sequence 1—5 was built up by stepwise elongation from its C-terminal to its N-terminal end. Here again, extensive use was made of the acyl chloride condensation. The two main sequences 1—5 and 6—9 were allowed to react in the presence of tetraethylpyrophosphite, and the resulting protected nonapeptide was subjected, without further purification, to reduction by sodium in liquid ammonia, followed by oxidation. The crude product thus obtained exhibited a biological activity of only 21 IU/mg. It was purified by counter-current distribution, followed by block electrophoresis and a second counter current distribution. The final material possessed a pressor activity of 220 IU/mg. In spite of its relatively low biological activity, it behaved as a single substance and was undistinguishable from the natural product on ion exchange chromatography and paper electrophoresis. Its amino acid composition was as expected and the ratio of its pressor,

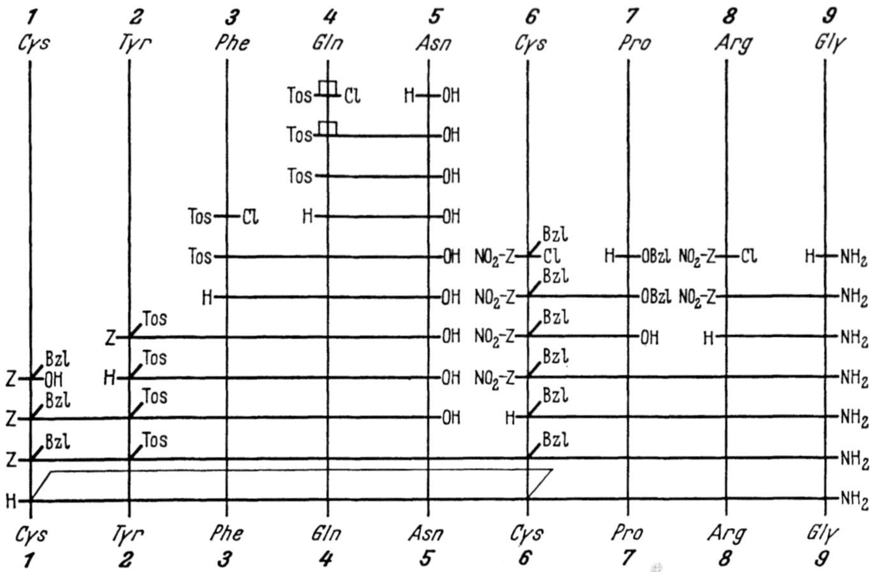

Fig. 10. Synthesis of vasopressin (DU VIGNEAUD et al., 1954; KATSOYANNIS et al., 1957)

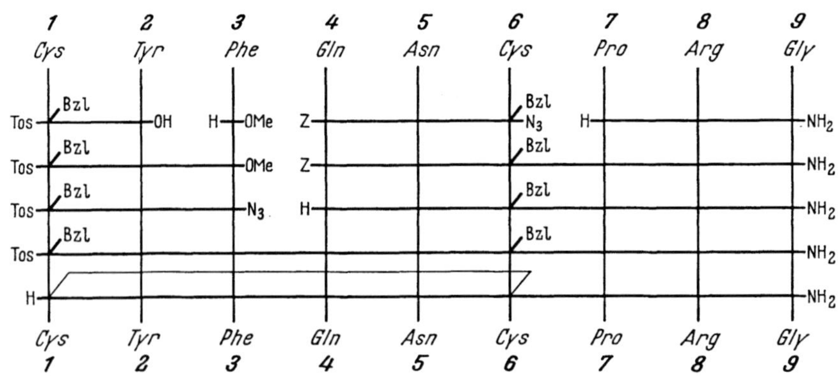

Fig. 11. Synthesis of vasopressin (DU VIGNEAUD et al., 1958)

antidiuretic and avian depressor activities was the same as for the natural product. It should be noted that this scheme of synthesis does not exclude racemisation of the asparagine residue which may explain why the product obtained exhibited only half the activity of the natural hormone.

In a second approach (DU VIGNEAUD et al., 1958), the same 3+(3+3) synthesis scheme was adopted (Fig. 11) as BOISSONNAS et al. (1955) had used for the synthesis of oxytocin. The condensation between the three main fragments, was effected by the azide method, this precluding the risk of racemisation. After removal of the protecting groups and establishment of the disulphide bridge by oxidation, the crude product exhibited a pressor activity of about 100 IU/mg. It was purified by counter-current distribution and yielded a material with 250

IU/mg. After an additional purification by electrophoresis on a cellulose block, vasopressin possessing about the same pressor activity as the natural product (i. e. 400 IU/mg) was obtained.

In a third approach (Studer and du Vigneaud, 1960) (Fig. 12) the guanido group of arginine was protected by the nitro group up to the penultimate step of the synthesis. The N-terminal hexapeptide was built up by the azide method

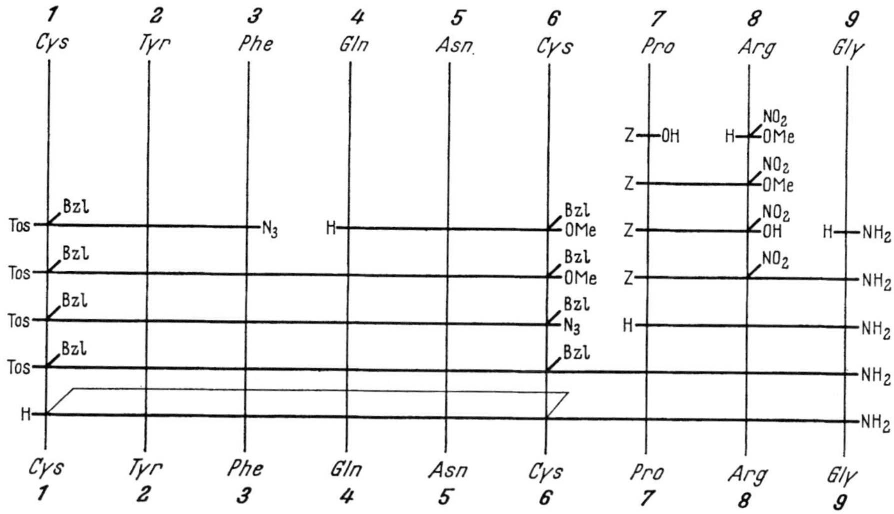

Fig. 12. Synthesis of vasopressin (Studer and du Vigneaud, 1960)

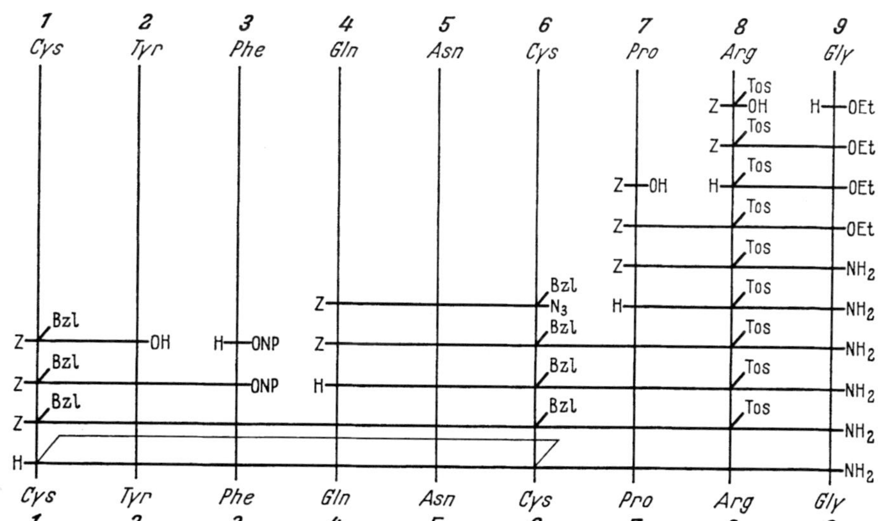

Fig. 13. Synthesis of vasopressin (Huguenin and Boissonnas, 1962)

according to the scheme 3+3. The azide of this hexapeptide was then condensed with the C-terminal tripeptide. This method of synthesis presents the advantage that the arginyl residue is introduced in a later step of the synthesis only. After treatment with sodium in liquid ammonia and oxidation with air, followed by purification by counter-current distribution and block electrophoresis, a vasopressin was obtained exhibiting a pressor activity of 350—400 IU/mg and identical in all other respects with the natural hormone.

In a fourth and more recent approach (Fig. 13), the guanido group of arginine was kept protected until the very last step of the synthesis (HUGUENIN and BOISSONNAS, 1962). The protecting group used in this instance was the tosyl group. The synthesis also followed the 3+(3+3) scheme. The median and C-terminal tripeptides were condensed by the azide method. The protecting group was removed from the N-terminal part of the hexapeptide obtained, which was then allowed to react either with the activated ester of the N-terminal tripeptide or with its azide. All the protecting groups of the nonapeptide obtained were cleaved off simultanousely by treatement with sodium in liquid ammonia. After oxidation and purification by counter-current distribution vasopressin with a pressor activity of 350 IU/mg was obtained. Shortly afterwards STUDER (1963a, b) obtained vasopressin independently in exactly the same way.

In a fifth and more recent approach to the synthesis of vasopressin (BODANSZKY et al., 1964) a quite different procedure was followed. A protected nonapeptide, having an ornithyl residue in position 8, was built up by stepwise backwards synthesis. The condensations were effected with the aid of activated p-nitrophenylesters, and the δ-amino group of ornithine was protected with a phthaloyl group. After the protected nonapeptide has been built up, the phthaloyl group was removed by hydrazinolysis, and the ornithyl residue was converted into an arginyl residue by guanidination. Removal of the other protecting groups and oxidation were performed in the classical way. After purification by ion-exchange chromatography and gel filtration, vasopressin with a pressor activity of approximatively 500 IU/mg was obtained.

E. Synthesis of Lysine-Vasopressin

The first synthesis of lysine-vasopressin was achieved at the same time when its structure was published (DU VIGNEAUD et al., 1953c). The biological activity of this first synthetic product was, however, fairly low. An improved version of this synthesis was described in greater detail a few years later (BARTLETT et al., 1956;

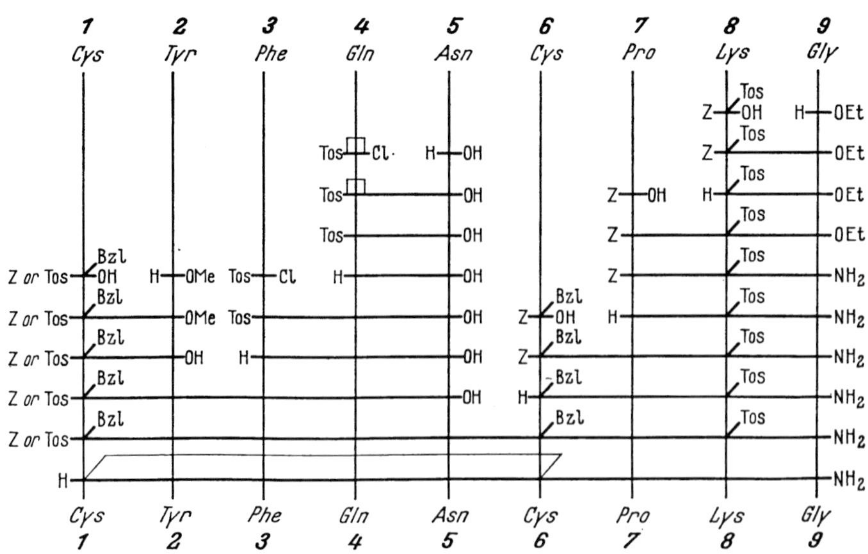

Fig. 14. Synthesis of lysine-vasopressin (BARTLETT et al., 1956; DU VIGNEAUD et al., 1957)

du Vigneaud et al., 1957). Two main sequences 1—5 and 6—9 were built up (Fig. 14), and then linked together. During the synthesis the basic and reactive ε-amino group of the lysine was protected by a tosyl group, which is stable enough to withstand the various manipulations of the synthesis and can be removed in the last step at the same time as the other protecting groups. Z-L-proline was allowed to react with H-Lys(Tos)-Gly-OEt in presence of phenylene chlorophosphite,

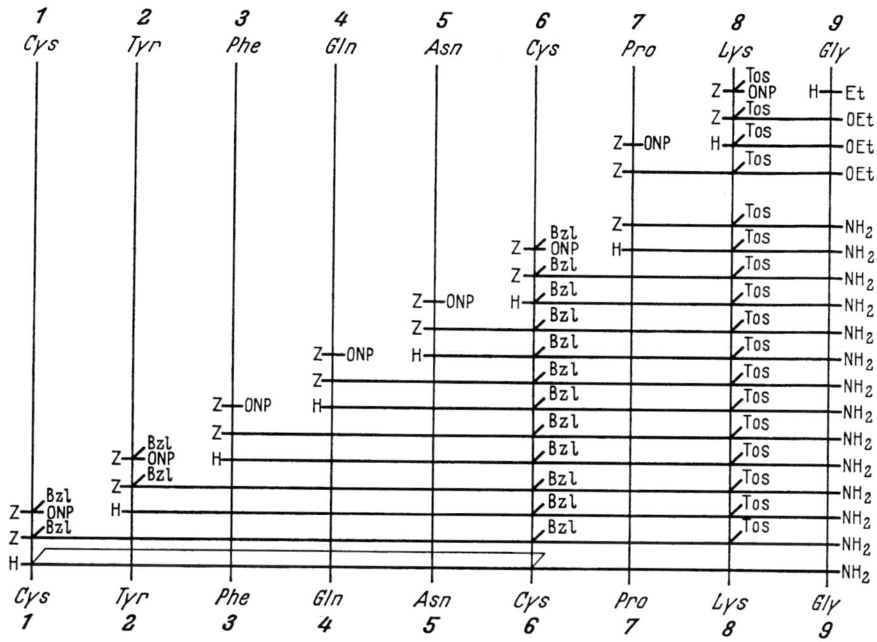

Fig. 15. Synthesis of lysine-vasopressin (Bodanszky et al., 1960)

yielding the c-terminal tripeptide ester. The Z group was removed by hydrobromic acid in acetic acid and the resulting tripeptide ester was coupled with Z-L-Cys(Bz)-OH in the presence of either tetraethylpyrophosphite or dicyclohexylcarbodiimide. In the next step the tetrapeptide ester was converted into the corresponding amide. The median tripeptide was built up by stepwise synthesis using the acyl chloride method. The n-terminal dipeptide was condensed with this median tripeptide by the mixed anhydride method. The two main fragments, 1—5 and 6—9, were then coupled together in the presence of a large excess of dicyclohexylcarbodiimide and yielded a crystalline protected nonapeptide. After removal of the protecting groups with sodium in liquid ammonia and subsequent oxidation with air, a crude material possessing a pressor activity of about 150—200 IU/mg was obtained. It was purified by counter-current distribution followed by block electrophoresis. The lysine vasopressin thus obtained exhibited a biological activity of 280 IU/mg and was identical with the natural product. Several steps of this synthesis as well as the purification of the end product were later still further improved (Meienhofer and du Vigneaud, 1960).

Bodanszky et al. (1960) have built up the protected nonapeptide of lysine, vasopressin by backwards stepwise addition of aminoacyl residues (Fig. 15). For the activation of the carboxyl function p-nitrophenylesters were used. The yield of each step (condensation and removal of the n-protecting group) was often greater than 90 %. The material obtained by this synthesis was purified by either cellulose-block electrophoresis, counter-current distribution or ion-exchange chromatography.

In another approach (BOISSONNAS and HUGUENIN, 1960) (Fig. 16) the 3+(3+3) scheme previously applied in the Boissonnas' synthesis of oxytocin was followed.

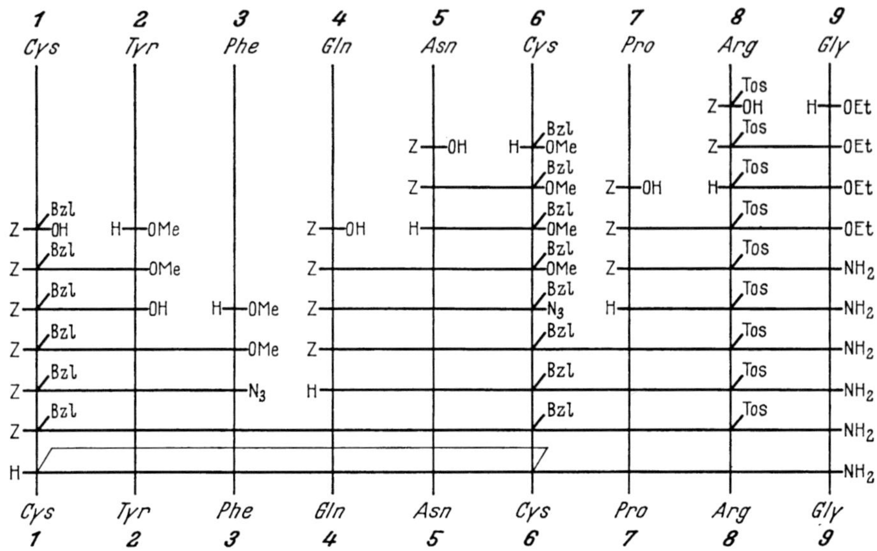

Fig. 16. Synthesis of lysine-vasopressin (BOISSONNAS and HUGUENIN, 1960)

Condensation by the azide method avoided the risk of racemisation. The final product after purification by counter-current distribution had a pressor activity of 270 IU/mg.

In a very novel synthesis of the protected nonapeptide (JOŠT, 1966), the main sequences, 2—5 and 6—9, were synthesised, and then coupled together by the azide method. Finally the activated ester of Z-Cys(Bz) was reacted with the octapeptide. This scheme of synthesis is especially convenient for the synthesis of analogues with modifications in positions 1 and 6.

F. Radioactive Vasopressins

Lysine-vasopressin randomly labelled with tritium was prepared by exposing the hormone to tritium gas (FONG et al., 1959, 1960). The material obtained exhibited a specific radioactivity of 300—400 microcuries/mg.

Lysine-vasopressin labelled in position 2 only was prepared by total synthesis using tritiated tyrosine (CARLSSON and SJÖHOLM, 1966). This material exhibited a specific radioactivity of 1800 microcuries/mg.

III. Vasotocin

A. Isolation

Structurally this hormone is intermediate between oxytocin and vasopressin, and has been found in birds, amphibians and fish. Its existence was first demonstrated pharmacologically in the posterior pituitary of the chicken (MUNSICK et al., 1959, 1960) and confirmed by isolation (CHAUVET et al., 1960b). Chicken acetonic postpituitary powder was extracted with cold 0.01 N sulphuric acid and horse neurophysin was added to the extract. The complex formed between neurophysin and the peptide hormones present in the extract was precipitated by addition of NaCl. After dissociation of the complex with trichloracetic acid, the peptide hormones were purified by ion-exchange chromatography on Amberlite IRC-50. A peptide possessing both pressor and oxytocic activity emerged from the column between oxytocin and vasopressin. On the basis of the amino acid composition of its hydrolysate (Cys_2, Tyr, Ile, Glu, Asp, Pro, Arg, Gly in equimolecular amounts), it was suggested (Chauvet et al., 1960b) that it might be identical with the vasotocin (Ile^3-Vasopressin), which had been obtained by synthesis two years earlier (Katsoyannis and du Vigneaud, 1958). The same group of authors also isolated vasotocin from the frog (Acher et al., 1960b) and from the bib cod (Acher et al., 1961) by the same method. Vasotocin was also isolated from the pollack (Heller and Pickering, 1961) and from the hake (Rasmussen and Craig, 1961). In this last instance, vasotocin was extracted from the fish pituitary with 0.25 M ammonium sulphate, precipitated with 1.25 M ammonium sulphate, and purified by counter current distribution and gel filtration on Sephadex G-25. The substance thus obtained exhibited the same biological properties as synthetic vasotocin (Katsoyannis and du Vigneaud, 1958).

B. Structure

Only in the case of vasotocin of fish origin has the structure been established by chemical examination (Acher, 1962). In parallel assays vasotocin, oxytocin and vasopressin were submitted to enzymatic degradation. Leucinaminopeptidase released tyrosine and isoleucine from both vasotocin and oxytocin, while tyrosine and phenylalanine were released from vasopressin under the same conditions. It was therefore concluded the N-terminal sequence of vasotocin was the same as that of oxytocin. Digestion with trypsin released glycinamide from vasotocin and vasopressin, whereas oxytocin remained intact. From these results it was concluded that the C-terminal sequence was the same as in vasopressin.

These degradation studies and identity of the biological properties of synthetic and natural vasotocin confirmed that vasotocin from natural sources had the following structure:

$$\text{H–Cys–Tyr–Ile–Gln–Asn–Cys–Pro–Arg–Gly–NH}_2$$

(disulphide bridge between the two Cys residues)

C. Synthesis

The first synthesis of vasotocin was achieved by Katsoyannis and du Vigneaud (1958, 1959) two years before this hormone was identified in nature. As these authors had already synthesised oxytocin and vasopressin, they linked together the N-terminal tripeptide (Z-Cys(Bz)-Tyr-Ile-N_3) used for the synthesis of oxytocin with the C-terminal hexapeptide (H-Gln-Asn-Cys(Bz)-Pro-Arg-Gly-NH_2) used in the synthesis of vasopressin (Fig. 17). After removal of the protecting groups with sodium in liquid ammonia and oxidation by air, the crude vasotocin was purified by counter-current distribution and electrophoresis on cellulose block.

Huguenin and Boissonnas (1962) performed another synthesis by condensing Tos-Cys(Bzl)-Tyr-Ile-ONP with H-Gln-Asn-Cys(Bzl)-Pro-Arg(Tos)-Gly-NH_2. In this scheme of synthesis the guanidino group of the arginine in position 8 is protected, this greatly facilitating the synthesis (Fig. 18). The crude material, obtained after removal of the protecting groups and formation of the disulphide bridge by oxidation with air, was easily purified by counter-current distribution. The activity of this preparation was twice as high as that of the product obtained by the American authors (Berde et al., 1962).

Bodanszky et al. (1964) have synthesised vasotocin by stepwise addition of N-protected amino acyl residues in their activated p-nitrophenylester form. In position 8, a N^{δ}phthaloyl-ornithyl residue was used. The phthaloyl group of the

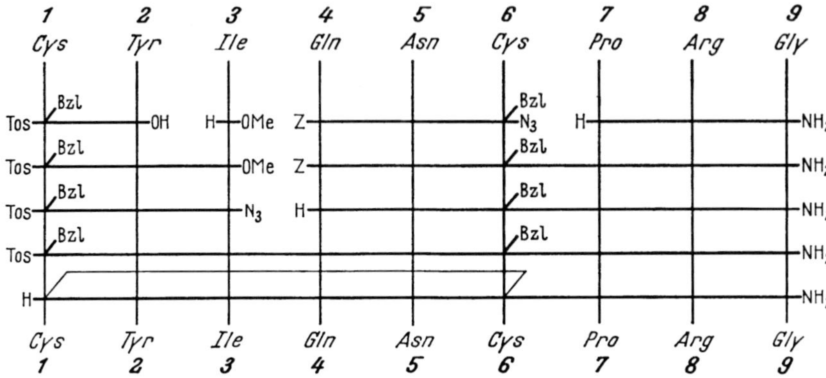

Fig. 17. Synthesis of vasotocin (du Vigneaud et al., 1958)

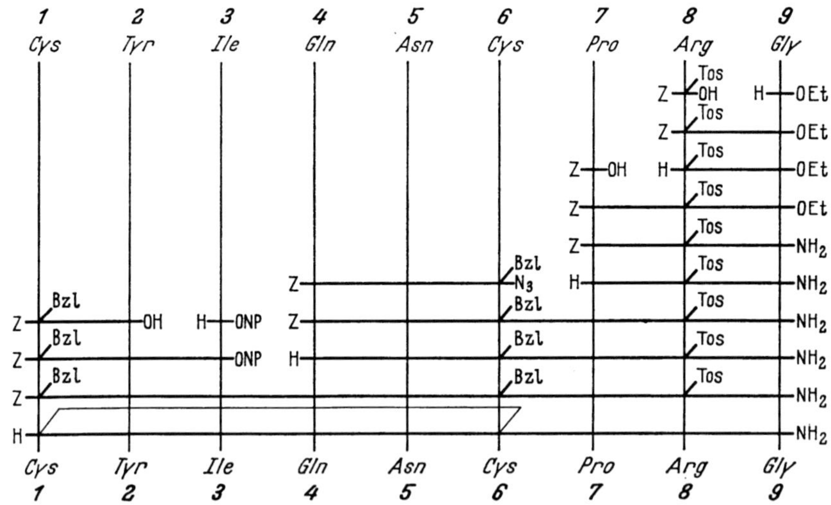

Fig. 18. Synthesis of vasotocin (Huguenin and Boissonnas, 1962)

protected nonapeptide was removed and the δ-amino group of ornithine was amidinated, in order to form an arginine residue. After treatment with sodium in liquid ammonia and oxidation, the crude material was purified by ion-exchange chromatography, followed by gel filtration. It exhibited a level of biological activity of the same order of magnitude as the material obtained by Katsoyannis and du Vigneaud (1958), i.e. it was about half as active as the product of Huguenin and Boissonnas (1962).

IV. Isotocin (Ichthyotocin)

A. Isolation and Elucidation of Structure

This hormone was isolated from some teleost fishes (Acher et al., 1962). The neurohypophysis was defatted with acetone and extracted with cold 0.01 N sulfuric acid. An active material, containing both isotocin and vasotocin in the form of their common complex with neurophysin, was precipitated on addition of sodium chloride. This protein-peptide complex was decomposed by treatment with trichloracetic acid and the peptidic fraction was purified by chromatography on Amberlite IRC-50 and paper. The material thus obtained was judged sufficiently pure for structural studies. Total hydrolysis yielded one mole of cystine, tyrosine, serine, aspartic acid, proline, glycine and two moles of isoleucine. Thus the amino acid content of isotocin differs from that of oxytocin in possessing serine and an additional isoleucine in place of glutamine and leucine. Leucinaminopeptidase caused the release of tyrosine and isoleucine as in oxytocin. Addition of more leucinaminopeptidase led to the release of serine, whereas, in the case of oxytocin, only a partial release of glutamine (due to the concurrent conversion to the pyrrolidone derivative) is observed.

On the basis of these results the following structure was proposed (Acher et al., 1962):

$$H\text{–}Cys\text{–}Tyr\text{–}Ile\text{–}Ser\text{–}Asn\text{–}Cys\text{–}Pro\text{–}Ile\text{–}Gly\text{–}NH_2$$

This structure was fully confirmed by total synthesis (Guttmann, 1962; Guttmann et al., 1962; Jöhl et al., 1963). The natural and the synthetic product exhibited the same ratios between their various biological activities.

B. Synthesis

In the first synthesis of isotocin (Guttmann, 1962) the C-terminal hexapeptide 4—9 was built up by the recurrent method, using mainly p-nitrophenylesters of protected amino acids (Fig. 19). The p-nitrophenylester of the tripeptide 1—3 was

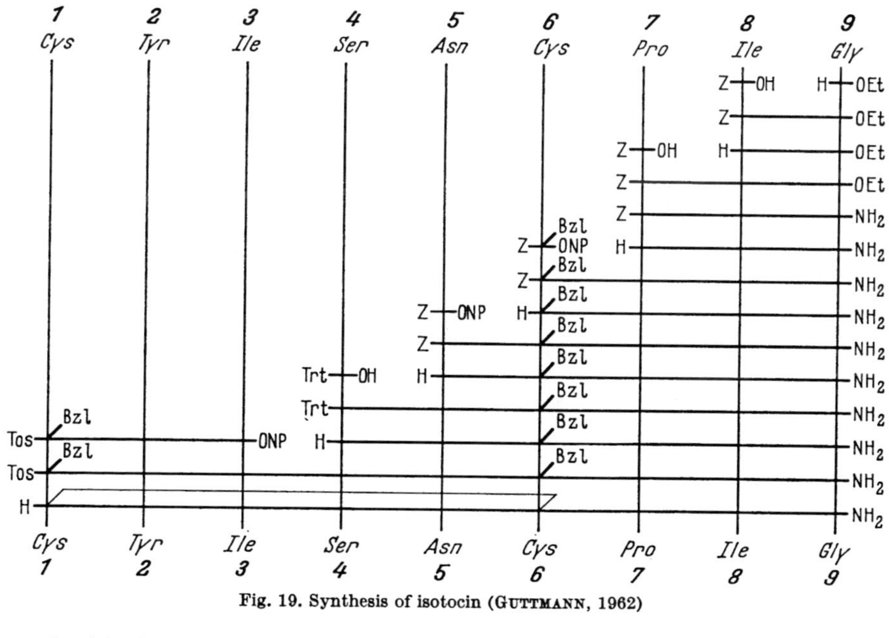

Fig. 19. Synthesis of isotocin (Guttmann, 1962)

reacted with the hexapeptide 4—9 and, after removal of the protecting groups of the nonapeptide with sodium in liquid ammonia, the disulphide bridge was established by air oxidation. After purification by counter-current distribution pure isotocin was obtained, thus making its full biological characterisation possible (Guttmann et al., 1962).

In a subsequent synthesis (JÖHL et al., 1963) (Fig. 20) the dipeptide 5—6 was condensed with the tripeptide 7—9 by the azide method. The pentapeptide obtained was condensed with the azide of the tetrapeptide 1—4, itself built up

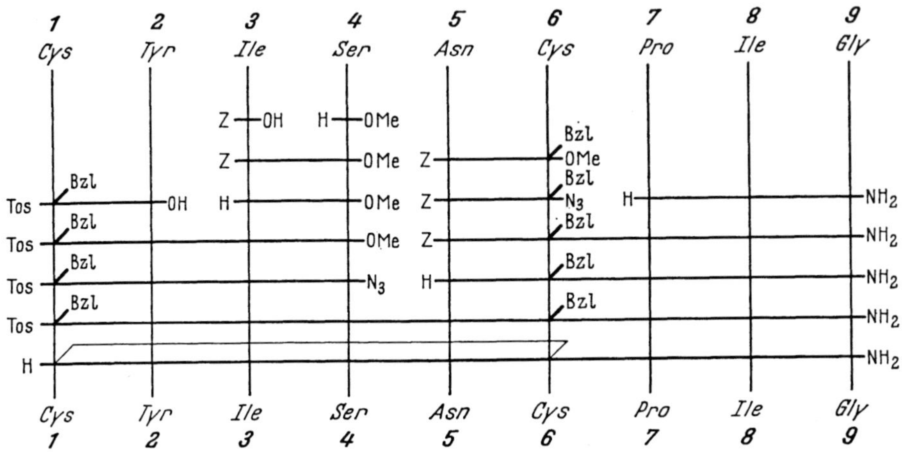

Fig. 20. Synthesis of isotocin (JÖHL et al., 1963)

by condensing two dipeptides using the dicyclohexylcarbodiimide method. The protecting groups were removed by treatment with sodium and liquid ammonia and the product resulting after oxidation with air was purified by counter-current distribution. The final product exhibited the same properties as that obtained by the first method.

V. Mesotocin

A. Isolation and Elucidation of Structure

Mesotocin was isolated from the posterior pituitary of frogs (ACHER et al., 1964). An acetonic powder of the posterior pituitary of Rana esculente was extracted with cold 0.01 N sulphuric acid and the oxytocic principle of the extract was salted out as a complex with neurophysin. The complex was dissociated by treatment with trichloracetic acid and the peptidic material purified by ion-exchange chromatography on Amberlite IRC-50.

On total hydrolysis the following amino acid composition was obtained: aspartic acid 0.92, glutamic acid 1.00, proline 1.10, glycine 1.27, cysteine 1.70, isoleucine 1.76 and tyrosine 0.72.

From the amino acid composition and chromatographic behaviour of mesotocin it was concluded that this hormone was most probably closely related to oxytocin and to isotocin. Parallel enzymatic studies were therefore undertaken with these three substances. The ratio of the aminoacids released from the three hormones on digestion with leucinaminopeptidase was established by the fingerprint method. On the basis of these results it was deduced that the N-terminal sequence of this new oxytocic hormone was identical with that of oxytocin i.e.: Cys-Tyr-Ile-Gln-Asn-Cys. The C-terminal sequence was deduced by partial hydrolysis of the product obtained on oxidising mesotocin with performic acid. This yielded a fragment which contained cysteic acid, proline and isoleucine and was identical in its chromatographic behaviour with the fragment $CySO_3$-Pro-Ile obtained by partial hydrolysis of oxidised isotocin. From these results it was concluded that mesotocin had the following structure (Acher et al., 1964):

H–Cys–Tyr–Ile–Gln–Asn–Cys–Pro–Ile–Gly–NH_2 (disulfide bridge Cys¹–Cys⁶)

Mesotocin was therefore identical with a synthetic analogue of oxytocin, Ile^8-oxytocin, which had already been synthetized three years earlier (Jaquenoud and Boissonnas, 1961).

B. Synthesis

As mentioned above the synthesis of mesotocin (Jaquenoud and Boissonnas, 1961) had in fact been accomplished before this hormone was identified in nature. The scheme of synthesis (Fig. 21) was the same as that followed by the

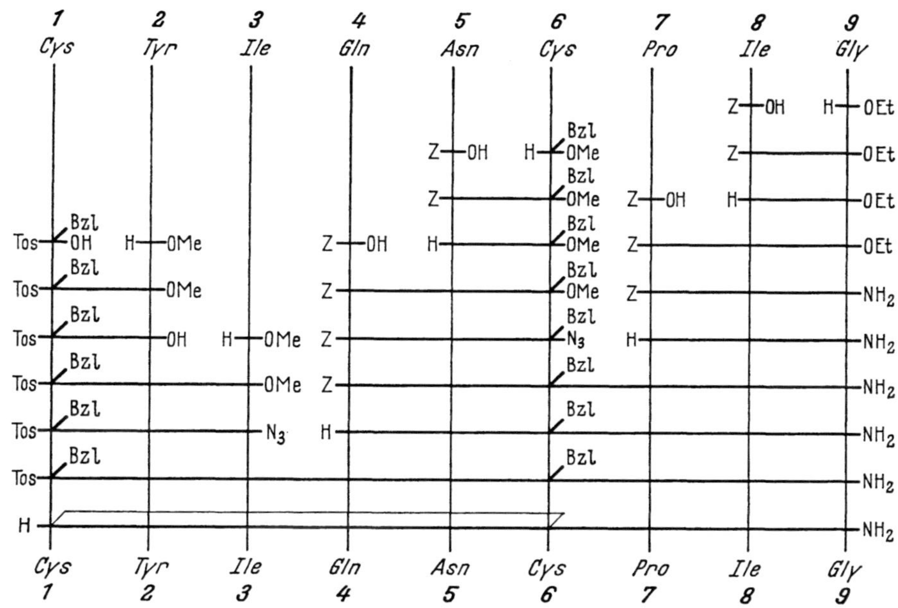

Fig. 21. Synthesis of mesotocin (Jaquenoud and Boissonnas, 1961)

same authors in their previous synthesis of oxytocin (Boissonnas et al., 1955), namely the 3+(3+3) scheme. The synthetic material was thoroughly purified by counter-current distribution, and its biological properties had been fully investigated (Berde and Konzett, 1960); the biological activities of the natural product itself have never been thoroughly studied.

VI. Glumitocin

Glumitocin was identified in a ray-fish, Raia clavata, and in a dog-fish, Squalus acauthias (Acher et al., 1965). From 8000 pituitaries of Raia clavata 60 mg of acetonic powder were obtained with extracted. This was dilute sulphuric acid. After adding neurophysin the protein-peptide complex was salted out by adding NaCl. After dissociating the complex with trichloroacetic acid the hormones were separated by ion-exchange chromatography. Total hydrolysis of the oxytocic fraction yielded equimolecular amounts of cystine, isoleucine, tyrosine, serine, aspartic acid, glutamic acid, proline and glycine.

Parallel degradation studies performed on this hormone, oxytocin and isotocin by leucinaminopeptidase led to the conclusion that its N-terminal sequence was Cys-Tyr-Ile-Ser-Asn. The material obtained after oxidation of the hormone with performic acid was submitted to the action of subtilisin and the fragments obtained were further degraded by partial hydrolysis. From their amino acid composition the C-terminal sequence of the hormone was deduced.

As a result of these studies the following structure was proposed:

$$\text{Cys–Tyr–Ile–Ser–Asn–Cys–Pro–Gln–Gly–NH}_2$$

This new hormone, which was called glumitocin, has not been synthesized hitherto.

It exhibits a rather low level of oxytocic activity, namely 8 IU/mg. In presence of magnesium ions this activity is increased ten fold.

References

Acher, R.: The comparative chemistry of neurohypophysial hormones. Symp. Zool. Soc. London **9**, 83—91 (1962).

—, and J. Chauvet: La structure de la vasopressine de boeuf. Biochim. biophys. Acta (Amst.) **12**, 487—488 (1953).

— — La structure de la vasopressine de boeuf. Biochim. biophys. Acta (Amst.) **14**, 421—429 (1954).

— —, and M.T. Chauvet: Les hormones neurohypophysiaires des mammifères: Isolement et caractérisation de l'oxytocine et de la vasopressine de la baleine (Balaenoptera physalus L.). Bull. Soc. Chim. biol. (Paris) **45**, 1369—1378 (1963).

— — —, and D. Crepy: Les hormones neurohypophysaires des poissons: Isolement d'une vasotocine du tacaud (*Gadus luscus* L.). Biochim. biophys. Acta (Amst.) **51**, 419—420 (1961).

— — — — Isolement d'une nouvelle hormone neurohypophysaire, l'isotocine, présente chez les poissons osseux. Biochim. biophys. Acta (Amst.) **58**, 624—625 (1962).

— — — — Phylogénie des peptides neurohypophysaires: Isolement de la mesotocine (Ileu^{8}-oxytocine) de la grenouille, intermédiaire entre la Ser^{4}-Ileu^{8}-oxytocine des poissons osseux et l'oxytocine des mammifères. Biochim. biophys. Acta (Amst.) **90**, 613—615 (1964).

— — — — Phylogénie des peptides neurohypophysaires: Isolement d'une nouvelle hormone, la glumitocine (Ser^{4}-Gln^{8}-oxytocine) présente chez un poisson cartilagineux, la raie (*Raia clavata*). Biochim. biophys. Acta (Amst.) **107**, 393—396 (1965).

— —, and M.T. Lenci: L'oxytocine et la vasopressine du cheval. Bull. Soc. Chim. biol. (Paris) **40**, 2005—2018 (1958a).

— — — Purification et structure de l'oxytocine et de la vasopressine du cheval. Biochim. biophys. Acta (Amst.) **31**, 545—548 (1959a).

— — — Purification et structure de l'oxytocine et de la vasopressine du mouton. Compt. Rend. **248**, 1435—1438 (1959b).

— — — Isolement de l'oxytocine du poulet. Biochim. biophys. Acta (Amst.) **38**, 344—345 (1960a).

— — —, F. Morel, and J. Maetz: Présence d'une vasotocine dans la neurohypophyse de la grenouille. Biochim. biophys. Acta (Amst.) **42**, 379—380 (1960b).

—, et Cl. Fromageot: Chimie des hormones neurohypophysaires. Ergebn. Physiol. **48**, 286—327 (1955).

—, A. Light, and V. du Vigneaud: Purification of oxytocin and vasopressin by way of a protein complex. J. biol. Chem. **233**, 116—120 (1958b).

Agishi, Y., and J.F. Dingman: Specific tritiation of oxytocin by catalytic deiodination. Biochem. biophys. Res. Commun. **18**, 92—97 (1965).

Bartlett, M.F., A. Joehl, R. Roeske, R.J. Stedman, F.H.C. Stewart, P.N. Ward, and V. du Vigneaud: Studies on the synthesis of lysine-vasopressin. J. Amer. chem. Soc. **78**, 2905—2906 (1956).

Berde, B., R. Huguenin, and E. Stürmer: The biological activities of arginine-vasotocin obtained by a new synthesis. Experientia (Basel) **18**, 444—445 (1962)

—, u. H. Konzett: Isoleucyl^{8}-Oxytocin, ein biologisch hochwirksames Polypeptid. Med. exp. (Basel) **2**, 317—322 (1960).

Beyermann, H. C., J. S. Bontekoe, and A. C. Koch: A synthesis of oxytocin. Rec. Trav. chim. Pays-Bas **78**, 935—946 (1959).

Bodanszky, M.: Synthesis of peptides by aminolysis of nitrophenyl esters. Nature (Lond.) **175**, 685 (1955).

—, J. Meienhofer, and V. du Vigneaud: Synthesis of lysine-vasopressin by the nitrophenylester method. J. Amer. chem. Soc. **82**, 3195—3198 (1960).

—, M. A. Ondetti, C. A. Birkhimer, and P. L. Thomas: Synthesis of arginine-containing peptides through their ornithine analogs. Synthesis of arginine vasotocin and L-histidyl-L-phenylalanyl-L-arginyl-L-tryptophylglycine. J. Amer. chem. Soc. **86**, 4452—4459 (1964).

—, and V. du Vigneaud: An improved synthesis of oxytocin. J. Amer. chem. Soc. **81**, 2504 to 2507 (1959a).

— — A method of synthesis of long peptide chains using a synthesis of oxytocin as an example. J. Amer. chem. Soc. **81**, 5688—5691 (1959b).

— — Synthesis of oxytocin by the nitrophenyl ester method. Nature (Lond.) **183**, 1324—1325 (1959c).

— — A new crystalline salt of oxytocin. Nature (Lond.) **184**, 981—982 (1959d).

Boissonnas, R. A., St. Guttmann, P.-A. Jaquenoud, and J.-P. Waller: Une nouvelle synthèse de l'oxytocine. Helv. chim. Acta **38**, 1491—1501 (1955).

—, and R. L. Huguenin: Synthèse de la Lys[8]-oxytocine (lysine-vasotocine) et nouvelle synthèse de la lysine-vasopressine. Helv. chim. Acta **43**, 182—190 (1960).

Carlsson, L., and I. Sjöholm: Synthesis of tritium-labelled oxytocin and lysine-vasopressin. Acta chem. scand. **20**, 259—260 (1966).

Chauvet, J., M. T. Lenci, and R. Acher: L'oxytocine et la vasopressine du mouton: Reconstitution d'un complexe hormonal actif. Biochim. biophys. Acta (Amst.) **38**, 266—272 (1960a).

— — — Présence de deux vasopressines dans la neurohypophyse du poulet. Biochim. biophys. Acta (Amst.) **38**, 571—573 (1960b).

Condliffe, P. G.: Partition chromatography of oxytocin and vasopressin. J. biol. Chem. **216**, 455—464 (1955).

Dudley, H. W.: Some observations on the active principles of the pituitary gland. J. Pharmacol. exp. Ther. **14**, 295—312 (1919).

Fong, C. T. O., I. L. Schwartz, E. A. Popenoe, L. Silver, and M. A. Schoessler: On the molecular bonding of lysine-vasopressin at its renal receptor site. J. Amer. chem. Soc. **81**, 2592—2593 (1959).

—, L. Silver, D. R. Christmas, and I. L. Schwartz: On the mechanisme of action of the antidiuretic hormone (vasopressin). Proc. nat. Acad. Sci. (Wash.) **46**, 1273—1277 (1960).

Guttmann, St.: Synthèse de la Ser[4]-Ileu[8]-oxytocine, une éventuelle hormone hypophysaire de certains poissons (Isotocine). Helv. chim. Acta **45**, 2622—2627 (1962).

— Use of the S-ethylcarbamoyl group for protection of the thiol function of cysteine. Proc. 6th European Symposium, Athens, September 1963, p. 11—19. Ed. by L. Zervas. Pergamon (1966).

— Synthèse du glutathion et de l'oxytocine à l'aide d'un nouveau groupe protecteur de la fonction thiol. Helv. chim. Acta **49**, 83—96 (1966).

—, B. Berde, and E. Stürmer: The synthesis and some pharmacological effects of serine[4]-isoleucine[8]-oxytocin, a probable neurohypophysial hormone. Experientia (Basel) **18**, 445—446 (1962).

Heaton, G. S., H. N. Rydon, and J. A. Schofield: The oxidation of some peptides of cysteine and glycine. J. chem. Soc. **1956**, 3157—3168.

Heller, H., and B. T. Pickering: Neurohypophysial hormones of nonmammalian vertebrates. J. Physiol. (Lond.) **155**, 98—114 (1961).

Huguenin, R. L., and R. A. Boissonnas: Synthèse de la Phe[2]-arginine-vasopressine et de la Phe[2]-arginine-vasotocine et nouvelles synthèses de l'arginine-vasopressine et de l'arginine-vasotocine. Helv. chim. Acta **45**, 1629—1643 (1962).

Irving, G. W., M. M. Dyer, and V. du Vigneaud: Purification of the pressor principle of the posterior lobe of pituitary gland by electrophoresis. J. Amer. chem. Soc. **63**, 503—506 (1941).

Jaquenoud, P.-A., and R. A. Boissonnas: Synthèse de la Ileu[8]-oxytocine et de la Val[8]-oxytocine, deux analogues de l'oxytocine modifiés dans la chaîne latérale.

Jöhl, A., A. Hartmann, and H. Rink: The synthesis of Ser[4]-Ileu[8]-oxytocin (Isotocin). Biochim. biophys. Acta (Amst.) **69**, 193—195 (1963).

Jošt, K.: A new synthetic route of oxytocin and vasopressin suitable for the preparation of analogues modified in position 6. Collection Czech. Chem. Commun. **31**, 2784 (1966).

Kamm, O., T. B. Aldrich, I. W. Grote, L. W. Rowe, and E. P. Bugbee: The active principles of the posterior lobe of the pituitary gland. J. Amer. chem. Soc. **50**, 573—601 (1928).

KATSOYANNIS, P.G., D.T. GISH, and V. DU VIGNEAUD: Synthetic studies of arginine-vasopressin: Condensation of S-benzyl-N-carbobenzoxy-L-cysteinyl-L-tyrosyl-L-phenylalanyl-L-glutaminyl-L-asparagine and its O-tosyl derivative with S-benzyl-L-cysteinyl-L-prolyl-L-arginylglycinamide. J. Amer. chem. Soc. **79**, 4516—4520 (1957).

—, and V. DU VIGNEAUD: Arginine-vasotocin, a synthetic analogue of the posterior pituitary hormones containing the ring of oxytocin and the side chain of vasopressin. J. biol. Chem. **233**, 1352—1354 (1958).

— — Arginine vasotocin. Nature (Lond.) **184**, 1465 (1959).

LAWER, H.C., S.P. TAYLOR, A.M. SWAN, and V. DU VIGNEAUD: Presence of glutamine and asparagine in enzymatic hydrolysates of oxytocin and vasopressin. Proc. Soc. exp. Biol. (N.Y.) **87**, 550—552 (1954).

LIGHT, A., and V. DU VIGNEAUD: On the nature of oxytocin and vasopressin from human pituitary. Proc. Soc. exp. Biol. (N.Y.) **98**, 692—696 (1958).

LINDNER, E.B., A. ELMQUIST, and J. PORATH: Gel filtration as a method for purification of protein-bound peptides, exemplified by oxytocin and vasopressin. Nature (Lond.) **184**, 1565—1566 (1959).

LIVERMORE, A.H., and V. DU VIGNEAUD: Preparation of high potency oxytocic material by the use of countercurrent distribution. J. biol. Chem. **180**, 365—373 (1949).

MAIER-HUESER, H., H. CLAUSER, P. FROMAGEOT, and P. PLONGERON: Préparation des hormones du lobe postérieur de l'hypophyse de boeuf. Biochim. biophys. Acta (Amst.) **11**, 252—257 (1953).

MEIENHOFER, J., and V. DU VIGNEAUD: Preparation of lysine-vasopressin through a crystalline protected nonapeptide intermediate and purification of the hormone by chromatography. J. Amer. chem. Soc. **82**, 2279—2282 (1960).

MÉNDEZ-BAUER, C.J., M.A. CARBALLO, H.M. CABOT, C.E. NEGREIROS DE PAIVA, and Y.H. GONZALES-PANIZZA: In: Oxytocin. Ed. by R. CALDEYRO-BARCIA and H. HELLER, p. 325. New York: Macmillan (Pergamon) 1961.

MUELLER, M.J., J.G. PIERCE, H. DAVOLL, and V. DU VIGNEAUD: The oxydation of oxytocin with performic acid. J. biol. Chem. **191**, 309—313 (1951).

MUNSICK, R.A., W.H. SAWYER, and H.B. VAN DYKE: Hormonal characteristics of the avian neurohypophysis. Fed. Proc. **18**, 110 (1959).

— — — Avian neurohypophysial hormones: Pharmacological properties and tentative identification. Endocrinology **66**, 860—871 (1960).

PHOTAKI, I.: Synthesis of N-protected oxytocins. Experientia (Basel) **20**, 487—488 (1964).

— A new synthesis of oxytocin using S-acyl cysteins as intermediates. J. Amer. chem. Soc. **88**, 2292—2299 (1966).

PIERCE, J.G., S. GORDON, and V. DU VIGNEAUD: Further distribution studies on the oxytocic hormone of the posterior lobe of the pituitary gland and the preparation of an active cristalline flavianate. J. biol. Chem. **199**, 929—940 (1952).

—, and V. DU VIGNEAUD: Preliminary studies on amino acid content of a high potency preparation of the oxytocic hormone of posterior lobe of the pituitary gland. J. biol. Chem. **182**, 359—366 (1950).

POPENOE, E.A., H.C. LAWLER, and V. DU VIGNEAUD: Partial purification and amino acid content of vasopressin from hog posterior pituitary glands. J. Amer. chem. Soc. **74**, 3713 (1952).

—, and V. DU VIGNEAUD: Degradative studies on vasopressin and performic acid-oxidized vasopressin. J. biol. Chem. **205**, 133—143 (1953).

— — A partial sequence of amino acids in performic acid-oxidized vasopressin. J. biol. Chem. **206**, 353—360 (1954).

PORATH, J.: Application of zone electrophoresis and cellulose in exchange chromatography to the fractionation of posterior pituitary hormones. Arkiv Kemi **11**, 259—274 (1957).

—, and A.V. SCHALLY: Gel filtration of posterior pituitary hormones. Endocrinology **70**, 738—742 (1962).

POTTS, A.M., and T.F. GALLAGHER: Cystine, tyrosine and arginine content of high potency pressor and oxytocic pituitary hormones. J. biol. Chem. **143**, 561—562 (1942).

— — Separation of oxytocic and pressor principles of posterior pituitary extracts. J. biol. Chem. **154**, 349—356 (1944).

RASMUSSEN, H., and L. CRAIG: The isolation of arginine vasotocin from fish pituitary glands. Endocrinology **68**, 1051—1055 (1961).

RESSLER, CH.: Inactivation of oxytocin suggesting peptide denaturation. Science **128**, 1281 to 1282 (1958).

RUDINGER, J., J. HONZL, and M. ZAORAL: An alternative synthesis of oxytocin. Collection Czech. Chem. Commun. **21**, 202—210 (1956).

RYCHLIK, I.: Oxytocin, Vasopressin and their structural analogues. Proc. 2nd Int. Pharmacological Meeting, Prague, 1963. Ed. by J. RUDINGER, p. 153. New York: Macmillan (Pergamon) 1964.

Saffran, M., B.V. Caplan, S. Mishkin, and B. Muhlstock: Use of percolation for the extraction of vasopressin. Endocrinology **70**, 43—46 (1962).
Sakakibara, S., Y. Nobuhara, Y. Shimonishi, and R. Kiyoi: A synthesis of oxytocin. Bull. chem. Soc. Japan **38**, 120—123 (1965).
Schally, A.V., nad R. Guillemin: Some biological and chemical properties of lysine-vasopressin dimer. J. biol. Chem. **239**, 1038—1041 (1964).
—, H.S. Lipscomb, and R. Guillemin: Chromatographic separation of oxytocin and vasopressin on carboxymethylcellulose. Biochim. biophys. Acta (Amst.) **31**, 252—254 (1959).
Sheehan, J.C., and J.P. Hess: A new method of forming peptide bonds. J. Amer. chem. Soc. **77**, 1067—1068 (1955).
Sjöholm, I.: Enzymic inactivation of oxytocin. Acta chem. scand. **18**, 889—898 (1964).
Smyth, D.G.: Reaction of cyanate with amino and hydroxyl groups; application to oxytocin. Acta Chim. Acad. Sci. Hung. **44**, 197—204 (1965).
Stehle, R.L., and A.M. Fraser: The purification of pressor and oxytocic hormones of the pituitary gland and some observations on the chemistry of the products. J. Pharmacol. exp. Ther. **55**, 136—151 (1935).
Studer, R.O.: Vergleich von synthetischem und natürlichem Arginin-Vasopressin. Chimia (Aarau) **17**, 22 (1963a).
— Vergleich von synthetischem und natürlichem Arginin-Vasopressin. Helv. chim. Acta **46**, 421—425 (1963b).
—, and V. du Vigneaud: Synthetic work related to arginine-vasopressin. J. Amer. chem. Soc. **82**, 1499—1501 (1960).
Sturm, K., R. Geiger u. W. Siedel: Verfahren zur Herstellung von Oxytocin. D.B.P. Nr. 1212533 (1966).
Tuppy, H.: The amino-acid sequence in oxytocin. Biochim. biophys. Acta (Amst.) **11**, 449—450 (1953).
— Polypeptides which affect smooth muscles and blood vessels, p. 49—58. Ed. by M. Schachter. New York: Macmillan (Pergamon) 1960.
— In: Oxytocin, p. 315—324. Ed. by R. Caldeyro-Barcia and H. Heller. New York: Macmillan (Pergamon) 1961.
—, u. H. Michl: Über die chemische Struktur des Oxytocins. Monatsh. Chem. **84**, 1011—1020 (1953).
—, u. H. Nesvadba: Über die Aminopeptidaseaktivität des Schwangerenserums und ihre Beziehung zu dessen Vermögen, Oxytocin zu inaktivieren. Monatsh. Chem. **88**, 977—988 (1957).
—, u. E. Wintersberger: Reinigung und Eigenschaften der Serum-Oxytocinase. Monatsh. Chem. **91**, 1001—1010 (1960).
Turner, R.A., J.G. Pierce, and V. du Vigneaud: The purification and the amino acid content of vasopressin preparations. J. biol. Chem. **191**, 21—28 (1951).
Velluz, L., G. Amiard, J. Bartos, B. Goffinet, and R. Heymès: Accès à l'oxytocine de synthèse, à l'aide d'intermédiaires S.N-tritylés. Bull. Soc. chim. Fr. **1956**, 1464—1467.
Vigneaud, V. du, M.F. Bartlett, and A. Joehl: The synthesis of lysine-vasopressin. J. Amer. chem. Soc. **79**, 5572—5575 (1957).
—, D.T. Gish, and P.G. Katsoyannis: A synthetic preparation possessing biological properties associated with arginine-vasopressin. J. Amer. chem. Soc. **76**, 4751—4752 (1954b).
— — —, and G.P. Hess: Synthesis of the pressor antidiuretic hormone, arginine-vasopressin. J. Amer. chem. Soc. **80**, 3355—3358 (1958).
—, H.C., Lawler and E.A. Popenoe. Enzymic cleavage of glycinamide from vasopressin and a proposed structure for this pressor-antidiuretic hormone of the posterior pituitary. J. Amer. chem. Soc. **75**, 4880—4881 (1953c).
—, Ch. Ressler, J.M. Swan, C.W. Roberts, P.G. Katsoyannis, and S. Gordon. The synthesis of an octapeptide amide with the hormonal activity of oxytocin. J. Amer. chem. Soc. **25**, 4879—4880 (1953a).
— — —, C.W. Roberts and P.G. Katsoyannis. The synthesis of oxytocin. J. Amer. chem. Soc. **26**, 3115—3121 (1954a).
— —, and S. Tripett. The sequence of amino acids in oxytocin, with a proposal for the structure of oxytocin. J. biol. Chem. **205**, 949—957 (1953b).
—, C.H. Schneider, J.E. Stouffer, V.V.S. Murti, J.P. Aroskar and G. Winestock. Tritiation of oxytocin by the Wilzbach method and the synthesis of oxytocin from tritium labelled leucine. J. Amer. chem. Soc. **84**, 409—413 (1962).
Ward, D.N., and R. Guillemin. A simple method for preparation of highly purified vasopressin. Proc. Soc. exp. Biol. (N.Y.) **96**, 568—570 (1957).
Yamashiro, D.: Partition chromatography of oxytocin on "Sephadex". Nature (Lond.) **201**, 76—77 (1964).
—, H.L. Aanning, and V. du Vigneaud: Inactivation of oxytocin by acetone. Proc. nat. Acad. Sci. (Wash.) **54**, 166—171 (1965).

The Influence of Enzymes on Neurohypophysial Hormones and Similar Peptides

HANS TUPPY

I. Introduction

Oxidizing, reducing and, particularly, proteolytic enzymes have proved capable of affecting oxytocin, vasopressin and related peptides. Their action has been studied for several reasons. Neurohypophysial hormones can be distinguished from each other and from unrelated biologically active compounds by their different susceptibility to enzymatic inactivation. Specifically acting enzymes are valuable tools in studies of hormone structure and structure-activity relationship. The occurrence, distribution and biological significance of enzymes, which may be involved in the metabolism of the neurohypophysial hormones under normal and pathological conditions, have of course been of particular interest. Enzymes may possibly play a physiological role in the release of the hormones from the sites of their synthesis or storage. Enzymes may influence the hormone levels in the circulation. Certainly, enzymes are involved in the breakdown of the hormones in various tissues. The insight into the role and mode of action of the enzymes involved in hormone metabolism has stimulated the synthesis of hormone analogues resistant to enzymatic attack and of hormone precursors which will release active hormones in enzyme-catalyzed reactions. Moreover, compounds have been studied which will either inhibit or activate the hormone-degrading enzymes and thus, it is hoped, enhance or depress, respectively, the action of the hormones themselves.

The following abbreviations are used in this review: ACTH (adrenocorticotropic hormone); CAP (cystine aminopeptidase); EDTA (ethylene diamine tetraacetate); GSH (glutathione); GSSG (oxidized form of glutathione); LAP (leucine aminopeptidase); β-MSH (β-melanocyte-stimulating hormone); $NADP^+$ (nicotinamide adenine dinucleotide phosphate); NADPH (reduced form of nicotinamide adenine dinucleotide phosphate); PCMB (p-chloromercuribenzoate).

II. Isolated Enzymes which Affect Neurohypophysial Hormones

A. Oxidizing and Reducing Enzymes

1. Tyrosinase and other Oxidases

The presence of tyrosine residues in the molecules of oxytocin and vasopressin renders the hormones susceptible to oxidation by tyrosinase, the reaction products being presumably dihydroxy or quinone derivatives. It has been reported that the uterotonic activity of crude posterior pituitary extracts and of partially purified oxytocin is destroyed by tyrosinase preparations from potatoes or mushrooms such as, e. g., *Psalliota campestris* (FREUDENBERG, WEISS, and BILLER, 1935; DE LA MAZA and CROXATTO, 1944; FRASER,1950). The destruction by tyrosinase of the pressor and antidiuretic activities of vasopressin preparations was recorded by CROXATTO and DE LA MAZA (1944) and by FRASER (1950).

More recently, BISSET (1962) carried out a careful study of the action of mushroom tyrosinase on synthetic oxytocin, synthetic vasopressin and, for the purpose of comparison, on bradykinin which does not contain tyrosine residues in its molecular structure. Under aerobic conditions, at pH 7.5, oxytocin and vasopressin were readily inactivated by the enzyme. Under the same conditions of incubation, tyrosinase did not affect the oxytocic activity of bradykinin. Oxytocin was inactivated less rapidly at pH 6.6 than at pH 7.5. At pH 3.9, neither oxytocin nor vasopressin were affected, whereas bradykinin was destroyed almost entirely. Thus, the inactivation of bradykinin was obviously due to the action of a contaminating enzyme other than tyrosinase present in the mushroom extracts. BISSET suggested that the difference between oxytocin and bradykinin in their reaction with tyrosinase preparations might find practical application in bioassay work as a means of identifying, and possibly separating, the two peptides in extracts of body fluids.

In the presence of enzyme inhibitors such as p-nitrophenol, ascorbic acid, or sodium diethyldithiocarbamate, and during incubation under anaerobic conditions, the inactivation of oxytocin by tyrosinase at pH 7.5 was blocked.

Upon incubation with tyrosinase, synthetic oxytocin underwent a parallel loss of its oxytocic and milk-ejecting activities, and synthetic vasopressin suffered a parallel loss of the pressor and antidiuretic activities. Treatment with tyrosinase, therefore, failed to dissociate the activities in either hormone.

The specific action of tyrosinase on the phenolic hydroxyl group in oxytocin and vasopressin is clearly indicated by the finding that the enzyme caused little or no inactivation of the hormone analogues, Phe^{2}-oxytocin and Phe^{2}-Lys^{8}-vasopressin, which lack phenolic hydroxyl groups. Nor was tyrosinase capable of abolishing the weak milk-ejecting potency of (O-Me)Tyr^{2}-oxytocin, a result which strongly suggested that the biological activity of (O-Me)Tyr^{2}-oxytocin was an inherent property of the hormone analogue and was not due to contamination by oxytocin which might have arisen as a by-product of the synthesis of its analogue.

Amine oxidase and diamine oxidase (histaminase) are unable to destroy oxytocin (PAGE, 1946). In the course of pregnancy, human blood plasma acquires a great capacity to inactivate both histamine and oxytocin. Although the increase in both activities appears to follow a similar time course, two different enzymes are involved.

2. *Glutathione-Insulin Transhydrogenase*

Dihydro-oxytocin, the open-chain derivative which can be obtained from oxytocin by chemical reduction of the disulphide bridge, is known to be biologically inactive. Recently, a purified enzyme, glutathione-insulin transhydrogenase, was found to be capable of attacking oxytocin and vasopressin, their dihydro derivatives being formed by reductive ring-opening (KATZEN and STETTEN, 1962; KATZEN, TIETZE, and STETTEN, 1963).

The enzyme, which was isolated from beef liver and purified so as to be homogeneous in the ultracentrifuge, catalyzes the transfer of hydrogen from GSH to the disulphide bonds of insulin. A spectrophotometric assay for glutathione-insulin transhydrogenase was developed in which the purified enzyme was coupled with purified glutathione reductase. In the presence of both enzymes and of glutathione, the reduction of insulin could be effected by NADPH and followed in the spectrophotometer at 340 $m\mu$. It was found that both oxytocin and vasopressin could replace insulin in this reaction, whereas several other compounds containing disulphide bonds, such as cystine, homocystine, lipoic acid and ribonuclease, were ineffective. It is possible that glutathione-insulin transhydrogenase or a similar enzyme plays a physiological role in the destruction of the neurohypophysial hormones in the liver (RYCHLIK, 1964), kidney (DICKER and GREENBAUM, 1958), uterus (AUDRAIN and CLAUSER, 1960) and elsewhere.

B. Proteolytic Enzymes

1. *Trypsin*

Trypsin is known to cleave peptide bonds which involve the carboxyl groups of the basic amino acids, lysine and arginine. It can be inferred from this specificity that the vasopressins and vasotocins which contain either arginine or lysine in their peptide chains, in contrast to oxytocin which does not, should be susceptible to tryptic hydrolysis. Indeed, many years before the molecular structures of the hypophysial hormones were elucidated, findings consistent with this inference were reported by CROXATTO, ALLIENDE, and CROXATTO (1942/1943b) and CROXATTO, CROXATTO, ILLANES, and SALVESTRINI (1942/1943). These authors found that the pressor activity, but not the oxytocic activity of posterior pituitary extracts was abolished by crystalline trypsin and suggested that this difference in susceptibility to trypsin of vasopressin and oxytocin could be made use of for the preparation of vasopressin-free pituitary extracts. Earlier results (DUDLEY, 1919; THORPE, 1926; FREUDENBERG, WEISS, and EYER, 1932; GULLAND and MACRAE, 1933b; VAN DYKE, CHOW, GREEP, and ROTHEN, 1942), which indicated that common preparations of trypsin were capable of inactivating the oxytocic as well as the pressor principle of neurohypophysial extracts, were obviously due to the action of contaminating enzymes. The susceptibility of pressor material to tryptic destruction has in recent years often been used as an enzymatic test indicating the presence of vasopressins or vasotocins (e. g., THORN and SILVER, 1957; THORN, 1959; MUNSICK, SAWYER, and VAN DYKE, 1960; HALLER, SACHS, SPERELAKIS, and SHARE, 1965).

The susceptibility of vasopressin and the resistance of oxytocin to the action of pure trypsin are retained in Van Dyke's protein, the complex formed by the neurohypophysial hormone peptides with the protein, neurophysin. After tryptic hydrolysis of Van Dyke's protein, the vasopressor activity was virtually destroyed, whereas the oxytocic activity was totally unaffected (ACHER and FROMAGEOT, 1955). Antidiuretic hormone which is present in rat serum in the form of a peptide-protein complex, is nevertheless as susceptible to trypsin as is standard vasopressin (THORN and SILVER, 1957).

Working with highly purified oxytocin, Lys^8-vasopressin and Arg^8-vasopressin, LAWLER and DU VIGNEAUD (1953) confirmed the previous findings which had indicated that the pressor activity of vasopressin was abolished by trypsin whereas the oxytocic activity of oxytocin was unaffected. They furthermore demonstrated that the small oxytocic activity of their pure vasopressin preparations, in contrast to the strong oxytocic activity of oxytocin, was susceptible to destruction by trypsin. This provided convincing evidence, in addition to the evidence previously obtained from analytical studies, that the oxytocic activity of the vasopressins was an intrinsic property of these pressor-antidiuretic principles and was not due to contamination by oxytocin. Similarly, BARNAFI, ROSAS, PEREDA, and CROXATTO (1962) offered the abolition by trypsin of the action of Lys^8-vasopressin on the renal excretion of sodium and potassium as evidence in favour of the inherent natriuretic and kaliuretic activity of this hormone.

The action of trypsin on Arg^8- and Lys^8-vasopressins was found to result in the liberation of glycine amide (DU VIGNEAUD, LAWLER, and POPENOE, 1953). Glycine amide was also released upon tryptic digestion of beef vasopressin previously oxidized with performic acid (ACHER and CHAUVET, 1953, 1954). Subsequently, vasopressins of several animal species such, e. g., as that of the horse and the fin whale (ACHER, CHAUVET, and LENCI, 1958, 1959; CHAUVET, CHAUVET, and ACHER, 1963), and arginine-vasotocin (Arg^8-oxytocin) (MUNSICK, SAWYER, and VAN DYKE, 1960; ACHER, 1963) were also subjected to tryptic hydrolysis, glycine amide being invariably released. The tryptic cleavage was of great value in the elucidation of the structure of the pressor hormones.

The oxytocic and milk-ejection activities of extracts prepared from the pituitary glands of various elasmobranch species were found to be resistant to the action of trypsin. This finding indicated that they were due neither to vasopressin nor to vasotocin, but rather to a peptide which does not contain a basic amino acid residue in its amino acid sequence (PERKS, DODD, and DODD, 1960; PERKS and SAWYER, 1965).

PREDDIE and SAFFRAN (1965) isolated from beef posterior pituitary tissue a large polypeptide which contains 48 amino acid residues in contrast to the 9 residues of oxytocin and vasopressin and exhibits a very weak oxytocic activity. This peptide was found to be susceptible to tryptic attack due to the occurrence in its amino acid sequence of four arginine residues and one lysine residue. Digestion by trypsin yielded five cleavage products, one of which contained N-terminal arginine and underwent a slow further cleavage, free arginine being released (PREDDIE, 1965).

2. *Chymotrypsin*

The susceptibility of oxytocin to the proteolytic action of chymotrypsin was first reported by CROXATTO, ALLIENDE, and CROXATTO (1942/1943b) and by CROXATTO, CROXATTO, ILLANES, and SALVESTRINI (1942/1943) and has since been confirmed repeatedly (DU VIGNEAUD, RESSLER, SWAN, ROBERTS, and KATSOYANNIS, 1954; HAWKER, WALMSLEY, ROBERTS, and ROBERTSON, 1959; GOLUBOW and DU VIGNEAUD, 1963; BARTH, PLIŠKA, and RYCHLÍK, 1967). Deamino-oxytocin was found to be broken down by α-chymotrypsin even more readily than was oxytocin. It was completely inactivated by the enzyme under conditions in which 30% of the activity of oxytocin still remained (GOLUBOW and DU VIGNEAUD, 1963). The chymotryptic inactivation of the hormone is occasioned by the proteolytic cleavage of the peptide bond which links the leucine and glycine residues in positions 8 and 9, respectively, glycine amide being released (BARTH, PLIŠKA, and RYCHLÍK, 1967). There was a close agreement between the rate of liberation of glycine amide from the hormone and the loss of its uterotonic activity. This enzymatic reaction was very sluggish, however, its rate being approximately 500 times slower than the release of glycine amide from vasopressin under the catalytic action of trypsin. The open-chain analogues, S. S'-dimethyldihydro-oxytocin and Ala^1-Ala^6-oxytocin, were attacked by chymotrypsin A at a much higher rate than oxytocin itself, the leucyl-glycine bond again being broken. Contrary to what one might have expected on the basis of the established specificity of chymotrypsin, the bond linking the tyrosine and isoleucine residues in positions 2 and 3 of the amino acid sequence was found to be resistant to attack by bovine chymotrypsin A both in oxytocin and in its open-chain analogues (BARTH, PLIŠKA, and RYCHLÍK, 1967). Porcine pancreatic chymotrypsin C acted on oxytocin in the same way as bovine chymotrypsin A, the leucyl-glycine bond being hydrolyzed (FOLK and COLE, 1965). When oxidized oxytocin was subjected to digestion by chymotrypsin C, however, the link between the glutamine and asparagine residues in positions 4 and 5 of the peptide chain was broken in addition to the leucyl-glycine bond.

Various investigators such as CROXATTO, ALLIENDE, and CROXATTO (1942/1943), CROXATTO, CROXATTO, ILLANES, and SALVESTRINI (1942/1943) and THORN and SILVER (1957) found that crystalline chymotrypsin was capable of destroying the pressor and antidiuretic principle of the mammalian posterior pituitary. BARTH, PLIŠKA, and RYCHLÍK (1967), however, who incubated Lys[8]-vasopressin with several times recrystallized bovine chymotrypsin A, could not observe a decrease of antidiuretic activity nor obtain chromatographic evidence of a fragmentation of this hormone. They suggest that the earlier findings which had indicated a destruction of vasopressin by chymotrypsin were due to traces of trypsin, which are present in most commercial chymotrypsin preparations. These authors emphasize that the loss of antidiuretic activity upon incubation of body fluids or tissue extracts with chymotrypsin (THORN, 1959; BARNAFI, ROSAS, PEREDA, and CROXATTO, 1962; DLOUHÁ, KRAUS, KŘEČEK, and PLIŠKA, 1965) was not really due to chymotrypsin and should not be considered valid evidence for the presence of vasopressin.

Recently, the preparation and the physiological properties of a Lys[8]-vasopressin dimer were reported (SCHALLY and GUILLEMIN, 1964; SCHALLY, BOWERS, KUROSHIMA, ISHIDA, CARTER, and REDDING, 1964). Chymotrypsin was used to distinguish between two possible configurations of the dimer, namely, between a cyclic parallel and a cyclic antiparallel structure (SCHALLY and BARRETT, 1965). Chymotryptic hydrolysis was found to result in the liberation of the α-amino groups of phenylalanine and glutamine residues which occupy positions 3 and 4 in the peptide chain of vasopressin. This indicated that vasopressin, in accord with its generally accepted specificity, had broken the bonds on the carboxyl side of the aromatic amino acid residues, tyrosine and phenylalanine, in positions 2 and 3. The amino acid composition of six fragments separated from the digestion mixture were determined and found to correspond to those expected for cleavage products of the antiparallel dimer.

The large posterior pituitary polypeptide isolated by PREDDIE and SAFFRAN (1965), which contains 48 amino acid residues, is readily cleaved by chymotrypsin both in its native and in the performic acid-oxidized state (PREDDIE, 1965). Peptide bonds involving the carboxyl groups of two tryptophan residues, one phenylalanine residue and one out of three leucine residues occurring in the amino acid sequence were found to be points of ready proteolytic attack by chymotrypsin. The structure of one of the chymotryptic cleavage products (AC-III),

Leu-Cys-Ser-Glu(NH_2)-Gly-Asp(NH_2)-Cys-Ala-Gly-Val,

which is derived from the carboxyl-terminal portion of the polypeptide, bears an obvious resemblance to that of oxytocin,

Cys-Tyr-Ile-Glu(NH_2)-Asp(NH_2)-Cys-Pro-Leu-Gly(NH_2).

The slight oxytocic activity of the large polypeptide can possibly be related to the similarity of its carboxyl-terminal portion with the cyclic peptide structure of oxytocin. There is circumstantial evidence indicating that the posterior pituitary hormones might be synthesized in the hypothalamus in the form of relatively inactive precursors which travel axonally towards the nerve endings in the posterior lobe and gain full biological activity by an enzyme-catalyzed loss of part of the molecule (SACHS and TAKABATAKE, 1964). The large pituitary polypeptide which can be degraded proteolytically to yield an oxytocin-like cyclic peptide is considered by PREDDIE (1965) to be a naturally occurring analogue of the hypothetical precursors of the neurohypophysial hormones.

3. Pepsin

Oxytocin is not inactivated by pepsin (FREUDENBERG, WEISS, and EYER, 1932; GULLAND and MACRAE, 1933b; CROXATTO, CROXATTO, and ALLIENDE, 1942; THORN and SILVER, 1957; HAWKER, WALMSLEY, ROBERTS, and ROBERTSON, 1959). Nor is the oxytocic activity present in Van Dyke's protein destroyed even upon prolonged treatment with pepsin (VAN DYKE, CHOW, GREEP, and ROTHEN, 1942). The neurohypophysial principle present in elasmobranch pituitaries, which is similar to oxytocin but not identical with it, was also found to be resistant to peptic digestion (PERKS, DODD, and DODD, 1960).

Vasopressin is not attacked by pepsin (THORN, 1959). In contrast, the corticotropin-releasing activity of hypothalamic extracts was found to be susceptible to destruction by pepsin. This provided evidence for the presence in such extracts of a corticotropin-releasing factor distinct from vasopressin (ROYCE and SAYERS, 1958).

4. Papain and Bromelain

FREUDENBERG, WEISS, and EYER (1932) noted that oxytocin was destroyed by papain. The previous failure by DALE and DUDLEY (1921) to observe an inactivation of the hormone by papain may have been due to the fact that these authors carried out their digestions in 0.1 M HCl, i. e. at a pH value far too low for optimum activity of the enzyme. GULLAND and MACRAE (1933a) showed that a commercial preparation of papain inactivated oxytocin extremely rapidly with a pH optimum of 7.4.

In experiments designed to prove the occurrence in oxytocin and vasopressin of asparagine and glutamine residues rather than of isoasparagine and isoglutamine residues, LAWLER, TAYLOR, SWAN, and DU VIGNEAUD (1954) allowed crystalline papain to act on the neurohypophysial hormones at pH 5.3. The digestion was carried out in the presence of hydrogen sulphide as an activator. Paper chromatography of the digests revealed several ninhydrin-positive cleavage products, two of which could be identified as asparagine and glutamine. Their amount in the papain hydrolyzate represented 20—30% of that theoretically derivable from the quantity of neurohypophysial hormone used. The occurrence of substantial amounts of free amino acids among the products of the papain-catalyzed hydrolysis clearly indicated the capability of this enzyme to bring about an extensive breakdown of oxytocin and vasopressin.

Bromelain, an enzyme with a specificity similar to that of papain, was reported not to degrade vasopressin (MARTIN, MOSS, and SMYTH, 1964). Chromatography of the incubation mixture provided no evidence of an hydrolytic liberation of free aminoacids or of lower peptides.

An unknown oxytocic substance accompanying oxytocin in extracts of blood could be distinguished from oxytocin by its unsusceptibility to the action of papain (HAWKER, WALMSLEY, ROBERTS, and ROBERTSON, 1959; HAWKER, 1961).

5. Aspergillus Oryzae Proteinase

A crystalline proteolytic enzyme from *Aspergillus oryzae* which ranks with trypsin among the most active gelatinolytic enzymes (CREWTHER and LENNOX, 1950) was used by DU VIGNEAUD, LAWLER, and POPENOE (1953) in their studies of the structure of Arg^8-vasopressin. This enzyme, like trypsin, catalyzed the hydrolysis of the arginyl bond and released glycine amide from the carboxyl-terminal end of the hormone molecule.

6. Bacillus Subtilis Proteinase

The enzyme subtilisin which is produced by a particular strain of *Bacillus subtilis* and is marked for its capability of transforming ovalbumin into plakalbumin (LINDERSTRØM-LANG and OTTESEN, 1949; GÜNTELBERG and OTTESEN, 1952), has been successfully used in the elucidation of the amino acid sequence of oxytocin. When performic acid-oxidized oxytocin was incubated with this proteinase, hydrolysis of the polypeptide chain occurred between the glutamine and asparagine residues in positions 4 and 5, between the leucine and glycine residues in positions 8 and 9 and, to a lesser degree, between the tyrosine and isoleucine residues in positions 2 and 3 (TUPPY, 1953; TUPPY and MICHL, 1953). When non-oxidized oxytocin was subjected to crystalline *B. subtilis* proteinase, the peptide bond linking Leu^8 and Gly^9 was broken exclusively, glycine amide being released (ACHER, CHAUVET, and LENCI, 1958, 1959). Performic acid-oxidized isotocin (Ser^4-Ile^8-oxytocin) was attacked by subtilisin between the Ser^4 and $Asp(NH_2)^5$ residues (ACHER, CHAUVET, CHAUVET, and CREPY, 1962). In oxidized glumitocin (Ser^4-$Glu(NH_2)^8$-oxytocin) subtilisin broke the peptide bonds between Ser^4 and $Asp(NH_2)^5$ and between $Glu(NH_2)^8$ and Gly^9 (ACHER, CHAUVET, CHAUVET, and CREPY, 1965).

7. *Pancreatic Carboxypeptidase*

The fact that the carboxyl-terminal amino acid residue in oxytocin and vasopressin carries a carboxamide rather than a free α-carboxyl group renders the neurohypophysial hormones unsusceptible to the action of carboxypeptidase. CROXATTO, CROXATTO, and RIOSECO (1945) were the first to point out that oxytocin and vasopressin are not affected by crystalline carboxypeptidase. In contrast, pepsitensin and angiotensin are readily inactivated by this enzyme, and so are anephrotensin (CROXATTO, PEREDA, and ZAMORANO, 1961) and the "unknown oxytocic substance" studied by HAWKER (1961).

The resistance towards carboxypeptidase of oxytocin, native vasopressin and performic acid-oxidized vasopressin was confirmed, respectively, by DU VIGNEAUD, RESSLER, and TRIPPETT (1953), THORN and SILVER (1957) and ACHER and CHAUVET (1954). When, however, oxytocin was first subjected to subtilisin and thereby deprived of its amidated carboxyl-terminal amino acid residue, glycine amide, a subsequent degradation by carboxypeptidase could be brought about, substantial amounts of the last but one amino acid residue, leucine, being released (ACHER, CHAUVET, and LENCI, 1958, 1959).

It was noted by HAWKER and ROBERTSON (1957, 1958) that in blood and hypothalamic extracts oxytocin is accompanied by another oxytocic substance which is rather similar to oxytocin in many respects. The susceptibility of this polypeptide to the action of carboxypeptidase was found useful in its differentiation from oxytocin (HAWKER, WALMSLEY, ROBERTS, and ROBERTSON, 1959; HAWKER, 1961; CROXATTO, PEREDA, and ZAMORANO, 1961).

The carboxyl-terminal portion of the sizeable posterior pituitary polypeptide which was discovered and isolated by PREDDIE and SAFFRAN (1965) is structurally similar to oxytocin. Under the action of carboxypeptidase, however, amino acids are readily liberated, because its carboxyl terminus, contrary to that of oxytocin and vasopressin, is not blocked by an amide group.

8. *Prolinase*

It was found by GULLAND and MACRAE (1933b) that a crude preparation of brewer's yeast prolinase was unable to inactivate oxytocin. This finding is accounted for by the internal position of the proline residue in the oxytocin molecule which, therefore, is inaccessible to the exopeptidase, prolinase.

9. *Kidney Leucine Aminopeptidase*

The best known among all aminopeptidases is leucine aminopeptidase (LAP) which has been isolated in highly purified form from swine kidneys (SPACKMAN,

Smith, and Brown, 1955). It is particularly active on peptides possessing amino-terminal leucine residues. Most amino acids other than leucine, however, can also be released, though more slowly, by the enzyme. LAP was shown to be capable of degrading hormonally active polypeptides such as, e.g., glucagon (Hill and Smith, 1959) and angiotensin (Elliott and Peart, 1957), the constituent amino acids being successively released from the amino terminus of the chain. In contrast, oxytocin was found to be attacked very slowly, even at high enzyme to substrate ratios (Hill and Smith, 1957). In dialyzates of the digestion mixture each amino acid present in the oxytocin molecule was found. Tyrosine and isoleucine, however, were recovered in less than stoichiometric quantities. Oxytocin shares the property of being exceptionally resistant to the action of renal LAP with a few other peptides likewise possessing a three-dimensional structure stabilized by disulphide bonds. In recent years, the action of high concentrations of LAP upon oxytocin and related neurohypophysial hormones was repeatedly used in studies of their amino acid sequence. When LAP was allowed to act on oxytocin or on mesotocin (Ile^8-oxytocin) the following result was obtained (Acher, Chauvet, Chauvet, and Crepy, 1964): There was a rapid initial release of the free amino acids, tyrosine and isoleucine, which occupy positions 2 and 3 in the amino acid sequence of the peptides, while the amino-terminal half-cystine residue remained attached to the peptide molecule via the disulphide bridge. Glutamine and asparagine which occupy positions 4 and 5, were set free only in small amounts. When, on the other hand, isotocin (Ser^4-Ile^8-oxytocin) was subjected to digestion by LAP, a heavy release of tyrosine, isoleucine and serine was observed, whereas asparagine appeared in smaller quantities. These findings were in agreement with the occurrence in isotocin of the amino-terminal amino acid sequence, Cys-Tyr-Ile-Ser-Asp(NH_2) (Acher, Chauvet, Chauvet, and Crepy, 1962, 1964). The incubation of glumitocin (Ser^4-Glu(NH_2)^8-oxytocin) with LAP gave results identical to those with isotocin (Acher, Chauvet, Chauvet, and Crepy, 1965): tyrosine, isoleucine, serine and asparagine were released sequentially. The amino-terminal sequences in vasotocin (Arg^8-oxytocin) and Arg^8-vasopressin, Cys-Tyr-Ile and Cys-Tyr-Phe, respectively, were also established using LAP as a degradative tool (Acher, 1963; Chauvet, Chauvet, and Acher, 1963).

In contrast to oxytocin, deamino-oxytocin turned out to be entirely resistant to LAP (Golubow and Du Vigneaud, 1963). Under conditions of incubation, in which 50% of the activity of oxytocin was destroyed by the enzyme, none of the activity of deamino-oxytocin was lost. This result is consistent with the known specificity of LAP, the action of which is restricted to substrates which contain a terminal amino acid residue with a free α-amino group.

Bartošek, Pliška, Rychlík, and Šorm (1964) partially purified an aminopeptidase from liver which they considered identical with kidney LAP on the basis of identical substrate specificity, kinetics of action, and other properties. According to their findings, the aminopeptidase is incapable of breaking down the neurohypophysial peptides as long as these are in their cyclic disulphide form. Only after opening of the ring by reductive cleavage of the disulphide bond will the hormones be attacked by the aminopeptidase, individual amino acids being sequentially released from the amino end of the open-chain derivatives.

10. Yeast Aminopeptidase

Gulland and Macrae (1933b) noted that oxytocin was destroyed by a crude preparation of yeast aminopolypeptidase and that this inactivation occurred optimally at pH 7.4. The authors surmised that the inactivation was not due to the aminopeptidase itself but rather to a contaminating enzyme present in the preparation. However, the ready destruction of oxytocin by yeast aminopeptidase was later confirmed by CROXATTO, CROXATTO, and ALLIENDE (1942) and CROXATTO, ALLIENDE, and CROXATTO (1942/1943a) who used an enzyme sample prepared by the method of JOHNSON (1941). The oxytocic hormone was destroyed at a neutral pH, provided that either cysteine or GSH was present as an enzyme activator. The activating effect of the sulphydryl compounds could be abolished by iodate. The results of these experiments led the authors to propose the hypothesis, which has since proved to be correct, that oxytocin is a polypeptide with a free terminal amino group. Vasopressin was also found to be destroyed by yeast aminopolypeptidase (CROXATTO, ILLANES, SALVESTRINI, and CROXATTO, 1942/1943). As in the case of oxytocin, the enzyme was active in the presence of cysteine or GSH and could be rendered inactive by iodate.

11. Human Pregnancy Plasma Oxytocinase

The destruction of oxytocin in the blood of pregnant women was discovered by FEKETE (1930, 1932). He found that the sera of pregnant women, in contradistinction to those of non-pregnant individuals, were capable of abolishing the uterus-stimulating activity of posterior pituitary extracts, the amount of oxytocin being directly related to the length of incubation with the sera. The enzymatic nature of the inactivation reaction was clearly established by WERLE and EFFKEMANN (1941). The principle responsible for the enzymatic destruction of oxytocin in pregnancy sera was called "oxytocinase" (WERLE, HEVELKE, and BUTHMANN, 1941). PAGE (1946, 1947), who studied the destruction of the commercial preparation, pitocin, in oxalated pregnancy plasma rather than in serum and adduced additional convincing evidence for the enzymatic character of the process, gave the enzyme the name "pitocinase". These terms are not satisfactory because, as we know, the enzyme concerned is not specific for oxytocin (pitocin), but will attack many peptide substrates other than oxytocin. Since, however, oxytocin was the first known and has continued to be considered a physiological substrate for this enzyme, the term "oxytocinase", which has now been widely used for more than two and a half decades, will be retained for the enzyme in the present review.

Biological and Chemical Assay Methods. In his pioneer investigations FEKETE (1930, 1932) followed the reduction of the oxytocic activity, which occurred upon incubation of neurohypophysial extracts with pregnancy sera, by assaying the residual oxytocin *in situ* on the gravid human uterus and *in vitro* on the isolated uterine horns of the guinea-pig and rat. The pregnant human uterus was again used by WOODBURY, AHLQUIST, ABREU, TORPIN, and WATSON (1946) for testing the loss of oxytocic activity suffered by pitocin and pitressin upon treatment with pregnancy blood. In most later work, the rat uterus was the test object (e.g. PAGE, 1946, 1947; WERLE, SEMM, and ENZENBACH, 1950; HAWKER, 1956; MELANDER, 1965). MÉNDEZ-BAUER and CARBALLO (1957) introduced an alternative biological method for assaying the residual hormone after incubation of oxytocin with biological fluids or tissue extracts containing oxytocinase. Their method is based on the rise of intramammary pressure in the lactating rabbit caused by intravenous injection of oxytocin and was successfully employed by MÉNDEZ-BAUER, CARBALLO, CABOT, NEGREIROS DE PAIVA, and GONZÁLEZ-PANIZZA (1961) and by RYDÉN and SJÖHOLM (1962).

A polarographic method for determining oxytocinase in blood serum was recently described by BARTIK and MICHNOVÁ (1966). After incubation of oxytocin with pregnancy serum, the polarographic wave due to oxytocin is decreased. The ratio of wave heights before and after incubation can be used as a measure for oxytocinase activity.

In 1957, TUPPY and NESVADBA provided evidence which indicated that the inactivation of oxytocin by the enzyme present in pregnancy serum was due to a proteolytic cleavage of the hormone molecule on the carboxyl side of its amino-terminal hemicystine residue. This finding suggested that oxytocinase had the specificity of an aminopeptidase. An aminopeptidase substrate containing, like oxytocin, amino-terminal hemicystine residues, *viz.* L-cystine di-β-naphthylamide, was shown to be susceptible to the hydrolytic action of pregnancy plasma oxytocinase and to be suited for the assay of this enzyme, particularly in blood serum. The β-naphthylamine released from L-cystine di-β-naphthylamide under the action of oxytocinase is diazotized and the resulting diazonium salt coupled with N-(1-naphthyl)ethylene diamine to yield a stable blue azo dye which can be readily measured colorimetrically at a wavelength of 565 mμ. This method employing L-cystine di-β-naphthylamide as a chromogenic substrate has in the past 10 years been widely used for the assay of oxytocinase (e.g. MÜLLER-HARTBURG, NESVADBA, and TUPPY, 1959; TITUS, REYNOLDS, GLENDENING, and PAGE, 1960; HASHIMOTO, 1961a; SJÖHOLM, YMAN, and SANDBERG, 1965; MELANDER, 1965; KLIMEK and PIETRZYCKA, 1961; HANSON and MANNSFELDT, 1967a; RYDÉN, 1966). Colour development takes 3—4 h when the assay procedure is performed as originally proposed by TUPPY and NESVADBA (1957). A modification introduced by BABUNA and YENEN (1966) reduces the time necessary for development of maximum colour to about 20 min. Another modification which renders the procedure still more proficient and lends itself to routine determinations of oxytocinase, consists in treating the enzyme-liberated β-naphthylamine with diazotized 3-chloro-4-nitroaniline (Echtrot 3 GL), followed by extraction of the red azo-dye into ethyl acetate and colorimetry at 546 mμ (HARDIE and RITCHIE, 1966). The amounts of oxytocinase required for the assay can be greatly reduced by measuring fluorometrically the β-naphthylamine liberated by the enzyme. The sensitivity of the fluorometric procedure is so high that as little as 50 μl of pregnancy serum will suffice for assaying its oxytocinase activity (ROTH, 1964).

The use of L-cystine di-β-naphthylamide as an oxytocinase substrate has the drawback that there are enzymes other than oxytocinase which may also catalyze its cleavage. Enzymes normally occurring in human sera are only slightly active towards this chromogenic substrate. In tissue extracts, however, enzymes other than oxytocinase with considerable activity towards L-cystine di-β-naphthylamide are usually present. A new chromogenic substrate, S-benzyl-L-cysteine β-naphthylamide, was shown to be cleaved by oxytocinase much faster than L-cystine di-β-naphthylamide and to be somewhat less susceptible to attack by aminopeptidases other than oxytocinase (TUPPY and WINTERSBERGER, 1964; WINTERSBERGER, MÜLLER-HARTBURG, and TUPPY, 1966; HANSON and MANNSFELDT, 1967a). The rate of cleavage by oxytocinase can be further increased by allowing the enzyme to act on this substrate in a solution containing 12—15% methyl cellosolve (TUPPY and WINTERSBERGER, 1964).

An oxytocinase substrate whose enzyme-catalyzed hydrolysis can be followed directly in the spectrophotometer is L-cystine di-p-nitroanilide (TUPPY, WIESBAUER, and WINTERSBERGER, 1962). This substrate has a negligible light extinction at 400 mμ, whereas p-nitroaniline liberated from it by oxytocinase exhibits a yellow colour and has a high extinction coefficient at 400 mμ. It was used by SEMM (1965) as a substitute for L-cystine di-β-naphthylamide. S-Benzyl-L-cystine p-nitroanilide was recently synthesized by HANSON and MANNSFELDT (1967a) and recommended as a chromogenic substrate useful for assaying oxytocinase in pregnancy serum. The p-nitroaniline released in the enzymatic reaction can not only be measured directly at 400 mμ, but can also be diazotized and coupled with

N-(1-naphthyl)ethylene diamine to give an azo dye which is measured in the colorimeter at 565 mμ.

Čihař, Beránková, Rychlík, and Šorm (1961) used S-benzyl-L-cysteinyl-tyrosine amide, S-benzyl-L-cysteinyl-glycine amide and similar peptide amides for assaying oxytocinase. After incubation with enzyme, the fragments were separated from each other by paper chromatography and their amounts evaluated by the ninhydrin reaction. These peptide amides, however, are readily attacked by LAP as well as by oxytocinase (Hanson and Mannsfeldt, 1967a) and are therefore less suitable for a differential assay of plasma oxytocinase.

Purification. First attempts to purify oxytocinase from human pregnancy plasma or serum involved salting out with ammonium sulphate (Werle, Hevelke, and Buthmann, 1941; Page, 1946; Werle, Semm, and Enzenbach, 1950; Dicker and Whyley, 1959a; Hashimoto, 1961a). From retroplacental serum 63% of the enzyme activity could be recovered in the protein fraction precipitating between 40 and 60% saturation of ammonium sulphate (Tuppy and Wintersberger, 1960).

An efficient further purification was achieved by fractionating a buffered solution of the ammonium sulphate precipitate with rivanol (Tuppy and Wintersberger, 1960) and removing both rivanol and inactive proteins by adsorption on bentonite. When the oxytocinase solution was subsequently chromatographed on a column of hydroxylapatite, contaminating proteins were retained to a considerable extent, whereas the enzyme quickly passed down the column. With retroplacental serum as the starting material an overall purification of oxytocinase of up to 4500fold was achieved (Tuppy, 1960; Tuppy and Wintersberger, 1960). Using the same procedure Goebelsmann and Beller (1965) obtained a 5200fold purification.

The high molecular weight of plasma oxytocinase is reflected in the behaviour of the enzyme in gel filtration experiments and can be utilized for separation purposes. Sjöholm (1964) showed that oxytocinase is only slightly retarded on Sephadex G-200 and is eluted shortly after the serum proteins, which have sedimentation coefficients of 10 S and above. Gel filtrations of retroplacental sera increased the specific activity of the enzyme by a factor of 4—5. Chromatography on Sephadex was successfully used by Goebelsmann and Beller (1965) for separating oxytocinase from an aminopeptidase which is present in all human sera and is particularly active on leucine β-naphthylamide.

Sjöholm, Yman, and Sandberg (1965) described a procedure for the large-scale purification of oxytocinase based on Cohn's method no. 10 for the fractionation of serum proteins with ethanol in the presence of zinc ions. When retroplacental serum was fractionated according to Cohn's method, the bulk of oxytocinase was obtained in the "precipitate IV+V". Stepwise elution of the precipitate with dilute ethanol containing ε-aminocaproate and acetate at increasing pH values gave a 75% yield of 50fold purified oxytocinase. A minor modification (Sjöholm and Yman, 1966a) resulted in an increase in the purification factor and the yield to about 65fold and 80%, respectively. Subsequent chromatography on hydroxylapatite led to a further 70—80fold purification. A final chromatography on DEAE-Sephadex yielded an oxytocinase preparation which was homogeneous in gel electrophoresis. In fact, two bands of active oxytocinase could be observed in the gels. It was shown, however, that these represented two different conformational forms of the same enzyme (Sjöholm and Yman, 1966b). The overall purification factor ranged from 6000—9000 depending on the oxytocinase content of the starting material. About 4 mg of purified oxytocinase were obtained from 1 litre of retroplacental serum.

The occurrence in pregnancy serum of more than one component with oxytocinase activity had been first observed by Page, Titus, Mohun, and Glendening (1961) who reported on the appearance of two bands of identical enzymatic specificity in vertical starch gel electrophoresis. Čihař, Beránková, Rychlík, and Šorm (1961) observed that the oxytocinase activity upon fractionation of pregnancy serum with alcohol was divided into two parts which behaved differently when subjected to chromatography on ECTEOLA cellulose. "Oxytocinase A", which was adsorbed quantitatively on this ion exchange material from a solution containing 0.01 M phosphate of pH 7 was purified approximately 400fold. "Oxytocinase B" was not adsorbed on ECTEOLA cellulose and was purified about 7fold by fractionating on a column of DEAE cellulose. Oxytocinase A and oxytocinase B did not differ in substrate specificity or susceptibility to inhibitors and were considered two forms of the same enzyme (Čihař, Beránková, Rychlík, and Šorm, 1961). Upon direct chromatography of unfractionated retroplacental serum on ECTEOLA cellulose, splitting of the enzyme peak into two could be observed (Tuppy and Wintersberger, 1964). Evidence for the presence of two forms of oxytocinase was also obtained by Sjöholm (1964) when he chromatographed retroplacental serum, which had been previously fractionated by gel filtration, on a column of DEAE cellulose. Two peaks of enzyme activity were obtained. The specific activity of the enzyme in the larger peak was 35—60 times greater than in serum. Barth, Pliška, Rychlík, and Šorm (1967), who subjected retroplacental serum to a fractionation procedure involving ethanol precipitation, gel filtration and chromatography on DEAE cellulose, obtained two separate enzyme species which they called 0-I and 0-II, both of which inactivated oxytocin. The specific activity of the major component, 0-II, was 3000 times higher than the oxytocinase activity in retroplacental serum. 0-I was unstable.

Stability. In neutral solutions, particularly in blood plasma or serum, oxytocinase shows a remarkable stability. Enzyme activity will remain unchanged for days, or even for several weeks, when pregnancy serum is stored in the cold unter sterile conditions (Werle, Hevelke, and Buthmann, 1941; Müller-Hartburg, Nesvadba, and Tuppy, 1959; Titus, Reynolds, Glendening, and Page, 1960; Hashimoto, 1961a). Oxytocinase activity was fully preserved in serum samples kept in the frozen or freeze-dried state for several months (Čihař, Beránková, Rychlík, and Šorm, 1961; Melander, 1965). Solutions of highly purified oxytocinase could also be stored in the refrigerator for several weeks without any noticeable loss of activity. When solutions of purified enzyme, however, were frozen and thawed or lyophilized, activity was abolished entirely or to a large extent (Tuppy and Wintersberger, 1960; Čihař, Beránková, Rychlík, and Šorm, 1961; Yman and Sjöholm, 1967).

Pregnancy serum does not lose oxytocinase activity to any significant extent when heated at 37° for 24 h (Čihař, Beránková, Rychlík, and Šorm, 1961; Melander, 1965). At 55—60° there is slow inactivation (Werle, Hevelke, and Buthmann, 1941; Dicker and Whyley, 1959a; Hashimoto, 1961a). Heating of sera at more elevated temperatures brings about rapid denaturation of the enzyme. Solutions of purified plasma oxytocinase exhibit a similar stability of enzymatic activity to moderate heating (Tuppy and Wintersberger, 1960).

At pH values ranging from 6—10, no inactivation was observed upon warming to 37° for 30 min. Above pH 11 and below pH 3.5, oxytocinase activity was completely lost. At pH values from 3.5 to 6, partial inactivation occurred (Yman and Sjöholm, 1967).

Treatment of pregnancy serum with a mixture of acetone and ether resulted in complete inactivation of oxytocinase (Werle, Hevelke, and Buthmann, 1941).

Fractional precipitation with ethanol, on the other hand, could be used with advantage for the purification of the enzyme. The presence in oxytocinase solutions of moderate amounts of water-miscible organic solvents may even enhance their enzymatic activity. An increase in activity by more than 50% was noted in solutions containing 10—15% (v/v) of methyl cellosolve (TUPPY and WINTERSBERGER, 1964).

Dialysis of pregnancy serum or of oxytocinase solutions does not impair the enzymatic activity (WERLE, HEVELKE, and BUTHMANN, 1941; HASHIMOTO, 1961a). This result indicates that oxytocinase does not contain an easily dissociable prosthetic group of low molecular weight which is essential for activity.

Antigenic Properties. When 4500fold purified oxytocinase suspended in complete Freund's adjuvant was repeatedly injected into rabbits, an antiserum was obtained which was capable of precipitating oxytocinase. Using Ouchterlony's technique of double-diffusion in agar gel only one precipitation line was obtained (TUPPY and WINTERSBERGER, 1960). The antigenicity of oxytocinase in rabbits and the appearance of a single line of precipitation in immunodiffusion experiments was confirmed by GOEBELSMANN and BELLER (1965).

Electrophoretic Behaviour. WERLE and SEMM (1956) subjected pregnancy serum to continuous vertical paper electrophoresis in a Michaelis buffer of pH 8.6 and found that oxytocinase migrated to the cathode side of serum albumin, its anodic mobility being a little faster than that of the α_1 globulins. After horizontal paper electrophoresis, approximately 20% of the enzyme activity was recovered in the albumin fraction, whereas 80% was found in the α_1 globulin band (WERLE and SEMM, 1956). HASHIMOTO (1961a) confirmed this result by showing that the enzymatic activities towards oxytocin (oxytocinase) and towards L-cystine di-β-naphthylamide ("cystine aminopeptidase" = CAP) were largely in the α_1 globulin fraction of the vertical paper electropherogram. RIAD and SCANDRETT (1962) who used cellulose acetate membranes as the support for the electrophoresis of human pregnancy serum, observed CAP activity both in the α_1 and α_2 globulins of the electropherogram rather than in a single sharply defined band. In horizontal starch gel electrophoresis of highly purified oxytocinase preparations one single aminopeptidase band was obtained, which represented oxytocinase and could be revealed using either L-cystine di-β-naphthylamide or, preferably, L-leucine β-naphthylamide as the chromogenic substrate (TUPPY, WIESBAUER, and WINTERSBERGER, 1963; SJÖHOLM and YMAN, 1966a). The pregnancy-specific aminopeptidase (oxytocinase) also appeared as a single band, in addition to another enzymecleaving L-leucine β-naphthylamide which occurs in all human sera irrespective of pregnancy, when human pregnancy sera or retroplacental sera were subjected to horizontal starch gel electrophoresis. In vertical starch gel electrophoresis of pregnancy sera, however, two additional enzyme bands were obtained by PAGE, TITUS, MOHUN, and GLENDENING (1961), both of which were capable of inactivating oxytocin and of cleaving the β-naphthylamides of L-cystine and L-leucine. On account of their ability to utilize L-cystine di-β-naphthylamide as a substrate, the enzymes were designated as cystine aminopeptidases 1 and 2, CAP_1 and CAP_2. CAP_1 migrated close to the fast α_2 globulin, whereas CAP_2 trailed the β_1 globulin (transferrin). Using both unfractionated retroplacental serum and highly purified oxytocinase preparations, SJÖHOLM and YMAN (1966a, b) confirmed the appearance of two separate aminopeptidase bands, CAP_1 and CAP_2, both in vertical starch gel and in polyacrylamide gel electrophoresis carried out at pH values of 8.2—9.6. CAP_2 was shown to predominate at pH 8.2—8.5, and CAP_1 at pH 9.0—9.6. At pH values of 7.2 and below, CAP_2 was to be seen exclusively, whereas at pH 10.4 only CAP_1 could be detected. Between pH 8.2 and 9.6, CAP_1 and CAP_2 are in a pH-dependent equilibrium. They can be slowly transformed into one another, the transformation of CAP_2 into CAP_1 being faster than the reverse process. CAP_1 and CAP_2 are considered to represent two different conformational species of the same enzyme with slightly different effective charges (Sjöholm and Yman, 1966b). Under physiological conditions, at pH 7.3—7.4, CAP_2 appears to be the only stable conformational form of oxytocinase.

Serum oxytocinase was shown to be a glycoprotein containing terminal N-acetyl-D-neuraminic acid residues which can be removed by treatment of the enzyme with *Vibrio cholerae* neuraminidase (Tuppy, Wiesbauer, and Wintersberger, 1963). The enzymatic release of the acidic carbohydrate residues results in a considerably lowered mobility of oxytocinase in horizontal starch gel electrophoresis (Tuppy and Wintersberger, 1964). Unexpectedly, the two conformational forms of oxytocinase, CAP_1 and CAP_2, yielded only one single enzyme species, CAP_N, when treated with neuraminidase (Sjöholm and Yman, 1966a). In all electrophoretic systems tried, including vertical starch-gel electrophoresis at pH values ranging from 5.9 to 10.4, CAP_N gave one single band which migrated somewhat more slowly than CAP_2 (Sjöholm and Yman, 1966a). Obviously, the sialic acid residues present in oxytocinase do not only provide negative charges to the enzyme molecules, but also play a significant role in establishing the conformational equilibrium between CAP_1 and CAP_2 (Sjöholm and Yman, 1966b). From the mobilities of CAP_2 and CAP_N in gel electrophoresis at various pH values, the isoelectric points of oxytocinase prior to and after removal of the sialic acid residues were deduced to be 3.7 and 4.5, respectively (Yman and Sjöholm, 1967).

Molecular Dimensions. Gel filtration was used by Yman and Sjöholm (1967) for evaluating the molecular weights and frictional ratios of oxytocinase and its neuraminidase-treated derivative. The molecular weights determined for the native and modified enzyme, 325,000 and 300,000, respectively, differed by about 8%, in accordance with the report of Tuppy, Wiesbauer, and Wintersberger (1963) on the amount of N-acetyl-D-neuraminic acid released from oxytocinase under the action of neuraminidase. The frictional ratios, 1.9 and 1.7, respectively, indicated that the molecules of oxytocinase are asymmetric and/or highly hydrated. The sedimentation constant, s_{20}, of oxytocinase was determined both at pH 10.4 and at pH 7.2, where the enzyme was believed to be predominantly in the CAP_1 and CAP_2 form, respectively (Sjöholm and Yman, 1966b). The s_{20} values obtained, 9.1 and 9.2 S, did not differ significantly and indicated that the reversible transformation of CAP_1 to CAP_2 did not involve a drastic change in molecular weight or molecular shape. The s_{20} for CAP_N is 9.6 S (Yman and Sjöholm, 1967). It is likely that the high molecular weight of oxytocinase is responsible for its failure to pass from the blood of pregnant women into the glomerular ultrafiltrate, or to pass through the placental barrier into the foetal circulation.

Enzyme Kinetics. Oxytocinase exhibits optimum activity in the neutral pH range. With oxytocin as the substrate, the optimum was found to be at about pH 7.0—7.5 (Rydén, 1966; Werle, Hevelke, and Buthmann, 1941; Hawker, 1956; Dicker and Whyley, 1959). When L-cystine di-β-naphthylamide and other synthetic arylamides were used as oxytocinase substrates, activity optima around or slightly above pH 7 were observed (Tuppy and Nesvadba, 1957; Melander, 1965; Rydén, 1966; Barth, Pliška, Rychlík, and Šorm, 1967; Hanson and Mannsfeldt, 1967a).

The rate of destruction of oxytocin by oxytocinase, or by diluted pregnancy serum or plasma, follows the kinetics of a first-order reaction (Page, 1946, 1947; Dicker and Whyley, 1959b; Méndez-Bauer, Carballo, Cabot, Negreiros de Paiva, and González-Panizza, 1961; Semm, 1961; Melander, 1965). It is directly proportional to the amount of enzyme present in the incubation mixture (WERLE, HEVELKE, and BUTHMANN, 1941), provided that the concentration of pregnancy plasma does not exceed 30% (MÉNDEZ-BAUER, CARBALLO, CABOT, NEGREIROS DE PAIVA, and GONZÁLEZ-PANIZZA, 1961) or 75 %(MELANDER, 1965). It is independent of the amount of oxytocin used. The velocity constant, k_1, of the reaction can be calculated from the half-life of destruction of oxytocin. 100 x k_1 has been recommended as the unit of oxytocinase activity (PAGE, 1946, 1947). Kinetic data reported by BELLER and GÖBELSMANN (1958, 1959) and by BELLER and SCHNIZ (1960), which seemed to contradict those expected for a first-order reaction, were subsequently not confirmed (MELANDER, 1965), The Michaelis constant, K_m, estimated according to the method of LINEWEAVER and BURK (1934) from the relationship between the reciprocals of the reaction velocities and the substrate concentrations, was found to be of the order of 10^{-5} M (MÉNDEZ-BAUER, CARBALLO, CABOT, NEGREIROS DE PAIVA, and GONZÁLEZ-PANIZZA, 1961; MELANDER, 1965). A recent study by SJÖHOLM and YMAN (1967) on the degradation by oxytocinase of tritiated oxytocin and vasopressin indicated that the Michaelis constants were 0.51×10^{-5} M and 1.07×10^{-5} M, respectively, and the maximum velocities were 0.12×10^{-5} and 0.18×10^{-5} moles per litre per min, respectively.

When synthetic substrates were employed for the assay of oxytocinase, it was generally attempted to use them in concentrations sufficiently great to saturate the enzyme in order to ensure zero order reaction kinetics and to obtain a linear progress curve. With L-cystine di-β-naphthylamide, saturation of the enzyme was achieved at above 0.25 mg/ml. When the enzyme concentrations were moderate and the incubation periods did not exceed 1 h, a linear relationship between enzyme level and rate of cleavage of substrate was obtained (TUPPY and NESVADBA, 1957; MELANDER, 1965). Deviations of the progress curve from linearity, which may occur when the enzyme level is high and the incubation time is prolonged, can be avoided by continuous shaking of the incubation mixtures, which will thereby be kept saturated with the moderately soluble substrate (RYDÉN, 1966). For the cleavage of L-cystine di-β-naphthylamide and L-leucine β-naphthylamide by oxytocinase, the K_m's were estimated to be 0.9×10^{-3} M and 1.6×10^{-3} M, respectively (HASHIMOTO, 1961a; YMAN and SJÖHOLM, 1967). These values are two orders of magnitude larger than the K_m for the oxytocinase-catalyzed cleavage of oxytocin. Considerably lower K_m values, *viz.* 0.50×10^{-5}M and 1.5×10^{-4} M, were determined for the hydrolysis by oxytocinase of L-cystine di-p-nitroanilide and L-leucine p-nitroanilide (TUPPY, WIESBAUER, and WINTERSBERGER, 1962).

Substrates of Plasma Oxytocinase. Oxytocin was the first and for many years the only known substrate for pregnancy plasma oxytocinase. The oxytocin solutions originally available for investigations of the enzyme were crude extracts of posterior pituitaries. Later, the destruction of hormonal activity by oxytocinase was verified using preparations of synthetic oxytocin. Some authors presented evidence which appeared to indicate that the oxytocic activity of partially purified neurohypophysial extracts was destroyed by the enzyme at a much greater rate than the oxytocic activity of commercial solutions of synthetic oxytocin (SEMM, 1957; DICKER and WHYLEY, 1960; MÉNDEZ-BAUER, CARBALLO, CABOT, NEGREIROS DE PAIVA, and GONZÁLEZ-PANIZZA, 1961). Other investigators failed to observe any difference between preparations of natural and synthetic oxytocin as regards their susceptibility to destruction by oxytocinase (BELLER and GÖBELSMANN, 1958; MELANDER, 1965). It is likely that impurities or preservatives present in some commercial preparations of synthetic oxytocin may act as enzyme inhibitors and thus may reduce the rate of enzymatic inactivation of the hormone (DICKER and WHYLEY, 1960).

Pregnancy plasma is capable of destroying enzymatically not only oxytocin but also vasopressin. In the course of pregnancy there is a similar progressive increase in the oxytocinase and "vasopressinase" activities of blood plasma. This led CROXATTO, VERA, and BÁRNAFI (1953) to assume that the same enzyme is involved in the inactivation of both hormones, oxytocin and vasopressin. The validity of this assumption was proved when highly purified plasma oxytocinase became available (TUPPY and WINTERSBERGER, 1960) and was found to inactivate vasopressin as readily and at approximately the same rate as oxytocin (STOKLASKA and WINTERSBERGER, 1959). GLENDENING, TITUS, SCHROEDER, MOHUN, and PAGE (1965) extended this finding by showing that both conformational forms of oxytocinase, CAP_1 and CAP_2, after separation by starch gel electrophoresis, would destroy oxytocin and vasopressin at similar rates. Additional evidence for the vasopressin-destroying potency of oxytocinase was recently provided by PLIŠKA, BARTH, and RYCHLÍK (1967) who demonstrated that plasma oxytocinase injected into laboratory animals was capable of decreasing *in vivo* the antidiuretic activity of lysine-vasopressin.

In order to elucidate the mechanism of the enzymatic inactivation of the neurohypophysial hormones by oxytocinase, TUPPY and NESVADBA (1957) incubated oxytocin with dialyzed pregnancy serum until the uterus-contracting potency of the hormone was nearly destroyed. From the incubation mixture, after deproteinization and oxidation by performic acid, substantial amounts of cysteic acid were isolated. This result indicated that oxytocinase is capable of breaking the peptide bond which links the amino-terminal hemicystine residue of oxytocin with the adjoining tyrosine residue, and thus exhibits the specificity of an aminopeptidase (TUPPY and NESVADBA, 1957; TUPPY, 1960). The susceptibility of vasopressin to oxytocinase is accounted for by the fact that vasopressin, like oxytocin, possesses a N-terminal hemicystinyl-tyrosine sequence. The view that oxytocinase is an aminopeptidase obtained strong support from the results of GOLUBOW, CHAN, and DU VIGNEAUD (1963) who showed that pregnancy serum which readily inactivated oxytocin was without effect on deamino-oxytocin. The lack of a free α-amino group in deamino-oxytocin renders this compound resistant to attack by plasma oxytocinase. This finding was recently confirmed by SEMM (1967).

The results which suggested that plasma oxytocinase was an aminopeptidase which released N-terminal hemicystine residues, led TUPPY and NESVADBA (1957) to synthesize L-cystine di-β-naphthylamide and to test it as a potential chromogenic oxytocinase substrate. This compound was indeed susceptible to hydrolysis by oxytocinase, β-naphthylamine being released which could be easily estimated colorimetrically. In the course of the purification of oxytocinase from retroplacental blood, the oxytocin-inactivating potency and the activity towards the synthetic substrate proved to be inseparable and to exhibit a constant ratio (STOKLASKA and WINTERSBERGER, 1959). Samples of unfractionated pregnancy serum and of highly purified enzyme, which exhibited an equal capability to cleave L-cystine di-β-naphthylamide, were also equally active in destroying oxytocin (TUPPY and WINTERSBERGER, 1960). The same electrophoretic components of pregnancy plasma which were capable of inactivating oxytocin and vasopressin, were also found to be responsible for the cleavage of L-cystine di-β-naphthylamide (GLENDENING, TITUS, SCHROEDER, MOHUN, and PAGE, 1965). Furthermore, the cleavage of the synthetic cystinyl compound by plasma from pregnant women could be inhibited by adding oxytocin to the incubation mixture. This showed that oxytocin and L-cystine di-β-naphthylamine were competing for the same enzyme (HASHIMOTO, 1961a; PAGE, TITUS, MOHUN, and GLENDENING, 1961). These results left no doubt, that L-cystine di-β-naphthylamide was indeed a substrate for oxytocinase.

Some L-cystinyl compounds other than L-cystine di-β-naphthylamide were subsequently shown to be also attacked by oxytocinase. L-Cystinyl-di-L-tyrosine amide, which contains the N-terminal dipeptide sequence of oxytocin and vasopressin, is hydrolyzed to cystine and tyrosine amide, when incubated with plasma oxytocinase (WINTERSBERGER and TUPPY, 1960; HANSON and MANNSFELDT, 1967a). L-Cystine di-p-nitroanilide has been recommended as a suitable chromogenic oxytocinase substrate, because the nitroaniline released under the action of the enzyme lends itself to colorimetry (TUPPY, WIESBAUER, and WINTERSBERGER, 1962).

BERÁNKOVÁ, RYCHLÍK, and ŠORM (1961) described the fission by pregnancy serum of a series of S-benzyl-L-cysteine peptides such as, e.g., S-benzyl-L-cysteinyl-tyrosine, S-benzyl-L-cysteinyl-phenylalanine, S-benzyl-L-cysteinyl-leucine, S-benzyl-L-cysteinyl-glycine and their respective amides. Using purified preparations of plasma oxytocinase, ČIHAŘ, BERÁNKOVÁ, RYCHLÍK, and ŠORM (1961) confirmed that from all these substrates the N-terminal amino acid, S-benzyl-L-cysteine, was released by the enzyme. Two fractions of plasma oxytocinase, which behaved differently upon chromatography, were found to be equally effective in cleaving S-benzyl-L-cysteine peptides.

Oxytocinase exhibits a definite optical specificity: S-benzyl-D-cysteinyl-L-tyrosine, in contradistinction to the corresponding L-cysteinyl derivative, is not appreciably attacked by the enzyme. In agreement with the known structural requirements of aminopeptidases, oxytocinase will not cleave S-benzyl-L-cysteinyl peptides unless the α-amino group of the N-terminal amino acid residue is free and the α-carboxyl group is joined to a primary amino group. Therefore, carbobenzoxy-S-benzyl-L-cysteinyl-tyrosine and S-benzyl-L-cysteinyl-L-prolyl-L-leucyl-glycine amide failed to be hydrolysed by plasma oxytocinase. It is not known, however, why S,S'-dibenzyl-dihydrooxytocin is resistant to attack by this enzyme (BERÁNKOVÁ and ŠORM, 1961).

Two chromogenic amide derivatives of S-benzyl-L-cysteine, *viz.* the β-naphthylamide (TUPPY and WINTERSBERGER, 1964; WINTERSBERGER, MÜLLER-HARTBURG, and TUPPY, 1966; HANSON and MANNSFELDT, 1967a) and the p-nitroanilide (HANSON and MANNSFELDT, 1967a) are among the best known oxytocinase substrates, their cleavage by the pregnancy enzyme being relatively fast and specific.

The enzymological studies reviewed so far clearly indicate that plasma oxytocinase behaves as a "cystine aminopeptidase" (CAP). It is capable of breaking peptide bonds which involve the carboxyl group of N-terminal L-hemicystinyl or S-benzyl-L-cysteinyl residues. However, the term CAP, which has been frequently used for oxytocinase (TITUS, REYNOLDS, GLENDENING, and PAGE, 1960; HASHIMOTO, 1961a, b; RIAD, 1962; SJÖHOLM, YMAN, and SANDBERG, 1965), must not be taken to indicate that N-terminal amino acid residues other than hemicystine or cysteine residues will not be released under the action of this enzyme.

In 1960, WINTERSBERGER and TUPPY showed that L-leucine β-naphthylamide and L-alanine β-naphthylamide were readily cleaved by plasma oxytocinase and were particularly suited for the detection of oxytocinase on electropherograms. It was observed that L-leucine β-naphthylamide was hydrolyzed by the enzyme some ten times faster than was L-cystine di-β-naphthylamide. GOEBELSMANN and BELLER (1965) reported that the rate of cleavage of L-leucine β-naphthylamide exceeds that of L-cystine di-β-naphthylamide by a factor of 11. The p-nitroanilides of L-leucine and glycine were also found to be hydrolyzed by oxytocinase, the rate of cleavage of the L-leucine derivative being several times higher than that of L-cystine di-p-nitroanilide (TUPPY, WIESBAUER, and WINTERSBERGER, 1962). The Michaelis constant, however, proved to be almost two orders of magnitude smaller for the p-nitroanilide of L-cystine ($K_m = 0.50 \times 10^{-5}$ M) than for the p-nitroanilides of glycine

($K_m = 0.65 \times 10^{-3}$ M) and L-leucine ($K_m = 0.15 \times 10^{-3}$ M), the difference indicating a marked affinity of oxytocinase for the L-cystinyl compound.

A systematic study of the action of oxytocinase on the β-naphthylamides of many different α-amino acids revealed that this aminopeptidase has a broad specificity (Tuppy, Wiesbauer, and Wintersberger, 1963). All the L-amino and imino acid β-naphthylamides tested were hydrolyzed by oxytocinase, though the rates of hydrolysis showed marked differences. The β-naphthylamide of L-leucine exhibited the best cleavability (=100), followed by the β-naphthylamides of L-phenylalanine (71), L-lysine (70), L-norleucine (60), L-alanine (55) and L-ornithine (45). The rates of cleavage of the β-naphthylamides of L-tyrosine, L-tryptophan, L-glutamine and L-asparagine were 10—20%, those of L-serine, L-histidine, glycine and L-cystine 5—10%, and those of L-proline, L-valine and L-isoleucine less than 5% of that determined for L-leucine β-naphthylamide. Thus, both neutral and charged aliphatic and aromatic N-terminal amino acid residues were liberated by oxytocinase. However, for amino acid β-naphthylamides to be hydrolyzed by the enzyme, their α-amino groups had to be unsubstituted and the α-carbon atom of the amino acid had to be in the L configuration. The β-naphthylamides of benzoyl-D, L-arginine and of D-leucine were entirely resistant to cleavage. Treatment of oxytocinase with neuraminidase, which resulted in the release of all the sialic acid residues present in the enzyme molecule, neither inactivated nor affected the specificity of oxytocinase. Apparently, the acidic carbohydrate residues are not essential for the enzymatic function of oxytocinase.

The observed broad substrate specificity, and particularly the susceptibility of L-tyrosine amide and L-tyrosine β-naphthylamide to hydrolysis by this enzyme (Wintersberger, Tuppy, and Stoklaska, 1960; Tuppy. Wiesbauer, and Wintersberger, 1963), suggested that the action of oxytocinase on the neurohypophysial peptides might not be limited to the cleavage of the terminal hemicystinyl bond, but might extend to the adjoining tyrosyl link or even further along the peptide chain. The experimental proof was provided by Sjöholm (1964) who subjected an oxytocinase-digest of oxytocin to thin-layer chromatography and could identify free tyrosine, a heptapeptide containing N-terminal isoleucine, and small amounts of free isoleucine. Recently, Sjöholm and Yman (1967) studied the enzymatic degradation of the neurohypophysial hormones in more detail using highly purified oxytocinase and samples of oxytocin and Lys⁸-vasopressin which were labelled with tritium in the tyrosine residues. Chromatography of the incubation mixtures showed that the disappearance of intact labelled oxytocin,

1 2 3 4 5 6 7 8 9
Cys-Tyr-Ile-Glu(NH_2)-Asp(NH_2)-Cys-Pro-Leu-Gly(NH_2),
(Cys 1 and Cys 6 joined by a bracket)

was accompanied by an initial rise in the amount of a tritiated nonapeptide,

2 3 4 5 6 7 8 9
Tyr-Ile-Glu(NH_2)-Asp(NH_2)-Cys-Pro-Leu-Gly(NH_2),
|
Cys
1

which obviously owed its formation to the cleavage of the bond between the N-terminal hemicystine residue and the adjoining tyrosine residue in the oxytocin molecule. The nonapeptide subsequently yielded free tritiated tyrosine and a nonradioactive octapeptide with N-terminal isoleucine. Further degradation by oxytocinase gave smaller amounts of free isoleucine, glutamine and asparagine. A similar result was obtained when oxytocinase was allowed to act an tritiated vasopressin. A labelled nonapeptide was initially formed which more slowly released ^{3}H-tyrosine. Upon prolonged incubation with oxytocinase, large amounts of phenylalanine and minor quantities of glutamine and asparagine were liberated. The degradation of oxytocin and vasopressin ceased with the appearance of the pentapeptides,

```
6   7   8   9                        6   7   8   9
Cys-Pro-Leu-Gly(NH2)    and    Cys-Pro-Lys-Gly(NH2),
 |                                    |
Cys                                  Cys
 1                                    1
```

respectively, which were resistant to further attack by oxytocinase. This finding is in agreement with the reported resistance of S-benzyl-Cys-Pro-Leu-Gly(NH_2) to hydrolysis by pregnancy serum (Beránková, Rychlík, and Šorm, 1961).

The lack of a narrow substrate specificity of oxytocinase instigated experiments in which the enzyme was allowed to act on peptides unrelated to oxytocin and vasopressin. Tuppy and Kreil (1962) used oxytocinase as a tool in the sequence determination of oligopeptides which had been obtained by tryptic hydrolysis of cytochrome c. Sjöholm and Yman (1967) showed that α-L-angiotensin and its amide could be extensively degraded by oxytocinase, the first five amino acids (Asp or Asp[NH_2], Arg, Val, Tyr and Val) being liberated. The remaining tripeptide, His-Pro-Phe, resisted further cleavage. Riniker and Schwyzer (1961) had previously made a similar observation when subjecting angiotensinamide to the action of LAP. Oxytocinase also resembled LAP in its failure to degrade β-L-angiotensin which differs from α-L-angiotensin in that the β-carboxyl rather than the α-carboxyl group of the N-terminal L-aspartic acid residue is involved in peptide linkage (Sjöholm and Yman, 1967).

Inhibitors and Activators of Pregnancy Plasma Oxytocinase. Numerous agents known to affect enzymes were tested for their action on the oxytocin-destroying potency of pregnancy plasma and on that of purified oxytocinase. It was hoped that specific inhibitors would help to gain a better insight into the mode of action of oxytocinase and might be used to differentiate if from other enzymes. Inhibitors which could be applied *in vivo* were searched for with particular emphasis because of their potential utilization in studies of the physiological role of oxytocinase.

Oxytocinase does not show the properties of a SH enzyme. Iodoacetate and iodoacetamide were of no effect (Page, 1946; Tuppy and Wintersberger, 1960; Hashimoto, 1961a). PCMB was found capable of inhibiting oxytocinase, but only in relatively high concentrations (Werle, 1960; Hashimoto, 1961a). Nitrogen mustard had no inhibitory action (Milani and Pinetti, 1951). L-Cystine and oxidized glutathione which impair the oxytocin-inactivating capability of some tissue extracts, produce no effect on pregnancy plasma oxytocinase (Semm, 1958; Čihař, Beránková, Rychlík, and Šorm, 1961; Hashimoto, 1961a). Nor was oxytocinase affected by oxidants such as potassium iodate, 2-methyl-naphthoquinone or hydrogen peroxide (Cespedes and Croxatto, 1949). Cytochrome c, however, was reported to be inhibitory (Croxatto and Cespedes, 1950).

Werle, Hevelke, and Buthmann (1941) found that L-cysteine and GSH were capable of increasing the oxytocin-destroying potency of pregnancy serum. Serum samples from men and nonpregnant women, which did not contain plasma oxytocinase, were enabled to destroy as much oxytocin and vasopressin as do pregnancy sera, when treated with thiol compounds such as L-cysteine, GSH and thiosorbitol (Werle, Hevelke, and Buthmann, 1941; Croxatto and Reyes, 1948; Croxatto, Cespedes, and Daza, 1951). H_2S and ascorbic acid were without effect. It is known that thiol compounds are capable of reducing oxytocin and that reduced oxytocin can be degraded by enzymes other than plasma oxytocinase. It is likely, therefore, that the effect of thiol compounds on the destruction of oxytocin in serum is not mediated by plasma oxytocinase. This interpretation is strengthened by results which were obtained in studies of the action of inhibitors on the cleavage of synthetic oxytocinase substrates. With S-benzyl-L-cysteine β-naphthylamide as the substrate, no activation of oxytocinase by cysteine could be observed (EL-KAMMAH and TUPPY, 1967). Nor could HASHIMOTO (1961a) obtain any evidence for an activation of the cleavage of L-cystine di-β-naphthylamide by oxytocinase in the presence of 10^{-4} to 10^{-3} M cysteine or glutathione.

The lack of inhibition of oxytocinase by semicarbazide suggested that the active centre of the enzyme did not contain carbonyl groups (WERLE, HEVELKE, and BUTHMANN, 1941; HASHIMOTO, 1961a). Recently, however, BARTH, PLIŠKA, RYCHLÍK, and ŠORM (1967) noted an inhibition of oxytocinase by dimedone (5×10^{-4} M) which was particularly effective at pH 7 and below, and they discussed the possible involvement of an aldehyde group in the active centre.

The esterase inhibitor, diisopropyl phosphorofluoridate, and some agents known to affect proteolytic enzymes such as trypsin inhibitor and trasylol, failed to inhibit oxytocinase (TUPPY and WINTERSBERGER, 1960; WERLE, HEVELKE, and BUTHMANN, 1941). It was found that puromycin was only slightly inhibitory to oxytocinase, whereas this antibiotic strongly affected an aminopeptidase other than oxytocinase present in human serum. The difference in the susceptibility of the aminopeptidases to inhibition by puromycin was exploited by WINTERSBERGER, MÜLLER-HARTBURG, and TUPPY (1966) to increase the specificity of the oxytocinase assay in the serum of pregnant women.

Among some pharmacologically active compounds tested for inhibitory action on oxytocinase, only quinine proved to be effective (MILANI and PINETTI, 1951). The question was raised by HASHIMOTO (1961a) whether the therapeutic use of quinine as an oxytocic agent might possibly be related to its inhibitory influence on oxytocinase.

A series of agents which are capable of binding alkaline earth metal ions (citrate, oxalate, fluoride and pyrophosphate) did not affect oxytocinase (WERLE, HEVELKE, and BUTHMANN, 1941; MILANI and PINETTI, 1951; TUPPY and WINTERSBERGER, 1960; HASHIMOTO, 1961a). Cyanide which is particularly effective in complexing heavy metal ions including copper and iron, failed to inhibit the enzyme (WERLE, HEVELKE, and BUTHMANN, 1941; MILANI and PINETTI, 1951). The chelating agents, 8-hydroxyquinoline and o-phenanthroline, however, which are known to bind zinc and other divalent cations, inhibited plasma oxytocinase immediately and completely in 10^{-3} M concentration (WERLE and SEMM, 1956; TUPPY and WINTERSBERGER, 1964). Inhibition by EDTA, first described by WERLE and SEMM (1956), proved to be a slow reaction which required prolonged incubation of the enzyme with the inhibitor in order to go to near completion (TUPPY and WINTERSBERGER, 1960; SEMM, 1963). It could be partially reversed by dialysis of the EDTA-containing enzyme samples (TUPPY and WINTERSBERGER, 1960) or by the addition of suitable amounts of divalent cations such as Mn^{++}, Co^{++}, Ni^{++}, Zn^{++} or Ca^{++} (WERLE and SEMM, 1956; HASHIMOTO, 1961a; BARTH, PLIŠKA, RYCHLÍK, and ŠORM, 1967). From these results the conclusion was drawn by WERLE and SEMM (1956) that plasma oxytocinase, like many other peptidases, required a divalent ion for its catalytic function. The inhibition by EDTA was frequently used to distinguish plasma oxytocinase from oxytocin-degrading tissue enzymes which appeared to be unaffected by this metal-chelating agent (SEMM, 1960; WERLE and SEMM, 1956). RYDÉN (1966), however, has recently pointed out that a clear distinction between plasma oxytocinase and tissue enzymes degrading oxytocin and L-cystine di-β-naphthylamide cannot be drawn with the help of EDTA, because there are some tissue enzymes which, like plasma oxytocinase, are liable to inhibition by this agent.

Many metal ions, particularly Cu^{++}, Cd^{++}, Zn^{++}, Co^{++}, Pb^{++}, Hg^{++} and Ag^{+}, were reported to be potent inhibitors of plasma oxytocinase. Fe^{++} and Mn^{++} are only slightly inhibitory, and Ca^{++} and Mg^{++} are without effect (WERLE, HEVELKE, and BUTHMANN, 1941; TUPPY and WINTERSBERGER, 1960; HASHIMOTO, 1961a; BARTH, PLIŠKA, RYCHLÍK, and ŠORM, 1967).

WERLE and SEMM (1956) reported that the degradation of oxytocin by pregnancy plasma oxytocinase was inhibited by protein fractions obtained from human serum by electrophoresis. A reduction in the oxytocinase activity of pregnancy serum of up to 25% was claimed to occur upon addition of serum from nonpregnant individuals (SEMM, 1958b). These findings, however, were not confirmed by other investigators (PAGE, 1946; MÜLLER-HARTBURG, NESVADBA, and TUPPY, 1959; HASHIMOTO, 1961a).

The oxytocinase-catalyzed hydrolysis of L-cystine di-β-naphthylamide is slowed down in the presence of oxytocin, because the peptide hormone and the synthetic substrate are competing for the same enzyme (PAGE, TITUS, MOHUN, and GLENDENING, 1961; HASHIMOTO, 1961a). The enzymatic cleavage of both oxytocin and L-cystine di-β-naphthylamide can be inhibited by L-cystinyl-di-L-tyrosine amide (WINTERSBERGER, TUPPY, and STOKLASKA, 1960). This compound which has in common with oxytocin the amino-terminal dipeptide sequence, is itself liable to attack by plasma oxytocinase and therefore acts as a competitive substrate. In the presence of an equimolar amount of L-cystinyl-di-L-tyrosine amide, the hydrolysis of L-cystine di-β-naphthylamide by plasma oxytocinase was reduced by approximately 50% and that of oxytocin by some 10%. The phenoxyethylamide, benzylamide, p-hydroxyanilide and tetrahydro-β-naphthylamide derivatives of L-cystine exhibited an inhibitory potency similar to that of L-cystinyl-di-L-tyrosine amide when tested on the oxytocinase-catalyzed cleavage of L-cystine di-β-naphthylamide (WINTERSBERGER, STOKLASKA, MOED, and VAN DIJK, 1964). A 100fold molar excess of such inhibitors was required in order to reduce the inactivation of oxytocin by plasma oxytocinase by 50—90%.

S-Benzyl-L-cysteinyl-L-tyrosine and its amide, and S-benzyl-L-cysteinyl-L-leucine, all of which are readily attacked by plasma oxytocinase, were reported by BERÁNKOVÁ, RYCHLÍK, and ŠORM (1959, 1960) to display a weak inhibitory effect on the enzymatic destruction of oxytocin. L-Cystinyl-bis-(L-prolyl-L-leucyl-glycine amide), S-benzyl-L-cysteinyl-L-prolyl-L-leucyl-glycine amide and S,S'-dibenzyl-dihydro-oxytocin, on the other hand, which are resistant to hydrolysis by oxytocinase, proved to be more powerful inhibitors of the inactivation of oxytocin by the pregnancy enzyme (BERÁNKOVÁ, RYCHLÍK, and ŠORM, 1959, 1960; BERÁNKOVÁ and ŠORM, 1961).

It was observed by the Czech investigators that some peptides which contained amino-terminal amino acid residues other than L-hemicystine or S-benzyl-L-cysteine, were also capable of counteracting the destruction of oxytocin by plasma oxytocinase. Glycyl-S-benzyl-L-cysteinyl-L-tyrosine amide and L-glutaminyl-L-asparaginyl-S-benzyl-L-cysteinyl-L-prolyl-L-leucyl-glycine amide, for instance, definitely inhibited the inactivation of the peptide hormone. It is an open question whether enzyme inhibition by these compounds was dependent on a prior enzymatic release of the N-terminal amino acid residues, which in these peptides precede the S-benzyl-L-cysteine residue (BERÁNKOVÁ, RYCHLÍK, and ŠORM, 1960). Dethio-oxytocin, a nonapeptide which contains neither hemicystine nor S-benzylcysteine residues, was found to be likewise a potent inhibitor of plasma oxytocinase (BERÁNková and Šorm, 1961). In this case, the basis for inhibition is apparently the overall structural resemblance between hormone and inhibitor rather than a close resemblance of the N-terminal sites. It has not been established whether dethio-oxytocin acts as a competitive inhibitor or as a competitive substrate when it retards the degradation of oxytocin by oxytocinase.

The cleavage of L-leucine p-nitroanilide by oxytocinase was found to be inhibited by Ala-Pro-Leu-Gly(NH_2) and Leu-Gly(NH_2) (Barth, Pliška, Rychlík, and Šorm, 1967). Various neutral and basic peptides present in thymus extracts will also interfere with the enzymatic activity of oxytocinase, presumably by competitive inhibition (Stoklaska and Wintersberger, 1962, 1963).

In 1948, Croxatto, Croxatto, and Reyes reported that angiotensin retarded the destruction of oxytocin and vasopressin by pregnancy sera. The inhibitory effect of angiotensin on plasma oxytocinase slowly disappeared in the course of the incubation. These results suggested that angiotensin, oxytocin and vasopressin were competitive substrates for oxytocinase. The recent demonstration by Sjöholm and Yman (1967) of a ready degradation of angiotensin by purified plasma oxytocinase gives support to the concept of a competition for this enzyme between angiotensin and the neurohypophysial hormones.

12. Phyto-Oxytocinase

Semm (1962a, b, c) tested the extracts of a great variety of plants for their capability of inactivating oxytocin. He found that approximately 80% of the leaves, roots and fruits tested yielded crude extracts which affected the hormone, some of them with remarkable efficiency. Aqueous extracts obtained from the seedlings of *Pisum sativum* and from the leaves of *Taraxacum officinale* were purified by extraction with ether and precipitation with acetone. Solutions suitable for further characterization of the oxytocin-inactivating principle were prepared by dissolving the acetone precipitate in water, lowering the pH to 5.6 by the addition of acetic acid, removing inactive insoluble material in the centrifuge, and finally adjusting the pH of the supernatant to 6.5. Upon lyophilization, a white powder was obtained which could be redissolved in water to give a highly active solution. The destruction of oxytocin was shown to be an enzymatic reaction which followed first-order kinetics. The enzyme concerned was termed "phyto-oxytocinase". It is remarkably stable. Heating at 57° caused slow inactivation. Dialysis against water did not impair enzyme activity. This result indicated that a freely dissociable cofactor of low molecular weight was not involved in the enzymatic reaction. Incubation of "phyto-oxytocinase" solutions with EDTA (1 mg/ml) reduced enzyme activity by more than 50%. The enzyme was considered by Semm to be a protease similar to the plasma oxytocinase of pregnant women, because partially purified preparations of the plant enzyme resembled the serum enzyme in cleaving L-cystine di-β-naphthylamide in addition to oxytocin. Biological and chemical assays in which oxytocin and L-cystine di-β-naphthylamide were used as the substrates, gave results which seemed to be in fair agreement. More recently, however, the plant extracts were shown to be capable of destroying deamino-oxytocin as readily as oxytocin (Semm, 1967), in contrast to plasma oxytocinase which is inactive against deamino-oxytocin (Golubow, Chan, and Du Vigneaud, 1963). This would indicate that the plant enzyme, unlike plasma oxytocinase, is not an aminopeptidase and that the cleavage of oxytocin and L-cystine di-β-naphthylamide by the plant extracts need not necessarily be due to the same enzyme. The activity of "phyto-oxytocinase" as determined with the help of L-cystine di-β-naphthylamide was found to be highest in the pH range of 6—7 (Semm, 1962). As indicated by its susceptibility to inhibition by metal-chelating agents, the enzyme is not identical with other known plant proteases such as, e.g., papain, ficin, bromelin and bromelain. No adverse reactions were observed when "phyto-oxytocinase" was administered to mice, guinea pigs, dogs and a rhesus monkey (SEMM, 1962c). A slightly toxic effect was noted in the hare. The capability of "phyto-oxytocinase" to inactivate oxytocin proved to be unimpaired in the presence of human serum. It was therefore hoped that the purified enzyme might be used therapeutically in obstetrics for the inactivation of oxytocin in the blood of pregnant women, the aim being to prevent premature labour (SEMM, 1962c). It should be emphasized, however, that repeated administrations of "phyto-oxytocinase" must be expected to lead to immunological accidents, since plant proteins tend to be strongly antigenic to the mammalian organism.

C. Hydrolases Other than Proteolytic Enzymes

Arginase

Neither oxytocin nor vasopressin are affected by arginase (GULLAND and MACRAE, 1933c; FRASER, 1950; DU VIGNEAUD, LAWLER, and POPENOE, 1953). The insusceptibility of Arg^{8}-vasopressin to the action of arginase is in agreement with the known specificity of this enzyme which will not attack peptide-bound arginine unless it occurs in the carboxyl-terminal position. When, however, Arg^{8}-vasopressin was first treated with trypsin and subsequently subjected to arginase action, a small amount of urea was liberated and could be detected in the digests (DU VIGNEAUD, LAWLER, and POPENOE, 1953). The prior tryptic release of glycine amide from Arg^{8}-vasopressin places the arginine residue into the carboxyl-terminal position and thereby renders it susceptible to attack by arginase.

III. Body Fluids and Tissues Capable of Enzymatically Inactivating Neurohypophysial Hormones

A. Blood

1. Plasma and Serum

Inactivation of Oxytocin in Plasma and Serum of Nonpregnant Humans. Most investigators failed to detect oxytocin-destroying activity in the serum and plasma of men and nonpregnant women (e.g., WERLE, HEVELKE, and BUTHMANN, 1941; DICKER and WHYLEY, 1959). Fetal blood serum and plasma were likewise found to be incapable of degrading oxytocin (WERLE and EFFKEMANN, 1941; PAGE, 1946; MÉNDEZ-BAUER, CARBALLO, CABOT, NEGREIROS DE PAIVA, and GONZÁLEZ-PANIZZA, 1961; WERLE, SEMM, and ENZENBACH, 1950). In careful determinations performed by PAGE (1946, 1947), however, traces of oxytocin-inactivating potency were detected in plasma samples from 22 nonpregnant women. The values varied with the phases of the normal menstrual cycle, so as to be very low during menstruation and somewhat higher about the time of ovulation. Oxytocinase assays in the plasma of normal men gave values which were still lower than those obtained for nonpregnant women. It was observed that in men taking 5 mg of stilboestrol daily, the mean value for oxytocin-inactivating ability was somewhat increased so as to reach about the level found in ovulating women. The plasma of patients suffering from jaundice likewise exhibited an elevated level of hormone-inactivating capacity. The occurrence in nonpregnancy plasma of traces of oxytocin-degrading activity was recently confirmed by MELANDER (1965). It is not known, however, whether these very low and fluctuating proteolytic activities are due to small traces of pregnancy plasma oxytocinase or to one or more proteases other than oxytocinase which may have a slight inactivating effect upon oxytocin. Starch gel electrophoresis did not provide evidence for the presence of pregnancy oxytocinase in the serum of nonpregnant individuals (WINTERSBERGER and TUPPY, 1960; PAGE, TITUS, MOHUN, and GLENDENING, 1961). This method may, however, be too insensitive to detect minute amounts of the enzyme.

The synthetic oxytocinase substrates, L-cystine di-β-naphthylamide and S-benzyl-L-cysteine β-naphthylamide, are slowly attacked by nonpregnancy sera (TUPPY and NESVADBA, 1957; MÜLLER-HARTBURG, NESVADBA, and TUPPY, 1959; TITUS, REYNOLDS, GLENDENING, and PAGE, 1960; HASHIMOTO, 1961b; RIAD, 1962; BONOW, CAROL, and WACHTEL, 1963; TUPPY and WINTERSBERGER, 1964; MELANDER, 1965; RYDÉN, 1966; HANSON and MANNSFELDT, 1967a). The very low CAP activity of nonpregnancy sera was found to be somewhat increased in some patients with liver diseases or advanced malignancies (MÜLLER-HARTBURG, NESVADBA, and TUPPY, 1959) and after operative trauma (KLIMEK, PIETRZYCKA, and GROCHOWSKI, 1962). The synthetic substrates are apparently more susceptible than oxytocin to the action of nonspecific aminopeptidases occurring in blood. The principal aminopeptidase of normal human serum, which efficiently cleaves L-leucine β-naphthylamide and L-alanine β-naphthylamide, displays a very slight but significant activity towards L-cystine di-β-naphthylamide (PAGE, TITUS, MOHUN, and GLENDENING, 1961). The latter substrate is hydrolyzed 74 times more slowly than L-leucine β-naphthylamide (GOEBELSMANN and BELLER, 1965). The pH optimum for the cleavage of L-cystine di-β-naphthylamide by nonpregnancy plasma is at pH 6.0 rather than at pH 7.3 where pregnancy plasma shows the strongest activity towards the synthetic substrates. It can be interferred from these findings that the hydrolysis of the naphthylamide substrates by nonpregnancy plasma is not due to plasma oxytocinase but rather to some other hydrolytic enzyme(s) (RYDÉN, 1966). HASHIMOTO (1961b) reported that the injection of oestradiol or progesterone into nonpregnant women did not cause an increase in the CAP activity of their sera. RYDÉN (1966), on the other hand, observed an augmentation of the CAP activity in serum following gestagen therapy. The enhanced enzyme activity, however, had a pH optimum around pH 6 and thus was not due to pregnancy oxytocinase whose pH optimum is at 7.3.

Inactivation of Vasopressin in Plasma and Serum of Nonpregnant Humans. The plasma from normal nonpregnant individuals does not destroy the vasopressor and antidiuretic activities of vasopressin (DICKER and TYLER, 1956; HAWKER, 1957; BARNES and SAWYER, 1960). Vasopressin is bound to protein, but not inactivated, when mixed with human plasma (ARIMURA and YAMAGUCHI, 1964). Human serum, on the contrary, contains considerable vasopressin-destroying activity (HELLER and URBAN, 1935; SCHOCKAERT and LAMBILLON, 1936a; WERLE and KALVELAGE, 1941; WERLE, 1960). Whole human serum, or Cohn fractions II and III prepared from it, will not only engage vasopressin in protein binding, but will in addition inactivate it (ARIMURA and YAMAGUCHI, 1964). CROXATTO, BADIA, and CROXATTO (1948) found that fibrinolysin, which fails to affect oxytocin, is capable of inactivating vasopressin. It is possible that the fibrinolytic activity of human sera is involved in the destruction of the pressor hormone.

Inactivation of Oxytocin in Plasma and Serum of Pregnant Women. FEKETE (1930, 1932) was the first to observe the striking capacity of pregnancy serum to destroy oxytocin. WERLE and his associates established that the principle responsible for this destruction was an enzyme, the activity of which showed a progressive rise during pregnancy. They could always detect it in the blood as early as in the second month of pregnancy and they found that there was maximum activity around term (WERLE, HEVELKE, and BUTHMANN, 1941; WERLE and EFFKEMANN, 1941). The change in plasma oxytocinase concentration from very early in pregnancy until after delivery was closely followed by PAGE (1946, 1947). His results indicated that during the first 4 months of human pregnancy the plasma concentration of this enzyme increased logarithmically in such a fashion that there was a 100% augmentation every 12 days. The highest level was found to be reached before and to be maintained during labour. Following delivery, the enzyme decreased logarithmically at the rate of about 25% per day and became undetectable within about 4 weeks.

Although all the workers in this field are agreed on the early appearance and the remarkable rise in activity of oxytocinase in the course of gravidity, there are considerable differences in results and opinion with regard to the details and the significance of the phenomenon.

Most but not all investigators found that oxytocinase measurements gave identical results irrespective of whether they were carried out with plasma or serum from the same donor. MÉNDEZ-BAUER and CARBALLO (1957), who performed biological oxytocinase assays, and TITUS, REYNOLDS, GLENDENING, and PAGE (1960) and HASHIMOTO (1961a), who made use of the synthetic oxytocinase substrate, L-cystine di-β-naphthylamide, for the enzyme estimations, failed to observe any difference in enzyme activity, when serum and plasma samples from the same gravid women were compared. FYLLING (1963), on the other hand, reported that oxytocinase values determined in plasma which was placed in siliconized glassware or in plastic material, tended to be lower than values determined in serum or in plasma exposed to unsiliconized glassware. Observations made by BELLER and GÖBELSMANN (1959) indicated that the oxytocinase activity of undiluted serum changed considerably during the first few hours after blood collection. Serum from women in the last month of pregnancy showed significantly higher oxytocinase values 3.5 h after blood collection than they did 1 h after collection, whereas earlier in pregnancy the enzyme activity in serum tended to decrease during this 2.5 h interval. The authors reported that oxytocinase assays in serum samples, which had been kept for 3.5 h rather than for only 1 h, gave results which were fairly reproducible and showed little scatter.

The increase in oxytocinase activity in women's plasma within a short time after conception led several investigators to test the possible value of oxytocinase assays for an early pregnancy diagnosis. PAGE (1947) reported that in women who are not jaundiced pregnancy can be diagnosed in this way 4 weeks after impregnation. Occasionally, elevated plasma oxytocinase values indicative of pregnancy were obtained as early as 2 weeks after conception (PAGE, 1946; WERLE, SEMM, and ENZENBACH, 1950). On the basis of more extensive experience, this pregnancy test was later reported to be 90% accurate three weeks after impregnation and unfailing 8 weeks after impregnation (WERLE and SEMM, 1951, 1955; SEMM, 1955). The early detection of pregnancy by means of oxytocinase assays was repeatedly confirmed (BELLER and GÖBELSMANN, 1959; DICKER and WHYLEY, 1959; MÉNDEZ-BAUER, CARBALLO, CABOT, NEGREIROS DE PAIVA, and GONZÁLEZ-PANIZZA, 1961). The biological oxytocin assays required for this test are so laborious, however, that the method is impracticable for routine purposes.

The use of L-cystine di-β-naphthylamide for the estimation of plasma oxytocinase is considerably simpler and much more accurate than the biological method (MÜLLER-HARTBURG, NESVADBA, and TUPPY, 1959; TITUS, REYNOLDS, GLENDENING, and PAGE, 1960). In early pregnancy, however, when the plasma oxytocinase level is still very low, the unspecific cleavage of L-cystine di-β-naphthylamide by aminopeptidases other than oxytocinase tends to obscure the as yet slow cleavage of this substrate by oxytocinase. A rise in the CAP values significantly above the nonpregnancy level could therefore be observed not earlier than after the 12th to 16th week of pregnancy (MÜLLER-HARTBURG, NESVADBA, and TUPPY, 1959; RIAD, 1962; MELANDER, 1965; BABUNA and YENEN, 1966). The determination of plasma oxytocinase by means of L-cystine di-β-naphthylamide has therefore been generally considered unsuitable for an early pregnancy diagnosis (TITUS, REYNOLDS, GLENDENING, and PAGE, 1960; RIAD, 1962; BONOW, CAROL, and WACHTEL, 1963; GOEBELSMANN and BELLER, 1965; MELANDER, 1965). Other more satisfactory tests are available which allow a reliable diagnosis of pregnancy a few weeks after conception.

The use of an alternative chromogenic substrate, S-benzyl-L-cysteine β-naphthylamide, which is hydrolyzed by pregnancy plasma at a considerably greater rate than is L-cystine di-β-naphthylamide, and the partial inhibition by puromycin of interfering enzymes present in nonpregnancy and pregnancy sera, have helped to render the chemical oxytocinase assay more efficient and more specific (TUPPY and WINTERSBERGER, 1964; WINTERSBERGER, MÜLLER-HARTBURG, and TUPPY, 1966). Plasma oxytocinase values determined in early stages of pregnancy with the help of this new chromogenic substrate are more accurate than the values obtained with L-cystine di-β-naphthylamide. The interference by enzymes other than oxytocinase, however, has not yet been entirely excluded.

PAGE (1946, 1947) suggested that the measurement of plasma oxytocinase, up to 16 weeks after conception, might be useful for estimating the week of pregnancy. He reported that the logarithm of enzyme concentration was increasing in a linear fashion with the week of pregnancy, the standard deviation being less than 1 week. During the later months of pregnancy, the scatter would become so great as to preclude an accurate prediction of the date of confinement. The value of biological oxytocinase assays for assessing the gestational age was confirmed and strongly emphasized by WERLE and SEMM (1955) and SEMM (1960). However, the results of a larger number of chemical oxytocinase determinations at different stages of pregnancy have revealed considerable individual variations and have led to the conclusion that this method does not give more than a rough estimate of gestational age (MÜLLER-HARTBURG, NESVADBA, and TUPPY, 1959; BONOW, CAROL, and WACHTEL, 1963).

Excepting the first trimester of pregnancy, where the chemical method of oxytocinase assay suffers from interference by unspecific aminopeptidases other than oxytocinase, a fair correlation has been found between the results of chemical oxytocinase estimations by means of L-cystine di-β-naphthylamide and the results of biological assays using oxytocin as the substrate (TITUS, REYNOLDS, GLENDENING, and PAGE, 1960; HASHIMOTO, 1961a; MELANDER, 1961, 1965).

PAGE (1946, 1947) originally reported that the overall increase in oxytocinase activity in women's plasma from the time of conception until term was more than a 1000 fold. This striking increment was derived from a comparison of the oxytocin-destroying capacity in weakly diluted nonpregnancy plasma and in highly diluted late-pregnancy plasma samples. The use of widely differing plasma dilutions in comparative oxytocinase assays, however, is likely to have resulted in an underestimation of low and an overestimation of high enzyme levels. Experiments carried out by MÉNDEZ-BAUER, CARBALLO, CABOT, NEGREIROS DE PAIVA, and GONZÁLEZ-PANIZZA (1961) have shown that a progressive dilution of pregnancy plasma brings about less than the expected decrease of oxytocinase activity. On that account, TITUS, REYNOLDS, GLENDENING, and PAGE (1960) consider the true increment of oxytocinase activity due to gravidity to be of the order of only 50—100 times. This value is in satisfactory agreement with the 60fold increase reported by WERLE and SEMM (1951) for the oxytocin-inactivating capacity of serum from the 8th week after conception until full term, and with the 15fold rise from the 13th week to the 38th week of pregnancy, which was reported by MÉNDEZ-BAUER, CARBALLO, CABOT, NEGREIROS DE PAIVA, and GONZÁLEZ-PANIZZA (1961).

The rate of hydrolysis of L-cystine di-β-naphthylamide in diluted serum buffered at pH 7.9 increases 25—30fold, on the average, in the course of pregnancy (MÜLLER-HARTBURG, NESVADBA, and TUPPY, 1959; TITUS, REYNOLDS, GLENDENING, and PAGE, 1960; KLIMEK and PIETRZYCKA, 1961; GOLUBOW, CHAN, and DU VIGNEAUD, 1963; BONOW, CAROL, and WACHTEL, 1963). When the enzyme assays were carried out at pH 7.3—7.4 instead of 7.9, the ratio between the average rates of hydrolysis of the chromogenic substrate in full-term pregnancy sera and in non-pregnancy sera was only 13—18 (TUPPY and NESVADBA, 1957; RIAD, 1962; RYDÉN, 1966). The increment of CAP activity occasioned by pregnancy is less, particularly when it is determined at the lower pH, than the increment of oxytocinase as determined by the biological assay method, because of the contribution to the CAP values of hydrolases other than oxytocinase which are present in nonpregnancy as well as in pregnancy sera and are somewhat more active at pH 7.3 than they are at pH 7.9. When the rise in oxytocinase activity during pregnancy was estimated using S-benzyl-L-cysteine β-naphthylamide as the substrate rather than L-cystine di-β-naphthylamide, a 30—50fold increase was observed (WINTERSBERGER, MÜLLER-HARTBURG, and TUPPY, 1966). This shows that, the higher the specificity of a substrate is for oxytocinase, the more closely will the activity increments observed during pregnancy approach those estimated by the biological method of oxytocinase assay.

Plasma oxytocinase attains the highest level during the last month of pregnancy and remains on a high level until after delivery (WERLE and EFFKEMANN, 1941; WERLE, HEVELKE, and BUTHMANN, 1941; PAGE, 1946; KANAZAWA, 1954; DICKER and WHYLEY, 1959; MÜLLER-HARTBURG, NESVADBA, and TUPPY, 1959; TITUS, REYNOLDS, GLENDENING, and PAGE, 1960; CENTARO, PERITI, and DE LAURENTIIS, 1961; MÉNDEZ-BAUER, CARBALLO, CABOT, NEGREIROS DE PAIVA, and GONZÁLEZ-PANIZZA, 1961; MELANDER, 1961, 1965; KLIMEK and PIETRZYCKA, 1961; HASHIMOTO, 1961b; RIAD, 1962; ZASZTOWT, 1963; BONOW, CAROL, and WACHTEL, 1963; SEMM and BERNHARD, 1963; BABUNA and YENEN, 1966). Indeed, in 1954, DICKER and TYLER (1956) had claimed that the capability of plasma to inactivate oxytocin diminished from mid-pregnancy towards term and that plasma taken around term usually failed to inactivate oxytocin. HILTON and JOHNSON (1959) presented data which suggested that the ability of plasma to destroy the oxytocic hormone decreased to zero or near zero in six out of nine women studied during the first stage of labour. A similar decline during the period of parturition was also reported by NAMIKI (1952). These reports raised considerable interest because they indicated that the onset of labour might be due, at least in part, to a diminishing interference of plasma oxytocinase with the action of oxytocin on the gravid uterus. Re-examination of the problem in many laboratories, however, failed to confirm the claims of any drastic decrease of plasma oxytocinase activity prior to delivery. The changes in oxytocinase activity which actually occur during the last weeks before term are small and irregular (HASHIMOTO, 1961b; MELANDER, 1965). The enzymatic activity may show a further increase (ZAMELLO and ZGLICZYNSKI, 1965), or may stay on a constant level (DICKER and WHYLEY, 1959; TITUS, REYNOLDS, GLENDENING, and PAGE, 1960), or may decrease by a few per cent (MÜLLER-HARTBURG, NESVADBA, and TUPPY, 1959; BELLER and SCHNIZ, 1960).

In labour and during delivery, significant changes in the oxytocinase activity of the plasma and serum appear to occur. MÜLLER-HARTBURG, NESVADBA, and TUPPY (1959) observed one or two oscillations of the enzyme level *sub partu* and ascribed them to rapidly occurring transient variations in the concentration of the plasma proteins. HASHIMOTO (1961 b) reported that in most parturient women the enzyme activity increased during labour, the maximum being attained when the placenta was expelled. In the majority of cases, where labour was induced by a prolonged infusion of oxytocin, a progressive rise in oxytocinase was found to take place (MÉNDEZ-BAUER, CARBALLO, CABOT, NEGREIROS DE PAIVA, and GONZÁLEZ-PANIZZA, 1961; HASHIMOTO, 1961 b). FYLLING (1963, 1964 a, b) who studied the influence upon the plasma oxytocinase level of oxytocin infusions and single intravenous oxytocin injections into parturient women, observed that the oxytocinase activity was significantly elevated one quarter of an hour following injection of 10 IU of oxytocin and then returned to the original value within about one hour. A few hours later, the values showed an upward trend again. The immediate response of the oxytocinase level to an injection of the oxytocic hormone was interpreted by FYLLING (1964 b) as a release of preformed enzyme into the circulation rather than an induced synthesis of enzyme under the influence of its substrate, oxytocin. However, the quick rise of the enzyme level may also be due to a transient change in the plasma protein concentration caused by the fall of blood pressure following the administration of a large dose of oxytocin (RYDÉN, 1966). RIAD (1966) frequently observed an increase in the plasma oxytocinase activity in patients who received an oxytocin infusion for induction of labour at term. The rise of enzyme level, which accompanied short unassisted labours and failed to occur in patients in whom the induction of labour failed, was ascribed to enzyme release from an intrauterine source due to vigorous myometrial activity.

KLIMEK (1964 a, b) reported that the increase in oxytocinase activity of the blood upon administration of oxytocin is much more marked earlier in pregnancy than it is towards term. The difference between the oxytocinase levels prior to and after oxytocin administration was found to be highest in mid-pregnancy and to disappear at the end of pregnancy. Estimations of oxytocinase levels in conjunction with oxytocin sensitivity tests were advocated by KLIMEK as the most reliable and precise method for estimating the term of pregnancy. According to DREWNIAK's experience (1964 a, b) this method allows of predicting the date of delivery with an accuracy of a few days, the average deviation being not more than 1.4 days.

In twin and triple pregnancies the plasma oxytocinase activities rise significantly above the corresponding values in singleton pregnancies (KANAZAWA, 1954; PAGE, TITUS, MOHUN, and GLENDENING, 1961; HASHIMOTO, 1961 b; MELANDER, 1965; ICHALIOTIS and LAMBRINOPOULOS, 1965). It was therfore suggested that oxytocinase determinations might be of diagnostic value in cases of suspected multiple pregnancies. The elevated oxytocinase levels are reflected not only in an enhanced CAP activity, but also in an increased LAP activity of the plasma samples (SCIARRA and BURRESS, 1960; LEWIS, 1962; MILLER, NAOR, MILKOVICH, and SCHMIDT, 1964).

After delivery, oxytocinase gradually disappears from the circulation. PAGE (1946) has reported that in puerperium the oxytocinase activity in plasma undergoes an exponential decrease at the rate of about 25% per day. A drop in the CAP level of approximately 60% within one week after delivery was observed by RIAD

(1962). Within 4—6 weeks *post partum* oxytocinase becomes undetectable (WERLE, HEVELKE, and BUTHMANN, 1941; WERLE and EFFKEMANN, 1941; PAGE, 1946; DICKER and WHYLEY, 1959b) and the CAP activity of the plasma returns asymptotically to the nonpregnancy level (MÜLLER-HARTBURG, NESVADBA, and TUPPY, 1959; HASHIMOTO, 1961b; RIAD, 1962).

The ready cleavage of L-leucine β-naphthylamide by plasma oxytocinase (WINTERSBERGER and TUPPY, 1960; GOEBELSMANN and BELLER, 1965) accounts for the finding that human pregnancy sera have a higher "leucine aminopeptidase" (LAP) (more correctly, leucine arylamidase) activity than sera from non-pregnant individuals (GREEN, TSOU, BRESSLER, and SELIGMAN, 1955; TUPPY and NESVADBA, 1957; BRAUN-FALCO and SALFELD, 1957; BRESSLER and FORSYTH, 1959; SIEGEL, 1959; ARST, MANNING, and DELP, 1959; BRESSLER, FORSYTH, and KLATSKIN, 1960; LEWIS, 1962; FYLLING, 1964). When nonpregnancy serum was subjected to paper electrophoresis and was stained for LAP, a single band was revealed in the α_1 globulin region. In late pregnancy sera an additional band was detected in the α_2 globulin fraction (SMITH, PINEDA, and RUTENBURG, 1962). Horizontal starch gel electrophoresis of sera from healthy nonpregnant individuals likewise showed only one LAP component, the band being in the postalbumin or fast α_2 globulin area. In sera from pregnant women, on the other hand, an additional band corresponding to oxytocinase was regularly encountered in the slow α_2 to β-globulin region (WINTERSBERGER and TUPPY, 1960; KOWLESSAR, HAEFFNER, and RILEY, 1961). PAGE, TITUS, MOHUN, and GLENDENING (1961), when subjecting pregnancy plasma to vertical starch gel electrophoresis, obtained three distinct LAP bands. The fastest moving component was the normal principal aminopeptidase which is found in all plasma samples from men and women. The two slower components were both capable of destroying oxytocin. They correspond to the conformational forms, CAP_1 and CAP_2, of oxytocinase which have recently been closely investigated by SJÖHOLM and YMAN (1966b). Results obtained by GLENDENING, TITUS, SCHROEDER, MOHUN, and PAGE (1965) indicate that the activities of the two oxytocinase components towards L-leucine β-naphthylamide account for the major part of the increase in LAP observed during human pregnancy.

Inactivation of Vasopressin in Plasma and Serum of Pregnant Women. In 1935, SCHOCKAERT and LAMBILLON found that pregnancy serum was antagonistic to the hypertensive action of neurohypophysial extracts. The inactivation of the pressor hormone was shown to be a time reaction. It was specific for vasopressin, other hypertensive agents such as adrenaline, sympathol and ephedrin remaining unaffected (SCHOCKAERT and LAMBILLON, 1936 a, b). The enzymatic nature of the reaction was established by WERLE and KALVELAGE (1941). These authors furthermore demonstrated that the capacity of serum to abolish the pressor action of vasopressin begins to increase about the second month of pregnancy and continues to rise until term. In puerperium the enzymatic activity diminishes slowly and approaches the low nonpregnancy level within a few weeks *post partum*. Fetal blood has a vasopressin-inactivating potency equal to that of nonpregnancy blood. DIECKMANN, EGENOLF, MORLEY, and POTTINGER (1950) reported that the antidiuretic effect of neurohypophysial extracts, like the pressor effect, was also abolished in the plasma of pregnant women from the 14th week of pregnancy through the early puerperium. These observations were confirmed and extended by McCARTNEY, VALLACH, and POTTINGER (1952); HAWKER (1956, 1957); DICKER and TYLER (1956) and BARNES and SAWYER (1960).

CROXATTO, VERA, and BÁRNAFI (1953) noticed that the progressive increase in the enzymatic activity responsible for the destruction of vasopressin in pregnancy serum closely parallels the rise in oxytocinase activity. This led the authors to assume that the same enzyme was involved in the inactivation of both hormones, oxytocin and vasopressin. This assumption received strong support from the work of STOKLASKA and WINTERSBERGER (1959) who found that highly purified oxytocinase was just as active towards vasopressin as it was towards oxytocin, and from that of GLENDENING, TITUS, SCHROEDER, MOHUN, and PAGE (1965) who demonstrated that the isozymes of oxytocinase, CAP_1 and CAP_2, were both capable of destroying oxytocin and vasopressin at similar rates. Plasma oxytocinase, however, cannot be responsible for all of the vasopressin-inactivating potency of human sera. Nonpregnancy sera, though virtually devoid of oxytocinase, nevertheless exhibit some "vasopressinase" activity (WERLE and KALVELAGE, 1941). Moreover, WERLE (1960) presented evidence which indicated that "vasopressinase", in contradistinction to oxytocinase, is not fully inhibited by EDTA. These findings can be accounted for by the occurrence in pregnancy serum of more than one vasopressin-degrading enzyme. One of the enzymes will be plasma oxytocinase, which is sensitive to EDTA and is highly augmented in pregnancy. The other enzyme(s) will be resistant to inhibition by EDTA and will presumably have such a specificity as to attack vasopressin but not oxytocin. Fibrinolysin and/or some other agent(s) with a trypsin-like specificity might be responsible for this part of the "vasopressinase" activity of human sera.

The Inactivation of Oxytocin and Vasopressin in Plasma and Serum in Pathological Disorders of Pregnancy. A high percentage of patients with preeclampsia and eclampsia are hypersensitive to the pressor action of vasopressin and show an increased sensitivity of the uterus during oxytocin infusion as compared to normal patients. Studies carried out by many investigators dealt with the problem whether this hypersensitivity might be due to a diminished inactivation of the neurohypophysial hormones in the blood. WOODBURY, AHLQUIST, ABREU, TORPIN, and WATSON (1946) and McCARTNEY, VALLACH, and POTTINGER (1952) found that toxaemia patients were capable of destroying oxytocin and vasopressin as rapidly as normal pregnant patients. PAGE (1946) and ARAGON (1948) observed a wide variation of oxytocinase values in the toxaemias. No correlation was found between enzyme level, the clinical course of toxaemias and the hypersensitivity of the patients to vasopressin (ARAGON, 1948; FYLLING, 1963). On the other hand, relatively low enzyme activities were frequently found in the blood of toxaemia patients when the chemical method using the synthetic substrate, L-cystine di-β-naphthylamide, was employed for the assay of oxytocinase (HASHIMOTO, 1961b; RIAD, 1962; SEMM and BERNHARD, 1963; BONOW, CAROL, and WACHTEL, 1963). A large-scale comparison between plasma samples from preeclamptic women with high blood pressure in labour and normal women in labour revealed that the difference in oxytocinase activity between the two groups was statistically significant (ICHALIOTIS and LAMBRINOPOULOS, 1964).

Conflicting results have been reported concerning the plasma oxytocinase activity in women with threatened or incomplete abortions. PAGE (1947), WERLE and SEMM (1951, 1955) and SEMM (1955, 1960) stated that in most cases of abortions the oxytocinase level was lower as compared to the normal levels at the corresponding stage of pregnancy. The enzyme level was claimed to rise following an oral or parenteral administration of gestagens such as allyloestrenol or 17-a-hydroxyprogesterone (SEMM, 1965).

Other authors, however, were unable to find a relationship between oxytocinase activity and abortions (KANAZAWA, 1954; MÜLLER-HARTBURG, NESVADBA, and TUPPY, 1959; PERITI, CENTARO, and DE LAURENTIIS, 1961; MELANDER, 1965). BABUNA and YENEN (1966) considered a decrease of the enzyme levels, if observed in serial determinations of oxytocinase in the same individual, to be an indication of disturbed placental function. Such a decrease was found in cases of toxaemia which resulted in foetal death.

After intrauterine foetal death, oxytocinase activity in maternal plasma may remain unchanged for some time, or may increase, or may start decreasing (SEMM, 1955; WERLE and SEMM, 1951; MÉNDEZ-BAUER, CARBALLO, CABOT, NEGREIROS DE PAIVA, and GONZÁLEZ-PANIZZA, 1961; HASHIMOTO, 1961b; KLEINER and VAN RYMENANT, 1964; MELANDER, 1965). Because of this variability of enzyme activity, determinations of oxytocinase are of little value in diagnosing foetal death *in utero*. Following abortions, the decline of oxytocinase concentration was found to be similar to that after normal delivery (PAGE, 1946). In some cases of therapeutic abortions, however, the decrease did not start until a few days after the intervention (MELANDER, 1965).

No obvious correlation exists between oxytocinase levels and deviations from the normal duration of pregnancy (KLIMEK, 1964). An increase in oxytocinase upon prolonged pregnancy was observed by some authors (SEMM, 1955; LAMBRINOPOULOS, 1964; BOROV, 1966), but could not be confirmed by others (STEPANKOVSKAYA, 1964; FYLLING, 1963).

A decrease of the oxytocinase activity was observed by KLIMEK (1964) in the blood of women with symptoms referred to as *post partum* hypothalamosis.

In cases of hydatidiform mole, low, normal and high values of plasma oxytocinase have been found (WERLE, SEMM and ENZENBACH, 1950; KANAZAWA, 1954; SEMM, 1957, 1958a, 1960, 1961; MÉNDEZ-BAUER, CARBALLO, CABOT, NEGREIROS DE PAIVA, and GONZÁLEZ-PANIZZA, 1961; HASHIMOTO, 1961b; PERITI, CENTARO, and DE LAURENTIIS, 1961b). An elevated oxytocinase activity was reported to occur in the blood of patients with choriocarcinoma (SEMM, 1955; BELLER and GÖBELSMANN, 1959a; HASHIMOTO, 1961b). SEMM (1955) considered this finding to be convincing evidence for the placental origin of oxytocinase. KANAZAWA (1954), however, was unable to detect plasma oxytocinase in cases of chorioepithelioma, and when PAGE, TITUS, MOHUN, and GLENDENING (1961) subjected the plasma of women with choriocarcinoma to starch gel electrophoresis, they could not detect the characteristic bands of plasma oxytocinase, CAP_1 and CAP_2. Nor could BRESSLER and FORSYTH (1959) and LEWIS (1962) observe an increase in LAP activity in the blood of patients with trophoblastic neoplasms.

Relation of Oxytocinase to the "Pregnancy Zone". In 1959, SMITHIES reported that in the serum of about 10% of women in late pregnancy or recently delivered a protein zone could be observed by starch gel electrophoresis which was absent from males and from nonpregnant women. This zone migrated as an a_2 globulin, its electrophoretic mobility being a little slower than that of the first haptoglobin 2—2 band. Using the same technique COOPER (1963) was able to detect the "pregnancy zone" in 86% of pregnant women. AFONSO and FARNHAM (1962) could make it out in 82% of parturient women and they observed that in the majority of cases it disappeared within 5 days to 8 weeks following delivery. PAGE, TITUS, MOHUN, and GLENDENING (1961) and AFONSO and FARNHAM (1962) drew the attention to the fact that the rate of migration of CAP_2, the form of oxytocinase which is stable at physiological pH values, is very similar to that of the "pregnancy zone".

Additional evidence for the presence in the blood of pregnant women of one or more substances which are absent from the blood of nongravid individuals was gained with the help of immunological techniques. MACLAREN, THORNES, ROBY, and REID (1959) showed that antisera obtained by injections of human pregnancy serum into rabbits, after proper absorption with nonpregnancy sera, contained antibody against at least one substance peculiar to pregnancy. This substance, which was demonstrated by means of Ouchterlony's immunodiffusion technique, proved to be different from choriongonadotropin. Wilken (1963) who made use of the same serological method, showed that this antigenic component could be detected in women's serum from the 6th week of pregnancy until about 2—3 weeks after delivery. It is undetectable in foetal blood and amniotic fluid. Immunoelectrophoresis indicated that it was an a_2 globulin, possibly an a_2 lipoprotein. Wilken considered the exclusive occurrence of this substance during pregnancy, its electrophoretic characterization as an a_2 globulin, and the antigenicity in the rabbit, which is in agreement with the antigenicity of oxytocinase as demonstrated by Tuppy and Wintersberger (1960) and by Goebelsmann and Beller (1965), strong arguments in favour of an identity of this serum component with oxytocinase. One point that Wilken believed to militate against the identity was his finding that the antigenic pregnancy factor did not vanish from the circulation until two to three weeks *post partum*, whereas oxytocinase, as Wilken mistakenly supposed, should disappear after expulsion of the placenta.

Further evidence for the identity of the pregnancy-specific antigenic a_2 globulin with oxytocinase was recently produced by Rittner (1966) who used an antiserum from a goat that had been immunized with pregnancy serum for immunodiffusion and immunoelectrophoretic studies. This investigator found that the antigenic principle could be detected in the sera of all women who were pregnant for three or more months. The concentration of this protein in serum was shown to increase with the age of pregnancy, although the individual values exhibited a marked scatter. The results obtained by the Ouchterlony technique indicated that the a_2 antigen was absent from the sera of 70 newborn babies tested, except for one. It was undetectable in the sera of pregnant animals such as hens, cows and pigs, but could be identified in the sera of various subhuman primates known to contain oxytocinase. It was shown that the antigenic a_2 globulin and Smithies' "pregnancy zone" occupy the same position on vertical starch gel electropherograms as does oxytocinase, which was located with the chromogenic substrate, L-leucine β-naphthylamide. These results strongly indicated that oxytocinase, or rather its CAP_2 component, and the pregnancy-specific antigenic a_2 globulin in the sera of humans and anthropoid apes are indeed identical.

Function of Oxytocinase in Pregnancy. There has been much speculation on the physiological significance of the increased oxytocinase activity in blood during pregnancy. A common hypothesis has been that this enzyme serves to regulate the oxytocin level in pregnancy plasma and may thereby prevent premature labour. This hypothesis, of course, implies the assertion that oxytocin is of importance in the initiation and maintenance of spontaneous labour.

Semm (1960, 1961), who has been the most ardent protagonist of this hypothesis, advanced the idea that the primate uterus was in particular need of a mechanism which could cope with high concentrations of endogenous oxytocin. The purpose of the high oxytocinase activity in late pregnancy blood should be to shield the uterus from premature stimulation, which might result in untimely labour, foetal death or rupture of the uterus. The effect of oxytocinase would be overcome at the end of pregnancy by an increased release of oxytocin from the neurohypophysis and by a sensitization of the uterine muscle to the stimulant action of the hormone.

Klimek (1964b) considered oxytocinase to be an adaptive enzyme the formation of which can be induced by oxytocin. It was claimed that a continuous increase in enzyme concentration during pregnancy indicates that increasing amounts of endogenous oxytocin are released from the pituitary gland. Women with high oxytocinase level in their plasma would therefore not require administration of exogenous hormone, or only single small doses of oxytocin, for the initiation of delivery. The ability of the organism to raise its plasma oxytocinase level under the influence of endogenous or exogenous oxytocin would be lost at the end of pregnancy as a result of a lowered adaptibility of the placenta, which was assumed to be the main source of oxytocinase. The oxytocin-oxytocinase equilibrium would then be shifted and labour could be initiated by small amounts of oxytocin.

There are several arguments which militate against an important role of oxytocinase in the regulation of the oxytocin level in pregnancy plasma:

1. When oxytocin is incubated with late-pregnancy blood at 37°, it takes the oxytocinase in the plasma 5—10 min to reduce the amount of hormone by one-half. Not more than 20 sec are required, on the other hand, for the transport of endogenous oxytocin from the neurohypophysis to the uterus. Within this short time less than 5% of the released oxytocin will be inactivated in the blood. It appears, therefore, that oxytocinase is unable to prevent the bulk of released oxytocin from reaching the target organ.

2. It has been said that oxytocinase, though being incapable of removing oxytocin quickly from the circulation, might hinder the hormone from staying at a high level over a longer period of time. However, there are other and more efficient mechanisms at work in the organism which are capable of quickly clearing oxytocin from the circulation. That is why the half-lives of injected oxytocin in the circulation are very similar for pregnant women and for human males, in spite of the fact that the latter do not possess oxytocinase whereas the former do. Nor does the clearance of oxytocin from the circulation of animals, the blood of which is not able to inactive oxytocin, differ appreciably from that found in humans.

3. One would expect that a factor which prevents premature labour should vanish or at least should exhibit a considerably decreased activity at the end of pregnancy. A significant decline of the oxytocinase activity, however, has not been found until after delivery. Nor does premature labour occur preferentially in patients with low oxytocinase levels.

In view of these facts, most investigators are agreed that the function of oxytocinase in human pregnancy is entirely obscure. When considering the possible role of this enzyme, one should keep in mind, however, that oxytocinase is not specific for oxytocin but will also attack vasopressin and other physiologically active peptides such as, e.g., angiotensin. It has therefore been proposed that the function of the enzyme might possibly be to protect the placental vessels from the constrictory action of vasopressin, or to contribute to the angiotensinase activity of pregnancy plasma and to help in this way to counteract pathological effects of the renin-angiotensin system (RYDÉN, 1966).

Inactivation of Oxytocin in Plasma and Serum of Animals. An oxytocin-destroying enzyme closely resembling that found in human pregnancy plasma was discovered in the pregnant rhesus monkey (WERLE, SEMM, and ENZENBACH, 1950). It was considered likely that the haemochorial placenta, which is common to subhuman primates and to man, is responsible for the appearance of plasma oxytocinase. No oxytocin-destroying activity, or only traces, were detected in the plasma of other nonpregnant or pregnant animals of the mammalian group such as cats, cows, horses, donkeys, sheep, pigs, dogs, rabbits, guinea-pigs, rats and mice (JONES and SCHLAPP, 1936; WERLE, HEVELKE, and BUTHMANN, 1941; PAGE, 1946; WERLE, SEMM, and ENZENBACH, 1950; WINKHAUS, 1954; SEMM, 1960; SAWYER, 1954; DICKER and WHYLEY, 1960; MANUNTA, 1960; MANUNTA and MARONGIU, 1961). In comparison with plasma, serum appears to inactive oxytocin somewhat more rapidly (HELLER, 1960).

In plasma and serum of pregnant women there is a fair correspondence between the oxytocinase and CAP activities, because the level of enzymes other than oxytocinase capable of cleaving cystine di-β-naphthylamide is very low. In animal sera such a close correlation between oxytocinase and CAP values does not necessarily exist. Hashimoto (1961b) observed a significant rate of cleavage of L-cystine di-β-naphthylamide in the serum of rats, rabbits, guinea-pigs and mice. It was noted that the CAP activity was approximately the same in non-pregnant and pregnant animals. Observations of Hanson and Mannsfeldt (1967a) indicated that the CAP level in rat serum tends to decrease in the course of pregnancy. The optimum for the cleavage of L-cystine di-β-naphthylamide by rat plasma was found to be about pH 6 (Rydén, 1966).

An increase in LAP activity similar to that observed in human serum during pregnancy, has not been found to occur in the serum of the pregnant bitch (Lettow and Jaeger, 1965). This is not surprising, since the rise in LAP activity in human pregnancy is due to the appearance of plasma oxytocinase, which is not present in the serum of pregnant mammals other than primates.

Ehrensing (1964) studied the occurrence of oxytocinase in the circulation of nonmammalian animals. He found that oxytocin-destroying activity was absent from the plasma of turtles and chickens, but that it was present in both male and female snakes. The level of oxytocinase in the plasma of the snake *Natrix rhombifera* was of the same order of magnitude as that in human plasma in the eighth month of pregnancy. CAP activity in plasma was high in all three species investigated, irrespective of whether or not they were capable of inactivating oxytocin. The CAP levels did not vary with sex or with the stages of the oestrous cycle. The absence of oxytocin-inactivating enzymes from the blood plasma of birds (chickens and pigeons) was also observed by Manunta and Marongiu (1961). In a recent paper by Suska-Brzezińska and Ewy (1965), on the other hand, significant oxytocin-destroying activity was claimed to be present in the serum of the domestic fowl, in addition to the CAP activity previously described by Ehrensing. The rates of cleavage of L-cystine di-β-naphthylamide in the serum of hens and in that of cocks were of the same order of magnitude. EDTA and 8-hydroxyquinoline acted as weak inhibitors. The authors presumed that the same enzyme was responsible for the cleavage of oxytocin and L-cystine di-β-naphthylamide and that it was similar to human pregnancy oxytocinase. This assumption, however, needs confirmation.

Inactivation of Vasopressin in Plasma and Serum of Animals. Larson (1938) observed that the antidiuretic activity of neurohypophysial extracts gradually disappeared when the extracts were incubated with blood of cats, dogs or rabbits. The enzyme responsible for the inactivation of vasopressin appeared to be contained in the serum. This followed from experiments of Heller and Urban (1935) which indicated that there was little difference between the inactivating potencies of dog serum and whole blood. The destruction of vasopressin by rat and dog serum was more recently tested by Dicker and Ginsburg (1950) and by Arimura and Yamaguchi (1964). In contrast to serum, heparinized blood or plasma from rats does not appear to affect vasopressin (Heller and Zaidi, 1957; Dicker and Ginsburg, 1950). It is likely, therefore, that the enzyme which degrades vasopressin is activated in the course of blood coagulation (Heller, 1960).

2. *Erythrocytes*

Oxytocin and vasopressin are not destroyed by intact red blood cells because they are unable to penetrate the erythrocyte wall. The influence of whole blood upon the neurohypophysial hormones does not differ from that exerted by blood plasma to any significant extent. Laked red blood cells of man, cat, horse and ox, however, have been found capable of destroying the pressor and oxytocic principles of neurohypophysial extracts (Jones and Schlapp, 1936; Croxatto, Traut-

MANN, and CROXATTO, 1943; PAGE, 1946; WERLE, SEMM, and ENZENBACH, 1950; WERLE and SEMM, 1956). The enzyme system involved in the destruction of the hormones is activated by cysteine and glutathione and inhibited by iodate which oxidizes cysteine and glutathione (CROXATTO, TRAUTMANN, and CROXATTO, 1943). The inactivation of oxytocin by haemolyzed human red cells differs from that effected by the plasma oxytocinase of pregnant women in being unaffected by the metal chelating agent, EDTA (WERLE and SEMM, 1956). SEMM and WIENDL (1962) investigated the cleavage by adult and foetal erythrocytes of the plasma oxytocinase substrate, L-cystine di-β-naphthylamide, in the belief that the enzyme estimated with the help of this chromogenic substrate was identical with the enzyme destroying oxytocin in the haemolysates. This assumption, however, was not justified. WINTERSBERGER and CHATTERJEE (1962) subjected the enzyme which hydrolyses L-cystine di-β-naphthylamide to a certain degree of purification and showed that it had no action on oxytocin. In haemolysates, contrary to what has been found for human pregnancy serum, oxytocin and L-cystine di-β-naphthylamide appear to be attacked by different enzymes. The enzyme destroying oxytocin may not be acting as an aminopeptidase. This is suggested by findings recently reported by SEMM (1967) which indicated that deamino-oxytocin, which is not susceptible to attack by aminopeptidases, is inactivated by haemolysates as readily as is oxytocin.

B. Urine

Cat urine does not destroy vasopressin (JONES and SCHLAPP, 1936). Neither oxytocin nor vasopressin are inactivated appreciably by human urine (WERLE and EFFKEMANN, 1941; WERLE and KALVELAGE, 1941). When, however, the proteins present in the urine of pregnant women were concentrated, some hormone-destroying activity (WERLE and EFFKEMANN, 1941) and the electrophoretic CAP bands characteristic of plasma oxytocinase became detectable (PAGE, TITUS, MOHUN, and GLENDENING, 1961). The leakage of plasma oxytocinase through the glomeruli was found to be more marked in patients with preeclampsia than in healthy pregnant women.

C. Kidney, Liver and Spleen

The mammalian kidney plays a prominent role in the clearance of oxytocin and vasopressin from the circulation. A minor part of the amount of hormone removed by the kidneys is excreted in the urine. The major part undergoes rapid inactivation in kidney tissue. DICKER and GREENBAUM (1954) suggested that the small amount of antidiuretic activity which is found in rat urine was not due to unmodified vasopressin but rather to a less active transformation product which, in contrast to vasopressin, was resistant to further enzymatic inactivation by kidney tissue. The presence in the urine of a modified form of vasopressin, however, could not be confirmed by GINSBURG, HELLER, and ZAIDI (1956). Many properties of the urinary antidiuretic substance were compared and found to be identical with those of vasopressin (THORN, 1959).

In addition to the kidneys, the splanchnic organs were found to take a significant part in the elimination of the neurohypophysial hormones from the blood. After bilateral nephrectomy the half-life of injected oxytocin and vasopressin in the circulation of rats was markedly increased. When the splanchnic area of the nephrectomized rats was then excluded from the circulation, the disappearance of vasopressin from the blood was further retarded and that of oxytocin was almost stopped (HELLER, 1960).

In 1935, Heller and Urban demonstrated that liver and kidney homogenates and extracts were capable of destroying enzymatically the antidiuretic activity of posterior pituitary extracts. Jones and Schlapp (1936) extended these findings by showing that both the pressor and the oxytocic hormones of the neurohypophysis were inactivated upon incubation with glycerol extracts of cat liver, kidney and spleen. Larson (1938) observed that the enzymatic process destroying the pressor hormone was more active in the liver and kidney of dogs and rabbits than in that of cats. The oxytocic principle was likewise inactivated when incubated with extracts of liver and kidney of cats, dogs or rabbits, liver being more active than kidney (Larson, 1939). It was suggested that the aminopolypeptidase activity present in the extracts was responsible for hormone destruction. Birnie (1953) found that cell-free extracts of rat liver tissue were more effective in destroying vasopressin than were extracts of kidney, spleen and other organs. Rudman, Malkin, Garcia, Di Girolamo, and Abell (1964), however, who studied the destruction of the adipokinetic activity of vasopressin upon incubation with homogenates of several organs of the rat and the rabbit, observed that rat kidneys and adrenals provided the preparations with the greatest enzymatic activity, liver and spleen being less potent. The oxytocin-destroying activities of kidney and liver homogenates from nonpregnant and pregnant rats were compared by Sawyer (1954), no significant change due to pregnancy being observed. Among the organs of the cow, the liver and the kidneys were found to have the highest oxytocin-inactivating power. The activity of spleen homogenates was considerably less than that of liver homogenates (Suska-Brzezińska, Golebska, and Ewy, 1965; Manunta, 1960). In many other animal species studied oxytocin was also found to be inactivated by liver tissue, whereas irregular results were obtained with spleen homogenates (Manunta and Marongiu, 1961). The presence in fresh human liver tissue of a potent vasopressin-inactivating system was first described by Birnie (1953). Human fetal kidney, liver and spleen were found to destroy oxytocin (Semm and Wiendl, 1962).

Extracts of hypertensive kidneys, which were capable of destroying angiotensin, were tested by Croxatto, Croxatto, and Alliende (1942) for their oxytocin-inactivating properties. Rapid destruction of the hormone was observed at pH 7, if cysteine or glutathione was added as an enzyme activator. Iodate reversed the activating effect of the thiol compounds (Croxatto, Alliende, and Croxatto, 1942/1943a). The enzyme present in kidney tissue extracts was ranked by Croxatto, Croxatto, and Sorolla (1942/1943) among the aminopeptidases. Purified renin preparations had no effect on oxytocin at pH 7 with or without cysteine (Croxatto, Croxatto, and Alliende, 1942). The pressor activity of posterior pituitary extracts was also destroyed by kidney extracts in the presence of cysteine, iodate again reversing the activating effect (Croxatto, Illanes, Salvestrini, and Croxatto, 1942/1943; Croxatto, 1942/1943; Croxatto, Trautmann, and Croxatto, 1943).

The inactivation of vasopressin by diseased or experimentally damaged liver tissue was investigated by Eversole, Birnie, and Gaunt (1949), Birnie, Blackmore, and Heller (1952) and Birnie (1953). When homogenates of mouse liver were incubated with vasopressin at pH 6.5, more antidiuretic material remained active in the case of liver homogenates from protein-deficient animals than from control animals. When extracts were made of liver taken from rats which had been given daily injections of carbon tetrachloride for 12 days, there was a sharp decline in the ability to inactivate vasopressin as compared with untreated controls. Extracts made of liver from rats which had been adrenalectomized showed a markedly decreased ability to inactivate vasopressin. These observations were consistent with the hypothesis that water retention observed after feeding on protein-deficient diets or following clinical and experimental liver damage was due, at least in part, to a decreasing rate of inactivation of the antidiuretic hormone by damaged liver tissue. The destruction of oxytocin was also found to be impaired in experimental liver cirrhosis (SCALABRINO and CARACRISTI, 1960). When cirrhosis was induced in the rabbit by administration of carbon tetrachloride, the power of liver homogenates to destroy oxytocin was reduced to approximately one-half (SCALABRINO, CARACRISTI, and PERITI, 1961).

The inactivation of vasopressin by rat kidney and liver slices was studied by DICKER and GREENBAUM (1954) who claimed that in both cases the antidiuretic activity of the hormone was not reduced to zero but reached a final level equivalent to 10—20% of the initial level. The addition of fresh kidney or fresh liver slices to a solution of vasopressin previously inactivated by kidney or liver slices resulted in no further decrease of the antidiuretic activity. However, the addition of fresh kidney slices to a solution of vasopressin previously inactivated by liver, or the addition of fresh liver slices to a solution of vasopressin previously inactivated by kidney, both resulted in a further decrease of the antidiuretic activity. The antidiuretic activity of urine collected from rats during and after infusion of vasopressin appeared to remain unchanged after incubation with kidney slices, but was destroyed by liver slices, and it was therefore ascribed to a hypothetical derivative enzymatically formed from vasopressin, rather than to vasopressin itself. These results, however, were not confirmed by GINSBURG, HELLER, and ZAIDI (1956).

SMITH and SACHS (1961) reported that highly purified arginine-vasopressin, when incubated in the presence of rat kidney slices, rapidly disappeared from the incubation medium, the process essentially following the kinetics of a first-order reaction. Optimum rate of hormone disappearance was observed over the range from pH 7 to pH 10. At 25°, the disappearance of vasopressin from the medium was not due to the presence of degradative enzymes leaking out from the tissue. When, however, the slices were incubated with vasopressin at 37°, instead of 25°, enzymes capable of inactivating the hormone were released from the cells into the medium. Diisopropyl phosphorofluoridate and EDTA did not affect the rate of loss of vasopressin from the incubation medium. PCMB and excess oxytocin caused inhibition. The vasopressin which disappeared from the medium could not be recovered from the kidney slices and had apparently undergone inactivation. This was confirmed by the use of ^{35}S-vasopressin prepared biosynthetically.

THORN and WILLUMSEN (1963) compared the inactivation of arginine-vasopressin and that of lysine-vasopressin upon incubation with slices of rat kidney and rat liver. The rate of inactivation of the two hormones by kidney slices was greater than that found in liver slices. Neither in kidney nor in liver slices was there a statistically significant difference between the amounts of arginine- and lysine-vasopressin inactivated per mg dry tissue. The short action of lysine-vasopressin observed after intravenous injection as compared with the much longer-lasting effect of arginine-vasopressin is therefore hardly due to a difference in the rate of enzymatic inactivation in liver or kidney tissue.

Attempts to identify the tissue elements in which vasopressin is inactivated were made by several authors. HELLER and ZAIDI (1957) incubated vasopressin with homogenates of "glomerular" and "tubular" fractions of rat kidney and noted that the inactivation was essentially due to tubular tissue. THORN and WILLUMSEN (1963) went one step further by studying the distribution of enzymes inactivating vasopressin in four different zones of the rat kidney. Slices from the outer cortex, inner cortex, outer medulla and papillary zones were all capable of destroying vasopressin, but the most marked hormone-inactivating potency was found in the papillary zone which is known to be the site of action of the antidiuretic hormone. It thus became apparent that the cellular site of vasopressin inactivation was located close to the site of action of the hormone.

The intracellular distribution of the vasopressin-inactivating enzyme system was investigated by Dicker and Greenbaum (1956). Homogenates of rat kidney were prepared in 0.25 M sucrose and separated into fractions in the centrifuge. There was a greater concentration of the enzymatic activity responsible for vasopressin destruction in the supernatant fraction than in a particulate fraction consisting mainly of mitochondria. No significant enzymatic activity could be detected in the nuclear fraction.

Dicker and Greenbaum (1958) subjected the particle-free supernatant of pig kidney homogenates to salt fractionation and found that the greatest inactivation of vasopressin occurred with the fraction which was precipitated between 40 and 50% saturation with ammonium sulphate at pH 8. The rate of inactivation of vasopressin by this enzyme fraction was diminished in the presence of oxygen. It was also decreased by cystine and oxidized glutathione, whereas cysteine and reduced glutathione were capable of enhancing it. p-Chloromercuribenzoate had an inhibitory action on the enzyme. The conclusion was drawn from these results that the enzyme inactivating vasopressin acted on the disulphide bond in the hormone molecule, reducing it to sulphydryl groups, and that the enzyme itself might be a sulphydryl enzyme with maximum activity in its SH form.

The antidiuretic activity of vasopressin, after having been destroyed by incubation with the kidney enzyme, could be restored only partially by addition of cystine or oxidized glutathione to the incubation mixture (Dicker, 1960). This finding was interpreted to indicate that a second enzyme was involved which irreversibly destroyed the vasopressin molecules the disulphide bonds of which had previously been ruptured by a reducing enzyme. The final inactivation of vasopressin was considered to be possibly due to an amidase, because the rate of disappearance of the antidiuretic activity of vasopressin upon incubation with the kidney enzyme fraction could be reduced by adding glutamine, asparagine and glycine amide (Dicker, 1960).

Inhibitors of the enzymatic inactivation of oxytocin by mouse liver slices and liver cell sap were studied by Beránková, Rychlík, and Šorm (1960). Cystine was found to be a potent inhibitor. A series of peptide fragments of the oxytocin molecule containing a cystinyl or a S-benzylcysteinyl residue (e.g., S,S'-dibenzyl-dihydrooxytocin, S-benzylcysteinyl-tyrosine, glutaminyl-asparaginyl-S-benzyl-cysteinyl-prolyl-leucyl-glycine amide, S-benzylcysteinyl-prolyl-leucyl-glycine amide, cystinyl-bis(prolyl-leucyl-glycine amide)) likewise acted as powerful inhibitors of oxytocin inactivation by the liver enzyme system. Dethio-oxytocin (alanyl-tyrosyl-isoleucyl-glutaminyl-asparaginyl-alanyl-prolyl-leucyl-glycine amide), however, a nonapeptide which does not contain cysteine or cystine residues, nevertheless was capable of interfering with the liver enzyme (Beránková and Šorm, 1961). This peptide, which structurally resembles oxytocin, appears to act as a competitive substrate when inhibiting oxytocin inactivation by liver cell sap. It was shown to be itself rapidly hydrolysed, free amino acids being successively released from the amino end of the peptide chain. The specificity of fission of the nonapeptide and of some shorter peptide fragments of the oxytocin molecule by liver cell sap suggested that the enzyme responsible for the cleavage of these substrates might be an aminopeptidase different from but similar to leucine aminopeptidase (Beránková, Rychlík, and Šorm, 1961).

Beránková, Rychlík, and Šorm (1960) confirmed the finding previously reported by Birnie (1953) that dialysis of tissue extracts leads to inactivation of the enzyme system destroying oxytocin. The activity of dialyzed liver extracts, however, was found to be restored by addition of reduced glutathione (RYCHLÍK, 1964). This observation and the susceptibility of the enzyme to inhibition by cystine led RYCHLÍK (1964) to consider the possibility that sulphydryl compounds might play a rôle in the inactivation of oxytocin by liver enzymes similar to that proposed by DICKER and GREENBAUM (1958) for the destruction of vasopressin in the kidney and by AUDRAIN and CLAUSER (1960) for the anaerobic inactivation of oxytocin in the uterus. The first step in the inactivation of oxytocin in liver extract was proposed to be a reductive rupture of the disulphide bond resulting in the formation of dihydro-oxytocin. The simultaneous oxidation of reduced glutathione was demonstrated by adding to the system NADPH and glutathione reductase. The reductive cleavage of oxytocin was thus coupled to the oxidation of NADPH to $NADP^+$, which could be followed spectrophotometrically by measuring the decreasing optical density at 340 mμ (RYCHLÍK, 1964).

$$\text{Oxytocin} + 2\ \text{G–SH} \xrightarrow[\text{}]{\substack{\text{glutathione-oxytocin}\\ \text{transhydrogenase}}} \text{dihydro-oxytocin} + \text{G–S–S–G}$$

$$\text{G–S–S–G} + \text{NADPH} + \text{H}^+ \xrightarrow[\text{}]{\substack{\text{glutathione}\\ \text{reductase}}} 2\ \text{G–SH} + \text{NADP}^+$$

The enzyme involved in the reductive cleavage of oxytocin was called glutathione-oxytocin transhydrogenase and was thought to be similar to, or even identical with, the insulin-reducing liver enzyme, glutathione-insulin transhydrogenase which had previously been shown to be capable of reducing oxytocin and vasopressin as well as insulin in the presence of glutathione (KATZEN and STETTEN, 1962; KATZEN, TIETZE, and STETTEN, 1963). The close relation between the catabolism of insulin and that of the neurohypophysial hormones is also indicated by the recent observation that the breakdown of insulin in rat kidney slices is depressed in the presence of oxytocin (CAMU and CONARD, 1966). It is noteworthy, however, that many years earlier, in 1957, HELLER and ZAIDI when studying the metabolism of antidiuretic hormone in rat kidney and liver, had already noticed the similarity between the fate of vasopressin and that of insulin and had pointed out that the possibility of a common metabolic pathway of these hormones should be the subject of further study.

Incubation of oxytocin with a dialyzed liver cell sap to which reduced glutathione, cysteine or mercaptoethanol had been added, resulted in the liberation of free amino acids. It was demonstrated by chromatography that cysteine, tyrosine and isoleucine, the first three amino acids in the peptide chain of reduced oxytocin, were released in a stepwise manner (RYCHLÍK, 1964). It thus became apparent that the inactivation of oxytocin by liver extract is a two-stage process. The first step, which consists in the reduction of the disulphide bond in oxytocin, is followed by a proteolytic attack on the peptide chain. The aminopeptidase responsible for the irreversible degradation of reduced oxytocin was partially purified from beef liver by precipitations with ammonium sulphate (40—60% saturation) and protamine and by chromatography on a column of DEAE-cellulose (BARTOŠEK, RYCHLÍK, and ŠORM, 1964; BARTOŠEK, PLIŠKA, RYCHLÍK, and ŠORM, 1964). The purified enzyme preparation exhibited optimum activity at pH 8.0—9.2. It could be inhibited by EDTA and activated by manganese and magnesium ions, whereas iodoacetamide was without effect. These properties indicated that liver aminopeptidase, like kidney leucine aminopeptidase (LAP), was a metallo-enzyme. Oxytocin was hydrolyzed neither by the liver tissue enzyme nor by LAP. Dihydro-oxytocin, S,S'-dimethyldihydro-oxytocin and dethio-oxytocin, on the other hand, were readily attacked by both enzymes. S-Benzylcysteinyl-tyrosine amide (JOŠT and RUDINGER, 1961) proved to be a suitable substrate for routine determinations of aminopeptidase activity. When the rates of cleavage of a series of S-benzylcysteinyl derivatives by the liver enzyme were compared with the rates of cleavage by LAP, a close correlation was found. It was therefore concluded that the liver tissue aminopeptidase, which is involved in the second stage of oxytocin inactivation, is likely to be identical with kidney LAP (BARTOŠEK, PLIŠKA, RYCHLÍK, and ŠORM, 1964).

D. Pancreas

In view of the wealth of enzymes occurring in this organ it is not surprising that extracts or slices of swine pancreas (WERLE and SEMM, 1956), mouse pancreas (BERÁNKOVÁ, RYCHLÍK, and ŠORM, 1959, 1960) and cow pancreas (SUSKA-BRZEZIŃSKA, GOLEBSKA, and EWY, 1965) were found to be capable of destroying oxytocin. The enzymes responsible for the inactivation of the hormone peptide were not affected by EDTA (WERLE and SEMM, 1956) and resembled the oxytocin-inactivating enzymes occurring in liver cell sap with regard to their susceptibility to inhibition by cystine and by some peptides containing cystinyl or S-benzylcysteinyl residues (BERÁNKOVÁ, RYCHLÍK, and ŠORM, 1960). The inactivation of oxytocin by mouse pancreas slices *in vitro* was found to be retarded in the presence of an amino acid mixture and to be enhanced by anaerobiosis and 2.4-dinitrophenol (LEBLOVÁ and RYCHLÍK, 1960).

E. Brain and Nervous Tissue

It is of particular interest that enzymes degrading oxytocin and vasopressin are present in the hypothalamus which is the very site of synthesis of the neurohypophysial hormones. The enzymes may possibly exert some control over the turnover of the hormones by varying the rate of their catabolism. In experiments designed to study hypothalamic hormone synthesis *in vitro*, the interference by such enzymes must be seriously taken into account.

HELLER and URBAN (1935) found that minced guinea-pig brain slightly inactivated vasopressin. Homogenates of rat brain and particularly rat hypothalamus were reported by ITOH and KIKUCHI (1959) not to affect vasopressin unless pyridoxal was added. Pyridoxal, however, would not appear to act as a cofactor of a hormone-degrading enzyme, but rather to have a direct impact upon the vasopressin molecule. As shown by HOOPER (1962), vasopressin is destroyed when incubated with pyridoxal even in the absence of any enzyme, a Schiff base being presumably formed.

The inactivation of the neurohypophysial hormones by homogenates of dog hypothalamus was intensively studied by HOOPER (1961b, 1962a). Both oxytocin and vasopressin were found to be destroyed when incubated with hypothalamic tissue homogenate at pH 7 and 37°. The enzymatic nature of the inactivation process was established by measuring the kinetics and the heat sensitivity of the system. The optimum pH for the inactivation of oxytocin and vasopressin was the same, the peak being between pH 7 and 8. The rate of destruction decreased with time and thus did not follow precisely that predicted by first-order kinetics. Oxytocin was destroyed approximately 2.8 times more rapidly than vasopressin. The rate of inactivation of oxytocin was reduced in the presence of vasopressin, and *vice versa*, indicating that oxytocin and vasopressin were substrates for the same enzyme. Enzyme activity was not inhibited by cyanide, fluoride and EDTA and therefore was likely to have no requirement for metal ions. The failure of iodoacetamide to inhibit the hypothalamic enzyme suggested that it did not possess thiol groups which were essential for activity. Diisopropyl phosphofluoridate did not inhibit significantly in millimolar concentration, but did so in 10 mM solution.

Enzymes capable of inactivating oxytocin also occur in parts of the central nervous system other than hypothalamus (Hooper, 1963a). Their distribution appears to correspond to regions containing a large number of nerve cells. No degradation of the neurohypophysial hormones was observed in dorsal roots, ventral roots and dorsal root ganglia.

The intracellular distribution of the enzymes inactivating oxytocin in dog hypothalamic tissue was investigated by subjecting homogenates to differential and density-gradient centrifugation (Hooper, 1962b). Enzyme activity was found to be associated with the supernatant and with the "mitochondrial" fraction which, beside mitochondria, contained lysosomes, neurosecretory material and myelin. The nuclear and microsomal fractions did not contain detectable amounts of enzymedestroying oxytocin. The "mitochondrial" fraction was further subdivided into three components by centrifuging in a gradient comprising 0.32, 0.8 and 1.2 M sucrose. When hypothalami from nonpregnant dogs were fractionated, most of the hormone-destroying activity was present in the heaviest layer of the "mitochondrial" fraction, whereas the layer containing particles of least density was devoid of detectable amounts of enzyme. With pregnant animals, an increase in particle-bound enzyme activity and a change in enzyme distribution were observed (Hooper, 1964). The activity was very low in the heavy fraction, whereas the activity in the lightest fraction, which was shown by electron microscopy to contain a heavy proportion of myelin threads, accounted for the major part of the particle-bound enzyme. This variation in enzyme distribution suggested that there was a change in the pattern of oxytocin metabolism in the hypothalamus during pregnancy.

A somewhat different picture was obtained when the intracellular distribution of enzymes destroying oxytocin was studied in rabbit hypothalamus (Hooper, 1966a). Enzyme activity was again detected in the supernatant and "mitochondrial" fractions of both nonpregnant and pregnant animals. The specific activity of the supernatant fractions was approximately three times that of the particle fraction. The particle-bound enzyme activity of the rabbit hypothalamus, however, was localized in the "intermediate-mitochondrial" fraction, whereas in dog hypothalamus it was associated with the "heavy-mitochondrial" fraction. The specific activity of the enzymes was found to rise during early pregnancy, the increase in enzyme concentration coinciding approximately with the period of blastocyst spacing in the uterus, after which it remained fairly constant at an elevated level until late pregnancy. The activity of the particulate fraction increased about 3.5fold, that of the supernatant enzyme increased somewhat less. Hooper (1966a) suggested that the increase in the activity of the hypothalamic enzymes inactivating oxytocin might be an index of increased hormone production in the hypothalamus at the time of blastocyst implantation.

A recent study (Hooper, 1966b) was devoted to the question of whether the release of oxytocin into the circulation triggered by parturition and by suckling might be correlated with an increased rate of hormone turnover at the site of its production in the hypothalamus. It was found that there was approximately three times as much activity in the supernatant fraction of the hypothalami of rabbits six hours after parturition as there was during late pregnancy. The particle-bound enzyme failed to increase during parturition. In lactating animals the high activity noted in the supernatant fraction after parturition was maintained until the third day *post partum*. Between the third and fifth days, the activity dropped to levels observed during late pregnancy, but stayed at these elevated levels for as long as 26 days *post partum*. In animals deprived of the suckling stimulus by removal of the litters shortly after delivery, the activity of the supernatant enzyme dropped rapidly and nonpregnant levels were attained by the seventh day. This led Hooper (1966b) to conclude that stimuli which cause a reflex release of oxytocin from the posterior pituitary gland will also bring about an augmented production and turnover of posterior pituitary hormones in the hypothalamus, this increase manifesting itself in an increased concentration of hypothalamic enzymes inactivating oxytocin.

Little information is available on the inactivation of neurohypophysial enzymes by human nervous tissue. Semm and Wiendl (1962) reported that foetal human brain was capable of destroying oxytocin and that, contrary to findings with all other human tissues tested, the enzyme(s) of the brain could be fully inhibited by the metal-chelating agent, EDTA.

F. Pituitary Gland

Surprisingly little is known about the enzymatic inactivation of the neurohypophysial hormones in the pituitary gland. When slices of the posterior lobe of hog or beef pituitary gland were incubated, gradual inactivation of the endogenous oxytocin was observed (Leblová and Rychlík, 1960). The rate of inactivation was decreased when a mixture of amino acids was present in the incubation mixture. Inactivation was considerably enhanced by anaerobiosis.

G. Lung

The available data on the degradation of neurohypophysial hormones by enzymes present in the lung are rather scarce. Extracts of foetal human lung tissue were found to destroy oxytocin (Semm and Wiendl, 1962), and both rabbit and rat lung homogenates were reported to inactivate the adipokinetic property of vasopressin (Rudman, Malkin, Garcia, Di Girolamo, and Abell, 1964).

H. Adipose Tissue

Rat adipose tissue homogenate contains an enzyme which destroys the adipokinetic activity of vasopressin, whereas homogenates of rabbit and guinea-pig adipose tissue are unable to inactivate this hormone (Rudman, Malkin, Brown, Garcia, and Abell, 1964; Rudman, Malkin, Garcia, Di Girolamo, and Abell, 1964). When slices of rat adipose tissue were incubated in a solution containing vasopressin, the adipokinetic activity rapidly disappeared from the incubation medium and there was no adipokinetic response of the tissue to vasopressin. In contrast, slices of adipose tissue from the rabbit or guinea-pig, which did not cause the disappearance of a detectable amount of activity from the medium, were responsive to vasopressin. Analogous observations were made for the adipokinetic activities of ACTH, β-MSH and pituitary fraction H. Thus, differences between species in responsiveness of their adipose tissue to hypophysial peptides appear to be related to differences in peptidase content of the fat cell.

The hormone-destroying activity of rat adipose tissue is reduced by freezing and thawing and abolished by freeze-drying. After centrifugation of tissue homogenates at $100000 \times g$, the major proportion of the activity was found in the water-insoluble triglyceride-rich cake and the minor proportion in the sedimented pellet. The adipose-tissue enzyme(s) attacking the hypophysial peptides appear to resemble the system which inactivates insulin (Di Girolamo, Rudman, Malkin, and and Garcia, 1965).

J. Cross-Striated and Heart Muscle

Larson (1938) found that posterior pituitary extracts lost their pressor activity when incubated at a neutral pH with muscle tissue from cats, dogs or rabbits.

In experiments carried out by DICKER and GREENBAUM (1956) rat muscle homogenate failed to effect an appreciable inactivation of vasopressin. Their finding that skeletal muscle only binds vasopressin without destroying it, was confirmed by HANKISS, KESZTHELYI, and DEMÉNY (1965). The Hungarian investigators found that rat heart muscle, on the contrary, was capable of inactivating vasopressin by an enzymatic process. The adipokinetic activity of vasopressin was reported by RUDMAN, MALKIN, GARCIA, DI GIROLAMO, and ABELL (1964) to be destroyed at a detectable rate by heart tissue from the rat and the rabbit.

A weak capacity of muscle tissue to inactivate oxytocin was first described by LARSON (1939). In rat skeletal muscle, however, SAWYER (1954) found considerable oxytocin-destroying activity which was in the same range as that encountered in uterine muscle, but did not increase during pregnancy. A significant level of "oxytocinase" activity was reported to occur in cow skeletal muscle (MANUNTA, 1960; SUSKA-BRZEZIŃSKA, GOLEBSKA, and EWY, 1965).

K. Intestine

An erepsin preparation obtained from the mucosa of the small intestine was found by DALE and DUDLEY (1921) to inactivate the pressor principle of neurohypophysial extracts. This was confirmed by LARSON (1938) who made the aminopeptidase component of dog intestinal mucosa responsible for vasopressin destruction. More recently, oxytocin inactivation was reported to be demonstrable in extracts of goat and cow intestine (WERLE, 1960; SUSKA-BRZEZIŃSKA, GOLEBSKA, and EWY, 1965). The relatively weak hormone-inactivating potency of such extracts is consistent with the experiments of GINSBURG and SMITH (1959) which indicated that the intestine was not an important organ of neurohypophysial hormone clearance.

L. Urinary Bladder

In the course of studies on the increased water permeability effected by neurohypophysial hormones in the bladder of amphibians, the observation was made that an ammonium sulphate extract of the bladder of the toad, *Bufo marinus*, was capable of inactivating oxytocin and its hormone analogues (KARLIN, 1963). This extract appeared to contain an aminopeptidase which differed in several respects from the oxytocinase encountered in human pregnancy plasma.

A different mechanism of action operates in the inactivation of vasopressin by a proteolytic enzyme which was isolated and purified from homogenates of toad bladder (CAMPBELL, THYSEN, and CHU, 1965). The enzyme was found to catalyze the cleavage of the lysyl-glycine peptide bond in lysine-vasopressin. Glycine amide was released from the rest of the hormone molecule, in which the disulphide bond remained intact. Although the specificities of trypsin and toad bladder protease were similar, their chromatographic properties were completely different. At present it is not clear whether the bladder enzyme is part of a specific regulatory mechanism for the inactivation of vasopressin or whether it has a more general function in the catabolism of a wide variety of peptide structures.

Some years ago, it was suggested by SCHWARTZ, RASMUSSEN, SCHOESSLER, SILVER, and FONG (1960) that the vasopressin-induced increase in the water permeability of the toad bladder may depend on the fixation of vasopressin to its receptor in the tissue by a thiol-disulphide interchange, and that possibly the dissociation of hormone from receptor may be effected by a disulphide reductase reaction. So far, however, experimental evidence for the existence of enzymes releasing neurohypophysial hormones from their receptor site in the bladder or in other organs is still lacking.

M. Uterus

Particular attention has been focussed on the occurrence of enzymes destroying oxytocin in uterine tissue, because it was considered possible that such enzymes may control the uterine action of circulating neurohypophysial hormone and prevent premature uterine activity during pregnancy.

Several investigators found that extracts prepared from pregnant human uterus at term and in labour possessed a marked ability to destroy oxytocin (Werle, Hevelke, and Buthmann, 1941; Carballo, 1961; Centaro, Periti, and De Laurentiis, 1961; Melander, 1965; Rydén, 1966). Dicker and Whyley (1960), however, failed to observe oxytocin inactivation by homogenates of human uterine strips removed during caesarian operations. The hydrolysis of L-cystine di-β-naphthylamide by extracts of human myometrium was studied by Melander (1965). Irrespective of whether the extracts were obtained from uteri of nonpregnant women, or of women in the 5th or in the last month of pregnancy, about the same levels of enzyme activity were observed which, on a weight basis, were lower than the specific activities of placental extracts. The enzyme activities responsible for the destruction of oxytocin and the cleavage of L-cystine di-β-naphthylamide had their optimum around pH 6 and were recovered almost exclusively in the soluble protein fraction of uterus homogenates (Rydén, 1966). As the rate of the enzymatic reactions decreased with time, it was suggested that the enzyme(s) involved were unstable.

In 1954, Sawyer reported that the capacity of the rat uterus to destroy oxytocin was characteristically dependent on the stage of pregnancy. Uteri from nonpregnant rats exhibited a fair degree of activity. In gravid uteri, in the period from about 7—21 days of pregnancy, a 4—8-fold increase in the ability to destroy oxytocin was claimed to occur. At delivery, or one day *post partum*, the enzyme activity of the rat uterus would have returned to the 7th day level. Based on the findings of a steady increase in the oxytocin-destroying activity of the uterus during pregnancy followed by a sharp decrease at the time of delivery, the hypothesis was advanced that this myometrial enzyme was part of a defence mechanism designed to prevent premature labour and delivery. Dicker and Whyley (1960) reported observations which lent support to this hypothesis. No oxytocin-destroying activity was found in nonpregnant rat myometrium, whereas the uterine muscle of the pregnant rat readily inactivated oxytocin. It was claimed that there was a steady increase in the rate of hormone inactivation from early pregnancy to a maximum at 21 days. These results, however, could not be confirmed by the recent work of Rydén (1966) who failed to find any significant difference between the oxytocin-degrading capabilities in myometrium of nonpregnant and pregnant rats. The ability to cleave L-cystine di-β-naphthylamide was even higher in nonpregnant rat uteri than it was in pregnant uterine muscle. The properties of rat myometrial cystine aminopeptidase closely resembled those of the corresponding enzyme in human uteri which was referred to above.

Homogenates of nonpregnant and pregnant rabbit uterus were also tested for their ability to destroy oxytocin. Dicker and Whyley (1960) reported that the rate of hormone inactivation effected by the myometrial homogenates decreased with progressing pregnancy and reached a minimum shortly before term. The assumption was made that the high level of oxytocin-destroying activity in the uterus, and its decrease as term approaches, were important factors in the preservation of uterine quiescene.

Manunta (1960) reported that oxytocin was slowly inactivated by cow uterus homogenates, the rate of destruction being considerably less than with homogenates of cow liver. Suska-Brzezińska, Golebska, and Ewy (1965), when testing various organs of the cow as to their ability to cleave oxytocin and L-cystine di-β-naphthylamide, found uterine tissue to be fairly active.

An important contribution to the problem of oxytocin inactivation in tissues has been made by Audrain and Clauser (1960) who observed that oxytocin, when incubated with rat uterine tissue under aerobic conditions, was not inactivated, whereas rapid irreversible destruction occurred under anaerobic conditions. The inactivation appeared to proceed in two steps. The uterine tissue would first cause a reversible reduction of the disulphide bridge in oxytocin. Then an irreversible inactivation would be effected by an enzyme system which was diffusing into the medium during incubation. It was pointed out that this enzyme might be a protease capable of cleaving reduced oxytocin while inactive toward nonreduced oxytocin, or it might act by catalyzing the irreversible formation of mixed disulphides. Similar experiments were carried out using organs other than the uterus, e. g. liver, kidney and diaphragm. In these cases, however, inactivation of oxytocin proceeded smoothly under both aerobic and anaerobic conditions, presumably because enzymes were present which were equally effective in cleaving oxytocin and reduced oxytocin.

N. Placenta

Enzymes in Human Placenta Degrading Oxytocin and Vasopressin. Werle, Hevelke, and Buthmann (1941) were the first to demonstrate oxytocin-destroying activity in placental extracts. Page (1946) subjected full-term human placentae to a brief extraction with saline and concluded from the activity of the extracts that, on a weight basis, the placental tissue was approximately one-half as potent in inactivating oxytocin as was full-term pregnancy plasma. Placental extracts which were several times more active than plasma samples obtained from the same women were prepared by Carballo and Méndez-Bauer (1957 b). Placental tissue taken from women at 30 weeks of pregnancy yielded extracts which were just as capable of inactivating oxytocin as those from full-term placental tissue.

Hawker (1956) showed that homogenates of human placenta destroyed both oxytocin and vasopressin. The pH optimum for the inactivation of oxytocin by placental extracts and by pregnancy plasma was found to be the same (pH 7—8). Rydén (1966) who studied the influence of pH on the degradation of oxytocin by homogenates of human placentae, observed two optima; one was at pH 6.0 and corresponded to the optimum for the destruction of oxytocin in several other tissues. The other and more prominent pH optimum was in the range from pH 7.0—7.5, where the plasma of pregnant women exhibits the highest oxytocinase activity. On the basis of inhibition studies Semm (1960) considered the oxytocin-degrading activity of placental extracts to be due to two different enzymes. One of them resembled plasma oxytocinase in being inhibited by EDTA, whereas the other one resisted the action of the complexing agent.

Hooper and Jessup (1959) subjected homogenates of human placentae to differential centrifugation in order to study the distribution of the enzymes which inactivate oxytocin and vasopressin. They found that the oxytocin-inactivating enzyme(s) occurred almost exclusively in the soluble protein fraction, whereas the vasopressin-degrading enzyme activity was associated predominantly with the mitochondrial and microsomal fractions. The mitochondrial and microsomal particles had to be treated with 0.5% sodium cholate at pH 8 followed by digestion with trypsin in order for the vasopressin-inactivating enzyme to be released (Hooper, 1960a). Maximum inactivation of oxytocin and vasopressin by placental homogenate was found to occur at pH 7.5—8.5 and pH 6.0—8.0, respectively (Hooper and Jessup, 1959; Hooper, 1960b). The authors reached the conclusion that in human placenta two separate systems were involved in the degradation of oxytocin and vasopressin. Both enzymes could be inhibited by copper ions. Silver and zinc ions, on the other hand, had a strong inhibitory effect on the oxytocin-degrading enzyme, whereas the vasopressin-inactivating enzyme was only slightly affected. Chelating agents such as EDTA, and thiol alkylating reagents such as iodoacetate and iodoacetamide, did not affect enzyme activity. The phosphorylating reagents, DFP and TEPP, however, completely inhibited the oxytocin-inactivating enzyme, while the vasopressin-destroying enzyme remained virtually unaffected (Hooper, 1959). The inhibition by EDTA of the vasopressin-inactivating principle of placenta extracts was confirmed by Vorherr and Hüskens (1963). Trasylol and ε-aminocaproate were found to be without inhibitory action.

Since plasma oxytocinase had been shown to be an aminopeptidase capable of hydrolyzing chromogenic substrates such as L-cystine di-β-naphthylamide and L-leucine β-naphthylamide, several investigators considered it of interest to study the cleavage of these aminopeptidase substrates by placental extracts. Riad (1962) homogenized washed human placentae with saline, centrifuged, and assayed the supernatants for CAP activity. Enzyme activity was found to be high. The concentration of the enzyme in placental tissue was estimated to be almost 4 times that in peripheral pregnancy plasma. The tissue, in contrast to the plasma, did not show an increase in aminopeptidase activity in the course of pregnancy. Melander (1965) compared the CAP activity of placentae from women in the fifth month of pregnancy with that of full-term placentae and found that the former was approximately one and a half times higher than the latter. Siegel (1959) reported that there was no increase in LAP activity per gram of placental tissue taken at different time intervals.

With L-cystine di-β-naphthylamide as the substrate Rydén (1966) observed a similar pH dependence of the enzymatic hydrolysis by placental extracts as with oxytocin: Enzyme activity was higher at pH 7.3 than at pH 6.0. A pH optimum above pH 7 is characteristic of plasma oxytocinase, whereas extracts of tissues other than placenta exhibit an activity optimum of about pH 6.

A crude preparation obtained from the soluble protein fraction of placenta extracts had the property of hydrolyzing esters of cystine and S-benzylcysteine. It was shown by Hooper (1961a) that, contrary to what might have been expected, this cystine esterase was not identical with oxytocinase.

The Placenta as the Possible Site of Origin of Pregnancy Plasma Oxytocinase. It is widely held that the placenta is the source of human plasma oxytocinase (Page, 1946; Kanazawa, 1954; Carballo and Méndez-Bauer, 1957b; Semm, 1958; Page, Titus, Mohun, and Glendening, 1961; Semm and Waidl, 1962; Rydén, 1966). There are good arguments in favour of this assumption:

1. Plasma oxytocinase has never been observed in a nonpregnant individual (Werle, Semm, and Enzenbach, 1950; Page, Titus, Mohun, and Glendening, 1961). After normal delivery and expulsion of the placenta the plasma oxytocinase activity immediately starts to decrease by an exponential function.

2. The absence of oxytocinase in foetal blood eliminates the foetus as a source of oxytocinase.

3. The blood concentration of oxytocinase roughly parallels the total mass of placenta. The highest oxytocinase values were encountered in multiple pregnancies (Page, Titus, Mohun, and Glendening, 1961; Miller, Naor, Milkovich, and Schmidt, 1964; Melander, 1965; Ichaliotis and Lambrinopoulos, 1965).

4. Placental extracts show a high enzymatic activity towards oxytocin and L-cystine di-β-naphthylamide (PAGE, 1946; HAWKER, 1956; CARBALLO and MÉNDEZ-BAUER, 1957b; HOOPER and JESSUP, 1959; RIAD, 1962; SEMM and WIENDL, 1962; SEMM, 1963; RYDÉN, 1966). One of the two pH optima of the enzymatic activity corresponds to the pH optimum of plasma oxytocinase (RYDÉN, 1966). The progress curve of the cleavage of L-cystine di-β-naphthylamide by placenta extracts was also quite similar to that obtained with human pregnancy plasma. Moreover, the extracts resembled pregnancy plasma in that their CAP activity was significantly inhibited upon addition of oxytocin (PAGE, TITUS, MOHUN, and GLENDENING, 1961).

5. When pregnancy plasma was subjected to paper electrophoresis, oxytocinase could be detected as a distinct LAP band in the α-2 globulin fraction. A LAP band with identical mobility was also found in placental extracts (SMITH and RUTENBURG, 1963). Using vertical starch gel electrophoresis, PAGE, TITUS, MOHUN, and GLENDENING (1961) could discern two bands in pregnancy sera with oxytocinase and CAP activity. The same oxytocinase bands could be demonstrated in some placental extracts.

There are arguments, however, which strongly militate against the placenta as the origin of plasma oxytocinase during pregnancy.

1. The oxytocinase level in plasma failed to decrease for a whole week following surgical removal of the placenta by vaginal hysterectomy (MELANDER, 1965).

2. In single pregnancies no correlation appears to exist between placental weight and plasma oxytocinase activity (SEMM, 1963; ICHALIOTIS and LAMBRINOPOULOS, 1965).

3. In placental homogenates the enzymes destroying oxytocin and vasopressin could be separated from each other. The placental oxytocinase was found to possess very little vasopressinase activity (HOOPER and JESSUP, 1959). Plasma oxytocinase, on the other hand, is capable of cleaving oxytocin and vasopressin at approximately the same rate (STOKLASKA and WINTERSBERGER, 1959; GLENDENING, TITUS, SCHROEDER, MOHUN, and PAGE, 1965). EDTA and other metal-chelating agents, while strongly inhibiting pregnancy plasma oxytocinase (WERLE and SEMM, 1956; TUPPY and WINTERSBERGER, 1960), had very little effect on the inactivation of oxytocin by placenta extracts (HOOPER, 1959). Conversely, diisopropyl phosphofluoridate completely inhibited the placental oxytocin-destroying activity (HOOPER, 1959), but had no effect on pregnancy plasma oxytocinase (TUPPY and WINTERSBERGER, 1960). Moreover, placenta extracts were found to inactivate deamino-oxytocin as readily as oxytocin (SEMM, 1967). Desamino-oxytocin, however, lacks a N-terminal amino group and is therefore resistant to the action of plasma oxytocinase and other aminopeptidases (GOLUBOW, CHAN, and DU VIGNEAUD, 1963; GOLUBOW and DU VIGNEAUD, 1963).

4. BECKMANN, BJÖRLING, and CHRISTODOULOU (1966 a, b) were unable to find a strict electrophoretic correspondence between enzymes with LAP activity in pregnancy plasma and in placenta extracts. Placenta extracts showed four different LAP enzyme zones none of which appeared to correspond to plasma oxytocinase. This led the authors to conclude that oxytocinase was probably not derived from the placenta. PAGE, TITUS, MOHUN, and GLENDENING (1961) were able to demonstrate two electrophoretic bands with CAP activity in human placental extracts and in pregnancy plasma, whereas no such band was detected in nonpregnancy plasma. However, not all the placental extracts showed CAP activity. The question was therefore raised whether the CAP bands, which did not regularly appear in the pherograms of the placenta extracts, might not have been due to contamination of placental tissue with maternal blood (RYDÉN, 1966).

5. KAZDA (1964) claimed that the oxytocinase levels were about three times higher in the intervillous blood than in the cubital blood of pregnant women. Other authors, however, were unable to find a difference between the levels of oxytocinase in uterine venous blood and systemic blood (e.g., WERLE and EFFKEMANN, 1941; RIAD, 1962), though such a difference has been established for many of the placental products including the enzyme, histaminase.

6. Oxytocinase is believed to be present in the "pregnancy zone", a protein fraction demonstrable by starch gel electrophoresis of pregnancy serum. However, the protein of the "pregnancy zone" was found not to cross-react immunologically with placental extracts. This points to the absence in such extracts of plasma oxytocinase (WILKEN, 1963).

Although none of these arguments may exclude the placenta as the site of production of plasma oxytocinase, "they indicate the need for further investigation of the problem. *In vitro* placental perfusion experiments, placental tissue culture and transplantation would be specially suitable for this purpose" (RIAD, 1962).

The investigators who believe plasma oxytocinase to be produced by the placenta consider the syncytiotrophoblast to be the most likely site of origin of the enzyme. The rise in oxytocinase activity in pregnancy blood follows the increase in syncytial mass rather than the increase in the cytotrophoblastic bulk (Langhans' cells) which diminishes markedly after midpregnancy (PAGE, TITUS, MOHUN, and GLENDENING, 1961). The plasma oxytocinase level parallels the concentration of the oestrogens, which are believed to stem from the syncytium, rather than the level of chorionic gonadotropin, which originates from the cytotrophoblast (PAGE, TITUS, MOHUN, and GLENDENING, 1961). In patients with choriocarcinoma having positive tests for chorionic gonadotropin the characteristic plasma oxytocinase bands were found to be absent. This was also interpreted to exclude the cytotrophoblast as the source of oxytocinase (PAGE, TITUS, MOHUN, and GLENDENING, 1961).

As plasma oxytocinase is capable of cleaving L-cystine di-β-naphthylamide and L-leucine β-naphthylamide, it was to be expected that the cells of origin of oxytocinase could be stained histochemically with the help of the chromogenic aminopeptidase substrates. SEMM and WAIDL (1962) and JAMES (1966) employed L-cystine di-β-naphthylamide in their attempt to localize oxytocinase histochemically and found the enzyme(s) cleaving this substrate to be most prominent in the syncytial layer of the trophoblast. PAGE, TITUS, MOHUN, and GLENDENING (1961) refer to histochemical work carried out by MERRILL which indicated the presence of intense activity in the syncytium. FUHRMANN (1959), however, failed to obtain evidence for more than very slight aminopeptidase activity in the syncytium of the placental villi.

Enzymes Degrading Oxytocin in the Placentae of Animals. Homogenates of placentae from pregnant rats and rabbits show a considerable capacity to destroy oxytocin. DICKER and WHYLEY (1960) reported that the ability of the placentae to inactivate the oxytocic hormone exceeds that of the uteri. SAWYER (1954), on the contrary, found that rat placentae, on a weight basis, were less potent than uterine muscle of pregnant rats. In rabbits, the rate of inactivation of oxytocin by homogenates of both placentae and uteri decreased in the course of pregnancy, reaching its minimum just before term (DICKER and WHYLEY, 1960).

The fact that the sera of pregnant animals (other than primates) fail to destroy oxytocin, whereas human pregnancy serum contains a high concentration of oxytocinase, and the supposition that the placenta is the source of human plasma oxytocinase, led RYDÉN (1966) to carry out a comparative study of the oxytocinase and cystine aminopeptidase activities in rat and human placentae. Differences in enzyme kinetics and pH optimum were noted. The progress curve for the degradation of oxytocin by rat placenta deviates from linearity due to an instability of the enzyme(s) involved, whereas the time course of oxytocin inactivation by human placenta appears to be linear. The cystine aminopeptidase activity present in homogenates of rat placenta has a pH optimum at pH 6, rather than at pH 7.4 where human placental extracts exhibit the highest activity toward L-cystine di-β-naphthylamide and toward oxytocin. The differences between the enzymatic properties of extracts from rat and human placentae were tentatively correlated with the absence of oxytocinase in rat and the presence of oxytocinase in human pregnancy blood.

HANSON and MANNSFELDT (1967c) compared the enzymatic hydrolysis by rat and human placenta extracts of a series of chromogenic substrates such as, e.g., L-cystine di-β-naphthylamide, S-benzyl-L-cysteine β-naphthylamide, S-benzyl-L-cysteine p-nitroanilide and L-leucine p-nitroanilide, which are all known to be substrates for plasma oxytocinase. Among the most clearcut and significant differences between rat and human placentae observed in this work were a lesser ability of rat placental extracts to cleave S-benzyl-L-cysteine β-naphthylamide and a much lower degree of inhibition of their CAP activity by EDTA. It was suggested that these differences reflect the presence in human placentae and the absence from rat placentae of the pregnancy-specific plasma oxytocinase.

O. Decidua, Foetal Membranes and Amniotic Fluid

MELANDER (1965) reported that extracts of human decidua contain enzymes which are capable of hydrolyzing L-cystine di-β-naphthylamide. It was assumed that these enzymes would also attack oxytocin. The CAP activity of the decidua extracts was almost as high as that of placenta extracts, and it was considered possible that the decidua might contribute to the inactivation of oxytocin in pregnant individuals. RYDÉN (1966) confirmed the occurrence of enzymes with CAP and oxytocin-destroying activity in human decidua. It was found that rat decidua contains similar enzymes and that the pH optimum for the enzymes is at pH 6.2, rather than at pH 7.3 where human pregnancy oxytocinase is most active. It appears unlikely, therefore, that the decidua may be a source of human pregnancy oxytocinase.

Rat foetal membranes possess a high specific activity of CAP and oxytocinase (RYDÉN, 1966). Maximum activity was noted at pH 6. There was no significant increase in enzyme levels in the course of pregnancy.

Human amniotic fluid appears to be free of oxytocinase activity and to contain no more than traces of CAP (MÜLLER-HARTBURG, NESVADBA, and TUPPY, 1959; HASHIMOTO, 1961b; RIAD, 1962).

P. Ovaries

Aqueous extracts of swine ovaries were found capable of destroying oxytocin both aerobically and anaerobically, the optimum activity being around pH 7 (FRIED and WÜST, 1954). Glutathione and cysteine failed to activate the ovarian enzyme system. Fractionation with ethanol in the cold resulted in a certain degree of purification. Loss of enzyme activity occurred upon dialysis. Storage at room temperature for 5 h, and even at 0° for 24 h, brought about a considerable decrease of enzymatic activity. This marked lability of the enzyme, as well as its unsusceptibility to inhibition by EDTA, is in contrast to the properties of pregnancy plasma oxytocinase which is rather stable during prolonged storage and liable to inhibition by metal-complexing agents (WERLE and SEMM, 1956).

Q. Mammary Gland and Milk

The disappearance of oxytocin from the blood of lactating rats is significantly faster than in non-lactating animals (Ginsburg and Smith, 1959). In nephrectomized lactating rats without splanchnic circulation the level of injected oxytocin decreased steadily, whereas in similarly treated non-lactating animals a constant level of oxytocin was reached (Heller, 1960). These results indicated that the mammary gland is involved in the clearance of oxytocin.

Werle and Maier (1954) reported that extracts of cow mammary gland were capable of inactivating oxytocin and vasopressin. The enzyme affecting vasopressin was rather stable, whereas that destroying oxytocin was inactivated when kept for 30 min at pH 5 or at pH 8.5 or when heated at 56° for 1 h. Cysteine and reduced glutathione increased the oxytocin-inactivating capacity of the extracts by several 100%. The oxytocin-inactivating enzymes from cow and goat udder could be inhibited by metal-chelating agents such as 8-hydroxyquinoline and EDTA, by cystine and by PCMB (Werle, 1960). The occurrence of an enzyme or enzymes in cow mammary gland capable of cleaving both oxytocin and L-cystine di-β-naphthylamide was noted in a recent study by Suska-Brzezińska, Golebska, and Ewy, 1965).

Colostrum of women and cows was found to have a low oxytocin- and vasopressin-cleaving activity which, however, could be markedly increased by the addition of cysteine (Werle, Hevelke, and Buthmann, 1941; Werle and Kalvelage, 1941; Werle, 1960). Milk was inactive unless sulphydryl compounds were added. The CAP activity of human milk was higher a few days *post partum* than it was one month later (Hashimoto, 1961b).

IV. The Action of Enzymes on Neurohypophysial Hormone Analogues and Precursors

The ability of human pregnancy plasma to inactivate oxytocin and vasopressin is due, at least to a large extent, to the action of an aminopeptidase, plasma oxytocinase, which splits the bond between the amino-terminal hemicystine residue and the adjoining tyrosine residue. In various tissue homogenates and extracts aminopeptidases were also found to be involved in the destruction of neurohypophysial hormones. This chapter will deal with analogues of oxytocin and vasopressin which had an altered susceptibility to aminopeptidases and were therefore expected to show a modified metabolic behaviour.

One group of analogues to be considered here are those which have been rendered resistant to aminopeptidase action by alteration of the amino-terminal hemicystine residue.

Deamino-oxytocin is not susceptible to attack by hog kidney LAP (Golubow and Du Vigneaud, 1963) and, contrary to oxytocin, by pregnancy plasma oxytocinase (Golubow, Chan, and Du Vigneaud, 1963). The question was raised whether the remarkably high activity of deamino-oxytocin on the pregnant human uterus *in situ* may be due to its resistance to oxytocinase (Saameli, 1964; Embrey, 1965; Althabe, Arnt, Branda, and Caldeyro-Barcia, 1966). There are arguments which contradict such a hypothesis. Deamino-oxytocin and oxytocin did not show differential persistence of their action on the human uterus (Saameli, 1964). During the 20 sec required for the transport of injected hormone from the arm vein to the uterus, the amount of oxytocin inactivated by pregnancy blood will be less than 5% (Althabe, Arnt, Branda, and Caldeyro-Barcia, 1966). Furthermore, oxytocinase is absent from the plasma of the pregnant cat in which deamino-oxytocin is nevertheless twice as potent as oxytocin as a stimulant of the uterus *in situ*. Thus, it appears that resistance to enzymatic inactivation is not a prime factor contributing to the enhanced potency of deamino-oxytocin.

In lactating women, on the third day of the puerperium, when the blood of the patients inactivated oxytocin but not deamino-oxytocin, the latter was found to have a milk-ejecting potency 1.5 times greater than oxytocin. Sixteen months later, when oxytocinase had completely disappeared from the blood, there was no significant difference in milk-ejecting potency between the two peptides (ALTHABE, ARNT, BRANDA, and CALDEYRO-BARCIA, 1966). A small part of the difference in potency observed during the early puerperium may possibly be due to the sensitivity of oxytocin, and the lack of sensitivity of deamino-oxytocin, to the action of plasma oxytocinase.

Deamino^{1}-lysine^{8}-vasopressin has higher antidiuretic, oxytocic and avian depressor activities than its parent compound, lysine-vasopressin. The possibility has been discussed by SCHWARTZ and LIVINGSTON (1964) that the enhanced biological activities could be due to prolonged survival of the deamino compound in the circulation or at the site of function due to its resistance to aminopeptidase attack. Retarded enzymatic degradation, however, cannot be responsible for all of the altered biological effects of deamino-vasopressin, since the mammalian pressor potency of the deamino compound is not enhanced but rather decreased as compared with that of its parent hormone.

(N-Me)Cys^{1}-oxytocin and D-Cys^{1}-oxytocin, both of which may be assumed to be resistant to degradation by aminopeptidases, were found to exhibit effects which were qualitatively indistinguishable from those of oxytocin itself (BERÁNKOVÁ-KSANDROVÁ, BISSET, JOŠT, KREJČÍ, PLIŠKA, RUDINGER, RYCHLÍK, and ŠORM, 1966). A protracted type of action could not be observed.

In a second group of analogues, resistance to aminopeptidase action was achieved by modifying the peptide bond which is cleaved by the enzyme. The sole representative of this group, (N-Me)Tyr^{2}-oxytocin, exhibited less than 1% of the oxytocic potency of oxytocin and was therefore not considered suitable for a more detailed study (HUGUENIN and BOISSONNAS, 1961).

In a third group of analogues, an additional amino acid or a short peptide chain was attached to the free amino group of the N-terminal hemicystine residue of oxytocin or of vasopressin (DU VIGNEAUD, FITT, BODANSZKY, and O'CONNELL, 1960; JOŠT, RUDINGER, and ŠORM, 1963; ZAORAL, PLIŠKA, ŘEŽABEK, and ŠORM, 1963; ZAORAL and ŠORM, 1964, 1965; KASAFIREK, JOŠT, RUDINGER, and ŠORM, 1965; KASAFIREK, RÁBEK, RUDINGER, and ŠORM, 1966). Compounds belonging to the third group produced a protracted effect in several *in vivo* tests. In many instances the protracted response was followed by tachyphylaxis and inhibition of subsequent responses. The protracted effect of these analogues appears to be due to the gradual enzymatic removal of the substituent group, causing continous liberation of active hormone. The term "hormonogen" was proposed to describe such compounds (RYCHLÍK, 1964; BERÁNKOVÁ-KSANDROVÁ, BISSET, JOŠT, KREJČÍ, PLIŠKA, RUDINGER, RYCHLÍK, and ŠORM, 1966).

The series of extended-chain analogues of oxytocin included glycyl-, sarcosyl-, L- and D-leucyl-, L-phenylalanyl-, L-prolyl-, glycyl-glycyl-, L-leucyl-L-leucyl-, and L-leucyl-glycyl-glycyl-oxytocin. Lysine-vasopressin was extended at the amino end by leucine, phenylalanine, tyrosine, tryptophan, proline, glycyl-glycine, leucyl-leucine, glycyl-proline, sarcosyl-glycine and glycyl-glycyl-glycine. In the series of oxytocin analogues, both the intensity of the biological response and its persistence were found to be dependent on the structure of the additional amino acid or peptide chain. Biological activity was higher for the leucyl- and phenylalanyl derivatives than for the glycyl derivatives. The prolongation of the effect, on the other hand, was found to be most pronounced in those extended-chain analogues in which glycine or a glycine peptide was the substituent, and least marked in those in which the substituent was leucine or phenylalanine. The index of persistence of the activity of the analogues is related to the specificity of leucine aminopeptidase. This enzyme as well as some other aminopeptidases are known to split leucyl and phenylalanyl derivatives much more rapidly than glycyl derivatives. Two analogues, sarcosyl- and D-leucyl-oxytocin, in which the terminal amino group of oxytocin was substituted by an amino acid which was not expected to be split by aminopeptidases *in vivo*, did not exhibit protracted or inhibitory effects. These findings provided indirect evidence for the involvement of enzymes in the action of hormonogens.

Direct evidence for the enzymatic release of hormone from hormonogens was obtained from *in vitro* incubation experiments (RYCHLÍK, 1964; BERÁNKOVÁ-KSANDROVÁ, RYCHLÍK, and ŠORM, 1964). When leucyl-oxytocin was incubated with dialysed liver cell sap, the oxytocic activity of the incubation mixture gradually increased. Concomitant with the rise in biological activity, leucine was liberated as revealed by chromatography. 15% of the biological activity and 35% of the amount of leucine expected by theory could be recovered in such experiments. When leucyl-oxytocin was incubated with human pregnancy serum, there was an initial rise in biological activity which was soon followed by a decrease. This finding could be accounted for by the fact that pregnancy plasma oxytocinase, contrary to dialysed liver cell sap, does not only remove the "extra" leucine residue from the amino end of oxytocin, but is also capable of inactivating oxytocin once it has been set free.

Within the past few years numerous "synthetic hormonogens" have been prepared and some of them have been studied with regard to their enzymatic conversion to neurohypophysial hormones. Investigations of this kind are valuable not only from a pharmacological point of view. They may also serve to stimulate the investigation of "physiological hormonogens". In recent years, evidence has accumulated which indicates that there may be precursors from which the neurohypophysial hormones arise in the organism (SACHS and TAKABATAKE, 1964; PREDDIE, 1965). It has not yet been established, however, whether enzymes are involved, and if so, which enzymes are active in the conversion of hormonogens to hormones.

References

ACHER, R.: Évolution moléculaire dans le domaine des hormones neurohypophysaires. VII Giornate Biochim. latine, p. 209—221 (1963).

—, et J. CHAUVET: La structure de la vasopressine de boeuf. Biochim. biophys. Acta (Amst.) **12**, 487—488 (1953).

— — La structure de la vasopressine de boeuf. Biochim. biophys. Acta (Amst.) **14**, 421—429 (1954).

— —, M. T. CHAUVET, et D. CREPY: Isolement d'une nouvelle hormone neurohypophysaire, l'isotocine, présente chez les poissons osseux. Biochim. biophys. Acta (Amst.) **58**, 624—625 (1962).

— — —, et D. CREPY: Phylogénie des peptides neurohypophysaires: Isolement de la mesotocine ($Ileu_8$-ocytocine) de la grenouille, intermédiaire entre la Ser_4-$Ileu_8$-ocytocine des poissons osseux et l'ocytocine des mammifères. Biochim. biophys. Acta (Amst.) **90**, 613—615 (1964).

— — —, et D. CREPY: Phylogénie des peptides neurohypophysaires: Isolement d'une nouvelle hormone, la glumitocine (Ser_4-Gln_8-ocytocine) présente chez un poisson cartilagineux, la raie (Raia clavata). Biochim. biophys. Acta (Amst.) **107**, 393—396 (1965).

— —, et M.-T. LENCI: L'ocytocine et la vasopressine du cheval. Bull. Soc. Chim. biol. (Paris) **40**, 2005—2018 (1958).

ACHER, R., J. CHAUVET, et M.-T. LENCI: Purification et structure de l'ocytocine et de la vasopressine du cheval. Biochim. biophys. Acta (Amst.) **31**, 545—548 (1959).

—, et C. FROMAGEOT: Chimie des hormones neurohypophysaires. Ergebn. Physiol. **48**, 285—327 (1955).

AFONSO, J.F., and N.G. FARNHAM: Studies of a new electrophoretic zone in labor and the puerperium and in newborn infants. Amer. J. Obstet. Gynec. **84**, 199—205 (1962).

ALTHABE, O., I.C. ARNT, L.A. BRANDA, and R. CALDEYRO-BARCIA: Comparison of the milk-ejecting potencies of oxytocin and deamino-oxytocin in lactating women. J. Endocr. **36**, 7—14 (1966).

AMES, R.G., and H.B. VAN DYKE: Thioglycollate inactivation of posterior pituitary antidiuretic principle as determined in the rat. Proc. Soc. exp. Biol. (N. Y.) **76**, 576—578 (1951).

ANASTAS'EVA, N.V.: Effect of pituitrin, quinine, proserine and phenatine on the activity of blood serum oxytocinase of pregnant female rabbits. Nauchn. Zap. Uzhgorodsk. Gos. Univ. **45**, 17—21 (1961).
Chem. Abstr. **59**, 15811 e (1963).

ARAGON, G.T.: An evaluation of plasma pitocinase determination in the toxemias of pregnancy. Amer. J. Obstet. Gynec. **55**, 961—966 (1948).

ARIMURA, A., and T. YAMAGUCHI: Serum protein-vasopressin binding and its influence on the pressor activity of the hormone. Jap. J. Physiol. **14**, 90—101 (1964).

ARST, H.E., R.T. MANNING, and M. DELP: Serum leucine aminopeptidase activity: Findings in carcinoma of the pancreas, pregnancy, and other disorders. Amer. J. med. Sci. **238**, 598—609 (1959).

AUDRAIN, L., et H. CLAUSER: Relation entre l'activité physiologique de l'ocytocine et l'état des son pont disulfure. Biochim. biophys. Acta (Amst.) **30**, 191—192 (1958).

— — Mécanisme de l'inactivation de l'ocytocine par le tissu utérin. Biochim. biophys. Acta (Amst.) **38**, 494—501 (1960).

BABUNA, C., and E. YENEN: Enzymatic determination of placental function. A rapid method. Amer. J. Obstet. Gynec. **95**, 925—934 (1966).

BARNAFI, L., R. ROSAS, T. PEREDA, and H. CROXATTO: Effect of vasopressin structural modifications on rat renal excretion of Na, K and water. Amer. J. Physiol. **202**, 593—596 (1962).

BARNES, A.C., and I.B. SAWYER: Measurements of vasopressinase in maternal and cord blood. Amer. J. Obstet. Gynec. **79**, 1053—1057 (1960).

BARTH, T., V. PLIŠKA, and I. RYCHLÍK: Chymotryptic and tryptic cleavage of oxytocin and vasopressin. Collection Czech. Chem. Commun. **32**, 1058—1063 (1967).

— — —, and F. ŠORM: Enzymic inactivation of oxytocin. V. Purification and some properties of enzymes from human retroplacental serum. Collection Czech. Chem. Commun. **32**, 2327—2336 (1967).

BARTIK, M., and E. MICHNOVA: Polarographic determination of oxytocinase and a contribution to the characteristics of aminopeptidases. Vet. Med. (Praha) **11**, 645—653 (1966).
Chem. Abstr. **66**, 43882 (1967).

BARTOŠEK, I., V. PLIŠKA, I. RYCHLÍK, and F. ŠORM: The inactivation of oxytocin in the liver. The proteolytic splitting. Probl. Evolyutsionnoi i Tekhn. Biokhim., Akad. Nauk SSSR, Inst. Biokhim., 276—286 (1964).

—, I. RYCHLÍK, and F. ŠORM: The inactivation of oxytocin in tissues. Proc. 2nd Int. Pharmacol. Meeting, Prague 1963, **10**, 185—188 (1964).

BECKMAN, L., G. BJÖRLING, and C. CHRISTODOULOU: Pregnancy enzymes and placental polymorphism. II. Leucine aminopeptidase. Acta genet. (Basel) **16**, 122—131 (1966a).

— — — Multiple molecular forms of leucine aminopeptidase in man. Acta genet. (Basel) **16**, 223—230 (1966b).

—, and M. GRIVEA: Variations in serum leucine aminopeptidase in pregnant women and in newborn children. Acta Paediat. Scand. **54**, 578—580 (1965).

BEHAL, F.J., R.D. HAMILTON, C.B. KANAVAGE, and E.C. KELLY: Studies on aminopeptidases in human blood. Arch. Biochem. **100**, 308—312 (1963).

BELLER, F.K., u. U. GÖBELSMANN: Der Abbau von natürlichem und synthetischem Oxytocin durch Oxytocinase. Klin. Wschr. **36**, 1005—1008 (1958).

— — Methodische Probleme der Serumoxytocinase-Bestimmung im Schwangerenserum. Acta endocr. (Kbh.) **31**, 467—480 (1959a).

— — Untersuchungen über die Serum-Oxytocinase. Bibl. Gynaec. (Basel) **20**, 174—178 (1959b).

—, u. H. SCHNIZ: Quantitative Probleme der Oxytozininaktivierung. Geburtsh. u. Frauenheilk. **20**, 563—569 (1960).

BERÁNKOVÁ, Z., I. RYCHLÍK, and F. ŠORM: Inhibition of oxytocin inactivation by some peptides. Experientia (Basel) **15**, 298—299 (1959).

Beránková, Z., I. Rychlík, and F. Šorm: Enzymic inactivation of oxytocin. I. Selective inhibitors of oxytocin inactivation. Collection Czech. Chem. Commun. **25**, 2575—2580 (1960).

— — — Enzymic inactivation of oxytocin. II. Fission of some peptide fragments of the oxytocin structure and their derivatives by pregnancy serum and liver cell sap. Collection Czech. Chem. Commun. **26**, 1708—1715 (1961).

—, and F. Šorm: Enzymic inactivation of oxytocin. III. Desthiooxytocin and S,S'-dibenzyldihydrooxytocin as oxytocinase inhibitors and substrates. Collection Czech. Chem. Commun. **26**, 2557—2561 (1961).

Beránková-Ksandrová, Z., G.W. Bisset, K. Jošt, I. Krejčí, V. Pliška, J. Rudinger, I. Rychlík, and F. Šorm: Synthetic analogues to oxytocin acting as hormonogens. Brit. J. Pharmacol. **26**, 615—632 (1966).

—, I. Rychlík, and F. Šorm: Oxytocin analogues with protracted effects. Proc. 2nd Int. Pharmacol. Meeting, Prague 1963, **10**, 181—183 (1964).

Birnie, J.H.: The inactivation of posterior pituitary antidiuretic hormone by liver extracts. Endocrinology **52**, 33—38 (1953).

—, K.E. Blackmore, and H. Heller: Changes in water diuresis and vasopressin inactivation in mice fed on protein deficient diets. Experientia (Basel) **8**, 30—31 (1952).

Bisset, G.W.: Effect of tyrosinase preparations on oxytocin, vasopressin and bradykinin. Brit. J. Pharmocol. **18**, 405—420 (1962).

— The effect on milk-ejecting activity of modifying two functional groups in oxytocin. In: Proc. 2nd Int. Pharmacol. Meeting, Prague 1963, **10**, 21—30 (1964).

Bonow, A., W. Carol, u. S. Wachtel: Die Bestimmung der Serum-Oxytocinase-Aktivität auf chemischem Wege. Zbl. Gynäk. **85**, 1537—1542 (1963).

Borov, V.I.: Activity of oxytocinase and cholinesterases at the end of pregancy and during labour. Akusherstwo i Ginekol. **42**, 39—42 (1966). Chem. Abstr. **65**, 17306f (1966).

Braun-Falco, O., u. K. Salfeld: Über das Verhalten der Leucinaminopeptidase-Aktivität im Blutserum und Blaseninhalt. II. Untersuchungen an Patienten mit Psoriasis, Neurodermatitis diffusa, Dermatitis, Ekzem und anderen Dermatosen. Arch. klin. exp. Derm. **205**, 103—111 (1957).

Bressler, R., and B.R. Forsyth: Serum leucine aminopeptidase activity in normal pregnancy and in patients with hydatidiform mole. New Engl. J. Med. **261**, 746—748 (1959).

— —, and G. Klatskin: Serum leucine aminopeptidase activity in hepatobiliary and pancreatic disease. J. Lab. clin. Med. **56**, 417—430 (1960).

Campbell, B.J., B. Thysen, and F.S. Chu: Peptidase catalyzed hydrolysis of antidiuretic hormone in toad bladder. Life Sci. **4**, 2129—2140 (1965).

Camu, F., and V. Conard: Effect de l'ocytocine sur l'inactivation de l'insuline par le rein de rat normal *in vitro*. Arch. int. Pharmacodyn. **162**, 247—252 (1966).

Carballo, M.A.: Discussion remark. In: Oxytocin. Ed. by R. Caldeyro-Barcia and H. Heller. Proc. Int. Symp., Montevideo **1959**, 343 (1961).

—, and C.J. Méndez-Bauer: Evolution of oxytocinase during pregnancy and induced labour. Proc. 2nd Uruguayan Congr. Obstet. Ginecol. **2**, 300—307 (1957a).

— — Placental origin of oxytocinase. Proc. 2nd Uruguayan Congr. Obstet. Ginec. **2**, 308—313 (1957b).

Centaro, A., P. Periti, and G. de Laurentiis: Oxytocin and oxytocinase activity of the blood and myometrium of women in labor. Riv. Ostet. Ginec. **16**, 297—326 (1961).

Cespedes, J., and H. Croxatto: Action of oxidants (thiol antagonists) on the oxytocinase activity of blood serum. Bol. Soc. Biol. Santiago **7**, 43—46 (1949).

Chauvet, J., M.-T. Chauvet, et R. Acher: Les hormones neurohypophysaires des mammifêres: Isolement et caractérisation de l'ocytocine et de la vasopressine de la balaine (*Balaenoptera physalus L.*). Bull. Soc. Chim. Biol. (Paris) **45**, 1369—1378 (1963).

Christlieb, M.: Über den Abbau von Oxytocin und Vasopressin *in vitro*. Arch. Exp. Pathol. Pharmakol. **194**, 44—51 (1940).

Čihař, M., Z. Beránková, I. Rychlík, and F. Šorm: Enzymic inactivation of oxytocin. IV. Characterization of purified preparations of serum oxytocinase. Collection Czech. Chem. Commun. **26**, 2632—2642 (1961).

Cooper, D.W.: A serum protein present in pregnant women. Nature (Lond.) **200**, 892 (1963).

Crewther, W.G., and F.G. Lennox: Preparation of crystals containing protease from *Aspergillus oryzae*. Nature (Lond.) **165**, 680 (1950).

Croxatto, H.: Hypertensinase action. Inactivation of hypertensin and pressor and oxytocic principles of the posterior pituitary in the organism. Rev. Med. Aliment. (Santiago) **5**, 259—271 (1942/1943).

—, J. Alliende, and R. Croxatto: Action of aminopolypeptidase of yeast and hypertensinase of kidney extracts on the oxytocic principle of the posterior pituitary. Rev. Med. Aliment. (Santiago) **5**, 228—229 (1942/43a).

Croxatto, H., J. Alliende, and R. Croxatto: Action of trypsin and chymotrypsin on the oxytocic principle of the posterior pituitary. Rev. Med. Aliment. (Santiago) **5**, 230—231 (1942/43b).

—, W. Badia, and R. Croxatto: Effect of fibrinolysin on oxytocin, vasopressin and hypertensinogen. Proc. Soc. exp. Biol. (N. Y.) **69**, 422—425 (1948).

—, and J. Cespedes: Action of cytochrome C on the oxytocinase and vasopressinase activity of blood serum. Bol. Soc. Biol. Santiago **7**, 54—57 (1950).

— —, and S. Daza: The effect of thiosorbitol on the inactivation of oxytocin and vasopressin by blood plasma. Bol. Soc. Biol. Santiago **8**, 96—100 (1951).

—, R. Croxatto, and J. Alliende: Destruction of oxytocin by the aminopeptidase of beer yeast and by extracts of hypertensive kidneys. Rev. Soc. argent. Biol. **18**, 441—453 (1942).

— —, G. Illanes, and H. Salvestrini: Action of chymotrypsin and trypsin on hypertensin and pressor and oxytocic principles of the posterior pituitary. Rev. Med. Aliment. (Santiago) **5**, 300—302 (1942/1943).

— —, and M. Reyes: The effect of hypertensin on the inactivation of oxytocin by the serum of pregnant women. Science **108**, 658—659 (1948).

— —, and M. Rioseco: Action of carboxypeptidase on pepsitensin, vasopressin and oxytocin. Rev. Soc. argent. Biol. **21**, 23—29 (1945).

—, C. Donoso, and R. Croxatto: Effect of amino acids on the inactivation of oxytocin by kidney hypertensinase extracts. Bol. Soc. Biol. Santiago **5**, 51—53 (1948a).

—, G. Illanes, H. Salvestrini, and R. Croxatto: Action of aminopolypeptidase and hypertensinase extracts from kidney on the pressor principle of the post-pituitary. Rev. Med. Aliment. (Santiago) **5**, 226—228 (1942/1943).

—, and J. de la Maza: Action of tyrosinase (extracts of *Psalliota Campestris*) on vasopressin. Bol. Soc. Biol. Santiago **2**, 46—48 (1944).

—, T. Pereda, and B. Zamorano: Oxytocic substances in blood serum. In: Oxytocin. Proc. Int. Symp., Montevideo **1959**, 412—424 (Publ. 1961).

—, and M. Reyes: Effect of cysteine and glutathione on the oxytocinase activity of blood plasma. Bol. Soc. Biol. Santiago **5**, 80—82 (1948).

—, R. Rosas, and L. Bárnafi: Effect of vasopressin and oxytocin on excretion of water and electrolytes (Na, Cl, and K) in the albino rat. Acta physiol. lat.-amer. **6**, 147—152 (1956).

—, A. Trautmann, and R. Croxatto: Destruction of hypertensin and the pressor and oxytocic principles of the posterior pituitary by extracts of red blood cells and kidney. Rev. Med. Aliment. (Santiago) **5**, 305—308 (1943).

—, C. Vera, and L. Bárnafi: Inactivation of antidiuretic hormone by blood serum of the pregnant woman. Proc. Soc. exp. Biol. (N. Y) **83**, 784—786 (1953).

Croxatto, R., H. Croxatto, and J. Sorolla: Aminopeptidase character of hypertensinase. Rev. Med. Aliment. (Santiago) **5**, 135—136 (1942/1943).

—, C. Donoso, and H. Croxatto: Effect of amino acids on the inactivation of vasopressin by kidney hypertensinase extracts. Bol. Soc. Biol. (Santiago) **5**, 54—56 (1948b).

Dale, H.H., and H.W. Dudley: On the pituitary active principles and histamine. J. Pharmacol. exp. Ther. **18**, 27—42 (1921).

Dicker, S.E.: The inactivation of vasopressin and of oxytocin, *in vitro*. In: Polypeptides which affect smooth muscles and blood vessels. p. 79—82. Ed. by M. Schachter. Proc. Symp., London **1959**, (Pub. 1960).

—, and M. Ginsburg: Some observations on the antidiuretic activity of rat serum. Brit. J. Pharmacol. **5**, 497—504 (1950).

—, and A.L. Greenbaum: The degree of inactivation of the antidiuretic activity of vasopressin by the kidneys and the liver of rats. J. Physiol. (Lond.) **126**, 116—123 (1954).

— — Inactivation of the antidiuretic activity of vasopressin by tissue homogenates. J. Physiol. (Lond.) **132**, 199—212 (1956).

— — The destruction of the antidiuretic activity of vasopressin by SH active compounds. J. Physiol. (Lond.) **141**, 107—116 (1958).

—, and C. Tyler: Inactivation of oxytocin and vasopressin by blood plasma of pregnant women. J. Obstet. Gynaec. Brit. Emp. **63**, 690—696 (1956).

—, and G.A. Whyley: Inactivation of oxytocin by plasma of pregnant women. J. Physiol. (Lond.) **146**, 33—34 P (1959a).

— — Inactivation of oxytocin by plasma of pregnant women. J. Obstet. Gynaec. Brit. Emp. **66**, 605—609 (1959b).

— — The role of oxytocinase during pregnancy in man and animals. Acta endocr. (Kbh.) **34**, (Suppl. **51**), 145 (1960).

Dieckmann, W.J., G.F. Egenolf, B. Morley, and R.E. Pottinger: The inactivation of the antidiuretic hormone of the posterior pituitary gland by blood from pregnant patients. Amer. J. Obstet. Gynec. **60**, 1043—1050 (1950).

DLOUHÁ, H., M. KRAUS, J. KŘEČEK, and V. PLIŠKA: Sensitivity of rats to vasopressin in the weaning period. Physiol. bohemoslov. **14**, 217—224 (1965).
DREWNIAK, K.: Evaluation of a biochemical method of determining the term of delivery. Ginek. pol. **35**, 27—32 (1964a).
— Clinical evaluation of the biochemical method of determining the term of delivery. In: Oxytocin and its analogues, p. 55—58. Ed. by R. KLIMEK and W. KROL. Polish Endocr. Soc., Krakow (1964b).
DUDLEY, H. W.: Some observations on the active principles of the pituitary gland. J. Pharmacol. exp. Ther. **14**, 295—312 (1919).
VAN DYKE, H. B., B. F. CHOW, R. O. GREEP, and A. ROTHEN: The isolation of a protein from the *pars neuralis* of the ox pituitary with constant oxytocic, pressor and diuresis-inhibiting activities. J. Pharmacol. exp. Ther. **74**, 190—209 (1942).
EHRENSING, R. H.: Plasma oxytocinase, cystine and leucine naphthylamidases of snake, turtle and chicken. Proc. Soc. exp. Biol. (N. Y.) **117**, 370—373 (1964).
EL-KAMMAH, B. M., and H. TUPPY: Unpublished experiments.
ELLIOTT, D. F., and W. S. PEART: The amino acid sequence in a hypertensin. Biochem. J. **65**, 246—254 (1957).
EMBREY, M. P.: The action of desamino-oxytocin on the human pregnant uterus. J. Endocr. **31**, 185—189 (1965).
EVERSOLE, W. J., J. H. BIRNIE, and R. GAUNT: Inactivation of posterior pituitary antidiuretic hormone by the liver. Endocrinology **45**, 378—382 (1949).
FEKETE, K.: Beiträge zur Physiologie der Gravidität. Endokrinologie **7**, 364—369 (1930).
— Gibt es während der Schwangerschaft ein aktives Hypophysen-Hinterlappenhormon im Blute? Endokrinologie **10**, 16—23 (1932).
— Beiträge zur Erklärung des Geburtseintrittes. Endokrinologie **12**, 183—192 (1933).
FOLK, J. E., and P. W. COLE: Chymotrypsin C. II. Enzymatic specificity toward several polypeptides. J. biol. Chem. **240**, 193—197 (1965).
FRASER, A. M.: The effect of arginase and of tyrosinase on the activity and composition of posterior pituitary extracts. Rev. canad. Biol. **9**, 54—61 (1950).
FREUDENBERG, K., E. WEISS u. H. BILLER: Notiz über Oxytocin. Z. Physiol. Chem. **233**, 172—173 (1935).
— —, u. H. EYER: Über Insulin und Pitutocin. Naturwissenschaften **20**, 685 (1932).
FRIED, R., u. L. WÜST: Über ein Oxytocin-abbauendes Ferment aus Schweineovarien. Naturwissenschaften **41**, 238 (1954).
FUHRMANN, K.: Kolorimetrische Bestimmung und histochemischer Nachweis der Aminopeptidase an Geweben weiblicher Genitalorgane. Zbl. Gynäk. **81**, 1105—1123 (1959).
FYLLING, P.: Serum and plasma oxytocinase activity during induction of labour. Acta obstet. gynec. scand. **42**, 227—239 (1963).
— Plasma oxytocinase activity, oestriol and pregnanediol excretion and the effect of induction of labour. Acta obstet. gynec. scand. **43**, 58—63 (1964a).
— Plasma oxytocinase activity following a single injection of pitocin. Acta obstet. gynec. scand. **43**, 103—106 (1964b).
— Serum and plasma leucine aminopeptidase activity during induction of labor. Scand. J. clin. Lab. Invest. **16**, 172—176 (1964c).
GINSBURG, M., H. HELLER, and S. M. A. ZAIDI: Re-appraisal of the evidence for the metabolic conversion of vasopressin into a less active derivative. Nature (Lond.) **178**, 803—804 (1956).
—, and M. W. SMITH: The fate of oxytocin in male and female rats. Brit. J. Pharmacol. **14**, 327—333 (1959).
DI GIROLAMO, M., D. RUDMAN, M. F. MALKIN, and L. A. GARCIA: Inactivation of insulin by adipose tissue. Diabetes **14**, 87—92 (1965).
GLENDENING, M. B., M. A. TITUS, S. A. SCHROEDER, G. MOHUN, and E. W. PAGE: The destruction of oxytocin and vasopressin by the aminopeptidases in sera from pregnant women. Amer. J. Obstet. Gynec. **92**, 814—820 (1965).
GOEBELSMANN, U., and F. K. BELLER: Separation of cystine-aminopeptidase and leucine-aminopeptidase and their determination in pregnant and nonpregnant women. Z. klin. Chem. **3**, 49—54 (1965).
GOLUBOW, J., W. Y. CHAN, and V. DU VIGNEAUD: Effect of human pregnancy serum on avian depressor activities of oxytocin and desamino-oxytocin. Proc. Soc. exp. Biol. (N. Y.) **113**, 113—115 (1963).
—, and V. DU VIGNEAUD: Comparison of susceptibility of oxytocin and desamino-oxytocin to inactivation by leucine aminopeptidase and α-chymotrypsin. Proc. Soc. exp. Biol. (N.Y.) **112**, 218—219 (1963).
GONZÁLEZ-PANIZZA, V. H., Y. SICA-BLANCO, and C. MÉNDEZ-BAUER: The fate of injected oxytocin in the pregnant woman near term. In: Oxytocin, p. 347—357. Ed. by R. CALDEYRO-BARCIA and H. HELLER. Proc. Int. Symp., Montevideo 1959 (1961).

GREEN, M.N., K.-C. TSOU, R. BRESSLER, and A.M. SELIGMAN: The colorimetric determination of leucine aminopeptidase activity with L-leucine-β-naphthylamide hydrochloride. Arch. Biochem. **57**, 458—474 (1955).

GULLAND, J.M., and T.F. MACRAE: The action of proteolytic enzymes on the oxytocic principle of the pituitary gland. Nature (Lond.) **131**, 470 (1933a).

— — The oxytocic hormone of the posterior lobe of the pituitary gland. III. The action of preparations of plant proteolytic enzymes. Biochem. J. **27**, 1237—1247 (1933b).

— — The oxytocic hormone of the posterior lobe of the pituitary gland. IV. The action of preparations of animal proteolytic enzymes, and some observations on the nature of the hormone. Biochem. J. **27**, 1383—1393 (1933c).

GÜNTELBERG, A.V., and M. OTTESEN: Preparation of crystals containing the plakalbumin-forming enzyme from *Bacillus subtilis*. Nature (Lond.) **170**, 802 (1952).

HALLER, E.W., H. SACHS, N. SPERELAKIS, and L. SHARE: Release of vasopressin from isolated guinea pig posterior pituitaries. Amer. J. Physiol. **209**, 79—83 (1965).

HANKISS, J.E., M. KESZTHELYI, and P. DEMÉNY: Inactivation of vasopressin by heart muscle. Tohoku J. exp. Med. **87**, 168—174 (1965).

HANON, F., and M. BRUNAUD: Determinism of uterine contraction at parturition. C. R. Soc. Biol. (Paris) **141**, 163—164 (1947).

HANSON, H., u. H.G. MANNSFELDT: Zur Aktivitätsbestimmung der Serum-Oxytocinase des menschlichen Schwangeren-Serums unter Verwendung chromogener Substrate. In prepn. (1967a).

— — Untersuchungen über die Angreifbarkeit von Serum-Oxytocinase-Substraten durch Gewebs-Enzyme („Gewebs-Oxytocinase") tierischer Organe. In prepn. (1967b).

— — Über die Humanplacenta als Synthese-Organ der schwangerschaftsspezifischen Serum-Oxytocinase des Menschen. In prepn. (1967c)

HARDY, S.M., and J.M. RITCHIE: Determination of serum oxytocinase (l-cystine-aminopeptidase) activity. Nature (Lond.) **209**, 76—77 (1966).

HASHIMOTO, T.: Studies on l-cystine-aminopeptidase. I. Biochemical aspect. J. Jap. obstet. gynaec. Soc. **8**, 87—95 (1961a).

— Studies on l-cystine-aminopeptidase. II. Clinical observations. J. Jap. obstet. gynaec. Soc. **8**, 96—104 (1961b)

HAWKER, R.W.: Inactivation of antidiuretic hormone and oxytocin during pregnancy. Quart. J. exp. Physiol. **41**, 301—308 (1956).

— Antidiuretic substance (ADS) in normal pregnancy and pre-eclamptic toxaemia. J. Endocr. **14**, 400—410 (1957).

— Oxytocin and an unidentified oxytocic substance in extracts of blood. In: Oxytocin, 425—436. Proc. Int. Symp., Montevideo 1959 (Publ. 1961).

—, and P.A. ROBERTSON: Oxytocin and lactation. J. clin. Endocr. **17**, 448—451 (1957).

— — Are there two oxytocic hormones? Med. J. Aust. **1958 I**, 671—672.

—, C.F. WALMSLEY, V.S. ROBERTS, and P.A. ROBERTSON: Further observations on oxytocin and oxytocic substance. Med. J. Aust. **1959** I, 460—461.

HELLER, H.: The metabolism and fate of the neurohypophysial principles. In: The neurohypophysis, p. 77—96. Ed. by H. HELLER. London: Butterworths Scientific Publications (1957).

— Inactivation of vasopressin and oxytocin *in vivo*. In: Polypeptides which affect smooth muscles and blood vessels, p. 59—69. Ed. by M. SCHACHTER. Proc. Symp., London **1959** (Pub. 1960).

—, and F.F. URBAN: The fate of the antidiuretic principle of postpituitary extracts *in vivo* and *in vitro*. J. Physiol. (London) **85**, 502—518 (1935).

—, and S.M.A. ZAIDI: The metabolism of exogenous and endogenous antidiuretic hormone in the kidney and liver *in vivo*. Brit. J. Pharmacol. **12**, 284—292 (1957).

HESS, R.: Arylamidase activity related to angiotensinase. Biochim. biophys. Acta (Amst.) **99**, 316—324 (1965).

HILL, R.L., and E.L. SMITH: Leucine aminopeptidase. VII. Action on long chain polypeptides and proteins. J. biol. Chem. **228**, 577—600 (1957).

— — Complete hydrolysis of glucagon by leucine aminopeptidase. Biochim. biophys. Acta (Amst.) **31**, 257—258 (1959).

HILTON, J.G., and R.F. JOHNSON: Changes in blood oxytocinase during parturition. Amer. J. Obstet. Gynec. **78**, 479—482 (1959).

HIRSCHFELD, J., and U. SÖDERBERG: Immuno-electrophoretic demonstration of precipitating components in sera from pregnant women. Nature (Lond.) **187**, 332—333 (1960).

HOOPER, K.C.: The action of inhibitors on enzymes from human placentae. J. Physiol. (London) **148**, 283—290 (1959).

— The preparation of soluble vasopressinase from human placenta. Biochem. J. **74**, 297—300 (1960a).

Hooper, K. C.: Some properties of enzymes destroying oxytocin and vasopressin. In: Polypeptides which affect smooth muscles and blood vessels, p. 83—86. Ed. by M. Schachter. Proc. Symp. (London) **1959** (Pub. 1960b).
— The preparation and properties of cystine esterase. Biochem. J. **78**, 409—412 (1961a).
— The catabolism of bradykinin, oxytocin, substance P and vasopressin by homogenate of dog hypothalamus. Biochem. J. **81**, 44 P (1961b).
— The catabolism of some physiologically active polypeptides by homogenate of dog hypothalamus. Biochem. J. **83**, 511—517 (1962a).
— The intracellular distribution of enzymes inactivating oxytocin in the dog hypothalamus. Biochem. J. **85**, 8 P (1962b).
— The enzymic inactivation of some physiologically active polypeptides by different parts of the nervous system. Biochem. J. **88**, 398—404 (1963a).
— The effect of pregnancy on the distribution of hypothalamic enzymes inactivating oxytocin. Biochem. J. **88**, 67 P (1963b).
— The distribution of hypothalamic peptidases in pregnant and non-pregnant dogs. Biochem. J. **90**, 584—587 (1964).
— Some observations on the behaviour of hypothalamic enzymes during the time of blastocyst implantation in the rabbit. Biochem. J. **99**, 128—132 (1966a).
— The metabolism of oxytocin during lactation in the rabbit. Biochem. J. **100**, 823—826 (1966b).
— and D. C. Jessup: The distribution of enzymes destroying oxytocin and vasopressin in human placentae. J. Physiol. (Lond.) **146**, 539—549 (1959).
Hopsu, V. K., S. Ruponen, and S. Talanti: Leucine aminopeptidase in the placenta of the rat. Acta histochem. (Jena) **12**, 305—309 (1961).
Huguenin, R. L., and R. A. Boissonnas: Synthèse de la (N-méthyl-Tyr)²-oxytocine. Helv. chim. Acta **44**, 213—231 (1961).
Ichaliotis, S. D., and Th. C. Lambrinopoulos: Preeclampsia associated with decrease in serum oxytocinase. Obstet. and Gynec. **24**, 659—661 (1964).
— — Serum oxytocinase in twin pregnancy. Obstet. and Gynec. **25**, 270—272 (1965).
Itoh, S., and T. Kikuchi: Inactivation of antidiuretic activity of vasopressin by hypothalamic tissue in the presence of pyridoxal. Jap. J. Physiol. **9**, 401—405 (1959).
James, N. T.: Histochemical demonstration of oxytocinase in the human placenta. Nature (Lond.) **210**, 1276—1277 (1966).
Johnson, M. J.: Isolation and properties of a pure yeast polypeptidase. J. biol. Chem. **137**, 575—586 (1941).
Jones, A. M., and W. Schlapp: The action and fate of injected posterior pituitary extracts in the decapitated cat. J. Physiol. (Lond.) **87**, 144—157 (1936).
Jošt, K., and J. Rudinger: Amino acids and peptides. XXXIV. Some peptides of S-benzylcysteine. Collection Czech. Chem. Commun. **26**, 2345—2354 (1961).
— —, and F. Šorm: Analogues of oxytocin exerting protracted biological effects. Collection Czech. Chem. Commun. **28**, 2021—2030 (1963).
Kanazawa, T.: Supplementary studies on blood pitocinase. J. Jap. obstet. gynaec. Soc. **1**, 42—72 (1954).
Karlin, A.: The *in vitro* release by the toad bladder of an inhibitor of oxytocin. Biochem. biophys. Res. Commun. **11**, 44—49 (1963).
Kasafirek, E., K. Jošt, J. Rudinger, and F. Šorm: Amino acids and peptides. LIV. Synthesis of further extended-chain analogues of oxytocin. Collection Czech. Chem. Commun. **30**, 2600—2608 (1965).
—, V. Rábek, J. Rudinger, and F. Šorm: Amino acids and peptides. LXVI. Synthesis of ten extended-chain analogues of lysine vasopressin. Collection Czech. Chem. Commun. **31**, 4581—4591 (1966).
Katzen, H. M., and D. Stetten: Hepatic glutathione-insulin transhydrogenase. Diabetes **11**, 271—280 (1962).
—, F. Tietze, and D. Stetten: Further studies on the properties of hepatic glutathione-insulin transhydrogenase. J. biol. Chem. **238**, 1006—1011 (1963).
Kazda, S.: Discussion remark. Proc. 2nd Int. Pharmacol. Meeting, Prague 1963, **10**, 150 (1964).
Kleiner, H., et M. van Rymenant: Détermination placentaire de l'ocytocinase sérique dans l'insuffisance et la mort fétale 'in utero'. Rev. franç. Étud. clin. biol. **9**, 321—323 (1964).
Klimek, R.: Discussion remark. Proc. 2nd. Int. Pharmacol. Meeting, Prague **1963**, **10**, 150 to 151 (1964a).
— Pregnancy and delivery in the light of studies on the oxytocin-oxytocinase system. In: Oxytocin and its analogues, p. 27—38. Ed. by R. Klimek and W. Krol, Polish Endocrinol. Soc., Krakow (1964b).
—, u. M. Pietrzycka: Biochemische Methode zur Bestimmung der Oxytocinase und ihre klinische Bewertung. Clin. chim. Acta **6**, 326—330 (1961).

Klimek, R., M. Pietrzycka, and J. Grochowski: The influence of operative trauma on blood levels of oxytocinase. Clin. chim. Acta **7**, 398—402 (1962).

Kowlessar, O.D., L.J. Haeffner, and E.M. Riley: Localization of serum leucine aminopeptidase, 5-nucleotidase, and nonspecific alkaline phosphatase by starch-gel electrophoresis: Clinical and biochemical significance in disease states. Ann. N. Y. Acad. Sci. **94**, 836—843 (1961).

Lambrinopoulos, T.C.: Prolonged pregnancy associated with increase in serum oxytocinase. Obstet. and Gynec. **23**, 780—782 (1964).

Larson, E.: Tolerance and fate of the pressor principle of posterior pituitary extract in anesthetized animals. J. Pharmacol. exp. Ther. **62**, 346—362 (1938).

— Fate of the injected oxytocic principle of posterior pituitary in anesthetized cats and dogs. J. Pharmacol. exp. Ther. **67**, 175—186 (1939).

Lawler, H.C., S.P. Taylor, A.M. Swan, and V. du Vigneaud: Prensence of glutamine and asparagine in enzymatic hydrolysates of oxytocin and vasopressin. Proc. Soc. exp. Biol. (N.Y.). **87**, 550—552 (1954).

—, and V. du Vigneaud: Enzymatic evidence for intrinsic oxytocic activity of the pressor-antidiuretic hormone. Proc. Soc. exp. Biol. (N. Y.) **84**, 114—116 (1953).

Leblová, S., and I. Rychlík: Inhibition of enzymic inactivation of oxytocin by amino acids. Collection Czech. Chem. Commun. **25**, 2926—2929 (1960).

Lettow, E., u. Ch. Jaeger: Bestimmung der Leucin-Aminopeptidase-Aktivität im Serum trächtiger Hündinnen. Zbl. Vet.-Med. **12**, 388—394 (1965).

Lewis, J.: Serum leucine aminopeptidase values in patients with trophoblastic tumors and in normal pregnancy. Amer. J. Obstet. Gynec. **84**, 1407—1411 (1962).

Linderstrøm-Lang, K., and M. Ottesen: Formation of plakalbumin from ovalbumin. C. R. Lab. Carlsberg, Ser. Chim. **26**, 403 (1949).

Lineweaver, H., and D. Burk: The determination of enzyme dissociation constants. J. Amer. chem. Soc. **56**, 658—666 (1934).

Mac Laren, J.A., R.D. Thornes, C.C. Roby, and D.E. Reid: An immunologic characteristic of the serum of normal pregnancy. Amer. J. Obstet. Gynec. **78**, 939—946 (1959).

Manunta, G.: On the inactivation of oxytocin in the cow. Boll. Soc. ital. Biol. Sper. **36**, 281—284 (1960).

—, and A. Marongiu: On the inactivation of oxytocin in Bos taurus, Equus caballus, Equus asinus, Ovis aries, Canis familiaris, Sus scrofa, Lepus cuniculus, Cavia cobaya, Mus norvegicus albinus, Mus musculus, Gallus gallus and Columbia livia. Boll. Soc. ital. Biol. Sper. **37**, 1—2 (1961).

Martin, G.J., J.N. Moss, and R.D. Smyth: Vasopressin potentiation and simulation by bromelain. Arch. int. Pharmacodyn. **152**, 445—449 (1964).

Martin, P.J., and H.O. Schild: Effect of thiols on oxytocin and vasopressin receptors. Nature (Lond.) **196**, 382—383 (1962).

— — Pharmacological antagonism between SH compounds and S-S polypeptides. Proc. 2nd Int. Pharmacol. Meeting, Prague 1963, **10**, 109—116 (1964).

De la Maza, J., and H. Croxatto: Action of tyrosinase on oxytocin. Bol. Soc. Biol. Santiago **2**, 23—26 (1944).

McCartney, C.P., F.J. Vallach, and R.E. Pottinger: Further studies on the inactivation of pitressin antidiuretic effect by the blood of pregnant women. Amer. J. Obstet. Gynec. **63**, 847—853 (1952).

Melander, S.: Plasma oxytocinase activity. A methodological and clinical study with special reference to pregnancy. Acta endocr. (Kbh.) **49**, Suppl. **96**, 1—94 (1965).

Melander, S.E.J.: Oxytocinase activity of plasma of pregnant women. Nature (Lond.) **191**, 176—177 (1961).

Méndez-Bauer, C.J.: In: Oxytocin, p. 342. Proc. Int. Symp., Montevideo **1959** (Pub. 1961).

—, and M.A. Carballo: Method for the quantitative determination of oxytocin. Proc. 2nd Congr. Urug. Obstet. Gynec. **2**, 291—299 (1957).

— —, H.M. Cabot, C.E. Negreiros de Paiva, and V.H. González-Panizza: Studies on plasma oxytocinase. In: Oxytocin, Proc. Int. Symp., Montevideo **1959**, 325—335 (Pub. 1961).

Milani, L.: Effect of pregnant blood serum on the uteromotor activity of the amniotic fluid. Boll. Soc. ital. Biol. Sper. **27**, 679—682 (1951).

—, and C. Pinetti: Pitocinase. I. Attempts to influence the inactivation of oxytocin by blood serum of the pregnant woman. Boll. Soc. ital. Biol. Sper. **27**, 1—4 (1951).

Miller, Z.B., E. Naor, L. Milkovich, and W.M. Schmidt: Serum levels of cystine aminopeptidase, leucine aminopeptidase, and alkaline phosphatase in single and twin pregnancies. Obstet. and Gynec. **24**, 707—715 (1964).

Müller-Hartburg, W., H. Nesvadba u. H. Tuppy: Die Anwendung einer chemischen Methode zur Bestimmung des Oxytocinasespiegels im Schwangerenserum. Arch. Gynäk. **191**, 442—456 (1959).

Munsick, R. A., W. H. Sawyer, and H. B. van Dyke: Avian neurohypophysial hormones: pharmacological properties and tentative identification. Endocrinology **66**, 860—871 (1960).

Nagatsu, I., L. Gillespie, J. M. George, J. E. Folk, and G. G. Glenner: Serum aminopeptidases, "angiotensinase", and hypertension. II. Amino acid β-naphthylamide hydrolysis by normal and hypertensive serum. Biochem. Pharmacol. **14**, 853—861 (1965).

Namiki, H. (1952), see Kanazawa (1954).

Page, E. W.: The value of plasma pitocinase determinations in obstetrics. Amer. J. Obstet. Gynec. **52**, 1014—1022 (1946).

— A blood test for estimating the week of pregnancy. Science **105**, 292—293 (1947).

—, M. A. Titus, G. Mohun, and M. B. Glendening: The origin and distribution of oxytocinase. Amer. J. Obstet. Gynec. **82**, 1090—1095 (1961).

Periti, P., A. Centaro, and G. de Laurentiis: Oxytocinase activity in the uterus of women in labor and in different conditions of pregnancy. Boll. Soc. ital. Biol. Sper. **37**, 453—455 (1961a).

— — — Oxytocinase in the blood of women in labor. Boll. Soc. ital. Biol. Sper. **37**, 455—457 (1961b).

Perks, A. M., M. H. I. Dodd, and J. M. Dodd: A neurohypophyseal principle in the elasmobranch pituitary. Nature (Lond.) **185**, 850—851 (1960).

—, and W. H. Sawyer: A new neurohypophyseal principle in an elasmobranch, *Raia ocellata*. Nature (Lond.) **205**, 154—156 (1965).

Pliška, V., T. Barth, and I. Rychlík: Effect of human serum oxytocinase on the antidiuretic action of lysine vasopressin and oxytocin in the rat. Experientia (Basel) **23**, 196—197 (1967).

Preddie, E. C.: Structure of a large polypeptide of bovine posterior pituitary tissue. J. biol. Chem. **240**, 4194—4203 (1965).

—, and M. Saffran: Isolation of a large polypeptide from bovine posterior pituitary powder. J. biol. Chem. **240**, 4189—4193 (1965).

Riad, A. M.: Studies on pregnancy serum cystine aminopeptidase activity 'oxytocinase'. J. Obstet. Gynaec. Brit. Emp. **69**, 409—416 (1962).

— Changes in pregnancy serum oxytocinase activity during oxytocin infusion and their physiological significance. J. Obstet. Gynaec. Brit. Cwlth **73**, 977—982 (1966).

—, and F. J. Scandrett: Distribution of cystine aminopeptidase activity (oxytocinase) in human pregnancy sera. Nature (Lond.) **193**, 372—373 (1962).

Riniker, B., u. R. Schwyzer: Die sterische Einheitlichkeit des synthetischen Val^5-Hypertensin II-Asp^1-β-amids. Helv. chim. Acta **44**, 658—667 (1961).

Rittner, Ch.: Über den immunologischen Nachweis von Aminopeptidasen, insbesondere der Oxytocinase (Cystinaminopeptidase). Z. Immun.-Forsch. **131**, 422—433 (1966).

Roth, M.: Fluorimetric assay of some peptidases. West European Symp. Clin. Chem. **4**, 10—17 (1964). Chem. Abstr. **63**, 2054 g (1965).

Royce, P. C., and G. Sayers: Corticotropin releasing activity of a pepsin labile factor in the hypothalamus. Proc. Soc. exp. Biol. (N.Y.) **98**, 677—680 (1958).

Rudman, D., M. F. Malkin, S. J. Brown, L. A. Garcia, and L. L. Abell: Inactivation of adrenocorticotropin, α- and β-melanocyte-stimulating hormones, vasopressin, and pituitary fraction H by adipose tissue. J. Lipid Res. **5**, 38—45 (1964).

— —, L. A. Garcia, M. di Girolamo, and L. L. Abell: Inactivation of the adipokinetic property of adrenocorticotropin, β-melanocyte-stimulating hormone, vasopressin and pituitary fraction H by tissues of the rat and rabbit. Endocrinology **75**, 867—876 (1964).

Rychlík, I.: Inactivation of oxytocin and vasopressin by tissue enzymes: a basis for the design of analogues. Proc. 2nd. Int. Pharmacol. Meeting, Prague 1963, **10**, 153—162 (1964).

Rydén, G.: Cystine aminopeptidase and oxytocinase activity in pregnancy. A comparative study in human and rat tissues. Acta obstet. gynec. scand. **45**, Suppl. 3 (1966).

—, and I. Sjöholm: Assay of oxytocin by rat mammary gland *in vitro*. Brit. J. Pharmacol. **19**, 136—141 (1962).

Saameli, K.: Quantitative comparison between oxytocin and four related neurohypophysial peptides on the human uterus *in situ*. Brit. J. Pharmacol. **23**, 176—183 (1964).

Sachs, H., and Y. Takabatake: Evidence for a precursor in vasopressin biosynthesis. Endocrinology **75**, 943—948 (1964).

Sasaki, N.: Antidiuretic substance in the bile. IX. The inactivation by a rat liver extract. Yamaguchi Igaku **9**, 116—117 (1960).

Sawyer, W. H.: Inactivation of oxytocin by homogenates of uteri and other tissues from normal and pregnant rats. Proc. Soc. exp. Biol. (N. Y.) **87**, 463—465 (1954).

Scalabrino, L., and R. Caracristi: Inhibitory action of liver homogenates *in vitro* toward oxytocin. Arch. Stud. Fisiopat. Ricambio **24**, 525—530 (1960).

Scalabrino, L., R. Caracristi, and P. Periti: Liver oxytocinase during experimental cirrhosis by carbon tetrachloride in the rabbit. Boll. Soc. ital. Biol. Sper. **37**, 450—452 (1961).
Schally, A.V., and J.F. Barrett: On the configuration of a lysine-vasopressin dimer. J. Amer. chem. Soc. **87**, 2497—2499 (1965).
—, C.Y. Bowers, A. Kuroshima, Y. Ishida, W.H. Carter, and T.W. Redding: Effect of lysine-vasopressin dimers on blood pressure and some endocrine functions. Amer. J. Physiol. **207**, 378—384 (1964).
—, and R. Guillemin: Some biological and chemical properties of a lysine-vasopressin dimer. J. biol. Chem. **239**, 1038—1041 (1964).
—, A.J. Kastin, J.F. Barrett, W.H. Carter, C.Y. Bowers, and W.F. White: On vasodepressor activity in the hypothalamus. Biochem. Pharmacol. **15**, 1805—1811 (1966).
Schockaert, J.-A., and J. Lambillon: Sur la présence d'une substance antagoniste de la vasopressine dans le sérum de femmes enceintes. C. R. Soc. Biol. (Paris) **119**, 1194—1197 (1935).
— — Observations complémentaires sur la substance antagoniste de la vasopressine dans le sérum de la femme enceinte. C. R. Soc. Biol. (Paris) **122**, 478—480 (1936a).
— — Spécificité de la substance inhibant l'action hypertensive de la vasopressine dans le sérum de la femme enceinte. C. R. Soc. Biol. (Paris) **122**, 481—484 (1936b).
Schwartz, I.L., and L.M. Livingston: Cellular and molecular aspects of the antidiuretic action of vasopressins and related peptides. Vitam. and Horm. **22**, 261—358 (1964).
—, H. Rasmussen, M.A. Schoessler, L. Silver, and C.T.O. Fong: Relation of chemical attachment to physiological action of vasopressin. Proc. nat. Acad. Sci. (Wash.) **46**, 1288 to 1298 (1960).
Sciarra, J.J., and D.A. Burress: Serum leucine aminopeptidase in twin pregnancy. Proc. Soc. exp. Biol. (N. Y.) **104**, 712—713 (1960).
Segura-Cardona, R.: Inhibition of angiotensin, bradykinin and oxytocin by extracts from several organs. Rev. esp. Fisiol. **20**, 27—35 (1964).
Semm, K.: Die klinische Bedeutung der Oxytocinasebestimmung. Klin. Wschr. **33**, 817—818 (1955).
— Der Abbau von synthetischem Oxytocin. Naturwissenschaften **44**, 424 (1957).
— Die Bildungsstätte der Serum-Oxytocinase. Arch. Gynäk. **191**, 57—64 (1958a).
— Oxytocin und Wehen. Fortschr. Geburtsh. Gynäk. **7**, 81—88 (1958b).
— Das Wehenproblem mit besonderer Berücksichtigung des Oxytocin-Oxytocinasehaushaltes. Z. Geburtsh. Gynäk., Suppl. **154**, 1—77 (1960).
— The significance of oxytocinase in pregnancy and labour. In: Oxytocin, p. 336—340. Proc. Int. Symp., Montevideo **1959**, (Pub. 1961).
— Der Abbau von Hypophysenhinterlappenhormon durch eine Phytooxytocinase. Naturwissenschaften **49**, 59 (1962a).
— Der Abbau von Hypophysenhinterlappenhormon durch pflanzliche Enzyme. Arzneimittel-Forsch. **12**, 252—260 (1962b).
— Der Abbau von Oxytocin durch menschliche und pflanzliche Enzyme. Geburtsh. u. Frauenheilk. **22**, 980—982 (1962c).
— Serum-Oxytocinase-Aktivität in der Placenta. Arch. Gynäk. **199**, 265—270 (1963).
— Oxytocin: Abbau durch Enzyme. Gynaecologia (Basel) **159**, 61—63 (1965).
— Anstieg der Serum-Oxytocinase-Aktivität im Blut nach 17-α-Hydroxyprogesteronkapronat- oder Allylöstrenol-Zufuhr. Arch. Gynäk. **202**, 459—461 (1965).
— Desamino-Oxytocin, ein von Schwangerenblut nicht inaktivierbares Wehenhormon. Geburtsh. u. Frauenheilk. **27**, 36—42 (1967).
—, and J. Bernhard: Zur Diagnostik des placentaren Stoffwechsels durch die Serum-Oxytocinase-Bestimmung im mütterlichen Blut. Arch. Gynäk. **199**, 271—278 (1963).
—, and E. Waidl: Histochemische Untersuchungen über die Serum-Oxytocinase-Bildung im menschlichen Trophoblasten. Z. Geburtsh. Gynäk. **158**, 165—171 (1962).
—, and H.-J. Wiendl: Über Oxytocin inaktivierende Gewebeextrakte. Zbl. Gynäk. **84**, 1669—1674 (1962).
Siegel, I.A.: Leucine aminopeptidase in pregnancy. Obstet. and Gynec. **14**, 488—490 (1959).
Sjöholm, I.: Enzymatic inactivation of oxytocin. Acta chem. scand. **18**, 889—898 (1964).
— Biochemical studies on oxytocin and oxytocinase. Acta pharm. Suecica **4**, 81—96 (1967).
—, and G. Rydén: Half-life of oxytocin and lysine-vasopressin in blood of rat at different hormonal stages. Acta pharm. Suecica **4**, 23—30 (1967).
—, and Å. Ryrfeldt: A procedure for determination of radioactive metabolites from tritiated oxytocin in tissues. Acta pharm. Suecica **4**, 77—80 (1967).
—, and L. Yman: Preparation of highly purified oxytocinase (cystine aminopeptidase) from retroplacental serum. Acta pharm. Suecica **3**, 377—388 (1966a).
— — Electrophoretic studies on oxytocinase (cystine aminopeptidase). Relation between electrophoretically found "isozymes". Acta pharm. Suecica **3**, 389—396 (1966b).

SJÖHOLM, I., and L. YMAN: Degradation of oxytocin, lysine-vasopressin, angiotensin II and angiotensin-II-amide by oxytocinase (cystine aminopeptidase). Acta pharm. Suecica **4**, 65—76 (1967).
— —, and F. SANDBERG: Purification of oxytocinase (cystine aminopeptidase) by ethanol fractionation. Acta pharm. Suecica **2**, 261—266 (1965).
SMITH, E.E., E.P. PINEDA, and A.M. RUTENBURG: Localization of serum leucine aminopeptidase activity by paper electrophoresis. Proc. Soc. exp. Biol. (N. Y.). **110**, 683—687 (1962).
—, and A.M. RUTENBURG: Electrophoretic behaviour of an aminopeptidase of human tissues and serum. Nature (Lond.) **197**, 800—801 (1963).
SMITH, M.W., and H. SACHS: Inactivation of arginine vasopressin by rat-kidney slices. Biochem. J. **79**, 663—669 (1961).
SMITHIES, O.: Zone electrophoresis in starch gels and its application to studies of serum proteins. Advanc. Protein Chem. **14**, 65—113 (1959).
SPACKMAN, D.H., E.L. SMITH, and D.M. BROWN: Leucine aminopeptidase. IV. Isolation and properties of the enzyme from swine kidney. J. biol. Chem. **212**, 255—269 (1955).
STEPANKOVSKAYA, G.K.: The role of oxytocic substances and enzymes destroying them in protracted gestations. Akush. i Ginek. **40**, 19—23 (1964). Chem. Abstr. **61**, 12465b (1964).
STOKLASKA, E., u. E. WINTERSBERGER: Zum Mechanismus des Oxytocin- und Vasopressin-Abbaues durch Schwangerenserum. Arch. Exp. Pathol. Pharmakol. **236**, 358—364 (1959).
— — Beeinflussung der Oxytocinaseaktivität durch Thymusextrakt. Wien. klin. Wschr. **74**, 944—946 (1962).
— — Über die Oxytocinasehemmstoffe im Thymusextrakt. Wien. klin. Wschr. **75**, 16—17 (1963).
SUSKA-BRZEZIŃSKA, E., and Z. EWY: Oxytocinase in hen serum. Bull. Acad. pol. Sci., Ser. Sci. Biol. **13**, 17—19 (1965).
—, M. GOLEBSKA, and Z. EWY: Biological and chemical determinations of tissue oxytocinase in cows. Acta physiol. pol. **16**, 151—158 (1965).
THORN, N.A.: Some chemical properties of antidiuretic material in the urine of rats. Acta endocr. (Kbh.) **32**, 128—133 (1959).
—, and L. SILVER: Chemical form of circulating antidiuretic hormone in rats. J. exp. Med. **105**, 575—583 (1957).
—, and N.B.S. WILLUMSEN: Inhibitory action of calcium on the inactivation of antidiuretic hormone by rat-kidney slices. Acta endocr. (Kbh.) **44**, 563—569 (1963).
THORPE, W.V.: Experiments on the chemical nature of the oxytocic principle of the pituitary gland. Biochem. J. **20**, 374—378 (1926).
TITUS, M.A., D.R. REYNOLDS, M.B. GLENDENING, and E.W. PAGE: Plasma aminopeptidase activity (oxytocinase) in pregnancy and labor. Amer. J. Obstet. Gynec. **80**, 1124—1128 (1960).
TUPPY, H.: The amino-acid sequence in oxytocin. Biochim. biophys. Acta (Amst.) **11**, 449 to 450 (1953).
— Enzymic inactivation and degradation of oxytocin and vasopressin. In: Polypeptides which affect smooth muscles and blood vessels, p. 49—58. Ed. by M. SCHACHTER. Proc. Symp., London **1959** (Pub. 1960).
— Biochemical studies of oxytocinase. In: Oxytocin, p. 315—324. Proc. Int. Symp., Montevideo **1959** (Pub. 1961).
—, u. G. KREIL: Über die beim tryptischen Abbau von Pferde-Cytochrom C entstehenden Peptide. Mh. Chem. **93**, 780—794 (1962).
—, u. H. MICHL: Über die chemische Struktur des Oxytocins. Mh. Chem. **84**, 1011—1020 (1953).
—, u. H. NESVADBA: Über die Aminopeptidaseaktivität des Schwangerenserums und ihre Beziehung zu dessen Vermögen, Oxytocin zu inaktivieren. Mh. Chem. **88**, 977—988 (1957).
—, U. WIESBAUER u. E. WINTERSBERGER: Aminosäure-p-nitroanilide als Substrate für Aminopeptidasen und andere proteolytische Fermente. Z. Physiol. Chem. **329**, 278—288 (1962).
— — — Über die Einwirkung von Neuraminidase auf die Serumoxytocinase. Mh. Chem. **94**, 321—328 (1963).
—, u. E. WINTERSBERGER: Reinigung und Eigenschaften der Serum-Oxytocinase. Mh. Chem. **91**, 1001—1010 (1960).
— — Investigations of pregnancy serum oxytocinase. Proc. 2nd Int. Pharmacol. Meeting, Prague 1963, **10**, 143—151 (1964).
DU VIGNEAUD, V., P.S. FITT, M. BODANSZKY, and M. O'CONNELL: Synthesis and some pharmacological properties of a peptide derivative of oxytocin: glycyloxytocin. Proc. Soc. exp. Biol. (N.Y.) **104**, 653—656 (1960).

du Vigneaud, V., H.C. Lawler, and E.A. Popenoe: Enzymatic cleavage of glycinamide from vasopressin and a proposed structure for this pressor antidiuretic hormone of the posterior pituitary. J. Amer. chem. Soc. **75**, 4880—4881 (1953).

—, C. Ressler, J.M. Swan, C.W. Roberts, and P.G. Katsoyannis: The synthesis of oxytocin. J. Amer. chem. Soc. **76**, 3115—3121 (1954).

— —, and S. Trippett: The sequence of amino acids in oxytocin, with a proposal for the structure of oxytocin. J. biol. Chem. **205**, 949—957 (1953).

Vorherr, H., u. G. Hüskens: Adiuretinabbau und Aminopeptidaseaktivität in Placentaextrakten. Klin. Wschr. **41**, 926—928 (1963).

Werle, E.: Discussion remark. In: Polypeptides which affect smooth muscles and blood vessels, p. 89—90. Ed. by M. Schachter (1960).

—, u. G. Effkemann: Über die oxytocinabbauende Fähigkeit des Schwangerenblutes. Arch. Gynäk. **171**, 286—290 (1941).

—, A. Hevelke u. K. Buthmann: Zur Kenntnis des oxytocinabbauenden Prinzips des Blutes. Biochem. Z. **309**, 270—282 (1941).

—, u. A. Kalvelage: Über die Vasopressin-inaktivierende Kraft des Blutes von Schwangeren und die Natur des inaktivierenden Prinzips. Biochem. Z. **308**, 405—412 (1941).

—, u. L. Maier: Über den Abbau von Oxytocin und Vasopressin durch Milchdrüsenextrakte der Kuh. Naturwissenschaften **41**, 380 (1954).

—, u. K. Semm: Aktivitätsbestimmung der Serum-Oxytocinase als Schwangerschaftsnachweis. Klin. Wschr. **29**, 544—545 (1951).

— — Methode zur Schwangerschaftsdiagnose mit Bestimmung des Alters der Frucht. Arch. Gynäk. **187**, 106—111 (1955).

— — Über die Oxytocinase des Schwangerenblutes. Arch. Gynäk. **187**, 449—457 (1956).

— —, u. R. Enzenbach: Über die Oxytocinase des Schwangerenblutes und der Erythrocyten. Arch. Gynäk. **177**, 211—217 (1950).

Wilken, H.: Die sogenannte „pregnancy zone", ein neuer Serumfaktor bei Schwangeren. Arch. Gynäk. **199**, 243—256 (1963).

Winkhaus, B.: Oxytocinase-Bestimmung bei Kühen unter Berücksichtigung der Bedeutung des Hormons Oxytocin bei der Milchentleerung und Geburtsauslösung. Vet. Med. Diss., München (1954).

Wintersberger, E., u. K.P. Chatterjee: Reinigung und Eigenschaften einer Aminopeptidase der menschlichen Erythrocyten. Mh. Chem. **93**, 1268—1278 (1962).

—, W. Müller-Hartburg u. H. Tuppy: Eine einfache Methode zur chemischen Bestimmung der Oxytocinaseaktivität in Schwangerenseren. Clin. chim. Acta **14**, 786—792 (1966).

—, E. Stoklaska, H.D. Moed, u. J. van Dijk: Substituierte Amide des Cystins als Inhibitoren des Oxytocinabbaues durch die Oxytocinase des Schwangerenserums. Rec. Trav. chim. Pays-Bas **83**, 1061—1068 (1964).

—, u. H. Tuppy: Zonen-Elektrophorese von Aminopeptidasen in Stärkegel. Mh. Chem. **91**, 406—411 (1960).

— —, u. E. Stoklaska: Über ein kompetitives Substrat der Oxytocinase. Mh. Chem. **91**, 577—581 (1960).

Woodbury, R.A., R.P. Ahlquist, B. Abreu, R. Torpin, and W.G. Watson: The inactivation of pitocin and pitressin by human pregnancy blood. J. Pharmacol. exp. Ther. **86**, 359—365 (1946).

Yano, F.: Antidiuretic substance in the bile. VI. The stability in some digestive juices and digestive enzymes. Yamaguchi Igaku **9**, 107—109 (1960).

Yman, L., and I. Sjöholm: Some physicochemical properties of oxytocinase (cystine aminopeptidase). Acta pharm. Suecica **4**, 13—22 (1967).

Zamello, J., and J.M. Zgliczynski: Blood peroxidase activity in women in the perinatal period. Ginek. pol. **36**, 147—151 (1965).

Zaoral, M., V. Pliška, K. Řežábek, and F. Šorm: Synthesis of two lysine-vasopressin analogues with protracted hormonal activity. Collection Czech. Chem. Commun. **28**, 747—749 (1963).

—, and F. Šorm: Preparation and biological activity of some new lysine vasopressin analogues. Proc. 2nd Int. Pharmacol. Meeting, Prague 1963, **10**, 167—171 (1964).

— — Amino acids and peptides LV. Synthesis of Gly-Cys[1]-lysine-vasopressin and Gly-Cys[1]-Tyr(Me)[2]-lysine vasopressin. Collection Czech. Chem. Commun. **30**, 2812—2816 (1965).

Zasztowt, O.: On the behaviour of oxytocinase during pregnancy. Roczn. Akad. Med. Marchlewskiego **9**, 3—7 (1963).

Bioassay Procedures for Neurohypophysial Hormones and Similar Polypeptides

E. STÜRMER

With 22 Figures

Introduction

The bioassay of active substances from the posterior pituitary is just as necessary today as it was 55 years ago when DALE and LAIDLAW introduced the guinea-pig uterus method. Unfortunately, what DALE and LAIDLAW regretfully admitted in 1912 is also valid: "There seems no prospect at present of the control of its (the posthypophysial extract's) efficiency by chemical methods", even though the complex octapeptide structure of the posthypophysial hormones has since been elucidated and confirmed by synthesis.

In latter years a number of excellent reviews has been published on the bioassay of the neurohypophysial hormones. (FITZPATRICK, 1961; SAWYER, 1961; THORP, 1962; SAWYER, 1966; BERDE and SAAMELI, 1966). For all that, the author of this chapter will endeavour to present the commonly used methods in all their details, so as to enable any competent animal experimenter to carry out successful assays on posthypophysial hormones without a long period of trial and error.

The scope of the methods described is governed by their importance for the standardisation of posthypophysial hormones in adequate concentration. The assaying of these hormones in minute quantities, e.g. in the blood and tissue fluids is dealt with by FITZPATRICK and BENTLEY. Thus the avian depressor method is of most interest, followed by the less exact assay methods employing the isolated rat uterus and the lactating mammary gland. Similarly, because of its greater importance, the bioassay of vasopressin by the rat blood pressure method is discussed more fully than the antidiuretic method.

The author's account of these methods and his general comments on their scope and limitations are based upon 6 years experience with them, during which time he has carried out several thousand oxytocin and several thousand vasopressin standardisation assays.

As the title of the chapter indicates, the standardisation of analogues and homologues of oxytocin and vasopressin is also touched upon. The assay method remains the same, of course, but difficulties occur for the following reason: Quantitative biological methods are only valid when used to compare identical substances, i.e. we must compare oxytocin with oxytocin and arginine^{8}-vasopressin with arginine^{8}-vasopressin. This requirement cannot be met when establishing the activity profiles of homologues and analogues of the posthypophysial hormones, since for these substances there is no identical standard. To characterise the oxytocic or the vasopressor/antidiuretic properties of an analogue or a homologue, such substances are generally compared with the International Standard. Provided the slopes of the dose-effect curves for standard and unknown do not differ too widely, reproducible values will be found within a defined dose range. All published data from comparisons of non-identical peptides should include details of the dose range and standard employed.

I. Standard Preparations for the Bioassay of Post-Hypophysial Hormones

A. The International Standard

The International Standard is a dry powder which is prepared from the fresh posterior lobes of ox pituitary glands by acetone extraction.

1. The Unit

The International Unit of pituitary (posterior lobe) extract is by definition the amount of oxytocin and vasopressin contained in 0.5 mg of the International Standard in use. This unit is sometimes referred to as the Voegtlin unit, presumably because the use of a posthypophysial powder as an international standard was first proposed by CARL VOEGTLIN in 1923 at the 1st International Conference of the Health Organisation of the League of Nations in Edinburgh. In terms of international units 1 mg of pure synthetic oxytocin has an oxytocic potency of 450 IU, or conversely 1 IU represents the oxytocic activity of 2.2 μg of pure synthetic oxytocin; 1 mg of pure synthetic arginine^8-vasopressin has a pressor potency of 400 IU, or conversely 1 IU represents the pressor or antidiuretic activity of 2.5 μg of pure arginine^8-vasopressin.

2. The History of the Standard Preparations

a) *Histamine and Potassium Chloride as Artificial Standards.* ROTH (1914a, b) of the Hygienic Laboratory of the Public Health Department in Washington worked out a method employing isolated uteri in which histamine was used as the standard for the bioassay of posthypophysial hormones. This method was subsequently adopted in U.S.P. IX (1916). It proved, however, to be unsatisfactory, and SPAETH (1918a, b) from the same laboratory suggested replacing histamine by potassium chloride. In thorough trials using isolated guinea-pig uteri BURN and DALE (1922) clearly demonstrated that neither histamine nor potassium chloride was suitable for use as a standard because the sensitivity of the organ to these artificial standards and to pituitary extract was subject to uncorrelated variation. They therefore suggested the use of an acid extract of fresh posterior pituitary lobes prepared under standardised conditions as a reference standard; moreover they showed that the posterior lobes could be dried at 40° C over phosphorus pentoxide without loss of activity.

b) *The 1st International Standard.* The first acetone-dried posterior pituitary powder was prepared by SMITH and MCCLOSKY (1924a, b) at the Hygienic Laboratory, Division of Pharmacology, in Washington in 1924. On the recommendation of CARL VOEGTLIN, at that time head of the Division of Pharmacology, this powder was accepted as the Posterior Pituitary Reference Standard for U.S.P. X and by the Health Organisation of the League of Nations at the Geneva Conference in 1925 as the International Standard. This Conference also took an important step in defining a unit of activity for postpituitary preparations as the activity of 0.5 mg of the dried standard material. On the recommendation of the Geneva Conference in 1925 and the Frankfurt Conference in 1928 any laboratory could prepare a dry powder by SMITH and MCCLOSKY's (1924) method and regard it as equipotent to the International Standard. Thus until 1935 the first internationally recognized standard was not a single powder stored and distributed from a central depot, but consisted of an unknown number of single preparations which had not always been shown to have the same biological activity (NELSON and MUNCH, 1925).

However, in October 1935 the Permanent Commission on Biological Standardisation of the Health Organisation of the League of Nations decided that it was necessary to establish a single International Posterior Pituitary Standard and adopted a powder which had been used as the British Standard for Pituitary (Posterior Lobe) Extract since 1926; this material had been prepared and kept at the National Institute for Medical Research, London, and had been shown to have the same biological activity as the SMITH and McCLOSKY preparation (Report of the Permanent Commission on Biological Standardisation, 1936).

c) *The 2nd International Standard.* The 2nd International Standard for Pituitary (Posterior Lobe) Extract superseded the first standard in 1942 (Department of Biological Standards, 1942/43). An assay performed previously on this material by an international team of experts had revealed that its oxytocic, vasopressor and antidiuretic activities were approximately 15% greater than those of the 1st International Standard (see Table 1). Nevertheless, the definition of the International Unit was not altered (see also GAUTIER, 1945/46). Elaborate precautions were taken to protect the standard from possible destruction during the war years (DALE, 1942).

d) *The 3rd International Standard.* The 3rd International Standard was established in 1957 and is still in use. In 1956 the WHO Expert Committee on Biological Standardization changed the name of the standard to the "3rd International Standard for Oxytocic, Vasopressor and Antidiuretic Substances". The word "substances" was used in spite of the recognised fact that vasopressor activity

Table 1. *Comparison of the activities of the 1st, 2nd and 3rd International Standards*

	Oxytocic %	Vasopressor %	Antidiuretic %
1st Standard	100	100	100
2nd Standard (in terms of 1st)	111	113	116.5
3rd Standard (in terms of 2nd)	92.7	92.8	93.7
3rd Standard (in terms of 1st)	102.9	104.9	109.2

BANGHAM and MUSSETT (1958).

and antidiuretic activity are due to the same peptide. The biological activities of the 3rd International Standard were compared with those of the 2nd International Standard in a joint international assay (BANGHAM and MUSSETT, 1958). The 3rd Standard was shown to be 7% less potent than the 2nd (see Table 1).

3. *The Potency of the 3rd International Standard*

The potency of the 3rd International Standard for Oxytocic, Vasopressor and Antidiuretic Substances (called for brevity the 3rd Standard) is 2.0 units/mg i.e. 1 unit equals 0.5 mg of the dry powdered material.

4. *Supply*

The 3rd Standard is kept for the WHO by the National Institute for Medical Research, Mill Hill, London N.W. 7, and is supplied in ampoules containing approximately 30 mg on request.

5. The Storage of the 3rd Standard

The standard ampoules should be stored in a refrigerator preferably at —10° C and in the dark immediately on receipt. Under these conditions the standard keeps indefinitely.

B. The U.S.P. Reference Standard

Besides the 3rd Standard there exists also the U.S.P. Posterior Pituitary Reference Standard.

1. The Potency of the U.S.P. Posterior Pituitary Reference Standard

The potency of the U.S.P. Reference Standard batch J is 2.4 units oxytocic activity per mg and 2.1 units vasopressor and/or antidiuretic activity per mg (see Table 2).

2. Supply

The U.S.P. Posterior Pituitary Reference Standard is obtainable upon request from U.S.P. Reference Standards, 46 Park Avenue, New York, N.Y. 10016. The ampoules contain about 100 mg dried ox post-pituitary.

3. Storage of the U.S.P. Reference Standard

Storage is as described in I.A.5.

Table 2. *Biological activities of the two post-pituitary standard powders*

	3rd International Standard for Oxytocic, Vasopressor and Antidiuretic Substances	U.S.P. Reference Standard, Batch J.
oxytocic activity	2 IU/mg	2.4 IU/mg
vasopressor and antidiuretic activity	2 IU/mg	2.1 IU/mg

C. Differences between the 3rd Standard and the U.S.P. Reference Standard

Since the 3rd Standard and the U.S.P. Reference Standard are not identical, differences may occur between the oxytocic, vasopressor or antidiuretic activity of the two. However, the U.S.P. Reference Standard Committee cooperates closely with WHO in order to minimise unavoidable differences in the actual units of potency.

D. Working Standard

Since the quantity of the 3rd Standard is limited, it is necessary for laboratories which perform bioassays regularly to establish their own standard.

1. Preparation of a Working Standard

A working standard may be prepared as follows: Ox pituitaries are removed in the slaughterhouse as soon as possible after death, freed from superfluous tissue and frozen. It is convenient to use a Dewar flask filled with dry ice (solid CO_2) and containing a thin-walled glass vessel to receive the pituitaries. The posterior lobes are dissected out cleanly in the laboratory. This is not very easily done unless the glands are allowed to thaw a little, since there is an optimum hardness at which separation from the rest of the pituitary is most readily accomplished. The posterior lobes are put into chilled acetone (4 ml acetone per posterior lobe) and left there for 3 h. The container is also cooled during this time. The acetone is then decanted and the posterior lobes are cut into small pieces and put into fresh acetone (same volume as for the first extraction). They remain there for 12 h (overnight). The acetone is decanted and the material is put into a desiccator over phosphorus pentoxide or calcium chloride. The dried material is then powdered in a mortar until it will pass through a mesh No. 40 sieve; it is then dried again for 12 h in the desiccator. The remaining fat is now extracted with fresh acetone in a Soxhlet apparatus for 3 h and the powder is dried to constant weight in a desiccator.

2. Storage of the Working Standard

The working standard can be kept in a desiccator in a refrigerator away from light, but it is more convenient to put it into glass ampoules. The amount of powder per ampoule will vary according to the needs of the laboratory (see I. E.); in general it will amount to 0.2—0.5 g. The filled ampoules are stood upright in the desiccator. The desiccator is evacuated and 24 h later is filled with dry air which has passed through a series of three wash bottles, the first and the third wash bottle containing concentrated sulphuric acid, the second containing phosphorus pentoxide spread uniformly on cotton-wool. The ampoules are now sealed as quickly as possible. Like the 3rd Standard they are stored at —10° C in the dark (see I.A.5).

3. Commercially Available Beef Acetone Dried Postpituitary Powder

It is simpler to purchase beef acetone dried postpituitary powder which is commercially available, e.g. from Armour Pharmaceutical Company, Kankakee, Illinois, USA. This commercial product is stored in a desiccator or in ampoules, as described, at —10° C.

4. Commercially Available Ampoules Containing Synthetic Oxytocin Solution

For the standardisation of oxytocin, commercially available ampoules containing oxytocin injection e.g. Syntocinon, may be used as the working standard. A number of ampoules from a single manufacturer's lot, kept in a refrigerator and re-assayed at intervals against the 3rd Standard can be used for a number of years as a working standard (Sawyer, 1966). It is necessary to establish the exact oxytocin activity of such ampoules before use as described in I.D.5., since the activity of such ampoule solutions may vary within the limits permitted by the pharmacopoeias: 85—120% (U.S.P. XVII), 90—111% (B.P. 1963).

5. Estimation of the Biological Activities of the Working Standard

The biological activities of the working standard (oxytocic activity and vasopressor or antidiuretic activity) must be carefully determined with reference to the 3rd Standard in at least 5—10 good experiments. In general, oxytocic activities attain a value of between 1200 and 1600 units/g acetone-dried powder. Commercial beef acetone-dried postpituitary powder from the Armour Pharmaceutical Company was found by the author to possess an oxytocic activity of 909 units/g for one batch (Batch No. CB 1340) and 1683 units/g for another batch (Batch No. X 79807, Stürmer, 1963). The main reason for this difference in biological activity from one batch of dried powder to another seems to be that the time between the death of the animals and the freezing of the glands cannot in practice be kept constant, and apparently, during this period loss of activity occurs.

As already mentioned, the oxytocin content and the vasopressin content of the working standard must be compared separately with the 3rd Standard, since postpituitary powder need not necessarily contain equal quantities of oxytocin and vasopressin. Thus the U.S.P. reference standard batch No. J is reported to possess an oxytocic activity of 2.4 units/mg and a pressor activity of 2.1 units/mg, and the posterior pituitary powder marketed by Armour, Batch No. X 79807, had an oxytocic activity of 1.68 units/mg and a vasopressor activity of 1.78 units/mg (STÜRMER, 1963).

E. Preparation of an Extract

In order to use the 3rd Standard or the laboratory working standard, an extract must be prepared. A portion of the standard material (not less than 10 mg and not more than 600 mg; normally the calculated amount that will be necessary for bioassay over the next 6 months) is weighed in a stoppered weighing bottle on a balance reading to 1 μg. The weighing process should be completed as quickly as possible since the standard powder is extraordinarily hygroscopic. GADDUM (1927) has shown that it gains some 10% of its own weight within 2—3 min. Moreover, owing to its low water content, the 3rd Standard readily assumes a strong electrostatic charge and is difficult to handle. It is, therefore, advisable to weigh out accurately a quantity of powder approximating to the calculated quantity, instead of attempting to arrive at the exact calculated weight by adding and removing powder. A burette is next filled with 0.25% acetic acid and adjusted to the mark. The standard powder is moistened with a few drops of acetic acid from the burette and transferred quantitatively to a hard-glass conical flask of appropriate size. The weighing glass must be rinsed several times with acetic acid from the burette, and the rinsings also added to the conical flask. Acetic acid is then run into the flask until the final volume corresponds to a concentration of 1 mg weighed powder per ml. The conical flask is now stoppered with grease-free cotton-wool or with a rubber bung with a condensation tube. The suspension is heated for 5 min in briskly boiling water, the contents of the flask being gently agitated all the time. The extract is then rapidly cooled under cold running water and filtered through a dry filter paper into a hard-glass vessel. The filtrate so obtained is an extract of the 3rd Standard or an extract of the working standard as the case may be. By definition, an extract of the 3rd Standard contains 2 units/ml.

1. Antimicrobial Treatment of the Extract Ampoules

The filtrate is put in hard-glass ampoules. When they have been sealed the ampoules are sterilised by heating for 3 min in a boiling water bath (as recommended in BP 1963) or by heating for 20 min in a current of steam on three successive days (as recommended in U.S.P. XVII).

2. Storage and Maximal Storage Time of Extract Ampoules

The standard extract ampoules or working standard extract ampoules are kept in a refrigerator for a period not exceeding 6 months. During this time the biological activity does not measurably decrease. When this storage period of 6 months has elapsed, it is not permissible to employ the ampoules for standardisation.

II. Bioassay Procedures

A. Introductory Remarks

The 3rd Standard and the working standard contain the active principles oxytocin and arginine[8]-vasopressin. The oxytocic activity of a posterior pituitary peptide must, generally speaking, be compared with the oxytocin component of the standard in a test set-up sensitive to oxytocin; the pressor activity of a peptide is determined by comparing it with the vasopressin component of the standard in a test set-up sensitive to vasopressin.

The set-ups most frequently employed for standardising the oxytocic activity of peptide solutions available in sufficient quantity and concentration are, in order of importance, the following:

1. The avian blood pressure test.
2. The isolated rat uterus test.
3. The test on the lactating mammary gland of the rabbit.

The set-ups most frequently employed for standardising vasopressin-like activity are, in order of importance:

1. The rat blood pressure test.
2. The rat diuresis test.

Other experimental set-ups described in the literature and in the pharmacopoeias are definitely less suitable for standardising peptide solutions.

B. The Chicken Depressor Method

1. The History of the Chicken Depressor Assay Method

PATON and WATSON (1912) observed a fall of blood pressure in birds (ducks) after intravenous injection of 0.5—1.0 ml of a posterior pituitary extract; this fall of blood pressure could not be eliminated by vagotomy or atropinisation. GADDUM (1928) and MORASH and GIBBS (1929) concluded from experiments on birds that the depressor effect was elicited by oxytocin. In 1939 COON described a quantitative method for the determination of oxytocin based on the depression of chicken blood pressure.

Further work on this method has been reported by SMITH (1942), SMITH and VOS (1943) and THOMPSON (1944). SMITH and VOS (1943) demonstrated that the depressor response in the chicken increases linearly with the logarithm of the injected dose of posthypophysial extract. THOMPSON (1944) adapted a method developed by VOS (1943) for the standardisation of ergonovine on the rabbit uterus to the chicken blood pressure test.

On November 1st, 1950, the Coon-Thompson method was adopted by U.S.P. XIV, replacing the *in vitro* test on the isolated guinea-pig uterus, described in previous US pharmacopoeias. In U.S.P. XV of December 15th, 1955, the chicken blood pressure method was slightly modified (1+2 dose assay instead of 1+3 dose assay). Thus in USA the chicken blood pressure method is the only officially recognised method for the standardisation of oxytocin.

In Great Britain the chicken blood pressure method acquired official status on September 1st, 1953, with the coming into force of BP 1953. In the latter, the method is listed first before the rat uterus method. Both methods replaced the *in vitro* test on the isolated guinea-pig uterus.

2. The Animal

A young, but full-grown, healthy White Leghorn rooster weighing between 1.8—2.3 kg (U.S.P. XVII: 1—2.5 kg; BP 1963; 1.1—2.3 kg) is selected. According to THORP (1962) Light Sussex birds are satisfactory, but Rhode Island Reds are of little use.

3. Anaesthesia

The bird is anaesthetised by i.m. injection of 200 mg/kg phenobarbitone sodium and is mounted for recording the blood pressure from the ischiatic artery.

Preparation and Administration of the 20% Phenobartitone Sodium Solution. 1 g phenobarbitone and 0.4 ml 1N NaOH are made up to 5.0 ml with distilled water. Dissolve by holding under hot water and allow to cool slowly to room temperature. The solution will keep for 1—2 days, after which time the substance crystallises out. The volume of solution injected is 1 ml per kg body weight. The injection is made bilaterally in the muscle on the inner side of the lower leg.

Sawyer (1961) prefers to use unanaesthetised birds, because he has frequently encountered difficulty in regulating anaesthesia. In his technique, the chickens are hooded and restrained in the dorsal recumbent crucifix position where they remain quiet for a number of hours. The blood vessels are cannulated under local anaesthesia. Whether the low sensitivity (a response usually being observed only to doses above 50 mU) is connected with the use of conscious animals has not been clarified. Nor is it clear whether the tachyphylaxia, which frequently occurs and which according to Sawyer (1961) is a serious problem with this method, is connected with the large intervals between injections (10 min) or with the absence of anaesthesia.

4. Exposure of the Ischiatic Artery

The bird is laid upon its right side. The left wing is tied up with the aid of a clip and the shoulder is supported on a board (14 × 10 × 2 cm) as shown in Fig. 1. In the two fields of operation outlined in black the feathers are carefully plucked. The femoral field is dealt with first. The left-hand edge of the photograph runs from the trocanter (left upper corner) to the knee joint (left lower corner) along the axis of the femur. Running diagonally from top right to bottom left is the border between an upper field with many feather follicles (pteryla) and a lower field free from follicles (apteria). The skin is divided along this border, marked in Fig. 2 with a black line, and since the skin is usually tough ,this can best be done with scissors. In so doing, care must be taken with the one or more vascular bundles which traverse the subcutaneous tissue across the path of the incision (Fig. 3). These vessels are exposed, ligated and cut. The biceps femoris is then reached; the fibres of this muscle run crosswise to the direction of the incision and are enclosed in a fascia. The fascia is cleanly divided in the direction of the skin incision and folded back to the left, the M. biceps femoris being separated from the M. semitendinosis. Fig. 4 shows the muscle together with the skin held on the left with two haemostats and pulled upwards. The ischiatic artery, vein and nerve are now clearly visible. The artery is cannulated in the usual way. Coon (1939) and U.S.P. XVII (1965) recommend that all lateral branches of the ischiatic artery should be ligated for a distance of approximately 2 cm proximally to the point of insertion of the cannula. This is a precaution which is intended to prevent anticoagulant fluid employed with the mercury manometer from finding its way into the circulation when a fall of blood pressure is elicited by injections of oxytocin. If a 0.3% heparin solution is employed instead of 5—8.5% sodium citrate solution (Coon, 1939; Thompson, 1944), this extra measure is unnecessary. Moreover, strain gauge transducers are finding increasing application for recording blood pressure and these function with hardly any displacement of volume.

5. The Blood Pressure Recording System

A narrow-bore mercury manometer is a cheap, reliable and perfectly adequate device for the bioassay (Condon, 1951); it is an aid to evaluating the findings if a one-limb, reservoir mercury manometer is used which gives a deflection of 1 mm per mm of blood pressure change. The best curves are still obtained with the aid of a mercury manometer writing on a smoked-drum kymograph, rotating at

Fig. 1

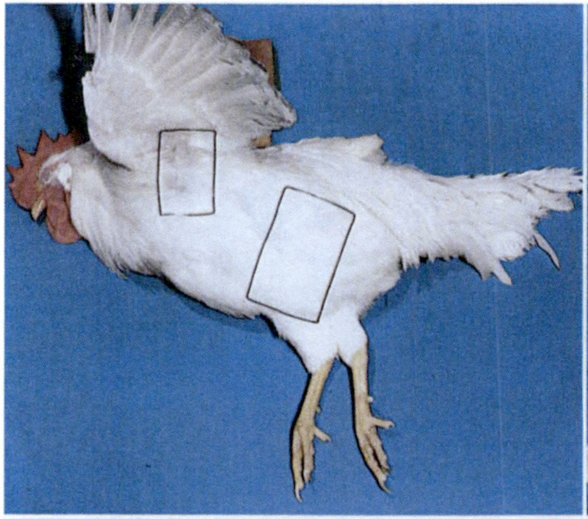

Fig. 2

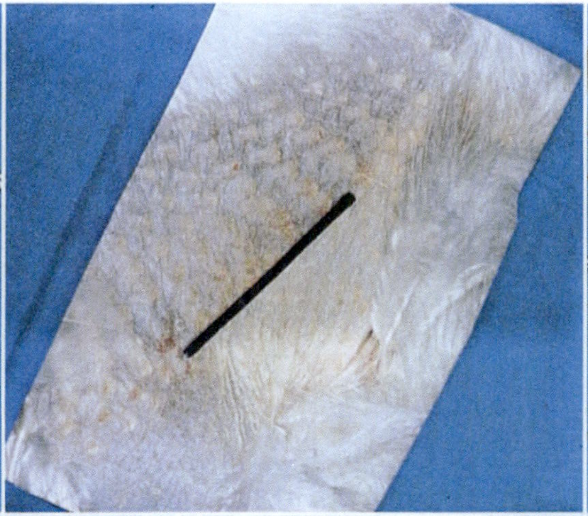

Fig. 3

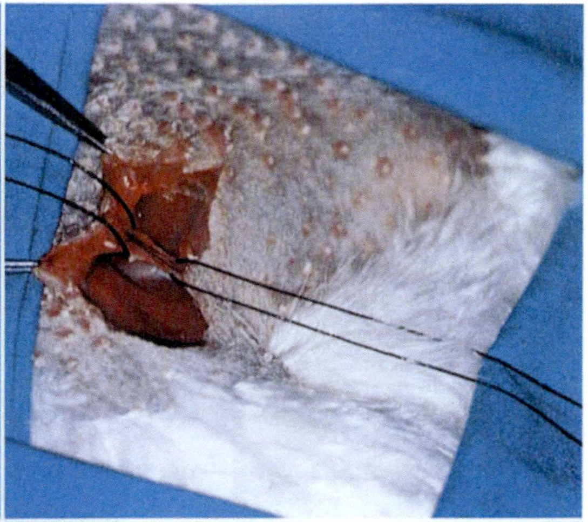

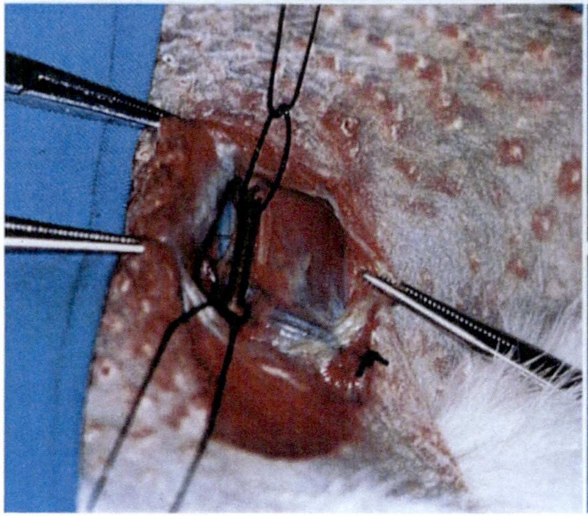

Fig. 4

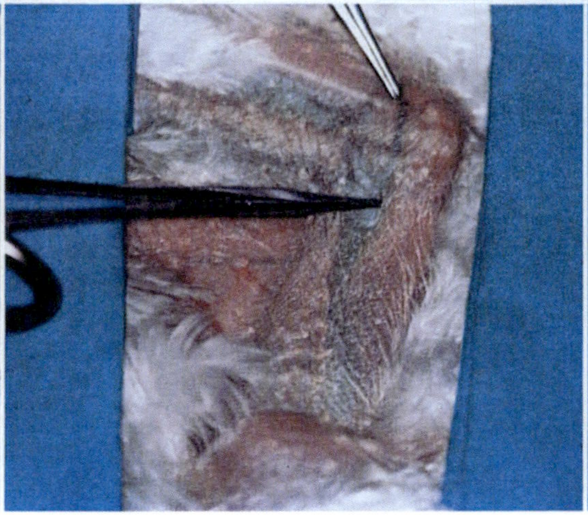

Fig. 5

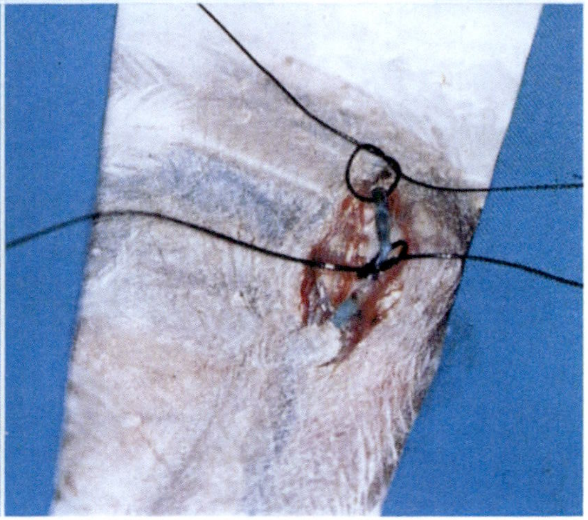

Fig. 6

Fig. 1. Rooster, anaesthetised with phenobarbitone sodium, 200 mg/kg, mounted in the typical position for exposure of the ischiatic artery and wing vein. The feathers are plucked in the rectangular areas outlined in black

Fig. 2. Rooster, field of operation, upper leg: exposure of the ischiatic artery. The border between the left upper area of the field with its many feather follicles (pteryla) and the right lower area devoid of follicles (apteria) is clearly visible. The incision is made along the black line

Fig. 3. Rooster, field of operation, upper leg: exposure of the ischiatic artery. Immediately beneath the skin a vascular bundle passes at right angles to the incision. It is cut between the two ligatures

Fig. 4. Rooster, field of operation, upper leg: exposure of the ischiatic artery. The fascia of the M. biceps femoris is divided in the direction of the skin incision, and the muscle is pulled aside with two haemostats. The ischiatic artery, vein and nerve are clearly visible. The ischiatic artery is slung on untied ligatures for cannulation

Fig. 5. Rooster, exposure of the wing vein. The vein which is to be cannulated runs between the tips of the two haemostats

Fig. 6. Rooster, exposure of the wing vein. The vein is exposed and ready for cannulation

---

2—3 mm/min. Any other pressure measuring or recording system may be used provided the trace per mm Hg of pressure change is at least 0.5 mm, and that individual pulsations are reproduced. If a mercury manometer is employed, the pressure in the system at the commencement of the assay should be set at 100—120 mm Hg.

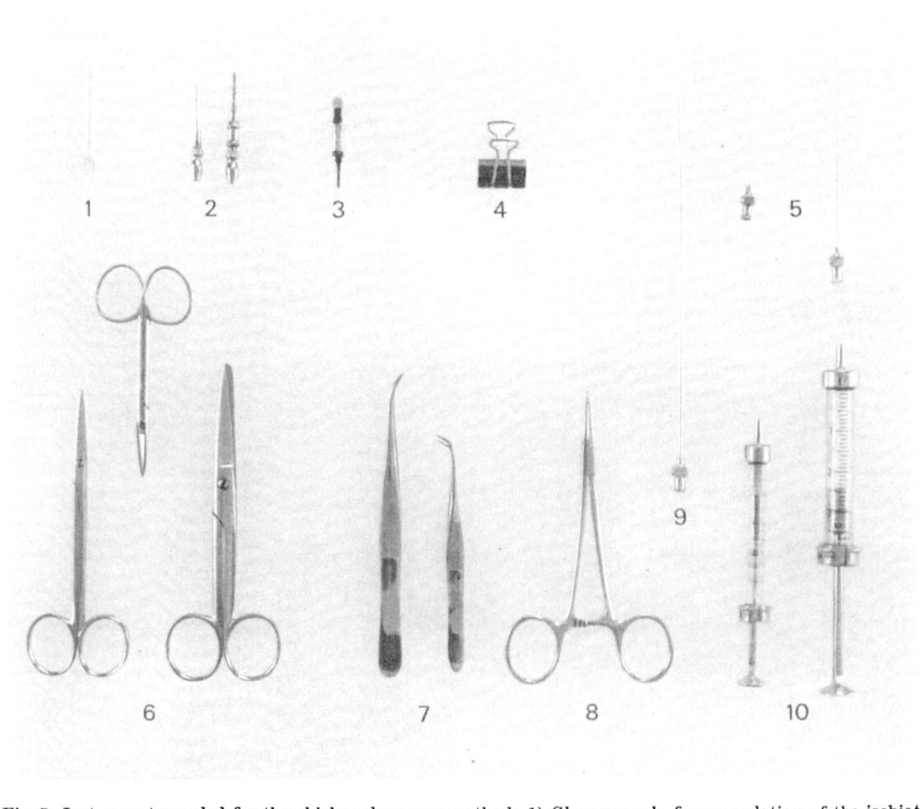

Fig. 7. Instruments needed for the chicken depressor method: 1) Glass cannula for cannulation of the ischiatic artery. The lower end is roughened with emery paper to ensure that the tubing to the manometer remains firmly attached (see also Fig. 8). 2) Metal cannula for cannulation of the wing vein. The cannula has a mandrin which reaches right to the tip. 3) Bull-dog forceps with narrow tips for clamping during cannulation. 4) Paper clip for tying up the wing. 5) Various cannulae. 6) Various types of scissors. 7) Fine curved forceps. 8) Halstead mosquito haemostat. 9) Long cannula for removing blood clots from the ischiatic artery cannula. 10) Syringes, the tuberculin syringe being used for the intravenous injection

6. *Exposure of the Wing Vein (Vena Cutanea Ulnaris)*

Fig. 5 shows the wing field, outlined in black in Fig. 1, here greatly enlarged and after removal of the feathers. The humerus runs vertically up the middle of the photograph. At the top the radius and ulna can be seen to make a right-angled bend to the left. Clearly visible through the skin and running between the points of the two haemostats is the wing vein (V. cutanea ulnaris) which is suitable for cannulation. The skin above the vein is cut with scissors. Over the vein there is an extraordinarily tough layer of connective tissue which is only divided at those places on the vein where the ligatures are to be tied (Fig. 6). The layer of connective tissue protects the thin-walled vein from damage during subsequent manipulations of the venous cannula. The venous cannula is tied in place in the usual way. Care should be taken to ensure that the cannula is accurately positioned along the axis of the vein. The cannula is supported on cloths.

7. *Instruments Employed in Making the Preparation*

Fig. 7 and 8 shows all the instruments required.

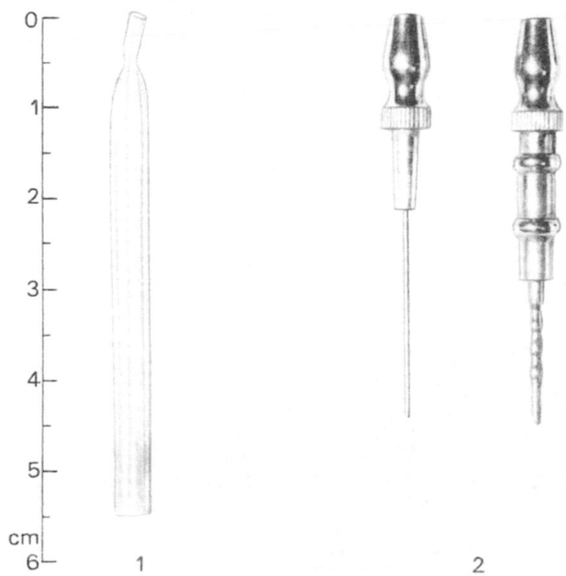

Fig. 8. Cannula 1 and 2 in Fig. 7 shown on a larger scale. 1) Glass cannula for cannulation of the ischiatic artery. Note that it has been roughened with emery paper at its lower end. 2) Mandrin (left) and assembled metal cannula for cannulation of the wing vein

8. *Test Procedure*

a) *Determining the Sensitivity of the Preparation.* Standard solution is diluted to a concentration of 100 mU/ml (1:20), and 0.20 ml, corresponding to 20 mU oxytocin, is injected rapidly i.v. The response should be a submaximal fall of blood pressure of about 20—40 mm Hg. If the response is less than 20 mm Hg the preparation is not very sensitive and after an interval of 3 min 0.4 ml of the standard dilution (40 mU) is injected. If the depressor response is again less than 20 mm Hg, a new standard dilution containing 500 mU/ml (1:4) is prepared, and 0.2 ml (100 mU) is injected. If the injection of 100 mU does not elicit a blood pressure fall of 20—40 mm Hg, the rooster is unsuitable for standardisation work, and a fresh bird must be anaesthetised and prepared.

In 100 unselected successive assays in the author's laboratory it was possible to commence with a dose of 20 mU in 83 assays and with a dose of 40 mU in 17.

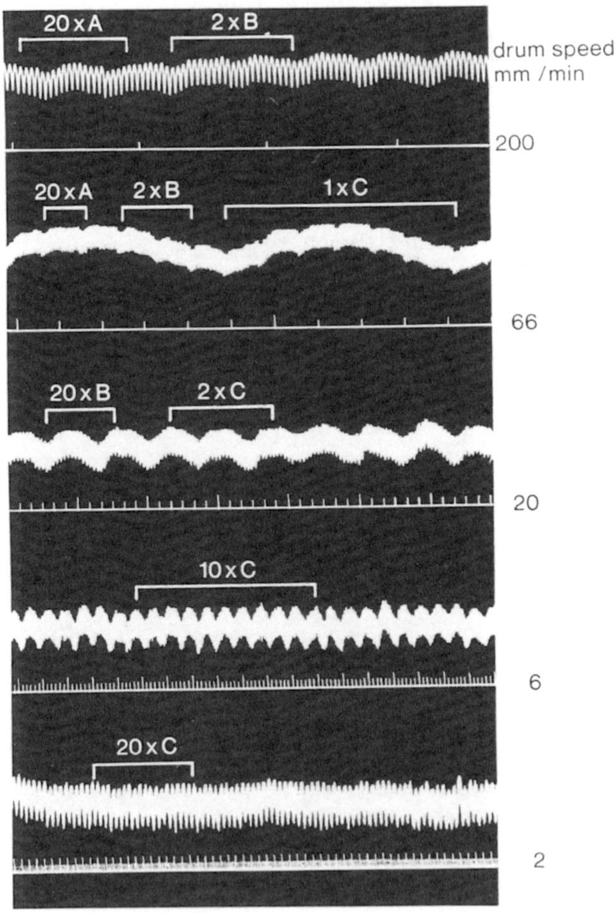

Fig. 9. Blood pressure of a rooster, recorded at different drum speeds. Time-base: short time markings = 10 sec; long time markings = 60 sec. For explanation see text

A decrease in sensitivity necessitated a change in dose level in 7 assays: 6 times from 20—40 mU, and once from 40—100 mU.

b) *The Volume of the Injection* should be not less than 0.15 ml (U.S.P. XVII: 0.15 ml; BP 1963: 0.14 ml) and not more than 0.5 ml (U.S.P. XVII: 0.5 ml; BP 1963: 0.4 ml).

c) *Timing the Injections.* The timing of the injections has an important influence on the quality of the assay. When the blood pressure tracing for a rooster is recorded with a high drum speed, 3 superimposed wave movements can generally be recognised (Fig. 9).

1. The systolic-diastolic pulsation corresponding to the heart rate of 100—200/min, the A-wave in Fig. 9.

2. A slower series of waves with a frequency of approx. 10—20/min, which is synchronous with the respiration — the B-wave in Fig. 9.

3. A slow wave with a frequency of about 1—1.5/min, probably due to central vasomotor tone. This is the C-wave in Fig. 9. With a low drum speed (2—3 mm/min) the C-wave is readily discernible (bottom tracing). In our experience it is important to ensure that the i.v. injections are always given when the C-wave is in the same phase; we prefer to inject at the point when the C-wave has just begun to fall after reaching a peak.

If a given dose of oxytocin is injected just after the C-wave has begun to descend after reaching a peak and then, about 3 min later, the same dose is injected when the C-wave is just beginning to rise after reaching a minimum, the depressor response to the injection given when the C-wave is falling is as much as 20% greater than the response to an injection administered when the wave is rising (STÜRMER, 1965).

Below it is stated that the interval between two injections is 3 min. In actual fact, this means that the investigator removes the mandrin from the wing vein cannula 2 min 45 sec after the last dose was injected, and inserts the tuberculin syringe for the next injection. At this stage he observes the C-wave. The injection is administered 3 min at the earliest after the previous injection at a point when the C-wave is in the same phase. In other words, injections are timed by the C-wave. A small proportion of roosters do not give a C-wave; in such cases injections are given at timed 3 min intervals. Roosters showing extrasystoles and roosters with a very irregular blood pressure do not give good results.

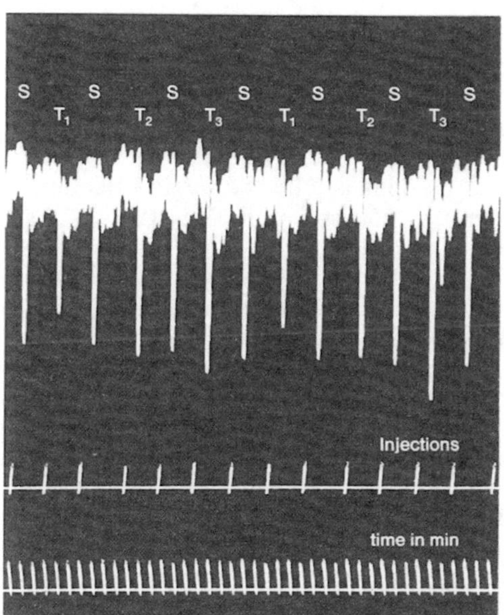

Fig. 10. Oxytocin-assay in the rooster. Representative section of an assay tracing

d) *Injection Sequence.* The injections are always administered according to a standard sequence: standard dose = S, test dose = T, standard dose = S, and so on throughout the whole assay, the standard dose being kept constant. Every test begins with a standard dose and ends with a standard dose (Fig. 10). If the standard dose has to be raised because of a falling off in the sensitivity of the preparation, the new series of injections begins and ends with the new standard dose. If the assay has to be interrupted (blood clot in the arterial cannula or other disturbances) injections are resumed starting with the standard dose, and if the last group of injections has not been completed, the last group of injections is repeated if not complete, i.e. if it does not make a S, T, S trio. Incomplete groups of injections, i.e. groups which do not begin and end with the injection of the standard dose, must be eliminated when computing the results.

e) *Dilution of the Test Solution.* In many cases one has some idea of the oxytocin content of the test solution. The latter is then diluted so as to give a solution which may be expected to contain 100 mU/ml. If the oxytocin content of the test solution is unknown, it must be determined in an approximate fashion in preliminary tests.

The first test dilution is selected so that the test dose (the volume of the injection being the same as for the standard dose) elicits the same depressor effect as the standard dose. The difference in activity between the standard and the test dose should be less than 10%. The more closely the activity of the test dose approximates to that of the standard dose, the better the results obtained. Once the equivalent dose of the test preparation has been found (T_2), the standard dose (S) is repeated, whereupon 4/5 of the volume of $T_2 = 80\%$ the dose T_2, is administered. This dose is T_1. After another dose of Standard (S) 6/5 of the volume of T_2, i.e. $T_2 + 20\%$ is injected. This dose is T_3. This is followed by an injection of Standard (S), and so on until 3 or more groups comprising S T_2 S T_1 S T_3 S are obtained, T_1, T_2, and T_3 being given in random order.

Table 3. *Assay report.*
No. St 8665, Rooster 2.25 kg, 200 mg/kg Na-Phenobarbitone i.m.

Dose No.	Preparation	Dose ml	Recorded response mm Hg	Dose No.	Preparation	Dose ml	Recorded response mm Hg
56*	S	0.2	22.5	67	S	0.4	37.5
57	T_2	0.2	21	68	T_1	0.32	32
58	S	0.2	20	69	S	0.4	39
59	T_3	0.24	27	70	T_3	0.48	48
60	S	0.2	18	71	S	0.4	33.5
61	T_1	0.16	15.5	72	T_2	0.4	32.5
62	S	0.2	19	73	S	0.4	28.5
63	T_2	0.2	18	74	T_3	0.48	41
64	S	0.2	16.5	75	S	0.4	27
65	S	0.4	48	76	T_1	0.32	22.5
66	T_2	0.4	45	77	S	0.4	30

* 55 doses had already been administered in two previous assays.
S = Laboratory working standard, T_1—T_3 = Test-solution.

f) *Decrease in Sensitivity.* If the depressor effect of the alternating standard doses decreases (tachyphylaxia) the dose of the standard can be raised from 20 mU up to 100 mU (the quotient S: T_{1-3} must remain constant). If the sensitivity decreases still further, the rooster is unsuitable and must be replaced.

g) *Measuring the Oxytocin Effect from the Tracings.* The depressor effects measured from the mean pressure to the point of minimum pressure, elicited by injection of the standard and test solution are measured to the nearest half or whole mm Hg and tabulated.

The report of an assay in which 10 doses of the unknown and 12 doses of the standard were administered is shown in Table 3.

In this assay the doses had to be increased in order to remain within the proper response range. The doses were increased starting with dose No. 65.

h) *Evaluation of the Results by Thompson's method* (*U.S.P. XIV, 1950*). In Thompson's method (1944) the results are evaluated from the data as described by Vos (1943) with one exception, namely that the reactions are not expressed as logarithms. Thompson (1944) showed with the results of 8 assays that conversion of the reactions to logarithms in the chicken blood pressure test offers no advantages. Tables 4 and 5 give details of the calculation as applied to the data from Table 3. In Table 4, columns 2 and 3, the logarithms of the doses have been multiplied by 10 in order to avoid negative logarithms. In columns 4 and 6 of

Table 4. *Analysis of the data in Table 3*

Dose No.	log. dose × 10 Standard X_s	Test X_t	4× recorded response Standard observed	Standard interpolated Y_s	Test Y_t	X $(X_s - X_t)$	Y $(Y_s - Y_t)$
56	0.301	—	90	—	—	—	—
57	—	0.301	—	85	84	0.0	+ 1
58	0.301	—	80	—	—	—	—
59	—	0.380	—	76	108	— 0.079	— 32
60	0.301	—	72	—	—	—	—
61	—	0.204	—	74	62	+ 0.097	+ 12
62	0.301	—	76	—	—	—	—
63	—	0.301	—	71	72	0.0	— 1
64	0.301	—	66	—	—	—	—
65	0.602	—	192	—	—	—	—
66	—	0.602	—	171	180	0.0	— 9
67	0.602	—	150	—	—	—	—
68	—	0.505	—	153	128	+ 0.097	+ 25
69	0.602	—	156	—	—	—	—
70	—	0.681	—	145	192	— 0.079	— 47
71	0.602	—	134	—	—	—	—
72	—	0.602	—	124	130	0.0	— 6
73	0.602	—	114	—	—	—	—
74	—	0.681	—	111	164	— 0.079	— 53
75	0.602	—	108	—	—	—	—
76	—	0.505	—	114	90	+ 0.097	+ 24
77	0.602	—	120	—	—	—	—

Table 5. *Analysis of the data in Table 3*

Parameter	Formula	Value
N	Number of doses of test material	10
S (X)	Sum of X	0.054
S (X^2)	Sum of X^2	0.04695
S (Y)	Sum of Y	— 86
S (Y^2)	Sum Y^2	7,509
S (XY)	Sum of X × Y	16.345
$\bar{x}$	S (X) / N	0.0054
$\bar{y}$	S (Y) / N	— 8.6
(x^2)	S (X^2) — $\bar{x}$ S (X)	0.046658
(y^2)	S (Y^2) — $\bar{y}$ S (Y)	6,769.4
(xy)	S (XY) — $\bar{x}$S (Y)	16.8094
b	(xy) / (x^2)	360.3
M	$\bar{x} - \bar{y}$ / b	0.02927
relative potency (%)	100 (Antilog. M)	107%
Reduced (y^2)	(y^2) — b (xy)	713.0
s^2	Reduced y^2 / N — 2	89.13
V (X)	$\frac{s^2}{b^2}\left\{\frac{\bar{y}^2}{b\,(xy)} + \frac{1}{N}\right\}$	0.00007704
s M	$\sqrt{V(X)}$	0.00877
Standard error	2.302 sM (100) (Antilog. M)	2.16 ≈ 2.2%

Table 4, the measured values have been multiplied by 4 to avoid the need for introducing decimals when interpolating the standard responses. If, as recommended by U.S.P. XVII, the results are measured from the tracings to the nearest whole mm, it suffices to multiply by a factor of 2 (the use of factors facilitates the calculation and does not affect the result in any way).

The potency of the unknown as determined in this assay is 107 ± 2.2% (standard error). In the author's laboratory any assay in which the standard error is 5% or more is rejected.

For the arithmetical work a calculating machine is used, with which squares can be obtained. If standardisation assays are carried out daily, it is expedient to programme the arithmetical operations for a computer. In the author's laboratory all calculations have been carried out by computer since 1964.

j) *Calculation of the Results by the U.S.P. XVII Method.* In U.S.P. XV (1955) and subsequent editions the prescribed method 1+3 assay was changed to a 1+2 assay. The alternation of standard and test injections remains unaltered, but test

Table 6. *Selected data from Table 3 arranged for analysis of data in accordance with U.S.P. XVII*

Dose No.	log dose × 10 Standard X_s	Unknown X_u	2 × mm recorded response* Standard observed	Standard interpolated Y_s	Unknown Y_u	x $X_u—X_s$	y $Y_u—Y_s$
58	0.301	—	40	—	—	—	—
59	—	0.380	—	38	54	+ 0.079	+ 16.0
60	0.301	—	36	—	—	—	—
61	—	0.204	—	37	31	— 0.097	— 6.0
62	0.301	—	38	—	—	—	—
67	0.602	—	75	—	—	—	—
68	—	0.505	—	76.5	64	— 0.097	— 12.5
69	0.602	—	78	—	—	—	—
70	—	0.681	—	72.5	96	+ 0.079	+ 23.5
71	0.602	—	67	—	—	—	—
73	0.602	—	57	—	—	—	—
74	—	0.681	—	55.5	82	+ 0.079	+ 26.5
75	0.602	—	54	—	—	—	—
76	—	0.505	—	57	45	— 0.097	— 12.0
77	0.602	—	60	—	—	—	—

* To eliminate the 0.5 values the recorded responses may be multiplied by 4.

injection T_2, i.e. the test dose equivalent to the standard, is omitted and the sequence of injections thus becomes: S, T_1, S, T_3, S, T_3, S, T_1, S, etc. In the assay given as an example in Table 3, test injections 57, 63, 66 and 72 would thus be omitted. Table 6 and 7 show details of the calculations according to U.S.P. XVII as applied to the data in Table 3.

The estimated potency is 110%, and the approximate confidence interval L is 0.243.

If L exceeds 0.20, the assay must be repeated or the number of sets of responses increased until the confidence interval of the combined results is 0.20 or less. Our example is a case in point (L = 0.243). Further injections would be necessary in order to raise the number of sets of responses (S, T, S) until L for the combined results was 0.2 or less. Normally 10—14 sets suffice.

k) *Assay Procedure According to BP 1963.* BP 1963 recommends the use of a 4-point assay method employing 2 standard doses and 2 test doses as described by SCHILD (1942) for the bioassay of histamine on the isolated guinea-pig ileum. This procedure has the advantage that the dose-effect curves for the standard and the test solution are both established by 2 points, and the 2 dose-effect curves can thus be shown to be parallel, this being a prerequisite for the quantitative comparison. The Thompson method described in detail above likewise employs 4 doses, but only 1 dose of the standard, so that the dose-effect curve of

Table 7. *Statistical analysis of data from Table 6 in accordance with U.S.P. XVII*

Parameter	Formula	Value
$\bar{x}$	average of all values of x $= \dfrac{S(x)}{n}$	—0.009
T_1	sum of differences y for the low dose = S (y low)	—30.5
T_2	sum of differences y for the high dose = S (y high)	+66.0
i	log interval between low and high dose	0.176
M'	log relative potency of the assay preparation $M' = \{i\,(T_1+T_2)/2\,(T_2-T_1)\} - \bar{x}$	0.04137
R	relative potency = antilog M' × 100	110.0%
	Calculation of the approximate confidence interval L.	
Σy^2	sum of the squares of y	1,846.75
f	number of sets	6
n	degrees of freedom = 2 (f—1)	10
s^2	error variance of a response unit $\dfrac{\left\{\Sigma y^2 - \dfrac{(T_1^2+T_2^2)}{f}\right\}}{n}$ $\dfrac{1{,}846.75 - \dfrac{930.25+4{,}356}{6}}{10} =$	96.571
t^2	square of Student's t for n = 10 degrees of freedom out of Table 9 p. 855 U.S.P. XVII	4.965
C	term measuring precision of the slope in a confidence interval $\dfrac{(T_2-T_1)^2}{\left\{(T_2-T_1)^2 - \dfrac{4\,(f+1)\,s^2\,t^2}{3}\right\}}$ $\dfrac{9{,}312.25}{9{,}312.25 - \dfrac{28 \cdot 96.571 \cdot 4.965}{3}}$	1.925
c'	constant for computing L $\dfrac{(4f-1)}{8\,(f+1)} = \dfrac{23}{56}$	0.411
L	approximate confidence interval $2 \cdot \sqrt{(C-1)\ (C \cdot M'^2 + c'\,i^2)}$ $2 \cdot \sqrt{0.925\,[(1.925 \cdot 0.0017)+(0.411 \cdot 0.031)]}$ $2 \cdot \sqrt{0.925\,(0.0033+0.0127)}$ $2 \cdot \sqrt{0.925 \cdot 0.016}$ $2 \cdot \sqrt{0.0148}$ $2 \cdot 0.12166$	0.243*

* In this example L exceeds 0.2. Therefore a second assay is necessary in order to increase the number of sets of responses until L for the combined results is 0.2 or less.

the latter is not established. This disadvantage of the assay set-up is of little account when oxytocin is being standardised. However, on comparing the activities of oxytocin (3rd Standard or working standard) with those of peptides possessing oxytocic properties but not identical with oxytocin in structure, errors can arise if the dose-effect curves do not have the same slope.

Nevertheless, the Thompson method has an important advantage over the 4-point method. It is a prerequisite of a comparative biological test in which a test preparation must respond to a series of doses of a standard and a test substance, that the animal preparation possess constant sensitivity. Since no test preparation ever fulfils this criterion, randomisation of the doses is applied with some success in order to counteract the sensitivity drift. When rapid and irregular changes in sensitivity occur, and this is precisely what happens in the chicken blood pressure method, randomisation falls down. Here recourse may be had to the method introduced by SMITH and VOS (1943) in which the effect of the doses of unknown is compared with the arithmetic mean of the effects elicited by doses of the standard preceding and following the dose of unknown. Rapid fluctuations in sensitivity are for the most part levelled out by taking the mean.

9. *Accuracy of the Chicken Depressor Assay*

In order to determine the accuracy attainable by this method THOMPSON (1944) reported the results of a blind assay study on 8 posterior pituitary extract solutions. The experiments on each of the 8 solutions involved a run of 12—17 doses of the unknown test solution. Each experiment was regarded as 2 separate and complete assays performed with a relatively small number of doses. The results are shown in Table 8. This shows the accuracy that may be expected when

Table 8. *Results of assays of "unknown" solutions*
THOMPSON (1944)

Assay No.	Number of unknown doses	True potency	Potency found	Standard error	% Error	% Standard error	% Error / % Std. error
1-a	6	80	80.4	2.1	0.5	2.6	0.19
1-b	6	80	83.5	6.6	4.4	7.9	0.56
2-a	7	75	71.2	1.3	5.1	1.8	2.84
2-b	6	75	75.7	4.2	0.9	5.5	0.16
3-a	8	120	112.9	3.1	5.9	2.8	2.11
3-b	9	120	119.5	5.4	0.4	4.6	0.09
4-a	8	100	105.2	8.2	5.2	7.8	0.67
4-b	7	100	102.0	5.8	2.0	5.7	0.35
5-a	8	110	113.7	4.8	3.4	4.2	0.81
5-b	7	110	117.6	4.7	6.9	4.0	1.71
6-a	8	110	110.5	3.5	0.5	3.2	0.16
6-b	7	110	114.6	1.6	4.2	1.4	3.00
7-a	8	90	90.5	7.1	0.6	7.8	0.08
7-b	7	90	87.8	3.0	2.4	3.5	0.69
8-a	8	80	79.3	2.5	0.9	3.1	0.29
8-b	7	80	86.4	4.1	8.0	4.7	1.70
Mean					3.2	4.4	

6—9 doses of unknown are employed in an assay. The maximum percentile error was 8.0, the average error being 3.2%. Regarding each experiment as a single assay, a value was calculated for each solution based upon 12—15 doses of unknown. The results obtained by THOMPSON (1944) in this way are shown in Table 9. The maximum error was 4.5%, and the average error was 2.7%.

In our experience, the method gives good results (standard error less than 5%) if the number of injections of the unknown solution is not less than 10. Table 10 shows the distribution of the standard errors in 100 successive unselected

Table 9. *Results of assays* of "unknown" solutions*

Assay No.	Number of unknown doses	True potency	Potency found	Standard error	% Error	% Standard error	% Error / % Std. error
1	12	80	82.4	1.2	3.0	1.4	2.14
2	13	75	73.2	1.9	2.4	2.5	0.96
3	17	120	116.4	3.4	3.0	3.0	1.00
4	15	100	103.3	6.1	3.3	5.9	0.56
5	15	110	115.0	3.2	4.5	2.7	1.67
6	15	110	112.6	2.1	2.4	1.9	1.14
7	15	90	89.3	3.6	0.8	4.0	0.20
8	15	80	81.8	2.3	2.3	2.8	0.82
Mean					2.7	3.0	

* Same assays as in Table 8 but each pair (a and b) combined and calculated as one assay. THOMPSON (1944)

Table 10. *Distribution of relative standard errors in 100 consecutive unselected oxytocin assays on chicken blood pressure performed by 5 different technicians*

% standard error range =	0—1	1.1—2	2.1—3	3.1—4	4.1—5	5.1—6	6.1—7	7.1—8
No. of assays =	1	28	34	23	6	6	1	1

mean standard error $\bar{x}_{100} = 2.9 \pm 1.2\%$ ($\pm$ standard deviation).

assays conducted in our laboratory by 5 different technicians. It will be seen from the Table that a standard error greater than 5% was observed in 8 of 100 assays, and that the mean relative standard error was 2.9% (standard deviation $= \pm 1.2$).

In 1957 ELMQUIST published a statistical analysis on 47 complete chicken blood pressure assays by the 4-point method (2 doses of standard and 2 doses of test solution). The purpose of her analysis was to ascertain the minimum number of elicited responses which are required to ensure limits of error between 80 and 125% in a 2×2 dose assay at $P = 0.05$ (calculation of errors by Holton's method, 1948). She found that 6 groups each of 4 doses were a minimum recommendation, assuming that the doses within the groups were given randomly. In addition, she showed that no appreciable increase in accuracy was obtained if the number of elicited responses exceeded 32, the curves asymptotically approaching 90—111%.

10. Discussion of the Method

The Coon-Thompson method, as THOMPSON stated in 1944, is "simple, rapid, economical and accurate". It may now be added that the method has proved its worth.

Without any great difficulty an investigator can prepare a chicken and carry out 3—5 complete assays, each of about 22 doses, in one day. Each assay takes about 1 h. In the intervals between assays, the sensitivity of the preparation generally rises again. It is rare that a chicken has to be rejected because it has too low a blood pressure, because tachyphylaxia develops or because the preparation is insufficiently sensitive.

LLOYD and PICKFORD (1961) have sought to analyse the depressor action of oxytocin on the chicken blood pressure pharmacologically. An augmented and prolonged depressor response to oxytocin was seen after atropine (1—2 mg i.v.), bretylium (6 mg i.v.), tetraethylammonium (8—10 mg i.v.) or decapitation, but not after decerebration, dihydroergotamine (1—1.3 mg i.v.) or dibenamine (5—20 mg i.v.). Reserpine (10 mg s.c. given in divided doses on 2 consecutive days) did not alter the response to oxytocin, and pretreatment of the animals with stilboestrol (50—100 μg/kg s.c. or i.m.) alone or in combination with progesterone (1 mg), caused, if anything, a greater depressor response to oxytocin.

The depressor reaction may still be elicited after exclusion of the splanchnic circulation (HOGBEN, 1925). BUÑAG and WALASZEK (1961), showed that there was a reduction in the amplitude of ventricular contractions after i.v. oxytocin injections in chickens, and that this depression was not significantly altered by atropine.

11. Factors Influencing the Results of the Chicken Blood Pressure Assay

a) *Vasopressin.* As early as 1939 COON reported that the presence of large amounts of vasopressin caused a secondary rise of blood pressure after the initial fall of pressure, this making it difficult to maintain the required time intervals between injections. However, this disturbance only occurs when the ratio of pressor to oxytocic activity is 2.5:1 or higher.

Coon's findings were confirmed and added to by SMITH (1942). He investigated mixtures of oxytocin and vasopressin with activity ratios ranging from 1:15 to 30:1 in comparative experiments on the chicken blood pressure and the isolated guinea-pig uterus. The chicken blood pressure method gave higher results for mixtures whose activity ratios ranged from 3.5:1 to 30:1. The discrepancy between the avian depressor and the isolated uterus method varied with the pressor: oxytocin ratio and for a ratio of 30:1 amounted to 350%. The two methods were in agreement for pressor: oxytocic ratios ranging from 1:15 to 3.5:1 (Fig. 11).

The standardisation of oxytocin preparations is, therefore, unaffected when the vasopressin: oxytocin ratio varies from 0:1 (synthetic oxytocin) to 1:1 (unseparated posthypophysial extracts such as the 3rd Standard). On the other hand, oxytocin assays on vasopressin solutions by the chicken blood pressure method must be expected to yield higher values than those obtained by the isolated uterus method. For this reason U.S.P. XVII has retained the obsolete isolated guinea-pig uterus method for standardising the oxytocin content of vasopressin solutions, and BP 1963 recommends the rat uterus method. As synthetic vasopressin which is absolutely free from oxytocin becomes increasingly widely used, there will be less and less need for this test.

Moreover, the chicken depressor method generally gives higher values than the isolated rat uterus method *in vitro* when determining the inherent oxytocic activity of pure synthetic arginine^8- or lysine^8-vasopressin and analogues with selective pressor activity. Chicken blood pressure method: arginine^8-vasopressin 60 $\pm$ 6 units/mg; lysine^8-vasopressin 40 $\pm$ 5 units/mg; isolated rat uterus *in vitro*; arginine^8-vasopressin approx. 20 units/mg; lysine^8-vasopressin 5.0 $\pm$ 0.5 units/mg (BERDE, BOISSONNAS, HUGUENIN, and STÜRMER. 1964).

b) *Ergometrine.* Ampoules containing 5 units of synthetic oxytocin and 0.5 mg Ergometrine Maleate B.P. (Syntometrine) have been found useful for the management of the third stage of labour. Since ergometrine influences arterial blood pressure it was necessary to investigate the effect of ergometrine on the avian oxytocic assay. BERDE and STÜRMER (1962) showed that the oxytocin content of the solution containing oxytocin and ergometrine in the above-

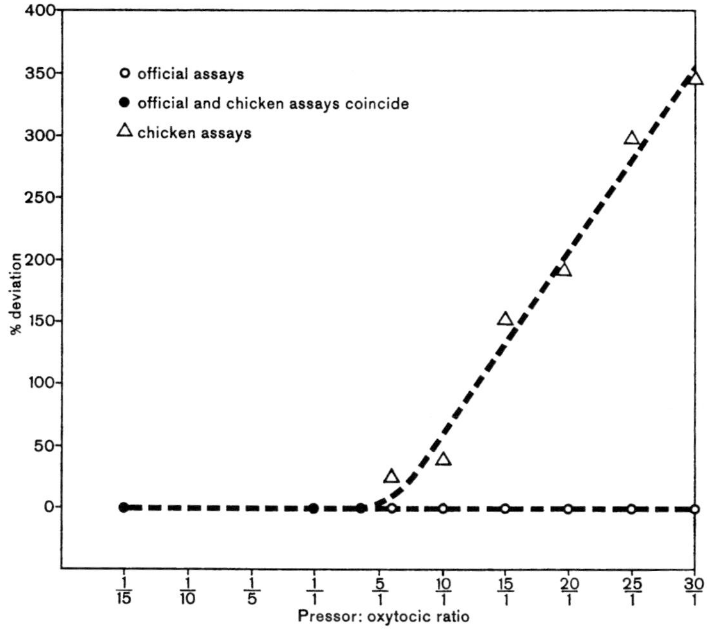

Fig. 11. Curve illustrating the percentage deviation of official (isolated guinea-pig) and chicken assay values of solutions with varying pressor-oxytocic ratios from the values calculated from the official potencies of the Pitocin and Pitressin from which they were prepared (SMITH, 1942)

Table 11. *The apparent oxytocin content of Syntometrine in different tests (the actual syntocinon content of Syntometrine is taken as 100%)*

Test	Value (%)	Note	
Rat uterus *in vitro*	119 ± 5	11	4-point-assays
	100 ± 15	5	
	138 ± 30	5	
	142 ± 27	8	
	171 ± 38	12	
	151 ± 28	10	
Chicken blood pressure — high sensitivity	100.5 ± 2.2	12	doses of unknown
	100.9 ± 2.8	12	
	102.6 ± 3.6	12	
	99.4 ± 3	10	
	101 ± 4.8	10	
Chicken blood pressure — low sensitivity	86 ± 3	10	doses of unknown
	71 ± 8	6	
	90 ± 4	6	
	76 ± 11	5	
Rabbit mammary gland *in situ*	107 ± 11	6	4-point-assays
	98 ± 10	4	
	102 ± 9	10	
	92 ± 7	5	
	104 ± 9	5	

BERDE and STÜRMER (1962).

mentioned ratio can be assayed with great accuracy by the chicken blood pressure method provided the rooster preparation is highly sensitive to oxytocin.

In 5 assays on highly sensitive chickens, i.e. chickens whose blood pressure fell by 30—50 mm Hg in response to 20 mU oxytocin, the maximum relative deviation from the actual potency was 2.6%, and the average deviation was 1.1% (see Table 11). The 2 μg of ergometrine injected along with the 20 mU of oxytocin does not counteract the vasodilatation provoked by the hormone. However, in higher doses the pressor effect of ergometrine attenuates the fall of blood pressure due to oxytocin. Thus, if the rooster has a low sensitivity, i.e. if 40—100 mU oxytocin are required to elicit a fall of blood pressure of 30—50 mm Hg, a lower oxytocin content than that actually present is measured, since the 4—10 μg ergometrine injected at the same time interferes with the depressor action of the hormone.

Table 11 illustrates clearly that the chicken blood presure test is superior to other oxytocin assay methods for determining oxytocin in the presence of ergometrine.

c) *Bradykinin.* Rocha e Silva (1960) stated that bradykinin was entirely without effect on the blood pressure of the chicken. This assertion was based on experiments with partially purified bradykinin. In 1960, Konzett and Stürmer showed that on administering high doses of pure synthetic bradykinin, a dose-dependent fall of arterial blood pressure was observed. The threshold dose was about 40—80 μg/kg. On a weight basis bradykinin is about 10,000 times less active than oxytocin. It is thus only in very exceptional cases that samples containing oxytocin will have a bradykinin content which is sufficiently high to influence the outcome of the assay.

d) *Acetylcholine.* Acetylcholine elicits a fall of blood pressure in the rooster. According to Konzett and Stürmer (1960) acetylcholine is some 1,000 times more potent than bradykinin and the latter is some 10,000 times less potent than oxytocin (w/w). Hence acetylcholine is about 10 times less active than oxytocin, and doses of 0.1 μg/kg or more will seriously interfere with an oxytocin assay. However, these are doses which might, in certain circumstances, occur in extracts. Therefore if the avian depressor assay must be employed for determining the oxytocin content of organ extracts, a purpose for which it is not primarily intended, the rooster must be adequately atropinised. Atropine in a dose of 1—2 mg i.v., which is reportedly sufficient to abolish all depressor responses to injected acetylcholine, augments and prolongs the response to oxytocin (Coon, 1939; Lloyd and Pickford, 1961).

e) *Serotonin and Tryptamine.* The influence of serotonin and tryptamine on chicken blood pressure has been investigated by Buñag and Walaszek (1961). In doses of 5—100 μg serotonin was depressor in 38 out of 46 roosters (83%), devoid of effect in 2 out of 46 (4%) and elicited a bizarre mixed depressor/pressor response in 6 out of 46 (13%). Tryptamine in doses of 50 μg—1.0 mg was depressor in 69 out of 71 roosters (97%) and pressor in 2 out of 71 (3 %). The characteristic response to an injection of either serotonin or tryptamine was an abrupt and short-lived dose-dependent fall in pressure commencing a few seconds after injection, i.e. a pattern of reaction similar to that seen after injection of oxytocin. An analysis of this reaction indicated that depressor response to serotonin and tryptamine is due not to a Bezold-Jarisch effect or to some other cholinergic mechanism, but involves histamine mediation (Buñag and Walaszek, 1962). The depressor action of 5-hydroxytryptamine on the blood pressure of the chicken has been adopted by Natoff and Lockett (1957) for assaying this compound according to a 4-point design.

f) *Histamine* in doses of 1 μg or more likewise elicits a depressor response. The hypotensive action of histamine is weaker, weight for weight, than that of acetylcholine. The reactions are dose-dependent, and have been satisfactorily employed for the bioassay of histamine (NATOFF and LOCKETT, 1957).

g) *Noradrenaline* elicits pressor responses in the chicken in doses around 1 μg. 1 μg (±) noradrenaline was equivalent in effect to 1.17 ± 0.08 μg (—) adrenaline in bioassays (NATOFF and LOCKETT, 1957). The dose-effect curves for the two drugs ran almost parallel.

h) *The Effect of Various Ions* on the oxytocin depressor response in the chicken was investigated by SMITH (1942). In a few experiments, he found that preliminary intravenous injection of potassium, sodium, calcium, zinc and cadmium compounds had no appreciable effect on subsequent injections of pituitary preparations.

The prior injection of 2 ml of roughly isotonic magnesium chloride solution containing 5 mg magnesium did not significantly affect the depressor response to U.S.P. posterior pituitary Standard solutions and Pitocin, but it markedly increased the depressor response to Pitressin injections (SMITH, 1942).

j) *Dichloroisoproterenol* (DCI), the classic antagonist to drugs acting on beta-adrenergic receptors, has been found to have a rather specific antagonistic effect on the depressor response to oxytocin in the chicken. A dose of 10 mg DCI per kg almost completely abolishes the depressor reaction to 10 mU/kg oxytocin and

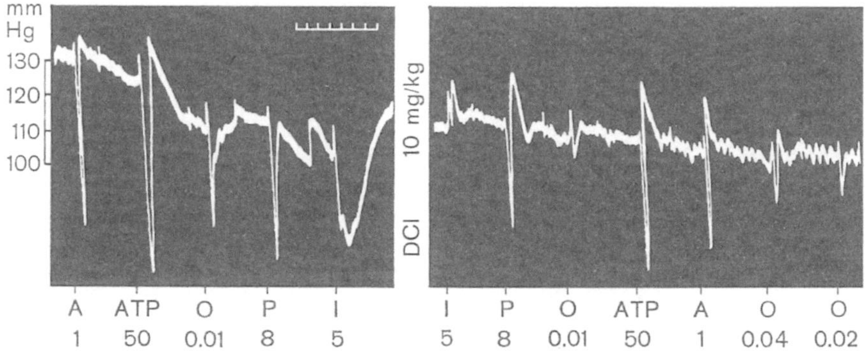

Fig. 12. The effect of DCI on arterial pressure responses of a chicken to various agonists. Chicken, 1.4 kg, ischiatic arterial pressure under phenobarbital anaesthesia. A, acetylcholine; ATP, adenosine triphosphate; O, oxytocin; P, substance P; I, isoproterenol. Doses of oxytocin and substance P expressed in units/kg; all other agonists as μg/kg. Time interval: 1 min. From WALASZEK, HUGGINS, and SMITH (1963)

to 5 μg/kg isoproterenol, but has no effect on the response to acetylcholine, ATP and substance P (Fig. 12). These findings suggest that oxytocin may exert its cardiovascular effect in the chicken mainly by a direct or indirect action on beta-adrenergic receptors (WALASZEK, HUGGINS, and SMITH, 1963).

k) *Adenosine triphosphate* (*ATP*), the co-enzyme playing an important patr in the transfer of phosphate bond energy, may be present in tissue extracts and body fluids. Its depressor action is about 40 times less than that of acetylcholine, and doses of approximately 5 μg/kg or more may seriously interfere with the results of an oxytocin assay. The depressor effect of ATP is not blocked by treatment of the rooster with dichloroisoproterenol (WALASZEK, HUGGINS, and SMITH, 1963).

l) *Substance P*. Tissue extracts, particularly extracts of the brain and intestines, may contain substance P. Substance P from horse intestine with an activity of 10—80 units/mg — very crude preparations, pure substance P from horse intestine having been shown to possess an activity of 120,000—140,000 units/mg,

(Boissonnas, Franz, and Stürmer, 1963; Vogler et al., 1963) — elicits dose-dependent biphasic depressor-pressor reactions in the chicken in doses of 1—16 units/mg. The depressor effect is not abolished by decapitation, bilateral cervical vagotomy, atropine or antihistamine drugs, hence it would appear to be mainly due to peripheral vasodilation. None out of 18 drugs examined for possible antagonism to substance P was found to have a specific substance P antagonistic effect in the chicken (Buñag and Walaszek, 1963).

C. Isolated Uterus Methods

In these methods isolated uterine muscle is suspended in modified Ringer's solution and the changes in length or tension in response to the unknown and standard preparations are recorded.

1. A Brief History of the Methods

Uterine muscle, the target organ for oxytocin and posthypophysial extracts, was first employed by Dale and Laidlaw in 1912 for standardising posthypophysial extracts, since the spinal cat customarily used at that time for standardisation was not satisfactory.

However, the guinea-pig uterus method included in U.S.P. X in 1926 and in B.P. VI in 1932 as a method of standardisation also failed to satisfy requirements as to reproducibility and accuracy (Hamilton and Rowe, 1916; Morell, Allmark, and Bachinski, 1940), and was superseded by the rat uterus method introduced by Beauvillain in 1943 and modified in 1948 by Holton. This method was adopted in the British Pharmacopoeia in 1953 as the second method after the chicken blood pressure assay, thus officially superseding the guinea-pig uterus method in Great Britain. In USA the guinea-pig uterus method was the officially recognised method for standardising oxytocin until October 1950, when it was superseded by the chicken blood pressure method with the coming into force of U.S.P. XIV on November 1st, 1950. It is still the official method for dertermining the oxytocin content of vasopressin solutions.

The rat uterus method is the best *in vitro* procedure for the determination of oxytocin. As a method it appears to be very simple; and its simplicity is frequently stressed in critical surveys on the standardisation of posthypohysial hormones (Sawyer, 1961; Thorp, 1962; Sawyer, 1966; Berde and Saameli, 1966). However, here a serious word of warning is called for: the number of sources of error in this test should not be underestimated, especially if the experimenter is not familiar with the technique of isolated organ investigations. The results may be influenced by extrinsic and intrinsic factors.

2. Extrinsic Factors

By extrinsic factors here are meant components of the unknown solutions which may simulate or inhibit an oxytocic response (contraction). When assaying organ extracts, as opposed to solutions of pure oxytocin, it must be borne in mind that such extracts may contain 5-hydroxytryptamine, acetylcholine, substance P, plasmakinins, angiotensin (see Schachter, 1960 for references), unidentified oxytocic peptides (Croxatto, Pereda, and Zamorano, 1961; Hawker, 1961), calcium or potassium ions (Bisset, 1961) which induce the rat uterus to contract; or, again, histamine or adrenaline may be present or the solution may have a low pH, and the uterus is then relaxed.

Bulbocapnine, an agent inducing experimental catatonia in laboratory animals, will potentiate oxytocin-induced contractions of isolated rat uterus in concentrations of 2—4 μg/ml (Walaszek, Huggins, and Smith, 1963). Ergometrine may also be regarded as an interfering extrinsic factor. When the oxytocin content of the combination preparation containing 5 units synthetic oxytocin and 0.5 mg ergometrine maleate (Syntometrine) is determined by the isolated rat uterus method, an erroneously high value is found for the oxytocin content. The avian blood pressure assay with a highly sensitive preparation and the assay on the mammary gland of the lactating rabbit yield correct values (BERDE and STÜRMER, 1962; see also Chapter II.B.11.b.). If facilities for carrying out these alternative assay methods are not available, the ergometrine must be extracted before the solution is assayed (SUND, 1963c). The use of organ bath solutions containing magnesium ions and added ergometrine, as proposed by SUND, (1963c) is hardly suitable for routine investigation work.

It follows, therefore, that a uterine contraction *in vitro* by no means indicates the presence of oxytocin. Thus the "oxytocic" activity of pure synthetic bradykinin *in vitro* is equal to that of oxytocin (KONZETT and STÜRMER, 1960).

The effect of some of the above-mentioned extrinsic factors can be eliminated by adding suitable specific antagonists to the organ bath solution. The level of interference by plasmakinins, substance P or angiotensin must be ascertained in parallel test set-ups highly sensitive to these peptides, since no specific antagonists are yet known.

If the method is confined in its application to the standardisation of synthetic oxytocin or posthypophysial extracts, the above-mentioned extrinsic factors can be largely ignored. The determination of the oxytocic activity of blood and tissue extracts is described in detail by FITZPATRICK and BENTLEY.

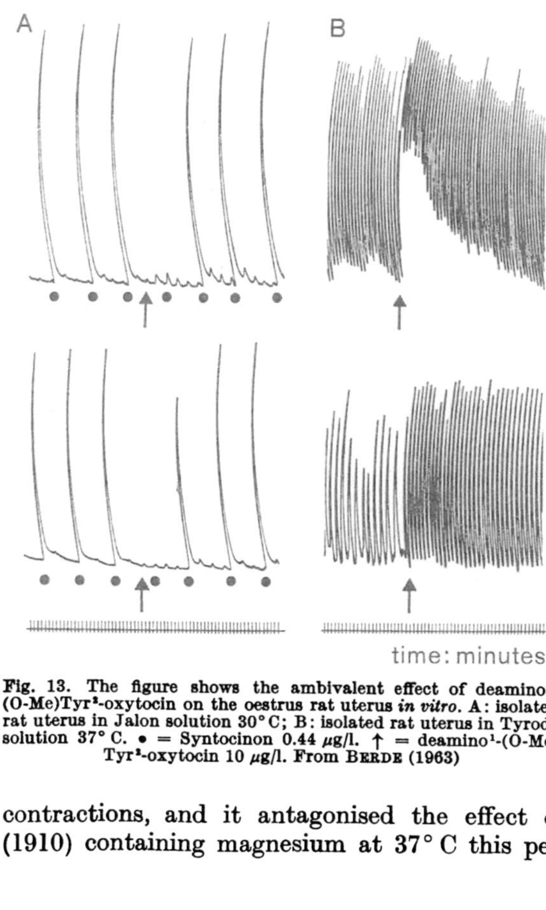

Fig. 13. The figure shows the ambivalent effect of deamino[1]-(O-Me)Tyr[2]-oxytocin on the oestrus rat uterus *in vitro*. A: isolated rat uterus in Jalon solution 30° C; B: isolated rat uterus in Tyrode solution 37° C. • = Syntocinon 0.44 μg/l. ↑ = deamino[1]-(O-Me) Tyr[2]-oxytocin 10 μg/l. From BERDE (1963)

3. *Intrinsic Factors*

The intrinsic factors reside in the experimental technique, the composition of the organ bath solution, the temperature of the organ bath, etc. The importance of these factors tends to be underestimated as it is not generally realised that changes in the ionic composition and temperature of the organ bath solution may alter the activity of a substance qualitatively as well as quantitatively. This is brought home forcibly by BERDE's (1963) investigations, on the action of deamino[1]-(O-Me) Tyr[2]-oxytocin on the isolated rat uterus (Fig. 13). In magnesium-free GADDUM solution (GADDUM, PEART, and VOGT, 1949) at 30° C the solution did not elicit contractions, and it antagonised the effect of oxytocin; in TYRODE solution (1910) containing magnesium at 37° C this peptide had an oxytocin-like effect.

The influence of these factors on the response of isolated uterine muscle are discussed at length by MUNSICK and need not concern us further here. The description of the actual technique given below should enable a beginner to arrive at useful results without a lengthy period of initiation.

4. The Rat Uterus Assay Procedure

a) *Selection and Pretreatment of the Rats.* Uteri appear to be most sensitive if taken from rats in pro-oestrus (FLATTERS, 1954; FITZPATRICK, 1961) or in oestrus (CHAN, O'CONNELL, and POMEROY, 1963). Suitable rats may be selected by vaginal smears. The British Pharmacopoeia 1963 recommends the use of the uteri from rats in the dioestrus stage. Rat uteri in the metoestrus stage are unsuitable, lacking sensitivity and possessing a low power of discrimination (FLATTERS, 1954). The female rats should weigh 120—200 g and should have been kept in segregation from the males, since pregnant or recently pregnant animals are not suitable (GADDUM, PEART, and VOGT, 1949).

If the experimenter is not familiar with the technique of preparing and diagnosing the oestrus phase in the rat and wishes to save himself the time-consuming daily check of vaginal smears from his rat colony, he may treat his animals with oestrogen, thus inducing permanent oestrus. It is generally recommended to administer an intramuscular injection of 25—50 μg/kg of an oily solution of stilboestrol dipropionate 17—18 h before the assay. We employ a 0.1% solution of oestradiol benzoate in arachis oil, administering 0.1 ml of this solution intramuscularly in the upper rear limbs of the rats 40 h before the commencement of the experiment, i.e. a total dose of 200 μg per animal.

Uterine sensitivity can be raised more than tenfold by repeated pretreatment of the rats with daily injections of stilboestrol for 3 days (FOLLET and BENTLEY, 1964), since as a result of this treatment the myometrium undergoes hypertrophy.

b) *Recording Set-up.* An organ bath containing 10 ml of solution is employed, there being no advantage in using smaller or bigger baths. The temperature of the bath is 28—32° C and is kept constant within 0.1° C with the aid of a thermostat. The load on the uterus should not exceed 1—2 g. The contractions are recorded isotonically, enlarged 4—5 times and recorded with a suitable linear writing lever (SCHILD, 1947; CAMBRIDGE and HOLGATE, 1955).

If the response is recorded isometrically, the dose-effect curves are not as steep as when recorded isotonically, i.e. on the one hand the power of discrimination of the uteri decreases, but on the other hand the permissible dose range is increased, hence there is less risk of straying beyond the maximum dose level. This advantage is dearly bought, quite literally so, in the financial outlay on equipment. However, the simple inexpensive isotonic method of recording, which, strictly speaking, is really a "semiisotonic" method (BERDE and SAAMELI, 1966) will render good service in skilled hands, although fundamentally it is inferior to the isometric method.

c) *Organ Bath Solution Free from Magnesium Ions.* Modified Locke solution containing only half the usual quantity of glucose and 1/4 the usual calcium content may be recommended (GADDUM, PEART, and VOGT, 1949). This solution differs from BEAUVILLAIN solution (1943) only in that it contains no magnesium chloride.

The formula is as follows:

	Mol. Weight	m-mol/l	g/l
NaCl	58.4428	153.9967	9.0
KCl	74.555	5.6334	0.42
$CaCl_2$	110.986	0.5406	0.06
$NaHCO_3$	84.00712	5.9519	0.5
Glucose	180.15894	2.7753	0.5

The weights given are for the anhydrous salts, all of which should be of analytical grade. It is convenient in practice to make up a concentrated stock solution.

The formula for a stock solution giving 200 litres of the solution ready for use is as follows:

NaCl	1800 g
KCl	84 g
$CaCl_2 \cdot 2\,H_2O$	15.9 g

made up to 10.0 litres with distilled water.

10 litres of solution ready for use are prepared as follows:

500 ml stock solution

+ 5 g $NaHCO_3$

+ 5 g glucose, made up to 10.0 litres with distilled water.

To oxygenate the solution in the organ bath, pure oxygen without CO_2 is employed (the formulation for another magnesium-free organ bath solution devised by Munsick (1960) is given in section II.C.4.d.).

Holton (1948), and after her many other authors, state that they used a modified Locke's solution or Jalon solution, but fail to indicate the composition of their solutions, leaving it to the reader to select a modified Locke's or Jalon's solution from those described in the literature. Other authors, commencing with van Dyke and Hastings (1928) indicate the ionic content of their solutions in mmol/litre, a practice followed also by Munsick (1960). Discrepancies are found when an attempt is made to convert the data in mmol into amounts of salt (see data by Sawyer, 1961 and Berde and Saameli, 1966), since exact data on the composition are not given and errors appear to have crept into the mmol values given.

Hence any description of method should always indicate the formulation of the organ bath solution. Moreover, it should always be stated whether the data refer to anhydrous substances or not. In the latter case, the water of crystallisation of the salts should also be declared.

d) *Bath Solutions Containing Magnesium Ions.* A van Dyke and Hastings solution (1928) modified by Munsick (1960) can be recommended for use as an organ bath solution containing magnesium ions.

The solution contains:

	molecular weight	mmol/l	g/l
NaCl	58.443	113.331	6.6234
KCl	74.555	6.088	0.4539
$CaCl_2$	110.986	0.5	0.0555
$MgCl_2$	95.218	0.5	0.0476
$NaHCO_3$	84.007	30.461	2.5589
Na_2HPO_4	141.959	0.818	0.1161
NaH_2PO_4	119.977	0.182	0.0218
Glucose	180.159	2.775	0.5

All the reagents should be of analytical grade and the weights given refer to the anhydrous salts.

The weights of salts given here differ in some cases from those in the composition of Munsick's solution stated in the literature (Sawyer, 1961; Berde and Saameli, 1966), but they indicate the exact composition of the solution as employed by Munsick (1967).

Munsick (1967) gives the following instructions for the use of the solutions in practice:

Stock solution I:

NaCl	120.67 g
$NaHCO_3$	46.62 g
KCl	8.27 g
Phenol red	135 ml of a 0.02% solution

ad 18,000 ml with distilled water.

Stock solution II (0.1636 M Na_2HPO_4 solution).
23.224 g Na_2HPO_4 (anhydrous)
dissolve in hot distilled water and make up to 1000 ml.

Stock solution III (0.0364 M NaH_2PO_4 solution).
5.023 g $NaH_2PO_4 \cdot 1\ H_2O$
ad 1000 ml with distilled water.

Keep solutions II and III in a refrigerator to avoid mould formation.

Stock solution IV (0.5 M $CaCl_2$ solution).
73.508 g $CaCl_2 \cdot 2\ H_2O$ ad 1000 ml distilled water.

Stock solution V (0.5 M $MgCl_2$ solution).
101.655 g $MgCl_2 \cdot 6\ H_2O$ ad 1000 ml distilled water.

1 litre of solution ready for use is prepared as follows:
988 ml stock solution I
+ 5 ml stock solution II
+ 5 ml stock solution III
equilibrate with 94% O_2 and 6% CO_2,
+ 1 ml stock solution IV
+ 1 ml stock solution V
+ 0.5 g glucose.

The solution in use is aerated with 94% O_2 and 6% CO_2.

Using stock solutions I—IV a magnesium-free solution can be prepared in the same fashion. Instead of stock solution V 1 ml distilled water is added. This magnesium-free solution can be recommended.

e) *Preparation of the Uterus.* The animal is killed with a blow to the head and bled by cutting the throat. Both horns of the uterus are removed and one horn is suspended between ligatures in the organ bath. The other horn may be kept in bath solution at room temperature for use later in the day. Great care must be taken not to stretch the preparation. After the uterus has been suspended it is left to relax for half an hour.

f) *Estimation of Sensitivity.* The 3rd Standard or substandard extract is diluted with 0.9% saline solution to give a solution containing 100 μU/ml. Commence by adding 0.2 ml (20 μU) to the organ chamber. The bath fluid is changed after the peak of the contraction is attained or after 60 sec. This is best done by overflow. If 20 μU elicits a large contraction the next dose should be 10 μU (0.1 ml of the 100 μU/ml solution). The doses are added at regular intervals, usually every three min, and are reduced or increased by a factor of 2 until the proper assay range (10—70% of maximum) is found. Normally the required dose range varies from 10—50 μU per ml.

g) *Dilution of the Test Solution.* The unknown solution is now tested. The assay should not be interrupted, i.e. the stimuli should still be applied at regular intervals (every three minutes). Often the investigator will have some idea of the possible oxytocin content of the unknown solution. In such a case the unknown is assumed to have a certain activity and is diluted accordingly, its effect being then compared with the doses of standard. The experienced investigator will generally rapidly arrive at the correct dilution range for the test solution, which should be diluted in such a way that equal volumes of standard and unknown solution elicit a closely similar response. Dosage overshoots should be avoided as far as possible, since they may upset the sensitivity of the system.

h) *The 4-Point Assay Procedure.* Once the dose ranges for standard and unknown solution have been established, the 4-point assay (Schild, 1942) can commence. In this procedure, a high and a low dose of standard and a high and a low dose of unknown are administered at random. The ratio of the high to the low dose of standard and, similarly, of the high to the low dose of the test solution is usually 4:3, but may be 3:2 or 8:5. For good results a total of 6—8 complete sets of 4-points (24—40 reactions) is usually necessary.

The response to each dose is measured in mm from the base line to the peak of the contraction.

j) *Statistical Evaluation of the Results.* The data are processed statistically by the method of Holton (1948) or by that described in B.P. 1963. The calculation with examples will be found in the sections dealing with the standardisation of vasopressin on the rat blood pressure.

k) *Other Methods of Evaluation.* Flatters (1954) describes a method of evaluation in which the mean effect of a dose of the unknown solution or standard solution is compared with a previously constructed dose-effect curve from which the oxytocin content of the unknown solution can be read off. Such a method falls short of present-day requirements, and is not admissible for the standardisation of oxytocin solutions.

A rather interesting method was proposed by Koll and Kaller (1952) for evaluation of assay results with posthypophysial extracts on the isolated guinea-pig uterus. This is a method in which the contraction maxima are recorded, while the base line is disregarded. The stimulating substance is not washed out of the organ bath after the contraction; it is allowed to act until a tonic end phase is reached in the contraction. The organ bath is then washed out thoroughly and the next dose in the 4-point assay programme is then added. The differences between the maxima are evaluated irrespective of the relaxed position of the uterus. This method was employed for the blind assay of 12 unknown solutions. All the results were within $\pm$ 5% of actual activity. No investigations have been carried out to ascertain whether this method can also be employed for the rat uterus.

l) *Some Practical Difficulties.*

α) Spontaneous Uterine Contractions. Spontaneous contractions interfere with the assay. Reducing the bath temperature by 1—2° C and/or shortening the interval between stimuli will sometimes suppress spontaneous contractility. If not another rat must be sacrificed; there is little point in trying the second horn of the uterus, since in general this will also display spontaneous contractions.

β) Low Uterine Sensitivity. If the uterus shows low sensitivity (failing to contract on adding 0.1 U), an attempt can be made to raise its sensitivity by increasing the bath temperature and extending the intervals between doses of substance.

m) *The Superflow Technique.* Reducing the volume of the bath will not raise the sensitivity of the isolated uterus, but it will reduce the total quantity of oxytocin required for a contraction.

In the superfusion method suggested by Gaddum (1953) the "bath" consists of nothing more than a drop of physiological solution which drips down the thread attaching the muscle to the writing lever at a steady flow rate of 1—5 ml per min. The superfused uterus in the pro-oestrus stage will react to oxytocin in concentrations as low as 2—8 μU/0.3 ml, and with it 4-point assays may be carried out with great precision (FITZPATRICK, 1961). Other authors have worked with rather higher oxytocin concentrations (10—20—200 μU/0.2 ml or more) (GINSBURG and SMITH, 1959; SIDDIQI and WALKER, 1960; SAWYER, 1966).

D. Milk Ejection Assay

There is now convincing evidence that the milk-ejection reflex consists of a neuro-hormonal arc, the efferent component of which is in all probability oxytocin released from the neurohypophysis into the blood stream. On reaching the mammary gland this hormone evokes a contraction of the myoepithelial, or basket cells, which force the milk out of the alveoli and smaller ducts. This process is known as milk-ejection or let-down, and is accompanied by a measurable rise in pressure (milk-ejection pressure) in the large milk ducts converging on the nipple (for literature see RICHARDSON, 1949; BERDE, 1959; TINDAL, BEYER, and SAWYER, 1963).

1. History of the Test

Since 1910 when OTT and SCOTT discovered that injection of an extract of pituitary posterior lobe into a lactating goat caused contraction of the udder glands and the discharge of milk, the milk-ejection phenomenon has been investigated by many authors. For assay purposes TURNER and COOPER (1941), used the unsuckled lactating rabbit. They estimated the minimal effective intravenous dose which would elicit a definite but minimal contraction of the mammary gland within 40 sec.

In 1952 CROSS and HARRIS demonstrated that the intensity of milk-ejection in the lactating rabbit was dependent on the dose of intravenously injected posterior pituitary extract (Pituitrin). The threshold dose was 5 mU, and 200 mU gave a maximal response. Using a float or piston recorder and a drum kymograph, CROSS and HARRIS (1952) measured the milk-ejection pressure in anaesthetised lactating rabbits through a glass cannula tied in a teat duct. Intravenous injections were given in the marginal vein of the ear. The use of the milk-ejection response as the basis of an assay method for oxytocin was established by VAN DYKE, ADAMSONS, and ENGEL (1955). Instead of a float or piston recorder, they employed the highly sensitive condenser microphone of a Sanborn electromanometer. By this modification an increase in sensitivity was obtained (isovolumetric technique, with negligible fluid displacement during pressure changes). For sensitive animals threshold doses of 0.5 mU have been reported, although the usual threshold dose is about 2—3 mU. A further modification of the method is described by BERDE and CERLETTI (1957), who used a strain gauge transducer (Statham Model P23B) and administered their intravenous injections into the jugular vein instead of the marginal ear vein.

2. The Animal

A healthy lactating rabbit with a body weight of 2—4 kg is selected on the 5th—21st day after parturition. Sensitivity does not seem to be correlated with body weight. The young must be left with the doe up to the day of the experiment to prevent involution of the mammary gland.

3. Anaesthesia

5 ml/kg of a 25% (w/v) urethane solution is injected subcutaneously (1.25 g/kg), and if necessary 10—25 mg pentobarbitone is injected intravenously into the marginal ear vein (0.2—0.5 ml nembutal sodium = 50 mg/ml). Deep even anaesthesia is essential, since otherwise sympatho-adrenal stimulation may cause transient inhibition of the response.

4. *Respiration*

The trachea is cannulated as a matter of routine. Artificial respiration is not normally necessary, but the rabbit must be ensured a good supply of oxygen, since hypoxia rapidly leads to irreversible damage to the myoepithelial cells and hence to a marked loss of sensitivity.

5. *Preparation*

The animal is fixed to the operating board in the supine position. One of the jugular veins is cannulated for intravenous injections and the carotid artery on the opposite side is cannulated for recording the blood pressure.

A dampened ligature is wound around a prominent teat, the tip of the teat is held with fine forceps, lifted up and cut off below the openings of the lactiferous ducts. A needle cannula with an external diameter of 0.9 mm is used for cannulation. The point of the needle is cut off and a groove is filed around the needle about 3 mm from the blunt end so that the needle can be firmly tied in the teat. This cannula is fixed opening downwards above the teat by means of a holder. The teat is now held with two pairs of forceps and carefully pulled over the cannula which drops into one of the 6 lactiferous ducts. The teat is securely tied in place around the skin overlying the groove in the needle cannula.

6. *Recording System*

The cannula is connected to a Statham Model P23BB strain gauge with a length of thick-walled polyethylene tubing. The tubing is filled with 1% (w/v) sodium citrate solution, care being taken to exclude air bubbles. From a syringe mounted on the second fitting of the transducer, 1—2 ml sodium citrate solution is injected into the mammary gland. If resistance is encountered, the cannula is not correctly inserted and must be reattached. The strain gauge is then raised vertically until the pressure in the system is zero. If the cannula is correctly positioned, the base line in the recording unit shows slight pressure fluctuations synchronous with the respiration. Spontaneous activity is observed only very rarely. The apparatus is so adjusted that a pressure change of 1 mm H_2O gives a trace of at least 1 mm on the recording unit.

7. *Test Procedure*

Injections of 3rd Standard and unknown solutions are given rapidly at regular intervals of 3 min in the external jugular vein. The injection volume is 0.1—0.5 ml. Each injection is washed in with an adequate volume of 0.9% NaCl solution.

A 2×2 dose assay procedure is employed. 2.5 and 4.0 mU doses of standard may be used. Equi-effective doses of the unknown solution are determined in the usual fashion. The sequence of injections is randomised.

A minimum of 4 groups (16 injections) is necessary for an assay. To estimate the biological activity of an unknown solution 4—8 assays on 2 different animals must be carried out. 100—120 injections can be administered to a good preparation.

If by error a high dose of oxytocin is administered, the pressure curve shows two peaks. The sensitivity of the preparation is transiently decreased by such an overshoot.

8. *Statistical Treatment*

The statistical treatment of the results is as described in the vasopressin assay on the rat blood pressure.

9. *Discussion of the Method*

The milk-ejection method is some 10—20 times more sensitive than the chicken blood pressure assay, but some 10—20 times less sensitive than the isolated rat uterus preparation. The test procedure is not too laborious, but a large rabbit colony must be kept if daily routine assays are to be carried out. The great advantage of the milk-ejection test is its relatively high specificity for posthypophysial hormones.

10. Substances which may Interfere with the Results

Most substances which are a troublesome source of interference in the chicken blood pressure and isolated rat uterus assays are without effect on the milk-ejection response to oxytocin. Thus histamine (20—150 μg base), 5-hydroxytryptamine (10—50 μg base) and acetylcholine are devoid of activity in this test (VAN DYKE, ADAMSONS, and ENGEL, 1955). However, adrenaline may inhibit the response to oxytocin. Bradykinin (0.01—10.0 μg i.v.) and angiotensin II (Val^5-angiotensin II-Asp-beta-amid, 0.5—500 μg i.v.) are also without effect according to BERDE and CERLETTI (1961), and the same applies to angiotensin I, anephrotoxin, pepsitensin, and pepsanurin (CROXATTO, PEREDA, and ZAMORANO, 1961). Substance P is also inactive (VAN DYKE, ADAMSONS, and ENGEL, 1955).

According to BERDE and STÜRMER (1962), oxytocin can still be determined by the rabbit milk-ejection assay procedure even if the oxytocin solution contains 0.1 mg ergometrine maleate per unit of oxytocin.

The method would be quite ideal if vasopressin did not also elicit an increase in milk-ejection pressure. True, unit for unit vasopressin is 6.1 ± 0.4 times less potent than oxytocin, but for assay purposes the oxytocin: vasopressin ratio must be known (CROSS and VAN DYKE, 1953).

11. Modifications of the Vivo Method

TINDAL and YOKOYAMA (1962), employed guinea-pigs instead of rabbits. Applying the substances intravenously, the standard doses were reduced to 0.3—0.9 mU (standard low dose) and 0.6—1.2 mU (standard high dose). The mean percentage error of nine 4-point assays was 3.0 ± 0.67. A further increase in sensitivity by a factor of 10—20 was achieved by administering the hormone solutions by close arterial injection into the blood supply of the mammary glands (FITZPATRICK, 1961; TINDAL and YOKOYAMA, 1962). In the guinea-pig, reliable assays with a percentage error of 3.7 ± 0.28 (mean of 7 assays) were carried out using intra-arterial oxytocin doses of 16—40 μU = standard low dose and 32—60 μU = standard high dose (TINDAL and YOKOYAMA, 1962; FITZPATRICK and WALMSLEY, 1962).

However, with the intra-arterial injection technique the superior specificity of the intravenous milk-ejection method is forfeited. Acetylcholine, 5-hydroxytryptamine and, in the guinea-pig but not in the rabbit, histamine can evoke a milk-ejection response. These false positive reactions can be limited by pretreatment of the animals with the appropriate antagonists (FITZPATRICK and WALMSLEY, 1962). False negative reactions occur after injection of adrenaline and/or noradrenaline which inhibit the milk-ejection effect. Pretreatment with dibenzyline eliminates this source of interference. Intra-arterial injections of bradykinin, angiotensin, anephrotoxin and pepsitensin do not provoke false positive reactions (FITZPATRICK and WALMSLEY, 1962; FITZPATRICK, MORRIS, and WALMSLEY, 1962). It has been reported that substance P will stimulate the mammary gland in large doses (FITZPATRICK, cited by SAWYER, 1966).

12. Reaction of Sucking Mice to the Better Milk Availability Induced by Oxytocin in the Mother

An indirect reaction to detect oxytocin was described by VORHERR in 1965. Lactating mice under aethanol anaesthesia were given increasing intravenous doses of oxytocin. The milk-ejection reaction thereby elicited leads to a change in the behaviour of the sucking young. They stretch out their hind limbs, reach upwards with their front limbs and pull vigorously at the teat. The threshold dose for this change of behaviour is around 0.13 mU/mouse. The method is unsuitable for use as a quantitative oxytocin assay procedure.

13. Cross-Circulation Technique in the Sheep

The reflex release of an oxytocic hormone in sheep has been studied by DEBACKERE, PEETERS, and TUYTTENS (1961), using a cross-circulation technique. In one ewe (the receptor) the intramammary pressure was recorded continuously, in the other, the donor, the genital organs were stimulated. The amount of hormone released by the donor's neurohypophysis evoked a milk-ejection pressure response in the receptor. This response was compared with that elicited by intravenously injected synthetic oxytocin and found to be of the order of 20—100 mU. This method is limited to larger animals and is not suitable for the standardisation of oxytocin.

14. In Vitro Methods

a) *Rabbit Mammary Strip.* Worthy of mention, but likewise unsuitable for routine assay work, are a few methods which make use of isolated mammary gland tissue.

In 1960 MENDEZ-BAUER, CABOT, and CALDEYRO-BARCIA described the use of lactating rabbit mammary strips *in vitro*. They obtained good discrimination in a dose range of 0.5—10 mU/ml and were able to show a linear relationship between oxytocin-concentration and response. The specificity of the reaction is claimed to be high, and the strips show no spontaneous activity. The sensitivity is of the same order as that of the intravenous *in vivo* assay, but less than that of the intra-arterial milk-ejection assay or the superfused rat uterus preparation.

The low specificity of rat mammary strips *in vitro* (see II. D. 14. b.) prompted MOORE and ZARROW (1965) to undertake new investigations on rabbit mammary strips. Under their experimental conditions the sensitivity range was 1—10 mU/ml, and over this range the dose-response curve was linear. Arg^8-vasopressin was found to have 15% of the stimulating activity of oxytocin. Histamine, 5-hydroxytryptamine, adrenaline, pilocarpine, ergonovine, insulin, relaxin, acetyl-strophanthidin, progesterone, DOCA and haemolysed human blood were without effect. Only substances with oxytocin-like structure and acetylcholine provoke effects, the latter was easily blocked by atropine which does not interfere with the action of oxytocin.

b) *Rat Mammary Strip.* In 1961 SMITH used strips of lactating rat mammary gland for assay purposes. In a series of five 4-point assays, each of 16 reactions, he obtained a mean percentage error of 3.9, and the mean fiducial limit ($P = 0.05$) was 15.3%. This preparation was shown to be more specific for oxytocin than the *in vivo* preparation, as the relative potency of $arginine^8$-vasopressin was only $3.2 \pm 0.24\%$ that of oxytocin unit for unit. The sensitivity of rat mammary strips is of the same order as that of rabbit mammary strips, i.e. 0.4—1.0 mU/ml.

In 1962 RYDÉN and SJÖHOLM confirmed the findings of SMITH (1961). The rat mammary strips reacted to as little as 0.005—0.1 mU/ml oxytocin. However, RYDÉN and SJÖHOLM (1962) also investigated the effect of other pharmacological agents on the rat mammary gland *in vitro* and found it to be highly sensitive to acetylcholine, adrenaline, noradrenaline and histamine, but less sensitive to 5-hydroxytryptamine. Moreover, acetylcholine considerably attenuated the response to simultaneously administered oxytocin. This lack of specificity greatly detracts from the value of the method.

c) *Rat Mammary Pieces.* Another technically very simple approach was followed by VAN DONGEN and HAYS (1966). Pieces of lactating rat mammary gland approximately 2 mm^3 in size were put in 0.01 ml oxytocin or unknown solution and observed through a dissecting microscope (magnification 15×). The time interval between exposure to oxytocin and the expulsion of milk was chosen as parameter. A linear relationship was found between log oxytocin-concentration and the log of this time interval over a concentration range of 10 mU — 0.1 m μU/ml. Since a volume of 0.01 ml was used, the actual amounts of oxytocin are 0.1 mU — 0.001 mμU. This is by far the most sensitive method for detecting oxytocin. However, this method is of low precision for assay purposes. In order to detect a tenfold difference in oxytocin concentration at a probability of 90% ($p = 0.1$), 13 or more observations are necessary. Because of this low power of discrimination, the method is unsuitable for oxytocin assay purposes. Moreover, the specificity of the effect elicited has not been investigated.

E. Immunobiological Methods

It is probable that immunobiological methods will attain high sensitivity coupled with high specificity for oxytocin. Thus, PERMUTT, PARKER, and UTIGER (1966) using a radio-immunoprecipitation method were able to detect 4 μU of unlabelled lysine[8]-vasopressin. The method described can presumably be readily adapted for oxytocin; the formation of antibodies to an oxytocin-albumin conjugate has already been demonstrated (HOLLÄNDER, FRANZ, and BERDE, 1966).

F. The Rat Blood Pressure Assay

1. History of the Test

The rat vasopressor assay was introduced by LANDGREBE, MACAULAY, and WARING (1946). To quote these authors: "The preparation is easy to set up, reliable, extremely sensitive and capable of good discrimination". An improvement in the method was introduced by DEKANSKI (1951, 1952), who pretreated the rats with adrenergic blocking agents to lower and stabilise the blood pressure. CHAUDHURY and JOPLIN (1960) employed pithed rat preparations (SHIPLEY and TILDEN, 1947) instead of anaesthetised rats for vasopressin assays and reported a 10 times greater sensitivity than with anaesthetised rats. According to SAWYER (1966) the pithed rat is as stable and as precise as a rat under urethane and responds to 400—800 μU vasopressin for assay purposes, this amounting to a 5-fold increase in sensitivity.

With the coming into force of U.S.P. XV on December 15, 1955, the rat blood pressure method was prescribed for vasopressin standardisation in USA; the method superseded standardisation of vasopressin on the blood pressure of the anaesthetised dog (U.S.P. XIV of November 1, 1950).

In Great Britain the rat blood pressure method received official recognition with the publication of the British Pharmacopoeia 1958 on September 1, 1958. It superseded the spinal cat blood pressure method of the previous British Pharmacopoeia 1953.

Hence in USA and Great Britain the rat blood pressure method is the only officially recognised method for the standardisation of vasopressin.

2. The Animal

A male albino rat, body weight 275—325 g (U.S.P. XVII) or about 300 g (BP 1958), is selected some 18 h prior to the assay.

3. *Pretreatment*

A 0.1% w/v solution of phenoxybenzamine is prepared and a dose of 1.0 ml/100 g rat body weight is injected slowly into a tail vein (U.S.P. XVII). The phenoxybenzamine solution is prepared as follows: 5 mg phenoxybenzamine hydrochloride (Dibenzyline) is dissolved in 0.1 ml ethanol. 1 drop of hydrochloric acid (35—38% w/w) is added and the solution is made up to 5 ml with 0.9% saline solution.

If the animal cannot be pretreated on the day preceding the assay, a 0.1% w/v solution of Dibenamine may be slowly injected via the femoral vein cannula in a dose of 0.1 ml/100 g body weight after the rat has been anaesthetised and prepared. The injection is repeated 10 min later and some 30 min afterwards the assay can be started. The Dibenamine solution is prepared in the same way as the solution of phenoxybenzamine.

The British Pharmacopoeia 1958 gives a general recommendation that the animal be pretreated with a suitable hypotensive agent such as hexamethonium tartrate.

In the author's laboratory the best results are obtained by pretreatment with intravenous phenoxybenzamine on the day before the assay; pretreatment with Dibenamine shortly before the commencement of the assay is not so good, but is acceptable; the author has no experience with hexamethonium.

The rat is pretreated with a sympathicolytic for the following reasons:

In an untreated rat intravenous injection of 0.1—0.5 ml 0.9% NaCl solution (the permitted volume of injection) elicits a pressor reaction. This reaction is completely prevented by means of a sympathicolytic (DEKANSKI, 1952).

Moreover, Dibenzyline and Dibenamine both abolish the usual pressor responses to adrenaline, noradrenaline, hydroxytyramine, nicotine and piperidine (DEKANSKI, 1951, 1952).

BARTELSTONE and NASMYTH (1965) have shown that infusion of a subliminal (pressor) dose of vasopressin (235—300 μU/kg/min) in the pithed rat leads to potentiation of the pressor reaction to intravenous injections of noradrenaline. In the light of similar findings for dogs, rats, cats and strips of isolated rat aorta, the authors conclude that endogenously liberated vasopressin may play a role in the responsiveness of vascular smooth muscle to endogenously liberated catecholamines. Conversely, it is conceivable also that endogenously released or exogenously administered catecholamines might influence the pressor effects of vasopressin, this being prevented by phenoxybenzamine blockade of the receptors.

Pretreatment with a sympathicolytic increases the sensitivity of the rats to vasopressin. The same phenomenon has also been observed in dogs (SUPEK et al., 1962).

Fig. 14. Rat mounted on the operating board in the dorsal position. The front paws are left free. The lines of incision are indicated by the black lines

Fig. 15. Rat, field of operation: neck. The trachea cannulated. Carotid artery prepared for cannulation

Fig. 16. Rat, field of operation: left upper hind leg. The inguinal ligament runs across the upper part of the field. The femoral artery and vein pass vertically downwards from under the ligament. Both give off a muscular branch to the left, and from them issue the superficial artery and vein which run to the right

Fig. 17. Rat, field of operation: left upper hind leg. The deep branch (superficial circumflex iliac artery and vein) are ready for tying off

Fig. 18. Rat, field of operation: left upper hind leg. The femoral vein is prepared for cannulation

Fig. 19. Rat, field of operation: left upper hind leg. Venous cannula tied in place

Fig.14

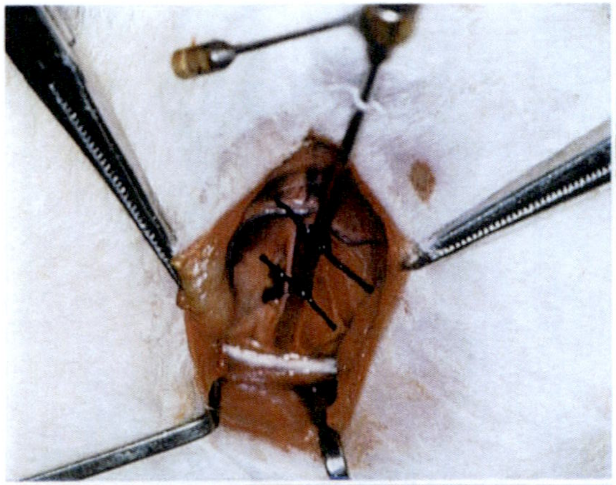

Fig. 15

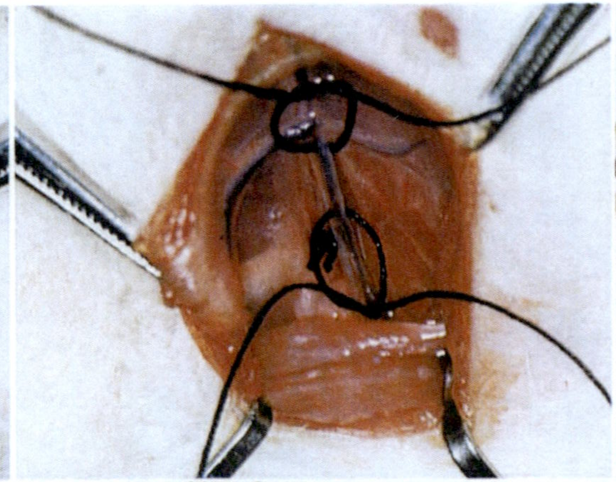

Fig. 16

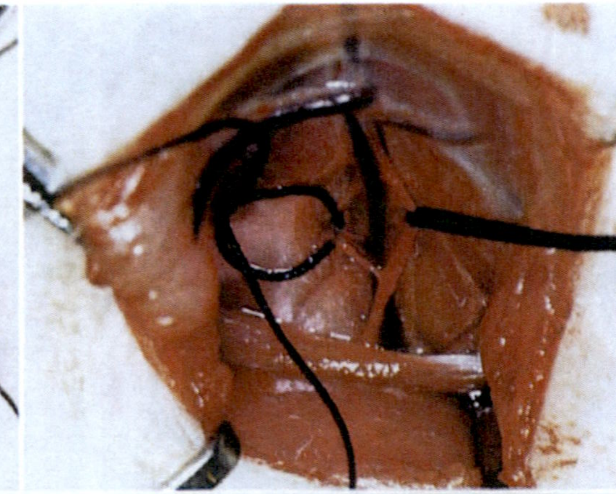

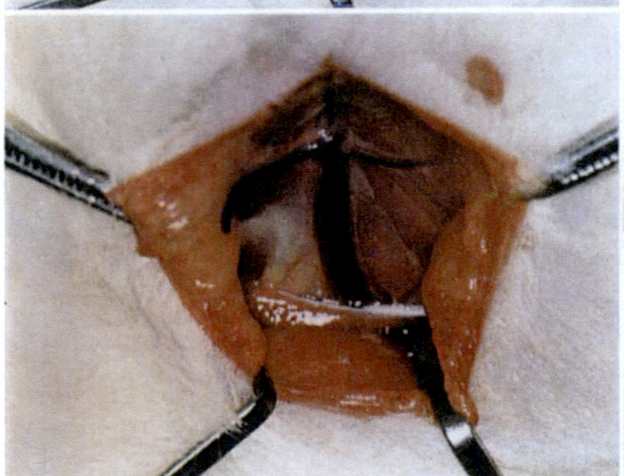

Fig. 17

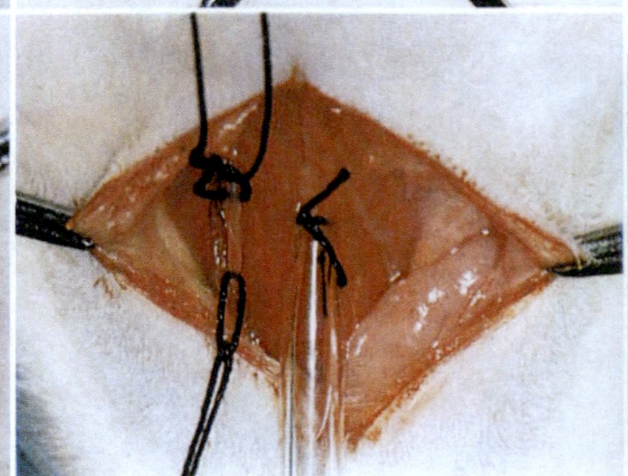

Fig. 18

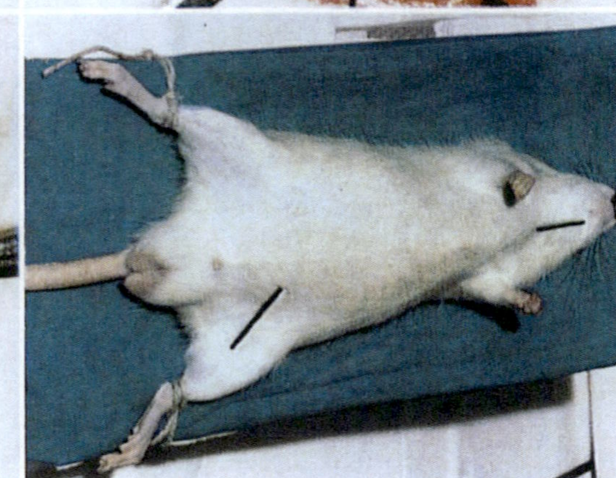

Fig. 19

4. *Anaesthesia*

On the day of the assay the rats are anaesthetised by subcutaneous injection of 0.7 ml/100 g body weight of a 25% w/v solution of urethane. The depth of anaesthesia necessary for preparation is attained within 45—60 min. Another method of anaesthesia which has also proved satisfactory is the intraperitoneal injection of 0.1 ml/100 g body weight of a solution prepared as follows: 25 g chlorobutanol is dissolved in 40 ml ethanol and the solution is made up to 100 ml by slowly adding warm distilled water with stirring (Pharmacopoea Nordica, 1960). With chlorobutanol the required depth of anaesthesia is attained in about 10 min.

5. *Operative Procedure*

The rat is mounted on a suitable operating board in the supine position by the teeth of the upper jaw and the two hind limbs. The front legs are not secured, this to facilitate spontaneous respiration. The trachea is first cannulated with a short glass or polythene tube about 2.5 mm in external diameter (the line of incision is shown in Fig. 14 and the trachea cannulated in Fig. 15). One carotid artery is then dissected for cannulation (Fig. 15). The femoral vein is then cannulated close to the inguinal ligament. Procedure: Skin incision in the left hind limb as shown in Fig. 14. The superficial epigastric (pudendal) vein is retracted to the right (Fig. 16) and the femoral vein is separated with a blunt instrument from the femoral artery in the direction of the inguinal ligament. Deep branches (superficial circumflex iliac artery and vein, Fig. 17) which issue from the femoral vessels must be located and tied off, otherwise bleeding may occur during cannulation. A short polythene cannula (described in the section on instruments) is tied into the femoral vein with two ligatures (Fig. 18 and 19) and the side arm of the cannula is joined to a 1 ml burette with a filling device by means of a short piece of rubber. The purpose of the burette is to wash in the active substance injected through the cannula. It is also possible to cannulate the jugular vein, but since the vagus nerves remain intact, manipulation of the cannula can lead to irritation. For this reason the femoral vein preparation is preferable.

After cannulation of the femoral vein the carotid cannula, which has an external diameter of approx. 1 mm and is filled with 1000 U/ml solution of heparin sodium, is now tied in and connected to a small-bore mercury manometer (Condon, 1951). It is better, but considerably more costly, to employ a strain-gauge transducer. When a mercury manometer is employed the pressure should be adjusted to 80 mm Hg.

The central and peripheral nervous system of the rat, including the two vagus nerves and the associated sympathetics remain intact. Artificial respiration is unnecessary and the animal need not be kept warm during the assay.

The latter recommendation is in line with the assay procedure described by Nielsen (1960), who makes no attempt to keep the body temperature constant but is at variance with the recommendation of U.S.P. XVII that the animal should be kept warm during its preparation and during the assay. In our experience the body temperature may fall to about 25° C during the assay without detriment to the sensitivity of the preparation. If the body temperature of rats anaesthetised with urethane is kept at the normal level (37° C), the blood pressure falls and the animals die before the assay can be completed (Stürmer, 1965).

Care should be taken when administering the injections, for which a tuberculin syringe is employed, to ensure that no air is injected since, in the rat, the tiniest air bubbles may lead to fatal embolism. The volume to be injected should be not less than 0.1 ml and should not exceed 0.5 ml.

6. *Instruments*

Fig. 20 shows the instruments and cannulas employed in the author's laboratory. The venous cannula for the femoral vein, shown on a larger scale in Fig. 21, has been found highly satisfactory. With it the injected solutions can be completely washed in and the cone of the cannula can be filled from below with 0.9% NaCl solution from the burette before the tuberculin syringe or stopper is put in place. This greatly reduces the risk of injecting air bubbles.

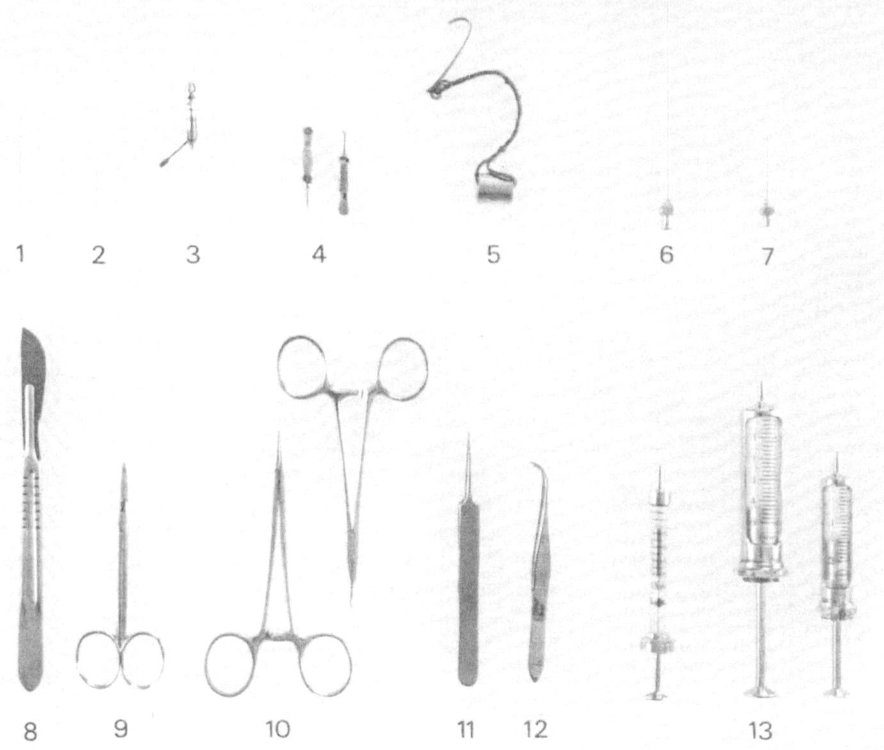

Fig. 20. Instruments: 1) Tracheal cannula, glass; 2) Cannula for the carotid artery, glass; 3) Cannula for the femoral vein, made from injection needles; 4) Bulldog clamps; 5) Weighted hook; 6, 7) Cannulas of various sizes; 8) Scalpel; 9) Fine scissors; 10) Halstead mosquito haemostats; 11) Watchmaker's forceps; 12) Fine curved forceps; 13) Various syringes

7. *The Test Procedure*

The test conforms to the 4-point assay design introduced by SCHILD (1942) for the bioassay of histamine. By a process of trial and error a low dose (S_1; T_1) and a high dose (S_2; T_2) of the standard (S) or unknown (T) dilution are determined, these being doses which elicit a rise of blood pressure greater than 20 mm Hg (S_1; T_1) and not exceeding 70 mm Hg (S_2; T_2). The time interval between injections remains the same at 12—15 min throughout the whole assay. The dose ratio (S_1:S_2 and T_1:T_2) depends upon the pressor effect elicited and normally lies between 1:2 and 3:5. If the pressor effects cannot be clearly discriminated with a dose ratio of 1:2, i.e. if double the dose (S_2; T_2) does not provoke a pressor response some 10—20 mm greater than that produced by the simple dose (S_1; T_1), the preparation is not suitable for assay purposes.

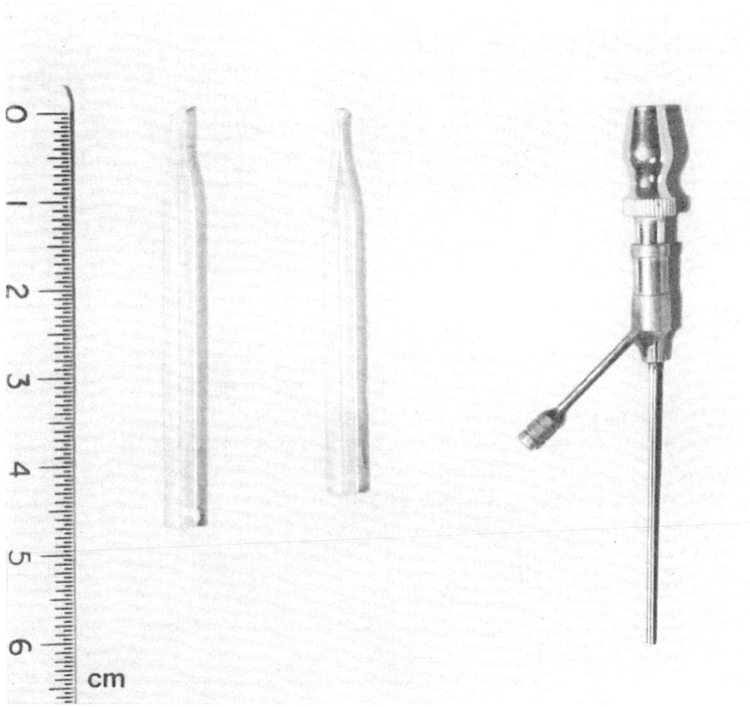

Fig. 21. Cannulas 1—3 from Fig. 21 shown on a larger scale. Instructions for making the venous cannula on the right: a hole is bored in the conical end of an ordinary injection cannula with blunted tip. A second cannula is soldered in place in this hole and serves as a side arm for washing in solution left in the cone and needle. Before the cannula is inserted in the vein a length of polyethylene tubing is pushed over the blunted tip

Table 12. *Report of an assay on two male rats*

S_1	d	S_2	d	T_1	d	T_2	d	
29	—1.1	55	2.7	31	0.6	54	—0.2	
35	4.9	51	—1.3	24	—6.4	54	—0.2	
21	—9.1	44	—8.3	26	—4.4	51	—3.2	
31	—0.9	50	—2.3	28	—2.4	50	—4.2	
30	—0.1	59	6.7	33	2.6	59	4.8	
28	—2.1	55	2.7	29	—1.4	53	—1.2	
29	—1.1	50	—2.3	29	—1.4	54	—0.2	
30	—0.1	49	—3.3	32	1.6	58	3.8	
32	1.9	55	2.7	37	6.6	56	1.8	
35	4.9	52	—0.3	35	4.6	54	—0.2	
30	—0.1	56	3.7	34	3.6	58	3.2	
31	0.9	52	—0.3	27	—3.4	49	—5.2	
$\bar{x}_{12} =$ 30.1		$\bar{x}_{12} =$ 52.3		$\bar{x}_{12} =$ 30.4		$\bar{x}_{12} =$ 54.2		$\Sigma d^2 = 592$

No. St 8723. Rat 1 = 300 g; rat 2 = 300 g.
Pretreatment: phenoxybenzamine i.v. 10 mg/kg 16 h, urethane s.c. 1.75 g/kg 1 h before the start of the assay.
S_1 = Standard low dose = 2.5 mU
S_2 = Standard high dose = 5.0 mU
Pressure reactions in mm Hg in 12 sets of 4-points (columns S_1, S_2, T_1, T_2); means ($\bar{x}_{12}$) and differences between the means and the individual values (d). Σd^2 = Sum of the squares of d.

The following procedure has proved successful with more than 90% of rats in the author's laboratory.

The 3rd Standard or substandard extract is diluted with 0.9% saline solution to a final concentration of 10 mU/ml. 0.25 ml corresponding to 2.5 mU vasopressin is injected as the standard low dose (S_1). This is washed in with 0.2 ml 0.9% saline solution from the burette, as is every injection throughout the assay. 15 min later 0.5 ml of the standard dilution corresponding to 5 mU vasopressin is injected (standard high dose = S_2). By trial and error equi-effective doses of the unknown dilution are determined (T_1 and T_2). The ratio T_1:T_2 must be exactly the same as the ratio S_1:S_2. Even if doses have to be reduced by half or doubled during the course of the assay, but this is very seldom necessary, the two ratios, S_1:S_2 and T_1:T_2, must remain the same.

a) *Sequence of Injections.* During the assay only very slight fluctuations in sensitivity occur. In general, the sensitivity increases during the first three hours of the assay, decreasing during the next three hours. To eliminate fluctuations in sensitivity, the sequence of injections is randomised. In accordance with U.S.P. XVII 4 pairs of injections are administered in random order, but the indicated sequence of the doses within pairs is maintained:

Pair 1: S_2 T_1. Pair 2: S_1 T_2. Pair 3: T_2 S_1. Pair 4: T_1 S_2.

Table 13. *Analysis of the data in Table 12*

Parameter	Formula	Value
I	log ratio of doses S_2/S_1	0.3010
E	difference in effect due to dose $= \frac{1}{2} \cdot (T_2 - T_1 + S_2 - S_1)$	23.0
F	difference in effect due to preparation $= \frac{1}{2} \cdot (T_1 + T_2 - S_1 - S_2)$	1.1
b	slope E/I	76.41
M	log potency ratio F/b	0.0144
% age potency	100 (antilog M)	103.4%
s^2	$\Sigma d^2/\Sigma\,(n-1) = 592/44$	13.4545
V	variance $s^2/n = 13.4545/12$	1.1212
t	at $P = 0.95$ with 44 degrees of freedom	2.02
$G/\sqrt{V(G)}$	$(T_2 - T_1 - S_2 + S_1)\,/\,\sqrt{4\,V} = 1.6/2.11773$ if this value is greater than that of t, the slopes are significantly different and the test invalid. 0.7555 is numerically less than 2.02 therefore the test is valid and the slopes not significantly different.	0.7555
B	$V/I^2 = 1.1212/0.090601$	12.375
g	index of significance of slope $B \cdot t^2/b^2 = 50.495/5{,}838$	0.008649
log fiducial limits if g is less than 0.1		
%	$2 \pm \frac{t}{b} \cdot \sqrt{V + BM^2}$	
	$= 2 \pm 0.02644 \cdot \sqrt{1.1212 + 12.375 \cdot 0.0002074}$	
	$= 2 \pm 0.02644 \cdot 1.06008$	2.028 — 1.972
fiducial limits %	antilog 2.028 — 1.972	106.7 — 93.8%
log fiducial limits if g exceeds 0.1		
%	$2 + \frac{g \cdot M}{1-g} \pm \frac{t}{b \cdot (1-g)} \cdot \sqrt{V \cdot (1-g) + BM^2}$ if g is greater than 1 the result is valueless. The fiducial limits of error of the estimated potency ($P = 0.95$) are not less than 66% and not more than 150% of the stated potency	

Pairs 1 and 2, Pairs 3 and 4, Pairs 1 and 3 as well as Pairs 2 and 4 each form a complete group of 4 injections (S_1, S_2, T_1, T_2). U.S.P. XVII lays down a total of 4 pairs of observations on 2 or more rats as a minimum; BP 1963 recommends a total of 4 or 5 groups (i.e. 16—20 injections). In the author's laboratory one experimenter tends 2 rats at a time, and in most cases it proves possible to administer 5—7 sets of 4 doses, i.e. a total of 20—28 injections per animal.

b) *Measuring the Recorded Reactions.* The pressor reactions — the distance from the mean pressure to the maximum pressure attained — are measured to the nearest mm Hg and tabulated. Two procedures may be followed in the statistical treatment of the measured values.

8. Statistical Treatment According to BP 1963

Table 12 shows the results of a 4-point assay on 2 rats (12 sets each of 4 points). Table 13 shows the statistical treatment of the results in this example.

9. Statistical Treatment According to U.S.P. XVII

The statistical treatment described in U.S.P. XVII differs fundamentally from that in BP 1963. Whereas in the latter the pressor reactions as such are the basis of the calculation, the U.S.P. XVII calculation is based upon the difference y between the increase in blood pressure after injection of the high dose and the increase after injection of the low dose of a pair of doses. This segregates the variation in sensitivity between pairs. In Table 14 the results of the example in Table 12 are arranged for evaluation in accordance with U.S.P. XVII. The statistical treatment of this example is illustrated in Table 15.

Table 14. *Data of the assay from Table 12 arranged for statisticat treatmenl according U.S.P. XVII*
Blood pressure rise (mm Hg) in dose pair no.

Set No.	1			2			3			4			Row totals $= T_r$
	S_2	T_1	y_1	S_1	T_2	y_2	T_2	S_1	y_3	T_1	S_2	y_4	
1	55	31	24	29	54	25	54	35	19	24	51	27	95
2	44	26	18	21	51	30	50	31	19	28	50	22	89
3	59	33	26	30	59	29	53	28	25	29	55	26	106
4	50	29	21	29	54	25	58	30	28	32	49	17	91
5	55	37	18	32	56	24	54	35	19	35	52	17	78
6	56	34	22	30	58	28	49	31	18	27	52	25	93
Column totals $= T_t$			$T_1 =$ 129			$T_2 =$ 161			$T_3 =$ 128			$T_4 =$ 134	$T =$ 552

10. Factors which may Influence the Results

a) *Hormones.* Female rats are unsuitable for vasopressin standardisation assays, since the vascular response of the rat to vasopressin varies with the concentration of ovarian hormones in the body (LLOYD, 1959a, b).

In male rats vasopressin sensitivity increases temporarily after castration (between the 5th and 10th day after orchidectomy). The dose of vasopressin required to raise the blood pressure of the rat 10 mm Hg was between 0.8 and 1.2 mU in untreated male rats and fell by a factor of 3—5 to 0.2—0.4 mU after castration (HONORÉ and LLOYD, 1961).

Injected intravenously, oxytocin does not affect the blood pressure of anaesthetised male rats in doses up to 100 mU (LLOYD, 1959a; HONORÉ and LLOYD, 1961).

Investigations by LLOYD (1959a, b), LLOYD and PICKFORD (1961), revealed a number of conditions under which oxytocin may have a pressor effect in the rat: oestrus and late pregnancy, administration of oestrogens alone or with

Table 15. *Analysis of data according U.S.P. XVII*

Parameter	Formula	Value
k	number of doses	4
f	number of sets	6
N	number of responses $= k \times f = 4 \times 6$	24
n	number of degrees of freedom $= (k - 1)(f - 1) = 3 \times 5$	15
R	ratio: standard dosage/unknown dosage	1
i	$\log (S_2/S_1) = \log (T_2/T_1) = \log (5/2.5) = \log 2$	0.301
T_a	$- T_1 + T_2 + T_3 - T_4 = - 129 + 161 + 128 - 134$	26
T_b	$T_1 + T_2 + T_3 + T_4 = 129 + 161 + 128 + 134$	552
M'	log relative potency $= i \cdot T_a/T_b = 0.301 \times \frac{26}{552}$	0.0142
R.P.	relative potency $= 100 \{\text{antilog}\,(M' + \log R)\}$	103.3%
T	sum of row totals $T_r = \Sigma T_r = \Sigma T_t = T_b$	552
s^2	error variance $= \frac{\Sigma y^2 - \Sigma T_r^2/k - \Sigma T_t^2/f + T^2/N}{n}$	
	$= \frac{\Sigma y^2 - \Sigma T_r^2/4 - \Sigma T_t^2/6 + T^2/24}{15}$	
	$= \frac{13{,}084 - 12{,}799 - 12{,}817 + 12{,}696}{15}$	10.933
t	value of t at n degrees of freedom with a probability $P = 0.95$ (from t-table)	2.131
t^2	$t \cdot t$	4.541
C	term measuring precision of the slope	
	$T_b^2/(T_b^2 - s^2 t^2 N) = \frac{552^2}{552^2 - 10.933 \times 4.541 \times 24}$	1.00393
	if C is negative, the slopes of standard and unknown are significantly different and the test is invalid. 1.00393 is positive, therefore the test is valid and the slopes not significantly different.	
L	confidence interval $= 2\sqrt{(C - 1)(CM'^2 + i^2)}$	
	$L^2 = 4(C - 1)(CM'^2 + i^2)$	
	$\frac{L^2}{4} = (C - 1)(CM'^2 + i^2)$	
	$= 0.00393 \times [1.00393 \times 0.0142^2 + 0.301^2]$	0.00035686
	$\frac{L}{2} = \sqrt{\frac{L^2}{4}} = 10^{-2}\sqrt{3{,}5686}$	0.01889
	$L = 2\,\frac{L}{2}$	0.0378
	if L exceeds 0.15 the assay is invalid.	
X_M	confidence limits for an estimated log potency	
	$= \log R + CM' \pm \frac{L}{2}$	
	$= 0.0 + 0{,}01426 \pm 0.0189$	0.99536—0.03316
R.P.	relative potency (with relative confidence limits)	103.3 (99—108)%

progesterone to male rats, pithing, bilateral vagotomy, decerebration, treatment with dihydroergotamine in a dose of 0.05—0.1 mg i.v., or 0.2 mg s.c. 2—3 h before the commencement of the assay, bretylium tosylate 1—2 mg i.v. or 2 mg s.c. $2^1/_2$ h before the assay, dibenamine given in 2 or 3 doses of 200 μg at 10 min intervals i.v., tetra-ethylammonium iodide, reserpine 0.5 mg s.c. daily for 2—4 days but not after atropine in a dose of 1—2 mg i.v. An enhanced pressor response to vasopressin by i.v. injection is observed in: females in oestrus, after pithing and decerebration, after treatment with dihydroergotamine, dibenamine, tetra-ethylammonium iodide and reserpine.

In practice male rats are used exclusively for standardisation, either anaesthetised after pretreatment with a sympathicolytic or as pithed rat preparations. In neither case is the possibility of interference by oxytocin excluded if the vasopressin solutions under investigation contain oxytocin. The 3rd Standard for example contains oxytocin. No investigations have been carried out to ascertain whether the pressor effects of oxytocin are of any significance in the dose range employed for standardisation (2.5—5 mU vasopressin). With an oxytocin: vasopressin ratio of 1:1 (3rd Standard) the doses of oxytocin administered along with the vasopressin are 10—20 times lower than the oxytocin doses employed by LLOYD and PICKFORD (1961). However, on standardising the vasopressin content of a purified oxytocin solution in which the oxytocin: vasopressin ratio is 20:1 or more, the doses of oxytocin administered simultaneously with the vasopressin are of the order of magnitude described. Further investigations are needed in order to clarify this question once and for all. If interference by oxytocin were of practical interest, e.g. as is vasopressin interference in the determination of oxytocin in the chicken blood pressure test, it would in all probability have come to light and have been described in the literature.

b) *Vasodilator Substances.* The intravenous infusion of acetylcholine 0.05 to 1.0 μg/min, isoprenaline 0.02—1.0 μg/min, 5-hydroxytryptamine 0.5—1.0 μg/min and histamine 2.5—5.0 μg/min lowered the blood pressure of the rat but did not alter the magnitude of the blood pressure response to vasopressin (LLOYD and PICKFORD, 1961).

c) *Preservatives.* U.S.P. XVII permits the addition of 0.5% chlorobutanol as a preservative to vasopressin solutions and extracts in ampoules with a declared vasopressin content of 10—20 U/ml, i.e. a maximum quantity of 5 mg chlorobutanol is present per 10 IU of the hormone. If 5 mU in 0.5 ml of vasopressin is injected as the unknown high dose, this volume of solution contains no more than 2.5 μg chlorobutanol. This dose does not influence the pressor effect of vasopressin. A dilator effect on isolated canine arteries is only observed with chlorobutanol doses of 100 μg/ml (SOMLYO, WOO, and SOMLYO, 1966).

d) *Histamine.* Postpituitary lobe powders may contain up to 1% of histamine acid phosphate equivalent by weight. The anaesthetised rat which has not been pretreated with a sympathicolytic agent gives the same response to a dose of pituitary extract before and after addition of histamine acid phosphate equivalent to 2% contamination of the original powder. Thus contamination with histamine to an extent likely to be encountered in commercial posterior pituitary powders will not affect the pressor assay in the anaesthetised rat. Spinal rats are very insensitive to histamine, but 0.05 mg will evoke a small rise of blood pressure without a preliminary fall (LANDGREBE, MACAULAY, and WARING, 1946).

e) *Tachyphylaxis.* After frequent successive doses, the response of spinal or anaesthetised cats to vasopressin progressively diminishes. This tolerance or tachyphylaxis persists for a period of $^1/_2$—1 h and is a function of the dose. The mechanism is not understood. In the rat injections can be made every 10—15 min without tolerance developing. A shorter interval between injections cannot be adopted because the blood pressure usually takes about 10 min to return to the base line. With a 15 min interval the rat blood pressure assay can be kept going for 12—15 h (Landgrebe, Macaulay, and Waring, 1946).

To overcome vasopressin tachyphylaxis in dogs Nash (1963) recommends administering about 8 mg/kg pyrogallol (1,2,3-trihydroxybenzene) which is claimed to prevent tachyphylaxis from occurring or to eliminate it if it does occur. This effect of pyrogallol is not due to inhibition of catechol o-methyltransferase by this substance.

f) *Lysine-vasopressin Dimers.* Under certain experimental conditions natural as well as synthetic vasopressin may polymerise to vasopressin-dimers (Schally and Guillemin, 1964). The blood pressure response of rats treated with phenoxybenzamine-urethane to these dimers was studied by Schally et al. (1964) and found to differ from the response to vasopressin monomer. The lysine^{8}-vasopressin dimers investigated, 1 "natural" and 1 synthetic dimer prepared by Guttmann (1962), elicited a pressor response which was slower in developing and lasted for much longer than that evoked by monomer. Moreover the specific pressor activity, i.e. the pressor activity in U/mg peptide material was found to be 11.31 U/mg for the natural dimer and 4.03 U/mg for the synthetic dimer. The dimers are therefore 20—70 times less active than the monomers and since they occur in ampoule solution only in minute amounts they will not interfere with the pressor assay of vasopressin solutions.

g) *Plasmakinins.* The occurrence of plasmakinins in postpituitary lobe extracts has not been described. However, if the rat blood pressure method is employed to determine the pressor activity of organ extracts or body fluids, such materials may contain plasmakinins under certain conditions. The plasmakinins bradykinin (kinin 9) and kallidin (kinin 10) lower the blood pressure of the rat in a dose-dependent fashion. The threshold dose for pure synthetic bradykinin is approximately 0.2 μg/kg rat body weight, corresponding to 0.06 μg/0.5 ml/300 g body weight rat (Konzett and Stürmer, 1960). Weight for weight kallidin is 3.3 times more potent than bradykinin (Stürmer and Berde, 1962; 1963). Thus in the rat the threshold dose for kallidin should be approx. 0.02 μg/0.5 ml/300 g body weight. Since the depressor effect of plasmakinins in the region of the threshold dose is very short-lived, and the pressor action of vasopressin lasts considerably longer, it may be assumed that in threshold doses the plasmakinins do not affect the outcome of the assay. Higher plasmakinin doses exert not only a more powerful, but also a more protracted fall of blood pressure and could counteract the effect of vasopressin, i.e. determination of vasopressin in plasmakinin-containing biological material would yield erroneously low values. Since at the present time no antagonists are known to the plasmakinins, it would be necessary in such cases to employ an assay method in which bradykinin had no effect, e.g. the antidiuretic assay in the rat.

h) *Angiotensin.* Like vasopressin, angiotensin exerts a pressor effect in the rat. There is no risk of interference from this source in the standardisation of synthetic vasopressin preparations and purified postpituitary extracts. However, the possibility of such interference cannot be excluded in the case of tissue extracts and body fluids. Here too recourse must be had to other test set-ups, since no antagonist is available.

j) *Substance P.* Intravenous administration of substance P generally elicits a brief fall in blood pressure due to peripheral vasodilatation. This effect, which occurs in all mammals, cannot be blocked by a specific antagonist and may, therefore, interfere with the vasopressin assay in rats.

G. Antidiuretic Assay

Determination of the antidiuretic effect of posthypophysial hormones is more time-consuming, more difficult and less accurate than standardisation of their pressor action on the rat blood pressure. On the other hand, the antidiuretic assay is extraordinarily specific and highly sensitive.

1. The History of the Antidiuretic Assay

The first quantitative and antidiuretic assays were carried out in dogs with bladder fistulae (Kestranek, Molitor, and Pick, 1925) and in human subjects (Bijlsma, Burn, and Gaddum, 1928). In 1930 Gibbs attempted to estimate the antidiuretic effect of posthypophysial extracts quantitatively in mice. The method described by Burn in 1931 has found wide use. It has been modified many times (Gilman and Goodman, 1937; Silvette, 1940; Krieger and Kilvington, 1940; Robinson and Farr, 1940; Ham, 1943; Birnie, Jenkins, Eversole, and Gaunt, 1949; Dicker and Ginsburg, 1950; Ginsburg, 1951; Stein, Jinks, and Mirsky, 1952; Berde, Doepfner, and Konzett, 1957).

2. Some Viewpoints on Method

a) *Administration of the Test Substances.* To-day it is generally agreed that the test substances must be administered intravasally (van Dyke, Adamsons, and Engel, 1955; Sawyer, 1966). Only by this route of administration is high sensitivity achieved, and the rapid return to the starting conditions permits standard and unknown injections to be given in a number sufficient for the needs of 3—6—point assay designs.

All the methods in which the posthypophysial hormones were injected subcutaneously suffered from a big drawback. The absorption of active substances from the subcutaneous tissues varies with the vaso-constrictor activity of the compounds injected. It emerged from our own investigations with analogues and homologues of vasopression (Berde, Boissonnas, Huguenin, and Stürmer, 1964; Huguenin, Stürmer, Boissonnas, and Berde, 1965; Stürmer, Huguenin, Boissonnas, and Berde, 1965) that vaso-constrictor activity did not necessarily parallel antidiuretic activity. Moreover, the active substances injected into the subcutaneous tissues are inactivated enzymatically to an unknown extent.

b) *Experimental Animal:* It is a relatively easy matter to make a choice on practical criteria among the animal species which are suitable for this assay method. If no well-trained bitches (Theobald, 1933; Samaan, 1935; Hare, Hickey, and Hare, 1941; O'Connor and Verney, 1942; Ames, Moore, and van Dyke, 1950; van Dyke, Adamsons, and Engel, 1955; Lauson and Bocanegra, 1961; Chan and Sawyer, 1962; Jaenike, 1963) or sheep (Cross, Thornton, and Tweddell, 1963) are available which will tolerate repeated gastric intubation and intravenous injections without reflex release of vasopressin, it is best to choose the rat, this being a cheap and suitable experimental animal (Jeffers, Livezy, and Austin, 1942). In most cases investigation of renal filtration by simultaneous determination of endogenous or exogenous creatinine clearance is dispensed with, so that it is no longer possible to say whether the antidiuretic effect is primarily due to increased reabsorption of water or is a secondary effect due to a reduced filtration rate (Hare, Hickey, and Hare, 1941; van Dyke, Adamsons, and Engel, 1955). Per kg of body weight, the dog and the rat are approximately equally sensitive to vasopressin (10—50 μU/kg). Thus, for the rat approx. 10—30 μU are employed per animal and injection, whereas for the dog approx. 250—500 μU are needed per animal and injection. It is seldom that more than one 4-point assay can be carried out in a dog in any one day (SAWYER, 1966); with rats it is usually possible to carry out three 4-point assays.

Because of the well-known lability of their renal circulation, rabbits are no longer employed (KESTRANEK, MOLITOR, and PICK, 1925; WALKER, 1939; FUGO and ARAGON, 1947; LINDQUIST and ROWE, 1949). Conscious water-loaded mice give a good diuretic response, but it is necessary to employ test and control groups, since only one dose can be administered per animal (NELSON and WOODS, 1934; HELLER and BLACKMORE, 1952).

c) *Anaesthesia:* In dogs, vasopressin assays are carried out without anaesthesia (THEOBALD, 1933; SAMAAN, 1935; HARE, HICKEY, and HARE, 1941; O'CONNOR and VERNEY, 1942; AMES, MOORE, and VAN DYKE, 1950; VAN DYKE, ADAMSONS, and ENGEL, 1955; LAUSON and BOCANEGRA, 1961; CHAN and SAWYER, 1962; JAENIKE, 1963). Methods have also been developed in which conscious rats are employed (GINSBURG and HELLER, 1953; JACOBSON and KELLOGG, 1956; HELLER, HERDAN, and ZAIDI, 1957; HUNTER, KALANT, and OGILVIE, 1959; GORDON and KALANT, 1960), but these were later abandoned in these same laboratories (HELLER and PICKERING, 1961; LEDERIS, 1961). Ethanol anaesthesia in rats has been found satisfactory, the ethanol serving also to block endogenous release of vasopressin (EGGLETON, 1942; STRAUSS, ROSENBAUM, and NELSON, 1950; VAN DYKE and AMES, 1951; DICKER, 1953; KLEEMAN, RUBINI, LAMDIN, and EPSTEIN, 1955; HELLER, 1960). However, it has been shown that painful stimuli and haemorrhage may trigger reflex antidiuresis even under ethanol anaesthesia (LITTLE and RADFORD, 1964; TATA and BUZALKOV, 1966).

For induction of anaesthesia and rapid attainment of the required state for the necessary operative manipulations it is customary to give ether in addition to alcohol. Since ether can stimulate endogenous release of vasopressin (AMES and VAN DYKE, 1952; DICKER, 1953) it is recommended to induce anaesthesia with Inactin (1-methyl-propyl)-thiobarbiturate sodium (WIRZ, 1956; SAWYER, 1961).

d) *Water load:* Procedures which ensure that the animals are under a constant water load are preferable to all methods in which water is given on one or several occasions to achieve hydration, since only a constant water load will ensure constant water diuresis. A constant water load may be maintained volumetrically by constant quantitative replacement of water corresponding to the volume of urine secreted, possibly allowing for insensible perspiration (BOURA and DICKER, 1953; DICKER, 1953; JACOBSON and KELLOGG, 1956; DETTELBACH, 1958; DE WIED, 1960; SHARE, 1961; WOLFMAN, MILLER, and COON, 1964; HEINTZ, DREWS, DREWS, and BRASS, 1964; TATA and GAUER, 1966). Alternatively, the water load may be kept constant by quantitative replacement of the loss in body weight due to excretion (SAWYER, 1958; SAWYER, 1961; BERDE and CERLETTI, 1961; DUFF, GRINELL, and KRAMAR, 1964). This latter method automatically compensates for extrarenal water loss also. In general, tap water at body temperature is employed for hydration. If 0.8% or stronger sodium chloride solutions are employed, administration of vasopressin elicits diuresis (SILVETTE, 1940).

The water is generally introduced directly into the stomach via a stomach tube, but intravenous infusion with normo- or hypotonic sodium chloride solutions has also been described (JACOBSON amd KELLOGG, 1956; CZACZKES, KLEEMAN, and KOENIG, 1964; HEINTZ, DREWS, DREWS, and BRASS, 1964; TATA and GAUER, 1966). The ethanol anaesthesia is maintained by adding a fixed percentage of ethanol to the water.

e) *Parameter:* Defining antidiuresis as a transient reduction in the quantity of urine produced in a given time, the task in hand is to measure this effect of vasopressin quantitatively. The volumetric method in which the drops of urine are counted is a very effective one, and with a few clever refinements of method it is possible to record drops with a constant volume of 5—7 μl (BERDE and CERLETTI, 1961; NIELSEN, 1965). Usually the number of drops excreted during a given collection period before injection of vasopressin is employed as the baseline value, and defined as 100% diuresis. After injection of vasopressin, the number of drops excreted in a collection period of the same duration is reduced. The deficit in number of drops excreted is expressed as a percentage of the number of drops excreted during the control period and is usually taken to be a measure of antidiuretic activity. Procedures in which the integral beneath the flow-curve is determined planimetrically or by calculation for a definite period before and

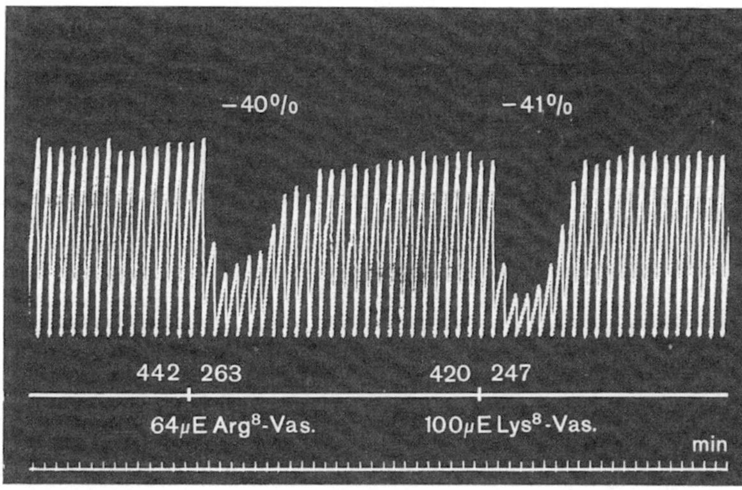

Fig. 22. Differences in the antidiuretic action of arginine⁸-vasopressin (3rd Standard) and synthetic lysine⁸-vasopressin on the hydrated, ethanol anaesthetized rat. The vertical lines indicate the diuresis in number of drops per minute. The number of drops for a 10 min period before and after intravenous injection is denoted by the appropriate sign. The decrease in diuresis for each 10 min period is calculated in %. Time given in minutes. From our calculations both arginine⁸- and lysine⁸-vasopressin appeared to exert an equal effect (i.e. —40% and —41% respectively). The latter substance exerting a somewhat quicker onset and shorter duration than arginine⁸-vasopressin.
However, the assessment of activity depends upon the specific criteria chosen. Thus if one considers the results in terms of maximum decrease, then clearly lysine⁸-vasopressin is the more active substance, but in terms of duration of effect, arginine⁸-vasopressin exerts the more sustained antidiuretic action.
(From BERDE and CERLETTI, 1961)

after injection are equally good. Both procedures can lead to false interpretations if, for example, the activity of lysine⁸-vasopressin is compared with the 3rd Standard. Apart from the fact that the dose-effect curves of the two substances differ significantly, their actions differ in quality (VAN DYKE, ENGEL, and ADAMSONS, 1956; SAWYER, 1958; NIELSEN, 1958; THORN, 1959; BERDE and CERLETTI, 1961; SAWYER, CHAN, and VAN DYKE, 1962). Fig. 22. If maximum antidiuretic activity is the yardstick, the activity relations arrived at will differ from those obtained by evaluating the excretory deficit over a given period of time. These difficulties will soon be eliminated since the international lysine⁸-vasopressin standard proposed in 1961 by BERDE and CERLETTI will be introduced in the not too distant future. Nevertheless, when determining the antidiuretic activity of homologues and analogues of vasopressin, the problem of comparing non-identical active substances remains, and a plea must be made for exact definition and description of the method of evaluation in investigations of this kind.

Owing to the increased tubular reabsorption of water in response to vasopressin, not only is the amount of urine excreted in a given time reduced, but the specific weight, electrical conductivity and chloride content of the urine increase, and its freezing point is proportionally depressed. These changes have also been made use of by various authors for the quantitative determination of vasopressin. None of the methods mentioned has proved superior to diret measurement of the antidiuretic effect.

Specific weight: THORN, 1957; BARATZ and INGRAHAM, 1959; RABASA and BERGMANN, 1964.

Depression of freezing point: CRAWFORD and PINKHAM, 1954.

Electrical conductivity: SAWYER, 1958; SAWYER, 1961; ALBERS and BRIGHTMAN, 1959; SHARE, 1961; SHARE and LEVY, 1962; YOSHIDA, MOTOHASHI, IBAYASHI, and OKINAKA, 1963.

Chloride content: DUFF, GRINELL and KRAMAR, 1964.

In the rat intravenous antidiuresis assay, a response is generally obtained with doses of approx. 10 μU. Some authors have achieved higher sensitivity (HELLER and ŠTULC, 1959: 0.625 μU; VORHERR and FRIEDBERG, 1959: 5 μU; CZACZKES, KLEEMAN, and KOENIG, 1964: 0.25 μU; HEINTZ, DREWS, DREWS, and BRASS, 1964: 0.1 μU; LITTLE and RADFORD, 1964: 2.5 μU; JONES and LEE, 1965: 2 μU; TATA and GAUER, 1966: 0.25 μU).

High sensitivity is also attained in the close arterial injection technique (HALLIDAY, 1966 cited by SAWYER, 1966: 1.5—3 μU).

Indeed, DUFF, GRINELL, and KRAMAR (1964) have reported routine assay of 0.005 μU arginine^8-vasopressin by intra-arterial injection in the tail artery of young rats.

3. *An Antidiuretic Assay Procedure*

Below is described in some detail a method which, for a relatively small outlay in effort and material, yields satisfactory results. Elsewhere in this volume FITZPATRICK and BENTLEY give a detailed report of an antidiuresis method which is designed for the determination of minute quantities of vasopressin rather than for the standardisation of the hormone which is the main topic under discussion in this chapter.

a) *The rat.* A group of about 20 healthy male rats, body weight 250 g, is selected.

b) *Pretreatment of the Rats.* By means of a stomach tube 10 ml of tap water at body temperature is introduced into the stomach of the rats every evening for 2—3 days. This training accustoms the animals to gastric intubation. On the evening before the assay, two rats are selected which can be intubated without showing signs of agitation. These animals are taken to the laboratory and are given drinking water ad libitum but no food. On the morning of the assay, both rats are given 5 ml of tap water at body temperature per 100 g body weight via a stomach tube.

c) *Anaesthesia.* 45 min after administration of the water the more placid rat is given 5 ml/100 g body weight of a 12% (v/v) ethanol solution via a gastric tube. Within 5—10 min, anaesthesia is usually so profound that preparation can be commenced. If necessary, ether can be given to provide a transiently more profound state of anaesthesia.

d) *Preparation.* The rat is fixed by its hind paws in a supine position on the operation board, the front limbs being left free. The skin of the lower abdomen is divided by means of a median incision down to the symphysis. The abdominal wall in the lower quadrant is divided along the linea alba, and the abdominal cavity is opened. A thread is looped around the upper pole of the bladder fundus, the thread being left long to permit manipulation of the bladder during the subsequent introduction of the catheter. A second thread is looped around the neck of the bladder. The posterior wall of the bladder is opened medially with a fine pair of scissors. Any parasites in the bladder are washed out with 0.9% sodium chloride solution at body temperature. A soft rubber catheter about 7 cm in length (Rüsch No. 7, external diameter 2.2 mm) is then introduced with the opening pointing downwards towards the trigonum and fixed in place by drawing the second thread tight so that the upper two-thirds of the bladder is eliminated. The catheter completely fills the neck of the bladder, leaving scarcely any bladder space capable of contracting or expanding. The penis is ligated near the root. A third ligature is tied around the catheter between the penis and the lower end of the skin incision, and the abdomen is closed with two sutures.

A polyethylene catheter (PE 10) filled with 0.3% heparin solution (w/v) is introduced into the jugular vein in the usual way, and inserted a distance of about 4 cm, almost to the heart. The trachea is exposed and a loop of thread placed around it. A thread is also placed around the oesophagus. The trachea is opened and a tracheal cannula tied in place. A rubber catheter (Rüsch No. 7, external diameter 2.2 mm) is passed through the mouth into the stomach (approx. 13 cm) and fixed in place with the thread which is looped around the oesophagus. The rat is then laid ventrally on the scales (see below), the stomach tube connected to an infusion pump, the bladder catheter connected to the Woulfe bottle of the drop counting system and the venous cannula fixed in place on a stand independent of the scales, so that the insertion of an injection syringe does not affect the scales.

e) *Apparatus*. The rat is fixed by its front paws on a cork plate in the ventral position. A thermometer is introduced into the rectum and fixed to the scales. The body temperature of the animals is kept between 37° and 38° C by means of a lamp mounted over the animal. The scales are then set at a weight which comprises the sum of the following:

1. Body weight of the rat +9%.
2. Weight of the tracheal cannula.
3. Weight of the thermometer.
4. Weight of the cork plate and adhesive tape.
5. Weight of the bladder and stomach catheters.
6. Weight of the venous catheter.

The infusion pump now infuses a solution of 2% ethanol (v/v) containing 5% glucose (w/v) until the scales are balanced. As soon as the rat loses 0.2 g weight by excretion of urine and insensible perspiration during the course of the assay, the scales are put out of balance. A photoelectric device on the pointer of the scales switches the infusion pump on, which then delivers 0.2 ml of the ethanol/glucose solution, thereby restoring the balance. With the aid of this simple feedback mechanism, the water balance and depth of anaesthesia are kept constant throughout the assay. Over the next 30 min, the rate of diuresis generally increases, levelling off at a high value (15 — over 40 drops/min).

The bladder catheter is connected to a train of two Woulfe bottles with a capacity of 500 ml, which are filled with a solution containing 50% ethanol (v/v) and 0.5% sodium chloride (w/v) and are free from bubbles. The overflow from the second bottle leads to a number 16 injection needle, whose tip has been cut off horizontally, and which delivers 160—180 drops per ml for the drop counter. The system is, of course, sensitive to fluctuations in temperature, hence the room temperature should be kept as near as possible constant.

The number of drops is recorded with a cumulative recorder, e.g. Thorp recorder. In addition, each drop is counted on a resetting impulse counter. With this counter the exact number of drops can be determined for any given period during the assay.

f) *The Test Procedure.* When diuresis, defined as the number of drops per given period of time, has attained a practically constant level, a count is made of the number of drops during a 10-min period. 20 or 40 μU of the standard preparation is then given by intravenous injection in the jugular vein. The volume of injection is 0.1 ml and every injection is washed in with 0.1 ml 0.9% sodium chloride solution. The drop counter is set back to 0, and the number of drops during the 10-min period after injection is determined. The deficit in number of drops serves as a measure of antidiuretic activity of the standard or unknown as the case may be, and is expressed as a percentage of the number of drops counted before injection (initial value). The injections are given at intervals of 25 min. Under favourable conditions, the preparation can be used for seven hours or longer. Often the sensitivity to antidiuretic hormone and to similar peptides increases at the beginning of the experiment. Standardisation assays are only started when the sensitivity of the preparations has attained a stable level. The doses chosen for standardisation are those inhibiting diuresis by 20—80%.

g) *4-Point Assay Design.* The 4-point procedure is suitable for antidiuresis standardisation work. The ratio of the standard low dose to the standard high dose (S_1:S_2) and of the unknown low dose to unknown high dose (T_1:T_2) should be at least 1:2, or better 1:2.5 or 1:3. Three sets, each of 4 points (12 injections) are administered to a rat, the sequence of injections being randomised. The results for 3 rats are grouped together and regarded as one assay. The statistical evaluation is as for the rat blood pressure assay.

h) *3-Point Assay Design.* In this procedure a dose of unknown is given between two identical doses of standard, i.e. the sequence of injections is standard, unknown, standard, unknown, standard, etc. The dose of unknown is varied according to a definite schedule. The following unknown:standard dose ratio has been found satisfactory: 1:1; 1.6:1; 2.5:1; 4:1; 6.4:1; 10:1. In certain circumstances the intervals can be reduced by introducing additional dose ratios; 1.25:1; 2:1; 3.2:1; 5:1; 8:1. The dose ratios are selected according to the response which the unknown solution elicits. A ratio of standard or unknown is first found in which the reaction to unknown is noticeably weaker than the reaction after injection of the standard doses before and after the unknown. The ratio of unknown to standard is then increased step by step as indicated above until the response to the unknown is definitely greater than that on injecting the standard. For each dose ratio within the range: definitely weaker to definitely stronger response to unknown, at least 5 sets of 3 injections are made for comparison. The comparison is qualitative rather than quantitative, i.e. the responses are compared to ascertain whether the unknown acts more powerfully or weaker than the standard in the given dose ratio. In most cases it is at once clear whether the response is stronger or weaker. If the responses are identical, $^1/_2$ reaction is tabulated as being stronger and $^1/_2$ reaction as being weaker. For each dose ratio of unknown:standard, the relative frequency of the reactions: unknown stronger than standard are indicated as a percentage of the total number of reactions with this dose ratio and transformed into probits. The dose ratios and their probit values are now plotted on probability paper, the dose ratios on the abscissa and the probit values on the ordinate. The points obtained are joined by the best straight line, and the dose ratio with which unknown and standard are equipotent is read off from the graph at probit 5. The approximate standard error is likewise obtained graphically by the method of Miller and Tainter (1944).

H. Immunological Methods

Immunological methods combine high sensitivity with high specificity. Permutt, Parker, and Utiger succeeded in detecting 4 μU of unlabelled lysine[8]-vasopressin using a radio-immuno-precipitation method in 1966. Immunological methods are at present confined to specialised laboratories and call for a great deal of costly apparatus. Whether they will come to replace the established blood pressure and antidiuretic methods in due course it is still too early to say.

J. Unsuitable Methods

The methods listed below are unsuitable for quantitative assaying of posthypophysial hormones, despite the fact that some of them are given in pharmacopoeias.

1. Unsuitable Methods for the Determination of Oxytocin

a) *In vitro assay on the isolated guinea-pig uterus* (U.S.P. XVII; Pharmacopoea Internationalis).

b) *In vitro assay on the cloacal end of the oviduct of the turtle* (Munsick, Sawyer, and van Dyke, 1960).

c) *In vitro assay on the isolated intestine of the tench, tinca vulgaris* (Ohnesorge and Rehberg, 1963).

d) *Assay on the crop glands of the pigeon* (Chaudhury and Chaudhury, 1952; Höhn, 1963; Mizuno and Meites, 1963).

e) *Assay based on intestinal inhibitory response* (Levy, 1963).

f) *Assay based on the behavioural response in sucking litter mice* (Vorherr, 1965).

2. Unsuitable Vasopressin Assay Methods

a) *In vitro assay on isolated toad bladders* (Edelman, Petersen, and Gulyassy, 1964; Natochin, Janáček, and Rybová, 1965).

b) *In vitro assay on the isolated guinea-pig colon* (Botting, 1965).

c) *Assay on the blood pressure of the spinal cat* (Pharmacopoea Internationalis).

d) *Assay on the antidiuretic response of rabbits* (Fugo and Aragon, 1947; Lindquist and Rowe, 1949).

e) *Assays on frogs and toads* (Brunn, 1921; Buchborn, 1955; Lauber, Eversole, and Childs, 1959; Pigeon and Epstein, 1963).

f) *Assay based on the instestinal inhibitory response* (Levy, 1963).

References

Albers, R.W., and M.W. Brightman: A major component of neurohypophysial tissue associated with antidiuretic activity. J. Neurochem. **3**, 269—276 (1959).

Ames, R.G., and H.B. van Dyke: Antidiuretic hormone in the serum or plasma of rats. Endocrinology **50**, 350—360 (1952).

—, D.H. Moore, and H.B. van Dyke: The excretion of posterior pituitary antidiuretic hormone in the urine and its detection in the blood. Endocrinology **46**, 215—227 (1950).

Arimura, A., and J.F. Dingman: Specific and sensitive assay method for vasopressin and oxytocin using glass-paper-chromatography. Nature (Lond.) **184**, 1874—1875 (1959).

Baïsset, A., et P. Monastruc: Le dosage de l'hormone antidiurétique. Rev. franç. Étud. clin. biol. **5**, 1030—1034 (1960).

Bangham, D.R., and M.V. Mussett: Third International Standard for Posterior Pituitary (Re-named Third International Standard for Oxytocic, Vasopressor and Antidiuretic Substances in 1956). Bull. Wld Hlth Org. **19**, 325—340 (1958).

Baratz, R.A., and R.C. Ingraham: Sensitive bioassay method for measuring antidiuretic hormone in mammalian plasma. Proc. Soc. exp. Biol. (N.Y.) **100**, 296—299 (1959).

BARTELSTONE, H.J., and P.A. NASMYTH: Vasopressin potentiation of catecholamine actions in dog, rat, cat, and rat aortic strip. Amer. J. Physiol. **208**, 754—762 (1965).
BEAUVILLAIN, A.: Titrage des préparations posthypophysaires par leur seuil d'action sur l'utérus isolé de rat adulte. C.R. Soc. Biol. (Paris) **137**, 284—285 (1943).
BENTLEY, P., and S. E. DICKER: Effects of transient changes of acidity on the isolated rat's uterus, with reference to the assay of oxytocic activity. Brit. J. Pharmacol. **10**, 424—428 (1955).
BENTLEY, P.J., and E. MCEVEN: The effects of ion changes on the contraction of the rat uterus stimulated by oxytocin. Brit. J. Pharmacol. **16**, 45—49 (1961).
— The potentiating action of magnesium and manganese on the oxytocic effect of some oxytocin analogues. J. Endocr. **32**, 215—222 (1965).
BERDE, B.: Recent progress in oxytocin research. Springfield, Ill.: Charles C. Thomas 1959.
— Unpublished data, 1963.
—, R. A. BOISSONNAS: Synthetic analogues and homologues of the posterior pituitary hormones. In: The Pituitary gland. Ed. by G.W. HARRIS and B.T. DONOVAN. London: Butterworths & Co. 1966.
— —, R. L. HUGUENIN, and E. STÜRMER: Vasopressin analogues with selective pressor activity. Experientia (Basel) **20**, 42—43 (1964).
—, et A. CERLETTI: Démonstration expérimentale de l'action de l'oxytocine sur la glande mammaire. Gynaecologia (Basel) **144**, 275—278 (1957).
— — Über die Wirkung pharmakologischer Oxytocindosen auf die Milchdrüse. Acta endocr. (Kbh.) **34**, 543—557 (1960).
— — Über die antidiuretische Wirkung von synthetischem Lysin-Vasopressin. Helv. physiol. Acta **19**, 135—150 (1961).
— — Prüfung von Bradykinin und Hypertensin an der Milchdrüse. Helv. physiol. Acta **19**, C 7 — C 10 (1961).
—, W. DOEPFNER, and H. KONZETT: Some pharmacological actions of four synthetic analogues of oxytocin. Brit. J. Pharmacol. **12**, 209—214 (1957).
—, R. HUGUENIN, and E. STÜRMER: The biological activities of arginine-vasotocin obtained by a new synthesis. Experientia (Basel) **18**, 444 (1962).
—, and K. SAAMELI: Evaluation of substances acting on the uterus. In: Methods in drug evaluation, p. 481—514. Ed. by P. MANTEGAZZA and F. PICCININI. Amsterdam: North-Holland Publ. Co. 1966.
—, and E. STÜRMER: The biological assay of oxytocin in the presence of ergometrine. J. Pharm. Pharmacol. **14**, 169—171 (1962).
BERGER, E., and J.M. MARSHALL: Interactions of oxytocin, potassium and calcium in the rat uterus. Amer. J. Physiol. **201**, 931—934 (1961).
BIJLSMA, U.G., J.H. BURN, and J.H. GADDUM: A comparison of the oxytocic, pressor and antidiuretic activities of commercial samples of pituitary extract. Quart. J. Pharm. Allied Sci. **1**, 493—508 (1928).
BIRNIE, J.H., W.J. EVERSOLE, W.R. BOSS, C.M. OSBORNE, and R. GAUNT: An antidiuretic substance in the blood of normal and adrenalectomized rats. Endocrinology **47**, 1—12 (1950).
—, R. JENKINS, W.J. EVERSOLE, and R. GAUNT: An antidiuretic substance in the blood of normal and adrenalectomized rats. Proc. Soc. exp. Biol. (N.Y.) **70**, 83—85 (1949).
BISSET, G.W.: The assay of oxytocin and vasopressin in blood and the mechanism of inactivation of these hormones by sodium thioglycollate. In: Oxytocin, p. 380—398. Symposium in Montevideo 1959. Ed. by R. CALDEYRO-BARCIA and H. HELLER. Oxford: Pergamon Press 1961.
BOISSONNAS, R.A., J. FRANZ, and E. STÜRMER: On the chemical characterization of substance P. Ann. N.Y. Acad. Sci. **104**, 376—377 (1963).
BOTTING, J.H.: An isolated preparation with a selective sensitivity to vasopressin. Brit. J. Pharmacol. **24**, 156—162 (1965).
BOURA, A., and S.E. DICKER: An apparatus for the maintenance of a constant water load and the recording of urine flow in rats. J. Physiol. (Lond.) **122**, 144—148 (1953).
BROTANEK, V., and S. KAZDA: Differences in the vasodepressor reaction to oxytocin in men and nonpregnant and pregnant women. Amer. J. Obstet. Gynec. **93**, 547—552 (1965).
BRUNN, F.: Beitrag zur Kenntnis der Wirkung von Hypophysenextrakten auf den Wasserhaushalt des Frosches. Z. ges. exp. Med. **25**, 170—175 (1921).
BUCHBORN, E.: Ein quantitativer biologischer Adiuretin-(Vasopressin-)Nachweis an der Kröte. Z. ges. exp. Med. **125**, 614—625 (1955).
BUÑAG, R.D., and E.J. WALASZEK: The depressor effect of serotonin and tryptamine on chicken blood pressure. J. Pharmacol. exp. Ther. **133**, 52—56 (1961).
— — The mechanism of serotonin and tryptamine induced vasodepression in the chicken. J. Pharmacol. exp. Ther. **135**, 151—155 (1962).
— — The cardiovascular effects of substance P in the chicken. Ann. N.Y. Acad. Sci. **104**, 437—448 (1963).

BURN, J.H.: Estimation of the antidiuretic potency of pituitary (posterior lobe) extract. Quart. J. Pharm. **4**, 517—529 (1931).

—, and H.H. DALE: Reports on biological standards. I. On the physiological standardization of the extracts of the posterior lobe of the pituitary body. Spec. Rep. Ser. Med. Res. Counc. London No. 69, p. 5—52 (1922).

—, D.J. FINNEY, and L.G. GOODWIN: Biological standardization, 2nd ed. London: Oxford University Press 1950.

CAMBRIDGE, G.W., and J.A. HOLGATE: Superfusion as a method for the study of drug antagonism. Brit. J. Pharmacol. **10**, 326—335 (1955).

CERLETTI, A., and W. DOEPFNER: Comparative study on the serotonin antagonism of amide derivatives of lysergic acid and of ergot alkaloids. J. Pharmacol. exp. Ther. **122**, 124—136 (1958).

CHAN, W.Y., M. O'CONNELL, and S.R. POMEROY: Effects of the estrous cycle on the sensitivity of rat uterus to oxytocin and desamino-oxytocin. Endocrinology **72**, 279—282 (1963).

—, and W.H. SAWYER: Natriuresis in conscious dogs during arginine-vasopressin infusion and after oxytocin injection. Proc. Soc. exp. Biol. (N.Y.) **110**, 697—699 (1962).

CHAUDHURY, R.R., and M.R. CHAUDHURY: Action of synthetic oxytocin on the crop gland of the pigeon. Nature (Lond.) **193**, 179—180 (1962).

—, and G.F. JOPLIN: Preliminary observations on the release of oxytocin and vasopressin in human subjects. J. Endocr. **21**, 125—128 (1960).

CLEGG, P.C.: The effect of adrenergic blocking agents on the guinea-pig uterus *in vitro*, and a study of the histology of the intrinsic myometrial nerves. J. Physiol. (Lond.) **169**, 73—90 (1963).

COHEN, A., R.A. HALL, B. HEATH-BROWN, M.W. PARKES, and A.H. REES: Oxytocic activity of basic (aminomethyl) derivatives of phenols and related compounds. Brit. J. Pharmacol. **12**, 194—208 (1957).

CONDON, N.E.: A modification of the conventional mercury manometer for blood pressure recordings. Brit. J. Pharmacol. **6**, 19—20 (1951).

COON, J.M.: A new method for the assay of posterior pituitary extracts. Arch. int. Pharmacodyn. **62**, 79—99 (1939).

CRAWFORD, J.D., and B. PINKHAM: An assay method for antidiuretic hormone based on a more specific response index. Endocrinology **55**, 521—529 (1954).

CROSS, B.A., and H.B. VAN DYKE: The effects of highly purified posterior pituitary principles on the lactating mammary gland of the rabbit. J. Endocr. **9**, 232—235 (1953).

—, and G.W. HARRIS: The role of the neurohypophysis in the milk-ejection reflex. J. Endocr. **8**, 148—161 (1952).

CROSS, R.B., W.M. THORNTON, and E.D. TWEDDELL: The effect of vasopressin on water and electrolyte excretion by the sheep. Aust. J. exp. Biol. med. Sci. **41**, 629—636 (1963).

CROXATTO, H., T. PEREDA, and B. ZAMORANO: Oxytocic substances in blood serum. In: Oxytocin, p. 412—424. Symposium in Montevideo 1959. Ed. by R. CALDEYRO-BARCIA and H. HELLER. Oxford: Pergamon Press 1961.

CZACZKES, J.W., C.R. KLEEMAN, and M. KOENIG: Physiologic studies of antidiuretic hormone by its direct measurement in human plasma. J. clin. Invest. **43**, 1625—1640 (1964).

DALE, H.H.: Wartime arrangements for international biological standards and the new standard for pituitary (posterior lobe) preparations. Brit. med. J. **1942 II**, 385—387.

—, and P.P. LAIDLAW: A method of standardising pituitary (infundibular) extract. J. Pharmacol. exp. Ther. **4**, 75—95 (1912).

DEBACKERE, M., G. PEETERS, and N. TUYTTENS: Reflex release of an oxytocic hormone by stimulation of genital organs in male and female sheep studied by a cross-circulation technique. J. Endocr. **22**, 321—334 (1961).

DEKANSKI, J.: A pressor substance in urine. Brit. J. Pharmacol. **6**, 351—356 (1951).

— The quantitative assay of vasopressin. Brit. J. Pharmacol. **7**, 567—572 (1952).

DETTELBACH, H.R.: A method for assaying small amounts of antidiuretic substances with notes of some properties of vasopressin. Amer. J. Physiol. **192**, 379—386 (1958).

DICKER, S.E.: Method for the assay of very small amounts of antidiuretic activity with a note on the antidiuretic titre of rat's blood. J. Physiol. (Lond.) **122**, 149—157 (1953).

— Release of vasopressin and oxytocin from isolated pituitary glands of adult and new-born rats. J. Physiol. (Lond.) **185**, 429—444 (1966).

—, and M. GINSBURG: Some observations on the antidiuretic activity of rat serum. Brit. J. Pharmacol. **5**, 497—504 (1950).

VAN DONGEN, C.G., and R.L. HAYS: A sensitive in vitro assay for oxytocin. Endocrinology **78**, 1—6 (1966).

DUFF, W.M., E.H. GRINELL, and J. KRAMAR: Ultrasensitive bioassay of vasopressin. Physiologist **7**, 120 (1964).

van Dyke, H. B., K. Adamsons, and S. L. Engel: Aspects of the biochemistry and physiology of the neurohypophysial hormones. Recent Progr. Hormone Res. **11**, 1—41 (1955).
—, and R. G. Ames: Alcohol diuresis. Acta endocr. (Kbh.) **7**, 110—121 (1951).
—, S. L. Engel, and K. Adamsons: Comparison of pharmacological effects of lysine and arginine vasopressins. Proc. Soc. exp. Biol. (N.Y.) **91**, 484—486 (1956).
—, and A. B. Hastings: The response of smooth muscle in different ionic environments. Amer. J. Physiol. **83**, 563—577 (1928).
Edelman, I. S., M. J. Petersen, and P. F. Gulyassy: Kinetic analysis of the antidiuretic action of vasopressin and adenosine-3',5'-monophosphate. J. clin. Invest. **43**, 2185—2194 (1964).
Eggleton, M. G.: The diuretic action of alcohol in man. J. Physiol. (Lond.) **101**, 172—191 (1942).
Elmquist, A.: Synpunkter på bestämning av felgränser vid biologisk styrkebestämning av oxytocin. Svensk. farm. T. **61**, 657—661 (1957).
Fielitz, C. A., V. H. Gonzalez-Panizza, and R. Caldeyro-Barcia: Effect of low concentrations of oxytocin on the uterine response to electrical stimulation. Acta physiol. lat.-amer. **10**, 201—204 (1960).
Fitzpatrick, R. J.: The estimation of small amounts of oxytocin in blood. In: Oxytocin, p. 358—377. Symposium in Montevideo 1959. Ed. by R. Caldeyro-Barcia and H. Heller. Oxford: Pergamon Press 1961.
—, A. Morris, and C. Walmsley: Oxytocin-like activity of the blood of cows in labour. XXII Int. Congr. Physiol. Sci. Leiden 1962. Proc. Vol. 2, Abstract No. 522.
—, and C. Walmsley: The concentration of oxytocin in bovine blood during parturition. J. Physiol. (Lond.) **163**, 13—14 P (1962).
Flatters, M.: Über die Vorzüge der Verwendung von Ratten-Uteri im Proöstrus zur Auswertung von Oxytocin. Arch. exp. Pathol. Pharmakol. **221**, 171—176 (1954).
Follett, B. K., and P. J. Bentley: The bioassay of oxytocin: increased sensitivity of the rat uterus in response to serial injections of stilboestrol. J. Endocr. **29**, 277—282 (1964).
Fuchs, A. R., and F. Fuchs: Spontaneous motility and oxytocin response of the pregnant and non-pregnant human uterine muscle *in vitro*. J. Obstet. Gynaec. Brit. Cwlth. **70**, 658—664 (1963).
Fugo, N. W., and G. T. Aragon: The utilization of an old technique for a sensitive antidiuretic assay. Fed. Proc. **6**, 330—331 (1947).
Gaddum, J. H.: The weighing of standard pituitary powders. Pharm. J. **119**, 580 (1927).
— Some properties of the separated active principles of the pituitary (posterior lobe). J. Physiol. (Lond.) **65**, 434—440 (1928).
— The technique of superfusion. Brit. J. Pharmacol. **8**, 321—326 (1953).
—, W. S. Peart, and M. Vogt: The estimation of adrenaline and allied substances in blood. J. Physiol. (Lond.) **108**, 467—481 (1949).
Garcia de Jalon, P.: El uso de las sales de magnesio en los ensayos de los extractos de lóbulo posterior de hipófisis. Farmacoter. act. **4**, 177—182 (1947).
—, J. Bayo Bayo y M. Garcia de Jalon: Sensible y nuevo método de valoración de adrenalina en útero aislado de rata. Farmacoter. act. **2**, 313—318 (1945).
Gauer, O. H., and P. S. Tata: Vasopressin studies in the rat. II. The amount of water reabsorbed by the rat kidney after a single i.v. injection of vasopressin: the vasopressin water equivalent. Pflügers Arch. ges. Physiol. **290**, 286—293 (1966).
Gautier, R.: The health organisation and biological standardisation. Quart. Bull. Hlth Org. L.o.N. **4**, 530—533 (1935).
— The health organisation and biological standardisation (second memorandum). Bull. Wld Hlth Org. **12**, 42—44 (1945/46).
Gibbs, O. S.: A practical test for the antidiuretic action of pituitary. J. Pharmacol. exp. Ther. **40**, 129—137 (1930).
Gilman, A., and L. Goodman: The secretory response of the posterior pituitary to the need for water conservation. J. Physiol. (Lond.) **90**, 113—124 (1937).
Ginsburg, M.: A method for the assay of antidiuretic activity. Brit. J. Pharmacol. **6**, 411—416 (1951).
—, and H. Heller: The antidiuretic assay of vasopressin by intravenous injection into unanaesthetized rats. J. Endocr. **9**, 267—273 (1953).
—, and M. W. Smith: The fate of oxytocin in male and female rats. Brit. J. Pharmacol. **14**, 327—333 (1959).
Gordon, E. R., and H. Kalant: Modification of the assay for small amounts of antidiuretic hormone. Canad. J. Biochem. **38**, 1380—1381 (1960).
Grindeland, R. E., and E. Anderson: Assay of vasopressin in blood. Fed. Proc. **23**, 150 (1964).
Guerne, J. M., et F. Stutinsky: Etude *in vivo* des variations de la sensibilité à l'ocytocine de l'utérus de la ratte cyclique. J. Physiol. (Paris) **53**, 357—358 (1961).

Gulyassy, P.F., and I.S. Edelman: Hydrogen-ion dependence of the antidiuretic action of vasopressin, oxytocin and deaminooxytocin. Biochim. biophys. Acta (Amst.) **102**, 185—197 (1965).

Guttmann, St.: Personal communication 1962.

—, B. Berde, and E. Stürmer: The synthesis and some pharmacological effects of serine[4]-isoleucine[8]-oxytocin, a probable neurohypophysial hormone. Experientia (Basel) **18**, 445 (1962).

Ham, G.C.: Reproducible diuresis and chloruresis for bioassay of antidiuretic activity. Proc. Soc. exp. Biol. (N.Y.) **53**, 210—213 (1943).

Hamburger, C.: Modification of the standardization of posterior pituitary extract after Dale's principle. Acta pharmacol. (Kbh.) **1**, 112—119 (1945).

Hamilton, H.C., and L.W. Rowe: Pituitary standardization. J. Lab. clin. Med. **2**, 120—129 (1916).

Hans Berteau, M.J., et R. Vanden Driessche: Extraction et dosage biologique de l'ocytocine hypophysaire, hypothalamique et plasmatique. Arch. int. Pharmacodyn. **132**, 481—482 (1961).

Hare, K., R.C. Hickey, and R.S. Hare: The renal excretion of an antidiuretic substance by the dog. Amer. J. Physiol. **134**, 240—244 (1941).

Hartley, P.: Report on the international biological standards maintained at the National Institute for Medical Research, Hampstead, London, on behalf of the Health Organisation of the League of Nations. Quart. Bull. Hlth Org. L.o.N.; Special Number: Biological Standardisation, p. 713—727 (1936).

Hawker, R.: Oxytocin and an unidentified oxytocic substance in extracts of blood. In: Oxytocin, p. 425—434, Symposium in Montevideo 1959. Ed. by R. Caldeyro-Barcia and H. Heller. Oxford: Pergamon Press 1961.

—, C.F. Walmsley, V.S. Roberts, J.K. Blackshaw, and J.C. Downes: Oxytocic activity of blood in parturient and lactating woman. J. clin. Endocr. **21**, 985—995 (1961).

Hawkins, D.F.: Acting agents on the uterus. In: Evaluation of drug activities: Pharmacometrics, p. 665—701. Ed. by D.R. Laurence and A.L. Bachrach. London: Academic Press 1964.

Heintz, R., E.F. Drews, G. Drews u. H. Brass: Untersuchungen über den Gehalt des menschlichen Plasmas an antidiuretischem Hormon mit einer verbesserten Methode zum Hormonnachweis. Klin. Wschr. **42**, 771—776 (1964).

Heller, H., and K.E. Blackmore: The assay of small amounts of antidiuretic activity by intravenous injections into mice. J. Endocr. **8**, 224—228 (1952).

—, G. Herdan, and S.M.A. Zaidi: Seasonal variations in the response of rats to the antidiuretic hormone. Brit. J. Pharmacol. **12**, 100—103 (1957).

—, and B.T. Pickering: Neurohypophysial hormones of nonmammalian vertebrates. J. Physiol. (Lond.) **155**, 98—114 (1961).

— —, J. Maetz, and F. Morel: Pharmacological characterization of the oxytocic peptides in the pituitary of a marine teleost fish (*Pollachius virens*). Nature (Lond.) **191**, 670—671 (1961).

Heller, J.: The physiology of the antidiuretic hormone. IV. The effect of certain anaesthetics on the antidiuretic activity of rat blood plasma. Physiol. bohemoslov. **9**, 283—288 (1960).

—, and J. Štulc: Physiology of the antidiuretic hormone. I. A simple titration method. Physiol. bohemoslov. **8**, 558—564 (1959).

Hogben, L.T.: Studies on the pituitary. V. The avine depressor response. Quart. J. exp. Physiol. **15**, 155—161 (1925).

Höhn, E.O.: Failure of oxytocin to produce a prolactin-like response in the pigeon's crop sac. J. Endocr. **26**, 177—178 (1963).

Holländer, L.P., J. Franz, and B. Berde: An attempt to produce antibodies to oxytocin and vasopressin. Experientia (Basel) **22**, 325—328 (1966).

Holton, P.: A modification of the method of Dale and Laidlaw for standardization of posterior pituitary extract. Brit. J. Pharmacol. **3**, 328—334 (1948).

Holzbauer, M., and M. Vogt: Modification by drugs of the response of the rat's uterus to adrenaline. Brit. J. Pharmacol. **10**, 186—190 (1955).

Honoré, L.H., and S. Lloyd: The effects of castration on the vascular response of male rats to posterior pituitary hormones. J. Physiol. (Lond.) **159**, 183—190 (1961).

Hsu, Y.-Ch.: The influence of the magnesium concentration in the Ringer's solution used for the assay of oxytocin in pituitary (posterior lobe) extracts. Quart. J. Pharm. **21**, 146—151 (1948).

Huguenin, R.L., E. Stürmer, R.A. Boissonnas, and B. Berde: Desamino-arginine-vasopressin, an analogue of arginine-vasopressin with high antidiuretic activity. Experientia (Basel) **21**, 68—69 (1965).

Hunter, J., H. Kalant, and J.C. Ogilvie: A simple method for the assay of small amounts of antidiuretic hormone. Canad. J. Biochem. **37**, 1215—1225 (1959).

Ishida, Y.: Studies of drug receptors on the plain muscle. III. Effect of hydrogen ion concentration upon ACh-, Ba-, and oxytocin-receptors of isolated rat uterus. J. Pharm. Soc. Japan **81**, 1717—1721 (1961).

Jacobson, H.N., and R.H. Kellogg: Isotonic NaCl diuresis in rats. Antidiuresis and chloruresis produced by posterior pituitary extracts. Amer. J. Physiol. **184**, 376—389 (1956).

Jaenike, J.R.: Acute effects of the administration of vasopressin during water diuresis in the dog. J. clin. Invest. **42**, 161—170 (1963).

Jeffers, W.A., M.M. Livezy, and J.H. Austin: Method for demonstrating the antidiuretic action of minute amounts of pitressin; statistical analysis of results. Proc. Soc. exp. Biol. (N.Y.) **50**, 184—188 (1942).

Jones, J.J., and J. Lee: The value of the pre-operated rat in the bioassay of vasopressin. J. Endocr. **33**, 329—330 (1965).

Kestranek, W., H. Molitor u. E.P. Pick: Über die Wirkungsstärke von Hypophysenextrakten, gemessen an ihren antidiuretischen Eigenschaften. Biochem. Z. **164**, 34—43 (1925).

Kleeman, C.R., M.E. Rubini, E. Lamdin, and F.H. Epstein: Studies on alcohol diuresis. II. The evaluation of ethyl alcohol as an inhibitor of the neurohypophysis. J. clin. Invest. **34**, 448—455 (1955).

Koll, W., u. H. Kaller: Die Auswertung von Hypophysenhinterlappen-Extrakten am isolierten Meerschweinchen-Uterus mit Hilfe der mittleren Kontraktionshöhen in der Endeinstellung. Arch. exp. Pathol. Pharmakol. **215**, 133—147 (1952).

Konzett, H., and E. Stürmer: Biological activity of synthetic polypeptides with bradykinin-like properties. Brit. J. Pharmacol. **15**, 544—551 (1960).

Krejčí, I., I. Poláček, B. Kupková, and J. Rudinger: Dose-response analysis of the action of some oxytocin analogues on the isolated uterus: the effect of ions. In: Oxytocin, vasopressin and their structural analogues, p. 117—123. Ed. by J. Rudinger. Oxford: Pergamon Press 1964.

Krieger, V.I., and T.B. Kilvington: Antidiuretic substance in urine in relation to normal and toxaemic pregnancy. Med. J. Aust. **1**, 575—585 (1940).

Kuschinsky, G., u. H. Vorherr: Über eine einfache russkymographische Methode zur fortlaufenden Blutdruckmessung an Mäusen und Ratten. Experientia (Basel) **13**, 298—299 (1957).

Landgrebe, F.W., M.H.I. Macaulay, and H. Waring: The use of rats for pressor assays of pituitary extracts, with a note on responses to histamine and adrenaline. Proc. roy. Soc. Edinb., B **62**, 202 (1946).

Lauber, J.K., W.J. Eversole, and W.A. Childs: The use of the toad for bioassay of mammalian antidiuretic hormone (vasopressin). Endocrinology **64**, 316—318 (1959).

Lauson, H.D., and M. Bocanegra: Clearance fo exogenous vasopressin from plasma of dogs. Amer. J. Physiol. **200**, 493—497 (1961).

Lederis, K.: Vasopressin and oxytocin in mammalian hypothalamus. Gen. comp. Endocr. **1**, 80—89 (1961).

Levy, B.: The intestinal inhibitory response to oxytocin, vasopressin and bradykinin. J. Pharmacol. exp. Ther. **140**, 356—366 (1963).

Lindquist, K.M., and L.W. Rowe: The antidiuretic activity of the posterior pituitary and its quantitative evaluation. J. Amer. pharm. Ass., sci. Ed. **38**, 227—231 (1949).

Little, J.B., and E.P. Radford: Bio-assay for antidiuretic activity in blood of undisturbed rats. J. appl. Physiol. **19**, 179—186 (1964).

Lloyd, S.: The vascular response of the rat during the reproductive cycle. J. Physiol. (Lond.) **148**, 625—632 (1959a).

— Changes in the vascular responses of the rat during pregnancy. J. Physiol. (Lond.) **149**, 586—592 (1959b).

—, and M. Pickford: The action of posterior pituitary hormones and oestrogens on the vascular system of the rat. J. Physiol. (Lond.) **155**, 161—174 (1961).

— — The persistence of a depressor response to oxytocin in the fowl after denervation and blocking agents. Brit. J. Pharmacol. **16**, 129—136 (1961).

Marshall, J.M.: Behavior of uterine muscle in Na-deficient solutions; effects of oxytocin. Amer. J. Physiol. **204**, 732—738 (1963).

Martin, P.J., and H.O. Schild: Effects of thiols on oxytocin and vasopressin receptors. Nature (Lond.) **196**, 382—383 (1962).

McGaughey, H.S., W.A. Scoggin, W.L. Johnson, and W.N. Thornton: Definition of the stimulatory response of isolated human uterine tissues. The effect of posterior pituitary extract, vasopressin, and oxytocin on pregnant and nonpregnant human myometrial samplings in *vitro*. Amer. J. Obstet. Gynec. **88**, 68—74 (1964).

Mendez-Bauer, C., H.M. Cabot, and R. Caldeyro-Barcia: A new test for the biological assay of oxytcoin. Science **132**, 299—300 (1960).

Miller, L.C., and M.L. Tainter: Estimation of the ED_{50} and its error by means of logarithmic-probit graph paper. Proc. Soc. exp. Biol. (N.Y.) **57**, 261—264 (1944).
Mizuno, H., and J. Meites: Failure of oxytocin to stimulate the pigeon crop gland. Nature (Lond.) **198**, 1209—1210 (1963).
Moore, R.D., and M.X. Zarrow: Contraction of the rabbit mammary strip in vitro in response to oxytocin. Acta endocr. (Kbh.) **48**, 186—198 (1965).
Morash, R., and O.S. Gibbs: The effect of pituitary on the bird. J. Pharmacol. exp. Ther. **37**, 475—480 (1929).
Morell, C.A., M.G. Allmark, and W.M. Bachinski: On the biological assay of the oxytocic activity of pituitary extract (posterior lobe). J. Pharmacol. exp. Ther. **70**, 440—449 (1940).
Munsick, R.A.: Effect of magnesium ion on the response of the rat uterus to neurohypophysial hormones and analogues. Endocrinology **66**, 451—457 (1960).
— Personal communication, 1967.
—, and S.C. Jeronimus: Effects of diethylstilboestrol and magnesium on the rat oxytocic potencies of some neurohypophysial hormones and analogues. Endocrinology **76**, 90—96 (1965).
—, W.H. Sawyer, and H.B. van Dyke: Avian neurohypophysial hormones: pharmacological properties and tentative identification. Endocrinology **66**, 860—871 (1960).
Myerscough, P.R., and H.O. Schild: Quantitative assays of oxytocic drugs on the human postpartum uterus. Brit. J. Pharmacol. **13**, 207—212 (1958).
Nash, C.B.: Pyrogallol and vasopressin tachyphylaxis. Experientia (Basel) **19**, 649—650 (1963).
Natochin, J.V., K. Janáček, and R. Rybová: The swelling of frog bladder cells produced by oxytocin. J. Endocr. **33**, 171—177 (1965).
Natoff, I.L., and M.F. Lockett: The assay of histamine, 5-hydroxytryptamine, adrenaline, and noradrenaline, on the blood pressure of the fowl. J. Pharm. Pharmacol. **9**, 464—468 (1957).
Nelson, E.E.: Concerning a standard for liquor hypophysis U.S.P.X. J. Amer. pharm. Ass. **13**, 426—433 (1924).
—, and J.C. Munch: The standard for assay of pituitary solution U.S.P.X. J. Amer. pharm. Ass. **14**, 22—23 (1925).
—, and G.G. Woods: The diuretic-antidiuretic activity of posterior pituitary extracts. J. Pharmacol. exp. Ther. **50**, 241—253 (1934).
Nielsen, A.T.: A note on the relative antidiuretic potency of beef and hog vasopressin. Acta endocr. (Kbh.) **29**, 561—564 (1958).
— Dissimilarity between arginine- and lysine-vasopressin in rat pressor assays. Acta endocr. (Kbh.) **35**, 299—311 (1960).
— On the antidiuretic activity of Phe^2-Lys^8-vasopressin in the rat. Acta endocr. (Kbh.) **49**, 312—318 (1965).
O'Connor, W.J.: The effect of section of the supraopticohypophysial tracts on the inhibition of water diuresis by emotional stress. Quart. J. exp. Physiol. **33**, 149—161 (1946).
—, and E.B. Verney: The effect of removal of the posterior lobe of the pituitary on the inhibition of water-diuresis by emotional stress. Quart. J. exp. Physiol. **31**, 393—408 (1942).
Ohnesorge, F.K., u. M. Rehberg: Der Darm der Schleie (Tinca vulgaris) als Pharmakologisches Versuchsobjekt. Arch. exp. Pathol. Pharmakol. **246**, 81—82 (1963).
Ott, I., and J.C. Scott: The action of infundibulin upon the mammary secretion. Proc. Soc. exp. Biol. (N.Y) **8**, 48—49 (1910).
Parisot, J., et P. Mathieu: Action des extraits de lobe postérieur d'hypophyse sur les organes à fibres musculaires lisses. C. R. Soc. Biol. (Paris) **76**, 225—226 (1914).
Patil, P.N., A. Tye, and J.W. Nelson: Vasopressin tachyphylaxis. J. pharm. Sci. **53**, 684—686 (1964).
Paton, D.N., and A. Watson: The actions of pituitrin, adrenalin and barium on the circulation of the bird. J. Physiol. (Lond.) **44**, 413—424 (1912).
Permutt, M.A., C.W. Parker, and R.D. Utiger: Immunochemical studies with lysine vasopressin. Endocrinology **78**, 809—814 (1966).
British Pharmacopoeia, London, Pharmaceutical Press 1932.
— London, Pharmaceutical Press 1953.
— London, Pharmaceutical Press 1963.
Pharmacopoea Internationalis, Editio prima, Vol. I WHO Chron. 1951.
Pharmacopoeia of the United States of America, IX. Revision. Philadelphia 1916.
— of the United States of America, X. Revision. Philadelphia 1925.
— of the United States of America, XIV. Revision. Easton 1950.
— of the United States of America, XV. Revision. Easton 1955.
— of the United States of America, XVII, Revision. Easton 1965

Pharmacopoea Nordica, Editio Svecica, Vol. IV, Biologiska metoder. Stockholm 1960.

Pigeon, G., and F.H. Epstein: Water uptake in the intact frog. Amer. J. Physiol. **204**, 217—221 (1963).

Pittenger, P.S., and A. Quici: Isolated uterus assay for pituitary extract. Notes on method of eliminating some difficulties encountered with the above method (Second paper). J. Amer. pharm. Ass., sci. Ed. **12**, 14—19 (1923).

Rabasa, S.L., and F. Bergmann: A method to measure the renal sensitivity to ADH in the rat. With a note on the effects of water deprivation. Acta physiol. lat.-amer. **14**, 89—93 (1964).

Reynolds, S.R.M.: Physiology of the uterus. P. B. Hoeber, Inc. New York 1939.

— Physiology of the uterus. 2nd ed., P.B. Hoeber, Inc., New York 1949.

Richardson, K.C.: Contractile tissues in the mammary gland, with special reference to myoepithelium in the goat. Proc. roy. Soc. B. **136**, 30—45 (1949).

Robinson, F.H., and L.E. Farr: The relation between clinical edema and the excretion of an antidiuretic substance in the urine. Ann. inter. Med. **14**, 42—54 (1940).

Rocha e Silva, M.: Biochemistry and pharmacology of bradykinin. In: Polypeptides which affect smooth muscles and blood vessels, p. 210—231. Ed by M. Schachter. Oxford, London, New York, Paris: Pergamon Press 1960.

Roth, G.B.: Pituitary standardization. A comparison of the physiological activity of some commercial pituitary preparations. Publ. Hlth Service, Hygienic Lab. Bull. No. 100 (1914a).

— A new standard for the determination of the strenght of pituitary extracts. J. Pharmacol. exp. Ther. **5**, 559—570 (1914b).

Rydén, G., and I. Sjöholm: Assay of oxytocin by rat mammary gland in vitro. Brit. J. Pharmacol. **19**, 136—141 (1962).

Saameli, K.: Quantitativer Vergleich zwischen Oxytocin und fünf verwandten Peptiden am menschlichen Uterus *in situ*. Arch. Gynäk. **202**, 55—59 (1964).

Samaan, A.: The effect of pituitary (posterior lobe) extract upon the urinary flow in non-anaesthetized dogs. J. Physiol. (Lond.) **85**, 37—46 (1935).

Sawyer, W.H.: Differences in the antidiuretic responses of rats to the intravenous administration of lysine and arginine vasopressins. Endocrinology **63**, 694—698 (1958).

— Biological assays for oxytocin and vasopressin. Meth. med. Res. **9**, 210—219 (1961).

— Biological assays for neurohypophysial principles in tissues and in blood. In: The pituitary gland, Vol. 3. Ed. by G.W. Harris and B.T. Donovan. London: Butterworths 1966.

—, W.Y. Chan, and H.B. van Dyke: Antidiuretic responses to neurohypophysial hormones and their synthetic analogues in dogs and rats. Endrocrinology **71**, 536—540 (1962).

Schachter, M.: Polypeptides which affect smooth muscles and blood vessels. London: Pergamon Press 1960.

Schally, A.V., C.Y. Bowers, A. Kuroshima, Y. Ishida, W.H. Carter, and T.W. Redding: Effect of lysine vasopressin dimers on blood pressure and some endocrine functions. Amer. J. Physiol. **207**, 378—384 (1964).

—, and R. Guillemin: Some biological and chemical properties of a lysine-vasopressin dimer. J. biol. Chem. **239**, 1038—1041 (1964).

Schild, H.O.: A method of conducting a biological assay on a preparation giving repeated graded responses illustrated by the estimation of histamine. J. Physiol. (Lond.) **101**, 115—130 (1942).

— pA, a new scale for the measurement of drug antagonism. Brit. J. Pharmacol. **2**, 189—206 (1947).

Schröder, R., u. D. Rott: Über die Bestimmung und das Verhalten von ADH im menschlichen Plasma. Klin. Wschr. **37**, 1175—1181 (1959).

Share, L.: Acute reduction in extracellular fluid volume and the concentration of antidiuretic hormone in blood. Endocrinology **69**, 925—933 (1961).

—, and M.N. Levy: Cardiovascular receptors in blood titer of antidiuretic hormone. Amer. J. Physiol. **203**, 425—428 (1962).

Shipley, R.E., and J.H. Tilden: A pithed rat preparation suitable for assaying pressor substances. Proc. Soc. exp. Biol. (N.Y.) **64**, 453—455 (1947).

Siddiqi, S., and J.M. Walker: Oxytocic activity of rabbit's blood applied directly to superfused rat uterus. J. Physiol. (Lond.) **152**, 381—390 (1960).

Silvette, H.: The influence of post-pituitary extract on the excretion of water and chlorides by the renal tubules. Amer. J. Physiol. **128**, 747—753 (1940).

Smith, B. jr., J.M. Coon, P. Fourt, and E.M.K. Geiling: A proposed modification in the official method for the assay of posterior pituitary solution. J. Amer. pharm. Ass., sci. Ed. **30**, 151—153 (1941).

Smith, M. I., and W. T. McClosky: I. Studies on the bioassay of pituitary extracts: Concerning the use of a desiccated infundibular powder as a standard in the physiological evaluation of pituitary extracts. Hyg. Lab. Bull. No. 138, 1—36 (1924a).
— — II. Some factors concerned in the deterioration of pituitary extracts. Hyg. Lab. Bull. No. 138, 38—49 (1924b).
— — Further studies on the bioassay of pituitary extracts. The action of the standard infundibular powder on the secretion of urine. J. Pharmacol. exp. Ther. **24**, 371—389 (1925).
Smith, M. W.: Some properties of rat mammary tissue. Nature (Lond.) **190**, 541—542 (1961).
Smith, R. B.: A comparison of the official and the chicken methods for the oxytocic bioassay of posterior pituitary preparations. J. Pharmacol. exp. Ther. **75**, 342—349 (1942).
—, and B. J. Vos: The biological assay of posterior pituitary solution. J. Pharmacol. exp. Ther. **78**, 72—78 (1943).
Somlyo, A.V., C.Y. Woo, and A.P. Somlyo: Effect of magnesium on posterior pituitary hormone action on vascular smooth muscle. Amer. J. Physiol. **210**, 705—714 (1966).
Spaeth, R. A.: The standardization of pituitary extracts. Publ. Hlth Serv., Hyg. Lab. Bull. No. 115 (1918a).
— Concerning a new method for the biological standardization of pituitary extract and other drugs. J. Pharmacol. exp. Ther. **11**, 209—219 (1918b).
Standard, I. International: Report of the permanent commission on biological standardization. Quart. Bull. Hlth Org. Special Number 572—573 and 582 (1936).
Standard, Department of Biological Standards, National Inst. for Med. Res.: Memorandum on the replacement of the substance of the international standard preparation for pituitary posterior lobe. Bull. Hlth Org. L. o. N. **10**, 89—93 (1942/43).
Stein, M., R. Jinks, and I. A. Mirsky: The bioassay of pitressin and antidiuretic substances in blood and urine. Endocrinology **51**, 492—503 (1952).
Strauss, M. B., J. D. Rosenbaum, and W. P. Nelson: The effect of alcohol on the renal excretion of water and electrolyte. J. clin. Invest. **29**, 1053—1058 (1950).
Stürmer, E.: Unpublished data 1963.
— Unpublished 1965.
—, and B. Berde: Kallidin und Bradykinin, vergleichende pharmakologische Untersuchungen. Arch. exp. Pathol. Pharmakol. **243**, 355—356 (1962).
— — A pharmacological comparison between synthetic bradykinin and synthetic kallidin. J. Pharmacol. exp. Ther. **139**, 38—41 (1963).
—, R. L. Huguenin, R. A. Boissonnas, and B. Berde: Deamino^1-phenylalanine^2-arginine^8-vasopressin: a peptide with highly selective antidiuretic activity. Experientia (Basel) **21**, 583—585 (1965).
Sund, R. B.: A sensitive method for estimation of ergometrine, based upon serotonin antagonism on isolated rat uterus. Acta pharmacol. (Kbh.) **20**, 233—242 (1963a).
— On the actions of ergometrine on isolated rat uterus in absence and presence of magnesium ions. Medd. norsk farm. Selsk. **25**, 89—96 (1963b).
— Assay of oxytocin in pharmaceutical solutions containing both oxytocin and ergometrine, by the isolated rat uterus method. Medd. norsk farm. Selsk. **25**, 101—114 (1963c).
Supek, Z., B. Uroić, V. Gjuriš, and N. Marijan: The effect of adrenergic blocking agents and of chlorpromazine on blood pressure increase by vasopressin and angiotensin. J. Pharm. Pharmacol. **14**, 284—287 (1962).
Tata, P. S., and R. Buzalkow: Vasopressin studies in the rat. III. Inability of ethanol anesthesia to prevent ADH secretion due to pain and hemorrhage. Pflügers Arch. ges. Physiol. **290**, 294—297 (1966).
—, and O. H. Gauer: Vasopressin studies in the rat. I. A sensitive bioassay for exogenous vasopressin. Pflügers Arch. ges. Physiol. **290**, 279—285 (1966).
Taubert, M., u. H. Henn: Untersuchungen über die Gewinnung und den Nachweis von Adiuretin im Blut. Aerztl. Forsch. **11**, I/86—92 (1957).
Theobald, G. W.: The alleged relation of hyperfunction of the posterior lobe of the hypophysis to eclampsia and the nephropathy of pregnancy. Clin. Sci. **1**, 225—239 (1933).
Thompson, R. E.: Biological assay of posterior pituitary. J. Pharmacol. exp. Ther. **80**, 373—382 (1944).
Thorn, N. A.: A densimetric method for assay of small amounts of antidiuretic hormone. J. exp. Med. **105**, 585—590 (1957).
— Effects of arginine-, lysine- and leucine-vasopressin on urinary osmolality and rate of urine flow in hydrated rats and dogs. Acta endocr. (Kbh.) **32**, 134—141 (1959).
— Antidiuretic hormones and their analogues. Studies of renal effects — assay — circulating form. Dan. med. Bull. **7**, 116—117 (1960).
Thorp, R. H.: Posterior pituitary hormones. In: Methods in hormone research, Vol. 2, Bioassay, p. 495—516. Ed. by R. I. Dorfman. New York: Academic Press. 1962.

TINDAL, J.S., C. BEYER, and C.H. SAWYER: Milk-ejection reflex and maintenance of lactation in the rabbit. Endrocrinology **72**, 720—724 (1963).

—, and A. YOKOYAMA: Assay of oxytocin by the milk-ejection response in the anaesthetized lactating guinea-pig. Endocrinology **71**, 196—202 (1962).

TURNER, C.W., and W.D. COOPER: Assay of posterior pituitary factors which contract the lactating mammary gland. Endocrinology **29**, 320—323 (1941).

TYRODE, M.V.: The mode of action of some purgative salts. Arch. int. pharmacodyn. **20**, 205—223 (1910).

VOGLER, K., W. HAEFELY, A. HÜRLIMANN, R.O. STUDER, W. LERGIER, R. STRÄSSLE, and K.H. BERNEIS: A new purification procedure and biological properties of substance P. Ann. N. Y. Acad. Sci. **104**, 378—389 (1963).

VOGT, M.: Vasopressor, antidiuretic, and oxytocic activities of extracts of the dog's hypothalamus. Brit. J. Pharmacol. **8**, 193—196 (1953).

VORHERR, H.: Eine neue Methode zum Oxytocin-Nachweis an der lactierenden Maus. Arch. exp. Pathol. Pharmakol. **251**, 123 (1965).

—, u. V. FRIEDBERG: Verbesserte Methode zum Adiuretin-Nachweis. Klin. Wschr. **37**, 1171—1175 (1959).

— — Die quantitative Bestimmung der Adiuretin-Inaktivierung durch Schwangerenblut. Klin. Wschr. **38**, 447—449 (1960).

VOS, B.J.: Use of the latent period in the assay of ergonovine on the isolated rabbit uterus. J. Amer. pharm. Ass., sci. Ed. **32**, 138—141 (1943).

WALASZEK, E.J., C.G. HUGGINS, and C.M. SMITH: Drugs that modify actions of pharmacologically active polypeptides. Ann. N. Y. Acad. Sci. **104**, 281—289 (1963).

WALKER, A.M.: Experiments upon the relation between the pituitary gland and water diuresis. Amer. J. Physiol. **127**, 519—540 (1939).

DE WIED, D.: A simple automatic and sensitive method for the assay of antidiuretic hormone with notes on the antidiuretic potency of plasma under different experimental conditions. Acta physiol. pharmacol. neerl. **9**, 69—81 (1960).

WIRZ, H.: Der osmotische Druck in den cortikalen Tubuli der Rattenniere. Helv. physiol. pharmacol. Acta **14**, 353—362 (1956).

WOLFMAN, E.F., R.L. MILLER, and W.W. COON: Bioassay for antidiuretic substances: Essentials of a constant water-loading apparatus. J. surg. Res. **4**, 75—81 (1964).

YOSHIDA, S., H. IBAYASHI, S. MURAKAWA, and K. NAKAO: Cerebral control of secretion of antidiuretic hormone: Effect of electrical stimulation of the prepyriform area on the neurohypophysis in the dog. Endocrinology **77**, 597—601 (1965).

—, K. MOTOHASHI, H. IBAYASHI, and S. OKINAKA: Method for the assay of antidiuretic hormone in plasma with a note on the antidiuretic titer of human plasma. J. Lab. clin. Med. **62**, 279—285 (1963).

The Assay of Neurohypophysial Hormones in Blood and Other Body Fluids

R. J. FITZPATRICK and P. J. BENTLEY

With 20 Figures

> Methods are good if they are accurate, rapid and simple, and bad if they are inaccurate, slow and need skill. That accuracy is necessary all are agreed. That speed in obtaining results is important is well known ... Few people recognise that methods are good in proportion as the technique is simple.
>
> J. H. BURN (1937)
> Biological Standardisation

Introduction

This section will be mainly orientated around the detection and measurement of oxytocin and vasopressin at low concentrations, such as may occur naturally in blood or urine. The choice of method in this type of work is influenced more by considerations of high sensitivity, by specificity and by simplicity than by limits of error. This contrasts with requirements of methods for estimating the oxytocic potency of posterior pituitary glands, or for the investigation of synthetic homologues of oxytocin, when in general there is no practical limit to the amount of active substance available and hence the sensitivity of the method is not of great importance, whereas the reliability of the estimate is of very great importance indeed. Assays are discussed from this point of view, e.g. pharmacopoeial standardisation, in the chapter by STÜRMER.

This account will describe methods which place emphasis on sensitivity and specificity, and due regard also will be paid to the problems of bioassay associated with the quantitative extraction of oxytocin and vasopressin from body fluids. In addition special comment will be made on the assay and identification of the neurohypophysial hormones present in the lower vertebrates.

That high sensitivity is of special importance stems from the high dilution at which neurohypophysial hormones occur in body fluids under physiological conditions. The magnitude of this dilution may be crudely estimated from observations of the minimum effective dose or infusion of the hormones in normal animals or man. THEOBALD, for instance, has shown that the intravenous injection of as little as 5 mU vasopressin (THEOBALD, 1934a, b) or the infusion of 2.5 mU/min of oxytocin (THEOBALD, GRAHAM, CAMPBELL, GANGE and DRISCOLL, 1948) produces in man antidiuretic or uterine-stimulant responses comparable to those attributed to endogenous release of the hormones under physiological conditions. Other workers describing the effect of single intravenous injections of very low doses have also reported responses to be indistinguishable from physiological activity (see FITZPATRICK, 1957 and 1966). Adopting this approach, final blood or plasma concentrations of the order of 10 μU per ml or 20 pica mols per litre, may be postulated as normal.

To merely demonstrate the presence of the polypeptides at these low concentrations requires sensitivity very much greater than that for pharmacopoeial assay. Furthermore, to measure such concentrations of the active substances with accuracy, requires bioassay preparations which not only respond to low concentrations but which respond with consistency in respect of time and of dose. In general the consistency of response in assays declines as threshold sensitivity is approached and it is under these circumstances that sensitivity and accuracy of estimate come to some extent in conflict.

The extreme dilution of the active substance in fresh body fluids may be overcome, at least when large species are under investigation, by concentrating and extracting relatively large volumes of blood or other fluid. This in turn poses problems of processing the fluid in such a manner that any oxytocin or vasopressin originally present is protected from enzymatic or other forms of inactivation. Furthermore, such concentration procedures must not themselves produce or liberate substances which interfere with the subsequent assays of hormones, whether by inhibition (as may occur with histamine) or by augmentation (as with the kinins or potassium salts). Fresh biological fluids, such as blood, urine or foetal fluids are frequently unsuitable substances for direct bioassay, even if unconcentrated, due to the presence of naturally occurring substances which interfere with the assay, either in a specific sense or in a non-specific toxic manner.

To eliminate the effect of all undesirable substances and in order to identify the active substance, it is frequently necessary to purify the solutions under investigation. The more complex the purification the greater and more variable are the quantitative losses so that simple procedures are usually to be preferred.

As a further check on identity and concentration of the active substance it is often necessary to assay an unknown solution against the corresponding standard polypeptide using more than one assay preparation. Thus the investigator in this field requires a multiplicity of methods and for this reason we include some methods that are not necessarily first choice.

I. Assay of Oxytocin

Although pharmacological responses to oxytocin may be obtained from body systems other than the uterus and mammary gland, most investigators have used these two organs as the basis of their assay preparations, no doubt in the expectation that the organs which are almost certainly the physiological targets for endogenous oxytocin are most likely to offer the optimum sensitivity and specificity. To a considerable extent this has proved justified, but neither preparation is specific for oxytocin and it is only recently that sensitive modifications of existing methods have been described. Uterine and mammary gland assays will be described in detail but before doing so brief mention of other preparations is made.

General and Responses in Sub-Mammalian Vertebrates

The vasodepressor action of oxytocin in the hen (Paton and Watson, 1912; Gaddum, 1928; Coon, 1939; Smith and Vos, 1943) has been well investigated and is the basis of some pharmacopoeial methods of assay. It is rapid and reasonably simple, but for investigations of the hormone content of body fluids it lacks specificity and is much too insensitive, requiring a dose of approximately 100 mU to produce a useful response (Smith and Vos, 1943; Elmqvist, 1957). It is discussed in detail in another chapter of this volume by Stürmer.

Oxytocin produces contractile responses of the uterus or oviduct of birds, reptiles, fishes (Fitzpatrick, 1966) and amphibia (Heller, Ferreri and Leathers,

1967), but although this is potentially a source of sensitive preparations it has not yet been exploited, apart from a few studies on the identification of oxytocin-like neurohypophysial hormones in the lower vertebrates (van Dyke, 1959; Heller and Lederis, 1960; Heller, 1966; Heller et al., 1967).

Similarly, although the effects of oxytocin on water or sodium transport across the skin or bladder of amphibia are well established, these actions have only been used as yet in comparative studies of the endogenous hormones characteristic of the lower vertebrates (Sawyer, 1960; Acher, Chauvet, Chauvet and Crepy, 1962; Follett, 1963; Sawyer and van Dyke, 1963; Bentley and Heller, 1964; Ferguson and Heller, 1965). This aspect is discussed in relation to the assay of all the relevant neurohypophysial hormones at the end of this chapter, page 264.

A. Assays Based on Uterine Response

The discovery of oxytocin is attributed to the pioneer observations of H.H. Dale who was the first to describe uterine contractions in response to a simple extract of bovine posterior pituitary glands. Dale's initial observations were made in 1906 on the uterus of the intact pregnant cat and confirmed on uteri from a variety of species including dog, rabbit and guinea-pig, "in all functional conditions" and *in vitro* as well as *in vivo* (Dale, 1909).

Subsequently, Dale and Laidlaw (1912) and Burn and Dale (1922) developed assays based on the use of the isolated guinea-pig uterus, being influenced in the choice of species partly by the cheapness and availability of guinea-pigs at that time but also by the absence of interfering spontaneous contractions when uteri from virgin animals were used in their specified physiological saline (see Table 5). Although this assay procedure involved matching by bracketing, and although its discrimination was poor by modern standards, it remained the basis of all methods of standardisation of oxytocin until relatively recently.

Several modifications of the guinea-pig method were suggested including those by Morrell, Allmark and Bachinski (1940) who developed a quantal method, using multiple strips from the same uterus, and that of Hamburger (1945) who attempted multiple point assays, each using several guinea-pig uteri. In recent years however the guinea-pig uterus has not been widely used due to its reputation of lack of sensitivity, slowness of contraction, great variability and inconvenience (Gaddum, 1938; Holton, 1948; Stewart, 1949, 1950; Waring and Landgrebe, 1950). It would however be wrong to disregard this tissue. Several preparations of high sensitivity and convenience have been described. The detailed statistical analysis by Quivy and Bertrand (1948) shows that both the error and the index of precision (Gaddum, 1953a) are as low with the guinea-pig as with the rat uterus method which has superceded it. This paper by Quivy and Bertrand has been very largely overlooked by later workers but should be studied in parallel with that published almost one year later by Holton (1948), in which the rat uterus assay is described in terms of the same statistical criteria as Quivy and Bertrand, that is, those outlined by Bliss and Marks (1939a and b) and by Schild (1942).

More recently Styles and Sullivan (1962) using a sophisticated recording technique with both rat and guinea-pig uteri reported similar sensitivity (25 μU/ml) and indices of precision (less than 0.1) for the two types of muscle. Rorie and Newton (1965), using a technique based on the measurement of intra-uterine pressure *in vitro* have reported assays with a sensitivity of 100 μU/ml for the guinea-pig uterus, which compares reasonably with general experience using the rat uterus.

Although recent claims that the isolated uterus of the oestrous hamster (Ellett, 1964) or of the pro-oestrous mouse (Sen Min, 1964) are as good or better than other isolated uteri for assay purposes, the uterine preparation most widely used for investigating oxytocin in body fluids is undoubtedly the isolated rat uterus which will now be described in detail.

1. The Isolated Rat Uterus Method

The convenience of using the isolated rat uterus is expressed both in the short time required for each assay, and in the simple management of animal colonies: this together with greater sensitivity under certain specified conditions has led to the establishment of the rat uterus assay as the standard procedure with which all other assays of oxytocin should be compared.

As described by HOLTON (1948) the uterus is removed from a non-pregnant rat of 120—200 g body weight killed by concussion, i.e. without anaesthetic. One horn is suspended in a 10 ml water-bath filled with modified Locke's solution and contractions of the longitudinal muscle recorded using an isotonic frontal-writing lever (SCHILD, 1944) magnifying at least four times and exerting a load on the uterus equivalent to 1.2 g. Under these conditions maximum contractions are of the order of 100 mm as recorded on the writing surface. Spontaneous uterine contractions are minimised by reducing the temperature to 32° C and by using GARCIA DE JALON's (1947) modification of Locke's solution, with reduced calcium and glucose, equilibrated with 95% oxygen and 5% carbon dioxide (see Table 5). Nevertheless spontaneous activity is not overcome in all cases.

Without delay, doses of oxytocin are added to the bath every 3—4 min. 60—90 sec may be allowed for each contraction to develop, then the bath fluid is changed (twice). By trial and error two doses of standard oxytocin solution are found which give widely differing contractions; the weaker response should be considerably supraminimal (say 10—20% or more of maximal) and the higher considerably submaximal (not more than 80% of maximal). Too much time spent on selection of doses at this stage is likely to lead to reduced sensitivity later in the assay. Once the standard doses are selected, two doses of Unknown solution producing comparable effects to those of the two Standard doses are selected. It is important that the ratio of doses of Unknown should be exactly the same as the ratio of doses of Standard, since the comparison of Standard with Unknown will ultimately be based on the assumption that response is proportional to the logarithm of dose (see chapter by STÜRMER).

The sequence of doses is that conventional to a 2 and 2 assay procedure; groups of 4 different doses are used, comprising high and low dose of Standard solution and high and low dose of Unknown solution; each dose is given once in each group, its position in each group being determined either by chance or preferably by a previously established pattern which avoids any repetition of the same pair of drugs being given in succession during the period of assay. For 4 groups, each of 4 observations, a Latin square programme is convenient (see BLISS and MARKS, 1939a). The conditions must be kept as nearly identical as possible for each dose and for this reason mechanical devices to control the cycle are convenient but not essential. The number of groups of 4 doses is optional depending upon the precision of assay required, in general the precision increasing with the numbers of groups. Rarely is it necessary to extend the number of groups to 8 (i.e. 32 doses), as described by HOLTON (1948). Indeed it is not uncommon to find that the condition of the isolated muscle deteriorates so fast and responses to all doses decrease so rapidly and irregularly, that this source of variation itself interferes with the precision of assay: prolongation of the assay becomes worthless or even disadvantageous. It is in any case frequently desirable when investigating biological fluids or tissue extracts, to tolerate a relatively high error of assay based on relatively few responses, if this enables the investigator to assay a large number of samples in a short period. In other investigations the number of responses for an assay may be limited by the small total volume of extracts available. In these and similar circumstances the number of groups (each of 4 responses) may be reduced to 3 or 4. Table 1 illustrates the variation in the magnitude of the error with prolongation of assay. In this assay, full details of which are given on pages 206—209, 60 contractile responses, comprising 15 groups each of 4 responses, were obtained.

Table 1. *Variations in reliability of a rat uterus assay in relation to number of observations*
Statistical evaluation by AUDREY MORRIS

Responses	Low Standard	High Standard	Low Unknown	High Unknown
1st four	62	114	62	107
2nd four	56	108	59	106
3rd four	52	110	54	109
4th four	49	110	49	107
5th four	46	105	43	106
6th four	40	104	42	104
7th four	37	105	34	103
8th four	31	98	33	97
9th four	26	93	29	97
10th four	24	92	24	91
11th four	22	88	21	86
12th four	19	85	21	84
13th four	16	83	17	83
14th four	15	82	14	80
15th four	13	77	13	74

Responses in millimetres

Responses	Fiducial limits	Maximum percentage error	Average regression coefficient = b	Index of precision = Sy/b = λ
First 8 only	0.926—1.035	5.676	163	0.01064
First 12 only	0.935—1.045	5.693	175	0.01699
First 16 only	0.940—1.037	5.007	178	0.01873
First 24 only	0.952—1.033	4.151	187	0.02028
First 32 only	0.955—1.029	3.840	196	0.02224
All 60	0.973—1.018	2.250	206.5	0.01854

The error is very low (2.2%) when all responses are taken into account but is still only 5% or 6% when only the first few groups of 4 responses are considered. For most work with blood and other body fluids such an error is quite acceptable and prolongation of the assay beyond the first 12 observations in this case would have been unnecessary for such purposes. It is particularly noteworthy that the index of precision (λ) has suitably low values when only small numbers of responses are studied and that this function does not vary systematically with prolongation of the assay.

It is interesting to note that the regression coefficient (the slope of the log. dose response curve) increased with prolongation of this assay, an indication that the deterioration of response with time, affected responses to low doses more than those to high doses, i.e. the curve became steeper.

2. *Modifications of the Isolated Uterus Method*

a) *Cumulative Dose Assays*

RUDINGER and KREJČÍ (1962), FOLLETT and BENTLEY (1964) and CHAN, SCHULTZ and DU VIGNEAUD (1966) have extended the cumulative dose procedure of Ariens and de Groot (1954) to oxytocin assays, with very considerable saving of time and inconvenience. This procedure differs from the conventional organ bath technique in that doses of oxytocin are added successively to the bath fluid without the fluid being changed. The concentration in the bath is increased logarithmically by doubling the dose at intervals of 1 min until a maximum response is obtained. The responses are seen as a series of contractions superimposed on each other until a maximum is attained, and from them a log. dose response curve can be constructed. The method is both reliable and rapid. If the rats are pretreated with oestrogen it is also very sensitive, responses being obtained to 25 μU/ml or less, as shown in Fig. 1.

The method, since it is based on a multipoint assessment of each dose response relationship is more complicated to interpret statistically than the conventional method and probably for this reason is still not in widespread use. Moreover, Rudinger and Krejčí (1962) also point out that with some uteri, spasm (contracture) may supervene before the series of contractions reach true maximum. However, for many of the investigations of a preliminary nature, which abound in work concerning tissue extracts, there is great merit in using this method for the sake of speed and convenience (Chan, Fear and du Vigneaud, 1967). If pretreatment with oestrogen is used the method offers the simplicity, reliability and accuracy of the isolated rat uterus with the sensitivity more usually achieved with less convenient mammary tissue assays, or superfusion assays on the isolated uterus.

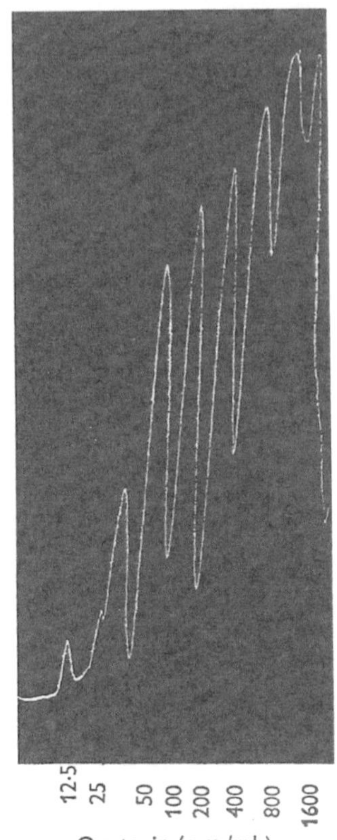

Fig. 1. Contractions of the isolated rat uterus in response to oxytocin using the cumulative dose procedure. The piece of uterus was taken from a rat which had received three injections of 100 μg stilboestrol at 24 h intervals. Note the high sensitivity of the uterus which responded to a dose of 12.5 μU oxytocin/ml. Volume of organ bath 2 ml (Follett and Bentley, 1964)

b) *Methods of Increasing Sensitivity*

The sensitivity of the isolated rat uterus to oxytocin is of the order of 50 μU/ml, or 10^{-10} molar, final concentration. If a 10 ml bath is used and if doses are administered in small volume (0.25 ml) this requires a concentration of oxytocin of about 1 mU/ml, or 2×10^{-9}, molar in the extract under investigation. Such sensitivity is inadequate for the estimation of physiological concentration of oxytocin in biological fluids. Modifications have been proposed which increase the sensitivity, but this is frequently complicated by decreased stability of the preparation and decreased correlation of dose with effect.

Sensitivity may be strictly interpreted in terms of the final *concentration* of oxytocin to which uterine muscle cells respond and in this sense the sensitivity of uterine muscle may be directly increased by hormonal or electrical influences. The sensitivity of an assay method may also be considered in terms of the total *dose* of oxytocin which is required for each response. The two interpretations are obviously related by a factor dependent on the dilution of the added dose by the bath fluid. Investigators working with tissue extracts are often more concerned with total dose of oxytocin required for a response rather than final concentration and accordingly modifications have been made to increase the sensitivity of the method by reducing the dilution within the organ bath. In some methods this dilution may be nil, that is, the uterus is directly exposed to, or immersed in, the prepared extract; the sensitivity of the method may then be further increased by decreasing the volume of extract to which the uterus is exposed.

Superfusion. GADDUM (1953b) reported that increased sensitivity of isolated smooth muscle was obtained if fluids were applied in small volume to the surface of a tissue which is otherwise suspended in air instead of being immersed in saline. The principle has been exploited with the rat uterus by SIDDIQI and WALKER (1960) and by FITZPATRICK (1961) for estimating the oxytocin concentration of blood and blood extracts.

The superfused preparation is a little more difficult to set up than a conventional organ bath. The tissue must be suspended in air in a jacketed chamber at about 32° C; the counter balance of the lever must be more carefully adjusted since the tissue is not immersed in fluid; prewarmed, physiological saline (or unextracted

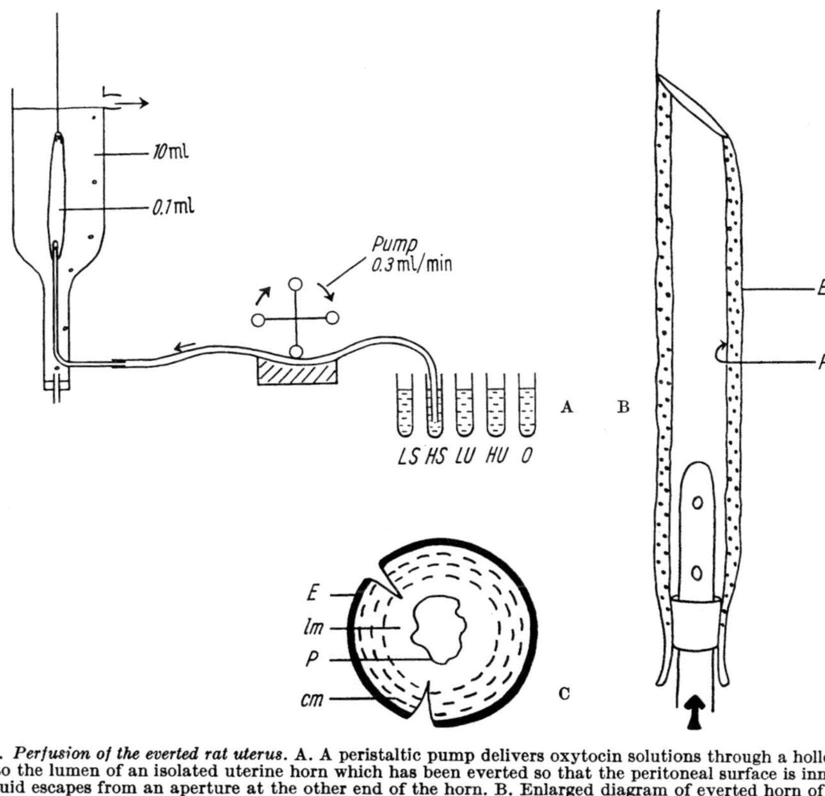

Fig. 2. *Perfusion of the everted rat uterus.* A. A peristaltic pump delivers oxytocin solutions through a hollow steel tube to the lumen of an isolated uterine horn which has been everted so that the peritoneal surface is innermost. The fluid escapes from an aperture at the other end of the horn. B. Enlarged diagram of everted horn of uterus: P = peritoneum; E = endometrium. C. Diagram of cross-section of everted horn of uterus to show relative positions of endometrium (E); circular muscle (cm); longitudinal muscle (lm) and peritoneum (P). The endometrium and circular muscle have been slit longitudinally

blood) is arranged to drop slowly over the tissue at about 3 ml/min; for assay of extracts this fluid is interrupted at regular intervals of from 1—3 min and a small volume (0.3 ml) of test solution is then allowed to drop on the tissue (also at 3 ml/min) and to soak in for up to 1 min before restarting the saline drip.

The superfused preparation at its best can be both extremely reliable and sensitive (such an example is given on pages 206—209) with detection of as little as 1 μU in 0.3 ml. There is however an increased incidence of spontaneous contractions, associated with the mechanical difficulty of regulating the drip system, and this is exaggerated if isometric rather than isotonic methods of recording are used. There is also a steep dose response relationship so that with an appreciable proportion of uteri there is such little difference between ineffective and maximally effective doses that comparison of Standard and Unknown is frustrating.

Eversion of Uterus. Sensitivity, expressed as dose administered, can obviously be increased by decreasing the size of the conventional organ bath, but this becomes impracticable for routine purposes below a volume of 1 or 2 ml. It is however possible to use the lumen of the uterus as its own organ bath; the lumen of one horn of the rat uterus has a volume of about 0.1 ml.

Oxytocin is not well absorbed from the endometrium. Accordingly the uterus is turned inside-out, so that the peritoneum becomes internal and the endometrium becomes external. (When this is done the endometrium embraces the muscle very tightly and it is advisable to slit the endometrium longitudinally to facilitate passage of fluid through the central lumen.) Krebs or a similar solution is perfused through the lumen of the everted uterus at the rate of 0.3 ml/min preferably using a peristaltic pump (see Fig. 2). The rate of passage of fluid is important. Simple injection by hand, or a high continuous rate of flow, sets off stretch reflexes (SETEKLEIV, 1964b) which interfere with the assay. We have found that for a rat uterus at pro-oestrus a flow rate of 0.3 ml/min is tolerated. This is about three times the effective volume of the uterine "lumen" (0.1 ml). In the assay this fluid is changed every third minute to a solution containing oxytocin which is perfused for 1 min. If the whole uterus is immersed in an organ bath, spontaneous contractions are negligible even at 37° C and without reduction of calcium concentration.

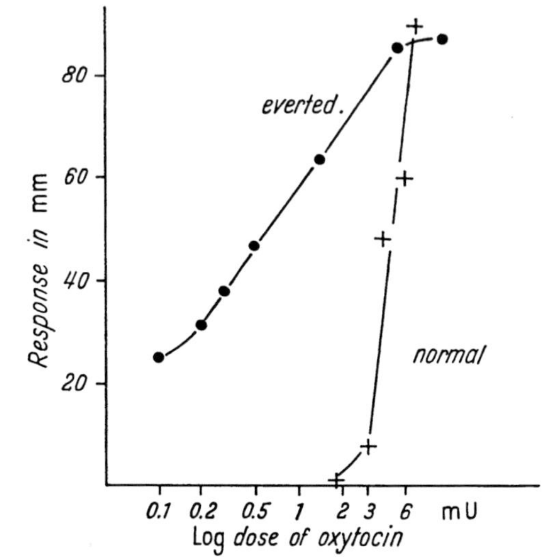

Fig. 3. Log dose response curves are compared for the two horns of the same rat uterus. One horn is suspended conventionally in an isolated organ bath of 10 ml; the other horn is everted and oxytocin solution is perfused through the lumen as in Fig. 2. Although the same dose is required by the two preparations for maximum contraction, the everted uterus is much more sensitive and shows good linearity over a much wider range of doses

Table 2. *Dose of oxytocin required to produce a measurable response from separate horns of the same rat uterus, in vitro, one horn being everted*

Rat	Preparation: Conventional 10 ml bath 0.3 ml dose	Preparation: Perfusion of everted uterus 0.3 ml dose	Dose ratio
A	1 mU	50 μU	20:1
B	1 mU	50 μU	20:1
C	2 mU	70 μU	30:1
D	3 mU	70 μU	45:1
E	3 mU	30 μU	100:1
F	2 mU	8 μU	250:1
G	3 mU	10 μU	300:1
	Geometric mean ratio		63:1

Contractions of the uterus are proportional to the concentration of oxytocin in the perfused fluid. The log. dose response curve is satisfactorily linear over a greater range of dose than with the conventional bath preparation or the superfused uterus (see Fig. 3). This wide range is of advantage when dealing with extracts of completely unknown strength.

The everted uterus preparation responds to a threshold dose of about 10 μU oxytocin and satisfactory assays can be obtained with doses of the order of 30 μU. If similar responses of the two horns of the same uterus are compared, one conventionally mounted and the other everted, the everted uterus is approximately 60 times more sensitive, as shown in Table 2.

The results obtained in four experiments, in each of which two solutions of known concentrations of oxytocin were assayed against each other, are given in Table 3. Results more than adequate for most investigations with tissue extracts

Table 3. *Statistical characteristics of four assays conducted on the everted rat uterus in vitro*

Assay	Number of observations n	True ratio ρ	Estimated ratio R	Fiducial limits* of R	Lambda** Sy/b	g***	Maximum % error
3.	12	1.0	1.0093	0.8908—1.1442	0.0379	.0316	13.4
1.	16	1.5	1.5535	1.408 —1.766	0.029	.0339	13.7
2.	16	0.8	0.8247	0.7195—0.9264	0.041	.0237	12.3
4.	28	1.25	1.1813	1.0369—1.3799	0.67	.0310	16.8

* Fiducial Limits at P = 0.05.
** Gaddum's Index of Precision.
*** Finney's Function $g = \frac{S^2y \quad t^2}{b^2(x-\bar{x})^2}$

were obtained with relatively few observations; they compare well with conventional rat uterine assays.

Composition of Bath Fluid. The action of oxytocin on the uterine muscle cell which is finally manifest as a contractile response, involves an initial depolarisation of the cell membrane, subsequent ionic redistribution particularly involving calcium ions, and consequential contraction of cellular actomyocin (COUTINHO and CSAPO, 1959; see also FITZPATRICK, 1966). Any factor which facilitates this sequence of events may improve the sensitivity of the tissue to oxytocin: it may also increase the frequency of spontaneous depolarisation and thus of spontaneous contractions. Increase in sensitivity (and in spontaneous contractions) are seen within limits, with increase in temperature and increase in calcium concentration in the bath fluid. A decrease of 30% in uterine contractions *in vitro* has been reported for a fall of 2° C (39° C to 37° C) by SETEKLEIV (1964a) and, for a decrease in calcium concentration (from 20% to 10% of normal Krebs solution), by WIQVIST, WIQVIST, FIELITZ and CALDEYRO-BARCIA (1962). In most assay procedures these relationships are exploited to control spontaneous contractions (by lowering the temperature or decreasing the calcium concentration) and this results in loss of sensitivity to oxytocin. (See BEAUVILLAIN, 1943; GARCIA DE JALON et al., 1945; GARCIA DE JALON, 1947; HOLTON, 1948, and CSAPO and CORNER, 1951b.) The calcium concentration should not however be lowered below. 8 mM or the loss in sensitivity to oxytocin becomes too great (COUTINHO and CSAPO, 1959; WIQVIST et al., 1962).

Variation in magnesium concentration has the opposite effect to that seen with calcium; increase in concentration up to about 10 mM magnesium increases uterine response to oxytocin (HSU, 1948). Adjustment of magnesium and calcium concentration have been used to improve *in vitro* uterine assays by numerous authors although usually in the guinea-pig rather than the rat (VAN DYKE and HASTINGS,

1928; FRASER, 1939; STEWART, 1949). The influence of magnesium concentration has been extended to the rat uterus by FIELITZ, GONZALEZ-PANIZZA and CALDEYRO-BARCIA (1960) and by MUNSICK (1960); the latter was able to exploit this effect not to increase sensitivity to oxytocin but to differentiate between oxytocin and its homologues found in submammalian vertebrates as described at the end of this chapter.

Three treatments to increase sensitivity of the myometrial cell have been reported; the influence of sex hormones, the application of electrical stimuli and the use of hyaluronidase.

Sex Hormone Administration. Oestrogens have long been known in many species to increase uterine reactivity, including reactivity to oxytocin. These hormones decrease the resting membrane potential so that it is more easily discharged either spontaneously or by depolarising substances, including oxytocin (KURIYAMA and

Table 4. *Sensitivity of isolated uteri to oxytocin after treatment in vivo with oestrogens*

Authors	Oestrogen	Administration		Species	Threshold concentration oxytocin
		Dose	Period		
STEWART (1949)	Stilboestrol	500 μg	12 days	guinea-pig	2 μU/ml
FITZPATRICK (1961)	Stilboestrol	50 μg/kg	overnight	rat	10 μU/ml
WIQVIST et al. (1962)	Oestradiol	50—100 μg/day	3 days	rat	10 μU/ml
STYLES and SULLIVAN (1962)	Oestradiol	25 μg	24 hours	rat	25 μU/ml
STYLES and SULLIVAN (1962)	Oestradiol	50 μg	24 hours	guinea-pig	25 μU/ml
FOLLETT and BENTLEY (1964)	Stilboestrol	100 μg/day	for 3 days	rat	25 μU/ml
FENDLER et al. (1963)	Oestrone	50 μg	for 4 days	rat	100 μU/ml

CSAPO, 1961; MARSHALL, 1959, 1962). Not surprisingly numerous authors have attempted to increase the sensitivity of uterine assays *in vitro* by administration of oestrogen usually in long acting bases (see Table 4).

However, oestrogens given in this manner are a relatively crude procedure, of uncertain latency and uncertain relationship to the endogenous oestrogen and progesterone secretion. It is not uncommon for the administration of oestrogen to produce such an unstable membrane potential that the assay is spoilt by spontaneous contractions or by the response to oxytocin assuming an all-or-none character. WIQVIST et al. (1962) claimed to have largely overcome the spontaneous activity associated with oestrogen treatment by removal of the ovarian tip of the uterus which acts as the pacemaker area in the oestrogènised uterus (MARSHALL, 1959).

Although administration of oestrogen may have some advantage for assays required infrequently at short notice, a more satisfactory general procedure is to exploit the natural balance of oestrogen and progesterone and to select animals when the endogenous sex hormone balance is optimal.

Parturient Uteri. The uterus is naturally most sensitive to oxytocin at parturition but few workers have attempted to exploit this sensitivity for assay purposes due to the high incidence of spontaneous activity and also to the complications of organising an animal colony on this basis. It is noteworthy however that COUTINHO (1964, 1966) has successfully used isolated uterine muscle from parturient rabbits. The spontaneous activity is controlled by reducing the temperature to 25° C and by regular electrical stimulation (see below). The difficulty of animal supply is largely overcome by storage of uterine segments, free of endometrium, in sodium-free glucose-rich Krebs solution at 4° C. This allows sensitivity to persist undiminished for at least 7—14 days. Such storage offers the added advantage for some investigators that the same rabbit myometrium may be used piecemeal for successive assays of a series of blood samples taken from one particular patient over a substantial period, e.g. throughout parturition.

Natural Oestrus. HOLTON indicated in her original description of the rat method that a relatively large proportion of uteri from rats chosen at random are unsuitable for assay due to lack of sensitivity or because of excess spontaneous activity. Successive workers have confirmed this. In addition they have noted the frequent incidence of uteri which appear to give all-or-none responses.

FLATTERS (1954) reported systematically upon the variation in sensitivity in relation to the ovarian cycle, in a paper which has been largely overlooked. She demonstrated quite clearly that uterine sensitivity to oxytocin is negligible in metoestrus but increases progressively in dioestrus and pro-oestrus, whilst in full oestrus the organ shows too much spontaneous activity to be useful. At the transition from pro-oestrus to oestrus although spontaneous contractions may be absent, the all-or-none type of response is common, and uteri frequently respond with maximal contraction to the mechanical stimulus of change of bath fluid especially after *sub-threshold* doses of oxytocin have been applied; this considerably interferes with assays when they are conducted at the sensitive end of the dose response curve, as is often the case when dealing with blood extracts. CHAN, O'CONNELL, and POMEROY (1963) have confirmed that oxytocin sensitivity in the rat is high at oestrus and pro-oestrus, that during dioestrus sensitivity falls to about half and in metoestrus to about one quarter of that at oestrus. SCHNEIDER and STUMPF (1953) and GUERNÉ and STUTINSKY (1961) also report that pro-oestrous and oestrous rats are more sensitive.

FLATTERS (1954) reported that the best conditions are at pro-oestrus when sensitivity is reasonably high (all such uteri gave 40% maximal response to 30 μU per ml at 32° C) but interfering spontaneous contractions are absent. At this stage the correlation of response with magnitude of dose is optimal for assay purposes and remains almost constant over periods of several hours. There was such remarkable consistency shown amongst uteri from different pro-oestrous animals, both as regards sensitivity and dose response relationship, that FLATTERS was able to construct a standard reference curve with the aid of which a large number of unknown extracts could be quickly and easily assayed over a short period of time.

Pro-oestrus in the rat lasts only a few hours and for our present purpose it is necessary that the rat is in pro-oestrus not merely on the day of assay but at the time it is sacrificed. To select such rats it is necessary to monitor a group of 12—20 each day, re-examining as close to the time of assay as possible those animals in whom pro-oestrus is to be expected that day, making the final choice within half an hour of the commencement of the assay. Such a regime poses formidable problems of colony management. These may however be reduced by exploiting present knowledge of the circadian rhythm of ovulation mechanisms.

It is now established that in the female rat the ovulation cycle, and hence pro-oestrus, is closely linked with a 24 hour rhythm (EVERETT and SAWYER, 1950; EVERETT, 1961; JÖCHLE, 1967). This rhythm is dependent at least in part upon the influence of light so that by controlling environmental light, control of the ovulation cycle may be developed. For instance, under a daily cycle of 14 hours light and 10 hours darkness, arranged conventionally about a working day, a very stable 4 or 5 day ovarian cycle can be observed with pro-oestrus typically in the early afternoon. If the timing of the artificial light period is changed relative to sidereal time, then the timing of the successive events of the ovarian cycle changes proportionately (EVERETT, 1961). Accordingly, it should be practicable in most rat colonies to so arrange an artificial light programme within the 24 hour day that pro-oestrus, or even a suitable sub-division of pro-oestrus, will occur in the majority of females at a specified time of day (such as 09.00 hours) convenient to the working timetable of any particular laboratory.

Hyaluronidase. A further attempt to improve sensitivity by drug treatment has been reported by FENDLER, ENDRÖCZI, and LISSÁK (1963) who demonstrated that hyaluronidase treatment increased sensitivity of the rat uterus to oxytocin (but

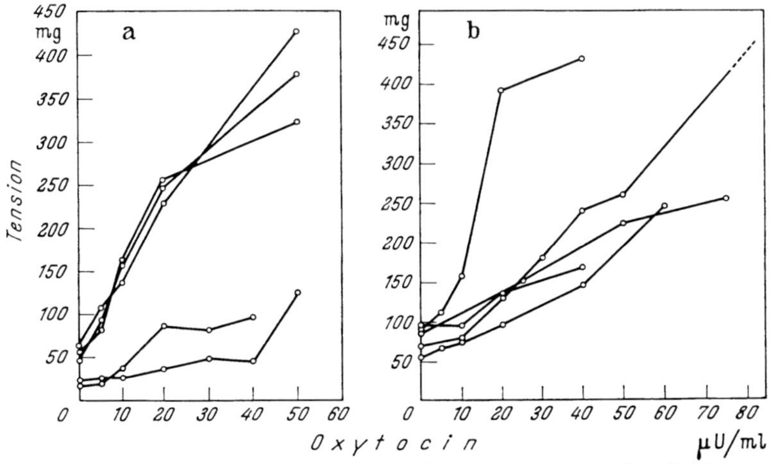

Fig. 4. Effects of oxytocin concentration on the response of the rat uterus to regular slightly suprathreshold electrical stimulation of constant strength. A = superfused at 2 ml/min; B = immersed in isolated organ bath (WIQVIST et al., 1962)

not to acetylcholine). A five- to tenfold increase in sensitivity was seen after 40 min exposure *in vitro* to a concentration of 3 IU per ml hyaluronidase ("Hyason" — Organon). An augmentation of similar magnitude was observed when hyaluronidase was administered to intact rats over 5 days (75 IU i.p. daily). The authors attribute the augmentor effect to increase in cell permeability to oxytocin. The reports are worth closer investigation to incorporate any advantage into *in vitro* assay procedures.

Electrical Stimulation. Some workers have advocated increasing the sensitivity and reactivity of isolated uterine muscle to oxytocin by subjecting the tissue to electrical stimulation. The strength, duration and frequency of stimuli suitable for work with isolated myometrium are given in considerable detail by CSAPO and GOODALL (1954). For modification of sensitivity to oxytocin the magnitude of stimulation should be adjusted to produce a small but consistent contraction of the tissue. Effects of oxytocin are then seen as increase in magnitude of these contractions. It is considered that the uterus is made up of functional units each of which obeys the all-or-none law, and each of which may have a different threshold of excitability (CSAPO and CORNER, 1951a, b; CSAPO, 1954). With a minimal suprathreshold of electrical stimulus few units are sufficiently excitable to respond, so that the magnitude of the total contractile effect is low. The effect of oxytocin in such a system is to lower the excitability of all fibres by decreasing the membrane potential. Consequently a larger proportion of muscle fibres respond to the standard electrical impulse, and a greater magnitude of contractile response is obtained.

The effects of electrical stimulation and of oxytocin, in so far as they each act on the membrane potential, may be considered as additive. Not only does oxytocin reduce the threshold to electrical stimulation but conversely electrical stimulation reduces the threshold to oxytocin, that is, it increases the sensitivity to oxytocin and this phenomenon may be used in assays. Surprisingly this has not been widely exploited.

FIELITZ et al. (1960) and WIQVIST et al. (1962) described such a method using the isolated rat uterus suspended in air at 28° C between two platinum wires at a resting tension of 0.1 g and superfused at 2 ml/min with Krebs solution with low (20%) calcium. Contractions which were recorded isometrically were induced electrically every 3 min. A voltage was chosen just sufficient to produce small regular contractions (usually between 3 and 12 volts) when applied for 10—15 sec at 50 cps. When standard suprathreshold responses were obtained to the electrical stimulation, the superfusion fluid was changed to one containing oxytocin. Clear augmentation of response is seen proportional to the concentration of oxytocin (see Fig. 4), over a range of 5—50 μU/ml, although the sensitivity depends on the concentration of calcium in the superfusion fluid. With higher concentrations of calcium, FIELITZ et al. (1960) obtained responses to 0.5 and 1.0 μU/ml but suffered from excessive spontaneous contractions.

STYLES and SULLIVAN (1962) have described this type of preparation using the rabbit, guinea-pig, and rat uterus immersed at 28° C in Krebs solution (calcium 0.25 mM). A stimulus of 15 volts for 5 sec (50 c/s) was applied at intervals of 1 min to two ring electrodes 6.5 cm apart and not in direct contact with the tissue. When oxytocin was added to the bath the uterus responded to, and discriminated between, doses of the order of 25 μU/ml which would not have been discriminated by the unstimulated tissue.

COUTINHO and CSAPO (1959) and COUTINHO (1964) have also described this phenomenon for isolated rabbit myometrium. According to COUTINHO (1964, 1966) the principle may be used for the assay of oxytocin and of oxytocin-like substances in human blood at the time of parturition. In COUTINHO's laboratory uterine muscle is removed under anaesthesia from a rabbit during the birth of a litter when the sensitivity is of course particularly high. For the assay a piece of myometrium about 0.5 cm wide by 3 cm long is suspended in a conventional waterbath in normal Krebs solution usually at 25° C to reduce spontaneous contractions. The lower end of the strip is in contact with a platinum electrode and the second electrode consists of a platinum ring approximately 1 cm diameter suspended in the Krebs solution, near to but not in contact with the upper end of the uterine strip. Isometric contractions are recorded with a strain gauge. At intervals of 1 min electrical stimuli at 60 cps and of 5 sec duration are applied at a potential of 1 volt per centimetre length of the strip. The voltage is adjusted by means of a variable resistance until contractions are 10—25% of maximal. When oxytocin is added to the bath fluid an increased amplitude of contraction is seen which is proportional to the final concentration of oxytocin in the bath, over a range of 5—25 μU/ml.

In all the modifications of the electrical stimulation method, referred to above, at least 10—15 min is required to observe and measure the response to each concentration of oxytocin. This is an important limitation to the usefulness of the procedure when many extracts have to be assayed over a short time, although this may be mitigated by running more than one preparation coincidentally and perhaps by incorporating the effect of hyaluronidase described above. Moreover this 10 min latency prevents the exploitation of the advantage of sensitivity of the superfusion principle, which relies essentially on the administration of a single very small volume of solution: when it is necessary to continue superfusion of an oxy-

Table 5. *Physiological saline solutions used in bioassays of oxytocin*

	Ref. 1	Ref. 2	Ref. 3	Ref. 4	Ref. 5	Ref. 6	Ref. 7	Ref. 8
millimols per litre								
NaCl	154.	113.	118.4	154.	113.	154.	136.8	136.8
KCl	5.64	6.20	4.74	5.64	6.20	5.64	2.69	2.69
$CaCl_2$	2.20	0.53	2.53	1.10	0.50	2.54	0.91	1.80
$MgCl_2$	0.05	1.00	0	0	0 or 0.5	0	0.99	1.05
$MgSO_4$	0	0	1.18	3.12	0	1.18	0	0
$NaHCO_3$	5.95	30.0	24.9	5.95	30.0	5.95	11.9	11.9
NaH_2PO_4	0	1.00	0	0	1.00	0	0	0.42
Na_2HPO_4	0		0	0		0	0.15*	0
KH_2PO_4	0	0	1.18	0	0	1.18	0	0
Glucose	2.78	0	11.11	5.56	2.78	5.56	5.56	1.0
Gas	air	5% CO_2	5% CO_2	5% CO_2**	5% CO_2	5% CO_2	5% CO_2	not gassed
pH	7.4	7.4	7.5	7.1	7.4	6.85	7.4	7.6
Grams per litre								
NaCl	9.0	6.60	6.9	9.0	6.60	9.01	8.0	8.0
KCl	0.42	0.46	0.35	0.42	0.46	0.42	0.2	0.2
$CaCl_2$	0.24	0.059	0.278	0.12	0.056	0.282	0.101	0.2
$MgCl_2$	0.005	0.096	0	0	0 or .05	0	0.094	0.1
$MgSO_4$	0	0	0.142	0.375	0	0.142	0	0
$NaHCO_3$	0.50	2.52	2.1	0.5	2.52	0.5	1.0	1.0
NaH_2PO_4	0	0.035***	0	0	0.035***	0	0	0.05
Na_2HPO_4	0	0.105***	0	0	0.105***	0	0.177*	0
KH_2PO_4	0	0	0.16	0	0	0.16	0	0
Glucose	0.50	0	2.00	1.00	0.50	1.00	1.00	1.00
Assay	uterus	uterus	uterus/ mammary gland	uterus	uterus	uterus	mammary gland	mammary gland

Weights given refer to anhydrous salts in all cases.
pH measured at 37° C after equilibrating with 5% CO_2 and 95% O_2.

References: 1. Burn and Dale (1922); 2. van Dyke and Hastings (1928); 3. Krebs and Henseleit (1932); 4. Garcia de Jalon (1947); 5. Munsick (1960); 6. Styles and Sullivan (1962); 7. Rydén and Sjöholm (1962); 8. van Dongen and Hays (1966a, b).

* Corresponding to 0.05 gms/l Na_2HPO_4, 12 H_2O not 5.0 gms as stated incorrectly in original publication (Sjöholm, 1967, personal communication).

** Gas composition not specified by original author.

*** As suggested by Bentley (1965).

tocin solution for 10 min, much the same total dose of oxytocin will be used for each observation as with conventional organ baths. This is confirmed by the observations of Wiqvist et al. (1962) that superfusion possessed little advantage (see Fig. 4).

3. The Uterus in Vivo

Attempts have been made to develop assay methods based on the uterine contractile response to oxytocin usually given intravenously. In general this response has been more difficult to evaluate than the milk-ejection response *in vivo*, and the uterine methods are relatively insensitive, lacking in specificity and precision. Apart from one important recent development in the laboratory of G. W. Bisset, the described methods are unlikely to be readily applicable to investigations of the oxytocin concentration in biological fluids. Accordingly they are mentioned only briefly.

Several species have been used including the cat, rat, rabbit, sheep, cow and man. ROBSON and SCHILD (1938a, b) used the cat uterus *in situ* for quantitative studies of the action of oxytocin and vasopressin, recording contractility by the Cushny myocardiograph. CLARY, CAMERON, and CRAVER (1951) also used anaesthetised cats but despite a more elegant method of recording intraluminal pressures and despite pretreatment with oestradiol, their sensitivity was no better and required doses of 50 mU oxytocin intravenously. BERDE and co-workers have improved the reliability and sensitivity of the procedure (BERDE, DOEPFNER, and KONZETT, 1957; BERDE and CERLETTI, 1964) but the method is not suitable for wide application to studies with body fluids.

For many years uterine responses of the rabbit uterus *in vivo* to oxytocin have also been studied quantitatively, usually by recording intra-uterine pressure (see REYNOLDS, 1949; CROSS, 1958a) but threshold sensitivity is relatively low in terms of the (intravenous) dose necessary, 1—5 mU. BERDE and CERLETTI (1958) and CROSS (1958b) have used the induction of labour in the rabbit for estimation of oxytocin, but although this must be considered useful for studies of identification or of structure-action relationships it is not a sensitive method (requiring doses of 100 mU or more), and necessitates large numbers of pre-parturient rabbits, the supply of which must be organised with great precision.

Although larger species such as sheep and cows have been used for this type of work (FITZPATRICK, 1960) they require doses too large for present considerations, and are too inconvenient.

Assays of oxytocin have also been conducted in women, usually when pregnant or post-partum (SCHILD, FITZPATRICK, and NIXON, 1951; BAINBRIDGE, NIXON, SCHILD, and SMYTH, 1956; CALDEYRO-BARCIA and POSEIRO, 1958; BERDE and SAAMELI, 1959; SAAMELI, 1963, and EMBREY, 1965). Although such assays can be as accurate as those conducted on the uteri of laboratory animals, the disadvantageous sensitivity and the ethical complications restrict them to work of direct clinical application, for which they are to be preferred over *in vitro* studies using human myometrium.

The Rat Uterus. It is only in the rat that oxytocin assays on the uterus *in situ* are likely to be useful in the investigation of biological fluids. BERDE et al. (1957) assayed oxytocin against four of its analogues in several preparations including the rat uterus *in vivo*. Their method of recording was very simple and the assay procedure was limited to a bracketing type of assay, the limits of error of which were not determined. Despite pre-treatment with oestrogen, these rats were relatively insensitive requiring doses of 50 mU or more intravenously. However GUERNÉ and STUTINSKY (1961) improved both method and sensitivity, and more recently BISSET, HALDAR, and LEWIN (1966) have described a much more reliable and sensitive method of considerable promise. Using the rat uterus *in situ* they have been able to overcome the disadvantages of low sensitivity, spontaneous activity and inferior reproducibility, customarily associated with this type of preparation by developing elegant technical procedures.

The contractile response of the uterus is measured as the increase in intraluminal fluid pressure, using a strain-gauge transducer. By incorporating a simple digital integrator into their recording system they are able to measure responses quantitatively, integrating amplitude, duration and frequency of contractions. A function of this parameter gives good regression with dose of oxytocin. Fig. 5 illustrates such responses to doses of 1—16 mU oxytocin, given intravenously.

In rats taken in early (vaginal) oestrus these authors find that spontaneous activity is not troublesome and that the uterus *in situ* is about as sensitive to intravenous oxytocin as the conventionally isolated rat uterus but considerably more specific. Sensitivity can be increased with responses to doses of 100 μU by retrograde arterial injection through a cannula passed up the contra-lateral iliac artery until the tip lies at the biforcation of the aorta.

Without doubt, the outstanding advantage of the Bisset method over the isolated uterus is the greater specificity to oxytocin. The isolated rat uterus is well recognised as a non-specific assay preparation responding to many substances at

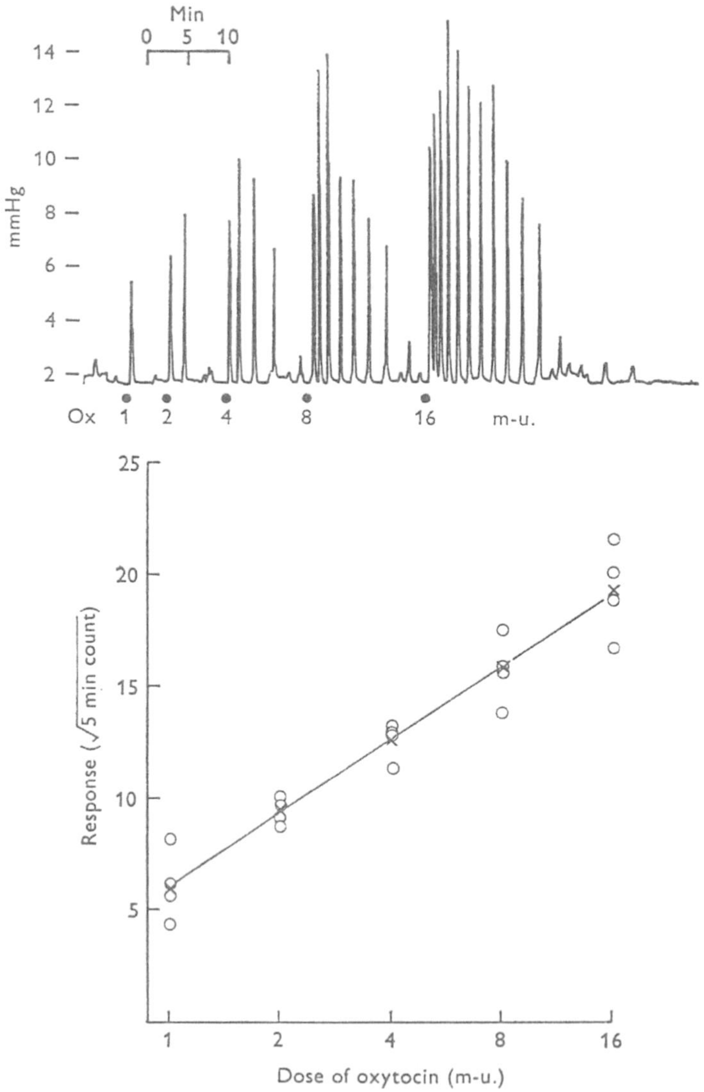

Fig. 5. *Above:* Responses, in mm Hg, of the rat uterus *in situ* to oxytocin administered intravenously. *Below:* Log dose response curve for oxytocin i.v. on rat uterus *in situ*. The response is expressed as a function of the integrated intra-uterine pressure changes over 5 min. Four injections for each of five doses are represented. Crosses represent means and circles individual responses (Bisset et al., 1966)

concentrations that may occur in blood and other extracts. Since specificity is largely a function of concentration Bisset et al. (1966) determined the threshold doses of several such substances *in vitro* and *in vivo* for the same uterine horn. They found that the ratio of doses for the two preparations is not constant but varies with the substance. The uterus *in situ* is as sensitive to oxytocin and vasopressin as the isolated uterus but less than half as sensitive to angiotensin, $^1/_{25}$th as sensitive to 5-hydroxytryptamine and $^1/_{400}$th as sensitive to bradykinin. Oxytocin is at least 10 times as potent as any other substance tested in its action on the uterus *in situ*. Furthermore the character of the uterine response to oxytocin is readily distinguishable *in vivo* from that of the other substances investigated, whereas this qualitative difference does not apply *in vitro*. This aids the detection of interfering substances in tissue extracts. They may also be detected *in vivo* by their coincident effect on the blood pressure, on which oxytocin, in the concentrations likely to occur in body fluids or extracts, is without effect.

A comparison of the sensitivity of uterine preparations to oxytocin both *in vitro* and *in vivo* is given in Table 6.

Table 6. *Sensitivity of uterine preparations to oxytocin*

Method	Threshold* Concen-tration**	Threshold* Dose**	Minimum concentration in solutions for assay**	References
A) In vitro				
1. perfused:				
rat (superfused)	15 μU	5 μU	15 μU/ml	FITZPATRICK (1961)
rat (everted)	30 μU	10 μU	30 μU/ml	FITZPATRICK (1967)
2. conventional bath, electrically stimulated:				
guinea-pig	3.3 μU/ml	33 μU	100 μU/ml	STYLES and SULLIVAN (1962)
rabbit	10 μU/ml	100 μU	300 μU/ml	COUTINHO (1966)
rat	25 μU/ml	250 μU	750 μU/ml	STYLES and SULLIVAN (1962)
3. conventional bath, unstimulated:				
guinea-pig	3 μU/ml	30 μU	100 μU/ml	STYLES and SULLIVAN (1962)
pro-oestrous rat	20 μU/ml	200 μU	600 μU/ml	FLATTERS (1954)
hyaluronidase rat	20 μU/ml	200 μU	600 μU/ml	FENDLER et al. (1963)
B) In vivo				
rat i.a.	—	5 μU	15 μU/ml	BISSET (1966)
rat i.v.	—	100 μU	300 μU/ml	BISSET (1966)
guinea-pig i.v.	—	1.5 mU	4.5 mU/ml	LINZELL (1955)
rabbit i.v.	—	2 mU	6 mU/ml	CROSS (1958a)

* Threshold taken as the minimum amount of oxytocin which consistently elicits a measurable response.

** For comparisons only it is assumed that doses are given in volumes of 0.3 ml and organ baths are of 10 ml capacity.
The references cited are usually those reporting the most sensitive modifications of specified preparations.

4. Example of Analysis of Assay at High Sensitivity

In an assay of oxytocin on the superfused rat uterus solutions were applied at intervals of 1 min in volume of 0.3 ml over 10 sec. Low dose of Standard was 2 μU oxytocin, and High dose of Standard 4 μU oxytocin. Similar solutions were used as Low dose Unknown and High dose of Unknown respectively so that the ratio of potency was 1.00.

Fifteen groups of four responses were studied, the sequence of doses within each group being randomised. The responses are given as contractions in mm, as recorded on a kymograph.

Group	Low Standard	High Standard	Low Unknown	High Unknown	Group Totals
1	62	114	62	107	345
2	56	108	59	106	329
3	52	110	54	109	325
4	49	110	49	107	315
5	46	105	43	106	300
6	40	104	42	104	290
7	37	105	34	103	279
8	31	98	33	97	259
9	26	93	29	97	245
10	24	92	24	91	231
11	22	88	21	86	217
12	19	85	21	84	209
13	16	83	17	83	199
14	15	82	14	80	191
15	13	77	13	74	177
Total	508	1454	515	1434	3911

The potency of the Unknown in terms of the Standard is calculated as described by Schild (1942) and Holton (1948).

$$\Sigma\ HS + \Sigma\ LS = 1962; \text{ mean response for Standard } = \bar{y}s = \frac{1962}{30} = 65.40$$

$$\Sigma\ HU + \Sigma\ LU = 1949; \text{ mean response for Unknown } = \bar{y}u = \frac{1949}{30} = 64.96$$

$$\begin{aligned} \Sigma\ HS + \Sigma\ HU &= 2888 \\ \Sigma\ LS + \Sigma\ LU &= 1023 \\ \hline \text{Total sum} &= 3911 \end{aligned}$$

Log ratio of doses $= d = \log 2 = 0.30103$

The average regression of response on log dose is b.

$$b = \frac{2888 - 1023}{30 \times 0.30103} = 206.5132$$

The logarithm of the ratio of Unknown to Standard is M

$$M = \frac{(1949 - 1962) \times 0.30103}{(2888 - 1023)} = (-.002098)$$

The arithmetic ratio of Unknown to Standard is R

$$R = \text{antilog } M = 0.995$$

The known true ratio of the solutions in this experiment is $= 1.000$

The estimate of the error of this ratio requires an analysis of the variance of the observations to eliminate known causes of variation; thus

Source of Variation	Sums of Squares of Deviations		Degrees of Freedom		Variance or Mean Square
Total		69344.983		59	
Groups	10744.23		14		767.445
Regression	57970.416		1		57970.416
Parallelism	12.15		1		12.15
S + U	2.816		1		2.816
Total 'Known' Deviations		68729.612		17	
Error (Residue)		615.371		42	14.652

sy $=$ Standard deviation of single observation $= \sqrt{14.652}$

Standard Error of M is obtained from formula

$$s^2_M = \frac{4\ S^2_Y}{n\ b^2} \left(\frac{M^2}{d^2} + 1\right)$$

substituting we obtain

$$s^2_M = \frac{4 \times 14.652}{60 \times (206.513)^2} \left[\frac{(0.002098)^2}{(0.3103)^2} + 1\right]$$

$$= 0.000022904 \times 1.0000487$$

$$s_M = 0.004786$$

The Fiducial Limits of $M = M \pm t \times s_M$

t for 42 degrees of freedom (at probability of $P = 0.05$) = 2.0181

Hence $t \times s_M = 0.009659$

Thus 95% fiducial limits of M =

M max = (—.002098) + .009659 = +.007561
M min = (—.002098) — .009659 = —.011757

and the 95% fiducial limits of R are given as

R max = antilog (.007561) = 1.018
R min = antilog (—.0011757) = antilog ($\overline{1}$.988243) = .973

B. Assays Based on Mammary Gland Response

There is an increasing tendency for the response of mammary gland myoepithelium to be used for assay of oxytocin in preference to that of the uterine myometrium. In general this is because the myoepithelium is thought to be more specific than the myometrium. This specificity, which however is not absolute and which may be species dependant, is of particular importance to investigations of body fluids which frequently contain substances capable of stimulating smooth muscle. This advantage of relative specificity must be judged against the greater inconvenience of the mammary preparations as compared with those of the isolated uterus. This inconvenience is most obvious with those mammary assay procedures which use intact anaesthetised animals but even with *in vitro* methods, using isolated strips of mammary gland, sophisticated strain gauges and equipment are necessary to record faithfully the small magnitude of response: moreover the animals for assay must be in a clearly defined stage of lactation, which requires a large and well organised animal breeding colony for all but the simplest of investigations. Accordingly many workers still find it desirable to retain simple uterine methods for the more routine assays in an investigation, with extension to the mammary gland as their facilities permit and when the identification of an active oxytocin-like substance in an extract becomes important. The two tissues should not be considered as strict alternatives but as complementing each other to an extent that will depend on the resources of the laboratory and on the precise details of the investigation.

The earliest suggestion that the mammary myoepithelium response could form the basis of an assay of oxytocin was that of TURNER and COOPER (1941). These authors reported that in lactating rabbits given oxytocin intravenously "within 20—40 sec there is an obvious contraction of the gland with a distension of the duct system radiating out from the nipple, which can be observed through the (shaven) skin". Responses were consistently obtained with doses of 1—2 mU oxytocin (Pituitrin or Pitocin). It is interesting that they obtained responses with 5 mU vasopressin (Pitressin) and also they were able to confirm the earlier reports of ELY and PETERSEN (1941) that fright could inhibit the mammary response to oxytocin, an effect attributed to the action of adrenaline. This early paper proposed an assay procedure based on serial dilution of biological material until no response was obtained. This did not find acceptance, but it is of interest that this subjective method of observation detected responses to doses of oxytocin as small or smaller than the later objective methods of VAN DYKE, ADAMSONS, and ENGEL (1955) and others.

Further work which drew attention to the exquisite sensitivity of the mammary myoepithelium to oxytocin was reported by LINZELL (1955), who observed with a dissecting microscope the alveolar contractions of the mammary gland in anaesthetised mice, rats, guinea-pigs and rabbits. The dorsal surface of the gland was exposed simply and oxytocin applied topically from a micro-syringe. Sensitivity varied enormously with typical responses to doses of 10^{-8} units (mouse) or 10^{-9} units (guinea-pig) but with extreme sensitivity of 2×10^{-14} units (guinea-pig).

This author also showed that other common pharmacological agents, including choline esters, histamine and 5-hydroxytryptamine, could cause alveolar contraction. However topical application was not developed as an assay method, probably because of its inconvenience and because it is difficult to interpret the response quantitatively in relation to dose.

1. Isolated Strips

The first workers to successfully measure the contractile response of an isolated strip of mammary tissue and to use it for the assay of oxytocin were MENDEZ-BAUER, CABOT and CALDEYRO-BARCIA (1960). They used rabbits from the 15th to 30th day of lactation to provide strips cut radially from teat to periphery of an abdominal gland (circa 5 × 3 × 35 mm). Strips were suspended in Tyrode's solution at 38° C, in a bath of small volume (1.5 ml) and isometric contractions recorded with sensitive strain gauges (Statham G7A ± 0.15 ounces). The tissue was put under initial tension equivalent to 50—100 mg. Exposure to oxytocin solutions elicited contractions exerting tensions of several hundred milligrams. The authors claimed that the linearity of the dose response relationship over a range of 0.5 to 10 mU/ml, its stability for many hours, together with the absence of spontaneous activity, represent considerable advantages over assays using isolated uteri. Furthermore their strips showed no response to fresh heparinised blood or plasma indicating better specificity than with the uterus, especially suitable for studies of body fluids.

The isolated rabbit mammary strip has been further studied by MOORE and ZARROW (1965) who give a more detailed account of the preparation including some minor modifications of technique. They confirmed the high specificity of this tissue showing not only that human blood from males or non-pregnant women (in contrast to blood from parturient women) is without effect, but that of 13 substances tested (including histamine, adrenaline and 5-hydroxytryptamine) only two, vasopressin and acetylcholine, produce oxytocin-like responses. The amount of acetylcholine required is large (2.5×10^{-5} g/ml) in relation to amounts to be expected in body fluids and extracts. Vasopressin has about 15% of the potency of oxytocin. Of the substances tested which failed to stimulate the myoepithelium, adrenaline, at 10^{-5} and 5-hydroxytryptamine at 10^{-2}, inhibit the response of the tissue to oxytocin, but only at concentrations unlikely to occur in biological fluids.

These authors also confirmed the relatively poor sensitivity reported by MENDEZ-BAUER et al. (1960) and reported a disappointing index of precision (λ) of 0.993. MANUNTA and ALBERGONI (1962) however reported a sensitivity of 100 μU/ml for this preparation.

Isolated mammary strip assays have also been developed using rat tissue by SMITH (1961), SJÖHOLM and RYDÉN (1962) and RYDÉN and SJÖHOLM (1962); the last of these accounts is particularly detailed. Strips of mammary tissue, excluding the teat area ($2 \times 4 \times 30$ mm) are suspended at 37—38° C in a small organ bath in Tyrode's or similar solution (see Table 5). These three authors reported favourably on the precision of the method, the fiducial limits of error at $P = 0.05$ being $\pm$ 10% (RYDÉN and SJÖHOLM) and $\pm$ 15% (SMITH): the index of precision, lambda, was relatively good at 0.115 (RYDÉN and SJÖHOLM). SMITH however differed from the Swedish authors in reporting relative insensitivity to oxytocin with requirements of 250 μU/ml and above: he suggested that superfusion would improve the sensitivity of the method. However, the present author (unpublished observations) has had little success with this modification due to the mechanical difficulties of measuring very small changes in tension when a drip superfusion is in operation, since each drop of perfusion fluid itself weighs about 50 mg. In contrast to SMITH, RYDÉN and SJÖHOLM were able to obtain measurable responses with only 5 μU/ml and the response remained proportional to dose up to 100 μU/ml. This increase in sensitivity is possibly attributable to the use of very sensitive recording gauges (SJÖHOLM and RYDÉN, 1962).

The rat gland differentiates between oxytocin and vasopressin better than the rabbit gland (SMITH, 1961) but in other respects is less specific, at least with the highly sensitive preparations described by RYDÉN and SJÖHOLM who report contractile responses to low concentrations of 10^{-11} of acetylcholine, adrenaline, noradrenaline and histamine. Responses were also obtained with somewhat higher concentrations of 5-hydroxytryptamine (10^{-8}). This is of considerable importance since many of these substances could occur in tissue extracts in the appropriate concentrations, and selective antagonists if available would be needed. Bradykinin and angiotensin, in concentrations up to 1 μg/ml have no measurable effect on this preparation (BROVETTO, OLHABERRY, GIOIA DE COCH, CODA, FIELITZ, CABOT, FRAGA, and COCH, 1967).

Response and recovery of both rat and rabbit mammary tissue is very slow *in vitro*, and only six observations can be made per hour. This is of consequence when a large number of extracts must be assayed in a short period of time but is otherwise not a great disadvantage since the magnitude of response is very stable over many hours. MOORE and ZARROW (1965) run two assays coincidentally to speed their results.

2. *Milk-Ejection in Vitro*

It is a common experience when conducting assays on isolated organs that the latent period, after application of oxytocin to the tissue but before the response becomes obvious, is proportional to the concentration of oxytocin. C.A. KEELE and colleagues in an unpublished communication to the British Pharmacological Society (1954) illustrated this for several polypeptides which stimulate smooth muscle, including oxytocin and the isolated uterus. However, the phenomenon had not been developed as a basis for assay until VAN DONGEN (1964) and VAN DONGEN and HAYS (1964 and 1966a) proposed an extremely sensitive assay procedure based on the relationship between concentration of oxytocin and the latent period of contraction of rat myoepithelial tissue.

Their procedure exploits the remarkable sensitivity of mammary tissue to topical application of oxytocin, described originally by LINZELL (1955) who observed contractions of the mammary gland alveoli to concentrations of oxytocin as low as 2×10^{-14} units per ml. Van Dongen and Hay's method is based on the microscopic observation of small isolated segments of lactating mammary gland, when placed individually in oxytocin solution: the time elapsing between immersion and the observation of the ejection of milk is the parameter used for assay purposes.

Pieces of mammary gland (approximately 2 mm cube) are obtained from an anaesthetised rat, beyond the third day of lactation. Care is taken to minimise connective tissue and large duct tissue. The young are removed from the mother at least 3 hours before, to ensure an adequate content of milk.

The small pieces of tissue are placed individually in a drop of Tyrode's solution containing oxytocin (or in blood plasma or in an appropriate extract) and observed through a dissecting microscope magnifying $15\times$; the latent period until the initiation of milk expulsion varies inversely with concentration of oxytocin; at 15° C the latent period is of the order of 50 sec for concentrations of 10^{-10} units oxytocin/ml but only about 13 sec for concentrations of 10 mU/ml. For assay purposes each standard or test solution is exposed to five pieces of mammary tissue and the mean latent period is the measure of response. To construct a standard curve, 5 solutions of oxytocin (differing in concentration in steps of 100-fold) are tested with 5 or 6 replicates at each dose. Standard curves may be obtained by using a series of solutions in which the concentration of oxytocin increases in geometric progression, between 10^{-10} to 10^{-2} units per ml (see Fig. 6).

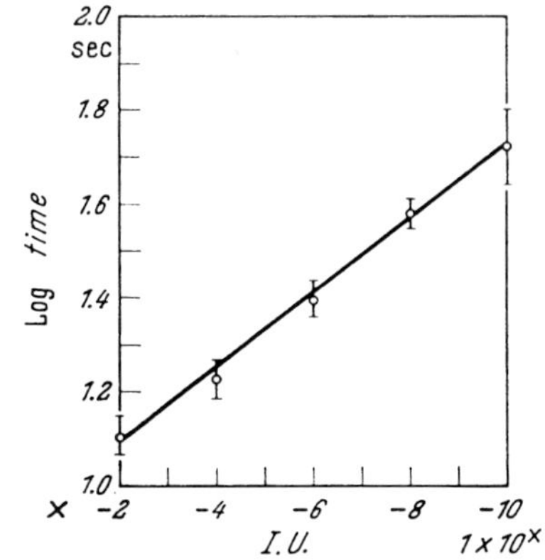

Fig. 6. Relationship between log oxytocin concentration (in units) and log time (in seconds) from exposure of isolated segments of rat mammary gland to oxytocin until milk-ejection is observed (VAN DONGEN and HAYS, 1966a)

The method has several advantages, but at least one disadvantage (low precision), and furthermore, judgement must be reserved in respect of specificity. The most impressive advantage is sensitivity. It is claimed that concentrations of 1×10^{-10} units/ml oxytocin can be measured and concentration 100 times less than this can be detected.

Since the volume of solution used for each observation is less than 0.1 ml (one drop) the amount of oxytocin detectable is less than 1×10^{-13} units, which is approximately 2×10^{-19} g or about 10^5 molecules. This must be approaching a situation in which relatively few molecules can be available for each receptor and in this sense may be near the ultimate obtainable sensitivity. At all events the method of assay is much more sensitive than any previously described. A modification of this method using slices instead of segments has confirmed this high sensitivity (ANDERSON, KUMARESAN, and TURNER, 1966).

A second advantage is that since the assay relationship is linear over a concentration range of 10^8 (a 100-million-fold change) observations can be made directly on body fluids without the complication of concentrating the fluid to suit the sensitivity of the assay. This is of very great benefit when the investigation concerns wide physiological variation in concentration of oxytocin in body fluids, the magnitude of which cannot be anticipated. The method should offer an enormous saving, not only in time but in reliability since such processing inevitably involves the risk of loss of oxytocin and the release of interfering substances.

This enormous range of concentrations over which detection is practicable represents a disadvantage for some purposes in that the slope of the regression is low. The second factor in the assay relationship — time — is not similarly stretched over a wide range and it follows that for a small increment in time, a wide range of concentrations is covered. Thus the discrimination of the assay is poor. The index of precision λ is greater than unity, which is not satisfactory for assay purposes. This limitation is recognised by the authors who indicate that no less than 13 observations for each solution are necessary to distinguish, with only 90% confidence, between tenfold differences in concentration. The procedure recommended (VAN DONGEN and HAYS, 1966a; ANDERSON et al., 1966) is to prepare and observe a series of 5 standard solutions of oxytocin in which the concentration varies geometrically in 100-fold steps (Fig. 6). This lack of precision is widely different from conventional assays which discriminate with greater reliability at concentration ratios, of high dose to low dose, of about 2:1 or less. Moreover with 5 concentrations each of Standard and Unknown and with five or six replications at each concentration the method becomes very time consuming and tedious, each assay requiring 2 hours or more. The tissue also deteriorates consequent on the prolonged maintenance *in vitro* after removal from the animal, so that repetition of an assay gives conflicting results (CLEVERLEY, 1966).

The published descriptions of the method do not offer evidence of specificity. It is probable that increase in sensitivity to oxytocin is accompanied by increase in sensitivity to other milk-ejecting substances, although not necessarily to the same degree. This point requires urgent investigation particularly in the light of the lack of specificity found with rat mammary gland *in vitro* by RYDÉN and SJÖHOLM (1962). Early reports already suggest that acetylcholine and 5-hydroxytryptamine may also induce milk-ejection responses *in vitro* as indeed one would expect from LINZELL's original observations (1955). More important is the observation that milk-ejection of brief latency has on a number of occasions been elicited with "blank" plasmas and even Tyrode's solution (CLEVERLEY, 1966). In this connection the greater specificity reported for rabbit mammary gland (MENDEZ-BAUER et al., 1960; MOORE and ZARROW, 1965) suggest that extension of the van Dongen and Hays method to rabbit tissue should be investigated.

It is obvious that the *in vitro* milk-ejection method is an appropriate choice for the initial estimation, within wide limits, of oxytocin in body fluids but that where greater precision and identification is required other assay methods will be needed for samples effectively screened by the van Dongen and Hays method. The range of concentrations of oxytocin expected in biological fluids is likely to be very wide, and impossible to anticipate, for instance during the successive stages of parturition. In these circumstances the *in vitro* milk-ejection assay is most advantageous as is well illustrated by the detection of a transient increase, of approximately one million-fold, in the milk-ejecting activity of bovine plasma during the expulsive phase of parturition (VAN DONGEN and HAYS, 1966b). Not least in importance in these particular experiments is the observation that there is negligible activity in plasma during the early stages of parturition and also in the bull during coitus (VAN DONGEN, 1964); the interpretation of this negative evidence cannot be confounded by any doubt of specificity.

3. Milk-Ejection in Vivo

The magnitude of the rise in intramammary pressure in response to oxytocin given intravenously was first developed as an assay method in the anaesthetised rabbit by CROSS and VAN DYKE (1953) and extended by VAN DYKE et al. (1955), by BERDE and CERLETTI (1957) and by GONZALEZ-PANIZZA, SICA-BLANCO and MENDEZ-BAUER (1961). LINZELL (1955) showed that it was also possible to record milk-ejection in response to intravenous oxytocin in the guinea-pig. This method is reliable but the rabbit requires threshold doses of about 3 mU oxytocin i.v. and this is not sufficiently sensitive for the investigation of biological fluids. A substantial increase in sensitivity was achieved by FITZPATRICK (1961) who introduced close arterial injection of oxytocin for milk-ejection assays in the rabbit. This permits the detection of about 150 μU oxytocin per dose and makes possible the estimation of the hormone in at least some blood extracts. In the rabbit, retrograde cannulation of the appropriate femoral artery is easy; the subcutaneous abdominal branch to the posterior mammary glands is large and its patency easily appreciated at all times. However, the rabbit possesses multiple mammary glands supplied posteriorly by the subcutaneous abdominal artery and anteriorly by the external thoracic artery. There is extensive anastomosis between these two arterial systems, and across the midline; this overlap of arterial supply is associated with variation in response to intra-arterial administration of oxytocin and with sub-optimal sensitivity. For this reason, and because the rabbit seems especially sensitive to interfering substances in plasma, the method has been superseded.

a) *The Guinea-Pig Preparation*

TINDAL and YOKOYAMA (1962) greatly improved the method by extending it to the guinea-pig which has only a single pair of mammary glands each with a discrete arterial supply, and their method is currently that with which other milk-ejection assays should be compared. It is accordingly given in detail, including modifications described by WALMSLEY (1963) and KNAGGS (1966).

For maximum sensitivity the guinea-pig should be primiparous and used for assay between the 2nd and 5th day of lactation, preferably on the 3rd or 4th day (not counting the day of parturition). A dietary supplement of 50 mg ascorbic acid each day after parturition is recommended albeit somewhat empirically. All pups are removed overnight to allow the glands to engorge with milk so that during the milk-ejection process and recovery, the system approaches an isometric condition which is further emphasised by strapping the external surface of the glands with heavy "Elastoplast".

The guinea-pig has only a single large teat duct so that cannulation of the teat is very much easier than in the rabbit which has numerous fine teat ducts. This means that wider bore cannulae may be used with consequent advantage in minimising manipulation of the gland and also in the efficiency of the transmission of pressure to recorders. Provided that the sphincter at the tip of the teat is cut off, a blunted hypodermic needle of 1.5 mm outside diameter may be introduced: it should be advanced gently to the base of the teat, where slight resistance may be felt before the tip of the cannula enters the small teat sinus. Ligature of the cannula in this position is facilitated if the cannula is provided with an annular groove or very fine ridge (of "Araldite" or similar resin). At this stage milk should ooze from the cannula especially if the gland is pressed gently. Connection is then made, via an air-free fluid-filled system, to transducers sensitive to pressure changes over the range 0—5 cm mercury, and the electrical transducer signal appropriately amplified and recorded.

It is important that the teat cannula should be supported firmly, in such a way that its height above the guinea-pig may be adjusted to give slight stretch to the teat: this minimises the risk of intermittent occlusion of the terminal aperture of the cannula by abutting against mammary tissue. A rack and pinion support is very convenient. Throughout the procedure the mammary gland should be handled with great delicacy since it is both responsive to mechanical stimulation and easily damaged (GROSVENOR, 1965).

If mammary engorgement is insufficient, or if too much milk is lost during the cannulation procedure, it is conventional to allow about 1 ml of an isotonic fluid such as saline or citrate to flow in by gravity. Fluid should not be forced in from syringes since this leads to alveolar rupture. The use of saline or citrate solutions has however been strongly criticised by GROSVENOR (1966) who recommends milk, serum or large molecular plasma-substitutes for this purpose (see below, under milk-ejection assay in the rat).

The myoepithelial response to oxytocin is seen as a rise of pressure of a few centimetres of water, the magnitude depending upon the dose (see Fig. 7). Initial hypersensitivity may be seen, capable of detecting 1 μU oxytocin i.a. but this usually disappears after 3 or 4 doses and thereafter the sensitivity remains constant for several

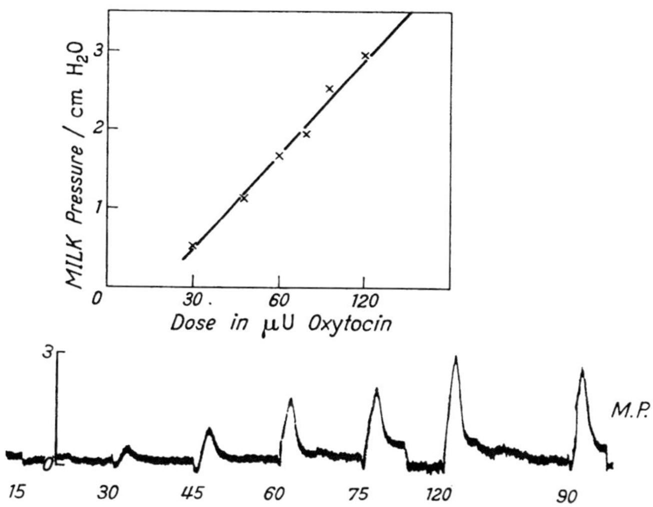

Fig. 7. Intra-mammary pressure responses in the guinea-pig, to close intra-arterial injection of synthetic oxytocin are shown as pressure recordings (below) and are plotted as a log dose-response curve (above). The relationship is satisfactorily linear for assay purposes. All doses are in microunits

hours provided the general condition of the animal is maintained. The latency of response is about 15 sec after i.v. injection but less than 5 sec after i.a. administration. Recovery usually has occurred within 1 min of injection and successive doses of pure solutions of oxytocin may be given every 2 or 3 min. Assays are conducted in a 2 and 2 pattern and with four groups each of four observations the percentage error of estimate is about 3% for intravenous assays ($P = 0.05$) TINDAL and YOKOYAMA (1962). The sensitivity of the intravenous assay is such that assays may be conducted with standard doses of 100—300 μU oxytocin, occasionally less (TINDAL and YOKOYAMA, 1962; WALMSLEY, 1963; KNAGGS, 1966). As with all intravenous assays the sensitivity can be increased by giving the oxytocin very rapidly so that the blood volume into which the dose is diluted during initial circulation, is minimised. Care must be taken, however, that deep anaesthesia is maintained since in moderate anaesthesia the rapid i.v. injection of saline may give spurious positive responses due presumably to stretch reflexes from the large veins. The intravenous method is most useful for many routine assays which do not require maximum sensitivity. It has the great advantage of requiring relatively little dissection time and little experience.

The maximum sensitivity is obtained with intra-arterial administration and assays may be conducted with doses of 15—60 μU: with a volume of injection of about 0.3 ml this corresponds to solutions for assay of approximately 50—200 μU/ml (see Table 7 which also gives estimates of reliability).

Table 7. *Assays of oxytocin on the mammary gland in vivo*

Species and route	Threshold dose (μU)	Lowest assay dose (μU)	Lowest assay concentration (μU/ml)	Index of precision λ	Error of estimate %	Fiducial limits P = 0.05	Ref.
Intra-arterial							
Rat	1—5	5—30	15—60	0.07	5.5	—	1
Rat	12.5	25	100	—	—	—	2
Mice	—	<70	—	—	—	—	2
Guinea-pig	1—10	15—60	50—200	0.08	3.7	±20%*	3
Guinea-pig	1—5	15—60	50—200	0.08	9.7	±26%	4
Guinea-pig	2—5	10—60	25—200	0.04—0.12	5.8*	±24%*	5
Rabbit	50	150	500	—	—	—	6
Intravenous							
Mouse	50	50—400	500	—	—	—	7
Rat	50	50—100	150—300	—	—	—	8
Rat	50	50—100	150—300	—	—	—	1
Rat	—	100	300	—	—	—	9
Rat	200	—	800	—	—	—	10
Guinea-pig	50	300	900	0.05	3%	—	3
Guinea-pig	50—100	100—600	300—2000	0.24—0.84	—	—	11
Guinea-pig	150	300	900	—	—	—	4
Rabbit	500	1000	2000	—	—	—	12
Man	—	10000	—	—	—	—	13
Man	250	1000	—	—	—	—	14
Man	1000	—	—	—	—	—	15

References: 1: Bisset (1966); 2: Vorherr et al. (1966, 1967); 3: Tindal and Yokoyama (1962); 4: Walmsley (1963); 5: Knaggs (1966); 6: Fitzpatrick (1961); 7: Vorherr (1965); 8: Grosvenor (1965); 9: Smelik (1966); 10: Vorherr et al. (1967); 11: Knaggs (1966); 12: Turner and Cooper (1941); 13: Beller et al. (1958); 14: Sica-Blanco et al. (1959); 15: Friedman (1960).

* Estimated from published figures.

For both the intravenous and intra-arterial methods of administration the reliability of the estimate is adversely affected by deterioration of the animal from any cause. In particular the presence of biologically active substances in the extracts of blood or other fluid causes rapid decline in sensitivity. This may be due to non-specific substances such as proteins or to more specific agents such as adrenaline, histamine and 5-hydroxytryptamine. Other substances may interfere by eliciting contractions of the myoepithelium. Some of these substances are shown in Table 8. Administration of antagonists such as dibenylene (1 mg), lysergic acid diethylamide (50 μg), mepyramine (10 μg) (Walmsley, 1963), in addition to atropine (1 mg), abolishes the effect of many of these substances but does not prevent "non-specific" deterioration nor the stimulant action of agents such as Substance P. Antagonists should be used with care and for specific investigations. Over enthusiastic or routine use of these potent drugs reduces the animals ability to maintain homeostasis and this is ultimately seen as a decrease in sensitivity and stability of the preparation.

Depth of anaesthesia is very critical. Freshly dissolved pentobarbitone sodium B.P. (free of preservatives) is given intraperitoneally at 50 mg/kg and thereafter supplemented as necessary with the same drug given intravenously, until spontaneous respiration just ceases. Respiration is subsequently maintained with a pump. Deeper anaesthesia than this is associated with loss of mammary gland sensitivity to oxytocin; lighter anaesthesia leads to erratic responses and to hypersensitivity of the gland, both to oxytocin and to other stimuli. In light anaesthesia the injection of saline either intra-arterially or intravenously if rapid enough, may elicit milk-ejection possibly by stimulating afferent pathways in the blood vessels which effect the release of endogenous oxytocin.

The effect of depth of anaesthesia on sensitivity is probably in part a reflection of changes in the tone of the mammary capillaries or of the pO_2 and pCO_2 in the mammary tissue which are critically related to optimal myoepithelial contraction (CROSS, 1955; LINZELL, 1955; CROSS and SILVER, 1961; HALPERN, BINAGHI, MAYER and BUGNARD, 1959). The oxygenation of the animal is very important and careful observation is necessary to avoid any cyanosis or any activation of the sympathetic nervous system. To avoid heat loss and fall of body temperature, which could lead to general vasoconstriction, including mammary vasoconstriction, it is essential to maintain the rectal temperature between 37—40° C, preferably with a thermostatically controlled operating table, supplemented if necessary by radiant heat over the mammary glands.

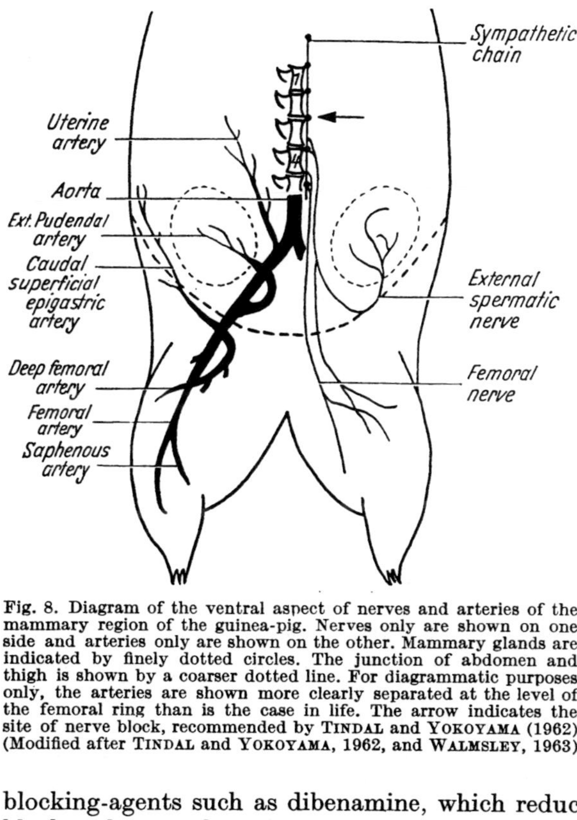

Fig. 8. Diagram of the ventral aspect of nerves and arteries of the mammary region of the guinea-pig. Nerves only are shown on one side and arteries only are shown on the other. Mammary glands are indicated by finely dotted circles. The junction of abdomen and thigh is shown by a coarser dotted line. For diagrammatic purposes only, the arteries are shown more clearly separated at the level of the femoral ring than is the case in life. The arrow indicates the site of nerve block, recommended by TINDAL and YOKOYAMA (1962) (Modified after TINDAL and YOKOYAMA, 1962, and WALMSLEY, 1963)

Since vasoconstriction is so important TINDAL (1960) and KNAGGS (1966) block sympathetic outflow by inducing paravertebral anaesthesia with the bilateral injection, of up to 2 ml 0.2% w/v nupercaine hydrochloride, between lumber spinal processes L_2 and L_3. This procedure is superior to the use of adrenergic alpha blocking-agents such as dibenamine, which reduces sensitivity. The use of beta-blockers has not been investigated in the guinea-pig (but see below for rat). All animals should be atropinised.

Arterial cannulation is effected, centripetally into either of the main arteries on the medial aspect of the thigh (the femoral or internal saphenous arteries). All other branches of the femoral arterial system, especially the deep femoral and caudal superficial epigastric, are identified and ligatured to limit the area of distribution of injected oxytocin, but no dissection should be undertaken within the abdominal cavity or of the inguinal abdominal wall. This is because the external pudendal artery, which supplies the mammary gland, arises from the external iliac artery as the latter passes through the femoral ring, and thereafter passes to the mammary gland, initially lying on the visceral aspect of the abdominal wall (see

Fig. 8). During the dissection, the artery selected for cannulation, must be freed from its accompanying nerve and vein and from connective tissue: it usually passes into spasm which renders cannulation impossible. This spasm is effectively relieved, immediately prior to cannulation, by soaking the area in a 1% solution of papaverine hydrochloride (TINDAL, 1960). During dissection of the femoral nerve, WALMSLEY floods the area with local anaesthetic to minimise reflexes causing mammary vasoconstriction. To facilitate intra-arterial injections and minimise the risk of injection of air bubbles into the mammary arterial system, it is recommended that the arterial cannula be connected to a three-way perspex tap of small dead space, such as that described by SIDDIQI and WALKER (1960).

As with all assays based on close arterial injection, the response may be affected by variation in dose (in units), in volume of administration, in concentration, and in speed of injection. With this particular assay the injected material will pass into the arterial pool in the iliac arteries and terminal aorta. If the volume of injection is large or the speed of injection excessive the response of the mammary gland will be less than expected, since a significant proportion of the injected dose will be lost down arteries to pelvic organs and to the contralateral iliac arterial system (as evidenced by weak responses of the contralateral mammary gland).

The volume of injected fluid (which preferably should be prewarmed to body temperature) should be between 0.2—0.4 ml and should not exceed 0.4 ml. The injection should not take longer than 4 sec, nor should it be given very rapidly (in less than 2 sec). A speed of 0.1 ml/sec is suitable (KNAGGS, 1966). Variation in total dose of oxytocin may be achieved by varying the volume of a constant concentration or by variation of concentration with volume of injection constant. Both methods have been successfully used (WALMSLEY, 1963, and KNAGGS, 1966), with similar precision, although the variation in volume with constant concentration is obviously the more convenient when solutions of unknown potency are being assayed.

b) *Milk-Ejection in the Rat*

Cannulation of the main teat duct in the rat is no more difficult than cannulation of one of the multiple teats ducts in the rabbit. Because of its small body size the rat offers advantages of sensitivity over most other laboratory animals, at least for assays involving intravenous injection. Moreover, it is very much easier and cheaper to maintain a regular supply of standard lactating females using rats rather than guinea-pigs. It is probable that milk-ejection assays in the rat will increase in popularity.

GROSVENOR has given a brief account of appropriate techniques (GROSVENOR, 1965; DE NUCCIO and GROSVENOR, 1967). Rats on or about the 4th day of lactation are used, under ether anaesthesia after atropine premedication (0.65 mg). The nipple tip of an abdominal mammary gland is removed and the duct cannulated with a fine stainless steel cannula connected to a pressure transducer by polyethylene tubing, filled with warm fat-free rat milk. The entire system, except the transducer, is filled with milk before insertion of the cannula into the nipple. After firmly tying the cannula in place, more milk is introduced into the system (0.15—0.7 ml) to fill the ducts and increase the pressure to 1 or 2 cm water above atmospheric. If rat milk (or rat serum, or cow milk) is used as fluid replacement, there is no subsequent fall in pressure as is seen when isotonic saline or citrate solutions are used, presumably because inorganic salts are not retained within the gland but the milk or serum proteins are. The basic intramammary pressure remains remarkably stable, which is of considerable advantage for assays. Moreover the leakage of milk from the distended gland into the surrounding connective tissue, which is presumably a reflection of a minor degree of damage and which is seen frequently in the guinea-pig (TINDAL and YOKOYAMA, 1962; KNAGGS, 1966) is not seen in the rat if milk is used to "top up" the fluid system (GROSVENOR, 1966).

The preparation is fairly stable for 1—2 hours under ether anaesthesia, but BISSET (1966) uses nembutal anaesthesia (35 mg/kg) with no loss of stability or sensitivity and most investigators would prefer this since ether is known to liberate endogenous neurohypophysial hormones (GINSBURG and HELLER, 1952; AMES and VAN DYKE, 1952; CHAUDHURY and WALKER, 1958). Depth of anaesthesia is critical in all oxytocin assays *in vivo* but it appears at present that this is less critical in the rat than in either the guinea-pig or rabbit. In general the preparation seems more robust and less fastidious than the guinea-pig. Sensitivity is good. According to DE NUCCIO and GROSVENOR (1967), SMELIK (1966) and BISSET (1966), 50—100 μU i.v. gives measurable responses; BISSET quotes a working range for assays of 100 to 300 μU i.v. When assays are based on intravenous injection the rat offers a minor technical advantage in that the jugular vein is much more easily dissected and cannulated than in the guinea-pig. This compensates for the greater difficulty of teat cannulation in the rat.

Intra-Arterial Injection in the Rat

BISSET (1966) has extended the principle of retrograde arterial injection to milk-ejection assay in the rat, with a gain in sensitivity of 15-fold as compared with intravenous assay. According to this worker the dissection of the area of the femoral artery is easier than in the guinea-pig and more like that in the rabbit: the appropriate artery to the posterior mammary glands arises from the femoral artery some distance (1 cm) distal to the femoral ring and then undulates in the superficial tissues to the mammary glands so that inspection is relatively easy: the major side branches of the femoral artery including the deep femoral are easily located and tied off. Papaverine solution is necessary to relax the artery immediately prior to cannulation. The technique of retrograde arterial injection is critical however, since the volume of the arterial tree is so small; BISSET recommends a consistent volume of 0.2 ml given at constant speed and pressure (ideally with an automatic device).

Responses appear in a few seconds as single peaks and last to 15—45 sec. The working range of doses for assay is 5—20 μU oxytocin. This is of the same high order of sensitivity as that reported by the Shinfield workers for the intra-arterial administration of oxytocin to the guinea-pig but it is achieved with less dependence on fastidious attention to certain details of technique, a feature of importance to some programmes of work. The index of precision is satisfactory at about 0.05.

The method is reasonably specific although milk-ejection responses are also given by intra-arterial administration of acetylcholine (0.01 μg), 5-hydroxytryptamine (0.1 μg), histamine (20 μg), angiotensin (10 μg) and bradykinin (0.1 μg). None of these are likely to complicate estimations of oxytocin in biological fluids, except possibly bradykinin. Adrenaline and nor-adrenaline interfere with subsequent mammary responses to oxytocin but this effect can be abolished by beta-adrenergic blocking agents (not alpha blockers surprisingly). In any case, if the blood pressure of the animal is monitored continuously it is easy to detect the presence of most biologically active substances by their effect on blood pressure, since oxytocin in concentrations likely to be present is without effect (BISSET, 1966). Other details of this assay are given in the Chapter by BISSET.

c) *Human Mammary Gland*

It is a relatively simple procedure to cannulate one of the numerous teat ducts of the nipple of a multiparous lactating woman and to record the milk-ejection pressure (SICA-BLANCO, MENDEZ-BAUER, SALA, CABOT, and CALDEYRO-BARCIA, 1959; FRIEDMAN, 1960; WIEDERMAN and STONE, 1962). Allowing for the difference in body weight the human myoepithelium is apparently more sensitive than that of the guinea-pig or rabbit; even so the minimum effective dose is of 250—500 μU given by rapid intravenous injection and doses of one or more milliunits are necessary for assays (BELLER, KRUMHOLZ, and ZEININGER, 1958; SICA-BLANCO et al., 1959). Although such assays have been conducted in lactating women conveniently and with precision (ALTHABE, ARNT, BRANDA, and CALDEYRO-BARCIA, 1966) they are too insensitive and too complicated by ethical considerations for the method to be used for other than clinical investigations such as the comparisons of different homologues and the effects of circulating oxytocinase (ALTHABE et al., 1966). It is possible to estimate the endogenous oxytocin in the circulation of women using this method: the milk-ejection responses of one mammary gland may be used to detect an oxytocin release when the other gland is suckled or during second stage labour, etc. and these responses may be matched with exogenous doses of oxytocin given intravenously. This is a crude form of assay but is superior to monitoring the uterus for this purpose because the mammary gland unlike the uterus, shows no spontaneous contractions, and moreover it is more sensitive.

4. Sucking Response

An interesting and sensitive technique has recently been described by VORHERR and colleagues (VORHERR, 1965; VORHERR, KLEEMAN, and GARIGAN, 1966; VORHERR, KLEEMAN, and LEHMAN, 1967) based upon the postural reaction of young mice or rats when the mother's milk is made available to them within the mammary gland by oxytocin injected into the mother. Lactating rats or mice (4th to 12th day post partum) are anaesthetised with 12% ethanol given orally (50 ml/kg) to supress endogenous release of oxytocin and vasopressin. At least half of each litter is removed overnight to ensure the presence of milk in the glands. At the beginning of each observation up to four of the young are allowed access to the mother and initially they lie quietly in a normal sucking posture. When oxytocin is injected a typical change in posture is seen within a well defined latent period. The young raise themselves on their hind legs and push against the mother with their forelegs until the nipple is stretched or is even dislodged from their mouths. This is presumably a response to a sudden increase in available milk. The smallest dose eliciting this effect in mice is about 130 μU, and in rats 200 μU, for intravenous administration (tail vein). If oxytocin is given by retrograde injection into the carotid artery (for the anterior glands) responses are seen with doses of 70 μU (mice) or 135 μU (rats) and this is reduced to 30 μU or less with retrograde injection into the femoral artery of *rats*. The recommended injection volume is 0.25 ml in the rat (but only 0.1 for mice), corresponding to a minimum concentration of 120 μU/ml in the solution for assay, so that this method is sufficiently sensitive to be considered for the determination of oxytocin in blood, at least when a relatively high concentration is expected as in second stage labour or after stimulation of the hypothalamic nuclei. This could be a useful confirmatory method for checking results found in other assays since the specificity is apparently good. Responses are elicited by oxytocin, vasopressin and by "unphysiologically high" concentrations of acetylcholine or of bradykinin but not by angiotensin, histamine, 5-hydroxytryptamine or adrenaline. No response was seen when venous plasma of non-pregnant women was administered although responses were seen when oxytocin was added to such plasma (100—200 μU/ml).

The limitation of the technique is that it is based on an all-or-none response. The same mother rat is offered to groups of only 4 pups at a time for each observation, so that repeat observations may be made at 10 min intervals until all teats have been sucked and depleted of milk. An initial dose of 25 μU i.a. is given and, depending on whether or not a response is seen in at least one pup, the next dose is halved (12.5 μU) or doubled (50 μU) and so on in geometric progression until the threshold is established.

The response can be expressed quantitatively in terms of the latency in seconds before the effect is seen, but although initial results indicate that the latency is inversely proportional to dose, there is inadequate differentiation between doses for this to form the basis of an assay. Clearly, even with replication using several

Table 8. *Specificity of mammary gland assays*

Species	Vasopressin	Acetylcholine	Histamine	5 HT.	Substance P	Angiotensin	Bradykinin	Plasmakinin	Pepsitensin	Anephrotensin	KCl	Whole blood	Whole plasma	References
In vitro mammary preparations														
Rabbit	.	+	0	0	.	.	.	.	.	.	.	0	.	1
Rabbit	.	.	.	.	.	.	.	.	.	.	.	0	0	2
Rat	.	+	+	+	.	.	.	.	.	.	.	.	.	3
Rat	.	.	.	.	.	0	0	.	.	.	.	.	.	4
In vivo mammary preparations														
topical application														
Mouse	+	+	+	+	.	.	.	.	.	.	.	.	.	5
suckling response														
Rat	+	+	.	0	.	0	0	.	.	.	.	.	0	6
i. v.		.02		300		5	5							
Rat	+	+	.	0	.	0	0	.	.	.	.	.	0	6
i. a.		.05		125		5	5							
milk-ejection														
Rabbit	.	.	.	.	.	0	0	.	.	.	.	.	.	7
i. v.														
G. pig	+	+	.	.	(+)	0	0	.	.	.	.	.	.	8
i. v.		5			1	25	10							
G. pig	+	+	+	+	.	.	.	.	0	0	.	0	0	9
i. v.			50	30										
Rat	.	+	0	+	.	+	+	.	.	.	.	.	.	10
i. a.		.01	20	0.1		10	0.1							
G. pig	+	.	.	.	+	0	0	0	0	0	0	0	0	9
i. a.					.005	2.5	0.1				40mEq			
G. pig	+	+	+	+	.	±	+	.	.	.	.	.	0	11
i. a.		.02	50	25		2	1							
isolated uterus														
Rat	+	+	(+)	+	+	+	+	+	+	+	+	+	+	
blood pressure														
i. v.	(+)	$\otimes$	$\otimes$	+	$\otimes$	+	$\otimes$	$\otimes$	+	($\otimes$)	$\otimes$	$\otimes$	$\otimes$	

Doses are given in micrograms

References: 1: MOORE and ZARROW (1965); 2: MENDEZ-BAUER et al. (1960); 3: RYDÉN and SJÖHOLM (1962); 4: BROVETTO et al. (1967); 5: LINZELL (1955); 6: VORHERR et al. (1967); 7: BERDE and CERLETTI (1961); 8: BISSET and LEWIS (1962); 9: WALMSLEY (1963); 10: BISSET (1966); 11: KNAGGS (1966).

+ = denotes milk-ejection, contraction, or hypertension.
$\otimes$ = denotes hypotension.
0 = denotes no milk-ejection with doses up to those listed of pure substances.

rats simultaneously, for a quantal assay the precision of this suckling method will be low in comparison with many of the assays described above.

5. *Specificity of Mammary Responses*

It was stated earlier that the mammary gland is more specific for oxytocin than is the uterus. This is well illustrated by Table 8 which lists the response of the mammary gland to a large number of active substances which may contaminate blood, urine and other biological fluids. It is important to note that *all* the substances listed will contract the isolated rat uterus. All authors are agreed that vasopressin produces milk-ejection in its own right and where it is important to differentiate between the neurohypophysial hormones this must be done by chemical or physical means.

Acetylcholine, 5-hydroxytryptamine and histamine also elicit milk-ejection, at least in some preparations, but only with concentrations unlikely to occur in body fluids or extracts, although this may not be true for all intra-arterial assays. These substances produce obvious blood pressure responses however, and moreover their effects may be competitively antagonised.

Of the polypeptides investigated, three, plasmakinin, pepsitensin and anephrotensin, which might be formed during extraction procedures, are apparently without effect on milk-ejection, at least in doses at least 10 times those which produce changes in systemic blood pressure in the laboratory animal under investigation. Angiotensin was found ineffective with some authors (apart from an after inhibition of the mammary gland) but two groups have reported milk-ejection following high doses (2 and 10 μg) given by the sensitive intra-arterial route. This is at least 20 times as great as the dose producing substantial hypertension after intravenous injection in the rabbit (BISSET and LEWIS, 1962), so that the presence of angiotension in quantities sufficient to cause milk-ejection would be revealed by coincident monitoring of the blood pressure: such concentrations are unlikely to occur in body fluids.

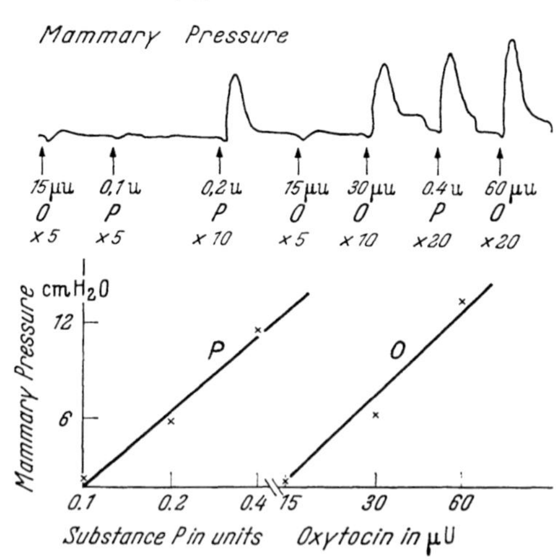

Fig. 9. *Above:* Intra-mammary pressure responses to intra-arterial administration of oxytocin (O) in micro units and substance P (P) in units. The Figs. x 5, x 10, x 20, refer to the attenuation of the recording galvanometer system. *Below:* Log dose-response relationship for oxytocin and substance P. There is no significant deviation from parallelism between the two curves

Substance P was found to cause milk-ejection by all investigators who studied this substance, in some cases in extremely small doses (5 ng). Although at this low dose, which is *less* than that necessary to produce hypotension, the milk-ejection effect is variable and confused with after inhibition. With higher doses not only is the effect consistent but the dose response curve for Substance P may parallel that to oxytocin (Fig. 9). This is of considerable importance since parallelism of dose response curves for standard and unknown solutions is usually considered good evidence of the identity of unknown with standard. Substance P is unlikely to be present in body fluids (as opposed to tissue extracts) but even so careful monitoring of blood pressure is necessary and chemical separation (for instance by chromatography) should be relied upon. Bradykinin is another polypeptide of importance as a potential contaminant. It is reported to produce responses only after intra-arterial administration of doses of 100 ng or more, but this amount must be considered as possible in blood extractions. Doses of this order would probably, but not invariably, produce obvious hypotension in the animal used for the assay but as with Substance P there is no effective antagonist and the chemical extraction procedure should be designed to separate any bradykinin from the oxytocin containing fraction.

It is worth reporting that histamine, angiotensin, 5-hydroxytryptamine and adrenaline, all produce decreased sensitivity to oxytocin, as do blood and blood plasma, and this effect may well limit the precision of assays if these substances persist through the extraction procedure.

II. Assay of Antidiuretic Hormones in Vertebrates

The measurement of neurohypophysial hormones in blood and urine is attended by special problems in that they are present in such small quantities as to be not detectable (unless extracted and concentrated) by more reliable assay procedures like that utilising the vasopressor effects of ADH in the rat (LANDGREBE, MACAULEY, and WARING, 1946; DEKANSKI, 1952). This latter assay procedure has been used to measure ADH in blood (200 ml) but only after concentration by the ion exchange chromatography method of WEINSTEIN, BERNE, and SACHS (1960) (see later). However even if concentration is performed the antidiuretic response (for instance in the rat) affords advantages since far smaller amounts of blood are needed to obtain amounts of hormone adequate for assay. Thus SHARE (1961) commences his extraction procedures with 10 ml blood and uses the antidiuretic response of the rat for assay of the ADH.

Mammalian Preparations

1. Antidiuresis in the Rat Detailed Account

The antidiuretic response of the rat to ADH can be used for estimation of neurohypophysial hormones which may or may not be extracted from the body fluids prior to their assay. Rather special techniques and precautions are necessary in order to be able to do this successfully especially if the ADH is not concentrated but injected directly as blood or urine. The assay procedure and its variations will be described in detail therefore.

Early attempts to measure the ADH in blood used the assay procedure of BURN (1931). Groups of rats were hydrated (5% of their body weight by gavage) and each group injected subcutaneously (s.c.) with standard and unknown quantities of ADH. The delay in the time to excrete 50% of the water load was taken as an index for calculations of the potency of the unknown. The sensitivity of this procedure was, however, only about 5 mU of ADH per rat. Increasing the hydration of the rats increases the sensitivity to ADH. KRIEGER and KILVINGTON (1940) and BIRNIE, JENKINS, EVERSOLE, and GAUNT (1949), for instance, hydrated their animals to about 12% of their body weight resulting in animals 5 or 6 times as sensitive as those used in the Burn assay.

The subcutaneous injection of preparations of vasopressin into rats may, however, lead to results which are qualitatively and quantitatively erroneous. NOBLE, RINDERKNECHT, and WILLIAMS (1939) noted that various extracts of body fluids may contain "augmentor" materials which delay the absorption of hormones from the site of injection and result in a falsely high estimate of the amount of hormone present. Such disparities led some workers to develop extraction procedures (see later) to remove such "augmentor" materials. Such augmentation, apparently, is not as likely to occur if in addition the extract is injected intraperitoneally (Noble, Plunkett, and Taylor, 1950). Birnie et al. (1949) used the intraperitoneal site of injection for unextracted materials (see also Lloyd and Lobotsky, 1950; Croxatto, Andrade, and Barnàfi, 1952; Stein, Jink, and Mirsky, 1952, and Crawford and Pinkham, 1954). However, as Noble et al. (1950) pointed out, i.p. injection of toxic materials present in extracts may give rise to great distress in the animal and this may lead to antidiuresis either directly or indirectly as a result of a release of endogenous hormones. Leaf and Mamby (1952) may have avoided the latter by using neurohypophysectomized rats but found the assay cumbersome. Ames and van Dyke (1952) compared the activities of various preparations of ADH by i.p. and intravenous injections and found that there may be a potentiation in activity as great as 25 times if the i.p. route of injection is used. Many of the reports of enormous concentrations of ADH in the blood (20—500 μU/ml compared with more acceptable figures of 1—100 μU/ml) when an i.p. assay procedure is used are discussed fully by van Dyke, Adamsons, and Engel (1955) who consider them erroneous and mainly the result of failure to use i.v. routes for administration of the hormone preparations. These conclusions are concurred with by Heller (1957), Sawyer (1961a), Walker (1961), Lauson (1960) and others.

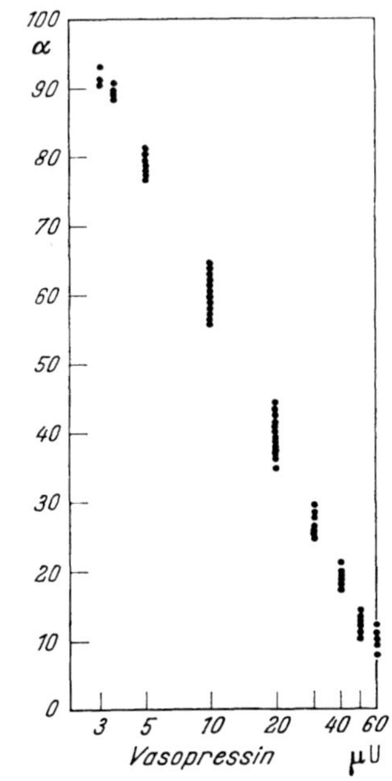

Fig. 10. Log dose-response regression line giving values for a (= antidiuretic effect). $a = \frac{b}{a} \times 100$ where number of drops (or increments of 0.1 ml) of urine excreted in the 10 min lasting from the 8th min before injection to 3rd min after injection is (a), and in the 10 min lasting from the 3rd to the 13th min after injection is (b). After 65 injections in 20 rats. Ordinate: values for a. Abscissa: log doses of vasopressin (μU/100 g). Note that there was no differential effect between 3 and 3.5 μU/100 g and between 50 and 60 μU/100 g (Dicker, 1953)

It is clear that reliable assays of ADH in blood and urine must be made using an i.v. method of administration of the hormone. A variety of animals (dogs, rabbits, man etc.) have been used but owing principally to their relatively large size, as compared with the rat, larger amounts of hormone are required. Thus, for the assay of small quantities of ADH, intravenous injection into rats or even smaller animals is theoretically desirable. Krieger and Kilvington (1940) modified the Burn rat assay and injected extracts into the tail vein. They continued to use rats in groups so that relatively large amounts of material were still required, though the objections to results based on s.c. and i.p. methods of assay would not apply to their work as it did to most of their contemporaries. Ginsburg and Heller (1953a) prepared rats for intravenous injection by inserting a cannula into the jugular vein on the day before the assay. They were thus able to give successive i.v. injections into the rats, which were hydrated with 3 doses of tap water each of 5% of body weight and were individually sensitive to 50 μU of ADH.

In 1942 Jeffers, Livezey, and Austin described a procedure to assay vasopressin in rats anaesthetized with ethanol (5% body weight 12% ethanol v/v). Ethanol depresses the release of endogenous ADH (Eggleton, 1942; van Dyke and Ames, 1951; Dicker, 1953) and thus one may hope (but see Ginsburg and Brown, 1956; Tata and Buzalkov, 1966) for an animal which is pharmacologically neurohypophysectomized and without the endogenous ADH which produces a less sensitive and less predictable preparation. This ethanol anaesthetised rat preparation of JEFFERS et al. (1942) was sensitive to 20 μU of ADH and was disinterred 10 years later by AMES and VAN DYKE (1952) who confirmed this sensitivity. DICKER (1953) modified the procedure and maintained the rat at a constant

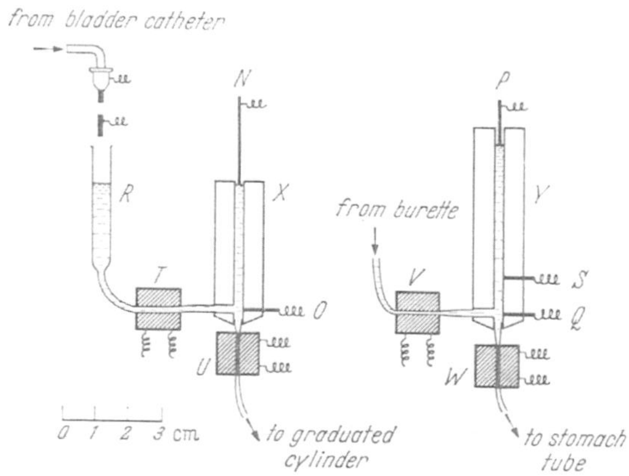

Fig. 11. Urine outflow (X) and water inflow (Y) meters. Drops falling from the needle accumulate in reservoir R. As converted telephone relay T is opened, water flows freely from R into Perspex tube X, until the meniscus makes contact with electrode N. T, U, V and W: converted telephone relays. N, O, P, S and Q: platinum electrodes. The height of both electrodes N and P can be varied. The volume of 'urine' (see text) is 'metered' between N and O; that of water, between P and S (BOURA and DICKER, 1953)

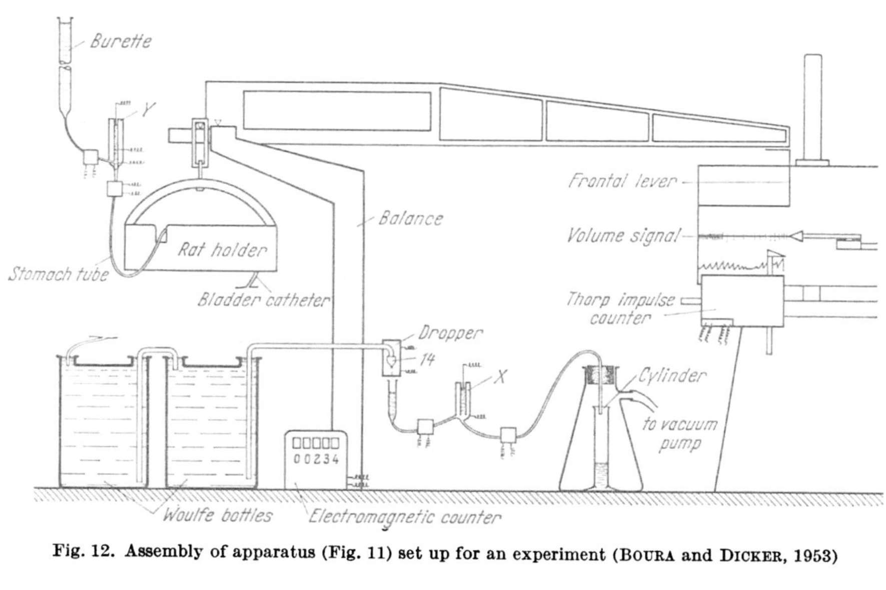

Fig. 12. Assembly of apparatus (Fig. 11) set up for an experiment (BOURA and DICKER, 1953)

level of hydration (equivalent to 8% of the body weight) so that it maintained a higher sensitivity for a longer period of time, reacting to 5—10 μU of ADH. The dose response relationship is illustrated in Fig. 10. BOURA and DICKER (1953) described an arrangement whereby the water load was maintained automatically and the urine flow recorded continuously by a drop recorder (see also DETTELBACH, 1958; ALBERS and BRIGHTMAN, 1959; DE WIED, 1960; SAWYER, 1961a; BERDE and CERLETTI, 1961; BISSET, 1962; DYBALL, LANE, and MORRIS, 1966). The arrangment used by BOURA and DICKER is shown in Fig. 11 and 12. Such modification of the procedure of JEFFERS et al. (1942) has been used widely with even further modifications in detailed technique which will be described later. Some of these changes result in preparations sensitive to even less than 1 μU of ADH (J. HELLER and STŮLC, 1959; CZACZKES, KLEEMAN, and KOENIG, 1964; MORAN, MILTENBERGER, SHUAYB and ZIMMERMAN, 1964, and TATA and GAUER, 1966) or in one instance to less than 0.1 μU (KRAMAR, GRINNELL, and DUFF, 1966). Endogenous antidiuretic hormone can be estimated by direct injection of the plasma or urine in which it is present or after isolation and concentration of the hormone (see later sections on blood and urine).

While the ethanol anaesthetised rat provides the most sensitive preparation for the assay of ADH even in the most experienced hands it is considered a capricious preparation and a 75% rate of success must be considered reasonable. In addition the sensitivity seems to vary somewhat between laboratories often for reasons not readily understood (see, for instance, J. HELLER and STŮLC, 1959, and JONES and LEE, 1965).

2. *Variations of Rat Antidiuresis Method*

A more detailed description of some of the differences in technique may help the reader to decide which assay is most suitable to his needs and also assist in "trouble shooting" problems with rats.

Size and Sex. In the original description of the assay JEFFERS et al. (1942) used female rats weighing about 200 g. Subsequently AMES and VAN DYKE (1952) used male animals while DICKER (1953) used females, in each case at about the same weight. It is not always clear why a certain sex is preferred. DETTELBACH (1958), who used females, found it necessary to ovariectomize them in order to overcome changes in sensitivity associated with the oestrous cycle. Other investigators who have used male rats include EISEN and LEWIS (1954), SHARE (1961), CZACZKES et al. (1964) and MORAN et al. (1964), while females were used by THORN (1957), BARATZ and INGRAHAM (1959), DE WIED (1960) and also by CZACZKES et al. (1964). J. HELLER and STŮLC (1959) appeared to have no preference and used either sex. One suspects that the choice is mostly associated with availability and the personal prejudice of the investigator, though DETTELBACH (1958), DE WIED (1960) and TATA and GAUER (1966) used females because their catheterization procedure is only possible in this sex. The possibility that differences in sensitivity occur in rats of opposite sex may be worth consideration.

The choice of the size of the rats may be partly dictated by availability but there is some evidence to suggest that it may be more directly important. Very young rats do not respond to antidiuretic hormone as well as adults but it is unlikely that anyone would consider using rats so young (less than 4 weeks). Old rats are often in poorer condition than their younger relatives and are not tolerant to the experimental procedures. In addition, large rats, by reason of their greater age, may not be reliable as assay animals: DICKER and NUNN (1958) compared antidiuretic assays using old white rats (about 350 days old, 325—415 g) with assays using younger animals (about 100 days, 210—270 g) and found that the older animals were unreliable and gave inaccurate results. Rats within the range of 200 to 300 g have generally been preferred, though SHARE (1961) and MORAN et al. (1964) used animals weighing up to 400 g; CZACZKES et al. (1964) on the other hand (see also TATA and GAUER, 1966; KRAMAR et al., 1966) used small animals weighing only 100—120 g. These investigators developed an unusually sensitive assay for ADH (0.25 to 1 μU per animal) and it seems likely that the low body weight of their animals may be contributing to this.

Anaesthesia and Hydration. The production (and maintenance) of ethanol anaesthesia in rats is usually carried out simultaneously with hydration and follows a fairly uniform procedure, though small modifications have been introduced. JEFFERS et al. (1942) administered, by gavage, a quantity of 12% ethanol equivalent to 5% of the body weight (see also AMES and VAN DYKE, 1952). This was followed in 30 min by 3% of the body weight of warm tap water. DICKER (1953) reversed this procedure and initially hydrated the rats (by gavage) with 5% of their body weight of warm tap water, following this in 45 min with the same dose of 12% ethanol solution in warm tap water: the hydration of the rats was maintained at a level equivalent to 8% of the body weight by continuous administration of 2% ethanol in tap water through an indwelling gavage tube. This procedure has been used often (see, for instance, THORN, 1957; SHARE, 1961; YOSHIDA, MOTOHASHI, IBAYASHI, and OKINAKA, 1963). Variations include the administration of 12% ethanol in two doses, each equivalent to 3% of the body weight, followed by 2% body weight of water, all doses 30 min apart (J. HELLER and STŮLC, 1959; CZACZKES et al., 1964). Maintenance of anaesthesia can also be carried out by i.v. infusion of 3% ethanol (MORAN et al., 1964) or i.p. injection of 25% ethanol (ALBERS and BRIGHTMAN, 1959). Individual investigators usually find the procedure which suits them and their rats best, and it is not possible or desirable to recommend any particular method.

The only major modification in the anaesthesia is that described by SAWYER (1961a). Anaesthesia is induced by i.p. injection of Inactin (sodium ethyl-1-methyl-propyl-thiobarbitone) at a dose of 7—10 mg/100 g. The necessary cannulae are then inserted under local procaine anaesthesia, the animals given a dose of 1.5% ethanol in 0.05% sodium chloride solution equivalent to 8% of their body weight and maintained at a constant level of hydration with this solution. THORN, SMITH, and SKADHAUGE (1965) use a slight variation of this procedure.

Administration of fluid is by gavage, using soft rubber catheters pushed down the oesophagus into the stomachs of animals previously starved for 12—18 hours. This can best be done with the aid of a wooden "gag" or by holding the animal firmly by the nape of the neck so that the teeth gape apart sufficiently so as not to cut into the catheter. Proper performance of this procedure without unduly stressing the rat is quite critical to the subsequent performance of the animal and to the establishment of a reasonable rate of urine flow (greater than 80 μl/min). If the animal is excessively stressed by the initial handling, or if it regurgitates fluid into the lungs, urine flow sufficient for the assay measurements will not occur. Thus many (DETTELBACH, 1958; DE WIED, 1960; MORAN et al., 1964; THORN et al., 1965 and others) prefer to "condition the rats", by gavaging them at intervals during a period of approximately two weeks prior to the assay. Whether this results in conditioning the rats or the investigators is not clear but either way the results appear to be favourable.

DICKER (1953) maintained the water load of the animals by leaving a thin polyethylene stomach tube in position, and passing water through this. Such a procedure has been widely used but due possibly to the irritation caused by the tube, and the tendency to vomit, regurgitation does sometimes occur; this together with the depression of the reflex that prevents fluid entering the lungs, will usually result in termination of the assay. If such regurgitation into the lungs occurs frequently it is advisable to perform a tracheotomy as a routine procedure at the beginning of each assay (see SAWYER, 1961a; THORN et al., 1965).

Alternatively some investigators prefer to maintain the state of hydration by infusing a saline dextrose solution through the jugular or tail vein (EISEN and LEWIS, 1954; MORAN and MILTENBERGER, 1963; CZACZKES et al., 1964; TATA and GAUER, 1966) or giving dilute saline intrarectally (ALBERS and BRIGHTMAN, 1959).

Collection of Urine. JEFFERS et al. (1942) laparotomised the rat while under ethanol anaesthesia (an additional small amount of ether is also sometimes used) and tied a cannula into the urinary bladder through which urine could be collected. This procedure has been used by AMES and VAN DYKE (1952), DICKER (1953) and THORN (1957) who took precautions to keep the urinary dead space minimal by ligating the bladder. This results in changes in urine flow being transmitted more rapidly and is particularly important if the index for response is one associated with changes in urine concentration (see later). Alteration in composition will only be seen in the simultaneously formed urine and will not be transmitted as are changes in volume. DETTELBACH (1958), DE WIED (1960) and TATA and GAUER (1966) used volume of urine as their index of response and simply inserted a catheter through the urethra into the bladder. DE WIED found that the laparotomy procedure resulted in failure of many rats subsequently to form reasonable volumes of urine and for this reason avoided it. J. HELLER and STŮLC (1959) reduced the urinary dead space and also avoided the surgical stress of the laparotomy on the day of the assay by making chronic fistulae of the ureters four days previous to the assay. CZACZKES et al. (1964) and KRAMAR et al. (1966) also used this procedure but JONES and LEE (1965) could not demonstrate that it made any difference to the sensitivity of the assay. It would be interesting to know if it had any influence on the number of assay failures, which can be as high as 30% (DE WIED, 1960 and personal observations — P. B.).

Injection Procedures. The intravenous route for the administration of the hormone preparations must be used but there is some variation in preferred sites for injection and the volumes administered.

HELLER (1956) noted that the volume of the injection given to a rat could influence the antidiuretic response. JEFFERS et al. (1942) originally suggested a standard volume of 0.5 ml and many investigators have similarly standardised the volume (for instance THORN, 1957, 0.5 ml; SAWYER, 1958, 0.2 ml; J. HELLER and STŮLC, 1959 and CZACZKES et al., 1964, 1 ml; MORAN et al., 1964, 0.2 ml) while others have taken care never to exceed a certain volume. It is clear that the volume of the injection should be kept minimal probably 0.5 ml or less and preferably should be standardized.

The site of i.v. administration may also be important and may influence the volume and composition of solutions that may be administered without directly affecting the reliability and sensitivity of the assays. JEFFERS et al. (1942) used the femoral vein (also DETTELBACH, 1958; NIELSEN, 1958; MORAN et al., 1964) while DICKER (1953), THORN (1957), SAWYER (1958) and BARATZ and INGRAHAM (1959) used the jugular. Others such as J. HELLER and STŮLC (1959), DE WIED (1960) and CZACZKES et al. (1964) administered solutions through one of the tail veins. Cannulation of the tail vein is usually considered a more difficult procedure than cannulation of the femoral or jugular vein but although it may be more traumatic for the investigator it is probably less so for the rat, so that it could be advantageous. In addition, solutions injected in this manner may be expected to equilibrate more completely before they reach "vital centres" so that non-specific effects due to changes in volume and to contaminants present in the extracts may not be as troublesome. On the other hand the hormone itself will suffer greater dilution before reaching its effector site, the kidney, so that there may be a drop in sensitivity.

A preparation of the rat, highly sensitive to ADH, has been described by KRAMAR et al. (1966) and which diverges in technique from previous assays in that injections are given through the tail *artery*. Antidiuresis to the injection of as little as 5 mμU (10^{-9} IU) of synthetic arg^8-vasopressin could be demonstrated though when Pitressin was used about 0.1 μU was required. It is difficult to understand the differences in response of these two preparations for while Pitressin may contain lys^8-vasopressin as well as arg^8-vasopressin such mixtures could not account for the observed differences. Before any definite conclusions about the sensitivity to the synthetic hormone can be drawn these results should be confirmed and the biological activity of the standard preparations tested by an independent assay such as that using the pressor effects in the rat.

Tachyphylaxis to ADH has been observed by some investigators (for instance DICKER, 1953; THORN, 1957) but was overcome by spacing the injections 50—60 min apart. Usually this is not difficult as a period such as this is often required for the urine volume to return to reasonable levels. DETTELBACH (1958) and DE WIED (1960), however, noted that this tachyphylaxis was not seen if injections were given through the femoral or tail veins, and DETTELBACH gave injections at 15 min intervals. The choice of the site for injection obviously must be decided according to the experience and needs of the individual investigator but the evidence strongly suggests that injections can be given more frequently via the femoral or tail vein than into the jugular.

Index of Response. The primary effect of antidiuretic hormone in rats is to decrease the urine volume and this is associated with secondary increases in concentration. Thus we have a choice, change in volume or in concentration, for an index of the response to the hormone.

Changes in urine volume have been widely used (JEFFERS et al., 1942; AMES and VAN DYKE, 1952; DICKER, 1953; SAWYER, 1958; DETTELBACH, 1958; J. HELLER and STŮLC, 1959; DE WIED, 1960, and CZACZKES et al., 1964). BOURA and DICKER (1953) described an electronically controlled system whereby the animals were maintained automatically at a constant level of hydration while the urine volume was continuously recorded with a drop counter (see also DETTELBACH, 1958; ALBERS and BRIGHTMAN, 1959; SAWYER, 1961a; BISSET, 1962; DYBALL et al., 1966).

THORN (1957) and BARATZ and INGRAHAM (1959) used changes in urine density as an index of the response but DE WIED (1960) found this unsatisfactory. THORN and his co-workers (SMITH and THORN, 1965; THORN et al., 1965) have subsequently used the osmotic concentration as an index. However SAWYER (1958) and J. HELLER and STŮLC (1959) point out the possibility that ethanol excreted in the urine of such rats would be expected to interfere with concentration measurements which depend on determination of freezing point or vapour pressure. The direct recording of conductivity of the urine as it leaves the ureter has been found by SHARE (1961) to give the most reliable measure of the hormone's effect. YOSHIDA et al. (1963) agree with SHARE and found the index of precision (λ) of the assay to be 0.08 if conductivity is used as the index of response compared with 0.24 if change in urine volume is substituted for it. Conductivity (see also ALBERS and BRIGHTMAN, 1959; MORAN et al., 1964) has the attraction of simplicity of determination and ease of continuous recording (see Fig. 13). However SAWYER (1958) compared conductivity with urine volume as an index of response and found that although they basically gave the same result there was a greater scatter in the results if conductivity was used for the calculation. The diverse experiences of different investigators about the most reliable parameter to use may be due do variations in technique and the reader should decide which is the most suitable and convenient parameter for his particular preparation.

Whichever index of response one uses the effect of the hormones in relation to a control response can be expressed in several ways. Urine volume, or a measure of its concentration for a period of about 5—20 min after the injection may be compared with a similar control period prior to injection. The urine volume after the injection is usually expressed as a percentage (or percentage reduction) of that of the control period (see, for instance, JEFFERS et al., 1942; DICKER, 1953; THORN, 1957; BARATZ and INGRAHAM, 1959, and DE WIED, 1960). Alternatively one can

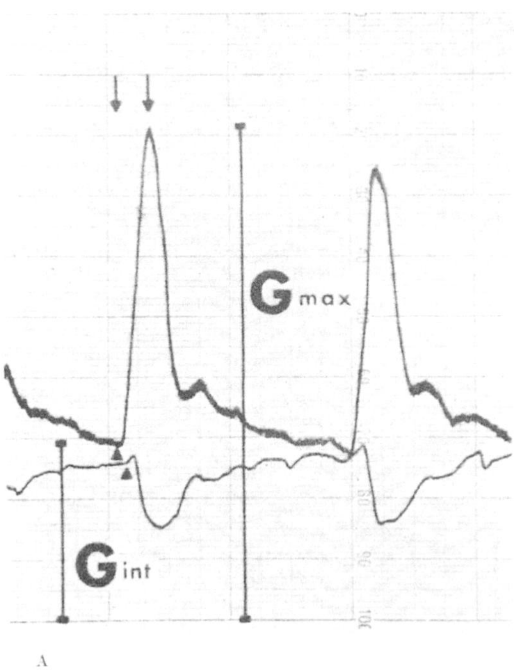

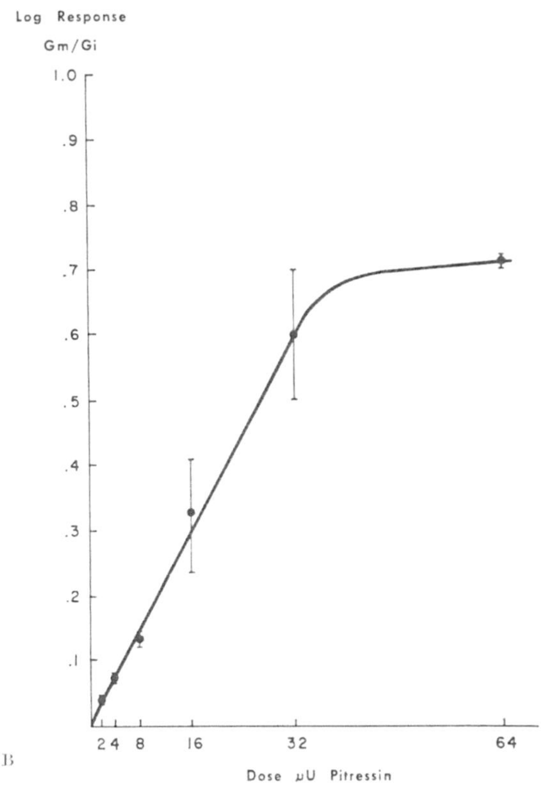

Fig. 13. *A*, Heavy line represents urine conductance. Light line represents urine flow. Triangle indicates time of injection of 12 µU of vasopressin in bioassay. Five-minute interval between time lines. *B*, Dose-response relationship of vasopressin (MORAN et al., 1964)

measure the area subtended under the curves of urine volume or conductivity for the duration of the antidiuretic effect and express the change in terms of the expected urine volume (or conductivity) for this period (KRIEGER and KILVINGTON, 1940; J. HELLER and STŮLC, 1959; SHARE, 1961; YOSHIDA et al., 1963, and TATA and GAUER, 1966). This, of course, takes into account not only the intensity of the effect over a short period but also its duration. If this method is used, particular care must be taken to ascertain that the unknown and standard preparation are the same material, as differences in their duration of action could affect the result. For instance arginine- and lysine-vasopressin have about the same intensity of effect in the rat but the duration of action of lysine-vasopressin is much less (NIELSEN, 1958; SAWYER, 1958) and this leads to statistically and biologically invalid comparisons.

A 2+2 assay design is usually used in bioassays for ADH using the ethanol anaesthetized rat but, owing to the long interval of time required between injections, it is often not possible to administer more than 8 doses of the hormone to any one rat (two 2+2 groups) and sometimes only one such group is obtainable. Accordingly the accuracy of the assay is reduced as compared with assays such as that using the blood pressure of the rat in which four such groups each of four injections, can easily be given. It appears that more injections can be given if the femoral vein route is used. DETTELBACH (1958) gave injections at 15 min intervals using this vein while NIELSEN (1958) found that it was possible to give the hormone at 30 min intervals and could perform assays using 12 injections (three groups of 2+2) on one rat. If it is desired to improve the accuracy of the assay duplicates can, of course, be done on different animals.

A three point assay design with probit evaluation, unknown being bracketed between two standards, has been found satisfactory by BERDE and CERLETTI (1961). This procedure considerably hastens the assay and is useful when rapid serial assays are being performed. A three point assay design was also found satisfactory by MORAN et al. (1964) but they added a number of refinements. It was established that the log response-dose relationship was linear between 0 and 20 μU of ADH. The response used in the calculation was the maximum conductance, following ADH injection, divided by the initial conductance. The response to the unknown was then bracketed between that of two standard ADH solutions and the procedure repeated 5 times. The calculations were carried out with an IBM 1620 computer, a procedure which can however be avoided by those in more penuric situations without loss in accuracy, but the classic (2+2) assay design is recommended.

Variation in Sensitivity Between Rats. Claims from different laboratories about the sensitivity and reliability of the ethanol anaesthetized rat for assay of ADH vary considerably. Even after allowing for differences in technique it is often difficult to understand the reasons for this. One must consider the possibility that nutritional and even genetic differences may be contributing. GINSBURG and HELLER (1953a) noted that by changing the diet and environmental temperature it was possible to increase the sensitivity of their rats about fourfold. They also reported that HELLER and SCHNIEDEN (unpublished observations) found considerable range in the sensitivity of rats in East Africa. Nutritional differences may influence the response of rats to ADH and GUGGENHEIM (1954), for instance, has found that thiamine deficiency results in the rats being more sensitive due to the relative inability of such animals to inactivate the hormone in the liver. In addition rats have been shown to be more sensitive to ADH during the spring and summer than at other times of the year (HELLER, HERDAN, and ZAIDI, 1957). Genetic effects have not yet been investigated but would provide some interesting excursions for an investigator well practised in the performance of these assays.

3. Antidiuresis in Other Species

Mouse. HELLER and BLACKMORE (1952) developed a procedure for the assay of ADH using unanaesthetized hydrated (15% of the body weight in three doses) mice which were given ADH preparations intravenously via the tail vein. Such mice are sensitive to from 10—50 μU ADH/10 g body weight but are of limited use since only 0.05 ml/10 g can be injected at one time. HELLER and BLACKMORE used this procedure to estimate ADH in the urine of newborn rats.

Dog. The dog has always been favoured for physiological and pharmacological investigations due largely to the fact that it can be trained to accept, without undue emotional responses, various undignified and unnatural procedures.

THEOBALD (1934a) and SAMAAN (1935) used bitches to assay ADH. The animals were unanaesthetized and were hydrated by gavage with 250 ml of water. Urine was collected by catheterization of the bladder and extracts injected intravenously. Bitches prepared in this way were sensitive to 0.25—0.5 mU of ADH. In 1941 this procedure was modified by HARE, HICKEY, and HARE (see also HARE, MELVILLE, CHAMBERS, and HARE, 1945), in order to assay ADH in blood and urine of untreated dogs. These investigators used bitches with surgical diabetes insipidus which were sensitive to 0.1—0.3 mU per animal. Volumes ranging from 0.1—100 ml could be injected without affecting the accuracy of the assay. The creatinine U/P concentration ratio was used as an index of the hormone effect, ruling out non-specific actions of substances that may alter the glomerular filtration rate. Substantially the same procedure was used by AMES, MOORE, and VAN DYKE (1950) to also estimate ADH in untreated blood and urine.

Dogs, unlike rats, are used repeatedly over periods of time which may extend over many months and even years. Thus sensitization to foreign materials may be expected to occur and HARE et al. (1945) reported an anaphylactic reaction in a dog used over a period of six weeks. DINGMAN (1957) used dogs with diabetes insipidus to estimate ADH in human blood and urine and he also noted one such reaction in his dogs.

Dogs exhibit different antidiuretic responses to the two antidiuretic hormones arginine- and lysine-vasopressin, the response to the latter only being about 15% of that to arginine vasopressin (VAN DYKE, ENGEL, and ADAMSONS, 1956). The dog is a useful preparation for identification of lysine-vasopressin of the Suinidae (pigs) (FERGUSON and HELLER, 1965).

For the assay of ADH present in untreated blood or urine, the apparent insensitivity of the dog (100—300 μU) compared with the ethanol-anaesthetized rat (1—10 μU) is substantially compensated for by the fact that larger volumes (up to 100 ml) can be injected into the dog (less than 1 ml in the rat). If adequate volumes of untreated blood or urine are available they probably could be assayed as easily in the dog as the rat.

Rabbit. Rabbits have one profound disadvantage and one great advantage for the assaying of ADH. Their prompt emotional responses to various stimuli can unpredictably affect urine flow but convenient veins are readily available (in the ear) into which injections can be made, a procedure which is of paramount importance for the accurate assay of ADH.

In 1939 WALKER used hydrated rabbits, "quietened" with a small dose of paraldehyde, to estimate ADH in whole blood and in extracts of urine. The animals were hydrated with 100 ml water, were sensitive to 0.2—0.5 mU ADH and could be given up to 5 ml of blood. FUGO and ARAGON (1947) and LINDQUIST and ROWE (1949) also used "quietened" rabbits (urethane and morphine) to assay ADH in human urine. The animals were initially hydrated to 5% of their body weight and this level of hydration was maintained by i.v. infusion of normal saline. The rabbits were sensitive to 0.1 mU of ADH.

GINSBURG and HELLER (1953a, b) used unanaesthetized rabbits to assay ADH in plasma. The rabbits were hydrated to the equivalent of 7.5% of their body weight and this was maintained by further doses of water. The sensitivity ranged from 32.5—125 μU/kg. Unfortunately only three doses of hormone could be administered in a day (compared with 8—12 in a rat) as the return of diuresis after ADH injection was slow.

The rabbit being an unpredictable creature is generally not considered very satisfactory for assay of ADH. Larger volumes of fluid can, however, be injected than in the rat so that it may afford a useful procedure on some occasions when plenty of dilute antidiuretic material is available.

Pig, Goat and Sheep. Animals which we generally consider of the "farm" rather than "laboratory" variety have been used to assay ADH.

Pigs were used by MUNSICK, SAWYER, and VAN DYKE (1958) to compare the antidiuretic activity of lysine- and arginine-vasopressins in this species. They used trained unanaesthetized pigs (15—20 kg) hydrated with one litre of water. The animals gave an antidiuretic response to doses of hormones ranging from 2—10 mU

Goats can also be used to measure ADH (ANDERSSON and PERSSON, 1958). Animals weighing 15—20 kg were given water equivalent to 15—20% of their body weight; they responded to doses of 2—6 mU of the hormone. ANDERSSON and PERSSON suggest that goats are easier to work with than dogs as they require no training and do not release ADH in response to emotional stimuli. This latter objection of course does not apply to dogs with diabetes insipidus.

The sheep has been used for assay of ADH in extracts of sheep urine by STACY and BROOK (1965). Animals weighing 30—35 kg were hydrated with 4—5 litres of water, and, when given i.v., 1 mU ADH could be detected.

The use of such exotic animals for routine assay of ADH will probably not develop far but in some circumstances they could prove useful. Measurement of ADH in the blood of such animals may be possible by direct transfusion from one animal to another.

Man. The presence of ADH in the blood of man has been detected and estimated by transfusion into suitably prepared human subjects. PAGE (1938) prepared women for assay procedures by hydrating them with 500 ml of water by mouth and infusing 800 ml of normal saline i.v. He then gave a transfusion of 500 ml of citrated blood and observed a small antidiuretic effect equivalent to less than 20 μU/ml ADH. BRUN, KNUDSEN, and RAASCHOU (1946) also transfused blood (200 to 400 ml) from men who had fainted, into hydrated human subjects. They demonstrated an antidiuresis which according to LEWIS (1953) would be equivalent to the injection of 1—2 mU of ADH. LEWIS also used human subjects (hydrated with 1 litre of water and 250 ml of 5% dextrose i.v.) and found them to respond to 1—2 mU ADH but the transfusion of 3—17 ml of human serum was without effect. DIEKMANN, EGENOLF, MORLEY, and POTTINGER (1950) assayed ADH, added to the plasma of pregnant women, on hydrated subjects (1800 ml of water over 2.5 hour period). Such subjects gave an antidiuretic response lasting 30—60 min when injected i.v. with about 40 mU ADH. BARNET, FORMAN, and LAUSON (1952) transfused 70—90 ml of blood from a child with nephrotic syndrome into another child with diabetes insipidus and found a concentration of ADH in the blood equivalent to less than 6 μU/ml.

A novel use of the observed inhibition of the neurohypophysis by ethanol (see rat assay) has been described in man by FERGUSON (1964). Medical students were fasted overnight and given 500 ml of beer (approx. 3.5% ethanol) for breakfast. On arrival at the laboratory they were given more beer so that they imbibed in total an amount equivalent to 2% of their body weight. An infusion of saline (60 drops a minute) was started and hormone injections given with this infusion. The state of hydration was maintained with more beer. This procedure was used to distinguish arginine- from lysine-vasopressin, the sensitivity being: arg^8-vasopressin 2.5—6 mU and lys^8-vasopressin 4—15 mU. The assay could only be extended for about 3 hours as the students become "uncomfortable" and the urine flow tended to decrease.

Man can thus be used to demonstrate the presence of ADH in body fluids though accurate routine assays do not seem to be feasible.

Fowl (Hen). Vasotocin has a pronounced antidiuretic effect when injected i.v. into chickens and this was used to aid identification of this hormone in birds (MUNSICK, SAWYER, and VAN DYKE, 1960). Conscious chickens were hydrated i.v. with hypotonic saline and 4 point (2+2) assays performed. SKADHAUGE (1964) has described in detail the establishment and maintenance of a diuresis in chickens and the effect of vasotocin. 20 hours prior to the experiment the hens weighing 2—2.5 kg were lightly sedated with 75—100 mg/kg phenobarbitone i.m. and were fasted.

Just before the experiment they received a priming dose (i.v. into a wing vein) of hypotonic saline (5% of isotonicity) of the following composition in mmol/l; NaCl 20, $NaHCO_3$ 30, and glucose 40. Subsequently a constant infusion (1.5 ml/min) of a more dilute solution was given. The composition of this later solution was mmol/l; NaCl 15, $NaHCO_3$ 20, and glucose 30. The urine was collected through small polyethylene funnels sewn over the ureters. The rate of flow was 0.6—1.2 ml/min and responses to vasotocin were obtained (i.v. leg vein) with from 7—50 $\times$ 10^{-9} g (1.6 to 11.6 mU pressor activity).

4. Factors which may Influence Antidiuresis Assays

The effects of pain and emotional stimuli on release of ADH has been dealt with in other parts of this book and it is obviously vital to avoid such stimuli in animals being used for assay purposes.

In addition a number of drugs and materials that occur in tissues either normally or as the result of experimental procedures could influence the antidiuretic responses of animals into which they are injected. These may promote endogenous release of ADH and include many anaesthetics such as ether, urethane and most barbiturates as well as substances such as nicotine and other cholinergic substances. Thus the use of these materials in experiments using antidiuresis assay animals is contraindicated or should be approached cautiously. Other materials potentially antidiuretic which are likely to occur naturally in tissue extracts or as a result of extraction procedures include histamine, 5-hydroxytryptamine (5-HT), ferritin and kinins.

Histamine is present in the hypothalamic-neurohypophysial region (see Robson and Stacy, 1962) and as noted by Waring and Landgrebe (1950) is a common contaminant of extracts of tissues from this area. Histamine has profound effects on the contractility of smooth muscle and when injected can release ADH (de Wied and Mirsky, 1959). Its effects on the assay of neurohypophysial hormones is, however, more likely to be troublesome in preparations using smooth muscles. No reports have been found of interference with assays depending on antidiuretic responses when the tissue extracts have been given i.v. but the possibility should be remembered. Histamine is excreted in urine and may be released into the circulation in certain stressful conditions. The extraction and dialysis procedures that are used to isolate the neurohypophysial hormones from blood and urine should remove any histamine. However when direct injections of urine or plasma are used to assay ADH the possibility of histamine interference should be considered. Thus Bocanegra and Lauson (1961) checked haemorrhagic dog plasma for histamine on the isolated guinea-pig ileum, and also showed that injections of as much as 10 μg of histamine i.v. into their assay dogs had no effects on the diuresis. De Wied and Mirsky (1959) found that 1 mg histamine i.p. had an antidiuretic effect in rats.

The possibility of 5-HT being present in extracts from the hypothalamic region should also be considered (see Robson and Stacy, 1962). No reports have been traced indicating it is troublesome in i.v. antidiuresis assays of neurohypophysial hormones extracted from such tissues. Extraction procedures for 5-HT usually involve its extraction into acetone and as neurohypophysial tissues are usually stored for at least 24 hours in acetone, prior to drying and extraction of the hormones, much of any 5-HT present would probably be removed. Any 5-HT present in blood or urine would probably be removed during the extraction procedures for ADH. In any event the amounts excreted in the urine are small and in blood it is principally present in the platelets so that if reasonable precautions are taken during collection and removal of the plasma it would not be expected to be troublesome.

When 5-HT is injected s.c. into rats, dogs, man, frogs and toads it has antidiuretic effects (ERSPAMER and OTTOLENGHI, 1950) but this is generally considered to be a result of pain at the injection site as i.v. injections into dogs or rats do not have an antidiuretic action (PAGE, 1954). AMES and VAN DYKE (1952) injected 4—6 μg 5-HT into their ethanol-anaesthetized rats while THORN and SILVER (1957) injected 7—30 μg/kg into the same preparation, without any effect on the diuresis. In addition 5-HT has been shown by BUCHBORN (1957) to have no effect when injected into the lymph sac of toads or to change the permeability of the isolated bladder of the bullfrog (ISHII, HIRANO, and KOBAYASHI, 1962).

Ferritin may be released into the circulation during shock and BAEZ, MAZUR, and SHORR (1952) have shown that this brings about a release of ADH and an antidiuresis in dogs. However GOLTNER and VORHERR (1959) have found it to be without such an effect when injected i.v. into rats unless very large doses were given. It does not affect the water metabolism of toads when injected into a lymph sac (BUCHBORN, 1957).

Kinins may be present in extracts of blood or in plasma as a result of extraction procedures or inadequate precautions during collection and these may be troublesome in assays using smooth muscle. If injected s.c. kinins may produce pain so it would not be surprising to observe an antidiuretic effect when they are administered in this way. However when using standard antidiuresis assays (i.v. injection) any expected effects of kinins would be mediated through their vascular actions and require amounts in excess of those expected in plasma or blood extracts: as with histamine and 5-HT the possibility of an effect should be considered, but BISSET and LEWIS (1962) have indicated that doses of up to 4 μg bradykinin are without effect on urine flow despite a fall in blood pressure of 30 mm Hg. With higher doses (8 μg) some transient antidiuresis accompanied by a more profound hypotension was seen and with even higher doses (16 μg) long lasting effects. Similarly with substance P, BISSET and LEWIS found that doses up to 6 units (0.2 μg) producing moderate hypotension (up to 25 mm Hg fall) elicited only transient and trivial antidiuresis. Higher doses (24 units) elicited profound hypotension (—70 mm Hg) and complete antidiuresis lasting over 20 min. These authors were able to demonstrate that moderate hypotension *per se* (produced with isoprenaline) is not accompanied by antidiuresis whereas more profound hypotension is accompanied by severe antidiuresis which lasts longer than the hypotension and which is presumably secondary to the fall in blood pressure. It would be interesting to know if this secondary effect were seen in hypophysectomised rats.

5. *Response of Isolated Smooth Muscle*

Oviduct of Hen and Turtle

The uterine (also called shell gland) portion of the hen oviduct contracts in the presence of neurohypophysial hormones and as with the rat uterus *in vitro* preparations can be used to measure the activity of these hormones. Such preparations have been described by MUNSICK et al. (1960) and HELLER and PICKERING (1961). A piece of the uterus about 2—3 cm long and 2—3 mm wide is obtained from a laying hen. It is suspended in a solution with a low calcium concentration and this, as with the rat uterus, assists the suppression of spontaneous contractions. MUNSICK et al. (1960) used VAN DYKE-HASTINGS solution (as for the rat uterus, see Table 5) but containing only 0.15 mM/l calcium and with 0.5 mM/l magnesium and 100 mg per cent of glucose. Magnesium was not included in the solution used by PICKERING and HELLER; the composition was g/l: NaCl 6.6, KCl 0.42, $CaCl_2$ 0.01, NaH_2PO_4 0.1, Na_2HPO_4 0.1 and $NaHCO_3$ 2.5. HELLER and PICKERING maintained the uterus at 40° while MUNSICK et al. kept it at 43°. Both recorded the contractions by classic isotonic procedures but subsequently MUNSICK (1964) recorded contractions isometrically with a strain gauge.

This preparation is not one of choice for measuring small amounts of neurohypophysial hormones but as explained in detail later has been particularly useful in aiding identification of vasotocin and distinguishing between lysine- and arginine-vasopressin.

Contractions of the cloacal end of the ovulating turtle oviduct were also used by SAWYER, MUNSICK, and VAN DYKE (1959) and MUNSICK et al. (1960) to help identify vasotocin. This was suspended in Frog-Ringer solution and the contractions recorded isotonically.

Very recently HELLER et al. (1967) have reported that the oviduct of the mud puppy (*Necturus maculosus*) contracts in response to vasotocin at concentrations as little as 1.2 nU/ml or 0.003 pg/ml. Sensitivity to other homologues including oxytocin is much less.

Terminal Colon of Guinea-Pig

Although it has long been known that the smooth muscle of the alimentary tract contracts in response to vasopressin it has been accepted until recently that this tissue was too insensitive to be used for assay of small concentrations of vasopressin. However, BOTTING in 1965 reported that the most proximal portion of the colon of the guinea-pig is more sensitive than the rest of the smooth muscle of the alimentary tract. When used as an isolated organ for assay purposes, the sensitivity is stated to vary from 1 μU/ml to 1 mU/ml and that with 2+2 assays the index of precision (λ) varies from 0.03—0.08. At its most sensitive this preparation could be useful in the investigation of the vasopressin content of biological fluids but published illustrations do not show a sensitivity greater than 100 μU/ml. Furthermore BOTTING states that sensitivity is decreased with tissue from females, old males, and also when low calcium solutions are used (to supress spontaneous contraction) which is not encouraging for workers looking for a consistently sensitive preparation. However, the desirability of developing a simple rapid procedure, of the appropriate sensitivity are so great that the method is worthy of further investigation, attempting modifications such as those described above for the isolated uterus (eversion, superfusion, electrical stimulation, hyaluronidase). The proximal colon preparation is not specific; it responds to oxytocin (but is at least 18 times less sensitive), to several analogues of the posterior pituitary hormones, and to acetylcholine, histamine, 5-hydroxytryptamine and angiotensin.

6. *Water and Sodium Metabolism in Amphibia*

Amphibia (frogs, toads, newts and salamanders) exhibit a variety of responses to the injection of their homologous hormones, such as arginine vasotocin, or hormonal analogues from other vertebrate groups, arginine- or lysine-vasopressin and oxytocin (see HELLER and BENTLEY, 1965). Intact frogs sitting in water increase in weight when injected with neurohypophysial extracts (BRUNN, 1921) and this is the combined result of an increase in water uptake through the skin, an increased rate of water reabsorption from the urinary bladder and decrease in urine formation by the kidney (see BENTLEY, 1963a). In addition there is an increase in sodium transport across the skin and bladder.

Intact Amphibia

Blood. Assay procedures utilising the response of the intact frog were described many years ago (BOYD and MACK, 1940; HELLER, 1941) and have been recently modified in order to determine ADH in human and rat blood plasma (BUCHBORN, 1955, 1956, 1957; LAUBER, EVERSOLE, and CHILDS, 1959) and to detect neurohypophysial hormones (principally arginine-vasotocin) in the circulation of dehydrated toads (SHOEMAKER, 1965). Such assays on intact frogs and toads are usually carried out on groups of about five animals, each member of different groups being injected (into a lymph sac) with control solutions or neurohypophysial hormones of known or unknown concentrations. The responses of the groups are compared either from dose-response curves taken from that particular assay or from ones established in previous experiments. The index of response varies and may be the total water uptake by the animal, the net gain of water (total water uptake minus urine loss) or inhibition of urine flow. BUCHBORN (1955, 1956, 1957) injected toads (*Bufo bufo*) with saline solutions equivalent to 5% of the body weight, containing known amounts of vasopressin or diluted plasma with an unknown ADH concentration. The percentage inhibition of diuresis for the two-hour-period following the injection, as compared with the three-hour-period before the injection, was taken as the index of the response. Using such a procedure BUCHBORN was able to detect as little as 0.05 μU ADH/10 g toad body weight. As the assay requires groups of five toads the overall minimal dose is about 10 μU. The response related to the log dose was linear over the range 10—1500 μU ADH. The assay is specific in that

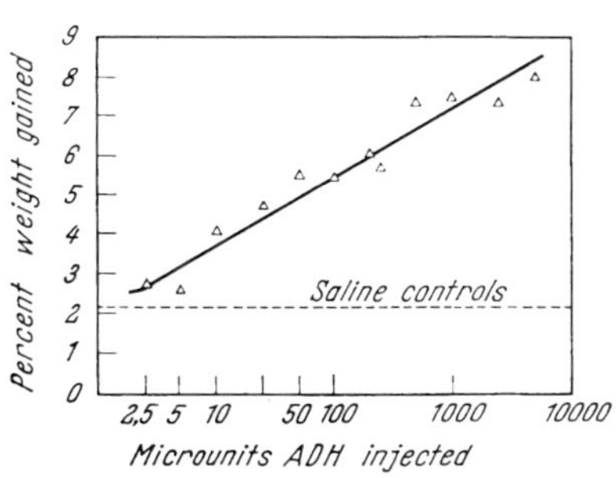

Fig. 14. Dose-response curve for *Bufo marinus* given various dosages of Pitressin. The abscissa is a logarithmic scale, 1 μU being 1 millionth of an International (pressor) unit. Each triangular point represents the mean response of five toads at the 3rd h after injection. The dashed line represents the average weight gain, after the same interval, of toads injected with saline only. (The zero point on the ordinate scale represents the mean hydrated weight, or pre-injection weight, of each toad; since the injected fluid constitutes 5% of the animal's body weight, every animal will be heavier at the next weighing. However, this net gain is gradually lost by animals who receive only saline; it is maintained or increased under the influence of ADH (LAUBER, EVERSOLE, and CHILDS, 1959)

oxytocin at these concentrations had no effect and neither did 5-hydroxytryptamine or ferritin. LAUBER et al. (1959) adapted this assay to the more widely available species *Bufo marinus*. They used the total gain in weight as the index of response and found a linear log dose response relationship over the range 5—5000 μU of arginine-vasopressin (see Fig. 14). They used this procedure to measure ADH in rat plasma.

Individual 2+2 type assays (high and low standards bracketing high and low doses of unknown) were not performed by BUCHBORN or LAUBER et al., the responses to the unknown being referred, with the aid of one standard, to the previously established linear response. BUCHBORN claims a reliability of $\pm$ 20% ($\lambda = 0.228$). Frogs and toads may show considerable variation in their sensitivities to neurohypophysial hormones so that it would be worthwhile to consider the use of the more traditional bioassay design. The assay procedure of BUCHBORN has been used by BANS and OLSEN (1959) and HOR, AVENHAUS, and BUCHBORN (1963) to determine ADH concentration in human plasma.

However the estimates of BUCHBORN of the ADH activity of human blood are 20—30 times higher than those found by other investigators using intravenous injection of plasma or blood extracts into rats (Table 9) so that use of this procedure must be considered with some caution (HELLER, 1957; SAWYER, 1961a, and WALKER, 1961). The reasons for the difference are not clear and if elucidated could have considerable interest, especially as BUCHBORN has ruled out interference by ferritin or 5-hydroxytryptamine. It is possible that, as suggested by HELLER (1957), some potentiation of the hormone action is occurring.

Tissue Extracts. In 1941 HELLER used assays on intact frogs in order to demonstrate the presence of a new hormone in the neurohypophysis of frogs. This subsequently proved to be arginine-vasotocin. Intact frogs were again used in 1959 by PICKERING and HELLER to help identify the hormone in a variety of lower vertebrates and the procedure is described in detail by HELLER and PICKERING (1961). Identification of hormones in lower vertebrates depends on a variety of assays (a "pharmacological profile", see SAWYER in this volume) and the response of the intact frog or toad has been used often. Frogs are kept in tap water to ensure that they are adequately hydrated at the beginning of an experiment. The frogs' urinary bladders are emptied by a combination of suprapubic pressure and catheterization, their skin is dried with a soft cloth and they are weighed. This procedure is repeated at hourly intervals. After 3 h the animals are injected with the hormone or control solutions and the weight gain (bladder empty) recorded each hour until it reaches a maximum value. Groups of 5 or 6 animals are usually used and the mean maximum weight increase of each group is used as the index of response. HELLER and PICKERING (1961) defined the unit of frog water balance activity as that exerted by 1 unit of synthetic oxytocin.

SAWYER (1961b) used assays utilizing the antidiuretic response of the bullfrog *Rana catesbiana* to aid identification of vasotocin. Male frogs weighing 300—700 g, were used (URANGA and SAWYER, 1960). 1—8 days before the experiments the ureters were cannulated after the animals had been anaesthetized with Tricaine-methanesulphonate (MS 222, Sandoz). The frogs were placed in water and urine was collected over 15 min periods. The solutions containing neurohypophysial hormones were injected into a lymph sac or i.v. through an implanted cannula. The median antidiuretic response for vasotocin using the lymph sac route is about 150×10^{-9}g/kg (35 mU pressor).

Arginine-vasotocin is the homologous neurohypophysial antidiuretic hormone in nearly all of the lower tetrapod vertebrates (see SAWYER this book) including the amphibia, and these animals usually show a far greater response to it than mammalian ADH (arginine- or lysine-vasopressin). Thus amphibian bioassay preparations may offer particular advantages for the detection and estimation of neurohypophysial hormones in non-mammalian vertebrates. SHOEMAKER (1965) used the response of the intact toads *Bufo valicens* and *B. cognatus* to detect neurohypophysial hormones in the circulation of the dehydrated toad *B. marinus*. The rates of water uptake and urine formation were measured and it was found that as little as 0.1 to 0.25 ml of plasma when injected (i.p.) into toads sitting in water resulted in a net water gain equivalent to 3—5% of their body weight.

Different species of amphibia may differ considerably in their relative and absolute responses to different hormone analogues (BENTLEY and HELLER, 1964; HELLER and BENTLEY, 1965) so that when planning to use such assays it is advisable to select a species carefully in relation to the specific hormones to be measured. Thus *Rana esculenta* is about 20 times as responsive to arginine-vasotocin as to arginine-vasopressin, while in *Bufo bufo* the former hormone is only slightly more active. On the other hand. *B. bufo* is far more responsive than *R. esculenta* to injection of all neurohypophysial hormones so far tested on it and for a similar response requires 10—20 times less arginine-vasotocin than *R. esculenta*. By selection of the species most sensitive to a hormone it may be possible to develop an assay based on the above procedures using intact amphibia and capable of measuring arginine-vasotocin in the circulation of lower vertebrates.

Isolated Skin and Bladder

Amphibian skin and urinary bladder survive for many hours *in vitro*. Water and sodium transport across such preparations of the skins and bladders of frogs and of toads is increased by neurohypophysial hormones and the responses given to the hormones can be used for their bioassay.

The effects of neurohypophysial hormones on water and sodium transport across the skin of frogs and toads were used by MOREL, MAETZ, and LUCARAIN (1958) to compare the biological activities of vasopressin and oxytocin. They used the method described originally by USSING and ZERAHN (1951). A piece of skin with a surface area of about 7 cm^2 is anchored between two lucite chambers each containing frog Ringer solution (or a modification of this) which is aerated. Sodium transport can be directly measured by using isotope procedures but this is not convenient. USSING and ZERAHN found that the current required to reduce to zero the normal electrical potential difference (p.d.) across the skin (up to about 100 mV but usually 20—50 mV) was equivalent to the net sodium transport when both are expressed in terms of coulombs. This current is called the short-circuit current and can easily be measured. Both sides of the skin are connected, through agar-Ringer or agar-KCl bridges and calomel cells, to a potential measuring device such as a voltmeter or potentiometer. Another pair of such bridges are connected, through silver-silver chloride cells, to a battery from which varying amounts of current can be drawn with the aid of a potentiometer. The current in this latter circuit can be measured with an instrument such as an ampere-meter. The current from the battery is applied in the direction opposing the normal p.d. which is then reduced to zero. The current required to do this is the short-circuit current. A

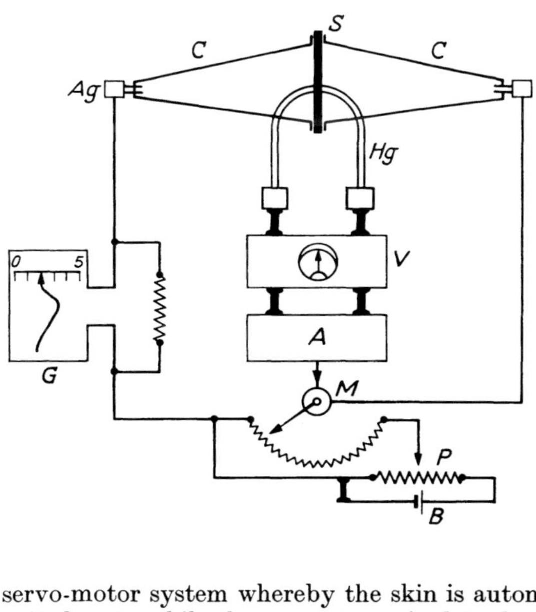

Fig. 15. Scheme for measuring the net flux of sodium across frog skin

Ag	Silver/Silver chloride electrodes
G	galvanometer and shunt
M	servo motor
A	amplifier
V	millivoltmeter of high impedance
Hg	Mercury/Calomel electrodes
S	strip of skin in plastic chamber
P	potentiometer
B	battery of 90 volts
C	plastic chamber

(After MAETZ, MOREL, et RACE, 1959)

servo-motor system whereby the skin is automatically maintained in a short-circuited state while the current required to do this is simultaneously recorded has been described by MAETZ, MOREL, and RACE (1959), and this is shown in Fig. 15.

A system for automatically short-circuiting and recording from six pieces of frog skin simultaneously is described in detail by MOREL, ODIER and LUCARAIN (1961).

The measurement of water transport in these preparations of amphibian skin is not as simple as that of sodium transport and depends on the maintenance of a constant level of fluid in a capillary attached to one, or both, sides of the bath. This is performed with the aid of a micrometer syringe. BOURGUET and JARD (1964) have described an automatic procedure for recording changes in volume in such a system. These methods have been used to measure the activities of vasotocin and its analogues (ACHER, CHAUVET, LENCI, MOREL, and MAETZ, 1960; BOURGUET and MAETZ, 1961) as well as to assist in the original identification of ichthyotocin (ser[4], Ile[8]-oxytocin) in teleost fish (HELLER, PICKERING, MAETZ, and MOREL, 1961).

The frog and toad bladder *in vitro* respond in the same manner as the skin when exposed to neurohypophysial hormones (LEAF, ANDERSON, and PAGE, 1958; BENTLEY, 1958) but less hormone is required, thus potentially providing a more sensitive assay method. It was found in the bladder of *Bufo marinus* that the responses were linear when related to the log dose for the range 10—100 μU/ml (Pituitrin) for water movement (BENTLEY, 1958) and 25—1000 μU/ml (Pitressin) for sodium (short-circuit current) transport (BENTLEY, 1960).

An assay procedure using changes in water transfer across the bladder has been described by SAWYER (1960). The bladder is prepared in the following manner (see BENTLEY, 1958; SAWYER, 1960): the bladder is dissected from the pithed or anaesthetized (MS 222) animal and rinsed in frog Ringer solution. It is tied to the end of a piece of glass tubing (serosal side facing outwards) and suspended in a bath of aerated frog Ringer solution. The inside is filled with dilute Ringer solution so that an osmotic gradient exists between the two sides. When neurohypophysial hormones are placed in the fluid bathing the serosal (outside) side, water passes out of the bladder and into the outer bathing solution. The amount of water moving in this way can be measured by weighing the bladder and its attached piece of glass tube on a highly damped balance. SAWYER developed this as a four point (2+2) assay design, an example of which is shown in Fig. 16. This assay has been used by a number of investigators to estimate neurohypophysial hormones in extracts from the neurohypophysis (for instance, ISHII et al., 1962; SAWYER and PICKFORD, 1963) and to aid in their identification (see SAWYER, 1961b).

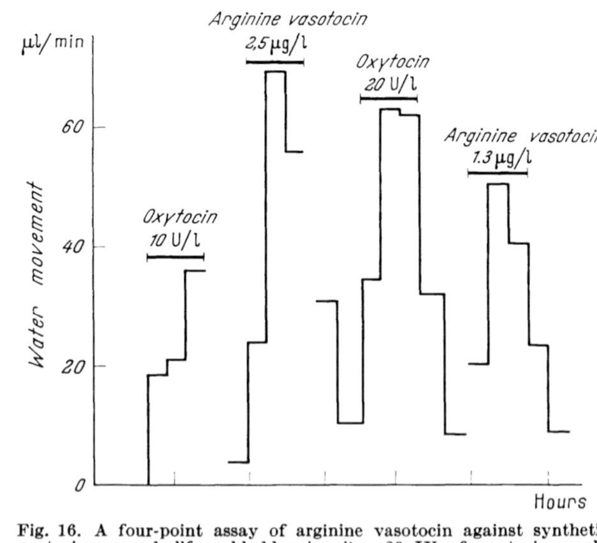

Fig. 16. A four-point assay of arginine vasotocin against synthetic oxytocin on a bullfrog bladder *in vitro*. 20 IU of oxytocin would represent approximately 55 μg of the pure peptide (SAWYER, 1960)

Changes in the short-circuit current across the frog or toad bladder can be detected more readily than changes in water transfer so that assays based on its measurement usually require less hormone. A method using a four point (2+2) assay design is described by BENTLEY (1963b). The preparation itself may be made in either of two ways. The bladder may be set up as a diaphragm between two lucite chambers as already described for the skin (LEAF et al., 1958). Alternatively the "bag" arrangement, as used to measure water transport, can be used but with normal undiluted frog Ringer solution on both sides (BENTLEY, 1960). Bridges made of agar KCl are made out of thin pieces of polyethylene tubing which can be placed in position on both sides of the bladder. The short-circuit current is measured in the same way as it is across the skin. Short-circuit current is recorded until the baseline is reasonably steady, the hormone preparation is then added to the fluid on the serosal surface and the short-circuit current measured continuously or at intervals for 15 min. The response is taken to be the mean increase in current during this period as compared with the baseline. The baseline for the 15 min period is calculated from the initial value and that seen 20 min after the hormone has to be removed. Another dose of hormone can then be tested. This assay preparation has been used to measure the activity of vasotocin in extracts from the neurohypophyses of lampreys (BENTLEY and FOLLETT, 1963) and to help identify vasotocin, ser^4, ile^8-oxytocin and ile^8-oxytocin in amphibia and fishes (FOLLETT and HELLER, 1964a, b) and lysine- and arginine-vasopressin in the Suiformes (FERGUSON and HELLER, 1965). A detailed description of the idiosyncrasies of the amphibian urinary bladder *in vitro* is given by BENTLEY (1966).

Assay of neurohypophysial hormones using either water movement (hydroosmotic) or sodium transport (natriferic) across the skin or bladder are not as accurate or convenient as more conventional assays using pressor, antidiuretic, oxytocin or galactobolic responses in mammals. However the naturally occurring hormone analogues often exhibit marked differences in their activities when tested on the amphibian skin or bladder and this may provide invaluable information for identifying them.

7. *Radioimmune Assay for Vasopressins and Oxytocin*

Radioimmune assays of protein and polypeptide hormones offer the possibility of considerable sensitivity as well as specificity and have been used with particular success to assay small amounts of insulin. There has, however, been some doubt as to the possibility of obtaining antibodies to polypeptides the size of neurohypophysial hormones though GILLILAND and PROUT (1965) have reported the production of antibodies to oxytocin in rabbits. Conjugations of the hormones to larger proteins have been used as antigens to produce antiserum. For example, PERMUTT, PARKER, and UTIGER (1966), with the aid of toluene diisocyanate or carbodiimide, conjugated bovine serum albumin with synthetic lysine-vasopressin (LVP): subsequent injection of these antigens into rabbits resulted in the production of antibodies to LVP. Antibodies to LVP and oxytocin were also produced by conjugating rabbit serum albumin with these hormones, using carbodiimide as a coupling agent, and injecting the complexes into rabbits (HOLLANDER, FRANZ, and BERDE, 1966).

A radioimmune assay for LVP has been described by PERMUTT et al. (1966). They obtained antibodies from rabbits and found that LVP formed soluble complexes with these. Radioiodinated-LVP (LVP-^{131}I) can be used to produce these associations. The amount of the bound labelled hormone can be measured by precipitating the complex with goat anti-rabbit γ-globulin serum and counting the radioactivity present after centrifuging and washing. The association of LVP-^{131}I and the antibody is inhibited by LVP in a linear manner when the log of the dose of LVP is related to the percentage radioactivity that can be precipitated. Thus a low percentage precipitation results from a high dose of non-radioiodinated LVP. Although the antibodies were clearly specific to LVP the association of LVP-^{131}I and the antibody was also inhibited by arginine-vasopressin so that it could also be assayed. The assay technique was sensitive to 4 μU of these antidiuretic hormones which is not as sensitive as the rat antidiuretic assay for ADH. The authors could not assay hormones in plasma samples and suggest that plasma may have non-specific inhibitory effects in the assay. Oxytocin was 4000 times less active than the vasopressin in inhibiting the association of LVP-^{131}I and the antibody.

Clearly further work will need to be done to develop such assays to a point of usefulness equalling or exceeding the bioassay procedures at present available but the possibility of doing this and being able to distinguish between the vasopressins and oxytocin is an attractive one.

III. Treatment of Blood and Other Fluids

A. Collection of Blood

Site. The neurohypophysial hormones are released into the jugular venous system. In some animals such as the sheep, horse, and rat they pass into the external jugular vein whilst in other species, such as man and the cat, drainage is via the internal jugular vein. The hormones are rapidly removed from the circulation so that large differences in the concentration of the hormones are seen, especially when jugular blood is compared with peripheral venous or arterial blood (Ames et al., 1950, for ADH in dogs; Dicker and Tyler, 1952, for ADH in children; Bisset, 1961, for ADH in adult man; Walmsley, 1963, for oxytocin in ruminants). Ginsburg and Heller (1953b) found in anaesthetised rats that the plasma concentration of ADH in mU/ml was 1.3 in external jugular vein; 1.2 in right heart; 0.27 in carotid artery and 0.1 in renal or hepatic vein. Similar regional differences were demonstrated in sheep and mice. Bisset and co-workers (1967) have recently reported considerable difference between ADH activity of peripheral venous blood (580 μU/ml) as compared with internal jugular blood (2250 μU/ml) during and after electrical stimulation of the hypothalamus in the cat. (For further discussion see Ginsburg, this volume).

In large animals such as horses, ruminants and dogs it is often possible to obtain blood samples directly from the external jugular vein with a minimum of excitement. Even so, it is advisable to practise local anaesthesia of vein puncture and to sample from an indwelling catheter to avoid the risk of the release of hormones during the period of sampling, due to the stimulus of the pain of needle puncture, or even to apprehension.

In small animals such as the rat, blood sampling is much more difficult. Collection of blood by heart puncture, even in anaesthetised animals, usually elevates the concentration of ADH. Rapid decapitation, which results in a sample predominantly from the carotid artery has often been used (Ames and van Dyke, 1952; Dicker, 1953; Robinson and MacFarlane, 1956; Baratz and Ingraham, 1959), but the concentration in the carotid artery is low and a correspondingly more sensitive assay is needed. Moreover every such blood sample is also a terminal one placing limitations on the experimental design. To avoid this, chronic catheters may be placed in blood vessels, such as the external jugular vein, prior to the acute experiment, making sampling less heroic and permitting repeat sampling in any one animal. Such sampling may still require the second jugular to be occluded to permit an adequate rate of blood flow and this is difficult in non-anaesthetised animals although they can be trained to accept appropriate gentle finger pressure without evident excitement. In man, sampling from an arm vein is usually a simple affair but all steps should be taken to avoid pain and apprehension. Blood cannot be obtained easily by venepuncture from the internal jugular vein but Caldeyro-

BARCIA and associates have devised a technique which approximates to this. They advance a catheter from an arm vein until the tip lies in the innominate vein close to the junction with the internal jugular. Before withdrawing each sample, arm cuffs are inflated to decrease the return of venous blood from the arms. These authors claim to obtain blood with much higher oxytocin activity than peripheral venous blood (COCH, BROVETTO, CABOT, FIELITZ, and CALDEYRO-BARCIA, 1965; see also BISSET and LEE, 1957, and BISSET, 1961).

Blood Loss. If relatively large volumes of blood are removed from an animal, an elevated concentration of ADH will result. GINSBURG and HELLER (1953b) found that blood loss equivalent to about 2.5 ml/100 g body weight in rats anaesthetized with ether resulted in a 10—15-fold increase in the concentration of ADH in plasma. GINSBURG and BROWN (1956 and 1957) extended these experiments to rats anaesthetized in a variety of ways and found that haemorrhage increased the circulating ADH levels as much as 100-fold, the release being related to decreases in blood pressure. Haemorrhage has the same effect in dogs (WEINSTEIN, BERNE, and SACHS, 1960).

BELESLIN, BISSET, HALDAR, and POLAK (1967) have shown that in anaesthetized cats there is a similar dramatic rise in ADH secretion (but *no* oxytocin secretion) after haemorrhage, and that this effect is almost certainly attributable to the fall in blood pressure rather than reduction in blood volume. However they also showed that the secretion of vasopressin long outlasts the brief period of hypotension, reaching a peak usually about 20 min after the haemorrhage and in many cases still demonstrable after approximately 1 hour. This has important implications in experiments in which hypotension may be induced either as a necessary part of the experimental programme (rapid blood withdrawal, vagal stimulation) or inadvertently, for instance by crude surgery or anaesthesia leading to haemorrhage or circulatory shock. A dramatic and persistent release of ADH by surgery has been clearly shown by MORAN et al. (1964).

Anaesthesia. Efforts to minimise the secretion of ADH associated with stress during blood collection by administering conventional general anaesthetics are not encouraging. Thus AMES and VAN DYKE (1952) found that blood collected from rats by heart puncture while they were under ether anaesthesia had an even higher concentration of ADH than blood collected in this manner without anaesthesia, while with ethanol it was less. DICKER (1953) found that the plasma of rats (blood collected by decapitation) had undetectable amounts of ADH if ethanol was used as an anaesthetic while with chloralose it was 30 μU/ml and with ether 200 μU/ml. Elevated ADH levels associated with haemorrhage were similar whether the anaesthetic was ether, a barbiturate or urethane but was less if ethanol was used and was undetectable with chloralose (GINSBURG and BROWN, 1956). In this respect it was perhaps fortunate that FERGUSON (1941) in his original work on reflex release of oxytocin used a mixture of chloralose and urethane.

Although experimental observations can and must be carried out under general anaesthesia, it should be remembered that results from such experiments may differ from the non-anaesthetized animal and this is especially so when the anaesthesia is light or variable, as with a volatile agent such as ether. Similarly, high concentrations of oxytocin (or ADH) found in clinical patients may be attributable to general anaesthesia (BISSET, LEE, and BROMWICH, 1956).

Technique of Sampling. When blood comes in contact with glass and similar surfaces, active substances such as kinins are formed rapidly by enzymatic action. Accordingly all cannulae, needles and glassware, including glass syringes, should be freshly coated with silicone (BISSET, 1961). This should be done with great care since the thin coating of silicone may be easily damaged and such damage cannot be detected. Wherever possible glassware should be replaced with polyethylene or polypropylene; nylon syringes are sometimes used instead of glass syringes, both for initial sampling and for transfer between containers at all stages of processing until protein precipitation is complete. Gentle handling of the blood is essential to avoid the liberation of other interfering substances (discussed below) which are consequent upon haemolysis, disruption of platelets and so on. Heparin should be used as anticoagulant, 10 units per ml final concentration. Over enthusiastic use of heparin should be avoided since high concentrations can interfere with assays for oxytocin (Walker, 1960).

In some investigations the stability of oxytocin and vasopressin in blood after withdrawal may be important. This is especially important with the blood of pregnant and parturient women, since such blood contains large quantities of oxytocinase and vasopressinase which rapidly inactivate the octa-peptides (see Tuppy this volume). This effect is minimised by cooling to 0° C immediately. One of the present authors (R.J.F.) in conjunction with Caldeyro-Barcia's group, devised a system whereby blood was withdrawn from women, not into a syringe, but into a long polythene tube immersed in melting ice in a vacuum flask (Mendez-Bauer, Fitzpatrick et al., 1960, see also Fitzpatrick and Walmsley, 1965). This tube was about 50 cm long, about 5 mm bore and held 10 ml. Blood taken into this tube at the bedside was maintained at 0° C (including centrifugation) until the moment of assay. Inactivation by oxytocinase, as judged by recovery of added oxytocin, was only 5% after 1 hour. Although in this instance the plasma was assayed without processing it would be quite practicable to use this method of collection prior to precipitation of protein or even separation on Sephadex gel at 0° C.

B. Assays on Unextracted Blood

For some investigations it is desirable to assay fresh blood, plasma or other body fluid without any form of processing. In so far as extraction procedures may liberate interfering substances or permit loss of existing oxytocin or vasopressin this approach has, on the surface, much to commend it. Comparison of ADH activity in human blood determined in unextracted and extracted samples is shown in Table 9 and gives comparable results.

Table 9. *Estimated ADH activity of human blood collected peripherally or from internal jugular under similar conditions and assayed (a) untreated and (b) after extraction*

untreated		extracted	
		Peripheral blood	
	μU/ml		μU/ml
MacFarlane and Robinson (1957)	<12	Bisset and Lee (1958)	<8
Brun et al. (1946) (man) calc. Lewis (1953) . . . . about	10	Robinson et al. (1957)	<12.5
Heller and Stŭlc (1960b)	1.5	Miltenberger and Moran (1963) .	2
Czaczkes et al. (1964)	1.1	Yoshida et al. (1963)	1.1
Buchborn (1957) (toad).	30	Moran et al. (1964)	0.6
		Internal jugular blood	
	μU/ml		μU/ml
Heller (1957)	<5—8	Lee and Bisset (1958)	6
Lauson (1960) (man)	<6		

Plasma values have been approximately corrected for whole blood.

Bisset and Lee, and Robinson et al. extracted with acid alcohol, the others by ion-exchange chromatography.

Assays all performed by i.v. injection into rats except where indicated.

However this is not always desirable. It may not be convenient to inject samples into an assay animal at the same time intervals as the samples are obtained from the donor, e.g., during parturition, so that some form of storage becomes essential. More important than this, however, is the false assumption that the antidiuretic or oxytocic activity of fresh blood or plasma is necessarily a true measure of the hormone content. Enhanced activity may be due to the presence of substances which themselves are antidiuretic or oxytocic (such as bradykinin) or diminished activity may be due to the presence of inhibitors of the assay preparation (such as adrenaline).

In relation to this, attention must be drawn to the observations of ARMSTRONG and STEWART (1960) which have been largely overlooked by those concerned with neurohypophysial polypeptides. These authors detected very high oxytocic activity in fresh human plasma, which appeared transiently at parturition, and was equivalent during the second stage of labour to several units of oxytocin per ml plasma when assayed without extraction on the rat uterus *in vitro*. The active substance was not oxytocin and behaved pharmacologically as a kinin: furthermore a parallel decrease was observed in blood kininogen, the substrate from which kinin is formed by enzymes such as plasmin. It should be noted that although the plasma samples were held in polythene at 0° C this activity was present and even increased during the first hour or two after sampling. No activity was detected in human plasma from non-parturient patients, when kept under similar conditions, nor in the plasma from parturient women if this plasma were held at 20° C. Presumably the rates of kinin formation and of kinin destruction (by kininase) are differentiated by cooling to 0° C so that formation exceeds destruction at least as long as there is an excess of the precursor kininogen. This observation is of considerable importance to those concerned with estimation of blood oxytocin (or ADH) at parturition, especially since it has usually been considered that kinin formation in plasma, contained in polythene vessels, is negligible at 0° C (ARMSTRONG, JEPSON, KEELE, and STEWART, 1957) and in fact these are precisely the conditions adopted by those investigating blood oxytocin in animals and man (FITZPATRICK and WALMSLEY, 1965; FOLLEY and KNAGGS, 1965; COCH et al., 1965). Fortunately these workers used extraction and assay procedures which would distinguish between oxytocin and kinins but clearly such differentiation must receive emphasis in future.

With such provisos in mind however, the assay of antidiuretic material in whole blood, serum or plasma can be performed by direct injection of the fluid (sometimes after appropriate dilution) into the animal used for assay.

When using whole blood, donor and recipient animals of the same species are preferred, at least when *in vivo* assay preparations are involved. Such investigations have been made in the rabbit (WALKER, 1939), the dog (AMES et al., 1950) and in man (BARNET et al., 1952). Nevertheless, for special purposes, assay animals of different species from donors may be used as for instance in the estimation in the rabbit of the oxytocin activity of blood taken serially from parturient women (MENDEZ-BAUER, FITZPATRICK et al., 1960; COCH et al., 1965). In this work the sensitivity of the assay animals deteriorated progressively and rapidly so that only bracketing assays were possible, but this was adequate for the purpose under investigation; moreover it provided a method of avoiding difficulties due to the presence of oxytocinase in the blood. With *in vitro* preparations for oxytocin assay there is more freedom: for instance SIDDIQI and WALKER (1960) superfused rabbit arterial blood over the rat uterus successfully and the isolated mammary gland of the rabbit may be used to measure oxytocin in blood or plasma, if present in high concentration (MENDEZ-BAUER et al., 1960; MOORE and ZARROW, 1965). WALMSLEY's (1963) procedure is to be commended for *in vivo* work. She assayed fresh plasma in lactating guinea-pigs, obtaining only approximate results because of the deterioration: active samples were subsequently reassayed with precision — and good agreement — after gel filtration, lyophilisation and chromatography.

Early assays measuring the ADH activity of plasma and serum were carried out by s.c. or i.p. injection into hydrated rats and this gave rise to some discrepancies in the results, in that the activity of serum did not appear to be the same as in plasma (DICKER and GINSBURG, 1950; GINSBURG and HELLER, 1951) although CROXATTO et al. (1952) did not find this to be so. These differences were resolved (see AMES and VAN DYKE, 1952; DICKER, 1953) by use of i.v. route of injection into rats when it became clear that materials in plasma and serum may interfere with the accuracy of assays for ADH using the s.c. or i.p. method of injection. Thus many of the original excessively high estimates of ADH in plasma using i.p. or s.c. injection must be rejected as discussed above.

Furthermore it is now recognised that when blood coagulates many active substances (kinins, 5-hydroxytryptamine and others) are liberated into the serum in concentrations with oxytocic and antidiuretic activity. Serum cannot be considered for direct assays.

Usually when plasma is to be used, blood is collected into heparinised tubes, preferably from heparinised donors and is then centrifuged: plasma may be injected for assay within 10 min. (When the blood is taken from pregnant primates however even this period is too long, due to the presence of inactivating enzymes, unless the blood is maintained at low temperature.) Plasma so prepared from a wide variety of species has been injected into ethanol anaesthetised rats for antidiuretic assays. BUCHBORN (1955, 1956, 1957) also injected diluted untreated plasma into the lymph sacs of toads for assay purposes. Limitations of such assays for ADH are based on the volume of injection (which is limited to 1 ml in the rat) and the corresponding sensitivity of the assay animal rather than on the presence of interfering substances.

The possibility of interference caused by substances present in plasma does not appear to have been reported in the i.v. rat assay but it may be wise to consider such a possibility. SHARE (1965) noted that the presence of 0.1% bovine plasma albumen in standard solutions of ADH injected into ethanol anaesthetised rats results in a potentiation of the antidiuretic activity 1.5 times, and it seems possible that this may also occur in plasma. However, CZACZKES et al. (1964) added ADH to plasma and found that when this was injected into rats recovery was close to 100% (see Table 9). Attempts to confirm that the material for assay is identical with ADH (for instance, inactivation by thioglycollate or enzymes) should be routinely performed.

When oxytocin assays are attempted with carefully prepared plasma the chief disadvantage is the progressive deterioration of the preparations, both *in vivo* and *in vitro*, and this prohibits the repetitive observations necessary for critical assays except where each observation is made on fresh pieces of tissue *in vitro* (VAN DONGEN and HAYS, 1966a). With each injection of plasma, intravenously or intraarterially, a fall in blood pressure is consistently observed and this is likely to reflect a progressive deterioration in the circulation in general and in the mammary gland in particular, leading to loss of sensitivity to oxytocin. There is also a high probability that this hypotensive response to plasma results in the release of hormones from the neurohypophysis, especially ADH (BELESLIN et al., 1967). In these circumstances, injections of plasma or blood cannot be considered as good methods. *In vitro* methods of assay are less vulnerable to the disadvantages of whole plasma but sensitivity is still a limitation, especially where wide physiological variations in hormone concentrations may be expected as with oxytocin in parturition (FITZ-

PATRICK and WALMSLEY, 1965), or in milk let-down (FOLLEY and KNAGGS, 1965). For such investigations, an assay method will only be of use for direct estimation of hormones in blood or plasma if response is proportional to dose over a range of concentrations of perhaps a million-fold: this is true of the VAN DONGEN and HAYS (1964, 1966a, b) method of assay, but of no other. There are other limitations to this particular assay, discussed earlier, but its outstanding advantage seems to be that it permits fresh blood and plasma to be used to good purpose.

Plasma containing ADH (or possibly oxytocin) can be stored to await assay but certain precautions should be taken. The optimal pH for stability of both octapeptides in aqueous solutions is about 3. For relatively short periods of time (1 h) and in the absence of semi-specific enzymes, inactivation is not great. Thus ADAMSONS, ENGEL, and VAN DYKE (1958) found that the concentration of endogenous ADH in dog plasma at pH 7.8 decreased only 30% in 48 h at 2° C. GINSBURG and HELLER (1953b) noted a reduction in rat plasma of about 50% in 20 h at 5° C. DETTELBACH (1958) acidified (pH 3) rat plasma, to which ADH had been added, brought it to the boil and stored it at —20° for 130 days without loss of activity. CZACZKES et al. (1964) measured the stability of endogenous ADH in human plasma and found that while it was stable at room temperature for 40 min there was some decrease in 1—2 h even if it was refrigerated. They found that the most satisfactory procedure was to divide the plasma into 1—2 ml samples, freeze it by dropping pebbles of solid CO_2 into the container and then to store it at —20°. After 17 days there was no detectable loss in activity. Very few workers have described storage of plasma prior to oxytocin assays, although much the same stability would be expected.

C. Extraction of Blood and Plasma

From what has been said above concerning the limitations of conducting assays on fresh plasma (or other biological fluids) it follows that some form of extraction must usually be practised. These may be simple and based on the separation of large molecular substances only (in which case the protein-free solutions must still be considered as possibly containing interfering substances) or they may be more complex in which case, after initial separation from protein, the hormones are "purified" by separation from other relatively small molecular substances, and from each other. With increasing complexity of purification, one must expect greater losses and the investigator must balance the good recoveries of simple methods against the disadvantages of assaying impure extracts.

The neurohypophysial hormones are thought to be transported in the blood, bound to protein in an easily dissociable form. There is considerable confusion on the magnitude of this binding which may well vary between species, and the account of GINSBURG (this volume) should be consulted.

Dialysis and Ultrafiltration

In 1924 SMITH and MCCLOSKY demonstrated that neurohypophysial hormones added to saline solutions can pass through dialysis membranes. This suggested that well tried dialysis procedures may be useful in extracting neurohypophysial hormones from body fluids. There is, however, considerable confusion in the literature as to whether or not the hormones present in blood or urine can pass across dialysis membranes. Thus early procedures for extraction from blood depended on the observation that the hormones pass through such membranes into the dialysate or ultrafiltrate while, in contrast to this, extraction from urine was dependant on their retention by such membranes (see later section). In addition it was found that neurohypophysial hormones added to urine passed through the membranes far more readily than the endogenous antidiuretic material, suggesting that the latter is bound to some larger molecule (see extraction of urine). To almost completely confuse the picture it was found that when neurohypophysial hormones are added to blood they do not necessarily dialyse readily from this medium.

Experiments using exogenous neurohypophysial extracts are inconsistent. In 1937 HELLER found that such extracts added to rabbit blood were not dialysable or ultrafiltratable and he reviewed the evidence previous to this which generally supported his conclusions (see, for instance, THEOBALD, 1934a; LEVITT, 1936). Neurohypophysial hormones added to human plasma have also been shown to pass relatively slowly across a dialysis membrane as compared with the observed fast rate when they are dissolved in a saline solution (HELLER, 1957). The effect of the dielectric constant of the solvent on the rate of passage of peptides across dialysis membranes, has been critically evaluated by CRAIG, HARFENIST, and PALADINI (1964).

Consideration of more recent experiments using the endogenous ADH present in blood unfortunately does not help us resolve the problem. Using rat serum THORN and SILVER (1957) and THORN (1959a) found that the hormone present did not pass through a collodion ultrafilter and that the active material, oxytocic as well as antidiuretic, moved electrophoretically with the beta-globulins. Dialysis against 0.2 N acetic acid (pH about 2.5) resulted in the hormones passing across the membrane indicating that this procedure apparently dissociated the complex. These experiments were confirmed by SMITH and THORN (1965). A somewhat similar complex formation in human plasma has been described by DINGMAN (1957) and ARIMURA and YAMAGUCHI (1964).

Experiments using dog plasma contrast with these observations. LAUSON (1960) and BOCANEGRA and LAUSON (1961) found that 75—80% of the antidiuretic material present was ultrafiltratable and presumably in the free state. More recently BROOK and SHARE (1966), also using dogs, carried out a careful series of experiments both *in vitro* and *in vivo* and characterized their material by cation-exchange chromatographic extraction prior to assay. They dialysed the blood of dogs in an *in vivo* system and recovered ADH in the dialysate and also found that *in vitro* it passed across dialysis membranes equally rapidly from blood or a saline-dextran solution. It is difficult to assess much of the evidence from earlier experiments, as relatively insensitive and sometimes unspecific assay procedures were used and the pH was not always clearly stated.

The use of dialysis procedures to separate ADH and oxytocin from blood cannot at present be recommended as it is uncertain if the hormones will pass across the membranes and if so in what quantity. There is too much uncertainty about species variation. In addition although the hormone may be separated from the plasma proteins the possibility that other small molecules, which could interfere with the assays, may also move in this way must be considered.

Alternative methods of extracting the hormones from blood have been developed and usually these involve the removal of protein from solution as the first, or in many cases the principle step. Usually deproteinisation involves either gel filtration or precipitation. Denaturing agents used include ethanol, acid ethanol, acetone, trichloroacetic acid and boiling water. In addition to retaining the hormones in solution, and removing the proteins which interfere with bioassay, these agents also denature those enzymes in blood which inactivate polypeptide hormones and also those enzymes which liberate interfering substances. Table 10 gives a summary of methods together with published estimates of recovery of added hormones.

Table 10. *Recoveries of vasopressin or oxytocin by various extraction procedures*

Material extracted	Extraction method	Purification	Concentration temperature	Elution fluid	Recovery ADH	Recovery Oxy.	Ref.
Blood	acid ethanol	dialysis	40° C max.	—	116%	101%	1
Blood	acid ethanol	dialysis	40° C max.	—	31%	35%	2
Blood	acid ethanol	dialysis	50° C max.	—	68%	77%	3
Blood	acid ethanol	dialysis	45° C max.	—	—	83%	4
Blood or Plasma	acetone	—	40° C max.	—	(<60%)	87%	5
Blood or Plasma	acetone	—	40° C max.	—	—	88%	6
Blood or Plasma	acetone	Sephadex	lyophilise — 70° C	water	—	74%	7
Blood	ethanol	—	55° C max.	—	69%	84%	8
Blood	ethanol	—	55° C max.	—	75%	78%	9
Plasma	water 100°C	dialysis	lyophilisation	—	—	55%	10
Blood	T.C.A. 15%	ion-exchanger	< 30° C	pyridine acetate	60%	—	11
Blood	T.C.A. 12.5%	ion-exchanger	—	pyridine acetate	40%	—	12
Blood	T.C.A. 12.5%	ion-exchanger	20° C	acid ethanol	80—90%	—	13
Plasma	T.C.A. 12.5%	ion-exchanger	50° C	acetic acid	89%	—	14
Plasma	T.C.A. 7.5%	1) ion-exchange 2) electro-phoresis	lyophilisation	1) aqueous pyridine 2) saline	—	35%	15
Plasma	—	Sephadex	lyophilise — 70° C	water	—	70%	7
Plasma	—	Sephadex	lyophilisation	water	—	85%	16
Blood	—	Sephadex	lyophilisation	water	—	74%	17
Sephadex Eluates	—	ion-exchanger	lyophilisation	ammon acetate	—	55%	17

References: 1: BISSET and WALKER (1954); 2: BISSET et al. (1956); 3: BISSET and LEE (1957); 4: BISSET (1961); 5: GINSBURG and SMITH (1959); 6: FITZPATRICK (1961); 7: WALMSLEY (1963); 8: BELESLIN et al. (1967); 9: BISSET et al. (1967); 10: COCH et al. (1965); 11: WEINSTEIN et al. (1960); 12: SHARE (1961); 13: MORAN et al. (1964); 14: YOSHIDA et al. (1963); 15: COCH et al. (1967); 16: FOLLEY and KNAGGS (1965); 17: KNAGGS (1966).

Acid Ethanol

In 1937 MELVILLE rejected dialysis and ultrafiltration as a basis for the extraction of the neurohypophysial hormones from blood and developed a method in which the proteins are precipitated with alcohol and the hormones remain in the supernatant fluid. This was based on the earlier recommendation of STEHLE (1933) that ethyl alcohol is the best solvent for the pressor and oxytocin principles of the gland, and on the success of MARX and SCHNEIDER (1934) who claimed to be able to measure 50 μU ADH per ml of blood using methyl or ethyl alcohol.

Melville's (1937) procedure, involved the addition of an excess (9 volumes) of 80% ethanol to heparinised blood. The mixture was acidified with N-sulphuric acid using Congo Red as external indicator. Subsequently the precipitate was filtered off, washed and the filtrate concentrated about tenfold. MELVILLE claimed a high rate of recovery but gave no figures.

Bisset and Walker (1954) and Bisset et al. (1956) modified Melville's procedure chiefly by concentrating to dryness at 40° C and by dialysing their extracts to remove potassium and 5-hydroxytryptamine liberated from cellular components of blood. Recoveries of added hormones were disappointing (35% for oxytocin; 31% for ADH). Nevertheless their method was used by other workers (Baïsset and Montastruc, 1957; Robinson, Hawker, and Robertson, 1957; Hawker, 1961). Bisset and Lee (1957) obtained better recoveries (oxytocin range 50 to 115%; ADH 47—90%) with a modification of the method in which concentration was effected more gently.

Their procedure, which should be regarded as the standard for acid alcohol, is as follows: 10 ml blood is collected in heparinised nylon or siliconed glass syringes to minimise the formation of kinins: it is then added to 9 volumes of 80% (v/v) ethanol in a polythene vessel, and N-sulphuric acid added until the solution turns Congo Red blue. The mixture is shaken vigorously, centrifuged immediately, and the supernatent concentrated *in vacuo*, to about 10 ml, at a maximum temperature of 50° C. (At this stage most of the alcohol has been removed leaving an aqueous solution, which evaporates much less readily.) This supernatent is placed in a vacuum dessicator, over phosphorus pentoxide, and is reduced to about 2 ml or less: the residue is subsequently dialysed for 45 min against tap water.

The limitations of the method relate to the production of substances which interfere with bioassay particularly on the uterus. These include agents released from whole blood cells, and also substances formed or extracted from plasma (Hawker and Robertson, 1958; Hawker, 1961). Some of these may be removed (for instance by dialysis) although this offers some risk of loss of hormones.

Because the acidification is effected with a non-volatile acid, the concentration of acid must increase to an unknown degree in the final stages of evaporation. It has been suggested tentatively by Fitzpatrick (1961) that this might produce from the small quantities of protein which remain in solution, biologically active peptides similar to those reported by Croxatto (1957) and Croxatto, Pereda, and Zamorano (1961) as being formed from protein by simple acidification procedures. In view of the success reported recently (see below) with acetic and trichloroacetic acids as plasma protein precipitants this suggestion now appears somewhat over cautious, but a change to a volatile acid for use with alcohol still seems reasonable.

Ethanol. Bisset has however resolved the problem by using non-acidified ethanol with good recoveries. With his co-workers (Bisset, Hilton, and Poisner, 1967) he has developed the following procedure.

Taking precautions against the formation of kinins, plasma is separated from blood cells and then treated with two volumes of absolute ethanol. The cells are washed with saline and the washings added to the plasma alcohol mixture which is then centrifuged (at 2900 gravity). The resulting supernatant is concentrated almost to dryness *in vacuo* at 55° C, the concentrate acidified (pH 3—5) and recentrifuged. The second supernatant is stored at 4° C until required for assay when it is neutralised with normal sodium carbonate. Recovery of milk-ejecting and antidiuretic activity after the addition of oxytocin (Syntocinon), vasopressin (Pitressin), or Standard Pituitary Posterior Lobe Extract, to human and cat blood corresponded to 77.6% $\pm$ 2.72 s.e. for oxytocin and 75.3% $\pm$ 2.91 for vasopressin. The range of hormone concentrations in blood from which recovery was attempted ranged from 40—20,000 μU/ml and recovery was good at low concentration as well as high.

Essentially similar results were obtained by Beleslin et al. (1967) using this method in Bisset's laboratory. These workers were able to show that no significant concentrations of interfering substances (bradykinin, 5-hydroxytryptamine, Substance P or catecholamines) appeared in their extracts.

Acetone. GINSBURG and SMITH (1959) and FITZPATRICK (1961) independently developed the use of acetone for the extraction of oxytocin from blood or plasma. Blood is collected with precautions against the formation of kinins and to it is added an excess (10 volumes) of dry acetone. The resulting protein precipitate is separated by centrifugation. The acetone is removed from the supernatant by evaporation in a stream of air at 37° C and the remaining fluid (mostly water) washed repeatedly with excess ether to remove traces of acetone and lipide materials which interfere with assay. Recoveries of oxytocin are as good or better than with the acid alcohol method. GINSBURG and SMITH recovered between 66 and 90% of hormone added to rat plasma and between 78—104% when added to whole rat blood. Their mean for all experiments was 87 ($\pm$ 2.7% s.e.: n = 13): the concentration of oxytocin added was 4 or 8 mU/ml.

FITZPATRICK (1961) attempted recoveries of a wide range of concentrations, from 8 μU/ml to 2.5 mU/ml in the plasma and blood of sheep and of man, whilst WALMSLEY (1963) extracted concentrations of 200—1000 μU/ml from equine and human blood: both these workers reported similar recoveries to those of GINSBURG and SMITH.

Although recoveries are satisfactory for oxytocin the method is unsatisfactory for vasopressin with recoveries always less than 60%, often very much less (GINSBURG and SMITH, 1959).

As with simple ethanol and acid ethanol extraction procedures, the acetone extracts may contain many substances which interfere with assay. WALMSLEY (1963) cleaned up her acetone extracts by gel filtration and paper chromatography. These are necessary procedures for work of any precision and are described later in this section.

In these experiments of the Bristol groups extraction was completed either without delay after sampling, or with storage at low temperature (—14° C; usually as protein free acetone solution). WALMSLEY (1963) has shown that losses are negligible with such storage over 1 week, but detected a fall of 20% over the second or third week. The method has become further suspect due to the recent demonstration by YAMASHIRO, ANNING, and DU VIGNEAUD (1965) that oxytocin (and also lysine-vasopressin and arginine-vasopressin) slowly combines with acetone to form a compound with very reduced biological activity (5%) and with different chromatographic mobility, to oxytocin. This inactivation is almost complete in 24 h at 25° C, with about 50% inactivation every 8 h. Clearly this reaction would contraindicate the use of the acetone method for experiments in which storage of the acetone extracts is uncontrolled. (WALMSLEY, 1963 encountered such a situation during an investigation in which oxytocin was found in the blood of one group of mares at parturition but not in another. For both groups large volumes of acetone extract were transported by road some 200 miles to the laboratory, with only primitive facilities for maintaining them at low temperature.) It is also speculative as to how fast such inactivation occurs at the temperature at which the acetone is evaporated off.

YAMASHIRO et al. (1965) indicate that the acetone-oxytocin compound is hydrolysed back to oxytocin and acetone by treatment with 0.1 N acetic acid at 100° C. Such a step could be added to the acetone method but would require close investigation before acceptance.

Hot Aqueous Acid. Although oxytocin and vasopressin for pharmacopoeal purposes have been traditionally extracted from posterior pituitary glands with dilute solutions of acetic acid at 100° C, such procedures have been rarely applied to biological fluids. BELL and MORRIS (1934) attempted this type of extraction using boiling mineral acid (as did THEOBALD, 1934a, b) but obtained unacceptably high values and the method was generally considered non-specific (BELL and ROBSON, 1935) and fell into disrepute. DETTELBACH (1958) was able to recover added ADH from plasma by boiling at pH 3. It is interesting therefore to note that COCH et al. (1965) at Montevideo have recently revived this procedure for the estimation of endogenous oxytocin in blood. The prime consideration of these authors was the rapid and certain inactivation of oxytocinase in the blood of pregnant women. Blood was collected from the region of the internal jugular vein and cooled to 0° C *during withdrawal*: plasma was separated at 0° C and then added to boiling water. This was adjusted to pH 5 with 0.1 N. HCl, the precipitated protein separated by centrifugation and small molecular substances removed by dialysis. Concentration was by freeze-drying and storage was effective in the dry state at 4° C or below. Of oxytocin added up to concentrations of 100 μU/ml, 55% was recovered. Somewhat surprisingly, in view of the results of BELL and MORRIS (1934), CROXATTO (1957) and CROXATTO et al. (1961), interfering substances did not cause trouble, at least in mammary gland assays.

Trichloroacetic Acid and Ion Exchange Resins. Trichloroacetic acid is a potent protein precipitant, which can be removed easily at a later stage by a variety of methods. In recent years it has been used in association with the subsequent absorption of the polypeptide hormones on to Amberlite columns. The use of ion-exchange chromatography for the purification and separation of neurohypophysial hormones was pioneered by TAYLOR in 1954, by LIGHT, ACHER, and DU VIGNEAUD (1957) and ACHER, LIGHT, and DU VIGNEAUD (1958). These peptides were found to be absorbed on to small columns of Amberlite CG-50 from which they could be eluted separately by use of concentration and pH gradients. ACHER et al. (1958) prepared extracts of neurohypophysial tissue by separating the peptides from proteins by precipitation of the latter with trichloroacetic acid and freeing the peptides of the trichloroacetic acid in an ion-exchange column (Amberlite AR-45).

These procedures were modified by WEINSTEIN et al. (1960) in order to extract ADH from large samples (100 ml) of blood. The procedure they used involved precipitation of blood protein with ice cold 15% trichloroacetic acid, removal of the trichloroacetic acid with ether, and after adjusting the pH to 4.5 with ammonium hydroxide passing the solution through a short ion-exchange column in the hydrogen form. ADH is retained on the column at this pH but is later eluted with a pyridine-acetic acid buffer, both components of which are volatile and removed during concentration *in vacuo*. These authors recorded a recovery rate of 60% (range 52 to 67%) using a concentration of 50 μU/ml and a pressor method of assay.

A year later SHARE (1961) described a slightly modified version, which he used for measurement of ADH in smaller volumes of blood, final assay being by antidiuresis in the rat. Share's method of extraction, which is very similar to that of WEINSTEIN et al. (1960) is given in detail:

1. 10—15 ml of blood is added to 4 volumes of 12.5% trichloroacetic acid at 0° C and mixture centrifuged. The precipitate is washed with 1 volume of 10% trichloroacetic acid and twice with half volumes of 5% trichloroacetic acid.
2. The washings and supernatant are filtered (No. 12 Whatman) and trichloroacetic acid removed by triple extraction with equal volumes of di-ethyl ether.
3. Solution adjusted to pH 4.5 with ammonium hydroxide.
4. Pass through ion-exchange column, 1 cm high × 1 cm diameter at a rate of 1 ml/min. (Amberlite, IRC-50 ground form XE-64 in hydrogen form, prepared according to HIRS, MOORE, and STEIN (1953) and washed successively with 30% pyridine/4% acetic acid, water, 2N hydrochloric acid and water.)

5. Wash column with 10 ml water and elute with 25 ml 30% pyridine/4% acetic acid, into flasks containing 3 mg l-cystine in 0.5 ml of 17.6% formic acid (to ensure stability of hormone) and evaporate to dryness *in vacuo*.

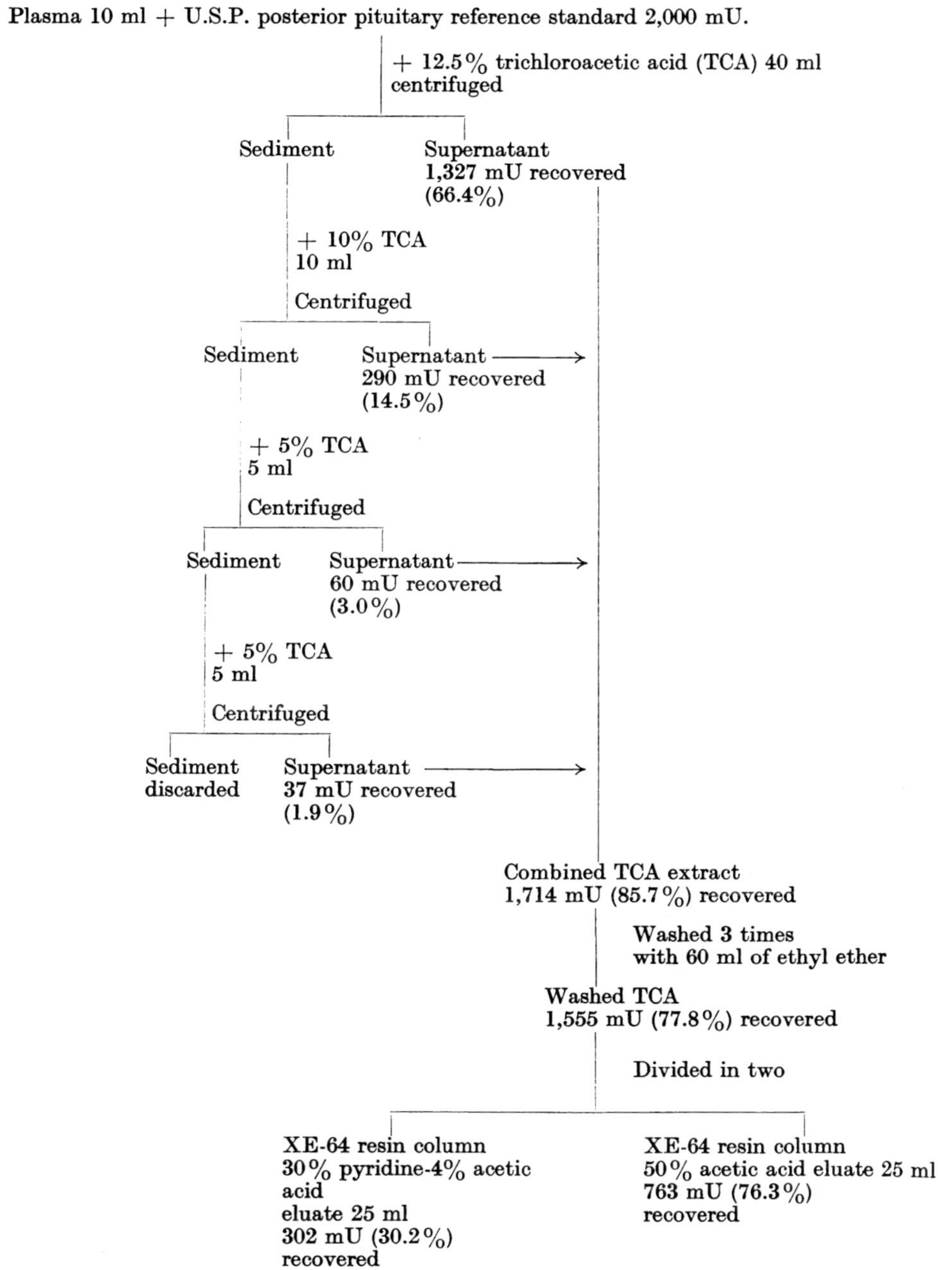

Fig. 17. The successive stages of the extraction of ADH from blood plasma is shown, with the recovery at each stage (YOSHIDA et al., 1963)

6. Traces of pyridine are removed by washing 5 times with water and concentrated *in vacuo*.

Using this procedure SHARE recovered only 40% of ADH added to whole blood but when he used plasma instead, he obtained 65% recovery (1965).

The procedure of SHARE has been used with small modifications chiefly with regard to materials used to elute the ADH from the column. Thus YOSHIDA et al. (1963) eluted the hormone with 50% acetic acid (see also DINGMAN, GONZALEZ-AUVERT, AHMED and AKIMURA, 1965; DINGMAN, AHMED, and GEORGE, 1966) and, as the hormone is stable in this solution, omitted addition of l-cystine to the final eluate. In an impressive step-by-step comparison using the two elution fluids pyridine-acetic acid and 50% acetic acid they found that considerable losses of ADH occurred during the washing procedures necessary to rid the eluate of pyridine (see Fig. 17). Using acetic acid they claim a recovery of 80—90%. The chromatographic procedures were performed at room temperature not 4° C as used by SHARE (see Fig. 17). MORAN et al. (1964) also used the method of SHARE but eluted the ADH with 70% ethanol acidified to pH 2 with hydrochloric acid and obtained recovery of 80—90%.

The material eluted from the ion-exchange column presumably contains a variety of peptides along with a certain amount of inorganic material (see DIXON and STACK-DUNNE, 1955). Further purification of the eluate has been carried out by DINGMAN et al. (1965) using chromatography on glass-fibre paper strip, impregnated with silicic acid. This procedure is described in detail by ARIMURA and DINGMAN (1959). For the purification of ADH they used a solvent system of butanol, ethanol and ammonium hydroxide (60:30:10) and for oxytocin n-amyl alcohol and acetic acid (80:5). Recovery was almost 100% after these procedures but nevertheless the method has not become popular.

COCH, FIELITZ, BROVETTO, CABOT, CODA, and FRAGA (1968) have used a similar method with trichloroacetic acid and Amberlite resin for studies on oxytocin in human plasma. After elution with aqueous pyridine, the eluates are lyophilised, and the residues taken up in a small volume of acetone water (2:1) and spotted on to suitably washed filter paper for electrophoresis (or partition chromatography). The electrophoresis strip of effective length 25 cm is carefully saturated with 3% acetic acid and sandwiched between two horizontal glass plates. Reservoirs of 3% acetic acid serve as conducting medium and an electric field of 10 volts per cm is applied along the strip for 2 h. A separate parallel strip is set up with synthetic oxytocin, and if necessary other peptides.

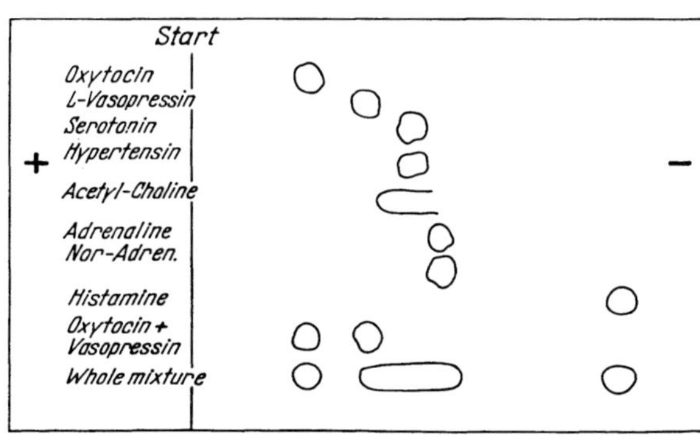

Fig. 18. Electrophoretic patterns demonstrating the migration of polypeptides and other substances on filter paper impregnated with 3% acetic acid: potential 10 volts/cm. Time 2 hours. (After BROVETTO et al., 1967)

The positions of the control spots are then visualised with iodine or with the procedure described by HELLER and LEDERIS (1958). Synthetic oxytocin migrates towards the cathode about 4.5 cm, well separated from vasopressin and other active substances which migrate faster as shown in Fig. 18. Sections (3 cm long) are removed from the parallel experimental strip and eluted by DENT'S (1947) method with Tyrode's solution. This elution procedure gives 100% recoveries, the electrophoresis separation gives 88% recoveries (with loads of 1—5 mU) BROVETTO et al. (1967). However, only 35% of oxytocin added to plasma and subjected to the whole procedure, was recovered (COCH et al., 1968) the greatest losses being during lyophilisation (40%) and on the ion-exchange column (35%). Nevertheless the results of the electrophoresis procedure are encouraging and merit further work.

ACHER, BEAUPAIN, CHAUVET, CHAUVET, and CREPY (1964) separated small quantities of hormones from neurohypophysial tissues by microchromatography on Amberlite (CG-50) columns eluted by gradients of concentration and pH. It may well be possible to modify such a procedure to isolate the hormones from blood in a relatively pure condition.

Gel Filtration. Dextran gels consisting of cross linked polysaccharide chains, almost inert chemically, have been used in column forms for separating substances widely differing in molecular weight. In general small molecules can diffuse into the particles whilst larger molecules are excluded by steric hindrance. When a suitable solvent flows through a column of such a gel it carries the large molecules through rapidly but the passage of smaller molecules is hindered to a degree inversely proportional to their molecular size.

Gels are available with different degrees of cross linkage and with corresponding different resolving power, expressed in terms of molecular size of solute. Sephadex G25 is the gel which has been used most widely for posterior pituitary hormones since it allows substances of M.W. 3500 and above — such as proteins — to pass with minor retention, but considerably hinders the passage of polypeptides of molecular weight 1000. Recently two new gels with higher degrees of cross linkage (G10 and G15) have become available which enable them to resolve compounds of lower molecular weight than G25. These permit fractionation up to M.W. 700 and 1500 respectively and may well displace or supplement G25 for this type of investigation.

Gel G25 has been used to separate oxytocin and vasopressin from protein in gland extracts (LINDNER, ELMQVIST, and PORATH, 1959; PORATH and SCHALLY, 1962) and oxytocin from the proteins in plasma (FITZPATRICK and WALMSLEY, 1962; KNAGGS, 1963; WALMSLEY, 1963; FITZPATRICK and WALMSLEY, 1965; FOLLEY and KNAGGS, 1965; KNAGGS, 1966).

The gel is initially swollen by mixing with saline (0.9%) and allowing to stand for several hours. It is then packed into a column (much as a chromatography column) with particular care to avoid creating channels or bubbles (see FLODIN, 1962). Relatively large columns (30 × 2 cm) are needed for use with plasma samples of 2 or more milliliters. WALMSLEY (1963) used polyethylene materials to support the column hoping to avoid the formation of kinins due to glass activation of blood enzymes, but she did not show whether this rather tedious precaution is necessary or even effective. KNAGGS (1966) obtained satisfactory results using glass supporting columns and reported no interfering substances detectable by i.a. milk-ejection assay. Maintaining the columns at low temperature is not an effective way of depressing enzyme reactions since the flow rate is greatly decreased, due apparently to increase in viscosity (KNAGGS, 1966).

Whilst proteins pass through the column as a band in advance of oxytocin or vasopressin, which themselves precede salts and some low molecular substances, simple gel columns do not generally allow separation of oxytocin from vasopressins or from other polypeptides such as bradykinin (but see FRANKLAND, HOLLENBERG, HOPE, and SCHACTER, 1966). All polypeptides should be considered as moving together and when it is necessary to establish the absence of extraneous polypeptides recourse is usually made to additional techniques such as chromatography.

Oxytocin and associated peptides leave the column diluted 5 or 10 times more than in the original plasma sample, and some method of concentration such as freeze drying is necessary. If the gel column is equilibrated and eluted with a saline solution this would have to be removed from the eluates by dialysis or other hazardous treatment, before lyophilisation, since high salt concentration would interfere with recovery of the hormones, with chromatography and with bioassay. Accordingly distilled water is used for equilibration of the gel and for elution, but this itself produces some complications. In the absence of salts, small quantities of basic aminoacids, such as arginine and histidine, and some proteins, including enzymes (which retain their activity), are strongly absorbed on to the gel, presumably by carboxyl groups in the gel (GLAZER and WELLNER, 1962; GELOTTE, 1966). The capacity of the gel is very low in this respect and they may be displaced readily by washing with 0.2 M sodium chloride.

Fortunately the absorptive effect does not appear to reduce the recovery of polypeptides seriously. Thus WALMSLEY (1963) recovered an average of 75% oxytocin (added to blood, plasma or saline) and KNAGGS (1966), recorded an average of 85% recovery for oxytocin added to plasma, and slightly less when added to blood.

However some degree of retention has been noted by HOPE, SCHACTER, and FRANKLAND (1964) and FRANKLAND et al. (1966) in the course of other experiments designed to separate oxytocin and vasopressin from the protein complex neurophysin. They found, using columns of Sephadex G25 made up in N-acetic acid, that not only could the protein be dissociated from the octapeptide hormones by elution with 0.05 N formic acid but that the two hormones were separated from each other, oxytocin preceding arginine-vasopressin. This separation cannot be attributed to a filtration effect due to a difference in molecular size, nor to molecular configuration since they appear in the wrong sequence. It is attributed to a greater affinity of the gel for arginine-vasopressin due to van der Waal's forces or to electrostatic attraction. This observation is stimulating for further work but as yet this separation has only been achieved in experiments using very large amounts of the peptides.

Recent developments of dextran gels which may have application to detection of hormones in blood, include thin layer techniques, the inclusion of ion-exchange in gel columns, and the production of gels which may be used with organic solvents.

Adsorption on to neurophysin. Recently PORTANOVA and SACHS (1967) have prepared a simple cellulose neurophysin resin which combines the advantages of the high specifity of neurophysin for oxytocin and vasopressin, with that of a solid phase adsorbent. Elution with 0.25 N acetic acid gave 90—100% recovery of microgram quantities of vasopressin.

D. Further Identification

Quantitative Interpretation of Assays. In many investigations it is desirable or essential to establish that the activity present in a body fluid (oxytocic, milk-ejecting, antidiuretic or pressor) is identifiable with a neurohypophysial hormone, endogenous or even exogenous. Although the specificity of a method of assay may provide some encouragement — as for instance with milk-ejection in preference to uterine assays for oxytocin — nevertheless none are specific.

The quantitative relationship of dose to effect may also be considered as serving to identify a substance: thus if an assay reveals that the dose response curve for an extract deviates significantly from parallelism with the corresponding curve for the pure hormone, then the activity of the extract is either due to another substance or to contamination with another substance. Tests for parallelism are then an essential part of assays but even when satisfactory they must not be taken as proof of identity since two substances may have the same dose response relationship (see Fig. 9). It is of course much less likely that such a similarity will apply to each of two totally different assay preparations and whenever sufficient material is available substances should be assayed on more than one preparation as proposed by GADDUM (1955) and exemplified for neurohypophysial hormones by HAWKER (1961) and SAWYER (1966a, b).

The identity of oxytocin in an extract can be more confidently interpreted by the use of recently developed competitive antagonists or inhibitors which are themselves inert or nearly inert (RUDINGER and KREJČÍ, 1962; CHAN et al., 1966). An illustration of such antagonism is shown in Fig. 19. Further aspects of identification by pharmacological assay procedures, particularly when one or more hormones are present in an extract simultaneously, are given in detail at the end of this chapter and are also discussed in chapters by RUDINGER and SAWYER.

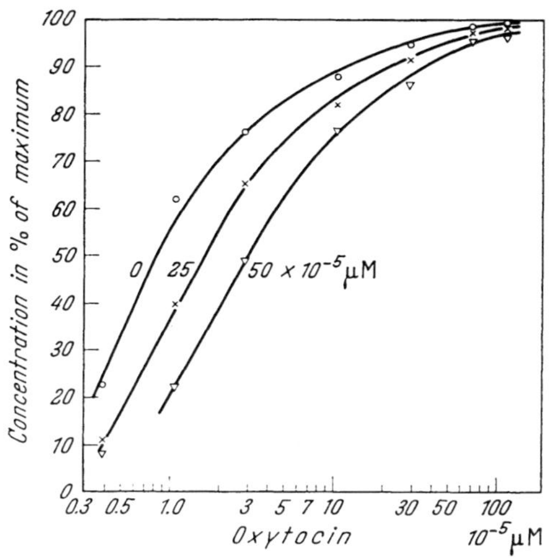

Fig. 19. The response of the rat uterus is shown in relation to concentration of oxytocin. In the presence of 1-l-pencillamine-oxytocin in stated concentrations (crosses and triangles) the response is inhibited (CHAN, FEAR, and DU VIGNEAUD, 1967)

Other procedures, to support the identity of a hormone thought to be present in an extract, include inactivation and chromatography. Inactivation has usually been effected by enzymes or sodium thioglycollate, both of which must be considered only semi-specific.

Inactivation. Freshly prepared sodium thioglycollate inactivates oxytocin and vasopressin due, according to VAN DYKE et al. (1942) to disruption of the disulphide bonds. This has been further studied for instance by BISSET (1961) who suggests that intermediate complexes may be formed with thioglycollates and other thiol-compounds. MARTIN and SCHILD (1962, 1965) have shown that although thioglycollate does destroy vasopressin and oxytocin, this is a slow process which is incomplete in the period of incubation usually adopted (30 min). However, a specific and reversible pharmacological antagonism between the hormones and thioglycollate occurs at the cell receptor level, the magnitude of antagonism depending on the concentration of thioglycollate. It is also shown by other thiol-compounds which do not disrupt the peptide molecule. The antagonism is effective on all *in vitro* preparations.

Since the site of inactivation of the hormones by thioglycollate, and the site of competitive antagonism each involve the S-S bridge in the polypeptides, it is apparent that this substance may also inactivate or antagonise other compounds with similar configuration and which may be present in tissue extract and contribute to their activity. FITZPATRICK (1961) for instance demonstrated that Substance P is also inactivated or antagonised by thioglycollate. The test must therefore be considered as non-specific although of course failure to affect the potency of an extract is some evidence of the absence of neurohypophysial hormones. It is also possible that other S-S compounds present could "protect" the hormones.

As proposed for an identity test (Ames et al., 1950; Vogt, 1953) extracts thought to contain neurohypophysial hormones are incubated for about 30 min at pH 7.4—8, with N/100 sodium thioglycollate *freshly prepared* as a Normal solution, from thioglycollic acid and sodium bicarbonate and added to the extract in the proportion of 1—100 volumes. However, this concentration of thioglycollate may interfere with the assay preparations themselves. A single application depresses many successive responses of the superfused uterus to small doses of synthetic oxytocin, unless the concentration is reduced to 0.002 M or less (Fitzpatrick, 1961). Martin and Schild (1962) have demonstrated similar relationships more elegantly for the isolated uterus in an organ bath. Even concentrations of 0.002 M given intra-arterially in guinea-pigs elicit abdominal (and possibly myoepithelial) contractions which interfere with oxytocin assays (Walmsley, 1963). It also may produce a non-specific antidiuresis (Sawyer, 1966a).

The thioglycollate test is, despite these limitations, still a widely used test especially for studies of antidiuretic hormone. Particular care should be paid to the conditions of incubation and assay, and to the inclusion of all relevant controls of any direct action of the thioglycollate on the assay tissue.

Inactivation by enzymes has also been exploited as a means of identifying active substances. The oxytocinase of human pregnancy plasma has been so used, particularly in studies directed at estimating the oxytocin content of human plasma, when it is a simple matter to take duplicate samples, one of which is suitably incubated to allow the enzyme to destroy oxytocin. This enzyme is apparently a somewhat specialised aminopeptidase and splits the oxytocin ring between the half cystine residue and the tyrosine component. It should not be considered specific, and in fact inactivates vasopressins as well (Tuppy, 1961).

Hawker and his associates in Queensland (Hawker and Robertson, 1958; Hawker, Walmsley, and Roberts, 1959; Hawker, 1961) have used this enzyme as one of a series to distinguish between on the one hand, their unknown oxytocic substance extracted from blood (animal as well as human) and on the other hand, oxytocin, vasopressin and a series of 10 other polypeptides including Substance P, bradykinin, hypertensin, pepsitocin. In addition to oxytocinase they used papain, pepsin, trypsin and chymotrypsin. For further details the original publications should be consulted but it may be noted here, for example, that trypsin inactivates vasopressin but not oxytocin. The use of such enzymes is not without snags. Sensitive preparations such as the superfused uterus respond to the presence of the enzymes themselves and care should be taken to control this source of error (Fitzpatrick, unpublished observation, 1967).

More elegant enzymatic degradation procedures have been proposed by Bisset (1962) and Beleslin et al. (1967) using purified tyrosinase at pH 7.5. This enzyme acts on the phenolic hydroxyl group in the molecules of oxytocin and both arginine and lysine vasopressin. Although the enzyme acts specifically on the tyrosyl residue at pH 7.5, at least some preparations of tyrosinase inactivate other polypeptides (for example bradykinin which does not contain tyrosine) although under different conditions (pH 3). This offers a method of distinguishing between activity in extracts due to the presence of oxytocin (or the vasopressins) and other polypeptides and it is recommended that whenever material permits it, duplicate incubations should be run at pH 7.5 and pH 3. The enzymes should be destroyed by boiling and the solutions neutralised before assay.

Chromatography. Ion-exchange and gel filtration columns have been mentioned above in relation to the demonstration of hormones in blood. In addition carboxymethyl cellulose columns and diethylamino ethyl cellulose Sephadex columns have been used to separate hormones in gland extracts especially those from the lower vertebrates: these are referred to at the end of this chapter. For the estimation of hormones in body fluids, chromatography has usually been confined to paper sheet procedures. This procedure was developed with reference to posterior pituitary hormones by HELLER and LEDERIS (HELLER and LEDERIS, 1958, 1959; HELLER, 1961; LEDERIS, 1961) and initially it was used to characterise pure substances and pituitary gland or hypothalamic extracts, i.e. when large amounts of activity were present. These authors tracked the position of their peptides by adopting the method of RYDON and SMITH (1952) for visualising a spot of synthetic oxytocin developed in parallel. Areas of paper corresponding to these reference spots are cut out and eluted in the usual way.

The procedure has been applied to the examination of blood and plasma extracts by FITZPATRICK and WALMSLEY (1962, 1965). Solutions are applied to Whatman No. I filter paper in multiple spots forming a horizontal band for the origin. After each application is dried more may be added, at the same spot, in order to load the paper with sufficient peptide to permit elution and detection, but this is a time-consuming procedure and likely to result in blurred lines of origin which of course will decrease the precision of the final separation. The sheets are developed for about 16 h (descending flow) at 18° C in a closed tank using as solvent system the organic phase of *freshly* prepared n-butanol-acetic acid-water, in the ratio of 5:1:4. After drying in a stream of warm air, which removes the traces of acetic acid, the reference areas are removed, the position of synthetic hormone visualised, and the main sheet cut into strips parallel to the line of origin. Each strip is eluted into a suitable saline solution and assayed.

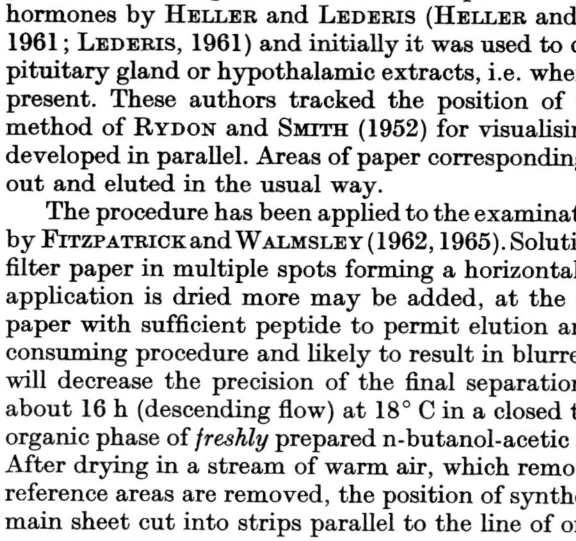

Fig. 20. Composite diagram representing the movement of various substances in sheet paper chromatography: Ox = oxytocin; AVT = arginine vasotocin; AVP = arginine vasopressin; LVP = lysine vasopressin; BK = bradykinin; A = angiotensin; P = substance P; 5HT = 5-hydroxytryptamine; Nor.Ad. = nor-adrenaline; H = histamine; X = milk-ejecting activity in plasma at parturition Solvent system: Butanol – Acetic Acid – Water: 5; 1; 4.

Using this procedure separation of oxytocin is good, since this substance migrates faster than most of the other substances under consideration (R_f 0.55—0.65). Lysine-vasopressin (R_f 0.1—0.16) and arginine-vasopressin (R_f 0.15—0.20) migrate much less and separation from interfering substances is less well defined. These relationships are well illustrated in Fig. 20, which is a composite representation of a chromatogram of neurohypophysial hormones and other active substances using the results of LEDERIS (1961), FITZPATRICK and WALMSLEY (1965) and COCH et al. (1965). Other solvent systems could be devised which would be more suitable for separation of the vasopressins (see ARIMURA and DINGMAN, 1959, and YAMASHIRO et al., 1965).

Paper chromatography is a tedious procedure requiring meticulous attention to detail. Losses may be considerable although with care recoveries of 65—90% can be expected. Some of the loss is probably associated with firm binding to the paper and before use this must be rigorously washed, preferably with acid ethanol, water and ethanol in succession. Furthermore the presence of proteins and salts in the solutions applied to the paper, greatly affect the R_f of the hormones and for this reason alone preliminary passage through a Sephadex gel is desirable.

ARIMURA and DINGMAN (1959) claim to have overcome the slowness and hazards of sheet filter-paper chromatography by using glass-fibre paper. Strips (6 $\times$ 15 cm) are impregnated with silicic acid, and dried in a dessicator. Two solvents are recommended with ascending development for only 30—50 min (butanol-ethanol-ammonium hydroxide in 60:30:10 ratio for vasopressin: n-amyl alcohol and acetic acid, 80:5 saturated with water, for oxytocin). Separation is said to be good. Recoveries of 1 mU quantities, after elution of appropriate strips in a physiological saline overnight, were between 90 and 100%. This method has as yet not become popular, possibly due to the difficulty of handling glass fibre paper, but if the results can be widely confirmed this would be a most useful technique.

E. Neurohypophysial Hormones in Lymph, Cerebrospinal Fluid, Foetal Fluids and Milk

Knowledge of the distribution of neurohypophysial hormones in the body is important when one is considering the metabolism of the hormone and the concentrations to be expected at target organ sites. Until recently detection outside of the vascular space had not been made. More sensitive assay procedures, concentration and extraction methods have made the measurement in the lymph possible, at least for ADH.

CZACZKES and KLEEMAN (1964) collected thoracic and cervical duct lymph from dogs and assayed it by direct injection in ethanol anaesthetised rats but could only find concentrations equivalent to less than 1 μU/ml, even though the plasma concentration was maintained above 700 μU/ml. Antidiuretic activity in the thoracic duct lymph of dehydrated and normal cats has also been measured (TATA et al., 1965) by direct injection into rats, and concentrations of about 1 μU/ml were found, equivalent to about 20% of the concentration in the plasma. This material, in contrast to that in plasma, lost 25% of its activity in 30—60 min. BROOK and SHARE (1966) collected thoracic and cervical duct lymph from dogs and extracted and concentrated it using the same method that SHARE (1961) used for blood. They found a concentration varying from 5—15 μU/ml in the thoracic duct fluid and 35—71 μU/ml in that from the cervical duct.

Studies of oxytocin in lymph have not been traced by the present reviewers, although it has been suggested some years ago (GINSBURG and SMITH, 1959) that the volume of distribution of oxytocin indicated passage beyond the extra cellular fluid compartment. This is further discussed by GINSBURG in this volume.

In 1936 LEVITT attempted unsuccessfully to demonstrate ADH in the spinal fluid of hypertensive subjects by the injection of 10 ml of this fluid s.c. into hydrated rabbits. He was unable to demonstrate any antidiuretic effect but further attempts using modern assay procedures would be worth consideration.

FRIEDMAN and FRIEDMAN (1933) refer to many earlier papers in which pressor, antidiuretic and oxytocin activity have been demonstrated in cerebro-spinal fluid and assumed to be due to the direct secretion from the gland into the fluid. In the light of the lack of specificity of the methods used by these workers they are not reviewed here and the interested worker is referred to the Friedmans' paper and to the review by HELLER and GINSBURG (1966). The Friedmans themselves attempted to overcome some of the disadvantages of earlier workers by using the fistulated rabbit uterus *in vivo* as test organ but the sensitivity was only 1 mU oxytocin i.v. They could find no oxytocin activity in fresh dog C.S.F., nor in human C.S.F. concentrated approximately 20—60 times (by a method using ethanol and dilute acetic acid successively and giving 80% recovery). This would indicate that if present oxytocin must be in a concentration of less than approximately 20 μU/ml. Vogt (1953) used more up to date methods of assay (isolated rat uterus; alcohol anaesthetised rat for ADH), of extraction (acid ethanol and concentration) and fo identification (thioglycollate and paper chromatography) but was not able to detect oxytocin or vasopressin-like activity.

Oxytocic substances have also been demonstrated in amniotic fluid but oxytocin itself has never been identified as such (Cuparencu, Grosu, Tomus and Idu, 1961; Hawkins, 1962). Most of this activity may be attributed to substances in the lipide fraction (Hanon, Coquoin-Carnot, and Piguard, 1961). Hawkins (1962) purified the active fraction chromatographically and obtained 4 distinct substances of a prostaglandin-like nature, which may be clearly distinguished from oxytocin (see Pickles and Fitzpatrick, 1966).

In investigations into the possible oxytocin content of foetal fluids not only must these substances and kinins be differentiated but in addition due regard must be given to the presence of uterine inhibitor substances, which are possibly due to the presence of the glycoprotein with these properties described by Stamm (1961). Karim (1966a, b) has reported that a substance which elicits contraction of uterine and other smooth muscle may be extracted by water from the arteries and veins of the human umbilical cord. The active substance has been distinguished from oxytocin, vasopressin and other known smooth muscle stimulants by a variety of pharmacological tests, by chromatography, electrophoresis and the action of enzymes. This substance has the characteristics of a lipid soluble unsaturated hydroxy acid.

Noddle (1962) has investigated whether that proportion of plasma clearance of oxytocin which may be attributed to the lactating mammary gland, is due to inactivation or to excretion. The milk of goats and cows when extracted by the acetone method (see above) produced contractions of the isolated uterus (superfused) but parallel assays on other isolated smooth muscle indicated that this was largely attributable to other peptides which may be similar to the kinins described in collostrum by Werle (1960). Oxytocin was stable when added directly to milk, but could only be detected in the milk after intravenous injection of enormous doses (up to 100 units).

F. Neurohypophysial Hormones in Urine of Mammals

Most of the reports published are concerned with ADH rather than oxytocin, probably because of the greater interest shown in the excretion of a substance which may be secreted over long periods, as distinct from one of which secretion is thought to be brief and intermittent. There is little reason to doubt that methods of extraction suitable for ADH will also be suitable for oxytocin.

Untreated Urine. It is usually considered necessary to extract, concentrate and purify urine, thought to contain neurohypophysial hormones, in order to eliminate the action of interfering substances. However, for preliminary investigations, when the concentration of hormone in urine is likely to be high and provided the material is given intravenously, extraction has not always been considered necessary. Hare et al. (1941) injected untreated dog urine i.v. into dogs with diabetes insipidus for the estimation of ADH. Human urine has also been administered in this way (Hare et al., 1945; van Dyke, Ames, and Plough, 1950) though an adverse reaction was noted by Hare et al. (1945) in some of the dogs. Ames et al.

(1950) and O'CONNOR (1951) also used this procedure in dogs. Direct injections of urine into rats have been made by many investigators (for instance, AMES and VAN DYKE, 1950; GINSBURG and HELLER, 1953c; DICKER, 1954; EISEN and LEWIS, 1954; CHAUDHURY, 1960).

GONZALEZ-PANIZZA et al. (1961) injected fresh human urine, from patients receiving macroinfusions of oxytocin (8 units/min i.v.), into rabbits and measured the oxytocin content by milk-ejection response. Normal urine does not elicit milk-ejection. Other workers have injected urine of animals directly into isolated organ baths and reported oxytocic activity (DALE, 1909; LARSON, 1939) but with such preparations normal constituents of urine may elicit oxytocic responses (GADDUM, 1955; HORTON, 1960).

Collection and Storage. While the urine is not always extracted prior to its administration certain precautions are usually taken, if it is not used absolutely fresh. In order to assure maximum stability of the hormones the urine is usually acidified to about pH 4 with acetic acid. THORN (1959b) found that when treated in this way it could be stored at 4° for 3 months with little loss in ADH activity. More stringent precautions, however, are to be preferred. EISEN and LEWIS (1954) froze the acidified material with dry ice and showed that it retained its ADH activity for several days: others have found storage of acidified urine in a deep freeze satisfactory (THORN and SMITH, 1965; STACY and BROOK, 1965). The urine may also be boiled and filtered as a preliminary to administration as well as to storage (see for instance, LARSON, 1939; KRIEGER and KILVINGTON, 1940; HARRIS, 1948; O'CONNOR, 1951; THORN and SMITH, 1965). This treatment presumably helps to precipitate any proteins present, rid the urine of volatile material such as ammonia and also sterilizes the material. The possibility that bacterial action on the urine may affect the activity in such preparations should be considered. Thus GILMAN and GOODMAN (1937) noted a loss in activity as a result of bacterial contamination and KRIEGER and KILVINGTON (1951) noted that faecal contamination of rat urine resulted in losses of the activity of post pituitary extracts which had been added to the urine. On the other hand KRIEGER, BUTLER, and KILVINGTON (1951) and CROXATTO et al. (1952) noted the appearance of materials with antidiuretic activity if bacteria were allowed to multiply in urine.

Extraction of Urine. Neurohypophysial hormones when present in urine are usually in low concentrations and may be accompanied by a variety of materials which may have undesirable actions when administered to animals or isolated organs. These not only include excretory by-products of various metabolic processes and substances such as the kinins (GADDUM, 1955; HORTON, 1960) but also various solutes which, if present in high osmotic concentrations, could influence the release of endogenous hormones in the assay animal. In addition, the injection of certain materials such as 5-hydroxytryptamine or kinins, especially by the subcutaneous or intraperitoneal routes, will result in pain or irritation which may also bring about endogenous ADH release. Contaminating materials may effect the rates of absorption of the hormone from the injection site (when not given intravenously) and so upset the accuracy of the assay (see for instance, NOBLE et al., 1939). Thus various attempts have been made to concentrate the urine and to rid it of undesirable contaminants prior to assay.

Dialysis. Dialysis and ultrafiltration through cellophane or collodion membranes are time honoured methods for separating large biological molecules from smaller ones particularly crystalloids. The use of dialysis for separating neurohypophysial hormones is, however, complicated by diverse views on whether they are loosely associated in urine with a protein, which could of course facilitate their retention by dialysis membranes.

GILMAN and GOODMAN (1937) dialysed acidified (pH 4) rat urine against water using cellophane membranes and showed that, while salts passed across the membrane the ADH activity was retained in the residue. Similar results were obtained by some investigators (AMES and VAN DYKE, 1950; AMES et al., 1950) but not by others; thus when posterior pituitary lobe extracts were added to various solutions, including urine, the hormone passed across the membranes (WALKER, 1939; SCHAFFER, CADDEN, and STANDER, 1941; HAM and LANDIS, 1942; DONALDSON, 1947).

However HAM and LANDIS (1942) showed that the endogenous antidiuretic material in human urine behaved differently from exogenous hormones of gland extracts in that it was largely retained by the dialysis membrane and could be concentrated by ultracentrifugation. They suggested that ADH present in urine is attached to some larger molecule. AMES et al. (1950) also found that endogenous ADH in acidified dog urine did not pass across dialysis membranes and showed that it could be concentrated by the ultracentrifuge. AUJARD, CSANYI, and LE BRETON (1954) found that the endogenous (but unidentified) oxytocic activity in rat urine was not dialysable. The early experiments of GILMAN and GOODMAN (1937) on rats were repeated by THORN (1959b) who found that small amounts of endogenous antidiuretic material were lost across the dialysis membrane but that the majority was retained. The antidiuretic material was identified as ADH by the criteria of inactivation by thioglycollate and trypsin digestion. The fact that THORN was able to measure small losses of endogenous ADH across the membrane was probably due to the fact that he had at his disposal a far more sensitive bioassay technique (ethanol anaesthetized rat) than was originally available.

Dialysis procedures to concentrate and purify urine for bioassay of ADH have been used widely, for instance: KRIEGER and KILVINGTON (1940), STUECK, LESLIS, and RALLI (1949), AMES and VAN DYKE (1950), KRIEGER et al. (1951), ITOH and KIMURA (1953) although others such as GROLLMAN and WOODS (1949) and NOBLE et al. (1950) found recoveries to be irregular.

When considering the separation of polypeptide hormones from urine by dialysis it is important to consider carefully the pH of the sample, the membrane thickness and the fact that, undoubtedly, small amounts of material may pass across the membrane. The losses during 3—4 h dialysis are probably small and may be balanced by the low recoveries obtained with more elaborate extraction procedures. However in some of the extraction procedures there is the advantage of more certain identification of the antidiuretic material with ADH.

The early and generally sustained dissatisfaction with dialysis procedures for concentration and purification of urine containing ADH has led to the development of a number of alternative methods.

Adsorption on to Collodion. In 1939 WALKER found that ADH could be adsorbed on to collodion. Urine brought to a pH 6—8 was filtered through collodion membranes from which it could be recovered by elution with 0.2 N hydrochloric acid. Recovery using this procedure was 81%. At a pH of 3 all the ADH passed into the ultrafiltrate. SCHAFFER et al. (1941) also used this procedure for measurement of antidiuretic material in human urine and obtained a 75% recovery.

Adsorption on to Zinc Ferrocyanide. NOBLE et al. (1939) demonstrated that various materials such as metal ions and materials present in extracts of blood and urine could delay the adsorption of ADH from subcutaneous sites of injection. They attempted to avoid this by extracting the antidiuretic hormone from the urine in the following manner: 100 ml of urine are brought to pH 5, 1 ml of 2N zinc sulphate is added and 1.125 ml of 2N potassium ferrocyanide added drop by drop with vigorous shaking. The mixture is cooled and centrifuged and the supernatant discarded. The precipitate is extracted three times with 25 ml portions of 80% ethanol containing 1% ammonia. This extract contains the ADH and is evaporated to a small volume *in vacuo* at 15° C and acidified. The solution is deep brown colour which can be further purified by precipitation of undesirable materials with 10 volumes of absolute ethanol. Recovery was 70—90% of the hormone added to urine. This procedure has been used to measure ADH in human urine after smoking (TAYLOR and WALKER, 1951, and BURN and SINGH GREWAL, 1951) and after exposure to high temperatures (HELLMAN and WIENER, 1953), haemorrhage, acceleration or fainting (NOBLE and TAYLOR, 1953). The recoveries of posterior pituitary extracts added to urine or saline mostly agree with the original claims; 81% (BURN and SINGH GREWAL, 1951), 80% (TAYLOR and WALKER, 1951), 109% (GOLDMAN and LUCHSINGER, 1956), 85% (NOBLE et al., 1950), but only 40% by BISSET and LEE (1958). The extraction has been discussed in detail by NOBLE et al. (1950) and NOBLE (1957). There is a high degree of impurity in the final extract and indeed GOLDMAN and LUCHSINGER (1956) experienced such a mortality rate in their rats that they resorted to further purification of their extracts with ether. NOBLE et al. (1950) rejected the subcutaneous route of injection due to the interference with "augmentor" materials present but found that the intra-peritonial route was satisfactory.

Antidiuretic material extracted from urine in this way has been identified chromatographically as arg^{8}-vasopressin (MAYER, 1960).

Adsorption on to Charcoal. GROLLMAN and WOODS (1949) used charcoal as an absorbant and eluted the antidiuretic material into glacial acetic acid. The following is the procedure used: urine is brought to pH 4.5—5 with acetic acid, 1 g of charcoal is added to every 100 ml of this acidified urine and the mixture agitated for several hours, left in an ice chest overnight and the supernatant discarded. The charcoal is washed with distilled water, suspended in glacial acetic acid (5 ml/g charcoal) and the mixture agitated for several hours. The acid is then separated and the ADH and other adsorbed materials precipitated by the addition of 10 volumes of equal parts ethanol and petroleum ether. The precipitate is removed by centrifugation, dried in a vacuum dessicator overnight and dissolved in distilled water ready for assay.

This procedure was used by ELLIS and GROLLMAN (1949) to demonstrate ADH in the urine of men, dogs and rats with various hypertensive conditions and also for demonstration of ADH in the urine of man (CLINE, COLE, and HOLDEN, 1953; STEIN et al., 1952; FALKNER, HAMMERSCHMIDT, and NEUMAYR, 1955).

The results of assays showing recovery of posterior pituitary lobe extracts from urine were not calculated by GROLLMAN and WOODS but the figures suggest a result of 90—100%. These results and the method have been strongly challenged by NOBLE (1957) and JESSUP, TAYLOR, and NOBLE (1957) who found after careful experiments that they could recover, at the most, only 10% of ADH added to urine. If 200 mU/100 ml ADH was added, recovery was negligible, while from 200 mU to 1 IU/ml, it was about 10%. In a step by step examination of the procedure they found 25% was not adsorbed on to the charcoal, 50% remained in the glacial acetic acid eluate and probably 15% remained on the charcoal. The error in the conclusions of GROLLMAN and WOODS has been ascribed by NOBLE to an error in their assay for the recovered antidiuretic hormone. It would thus seem that this method is not to be recommended.

Adsorption on to Cation Exchange Materials. ORR and SNAITH (1959) adsorbed antidiuretic material in urine on to a column of ZeoKarb 226 buffered at pH 4 and eluted it with acid alcohol. The recovered material satisfied the usual pharmacological and chromatographic criteria indicating that it was ADH.

A similar procedure was used by STACY and BROOK (1965) to isolate ADH from sheep urine. They modified the procedure of SHARE (1961) used to extract ADH from the blood (see section on extraction of blood). To deal with larger volumes of fluid (500 ml), urine acidified to pH 4.5 with glacial acetic acid was passed down a column of Amberlite CG-50 (hydrogen form) and eluted with pyridine acetate. The procedure was, however, modified. RUCH (1967) has also used Amberlite CG-50, in a larger column (5 × 12 cm) capable of dealing with 500 ml volumes of acidified, filtered, urine at 3 ml/min. Elution was with 50% acetic acid, followed by concentration *in vacuo*, and recovery of added ADH was approximately 75%. Extracted endogenous antidiuretic activity was inactivated by prolonged incubation (4 h) with sodium thioglycollate at pH 8.5.

These methods exploiting the developments of cation exchange resins would appear to be preferable to use of the older adsorption materials in that a purer preparation of the hormone is obtained more economically and elution can be made more selective.

Extraction with Phenol. NOBLE and his collaborators were not completely satisfied with the zinc ferrocyanide adsorption method for extraction of ADH in urine principally because it contained such a large quantity of contaminants. Subsequently they developed a new procedure (JESSUP, CARROLL, and NOBLE, 1956 and 1961) whereby the urine at pH 5 is concentrated five times and then extracted three times with equal volumes of phenol solution saturated with water. The ADH activity passes into the phenol from which it may be recovered by the addition of 3 volumes of diethyl ether, and back-extraction with water. The aqueous fraction is reduced to dryness and extracted with ethanol to remove impurities. The recovery of added post pituitary extracts was 85—90% and the final extract contained only one seventh of the impurities present after using the zinc ferrocyanide adsorption method. This procedure was also shown to extract ADH added to the blood with a recovery of 70—80%.

Excretion of Tritiated Hormones in Urine. Labelled forms of neurohypophysial hormones have been made and in the future may become increasingly available for experimental work although they are extremely expensive to prepare. TOWBIN and FERREL (1963) found that recovery of tritiated vasopressin from the urine correlated well with the radioactivity present suggesting that it could be used as a measure of hormone content.

Oxytocin, synthesised to include tritium labelled leucine has been administered to rats in large doses (0.1—15 units i.v.) and its distribution and excretion studied by AROSKAR, CHAN, STOUFFER, SCHNEIDER, MURTI, and DU VIGNEAUD (1964). Excretion into urine was very rapid — most activity appearing within 5—10 min but the total radioactivity recovered was only 20% of that administered. Parallel bioassay (on chicken vaso-depressor method) indicated that only 10% of the original biological activity was retained. The excess radioactivity is attributed to metabolic products undetectable by the bioassay.

IV. Assay of Neurohypophysial Hormones in the Suiformes and Non-Mammalian Vertebrates

The most satisfactory assays for neurohypophysial hormones were developed for the measurement of mammalian oxytocin and arginine-vasopressin and have been applied both to the measurement of these hormones in the quantities available in neurohypophysial tissue extracts and the relatively smaller amounts in the blood and urine. These methods have generally been applied with considerable success to the lower vertebrates but additional problems have arisen. Firstly several new hormones with different pharmacological activities have been discovered and secondly the quantities available are usually not as great as in mammals. The latter is influenced by two factors; the lower vertebrates that have been used are usually smaller in size so that on a unit body weight bases they would not be expected to contain as much hormone and in addition the fishes appear to have far less stored neurohypophysial hormone (on a body weight basis) than the tetrapods (see FOLLETT, 1963). The problem of accurate identification and measurement of the neurohypophysial hormones in the blood and urine have not yet been tackled in lower vertebrates. Even the circulating levels of lysine-vasopressin in the Suiformes seems to have been neglected. With the demonstration of a great diversity in the occurrence of lysine- and arginine-vasopressin in this mammalian group (FERGUSON and HELLER, 1965) and the obvious questions as to the genetic reasons for this, it is possible that interest in determining and identifying the vasopressins in the blood and urine of this group may be initiated. Previous methods for identifying whether an animal is a lysine- or arginine-vasopressin type (or even both) have depended on extraction of these hormones from the neurohypophysis; usually a terminal procedure. Identification in blood or urine could circumvent this and leave the animal available for breeding experiments. In addition, circulating neurohypophysial hormones in non-mammalian vertebrates may become of interest when a serious effort is made to decide their physiological function especially that in the fishes. Thus the determination of neurohypophysial hormones in the blood and urine of Suiformes and lower vertebrates is of potential interest but the discussion of suitable methods must be regarded largely as conjectural and theoretical.

A. Assay Methods — Index of Sensitivity 'S'

Apart from lysine-vasopressin in the Suiformes a number of analogues of mammalian arginine-vasopressin and oxytocin have been pharmacologically and chemically identified in lower vertebrates (see SAWYER this book). These are Arg^8-oxytocin (vasotocin, AVT), Ser^4-Ile^8-oxytocin (ichthyotocin, isotocin), Ile^8-oxytocin (mesotocin) and ser^4-glu^8-oxytocin (glumitocin). Others probably exist but have not yet been positively identified. The neurohypophysial peptides seem to have similar intrinsic activities in that they are fundamentally not very discriminating about the target organs which they can exite though they differ greatly in their potency at these sites. For instance mammalian oxytocin has an antidiuretic effect but only about 1% as great as arginine-vasopressin (ADH). In the same way vasotocin, although it is only found in lower vertebrates, has pronounced antidiuretic effects on mammalian kidneys, can stimulate the uterus and has a galactobolic action on the mammary gland. Thus one can consider the use of mammals for the assay of hormones that only occur in non-mammals and the converse of course also applies. The mammalian bioassay preparations have been well characterised over many years and some have a high degree of sensitivity to hormones from other species.

In Table 11 we have described the biological activity of the various neurohypophysial hormones in terms of the various assay preparations. While it is difficult to state unequivocally the sensitivity of these preparations to hormones we have substituted a figure (based on our personal opinion) for each assay. Such values are in terms of units of arginine-vasopressin for the rat antidiuretic assay and units of oxytocin for the others. If these estimates vary from the reader's he can substitute his own values. By dividing the activity of the hormone in IU/mg for any assay by the sensitivity of that assay in μU we arrive at a figure which we will term the "Index of Sensitivity". The higher this index the more useful the assay will be for detecting a particular hormone. Other factors such as reliability and accuracy obviously also will have to be taken into account before selecting the best assay for a particular hormone. The discrimination of an assay for one hormone compared with another can be seen from the relative activities of each hormone in that assay.

Table 11. *Activities of naturally occurring neurohypophysial hormones and their indices of sensitivity 'S'*

Hormone	*Rat antidiuretic*		*Rat uterus oxytocic*						*Mammary gland galactobolic*	
			Without magnesium			With magnesium				
	Activity U/mg	Index 'S'	Activity U/mg	Ind. 'S' (a)	(b)	Activity U/mg	Ind. 'S' (a)	(b)	Activity U/mg	Index 'S'
Arg^{8}-vasopressin	400[1]	*40*	20[1]	2	1	34[2]	3	1	70[1]	3
Lys^{8}-vasopressin	250[1]	*25*	5[1]	1	1				60[1]	3
Arg^{8}-oxytocin	186[3]	*19*	139	14	1	264[4,5]	26	5	100[1]	5
Oxytocin	5	1	450[1]	45	9	450[3,4]	45	9	450[1]	*18*
Ser^{4}-Ile^{8}-oxytocin	1[7]	1	150[7]	15	3	420[8,9]	42	9	300[7]	*12*
Ile^{8}-oxytocin	1[1]	1	289[1]	29	6	375[6]	38	8	328[1]	*14*

Assumed sensitivities of the assays: rat antidiuretic 10 μU; rat uterus (a) superfused 10 μU and (b) 2—3 ml bath 50 μU; mammary gland assay 25 μU.

References: 1: BERDE (1963); 2: VAN DYKE, SAWYER, and OVERWEG (1963); 3: Calculated from SAWYER, CHAN, and VAN DYKE (1962) using estimates of potency of more recent preparations; 4: MUNSICK (1960); 5: BENTLEY (1965); 6: FOLLETT and HELLER (1964b); 7: GUTTMANN, BERDE, and STÜRMER (1962); 8: SAWYER and VAN DYKE (1963); 9: FOLLETT and HELLER (1964a).

Vertebrates usually possess more than one neurohypophysial hormone and assays of hormones may be undertaken in the presence of other hormones or may require prior separation. In many instances, as for example oxytocin and vasopressin in mammals or vasotocin and oxytocin-like hormones in lower vertebrates, there is an assay available with a sufficiently great discrimination for at least one of these hormones, thus making their separation unnecessary. For example the pressor or antidiuretic assay on the rat is highly specific for vasopressins and vasotocin which can be measured using either of these assays. Vasotocin also has oxytocic activity but the amount in relation to the pressor-antidiuretic activity is known and can be subtracted from the total oxytocic activity of the sample, leaving an amount related to the other oxytocic hormone that may be present. In some instances sufficiently specific assays are not always available or suitable so that separation of the hormones prior to their assay is desirable. This occurs, for instance, with arginine- and lysine-vasopressin in Suiformes (FERGUSON and HELLER, 1965) and hormones with predominant oxytocic activities in some elasmobranchs (HELLER and ROY, 1965). In many instances the identity of the hormones in a particular species is unknown and SAWYER (1961b) developed ingenious combinations of assays from which the identity of certain hormones in such mixtures could be inferred. However, this is not always simple or feasible when, for instance, oxytocin-like peptides of rather similar activity are present (SAWYER, 1964). Positive identification and measurement will then depend on prior separation of the hormones by chemical methods. These procedures (see over) mostly involve paper chromatography (HELLER and LEDERIS, 1958; ARIMURA and DINGMAN, 1959), thin layer chromatography (FERGUSON, 1965) and column chromatography on various materials such as the ion-exchange resin Amberlite (ACHER et al., 1958).

1. *Lys⁸-Vasopressin*

Lysine-vasopressin (LVP) occurs in the Suiformes, the pigs, peccaries and hippopotamus. It may occur together with oxytocin or oxytocin and arginine-vasopressin (AVP). Details of the distribution in a large number of species are given by FERGUSON and HELLER (1965).

If the identity of the hormone is established and a reasonable amount of material is available it is best assayed for its pressor activity in the rat. If only a small quantity is provided the rat antidiuretic assay can be used. This is satisfactory for the assay of lysine-vasopressin (BERDE and CERLETTI, 1961) but there are a number of disadvantages if arginine-vasopressin is used as the reference standard. The two hormones have different periods of action, that of arginine-vasopressin being more sustained, thus making the choice of an index of response critical. If the maximum intensity of the antidiuresis is used as the index of response the dose response curve for the two analogues is not parallel (BERDE and CERLETTI, 1961; SAWYER, CHAN, and VAN DYKE, 1962). Synthetic LVP is available commercially and there is no reason why it should not be used as a reference standard in this and any other assays of identified LVP. The results can be given in terms of the standard units (pressor) or converted into micrograms. If LVP is present in a mixture with oxytocin separation is unnecessary and the usual assay procedures are sufficiently specific so as not to be significantly influenced by this hormone. However if AVP is also present separation is essential prior to assay.

Determination of LVP in blood and urine does not appear to have been undertaken but as suggested earlier may be a potentially useful procedure. If AVP is absent from the extracts the methods already described for arginine-vasopressin should be applicable but if present the hormones would have to be separated.

At present the main use for assays of LVP is to aid in its identification and distinction from AVP. There are several assays which are useful for this. The unknown vasopressin preparation is first assayed for its pressor activity in the rat. Its activity is then compared in different assays with a known sample of AVP or LVP (preferably both), the pressor activity of each extract being used as a basis for the comparison. If the maximum intensity of the antidiuresis in the rat is taken as the index of response, then LVP only has 60—70% of the activity (for each pressor unit) of AVP (SAWYER, 1958; THORN, 1959c; SAWYER et al., 1962). However, as the dose response lines for the two hormones converge the assay is difficult in that the differences observed will depend on which part of these curves are being used for calculation of the relative potency. Redesign of this assay using synthetic LVP as the standard may be possible. The dog antidiuretic assay affords a better method as the response to LVP is only 15% of that to AVP and such problems as occur with the rat assay do not seem to arise (VAN DYKE et al., 1956).

The hen oviduct (or "uterus") assay also provides a means for discriminating between the hormones, as AVP is about 8—10 times as active in contracting this organ as LVP (VAN DYKE, 1959). This assay was used by HELLER and LEDERIS (1960) to assist identification of LVP in the hippopotamus. Lysine-vasopressin and oxytocin may be separated prior to assay on hen uterus as the hormones have similar actions on this organ. However if the assays are performed in relation to the pressor activity present in the standards and extract this is probably not necessary; the conclusions to be drawn from the results should still be obvious. Thus if oxytocin is present in similar amounts to LVP the total hen uterus activity present will be double that if LVP was present alone but this will still only be about one fifth of the activity expected if AVP were present. In the presence of AVP the effects of oxytocin at its usual concentrations will be negligible in relation to the error of the assay.

HELLER (1963) described assays which could distinguish LVP from AVP and in addition to the above showed that assays on intact toads, newts and salamanders gave responses sufficiently different so as to aid identification. The dose response curves for water retention of *Bufo bufo*, *Rana esculenta*, *Triturus alpestris* and *Ambystoma maculosus* injected with various hormones, including AVP and LVP are given by HELLER and BENTLEY (1965) and BENTLEY and HELLER (1964).

More recently FERGUSON and HELLER (1965) have utilised the toad bladder natriferic (sodium transport) assay for distinguishing LVP and AVP, the latter hormone being about 10 times more active than the former. The hormones must be separated as oxytocin will significantly influence the response of the toad bladder. This method is, however, convenient, reliable and reasonably economic regarding the amount of material required.

Arginine-vasopressin is two to three times more active in producing an antidiuresis in man than LVP (equal pressor units) (DICKER and EGGLETON, 1961). FERGUSON (1964) used men (medical students) as bioassay preparations to distinguish these hormones but does not recommend it (personal communication) as the assays are technically more difficult to perform than those using the toad bladder natriferic response.

2. Arg^8-Oxytocin (Vasotocin)

Vasotocin (AVT) occurs in birds, reptiles, amphibians and fishes and may be present together with oxytocin (birds), oxytocin or Ile^8-oxytocin (reptiles, amphibians and lungfishes) and Ser^4-Ile^8-oxytocin (Actinopterygian fishes) (see SAWYER this vol.).

If reasonable amounts of AVT are available the assay of choice is the measurement of its pressor activity in the rat or if less hormone is available the rat antidiuretic assay. Both procedures are sufficiently specific to allow bioassay in the presence of the oxytocic hormones that may accompany it. If the AVT has been separated or is present alone it can be assayed for oxytocic activity on the rat uterus. Addition of magnesium (0.5 mM) to the fluid bathing the uterus will improve its sensitivity to the AVT 1.9 times (MUNSICK, 1960; BENTLEY, 1965) while (0.1 mM) manganese will improve it 3.3 times (BENTLEY, 1965). The standard hormone preparations used have been AVP for the rat pressor and antidiuretic assays and oxytocin for the rat uterus. These appear to be satisfactory in that there are no reports suggesting that the dose response lines are not parallel. However such a possibility should be kept in mind and if available it would be preferable to use synthetic AVT as a standard.

Measurement of AVT in blood and urine does not appear to have been reported but the well established procedures for AVP determination in mammals are probably applicable providing, of course, that the amount in the circulation of these lower vertebrates is comparable. From Table 11 it can be seen that the most sensitive and specific assay is that using antidiuresis in the rat.

Similarly as with LVP, a variety of assays are used for the pharmacological identification which can be made with reasonable accuracy by comparing the rat pressor (or antidiuretic) and oxytocin activity. In synthetic AVT this is present in the ratio 5 pressor-antidiuretic units/3 oxytocic units. Preparations suspected of containing AVT can be standardised either by rat pressor (or antidiuretic) assay or by measuring its oxytocic activity on the rat uterus. Assays can then be performed and comparison with AVT made in terms of equal amounts of pressor or oxytocic activity. The hen uterus is thus 12—30 times as sensitive to AVT as AVP/rat pressor unit and 220—550 times as sensitive to AVT as oxytocin/rat uterus oxytocic unit (calc. from MUNSICK et al., 1960; HELLER and PICKERING, 1961). In the same way assays based on water transfer across the isolated bladder of the frog *Rana catesbiana* indicate that AVT is 210 times as active as oxytocin and about 2500 times as active as AVP (calc. from Sawyer, 1960). When assayed by water retention on frogs (*Rana temporaria*) AVT was about 65 times as active as oxytocin/rat oxytocic unit (Heller and Pickering, 1961). Recently it has been reported that the oviduct of the mud puppy (*Necturus maculosus*) is very much more sensitive to AVT (1.2 nU/ml) than to oxytocin (Heller et al., 1957).

Changes in sodium transport (natriferic activity) across the skin and bladder of frogs and toads are also used to assist in identification of vasotocin (for instance, Acher et al., 1960; Follett and Heller, 1964a, b), AVT always being far more active than any other neurohypophysial hormones.

Assays using intact or isolated preparations of amphibia may show considerable species variation in the magnitude of the differences in response to different hormones including AVT. Thus the differences between AVP and AVT as measured by the water retention response of the toad *Bufo bufo* are not nearly as great as in *Rana esculenta* (Heller and Bentley, 1965). Obviously care should be taken to find out the characteristic responses to hormones for each species before using it for such assay procedures.

As already described the rat uterus oxytocic activity of AVT is potentiated 1.9 times relative to oxytocin in the presence of 0.5 mM magnesium, or 3.3 times in 0.1 mM manganese. In birds oxytocin is present along with vasotocin and it may be practicable to assay both activities using a single preparation of the rat uterus with magnesium or manganese present on one occasion and absent on another. The vasotocin present will potentiate relative to the oxytocin and the increase in activity will be related to the amount of AVT present. This can be calculated from the known potentiation of this hormone. The success of such a system will be dependant on the accuracy of the assays and the relative amounts of the two hormones present.

3. *Ser^4-Ile^8-Oxytocin (Ichthyotocin, Isotocin)*

Serine^4-isoleucine^8-oxytocin is present in actinopterygian fish accompanied on all occasions by AVT.

The sensitivities of the different assay preparations to this hormone are given in Table 11. If the hormone has been separated from AVT the usual assays for oxytocic activity on the rat uterus are preferable. The sensitivity of the hormone is potentiated 2.8 times by the presence of 0.5 mM magnesium in the organ bath fluid (Follett and Heller, 1964a; Sawyer and van Dyke, 1963) and this provides a sensitive and reliable method for assay of smaller amounts of the hormone. Alternatively the galactobolic assay may be considered in the context of the purity and quantity of the hormone available.

There is no single specific assay which allows the estimation of Ser^4-Ile^8-oxytocin in the presence of AVT as both hormones have oxytocic and galactobolic activity and it is not feasible to assay the former hormone in any other way. However measurement can be made by using dual assays, rat pressor or antidiuretic for AVT and rat uterus oxytocic for the total oxytocic activity present. The oxytocic or galactobolic activity associated with the pressor-antidiuretic activity of AVT is known and can be subtracted from the total leaving that which is due to the Ser^4-Ile^8-oxytocin.

Determination of Ser^4-Ile^8-oxytocin in blood or urine has not been reported. It should be possible to extract, separate and concentrate the hormone using the usual chromatographic methods and then to assay the Ser^4-Ile^8-oxytocin on a uterus or mammary gland preparation. If only mixtures of hormones are available a dual assay will again be necessary, the mammary gland to assay the galactobolic activity, the rat antidiuretic procedure being used to measure the AVT thus making subtraction of its galactobolic component possible.

Pharmacological identification of Ser⁴-Ile⁸-oxytocin is performed utilising several assays. As already mentioned the oxytocic activity relative to oxytocin is potentiated 2.8 times by the presence of 0.5 mM magnesium in the bath fluid and this figure so far appears to be specific to this hormone. When assayed on the frog bladder (water or natriferic) it is 30 times less active (unit for unit of oxytocic activity) than oxytocin (FOLLETT, 1963; SAWYER and VAN DYKE, 1963) and 40 times less active than Ile⁸-oxytocin (frog bladder natriferic, FOLLETT and HELLER, 1964b). Its ratio of activity galactobolic assay/rat uterus assay is 2.5 (SAWYER and VAN DYKE, 1963; FOLLETT and HELLER, 1964a) and fowl blood depressor/rat uterus 2.4 (FOLLETT and HELLER, 1964a). In addition the natriferic response of the frog skin is very much smaller than that expected from oxytocin (HELLER et al., 1961).

4. *Ile⁸-Oxytocin (Mesotocin)*

Ile⁸-oxytocin occurs in at least one reptile, some amphibians, lungfishes and a Brachiopterygian fish. Arginine-vasotocin is also present in all these instances.

This hormone is rather similar to oxytocin in its pharmacological properties and if sufficient material is available may be best assayed for its oxytocic activity on the rat uterus. In instances when it has not been separated from AVT the AVT oxytocic component can be calculated and separated by also performing rat pressor or antidiuretic assays.

This hormone has not yet been assayed in blood or urine but the procedures suggested for oxytocin (oxytocic or galactobolic) should be suitable if it is present in similar amounts as in mammals. If AVT is present it will also have to be assayed since it contributes a significant amount of the oxytocic or galactobolic activity present and the appropriate adjustments will have to be made. Separation from AVT should be possible by adapting the well tried chromatographic and elution procedures that are used for mammalian blood.

Although the pharmacological properties of Ile⁸-oxytocin are rather similar to oxytocin there are significant differences which are used to distinguish it from similar peptides. The most noteworthy is the ratio hen blood pressure depressor/rat uterus oxytocic which is 1.56 compared with unity for oxytocin (oxytocin is the standard for both assays) and 2.4 for Ser⁴-Ile⁸-oxytocin (FOLLETT and HELLER, 1964b). In addition the ratio rat uterus oxytocic plus Mg^{2+}/rat uterus oxytocin minus Mg^{2+} is 1.33 and the hen oviduct oxytocic/rat uterus oxytocic plus Mg^{2+} is 0.0036 compared with 0.11 for oxytocin (MUNSICK, 1966). The frog bladder natriferic activity is increased 1.4 times relative to its rat uterus oxytocic activity (FOLLETT and HELLER, 1964b).

5. *Ser⁴-Gln⁸-Oxytocin (Glumitocin)*

Using the procedure of gradient elution from Amberlite columns ACHER, CHAUVET, CHAUVET, and CREPY (1965) have separated and described the structure of a hormone present in the neurohypophysis of the elasmobranch fish *Raia clavata*.

This hormone, like isotocin or ichthyotocin, has serine present at position 4 but instead of isoleucine at position 8 has glutamine. It has weak oxytocic activity (about 8 units/μM) which is increased about 10 times when assayed using the rat uterus bathed in a solution containing 0.5 mM mangesium in addition to the usual constituents. This potentiation in activity clearly distinguishes this hormone from all other known neurohypophysial hormones and probably provides the most convenient procedure for its assay.

Heller and Roy (1965) also described the pharmacological properties of two neurohypophysial peptides which they isolated by paper chromatographic procedures from the pituitary of *Raia clavata*. Glumitocin is probably identical with their "slow moving fraction" which had a ratio of oxytocic activity rat uterus minus Mg^{2+}/rat uterus plus Mg^{2+} of 6.14 ± 0.9. In addition this peptide also showed a ratio of activity hen blood pressure depressor/rat uterus oxytocic minus Mg^{2+} of 7.2 and galactobolic/rat uterus oxytocic minus Mg^{2+} of 1.8. More highly purified preparations may give ratios which differ slightly from these values.

Both Heller and Roy, and Acher et al. (1965) identified a second neurohypophysial fraction the structure of which is not yet positively known but which has some pharmacological properties similar to those of vasotocin.

B. Separation Procedures

A detailed description of these procedures is not germane to this chapter but some examples of their uses and applications are given below. Paper chromatography can be used for separation of mammalian vasopressins (arginine and lysine) and oxytocin (Heller and Lederis, 1958; Arimura and Dingman, 1959), and the separation of AVT from oxytocin-like hormones in amphibians, reptiles and fish (Pickering and Heller, 1959; Heller and Pickering, 1961; Sawyer and Pickford, 1963; Follett and Heller, 1964a, b). This method has also been used to separate AVT and oxytocin in birds (Munsick et al., 1960). Thin layer chromatography on carboxymethylcellulose (CMC) can separate arginine- and lysine-vasopressin as they occur in Suiformes (Ferguson and Heller, 1965). Column chromatography on an ion-exchange resin (Amberlite) separates mammalian hormones (Acher et al., 1958), Ser^4-Ile^8-oxytocin from AVT in teleost fish (Heller and Pickering, 1961; Heller et al., 1961; Acher et al., 1962) and vasotocin from Ile^8-oxytocin in frogs (Acher et al., 1964; Acher, Chauvet, Chauvet, and Crepy, 1964). Carboxymethylcellulose is also used for column chromatography and separates AVT from Ser^4-Ile^8-oxytocin in teleost fish (Sawyer and van Dyke, 1963) AVT from oxytocin or Ile^8-oxytocin in reptiles and amphibians (Munsick, 1966) and oxytocin from vasopressins in Suiformes (Ferguson and Heller, 1965). Another ion-exchange ("exclusion") material that can be used for column chromatography is diethylaminoethylcellulose, DEAE-Sephadex (Porath and Lindner, 1961; Porath and Schally, 1962). Tissue extracts can be "cleaned" and prepared for subsequent separation procedures by "gel filtration" (Lindner, Elmqvist, and Porath, 1959; Sawyer and van Dyke, 1963; Follett and Heller, 1964a).

References

Acher, R., R. Beaupain, Jacqueline Chauvet, M.T. Chauvet, and D. Crepy: The neurohypophysial hormones of the amphibians. Comparison of the hormones of *Rana esculenta* and *Xenopus laevis*. Gen. comp. Endocr. **4**, 596—601 (1964).

—, Jacqueline Chauvet, M.T. Chauvet: Phylogénie des peptides neurohypophysaires. Isolement de la mesotocine (Ileu-ocytocine) de la grenouille, intermédiaire entre la ser⁴-Ileu⁸-ocytocine des poissons oisseux et l'ocytocine des mammiferes. Biochim. biophys. Acta (Amst.) **90**, 613—615 (1964).

— — — Phylogénie des peptides neurohypophysaires. Isolation d'une nouvelle hormone, la glumitocin (Ser^4-Glu^8-ocytocine) presente chez un poisson cartilaineux, la Raia (*Raia clavata*). Biochim. biophys. Acta (Amst.) **107**, 393—396 (1965).

— — —, et D. Crepy: Isolement d'une nouvelle hormone neurohypophysaire, l'isotocine, présente chez les poissons oisseux. Biochim. biophys. Acta (Amst.) **58**, 624—625 (1962).

— —, et Marie-Therese Lenci: L'ocytocine et la vasopressine de cheval. Bull. Soc. Chim. biol. (Paris) **40**, 2005—2018 (1958).

— — —, F. Morel, et J. Maetz: Presence d'une vasotocine dans la neurohypophyse de la grenouille (*Rana esculenta* L.). Biochim. biophys. Acta (Amst.) **42**, 379—380 (1960).

ACHER, R., A. LIGHT, and V. DU VIGNEAUD: Purification of oxytocin and vasopressin by way of a protein complex. J. biol. Chem. **233**, 116—120 (1958).
ADAMSONS, K., jr., S.L. ENGEL, and H.B. VAN DYKE: The stability of natural and synthetic neurohypophysial hormones *in vitro*. Endocrinology **63**, 679—687 (1958).
ALBERS, R.W., and M.W. BRIGHTMAN: A major component of neurohypophysial tissue associated with antidiuretic activity. J. Neurochem. **3**, 269—276 (1959).
ALTHABE, O., jr., I.C. ARNT, L.A. BRANDA, and R. CALDEYRO-BARCIA: Comparison of the milk-ejecting potencies of oxytocin and deamino-oxytocin in lactating women. J. Endocr. **36**, 7—14 (1966).
AMES, ROSE G., and H.B. VAN DYKE: Antidiuretic hormone in the urine and pituitary of the kangaroo rat. Proc. Soc. exp. Biol. (N.Y.) **75**, 417—420 (1950).
— — Antidiuretic hormone in the serum and plasma of rats. Endocrinology **50**, 350—360 (1952).
—, D. MOORE, and H.B. VAN DYKE: The excretion of posterior pituitary antidiuretic hormone in the urine and its detection in the blood. Endocrinology **46**, 215—227 (1950).
ANDERSON, R.R., P. KUMARESAN, and C.W. TURNER: Bioassay for oxytocic activity in posterior pituitary glands of cattle and rats. J. Animal Sci. **25**, 917—918 (1966).
ANDERSSON, B., and N. PERSSON: Intravenous assay of antidiuretic hormone using the goat. Acta physiol. scand. **42**, 257—261 (1958).
ARIËNS, E.J., and W.M. DE GROOT: Affinity and intrinsic activity in the theory of competitive inhibition. Arch. int. Pharmacodyn. **99**, 193—205 (1954).
ARIMURA, A., and J.F. DINGMAN: Specific and sensitive assay method for vasopressin and oxytocin using glass paper chromatography. Nature (Lond.) **184**, 1874—1875 (1959)..
—, and J. YAMAGUCHI: Serum protein-vasopressin bindings and its influence on the pressor activity of the hormone. Jap. J. Physiol. **14**, 90—101 (1964).
ARMSTRONG, DESIRÉE A.J., J.B. JEPSON, C.A. KEELE, and J.W. STEWART: Pain producing substances in human inflammatory exudates and plasma. J. Physiol. (Lond.) **135**, 350 (1957).
—, and J.W. STEWART: Spontaneous plasma kinin formation in human plasma, collected during labour. Nature (Lond.) **188**, 1193 (1960).
AROSKAR, J.P., W.Y. CHAN, J.E. STOUFFER, C.H. SCHNEIDER, V.V.S. MURTI, and V. DU VIGNEAUD: Renal secretion and tissue distribution of radio-activity after administration of tritium labelled oxytocin to rats. Endocrinology **74**, 226—234 (1964).
AUJARD, C., E. CSANYI, et E. LE BRETON: Recherches sur l'activité ocytocique des urines. Arch. Sci. physiol. **9**, 71—82 (1954).
BAEZ, S., A. MAZUR, and E. SHORR: Role of the neurohypophysis in ferritin induced antidiuresis. Amer. J. Physiol. **169**, 123—133 (1952).
BAINBRIDGE, M.N., W.C.W. NIXON, H.O. SCHILD, and C.N. SMYTH: Synthetic oxytocin. Brit. med. J. **1**, 1133—1135 (1956).
BAÏSSET, A., et P. MONTASTRUC: Polyurie par distension auriculaire chez le chien; role de l'hormone antidiuretique. J. Physiol. (Paris) **49**, 33—36 (1957).
BANS, H.W., u. J.M. OLSEN: Das antidiuretische Prinzip (ADH) und die Osmolalität im Serum bei der Adipositas. Acta endocr. (Kbh.) **31**, 426—432 (1959).
BARATZ, R.A., and R.C. INGRAHAM: Sensitive bioassay method for measuring antidiuretic hormone in mammalian plasma. Proc. Soc. exp. Biol. (N.Y.) **100**, 296—299 (1959).
BARNET, H.L., C.W. FORMAN, and H.D. LAUSON: The nephrotic syndrome in children. Advanc. Paed. **5**, 53—128 (1952).
BEAUVILLAIN, A.: Titrage des préparations post-hypophysaires par leur seuil d'action sur l'utérus isolé de rat adulte. C.R. Soc. Biol. (Paris) **137**, 284—285 (1943).
BELESLIN, D., G.W. BISSET, JAYA HALDAR, and R.L. POLAK: The release of vasopressin without oxytocin in response to haemorrhage. Proc. roy. Soc. B **166**, 443—458 (1967).
BELL, G.H., and S. MORRIS: The oxytocic property of the blood of the cow. J. Physiol. (Lond.) **81**, 63—69 (1934).
—, and J.M. ROBSON: Oxytocic properties of blood extracts and their physiological significance. J. Physiol. (Lond.) **84**, 351—361 (1935).
— — The effect of certain hormones on the activity of the uterine muscle of the guinea-pig. J. Physiol. (Lond.) **88**, 312—317 (1936).
BELLER, F.K., K.H. KRUMHOLZ u. K. ZEININGER: Vergleichende Oxytocin-Bestimmungen gemessen durch den lactogogen Effect der Milchdrüse. Acta endocr. (Kbh.) **29**, 1—8 (1958).
BENTLEY, P.J.: The effects of neurohypophysial extracts on water transfer across the wall of the isolated urinary bladder of the toad *Bufo marinus*. J. Endocr. **17**, 201—209 (1958).
— The effects of vasopressin on the short circuit current across the wall of the isolated bladder of the toad, *Bufo marinus*. J. Endocr. **21**, 161—170 (1960).
— Neurohypophysial function in amphibians and reptiles. Symp. Zool. Soc. (Lond.) **9**, 141 to 152 (1963a).

Bentley, P. J.: A method for the detection and estimation of small amounts of arginine vasotocin. J. Endocr. **26**, 295—296 (1963b).
— The potentiating action of magnesium and manganese on the oxytocic effect of some oxytocin analogues. J. Endocr. **32**, 215—222 (1965).
— The physiology of the urinary bladder of Amphibia. Biol. Rev. **41**, 275—316 (1966).
—, and B.K. Follett: Kidney function in a primitive vertebrate, the cyclostome *Lampetra fluviatilus*. J. Physiol. (Lond.) **169**, 902—918 (1963).
—, and H. Heller: The action of neurohypophysial hormones on the water and sodium metabolism of urodele amphibians. J. Physiol. (Lond.) **171**, 434—453 (1964).
Berde, B.: Pharmacologie des hormones neurohypophysaires et leurs analogues synthetiques. Paris: Masson 1963.
—, et A. Cerletti: Demonstration experimentale de l'action de l'ocytocine sur la glande mammaire. Gynaecologia (Basel) **144**, 275—278 (1957).
— — Quantitative comparison of substances related to oxytocin. A new test. Acta endocr. (Kbh.) **27**, 314—324 (1958).
— — Über die antidiuretische Wirkung von synthetischem Lysin-Vasopressin. Helv. physiol. pharmacol. Acta **19**, 135—150 (1961).
— — Medizinische und biologische Aspekte von Arbeiten mit synthetischen Peptiden von neurohypophysanem Typus. Klin. Wschr. **42**, 1159—1165 (1964).
—, W. Doepfner, and H. Konzett: Some pharmacological actions of four synthetic analogues of oxytocin. Brit. J. Pharmacol. **12**, 209—214 (1957).
—, and K. Saameli: The action of the synthetic polypeptide valyl-oxytocin on the human uterus *in vitro* and *in vivo*. Acta endocr. (Kbh.) **32**, 391—398 (1959).
Birnie, J.H., R. Jenkins, W.J. Eversole, and R. Gaunt: An antidiuretic substance in the blood of normal and adrenalectomized rats. Proc. Soc. exp. Biol. (N.Y.) **70**, 83—85 (1949).
Bisset, G.W.: The assay of oxytocin and vasopressin in blood and the mechanism of inactivation of these hormones by sodium thioglycollate. In: Oxytocin, pp. 380—398. Ed. by R. Caldeyro-Barcia and H. Heller. London: Pergamon Press 1961.
— Effect of Tyrosinase preparations on oxytocin, vasopressin and bradykinin. Brit. J. Pharmacol. **18**, 405—420 (1962a).
— Synthetic analogues of oxytocin acting as antagonists. J. Physiol. (Lond.) **165**, 69P—71P (1962b).
— Personal communication (1966).
—, Jaya Haldar, and J.E. Lewin: Actions of oxytocin and other biologically active peptides on the rat uterus. In: Endogenous Substances affecting the Myometrium. Memoir 14 Soc. for Endocrinology. Ed. by V. Pickles and R.J. Fitzpatrick. C.U.P. (Lond.) (1966).
—, S.M. Hilton, and A.M. Poisner: Hypothalamic pathways for independent release of vasopressin and oxytocin. Proc. roy. Soc. B **166**, 422—442 (1967).
—, and J. Lee: An improved method for extracting oxytocic and antidiuretic hormones from blood. Lancet **1957 I**, 1173—1174.
— — Antidiuretic activity in the blood after stimulation of the neurohypophysis in man. Lancet **1958 II**, 715—719.
— —, and A.F. Bromwich: Oxytocic and antidiuretic activity in blood from internal jugular vein in man. Lancet **1956 II**, 1129—1132.
—, and G.P. Lewis: A spectrum of pharmacological activity in some biologically active peptides. Brit. J. Pharmacol. **19**, 168—182 (1962).
—, and J.M. Walker: Assay of oxytocin in blood. J. Physiol. (Lond.) **126**, 588—595 (1954).
Bliss, C.I., and H.P. Marks: The biological assay of insulin. I. General considerations directed to increasing the precision of the curve relating dosage and graded response. Quart. J. Pharm. **12**, 82—110 (1939a).
— — The estimation of drug potency from a graded response. Quart. J. Pharm. **12**, 182—205 (1939b).
Bocanegra, M., and H.D. Lauson: Ultrafiltratability of endogenous antidiuretic hormone from plasma of dogs. Amer. J. Physiol. **200**, 486—492 (1961).
Botting, J.H.: An isolated preparation with a selective sensitivity to vasopressin. Brit. J. Pharmacol. **24**, 156—162 (1965).
Boura, A., and S.E. Dicker: An apparatus for the maintenance of a constant water load and the recording of urine flow in rats. J. Physiol. (Lond.) **122**, 144—148 (1953).
Bourguet, J., et S. Jard: Un dispositif automatique de mesure et d'enregistrement du flux net d'eau à travers la peau et la vessie des amphibiens. Biochim. biophys. Acta (Amst.) **88**, 442—444 (1964).
—, et J. Maetz: Arguments en faveur de l'indépendance des mécanismes d'action de divers peptides neurohypophysaires sur le flux osmotique d'eau et sur le transport actif de sodium au sein d'un même recepteur; études sur la vessie et la peau de *Rana esculenta* L. Biochim. biophys. Acta (Amst.) **52**, 552—565 (1961).

BOYD, E.D., and E.G. MACK: A method for assaying pituitary water retention principle. Endocrinology **26**, 153—159 (1940).
BROOK, A.H., and L. SHARE: On the question of protein binding and diffusability of the circulating antidiuretic hormone in the dog. Endocrinology **78**, 779—785 (1966).
BROVETTO, J., J. OLHABERRY, M.N. GIOIA DE COCH, H. CODA, C. FIELITZ, H.M. CABOT, A. FRAGA, and J.A. COCH: Chromatographic and electrophoretic separation of oxytocin from the substances that interfere with its biological assay on the isolated rat mammary gland. J. Endocr. **38**, 355—356 (1967).
BRUN, C., E.O.E. KNUDSEN, and F. RAASCHOU: Kidney function and circulatory collapse. Postsyncopal oliguria. J. clin. Invest. **25**, 568—574 (1946).
BRUNN, F.: Beitrag zur Kenntnis der Wirkung von Hypophysenextrakt auf den Wasserhaushalt des Frosches. Z. ges. exp. Med. **25**, 170—187 (1921).
BUCHBORN, E.: Ein quantitativer biologischer Adiuretin-(Vasopressin)-Nachweis an der Kröte. Z. ges. exp. Med. **125**, 614—625 (1955).
— Adiuretin und Serum-Osmolarität. Klin. Wschr. **34**, 953—957 (1956).
— Plasma level of antidiuretic hormone and serum osmolarity in normal human adults. Endocrinology **61**, 375—379 (1957).
BURN, G.P., and R. SINGH GREWAL: The antidiuretic response to and excretion of pituitary (posterior lobe) extract in man, with reference to nicotine. Brit. J. Pharmacol. **6**, 471—482 (1951).
BURN, J.H.: Estimation of antidiuretic potency of pituitary (posterior lobe) extract. Quart. J. Pharm. **4**, 517—529 (1931).
— Biological Standardisation. London: O.U.P. (1937).
—, and H.H. DALE: On the physiological standardisation of extracts of the posterior lobe of the pituitary body. Reports on biological standards. M.R.C. Special reports ser. no. 69, pp. 1—52 (1922).
CALDEYRO-BARCIA, R., and J.J. POSEIRO: Oxytocin and contractility of the pregnant human uterus. Ann. N.Y. Acad. Sci. **75**, 813—830 (1958).
CHAN, W.Y., R. FEAR, and V. DU VIGNEAUD: Endocrinology **81**, 1267—1277 (1967).
—, M. O'CONNELL, and S.R. POMEROY: Effects of the estrous cycle on the sensitivity of rat uterus to oxytocin and deamino-oxytocin. Endocrinology **72**, 279—282 (1963).
—, H. SCHULTZ, and V. DU VIGNEAUD: Some pharmacological studies on I-l-penicillamine-oxytocin and l-deamino-penicillamine-oxytocin: two potent oxytocin inhibitors. 3rd Int. Pharmacological Congr., Abst. 449 (1966).
CHAUDHURY, R.R.: Formation and excretion of ADH in Indian subjects. Clin. Sci. **19**, 641 to 644 (1960).
—, and J.M. WALKER: The release of neurohypophysial hormones in the rabbit by anaesthetics and by haemorrhage. J. Physiol. (Lond.) **143**, 16P (1958).
CLARY, M.L., A. CAMERON, and B.N. CRAVER: Influence of female hormones on motility of cat's uterus and its responses to oxytocics. Proc. Soc. exp. Biol. (N.Y.) **77**, 778—783 (1951).
CLEVERLEY, JACQUELINE: Personal communication (1966).
CLINE, T.N., J.W. COLE, and W.D. HOLDEN: Demonstration of an antidiuretic substance in the urine of postoperative patients. Surg. Gynec. Obstet. **96**, 674—676 (1953).
COCH, J.A., J. BROVETTO, H.M. CABOT, C.A. FIELITZ, and R. CALDEYRO-BARCIA: Oxytocin equivalent activity in the plasma of women in labor and during puerperium. Amer. J. Obstet. Gynec. **91**, 10—17 (1965).
—, C. FIELITZ, J. BROVETTO, H.M. CABOT, H. CODA, and A. FRAGA: Isolation and estimation of oxytocin from the blood of puerperal women during suckling. J. Endocr. **40**, 137—144 (1968).
COON, J.M.: A new method for the assay of posterior pituitary extracts. Arch. int. Pharmacodyn. **62**, 79—99 (1939).
COUTINHO, E.M.: Hormone induced ionic regulation of labor. Symposium 31, part II. Proc. 2nd Int. Congr. of Endocrinology, London. Excerta Medica (Lond.) (1964).
— Personal communication (1966).
—, and A. CSAPO: The effect of oxytocics on the 'calcium deficient' uterus. A measure of oxytocic potency. J. gen. Physiol. **43**, 13—27 (1959).
CRAIG, L.C., E.J. HARFENIST, and A.C. PALADINI: Dialysis studies 7. Behaviour of angiotensin, oxytocin, vasopressin and some of their analogues. Biochemistry **3**, 764—769 (1964).
CRAWFORD, J.D., and B. PINKHAM: An assay method for antidiuretic hormone based on a more specific response index. Endocrinology **55**, 521—529 (1954).
CROSS, B.A.: The hypothalamus and the mechanism of sympathetico-adrenal inhibition of milk-ejection. J. Endocr. **12**, 15—28 (1955).
— The motility and reactivity of the oestrogenized rabbit uterus *in vivo*; with comparative observations on milk-ejection. J. Endocr. **14**, 237—260 (1958a).
— On the mechanism of labour in the rabbit. J. Endocr. **16**, 261—271 (1958b).
—, and H.B. VAN DYKE: The effects of highly purified pituitary principles on the lactating mammary gland of the rabbit. J. Endocr. **9**, 232—235 (1953).

CROSS, B.A., and I.A. SILVER: Mammary oxygen tension and the milk-ejection mechanism. J. Endocr. **22**, xxxiii (1961).
CROXATTO, H.: Polypeptides with posterior pituitary-like activities. In: The Neurohypophysis, pp. 51—64. Ed. by H. HELLER. London: Butterworths 1957.
—, F. ANDRADE, and L. BARNÀFI: Antidiuretic action of human plasma. Acta physiol. lat.-amer. **2**, 142—150 (1952).
—, T. PEREDA, and B. ZAMORANO: Oxytocic substances in blood serum. In: Oxytocin, pp. 412—424. Ed. by R. CALDEYRO-BARCIA and H. HELLER. London: Pergamon Press 1961.
CSAPO, A.: Dependence of isometric tension and isotonic shortening of uterine muscle on temperature and on strength of stimulation. Amer. J. Physiol. **177**, 348—354 (1954).
—, and G.W. CORNER: *In vitro* contracture of pseudopregnant uterine muscle contrasted with estrous motility. Endocrinology **49**, 349—368 (1951a).
— — Shortening of uterine muscle at different temperatures. Proc. Soc. exp. Biol. (N.Y.) **78**, 266—269 (1951b).
—, and M. GOODALL: Excitability, length tension relation and kinetic of uterine muscle contraction in relation to hormonal status. J. Physiol. (Lond.) **126**, 384—395 (1954).
CUPARENCU, B., L. GROSU, L. TOMUS, e V. IDU: Cercetari experimentale asupra principiului ocitocic placentar. Fiziol. Revista Soc. Stüntelor Med. Romina **1**, 49—53 (1961).
CZACZKES, J.W., and C.R. KLEEMAN: The effects of various states of hydration and plasma concentration on the turnover of antidiuretic hormone in mammals. J. clin. Invest. **43**, 1649—1658 (1964).
— —, and M. KOENIG: Physiological studies of antidiuretic hormone by its direct measurement in human plasma. J. clin. Invest. **43**, 1625—1640 (1964).
DALE, H.H.: On some physiological actions of ergot. J. Physiol. (Lond.) **34**, 163—206 (1906).
— The action of extracts of the pituitary body. Biochem. J. **4**, 427—447 (1909).
—, and P.P. LAIDLAW: A method of standardising pituitary (infundibular) extracts. J. Pharm. Pharmacol. **4**, 75—95 (1912).
DEKANSKI, J.: The quantitative assay of vasopressin. Brit. J. Pharmacol. **7**, 567—572 (1952).
DENT, C.E.: The amino-aciduria in Fanconi Syndrome. A study making intensive use of techniques based on paper partition chromatography. Biochem. J. **41**, 240—253 (1947).
DENUCCIO, D.J., and C.E. GROSVENOR: Effect of suckling and hormones on contractility of involuting rat mammary gland. Amer. J. Physiol. **212**, 149—156 (1967).
DETTELBACH, H.R.: A method for assaying small amounts of antidiuretic substances with notes on some properties of vasopressin. Amer. J. Physiol. **192**, 379—386 (1958).
DICKER, S.E.: Method for the assay of very small amounts of antidiuretic activity with a note on the antidiuretic titre of rat's blood. J. Physiol. (Lond.) **122**, 149—157 (1953).
— The fate of the antidiuretic activity of pitressin in rats. J. Physiol. (Lond.) **124**, 464—475 (1954).
—, and M.G. EGGLETON: Renal excretion of hyaluronidase and calcium in man during the antidiuretic action of vasopressin and some analogues. J. Physiol. (Lond.) **157**, 351—362 (1961).
—, and M.G. GINSBURG: Some observations of the antidiuretic activity of rats serum. Brit. J. Pharmacol. **5**, 497—504 (1950).
—, and J. NUNN: Antidiuresis in adult and old rats. J. Physiol. (Lond.) **141**, 332—336 (1958).
—, and C. TYLER: Antidiuretic titre of blood from internal jugular vein of children. J. Physiol. (Lond.) **117**, 28—29 P (1952).
DIEKMANN, W.J., G.F. EGENOLF, B. MORLEY, and R.E. POTTINGER: The inactivation of the antidiuretic hormone of the posterior pituitary gland by blood from pregnant patients. Amer. J. Obstet. Gynec. **60**, 1043—1049 (1950).
DINGMAN, J.F.: Hypothalamus and the endocrine control of sodium and water metabolism in man. Amer. J. med. Sci. **235**, 79—99 (1957).
—, A.B. AHMED, and B.C. GEORGE: Oxytocin secretion in normal and hypopituitary subjects. Abstract 145 of 48th meeting of the Endocrine Society (U.S.A.), p. 99 (1966).
—, C. GONZALEZ-AUVERT, A.B.J. AHMED, and A. AKIMURA: Plasma antidiuretic hormone in adrenal insufficiency. J. clin. Invest. (proc.) **44**, 1041 (1965).
DIXON, H.B.F., and M.P. STACK-DUNNE: Chromatographic studies on corticotrophin. Biochem. J. **61**, 483—495 (1955).
DONALDSON, W.: The dialyzability of the pressor and antidiuretic activities of vasopressin. J. clin. Invest. **26**, 1023—1025 (1947).
DYBALL, R.E.J., G.J. LANE, and R.G. MORRIS: A simplified automatic device for the performance of antidiuretic assays. J. Physiol. (Lond.) **186**, 43P (1966).
DYKE, H.B. VAN: The nature of the vasopressins and their secretion. Proc. XXI Int. Congr. Physiol. Buenos Aires, Symposia, pp. 61—70 (1959).
—, K. ADAMSONS, Jr., and S.L. ENGEL: Aspects of the biochemistry and physiology of the neurohypophysial hormones. Recent Progr. Hormone Res. **11**, 1—41 (1955).

DYKE, H. B., VAN, and ROSE G. AMES: Alcohol diuresis. Acta endocr. (Kbh.) **7**, 110—121 (1951).
— —, and I. C. PLOUGH: Excretion of antidiuretic hormone in urine of patients with cirrhosis of the liver. Trans. Ass. Amer. Phycns **63**, 35—38 (1950).
—, B. P. CHOW, R. O. GREEP, and A. ROTHEN: The isolation of a protein from the pars neuralis of the ox pituitary with constant oxytocic pressor and diuresis-inhibiting activity. J. Pharmacol. exp. Ther. **74**, 190—209 (1942).
—, S. L. ENGEL, and K. ADAMSONS, Jr.: Comparison of pharmacological effects of lysine and arginine vasopressin. Proc. Soc. exp. Biol. (N.Y.) **91**, 484—486 (1956).
—, and A. B. HASTINGS: The responses of smooth muscle in different ionic environments. Amer. J. Physiol. **83**, 563—577 (1928).
—, W. H. SAWYER, and N. I. A. OVERWEG: Pharmacological activities of the 8-citrulline analogues of oxytocin and vasopressin. Endocrinology **73**, 637—639 (1963).
EGGLETON, M. G.: The diuretic action of alcohol in man. J. Physiol. (Lond.) **101**, 172—191 (1942).
EISEN, V. D., and A. A. G. LEWIS: Antidiuretic activity of human urine after surgical operations. Lancet **1954 II**, 361—364.
ELLETT, M. H.: Variations in the oxytocic content of the posterior pituitary abstract during the oestrus cycle in the golden hamster (Mesocritetus Aurabus). Dissertation Abstr. (Physiol.) **25**, Nov. 1964, No. 5. Diss. No. 64—11,598, p. 3076.
ELLIS, M. E., and A. GROLLMAN: The antidiuretic hormone in the urine of experimental and clinical hypertension. Endocrinology **44**, 415—419 (1949).
ELMQVIST, A.: Synpunkter pa bestamning av felgranser vid biologisk styrkebestaming av oxytocin. Svensk. farm. T. **61**, 657—661 (1957).
ELY, F., and W. E. PETERSEN: Factors involved in the ejection of milk. J. Dairy Sci. **24**, 211—223 (1941).
EMBREY, M. P.: Action of desamino-oxytocin on the human pregnant uterus. J. Endocr. **31**, 185—189 (1965).
ERSPAMER, V., and A. OTTOLENGHI: Antidiuretic action of enteramine. Experientia (Basel) **6**, 428 (1950).
EVERETT, J. W.: The mammalian female reproductive cycle and its controlling mechanisms. In: Sex and Internal Secretions, Vol. I, pp. 497—555. Ed. by W. C. YOUNG. Baltimore: WILLIAMS and WILKINS (1961).
—, and C. H. SAWYER: A 24-hour periodicity in the "L.H. release apparatus" of female rats, disclosed by barbiturate sedation. Endocrinology **47**, 200—217 (1950).
FALKNER, R., M. HAMMERSCHMIDT, and A. NEUMAYR: The urinary output of antidiuretic substances in man during therapy of liver cirrhosis with a total-liver-extract. Acta med. scand. **151**, 473—480 (1955).
FENDLER, K., E. ENDRÖCZI u. K. LISSÁK: Einfluß der Hyaluronidase auf die Oxytocin-Empfindlichkeit des Rattenuterus *in vitro* und *in vivo*. Endokrinologie **44**, 153—156 (1963).
FERGUSON, D. R.: Neurohypophysial hormones in mammals. M.D. thesis, University of Bristol, pp. 63—64 (1964).
— Separation of mammalian neurohypophysial hormones by thin-layer chromatography. J. Endocr. **32**, 119—120 (1965).
—, and H. HELLER: Distribution of neurohypophysial hormones in mammals. J. Physiol. (Lond.) **180**, 846—863 (1965).
FERGUSON, J. K. W.: A study of the motility of the intact uterus at term. Surg. Gynec. Obstet. **73**, 359—366 (1941).
FIELITZ, C. A., V. H. GONZALEZ-PANIZZA, and R. CALDEYRO-BARCIA: Effect of low concentrations of oxytocin on the uterine response to electrical stimulation. Acta physiol. lat.-amer. **10**, 201—204 (1960).
FITZPATRICK, R. J.: On oxytocin and uterine function. In: The Neurohypophysis, pp. 203—217. Ed. by H. HELLER. London: Butterworths 1957.
— The reactivity of the ruminant uterus to posterior pituitary hormones. J. comp. Path. **70** 36—58 (1960).
— The estimation of small amounts of oxytocin in blood. In: Oxytocin, pp. 358—377. Ed. by R. CALDEYRO-BARCIA and H. HELLER. London: Pergamon Press 1961.
— The posterior pituitary gland and the female reproductive tract. In: The Pituitary Gland, Vol. 3, pp. 453—504. Ed. by G. W. HARRIS and B. T. DONOVAN. London: Butterworths 1966.
— Unpublished observations (1967).
—, and C. F. WALMSLEY: The concentration of oxytocin in bovine blood during parturition. J. Physiol. (Lond.) **163**, 13P—14P (1962).
— — Release of oxytocin during parturition. In: Advances in Oxytocin Research, pp. 51—73. Ed. by J. H. M. PINKERTON. London: Pergamon Press 1965.
FLATTERS, MARTHA: Über die Vorzüge der Verwendung von Rattenuteri im Proöstrus zur Auswertung von Oxytocin. Arch. Exptl. Pathol. Pharmakol. **221**, 171—176 (1954).

Flodin, P.: Dextran gels and their applications in gel filtration. Pharmacia, Uppsala, Sweden (1962).

Follett, B.K.: Mole ratios of the neurohypophysial hormones in the vertebrate neural lobe. Nature (Lond.) **198**, 693—694 (1963).

—, and P.J. Bentley: Bioassay of oxytocin. Increased sensitivity of the rat uterus in response to serial injections of stilboestrol. J. Endocr. **29**, 277—282 (1964).

—, and H. Heller: The neurohypophysial hormones of bony fishes and cyclostomes. J. Physiol. (Lond.) **172**, 74—91 (1964a).

— — The neurohypophysial hormones of lungfishes and amphibians. J. Physiol. (Lond.) **172**, 92—106 (1964b).

Folley, S.J., and G.S. Knaggs: Oxytocin levels in the blood of ruminants with special reference to the milking stimulus. In: Advances in Oxytocin Research, pp. 37—50. Ed. by J.H.M. Pinkerton. London: Pergamon Press 1965.

Frankland, B.T.B., M.D. Hollenberg, D.B. Hope, and B.A. Schacter: Dissociation of oxytocin and vasopressin from their carrier protein by chromatography on Sephadex G-25. Brit. J. Pharmacol. **26**, 502—510 (1966).

Fraser, A.M.: Effect of Mg on response of uterus to posterior pituitary hormones. J. Pharmacol. exp. Ther. **66**, 85—94 (1939).

Friedman, E.A.: Direct measurement of milk-ejection pressure in unanaesthetised lactating humans. Amer. J. Obstet. Gynec. **80**, 119—123 (1960).

Friedman, Gertrude S., and M.R. Friedman: An examination of cerebrospinal fluid for oxytocic activity as tested by the rabbit uterine fistula preparation. Amer. J. Physiol. **103**, 244—254 (1933).

Fugo, N.W., and G.T. Aragon: The utilization of an old technique for a sensitive antidiuretic assay. Fed. Proc. **6**, 330—331 (1947).

Gaddum, J.H.: Some properties of the separated active principles of the pituitary (posterior lobe). J. Physiol. (Lond.) **65**, 434—440 (1928).

— Error of oxytocic assay of post-pituitary extracts. Quart. J. Pharm. **11**, 697—699 (1938).

— Bioassays and mathematics. Pharmacol. Rev. **5**, 87—134 (1953a).

— The technique of superfusion. Brit. J. Pharmacol. **8**, 321—326 (1953b).

— The pharmacological analysis of tissue extracts. In: Polypeptides which stimulate Smooth Muscle, pp. 1—6. Ed. by J.H. Gaddum. London: E. and S. Livingstone 1955.

Garcia de Jalon, P.: El uso de las sales de magnesio en los ensayos de los extractos de lóbulo posterior de hipófisis. Farmacoter. act. **4**, 177—182 (1947).

—, J. Bayo Bayo, y M. Garcia de Jalon: Sensible y nuevo método de valoracion de adrenalina en utero aislado de Rata. Farmacoter. act. **11**, 313—318 (1945).

Gelotte, B.: Studies in gel filtration. Sorption properties of the bed material Sephadex. J. Chromatog. **3**, 330—342 (1960).

Gilliland, P.F., and T.E. Prout: Immunologic studies of octapeptides. II. Production and detection of antibodies to oxytocin. Metabolism **14**, 918—923 (1965).

Gilman, A., and L. Goodman: The secretory response of the posterior pituitary to the need for water conservation. J. Physiol. (Lond.) **90**, 113—124 (1937).

Ginsburg, M., and L.M. Brown: Effect of anaesthetics and haemorrhage on the release of neurohypophysial antidiuretic hormone. Brit. J. Pharmacol. **11**, 236—244 (1956).

— — The effects of haemorrhage and plasma hypertonicity on the neurohypophysis. In: The Neurohypophysis, pp. 109—124. Ed. by H. Heller. London: Butterworths 1957.

—, and H. Heller: Antidiuretic activities in plasma and serum. J. Physiol. (Lond.) **115**, 43 P (1951).

— — (Cited by H. Heller): The influence of the suprarenal cortex on mineral and water metabolism. In: The Suprarenal Cortex, pp. 187—199. Ed. by J.M. Yoffey. London: Butterworths 1952.

— — The antidiuretic assay of vasopressin by intravenous injection into unanaesthetised rats. J. Endocr. **9**, 267—273 (1953a).

— — Antidiuretic activity in blood from various parts of the cardiovascular system. J. Endocr. **9**, 274—282 (1953b).

— — The clearance of injected vasopressin from the circulation and its fate in the body. J. Endocr. **9**, 283—291 (1953c).

—, and M.W. Smith: The fate of oxytocin in male and female rats. Brit. J. Pharmacol. **14**, 327—333 (1959).

Glazer, A.N., and D. Wellner: Absorption of proteins on 'Sephadex'. Nature (Lond.) **194**, 862—863 (1962).

Goldman, R., and E.B. Luchsinger: Relationship between diurnal variations in urinary volume and the excretion of antidiuretic substance. J. clin. Endocr. **16**, 28—34 (1956).

Goltner, E., u. H. Vorherr: Die Wirkung des Ferritins auf den Blutdruck und die Diurese der Ratte. Z. ges. exp. Med. **132**, 359—365 (1959).

GONZALEZ-PANIZZA, V.H., Y. SICA-BLANCO, and C. MENDEZ-BAUER: The fate of injected oxytocin in the pregnant woman near term. In: Oxytocin, pp. 347—357. Ed. by R. CALDEYRO-BARCIA and H. HELLER. London: Pergamon Press 1961.
GROLLMAN, A., and B. WOODS: A new procedure for the determination of the antidiuretic principle in the urine. Endocrinology **44**, 404—414 (1949).
GROSVENOR, C.E.: Contraction of lactating rat mammary gland in response to direct mechanical stimulation. Amer. J. Physiol. **208**, 214—218 (1965).
— Personal communication (1966).
GUERNÉ, J.M., et F. STUTINSKY: Etude in vivo des variations de la sensibilité à l'ocytocine de l'uterus de la ratte cyclique. J. Physiol. (Paris) **53**, 357—358 (1961).
GUGGENHEIM, K.: Effect of posterior pituitary hormone on water metabolism in thiamine deficiency. Metabolism **3**, 44—48 (1954).
GUTTMANN, S., B. BERDE, and E. STÜRMER: The synthesis and some pharmacological effects of serine^4-isoleucine^8-oxytocin, a probable neurohypophysial hormone. Experientia (Basel) **18**, 445—446 (1962).
HALPERN, B.N., R. BINAGHI, L. MAYER, and C. BUGNARD: The mechanism of the inhibition by carbonic acid of the smooth muscle contraction produced by histamine and oxytocin. Brit. J. Pharmacol. **14**, 19—25 (1959).
HAM, G.C., and E.M. LANDIS: A comparison of pituitrin with the antidiuretic substance found in human urine and placenta. J. clin. Invest. **21**, 455—470 (1942).
HAMBURGER, C.: Modification of the standardization of posterior pituitary extract after Dale's principle. Acta pharmacol. (Kbh.) **1**, 112—119 (1945).
HANON, F., M. COQUOIN-CARNOT, and P. PIGUARD: The amniotic fluid. Gynéc. et Obstét. **60**, 211—236 (1961).
HARE, K., R.C. HICKEY, and R.S. HARE: The renal excretion of an antidiuretic substance by the dog. Amer. J. Physiol. **134**, 240—244 (1941).
—, E.V. MELVILLE, G.H. CHAMBERS, and R.S. HARE: The assay of antidiuretic material in blood and urine. Endocrinology **36**, 323—331 (1945).
HARRIS, G.W.: The excretion of an antidiuretic substance by the kidney after electrical stimulation of the neurohypophysis in the unanaesthetized rabbit. J. Physiol. (Lond.) **107** 430—435 (1948).
HAWKER, R.W.: Oxytocin and an unidentified oxytocic substance in extracts of blood. In: Oxytocin, pp. 425—434. Ed. by R. CALDEYRO-BARCIA and H. HELLER. London: Pergamon Press 1961.
—, and P.A. ROBERTSON: Some properties of an oxytocic substance found in blood extracts. Endocrinology **63**, 242—249 (1958).
—, CHRISTINE F. WALMSLEY, and VIVIENNE S. ROBERTS: Further observations on oxytocin and oxytocic substance. Med. J. Aust. **1**, 460—461 (1959).
HAWKINS, D.F.: Oxytocic lipids in human amniotic fluid. Nature (Lond.) **194**, 975—976 (1962).
HELLER, H.: The state in the blood and the excretion by the kidney of the antidiuretic principle of posterior pituitary extracts. J. Physiol. (Lond.) **89**, 81—95 (1937).
— Differentiation of an (amphibian) water balance principle from the antidiuretic principle of the posterior pituitary gland. J. Physiol. (Lond.) **100**, 124—141 (1941).
— The hormonal control of water and salt-electrolyte metabolism with special reference to higher vertebrates. Mem. Soc. Endocrinol. **5**, 25—37 (1956).
— The state and concentration of the neurohypophysial hormones in the blood. In: CIBA Foundation Colloquium, Vol. 11, pp. 3—14. Ed. by G.E.W. WOLSTENHOLME and E.C.P. MILLAR (1957).
— Occurrence, storage and metabolism of oxytocin. In: Oxytocin, pp. 3—23. Ed. by R. CALDEYRO-BARCIA and H. HELLER. London: Pergamon Press 1961.
— Pharmacology and distribution of neurohypophysial hormones. Symp. Zool. Soc. (Lond.) **9**, 93—106 (1963).
— Hormone content of the hypothalamo-neurohypophysial system. In: Recent studies on the Hypothalamus. Brit. med. Bull. **22**, No. 3 (1966).
—, and P.J. BENTLEY: Phylogenetic distribution of the effects of neurohypophysial hormones on water and salt metabolism. Gen. comp. Endocr. **5**, 96—108 (1965).
—, and E.K. BLACKMORE: The assay of small amounts of antidiuretic activity by intravenous injections into mice. J. Endocr. **8**, 224—228 (1952).
—, ELENA FERRERI, and D.H.G. LEATHERS: The effect of neurohypophysial hormones on the amphibian oviduct. J. Endocr. **37**, xxxix (1967).
—, and M. GINSBURG: Secretion, metabolism and fate of the posterior pituitary hormones. In: The Pituitary Gland, Vol. 3, pp. 330—373. Ed. by G.W. HARRIS and B.T. DONOVAN. London: Butterworths 1966.
—, G. HERDAN, and S.M.A. ZAIDI: Seasonal variations in the response of rats to antidiuretic hormone. Brit. J. Pharmacol. **12**, 100—103 (1957).

HELLER, H., and K. LEDERIS: Paper chromatography of small amounts of vasopressins and oxytocins. Nature (Lond.) **182**, 1231—1232 (1958).
— — Maturation of the hypothalamo-neurohypophysial system. J. Physiol. (Lond.) **147**, 299—314 (1959).
— — Posterior pituitary hormones of the hippotamus. J. Physiol. (Lond.) **151**, 47—49P (1960).
—, and B.T. PICKERING: Neurohypophysial hormones of non-mammalian vertebrates. J. Physiol. (Lond.) **155**, 98—114 (1961).
— —, J. MAETZ, and F. MOREL: Pharmacological characterisation of the oxytocic peptides in the pituitary of a marine teleost fish (*Pollachius virens*). Nature (Lond.) **191**, 670—671 (1961).
—, and B.P. ROY: Elasmobranch neurohypophysial hormones. J. Physiol. (Lond.) **177**, 50—51P (1965).
HELLER, J., and J. STŮLC: Physiology of the antidiuretic hormone. I. A simple titration method. Physiol. bohemoslov. **8**, 558—564 (1959).
— — Physiology of the antidiuretic hormone. II. The antidiuretic activity of normal human plasma. Physiol. bohemoslov. **9**, 5—12 (1960a).
— — Physiology of the antidiuretic hormone. III. The antidiuretic activity of plasma in normal and dehydrated rats. Physiol. bohemoslov. **9**, 93—98 (1960b).
HELLMAN, I.Z., and J.S. WIENER: Antidiuretic substance in urine following exposure to high temperatures. J. appl. Physiol. **6**, 194—198 (1953).
HIRS, C.H.W., S. MOORE, and W.J. STEIN: A chromatographic investigation of ribonuclease. J. biol. Chem. **200**, 493—506 (1953).
HOLLANDER, L.P., J. FRANZ, and B. BERDE: An attempt to produce antibodies to oxytocin and vasopressin. Experientia (Basel) **22**, 325—329 (1966).
HOLTON, PAMELA A.: A modification of the method of Dale and Laidlaw for standardisation of posterior pituitary extract. Brit. J. Pharmacol. **3**, 328—334 (1948).
HOPE, D.B., B.A. SCHACTER, and B.T.B. FRANKLAND: Dissociation of oxytocin, vasopressin and neurophysin by gel filtration. Biochem. J. **93**, 7P (1964).
HOR, G., H. AVENHAUS u. E. BUCHBORN: ADH Plasmaspiegel und -verteilungsraum nach exogener Zufuhr von ADH am Menschen. Klin. Wschr. **41**, 366—371 (1963).
HORTON, E.W.: Urinary kinin. In: Polypeptides which affect Smooth Muscles and Blood Vessels. pp. 263—271. Ed. by M. SCHACHTER. London: Pergamon Press 1960.
HSU, YU-C.: Influence of magnesium concentration in Ringer's solution for assay of oxytocin in pituitary (posterior lobe) extracts. Quart. J. Pharm. **21**, 146—151 (1948).
ISHII, S., T. HIRANO, and H. KOBAYASHI: Neurohypophysial hormones in the avian median eminence and pars nervosa. Gen. comp. Endocr. **2**, 433—440 (1962).
ITOH, S., and M. KIMURA: Occurrence of antidiuretic substance in human urine after heavy sweating. Jap. J. Physiol. **3**, 277—278 (1953).
JEFFERS, W.A., M.M. LIVEZEY, and J.H. AUSTIN: A method for demonstrating an antidiuretic action of minute amounts of pitressin. Statistical analysis of results. Proc. Soc. exp. Biol. (N.Y.) **50**, 184—188 (1942).
JESSUP, D.C., K.K. CARROLL, and R.L. NOBLE: A new method for the extraction of posterior lobe antidiuretic hormone from body fluids. Rev. canad. Biol. **15**, 260—261 (1956).
— — — Recovery of vasopressin from urine and blood by phenol extraction. Canad. J. Biochem. **39**, 1647—1649 (1961).
—, N.B.G. TAYLOR, and R.L. NOBLE: A comparison of methods for extracting pituitary antidiuretic substance from urine. Endocrinology **60**, 6—12 (1957).
JÖCHLE, W.: The circadian rhythm in female reproduction. In: Reproduction in the Female Mammal pp. 267—284. Ed. by G.E. LAMMING and E.C. AMOROSO. London: Butterworths 1967.
JONES, J.J., and J. LEE: The value of the preoperated rat in the bioassay of vasopressin. J. Endocr. **33**, 329—330 (1965).
KARIM, S.M.M.: A smooth muscle contracting substance in extracts of human umbilical cord. J. Pharm. Pharmacol. **18**, 519—530 (1966a).
— A smooth muscle contracting substance in extracts of human umbilical cord. Nature (Lond.) **211**, 425 (1966b).
KNAGGS, G.S.: Blood oxytocin levels in the cow during milking and in the parturient goat. J. Endocr. **26**, xxiv (1963).
— Blood oxytocin levels in relation to lactation and reproduction. Ph. D. Thesis, University of Reading (1966).
KRAMÁR, J., E.H. GRINNELL, and W.M. DUFF: Observations on the diuretic activity of antidiuretic hormone. Amer. J. med. Sci. **252**, 87—95 (1966).
KREBS, H.A., u. K. HENSELEIT: Untersuchungen über die Harnstoffbildung im Tierkörper. Hoppe-Seylers Z. physiol. Chem. **210**, 33—66 (1932).

KRIEGER, V.I., H.M. BUTLER, and T.B. KILVINGTON: Antidiuretic substance in the urine during pregnancy and its frequent association with bacterial growth. J. Obstet. Gynaec. Brit. Emp. **58**, 5—17 (1951).

—, and T.B. KILVINGTON: Antidiuretic substance in urine in relation to normal and toxaemic pregnancy. Med. J. Aust. **1**, 575—585 (1940).

— — The failure to detect antidiuretic substance in the blood and urine of dehydrated rats. Aust. J. exp. Biol. med. Sci. **29**, 77—84 (1951).

KURIYAMA, H., and A. CSAPO: A study of the parturient uterus with the microelectrode technique. Endocrinology **68**, 1010—1025 (1961).

LANDGREBE, F.W., MARGARET H.I. MACAULEY, and H. WARING: The use of rats for pressor assays of pituitary extracts, with a note on response to histamine and adrenaline. Proc. roy. Soc. Edinb. B **62**, 202—210 (1946).

LARSON, E.: Fate of injected oxytocic principle of posterior pituitary in anesthetized cats and dogs. J. Pharm. Pharmacol. **67**, 175—186 (1939).

LAUBER, J.K., W.J. EVERSOLE, and W.A. CHILDS: The use of the toad for bioassay of mammalian antidiuretic hormone. Endocrinology **64**, 316—318 (1959).

LAUSON, H.D.: Vasopressin and oxytocin in the plasma of man and other mammals. In: Hormones in Human Plasma. Nature and Transport, pp. 225—293. Ed. by H.N. ANTONIADES. Boston: Little, Brown & Co. 1960.

LEAF, A., J. ANDERSON, and L.B. PAGE: Active sodium transport by the isolated toad bladder. J. gen. Physiol. **41**, 657—668 (1958).

—, and A.R. MAMBY: The normal antidiuretic mechanism in man and dog; its regulation by extracellular fluid tonicity. J. clin. Invest. **31**, 54—71 (1952).

LEDERIS, K.: Vasopressin and oxytocin in the mammalian hypothalamus. Gen. comp. Endocr. **1**, 80—89 (1961).

LEE, J., and G.W. BISSET: The secretion of neurohypophysial hormones in man with special reference to liver disease. Proc. roy. Soc. Med. **51**, 361—362 (1958).

LEVITT, G.: The problem of an antidiuretic substance in the blood of patients with eclampsia and other hypertensive diseases. J. clin. Invest. **15**, 135—141 (1936).

LEWIS, A.G.: Observations on the antidiuretic substance in human serum. J. clin. Endocr. **13**, 769—772 (1953).

LIGHT, A., R. ACHER, and V. DU VIGNEAUD: Ion exchange chromatography of purified posterior pituitary preparation. J. biol. Chem. **228**, 633—641 (1957).

LINDNER, E.B., A. ELMQVIST, and J. PORATH: Gel filtration as a method for purification of protein bound peptides exemplified by oxytocin and vasopressin. Nature (Lond.) **184**, 1565—1566 (1959).

LINDQUIST, K.M., and L.W. ROWE: The antidiuretic activity of the posterior pituitary and its quantitative evaluation. J. Amer. pharm. Ass. **38**, 227—231 (1949).

LINZELL, J.L.: Some observations on the contractile tissue of the mammary glands. J. Physiol. (Lond.) **130**, 257—267 (1955).

LLOYD, C.W., and J. LOBOTSKY: Serum antidiuretic substances and urinary corticosteroid in the human. J. clin. Endocr. **10**, 318—329 (1950).

MACFARLANE, W.V., and K.W. ROBINSON: Seasonal changes in plasma antidiuretic activity. J. Physiol. (Lond.) **135**, 1—11 (1957).

MAETZ, J., F. MOREL, et B. RACE: Mise en évidence dans la neurohypophyse de *Rana esculenta* L. d'un facteur hormonal nouveau stimulant le transport actif de sodium à travers la peau. Biochim. biophys. Acta (Amst.) **36**, 317—326 (1959).

MANUNTA, G., e V. ALBERGONI: Sulla contrazione *in vitro* del mioepitelio mammario di coniglia ed oxytocina. Boll. Soc. ital. Biol. sper. **38**, 1263—1265 (1962).

MARSHALL, JEAN M.: Effects of estrogen and progesterone on single uterine muscle fibres in the rat. Amer. J. Physiol. **197**, 936—942 (1959).

— Regulation of activity in uterine smooth muscle. Physiol. Rev. **42**, Symposium on smooth muscle, pp. 213—227 (1962).

MARTIN, P.J., and H.O. SCHILD: Pharmacological antagonism of oxytocin and vasopressin by thiol compounds. J. Physiol. (Lond.) **163**, 51P (1962).

— — The antagonism of disulphide polypeptides by thiols. Brit. J. Pharmacol. **25**, 418—431 (1965).

MARX, H., u. K. SCHNEIDER: Untersuchungen zur Diurese. Über den Nachweis antidiuretischer Substanzen im Blute. Arch. exp. Pathol. Pharmakol. **176**, 24—28 (1934).

MAYER, F.S.: Identification of the antidiuretic substance in human urine. Acta endocr. (Kbh.) **35**, 568—574 (1960).

MELVILLE, K.I.: Antidiuretic pituitary substance in blood with special reference to toxaemia in pregnancy. J. exp. Med. **65**, 415—429 (1937).

MENDEZ-BAUER, C., H.M. CABOT, and R. CALDEYRO-BARCIA: A new test for the biological assay of oxytocin. Science **132**, 299—300 (1960).

MENDEZ-BAUER, C., R.J. FITZPATRICK, H.M. CABOT, L. BRANDA, L. ESCARCENA, C. FIELITZ, V.H. GONZALEZ-PANIZZA, J.A. COCH, J.J. POSEIRO, Y. SICA-BLANCO, N. SALA, H. ALVAREZ, C. GOMEZ-ROGERS, R. FERNANDEZ, E. COBO, y R. CALDEYRO-BARCIA: Potencia eyectolactea del plasma humano durante el embarazo, parto y puerperio. Tercer. Congreso Uruguayo de Ginecotocologia Tomo II, pp. 307—312 (1960).

MILTENBERGER, F.W., and W.H. MORAN: Peripheral blood levels of vasopressin (ADH) during surgical procedures. Surg. Forum **15**, 54—55 (1963).

MOORE, R.D., and M.X. ZARROW: Contraction of the rabbit mammary strip *in vitro* in response to oxytocin. Acta endocr. (Kbh.) **48**, 186—198 (1965).

MORAN, W.H., and F.W. MILTENBERGER: Use of the intravenous route for maintenance of water balance in the alcoholized rat bioassay of vasopressin. Fed. Proc. **22**, 386 (1963).

— —, W.A. SHUAYB, and B. ZIMMERMANN: The relationship of antidiuretic hormone secretion to surgical stress. Surgery **56**, 99—108 (1964).

MOREL, F., J. MAETZ, et C. LUCARAIN: Action des deux peptides neurohypophysaires sur le transport actif de sodium et le flux d'eau à travers la peau de divers éspèces de Bactraciens Anoures. Biochim. biophys. Acta (Amst.) **28**, 619—626 (1958).

—, M. ODIER, et C. LUCARAIN: Un Dispositif de Mesures multiples et simultanees du Transport actif de Sodium a travers plusieurs Regions d'une meme Peau de Grenouille. J. Physiol. (Paris) **53**, 757—762 (1961).

MORRELL, C.A., M.G. ALLMARK, and W.M. BACHINSKI: On the biological assay of the oxytocic activity of pituitary extract (posterior lobe). J. Pharm. Pharmacol. **70**, 440—449 (1940).

MUNSICK, R.A.: Effect of magnesium ion on the response of the rat uterus to neurohypophysial hormones and analogues. Endocrinology **66**, 451—457 (1960).

— Neurohypophysial hormones of chickens and turkeys. Endocrinology **75**, 105—112 (1964).

— Chromatographic and pharmacologic characterization of the neurohypophysial hormones of an amphibian and a reptile. Endocrinology **78**, 591—599 (1966).

—, W.H. SAWYER, and H.B. VAN DYKE: The antidiuretic potency of arginine and lysine vasopressin in the pig with observations on porcine renal function. Endocrinology **63**, 688—693 (1958).

— — — Avian neurohypophysial hormones pharmacological properties and tentative identification. Endocrinology **66**, 860—871 (1960).

NIELSEN, A.T.: A note on the relative antidiuretic potency of beef and hog vasopressin. Acta endocr. (Kbh.) **29**, 561—564 (1958).

NOBLE, R.L.: The excretion of posterior pituitary principles in the urine. In: The Neurohypophysis, pp. 97—106. Ed. by H. HELLER. London: Butterworths 1957.

—, E.R. PLUNKETT, and N.B.G. TAYLOR: Factors affecting the control of the pituitary gland. Recent Progr. Hormone Res. **5**, 263—301 (1950).

—, H. RINDERKNECHT, and P.C. WILLIAMS: The apparent augmentation of pituitary antidiuretic action by various retarding substances. J. Physiol. (Lond.) **96**, 293—301 (1939).

—, and N.B.G. TAYLOR: Antidiuretic substances in human urine after haemorrhage, fainting, dehydration and acceleration. J. Physiol. (Lond.) **122**, 220—237 (1953).

NODDLE, B.A.: Metabolism of oxytocin in the mammary gland. XXII Int. Congress of Physiclogical Sciences, Leiden. Comm. 523. Excerpta Medica Foundation (1962).

O'CONNOR, W.J.: The role of the neurohypophysis of the dog in determining urinary changes, and the antidiuretic activity of urine, following the administration of sodium chloride or urea. Quart. J. exp. Physiol. **36**, 21—48 (1951).

ORR, J., and A.H. SNAITH: A method for the estimation of antidiuretic hormone in urine. J. Endocr. **18**, xvi (1959).

PAGE, E.W.: The effect of eclamptic blood upon the urinary output and blood pressure of human recipients. J. clin. Invest. **17**, 207—218 (1938).

PAGE, I.H.: Serotonin (5-hydroxytryptamine). Physiol. Rev. **34**, 563—588 (1954).

PATON, D.N., and A. WATSON: The actions of pituitrin, adrenalin and barium on the circulation of the bird. J. Physiol. (Lond.) **44**, 413—424 (1912).

PERMUTT, M.A., C.W. PARKER, and R.D. UTIGER: Immunochemical studies with lysine vasopressin. Endocrinology **78**, 809—814 (1966).

PICKERING, B.T., and H. HELLER: Chromatographic and biological characteristics of fish and frog neurohypophysial extracts. Nature (Lond.) **184**, 1463—1464 (1959).

PICKLES, V.R., and R.J. FITZPATRICK (Editors): Endogenous Substances affecting the Myometrium. Mem. Soc. Endocrinol. No. 14. London: Cambridge University Press 1966.

PORATH, J., and E.B. LINDNER: Separation methods based on molecular sieving and ion exclusion. Nature (Lond.) **191**, 69—70 (1961).

—, and A.V. SCHALLY: Gel filtration of posterior pituitary hormones. Endocrinology **70**, 738—742 (1962).

PORTANOVA, R., and H. SACHS: A specific Adsorbent for Vasopressin: The Purification of Labeled Hormone. Endocrinology **80**, 527—529 (1967).

QUIVY, D., et I. BERTRAND: Dosage biologique des agents contracturants du muscle lisse. Lobe póstérieur d'hypophyse et histamine. Traitement des données expérimentales. Arch. int. Pharmacodyn. **75**, 353—361 (1948).

REYNOLDS, S. R. M.: Physiology of the Uterus. 2nd ed. New York: Hoeber 1949.

ROBINSON, K. W., R. W. HAWKER, and P. A. ROBERTSON: Antidiuretic hormone (ADH) in the human female. J. clin. Endocr. **17**, 320—322 (1957).

—, and W. V. MACFARLANE: The influence of environmental temperature on the level of plasma antidiuretic substance in the rat. Aust. J. biol. Sci. **9**, 130—138 (1956).

ROBSON, J. M., and H. O. SCHILD: Response of cat's uterus to hormones of posterior pituitary lobe. J. Physiol. (Lond.) **92**, 1—8 (1938a).

— — Effect of drugs in blood flow and the activity of the uterus. J. Physiol. (Lond.) **92**, 9—19 (1938b).

—, and R. S. STACY (Editors): Pharmacologically active substances in the central nervous system. In: Recent Advances in Pharmacology, 3rd ed., pp. 1—41. London: Churchill 1962.

RORIE, D., and M. NEWTON: New method for the quantitative estimation of oxytocin. Anat. Rec. **151**, 407 (1965).

RUCH, W.: Estimation of antidiuretic hormone in the urine of healthy subjects and patients with inappropriate secretion of vasopressin (Schwarter-Bartler Syndrome). Acta Endocr. (Kbh.) **54**, 113—121 (1967).

RUDINGER, J., and I. KREJČÍ: Dose-response relations for some synthetic analogues of oxytocin, and the mode of action of oxytocin on the isolated uterus. Experientia (Basel) **18**, 585—588 (1962).

RYDÉN, G., and I. SJÖHOLM: Assay of oxytocin by rat mammary gland *in vitro*. Brit. J. Pharmacol. **19**, 136—141 (1962).

RYDON, H. N., and P. W. G. SMITH: A new method for the detection of peptides and similar compounds on paper chromatograms. Nature (Lond.) **169**, 922—923 (1952).

SAAMELI, K.: An indirect method for the estimation of oxytocin blood concentration and half-life in pregnant women near term. Amer. J. Obstet. Gynec. **85**, 186—192 (1963).

SAMAAN, A.: The effect of pituitary (posterior lobe) extract upon the urinary flow in non-anaesthetized dogs. J. Physiol. (Lond.) **85**, 37—46 (1935).

SAWYER, W. H.: Differences in the antidiuretic responses of rats to the intravenous administration of lysine and arginine vasopressins. Endocrinology **63**, 694—698 (1958).

— Increased water permeability of the bullfrog (*Rana catesbiana*) bladder *in vitro* in response to synthetic oxytocin and arginine vasotocin and to neurohypophysial extracts from non-mammalian vertebrates. Endocrinology **66**, 112—120 (1960).

— Biological assays for oxytocin and vasopressin. Meth. med. Res. **9**, 210—219 (1961a).

— Comparative physiology and pharmacology of the neurohypophysis. Recent Progr. Hormone Res. **17**, 437—465 (1961b).

— Vertebrate neurohypophysial principles. Endocrinology **75**, 981—990 (1964).

— Biological assays for neurohypophysial principles in tissues and in blood. In: The Pituitary Gland, Vol. III, pp. 288—306. Ed. by G. W. HARRIS and B. T. DONOVAN. London: Butterworths 1966a.

— Neurohypophysial principles of vertebrates. In: The Pituitary Gland, Vol. III, pp. 307—329. Ed. by G. W. HARRIS and B. T. DONOVAN. London: Butterworths 1966b.

—, W. Y. CHAN, and H. B. VAN DYKE: Antidiuretic responses to neurohypophysial hormones and some of their synthetic analogues in dogs and rats. Endocrinology **71**, 536—540 (1962).

—, and H. B. VAN DYKE: Isolation of the oxytocin-like principle of a teleost fish (*Pollachius virens*) and comparison of its properties with those of synthetic 4-serine, 8-isoleucine oxytocin. Endocrinology **73**, 394—396 (1963).

—, R. A. MUNSICK, and H. B. VAN DYKE: Pharmacological evidence for the presence of arginine vasotocin and oxytocin in neurohypophysial extracts from cold blooded vertebrates. Nature (Lond.) **184**, 1464—1465 (1959).

—, and GRACE E. PICKFORD: Neurohypophysial principles of Fundulus heteroclitus: characteristics and seasonal changes. Gen. comp. Endocr. **3**, 439—445 (1963).

SCHAFFER, N. K., J. F. CADDEN, and H. J. STANDER: Measurement of the antidiuretic activity as applied to eclamptic urine and properties of antidiuretic substances in rat urine, pituitary and beef liver. Endocrinology **28**, 701—706 (1941).

SCHILD, H. O.: A method for conducting a biological assay on a preparation giving repeated graded responses illustrated by the estimation of histamine. J. Physiol. (Lond.) **101**, 115 to 130 (1942).

— An approximately linear and isotonic frontal writing lever. J. Physiol. (Lond.) **103**, 36P (1944).

—, R. J. FITZPATRICK, and W. C. W. NIXON: Activity of human cervix and corpus uteri. Their response to drugs in early pregnancy. Lancet **1951 I**, 250—253.

SCHNEIDER, W., u. C.L. STUMPF: Über den Einfluß des Sexualcyclus auf Hypophysenhinterlappenextrakt-Auswertungen nach der Methode von P. HOLTON. Arch. int. Pharmacodyn. **94**, 406—415 (1953).

SEN-MIN, WANG: A bioassay method for pituitary (posterior lobe) extract using the mouse uterus. Acta pharmaceutical. Sin. (**11** No. 9), 626—628 (1964).

SETEKLEIV, J.: Uterine motility of oestrogenised rabbit. I. Isotonic and isometric recording *in vivo*. Influence of anaesthesia and temperature. Acta physiol. scand. **62**, 68—78 (1964a).

— Uterine motility of oestrogenised rabbit. II. Response to distension. Acta physiol. scand. **62**, 79—93 (1964b).

SHARE, L.: Acute reduction in extracellular fluid volume and the concentration of antidiuretic hormone in blood. Endocrinology **69**, 925—933 (1961).

— Effects of carotid occlusion and left atrial distension on plasma vasopressin titer. Amer. J. Physiol. **208**, 219—223 (1965).

SHOEMAKER, V.A.: The stimulus for the water balance response to dehydration in toads. Comp. Biochem. Physiol. **15**, 81—88 (1965).

SICA-BLANCO, Y., C. MENDEZ-BAUER, N. SALA, H.M. CABOT, y R. CALDEYRO-BARCIA: Nuevo metodo para el estudio de la funcionalidad mamaria en la mujer. Arch. Ginec. Obstet. **17**, 63—72 (1959).

SIDDIQI, S., and J.M. WALKER: Oxytocic activity of rabbit's blood applied directly to superfused rat uterus. J. Physiol. (Lond.) **152**, 381—390 (1960).

SKADHAUGE, E.: Effects of unilateral infusion of arginine-vasotocin into the portal circulation of the avian kidney. Acta endocr. (Kbh.) **47**, 321—330 (1964).

SJÖHOLM, I.: Personal communication (1967).

—, G. RYDÉN: Improved method for quantitative estimation of oxytocin. Nature (Lond.) **193**, 77—78 (1962).

SMELIK, S.M.: Personal communication (1966).

SMITH, M.I., and W.T. MCCLOSKY: On the dialysis of the physiologically active constituents found in the infundibulum. J. Pharmacol. exp. Ther. **24**, 391—403 (1924).

SMITH, M.W.: Some properties of rat mammary tissue. Nature (Lond.) **190**, 541—542 (1961).

—, and N.A. THORN: The effect of calcium on protein binding and metabolism of arginine vasopressin in rats. J. Endocr. **32**, 141—151 (1965).

SMITH, R.B., jr., and B.J. VOS: The biological assay of posterior pituitary solution. J. Pharm. Pharmacol. **78**, 72—78 (1943).

STACY, B.D., and A.H. BROOK: Antidiuretic hormone activity in sheep after feeding. Quart. J. exp. Physiol. **50**, 65—78 (1965).

STAMM, O.: Extraction and isolation of a placental hormone with an inhibiting effect on the uterus. Experientia (Basel) **17**, 506—507 (1961).

STEHLE, R.L.: New method for separating pressor and oxytocic substances from posterior lobe of pituitary gland. J. biol. Chem. **102**, 573—590 (1933).

STEIN, M., R. JINK, and I.A. MIRSKY: The bioassay of pitressin and antidiuretic substances in blood and urine. Endocrinology **51**, 492—503 (1952).

STEWART, G.A.: An examination of factors affecting the precision of the assay of the oxytocic hormone in posterior pituitary lobe preparations. J. Pharm. Pharmacol. **1**, 436—453 (1949).

— The assay of posterior pituitary lobe extracts. Analyst **75**, 542—549 (1950).

STUECK, G.H., S.H. LESLIS, and E. RALLI: Preliminary observations on the antidiuretic substances recovered from the urines of patients with cirrhosis of the liver. Endocrinology **44**, 325—332 (1949).

STYLES, P.R., and T.J. SULLIVAN: Measurement of uterine activity *in vitro* by integrating muscle tension. Brit. J. Pharmacol. **19**, 129—135 (1962).

TATA, P.S., and R. BUZALKOV: Vasopressin studies in the rat. III. Inability of ethanol anaesthesia to prevent ADH secretion due to pain and haemorrhage. Pflügers Arch. ges. Physiol. **290**, 294—297 (1966).

—, and O.H. GAUER: Vasopressin studies in the rat. I. A sensitive bioassay for exogenous vasopressin. Pflügers Arch. ges. Physiol. **290**, 279—285 (1966).

—, J. HELLER u. O.H. GAUER: Über die antidiuretische Aktivität in der Lymphe von Katzen. Pflügers Arch. ges. Physiol. **283**, 222—229 (1965).

TAYLOR, N.B.G., and J.M. WALKER: Antidiuretic substance in human urine after smoking. J. Physiol. (Lond.) **113**, 412—418 (1951).

TAYLOR, S.P., jr.: Ion exchange chromatography of oxytocin, arginine-vasopressin and lysine-vasopressin. Proc. Soc. exp. Biol. (N.Y.) **85**, 226—228 (1954).

THEOBALD, G.W.: The repetition of certain experiments on which Moliter and Pick base their water centre hypothesis and the effect of afferent nerve stimuli on water diuresis. J. Physiol. (Lond.) **81**, 243—254 (1934a).

— The alleged relation of hyperfunction of the posterior lobe of the hypophysis to eclampsia and the neuropathy of pregnancy. Clin. Sci. **1**, 225—239 (1934b).

THEOBALD, G.W., A. GRAHAM, J. CAMPBELL, P.D. GANGE, and W.J. DRISCOLL: The use of post pituitary extract in physiological amounts in obstetrics. Brit. med. J. **1948 II**, 123—127.

THORN, N.A.: A densimetric method for assay of small amounts of antidiuretic hormone. J. exp. Med. **105**, 585—590 (1957).

— Binding *in vitro* of highly purified arginine vasopressin and synthetic oxytocin to rat serum globulin. Acta endocr. (Kbh.) **30**, 472—476 (1959a).

— Some chemical properties of antidiuretic material in the urine of rats. Acta endocr. (Kbh.) **32**, 128—133 (1959b).

— The effect of arginine-, lysine- and leucine-vasopressin on urine osmolality and rate of urine flow in hydrated rats and dogs. Acta endocr. (Kbh.) **32**, 134—141 (1959c).

—, and L. SILVER: Chemical form of circulating antidiuretic hormone in rats. J. exp. Med. **105**, 575—583 (1957).

—, and M.W. SMITH: Renal excretion of synthetic arginine vasopressin injected into dogs. Acta endocr. (Kbh.) **49**, 388—392 (1965).

— —, and E. SKADHAUGE: The antidiuretic effect of intravenous and intracarotid infusion of calcium chloride in hydrated rats. J. Endocr. **32**, 161—165 (1965).

TINDAL, J.S.: Personal communication (1960).

—, and A. YOKOYAMA: Assay of oxytocin by the milk-ejection response in the anaesthetized lactating guinea-pig. Endocrinology **71**, 196—202 (1962).

TOWBIN, E.C., and C.B. FERRELL: Stop flow study of renal excretion of tritiated vasopressin. Physiologist **6**, 288 (1963).

TUPPY, H.: Biochemical studies of oxytocinase. In: Oxytocin, pp. 315—324. Ed. by R. CALDEYRO-BARCIA and H. HELLER. London: Pergamon Press 1961.

TURNER, C.W., and W.D. COOPER: Assay of posterior pituitary factors which contract the lactating mammary gland. Endocrinology **29**, 320—323 (1941).

URANGA, J., and W.H. SAWYER: Renal responses of the bullfrog to oxytocin, arginine vasotocin and frog neurohypophysial extract. Amer. J. Physiol. **198**, 1287—1290 (1960).

USSING, H.H., and K. ZERAHN: Active transport of sodium as the source of electric current in the short circuited isolated frog skin. Acta physiol. scand. **23**, 110—117 (1951).

VAN DONGEN, C.G.: A bioassay for oxytocic activity in biological fluids and its use in certain phases of reproductive physiology. Dissertation Abstr. (Physiol.) **25**, Diss. No. 65-3688, p. 6726 (1965).

—, and R.L. HAYS: Bioassay for oxytocic activity in untreated blood plasma. J. Animal Sci. **23**, 1229 (1964).

— — A sensitive *in vitro* assay for oxytocin. Endocrinology **78**, 1—6 (1966a).

— — Oxytocic activity in unextracted blood plasma during calving. J. Reprod. Fertil. **11**, 317—323 (1966b).

VOGT, MARTHE: Vasopressor, antidiuretic and oxytocic activities of extracts of the dog's hypothalamus. Brit. J. Pharmacol. **8**, 193—196 (1953).

VORHERR, H.: Eine neue Methode zum Oxytocin-Nachweis an der lactierenden Maus. Arch. Exptl. Pathol. Pharmakol. **251**, 123 (1965).

—, C.R. KLEEMAN, and A. CARIGAN: New method for the estimation of oxytocin using lactating mice and rats. (Program abstracts of 48th Meeting of Endocr. Soc., U.S.A., 20—22 June, 1966. Abstract 146 p. 99.)

— —, and E. LEHMAN: Oxytocin induced stretch reaction in suckling mice and rats. A semiquantitative bioassay for oxytocin. Endocrinology **81**, 711—715 (1967).

WALKER, A.M.: Experiments upon the relation between the pituitary gland and water diuresis. Amer. J. Physiol. **127**, 519—540 (1939).

WALKER, J.M.: Oxytocin and vasopressin. Measurement in body fluids. In: Polypeptides which affect Smooth Muscles and Blood Vessels, pp. 36—41. Ed. by M. SCHACHTER. London: Pergamon Press 1960.

— Vasopressin. In: Hormones in Blood, pp. 165—173. Ed. by C.H. GRAY and A.L. BACHARACH. London: Academic Press 1961.

WALMSLEY, CHRISTINE F.: The concentration of oxytocin in blood in relation to reproduction. M.Sc. Thesis, University of Bristol (1963).

WARING, H., and F.W. LANDGREBE: Hormones of the posterior pituitary. In: The Hormones, Vol. II, pp. 427—514. Ed. by G. PINCUS and K.V. THIMMAN. New York: Academic Press 1950.

WEINSTEIN, H., R.M. BERNE, and H. SACHS: Vasopressin in blood: effect of haemorrhage. Endocrinology **66**, 712—718 (1960).

WERLE, E.: Kallikrein, kallidin and related substances. In: Polypeptides which affect Smooth Muscles and Blood Vessels, pp. 199—209. Ed. by M. SCHACHTER. London: Pergamon Press 1960.

WIED, DE D.: A simple automatic and sensitive method for the assay of antidiuretic hormone with notes on the antidiuretic potency of plasma under different experimental conditions. Acta physiol. pharmacol. neerl. **9**, 69—81 (1960).

—, and I. A. MIRSKY: The action of hydrocortisone on the antidiuretic and adrenocorticotrophic response to noxious stimuli. Endocrinology **64**, 955—966 (1959).

WIEDERMAN, J., and M. L. STONE: Effect of oxytocin on myoepithelium of the breast. J. appl. Physiol. **17**, 539—542 (1962).

WIQVIST, N., I. WIQVIST, C. A. FIELITZ, and R. CALDEYRO-BARCIA: Effects of oxytocin on the uterine response to electrical stimulation. Acta endocr. (Kbh.) **41**, 161—169 (1962).

YAMASHIRO, D., H. L. ANNING, and V. DU VIGNEAUD: Inactivation of oxytocin by acetone. Proc. nat. Acad. Sci. (Wash.) **54**, 166—171 (1965).

YOSHIDA, S., K. MOTOHASHI, H. IBOYASHI, and S. OKINAKA: Method for the assay of antidiuretic hormone in plasma with a note on the antidiuretic titer in human plasma. J. Lab. clin. Med. **62**, 279—285 (1963).

Production, Release, Transportation and Elimination of the Neurohypophysial Hormones

MICHAEL GINSBURG

With 26 Figures

The Hypothalamo-Neurohypophysial Neurosecretory System

At first the term 'neurosecretion' was used in the description of neurones that contained particles resembling secretory granules (SCHARRER and SCHARRER, 1940). Since then, advancing knowledge of neuronal structure and function, in particular the discovery by electron microscopy of synaptic vesicles and other inclusions containing transmitter substances and the demonstration that neurosecretory neurones transmit action potentials, has led to a narrowing of the distinction between neurosecretory and other neurones and to a tendency to make the definition more restrictive.

SCHARRER and BROWN (1962) remark that the term "should not be indiscriminately applied to nerve cells in general simply on the basis of the presence of granular cell inclusions, or to signify the release by neurones of active substances", but there is no general agreement as to what does constitute a neurosecretory cell. Fortunately, the neurohypophysial system exhibits all the essential characteristics of neurosecretion and therefore it is unlikely that, regardless of the outcome of current debate, the designation of the neurohypophysis as a neurosecretory system will be changed. The criteria proposed by B. SCHARRER (1959) for neurosecretory neurones are (a) they elaborate secretory material demonstrable by histological techniques, (b) they release physiologically active substances which affect organs lying distant from the central nervous system, thus playing an important role in neuroendocrine integration, and (c) they can receive stimuli from other neurones; their axons do not synapse with other neurones, muscles or exocrine glands but usually end on blood vessels. The hypothalamo-neurohypophysial system satisfies each of these criteria.

The idea that neurones could elaborate hormones was first established firmly by a series of papers from BARGMANN and his colleagues (BARGMANN, 1949, 1951; BARGMANN and SCHARRER, 1951; HILD, 1951; HILD and ZETLER, 1951, 1953), in which the staining characteristics of the neural lobe and the supraoptic and paraventricular nuclei were correlated with the functional state of the system and its hormone content. Prior to 1949 the prevailing view, first expressed by BUCY (1932), was that the hormones of the neurohypophysis were secreted by pituicytes. This was supported by the observation that in rats deprived of water, osmiophilic granules accumulated in pituicytes, (GERSH, 1939). Although the occurrence of fat droplets and increased mitotic activity in pituicytes in states known to deplete the neurohypophysis of its hormones have been reported more recently (SELYE and HALL, 1943; CHAMBERS, 1945; LEVEQUE and SMALL, 1959; DUCHEN, 1962), the functional significance of these changes even now is not known. It has been suggested (LEVEQUE and SMALL, 1959) that pituicytes might secrete a releasing factor that acts upon the neurones to liberate the hormones.

The presence of small amounts of hormone activity in median eminence and neural stalk was known from early work (VAN DYKE, 1926; SATO, 1928) and in 1938, RANSON and his co-workers (FISHER, INGRAM, and RANSON, 1938) clearly demonstrated that in order to produce experimental diabetes insipidus it was necessary to make lesions proximally in the neural stalk, or to destroy, bilaterally, the supraoptic nuclei, both procedures causing atrophy of the neural lobe. These observations are not compatible with the pituicyte hypothesis. In 1938, also, RASMUSSEN noted the numerous fine nerve fibres in the neural lobe and he suggested that the hormones were liberated from the nerve terminals.

However, the significance of these contributions was not apparent until the work of the anatomists at Kiel was reported. This depended on the exploitation of a modification by BARGMANN (1949) of the chrome-alum haematoxylin stain of GOMORI (1941). The close relationship between the activity of the supraoptic and paraventricular nuclei and the neural lobe was demonstrated by the combined use of hormone assay methods and the staining procedure (ORTMANN, 1951; HILD and ZETLER, 1953a and b). In some species, particularly in the dog, large amounts of the Gomori positive neurosecretory material were found in the supraoptic and paraventricular nuclei and when the pituitary stalk was divided, neurosecretory material accumulated above the cut (HILD and ZETLER, 1953b).

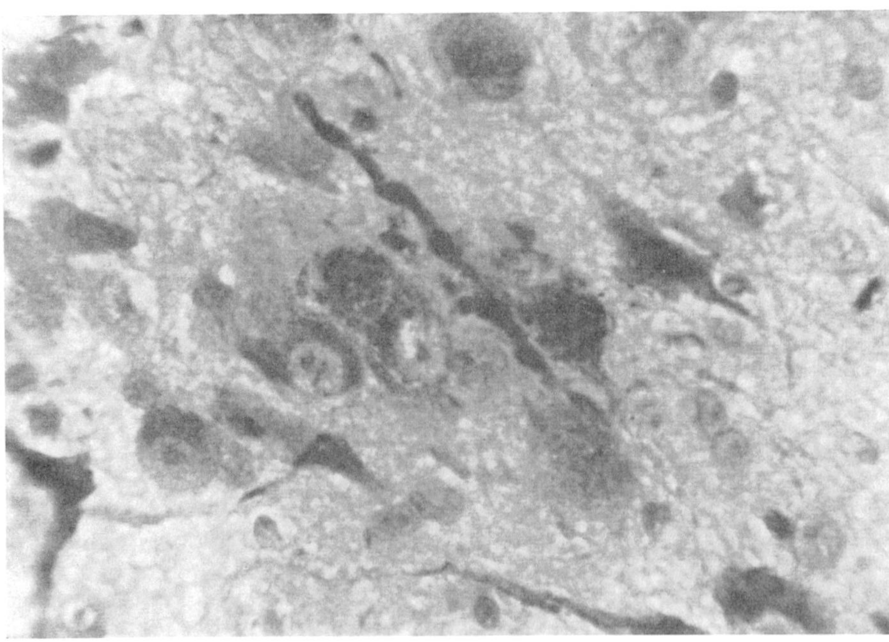

Fig. 1. Paraventricular nucleus of cat stained with chrome alum haematoxylin (× 410). Neurosecretory material in cell bodies and in beaded fibres. Reproduced by courtesy of Professor J. C. SLOPER. Int. Rev. Cytol. 7, 337—389 (1958)

When dogs were subjected to chronic dehydration and subsequently allowed access to water, changes in oxytocin and vasopressin content of the neural lobe ran more or less parallel to changes in the content of neurosecretory material (HILD and ZETLER, 1953a).

The correlation between the amounts of stainable substance in the neural lobe and the state of hydration has been confirmed by many groups of workers, some using more selective staining methods (KOVACS et al., 1954; BARNETT, 1954;

Adams and Sloper, 1956; Andersson and Jewell, 1957; Howe and Jewell, 1959). Changes in neurosecretory material in the neural lobe during lactation have been studied extensively and the situation is confused by differences between species although there is general agreement that the amount of neurosecretory material is reduced as is the hormone content of the gland. In the rat, neurosecretion in the neural lobe decreases considerably as does the stainability of the supraoptic and paraventricular nuclei (Stutinsky, 1953; Rinne, 1960), while in the mouse, although neurosecretion in the neural lobe decreases there is apparently no change in the hypothalamic nuclei (Brightman, 1955). However, the parallelism between neurosecretory material content is not maintained when acute rather than chronic stimulation of hormone release is involved (see p. 289).

These findings gave support to the proposal of Bargmann and Scharrer (1951) that the neurosecretion was related to the hormones and was synthesised in the cell bodies of neurones in the paraventricular and supraoptic nuclei; that the neurosecretion migrates in the form of droplets and strings of beads (Fig. 1) along the axons of the hypothalamo-neurohypophysial tract and finally accumulates in the posterior pituitary. This hypothesis has been confirmed, in general outline, in almost all recent studies.

1. The Nature of Neurosecretory Material

The original methods for staining neurosecretory material, aldehyde-fuchsin and chrome-alum haematoxylin are non-specific. Since they stain mucopolysaccharides it was thought that neurosecretory material might be mucoprotein (Schiebler, 1951, 1952). However, it could be shown (Howe and Pearse, 1956) that it contained neither lipid nor carbohydrate, and that treatment with pepsin and trypsin digests the neurosecretory material (Rinne, 1960). The claim of Hild and Zetler (1953b) that extraction with lipid solvents removed stainable substances without extracting hormone activity from neural lobes has not been substantiated by Sloper (1954, 1955) who was able to show that the original observation was due to a difference between the treatments accorded to the parts of the neural lobe set aside for assay and for histological examination.

The chrome-alum haematoxylin method for staining neurosecretory material becomes more selective when a preliminary stage of oxidation is employed and more specific methods have been developed that stain SS and SH groups, such as the performic acid-alcian blue method of Sloper and his colleagues (Adams and Sloper, 1956) and the dihydroxy-dinaphthyl-disulphide reaction (Barnett and Seligman, 1952; Barnett, 1954). It is believed that the significant effect of preliminary oxidation, is the conversion of cystine and cysteine to cysteic acid which takes part in the staining reactions.

Thus the evidence points to the conclusion that the stainable neurosecretory material is a protein or peptide rich in cystine or cysteine. The obvious candidates for this role are the neurohypophysial hormones themselves and Rodeck (1959a and b) has shown that various preparations of neurohypophysial hormones, including synthetic oxytocin, give the appropriate histochemical reactions when embedded and fixed in agar.

Another candidate for the role of neurosecretory material is the carrier protein neurophysin which also has a high content of cystine (Block and van Dyke, 1952; Hope et al., 1966; Ginsburg, Jayasena, Pickering, and Thomas, 1966) and has been shown to stain after treatment with the Gomori (Acher, 1958) and alcian blue techniques (Ginsburg and Ireland, 1965). There is an apparent discrepancy in that after acute stimulation of neurohypophysial hormone secretion the stainable neurosecretory material disappears from the neural lobe to a much greater extent than the hormone content. Very rapid depletion of neurosecretory material in rat neurohypophysis occurs within a few minutes of a moderately painful stimulus (ROTHBALLER, 1953; MONACI and NOCENTINI, 1955; DE GROOT and HARTFIELD, 1960). It is difficult to imagine that significant depletion of the hormone store occurs in such a short time and MOSES, LEVEQUE, GIAMBATISTA, and LLOYD (1963) have shown that a stressful stimulus (injection of formalin) does not noticeably deplete the gland of vasopressin, although the depletion of neurosecretory material is clear 5—15 min after the stimulus. Similarly, DRAGER and RENNELS (1955) have pointed out that the presence of neurosecretory material is not a good index of the amounts of oxytocin present and although lactation influences both neurosecretory material and oxytocin content in the same general direction the changes in the two parameters are not synchronous (RENNELS, 1958).

While these observations are important as a cautionary influence it should be stressed that the quantitative correlation between staining intensity and the amount of stainable material has not been resolved. The physico-chemical state of the hormone carrier complex very probably alters when the gland is stimulated and the possibility that this involves changes in conformation that affect stainability should be considered.

2. The Intra-Neuronal State of the Neurohypophysial Hormones

There are many published accounts of the electron microscopic ultrastructure of the neural lobe of the neurohypophysis in mammals (PALAY, 1955, 1957; BARGMANN and KNOOP, 1957; GREEN and MAXWELL, 1959, 1964; FUJITA and HARTMANN, 1961; HOLMES and KIERNAN, 1964; LEDERIS, 1965; BARER and LEDERIS, 1966 and many others) in fish (PALAY, 1960; LEDERIS, 1962) and amphibia (GERSCHENFELD, TRAMEZZANI, and DE ROBERTIS, 1960).

The main mass of the neural lobe of the neurohypophysis comprises unmyelinated nerve fibres, interspersed by pituicytes that are considered to be of neuroglial type. Occasionally, myelinated nerve fibres are seen. Many of the nerve fibres end in dilatations or swellings close to the capillaries but are separated from them by a perivascular space lined by a basement membrane. Other swellings are found along the course of nerve fibres and are not necessarily in close relation to capillaries. Neural swellings vary considerably in size; they are usually larger than 0.5 μ in diameter and there appears to be a more or less continuous gradation in size up to several μ in diameter. The larger bodies were recognised by early histologists as Herring bodies. The common feature of the swellings is that they contain large numbers of granules of the order of 100 mμ in diameter. According to BARER and LEDERIS (1966) myelinated nerve fibres in the neural lobe also contain large numbers of these granules. The particles, known as elementary or neurosecretory granules are membrane limited and in experiments where precautions are taken to avoid stimulation of neurohypophysial hormone secretion, most of them contain osmiophilic material that imparts an electron dense appearance to the core of the particle. Most sections of neural swellings contain mitochondria that are often irregular in shape and unusually electron dense. At swellings close to a perivascular space numbers of smaller particles, about 20—30 mμ in diameter are seen and are similar in appearance to synaptic vesicles though the resemblance is not necessarily a token of the identity of these particles. The parts of the nerve fibre connecting nerve swellings are usually devoid of granules and mitochondria but contain parallel strands of fibrils or tubules. In transverse section the tubules are 20 mμ in diameter and it is difficult to trace them in the nerve swellings.

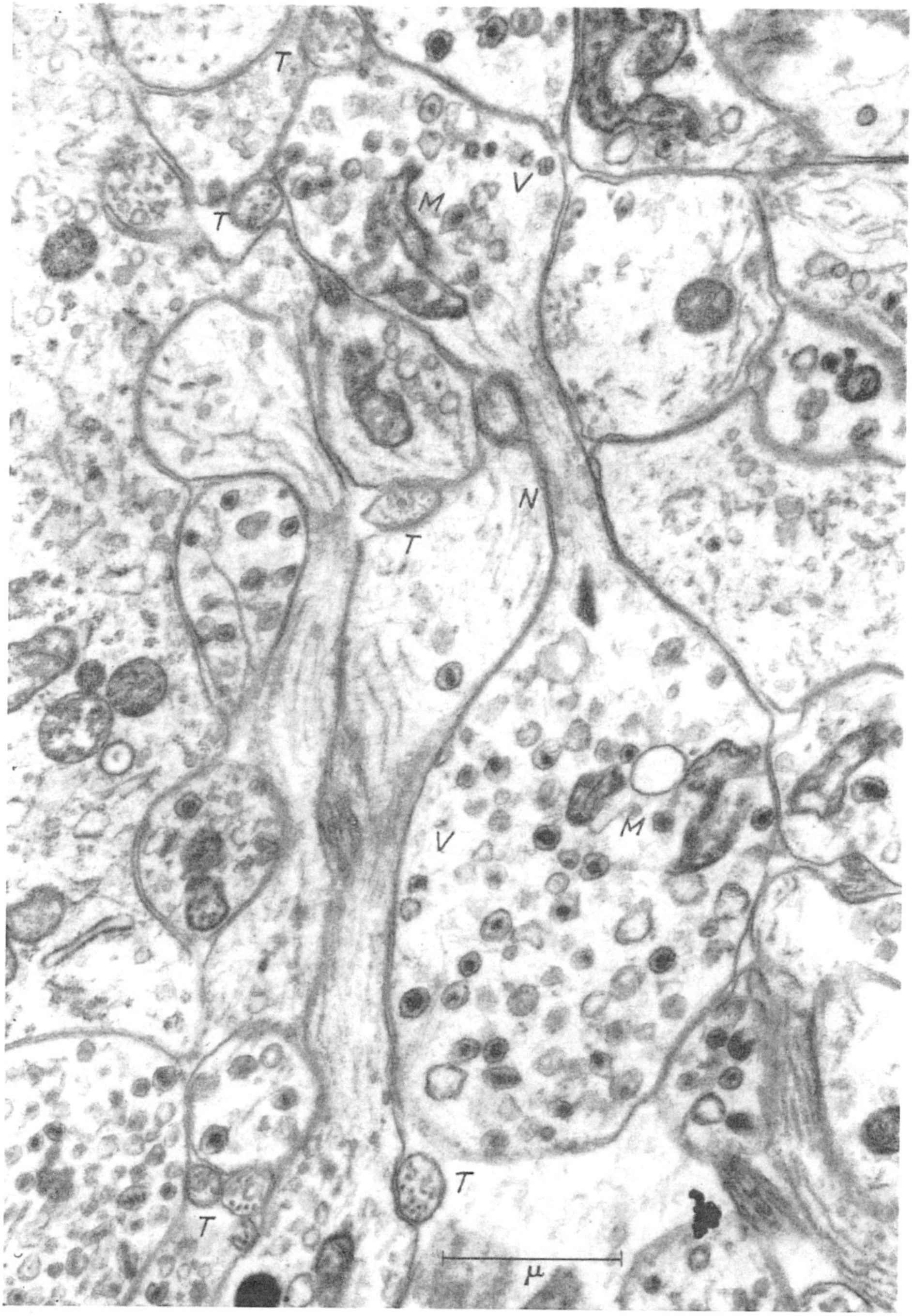

Fig. 2. Nerve fibres and neural swellings in a normal rabbit neural lobe. Swellings contain neurosecretory granules (V) and mitochondria M and are joined by a narrow nerve fibre N. Reproduced with permission from BARER and LEDERIS. Z. Zellforsch. **75**, 201—239 (1966)

The ultrastructure of the cell body of the neurosecretory neurones has not been studied as extensively as the structure of the neural lobe. This applies particularly to mammalian material for which there are special problems of fixation and preservation of nervous tissue for electron microscopy (SLOPER, 1965), and thus the most successful preparations have been obtained with hypothalami of fish (PALAY, 1960; LEDERIS, 1962; FOLLENIUS, 1963) and amphibia (GERSCHENFELD et al., 1960; BERN, NIKIOSHI, and HAGEDORN, 1962). More recently, MURAKAMI (1962) and SLOPER and BATESON (1965) have published descriptions of the ultrastructure of the supraoptic nuncleus in mouse, rat and dog.

In the neuronal cell body in the goldfish, PALAY (1960) distinguishes between the central and peripheral zones. The endoplasmic reticulum studded with ribosomes is distributed at the margin of the cell extends only a little way down the first part of the neurosecretory process and is absent from the nerve fibres and endings of the neural lobe. The virtual restriction of the sites of protein synthesis to the cell body is the usual condition in neurones (WAELSCH and LAJTHA, 1961) and since the neurosecretory products are peptides this is a point of particular significance to the site and mode of synthesis of the hormones.

The central zone contains the nucleus, many mitochondria and the Golgi complex which is composed of close packed curved masses of agranular membrane. In addition there are three main categories of droplets, (1) multivesicular bodies that occur in other neurones, about 1 μ in diameter and that contain 5—20 small vesicles, (2) large electron dense granules also about 1 μ in diameter and (3) small electron dense granules (0.1 μ in diameter).

The distribution of the diameters of electron dense inclusions in the neural lobe in the supraoptic nucleus of the dog is shown in Fig. 3.

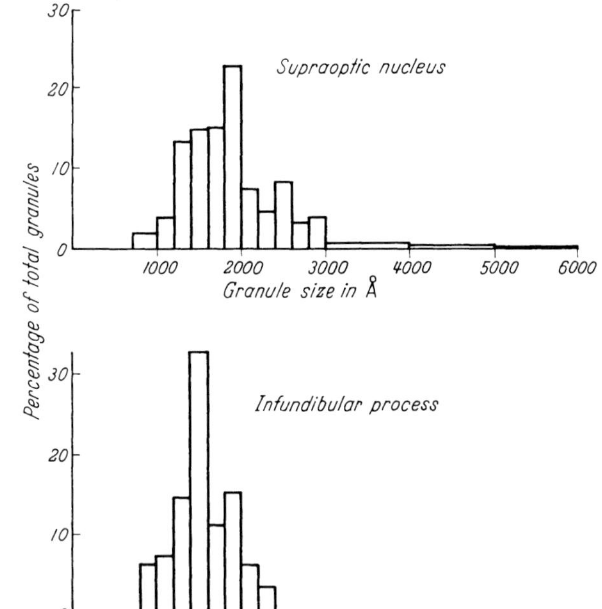

Fig. 3. Distribution of the diameters of electron dense inclusions in the supra-optic nucleus and in nerve endings of the neural lobe (infundibular process) in a dog. Reproduced with permission from SLOPER and BATESON. J. Endocr. 31, 139—150 (1965)

Most of the particles in the cell body are of a size that lies within the range of the neurosecretory granules seen in the neural lobe. It is believed that smaller granules in the cell body, if not identical with the neurosecretory granules, are at least their precursors. The large particles occur only in the cell body and are much less abundant. In the dog there appears to be a gradation of size between the large and small bodies, in contrast to the mouse (MURAKAMI, 1965) and goldfish (PALAY, 1960). PALAY (1960) and BERN (1963) hold the view that the large electron dense particles are not concerned with the neurosecretory process and suggest that the smaller particles are formed from the cisternae of the Golgi complex (Fig. 4). A contrary view is taken by LEDERIS (1964) who thinks that the neurosecretory granules might be formed by budding off from the larger vesicles. Two other proposals have been made to account for the genesis of the

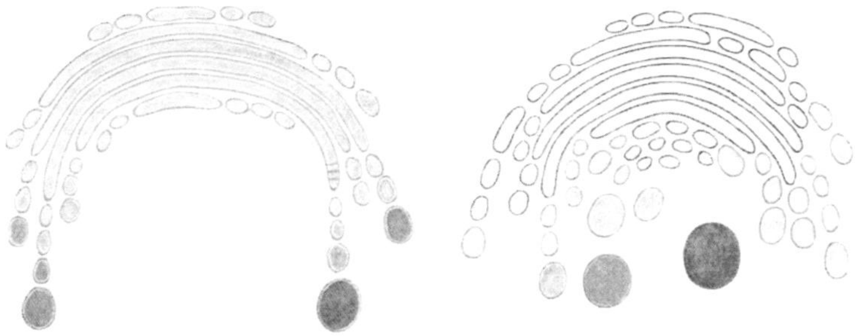

Fig. 4. Possible modes of formation of elementary neurosecretory granules by the Golgi apparatus. Diagram on left represents the appearance of electron dense material with Golgi lamellae and the formation of membrane-limited granules by budding. Diagram on right represents formation of electron-lucent vesicles and their subsequent transformation into electron-dense granules. Reproduced with permission from Bern. In: The General Physiology of Cell Specialisation. Ed. by D. MAZIA and A. TYLER. New York: McGraw Hill 1963

neurosecretory granules. KNOWLES (1958) and GREEN and MAXWELL (1959) have suggested that they might originate from mitochondria while DE ROBERTIS and his colleagues (DE ROBERTIS, 1964; GERSCHENFELD et al., 1960) suggest that the neurosecretory particles are formed by budding from "neuroprotofibrils".

According to GERSCHENFELD et al. (1960) the neurosecretory granules in the toad undergo alterations in size during transport towards the nerve terminals the mean diameter increasing from 62 mμ in axons at a point proximal to the median eminence to 150 mμ in axons near the nerve terminals and decreasing slightly to 115 mμ in the terminals themselves. DE ROBERTIS (1964) believes that these observations indicate "that secretory granules are being formed along the axon in the hypothalamic region" and that "there is progressive synthesis of material (hormone) along the axon".

However, as pointed out above, the data of SLOPER and BATESON (1965) does not show any difference in size distribution of neurosecretory granules between cell body and nerve terminal in dogs and there is no striking difference in size of granules in the axons at different levels in cat (GREEN and VAN BREEMAN, 1955) or pigeon (OOTA and KOBAYASHI, 1962).

The conclusion that the neurosecretory granules are the particles that contain the main intracellular store of neurohypophysial hormone is based principally on evidence obtained by differential centrifugation of neural lobe homogenates. The first experiments of this type were carried out by SCHIEBLER (1952) in which he obtained from neural lobes of cattle a granular fraction rich in neurosecretory material as indicated by staining by the chrome-alum haematoxylin method. Since the fraction also contained succinic dehydrogenase activity a relationship to mitochondria was suggested. A similar conclusion was reached by PARDOE and WEATHERALL (1955) in experiments with homogenates of rat neural lobe which showed that the hormone activities were associated with particles with sedimentation characteristics similar to mitochondria and that, by light microscopy, the presence of mitochondria could be demonstrated in the hormone rich pellets.

In subsequent investigations in which the study of the distribution of hormone activity among the sediments obtained by differential centrifugation of neural lobe homogenates in sucrose media has been coupled with electron microscopy of the pellets and distribution of biochemical markers for different cell organelles, the hormone rich sediment has been shown to be composed of particles

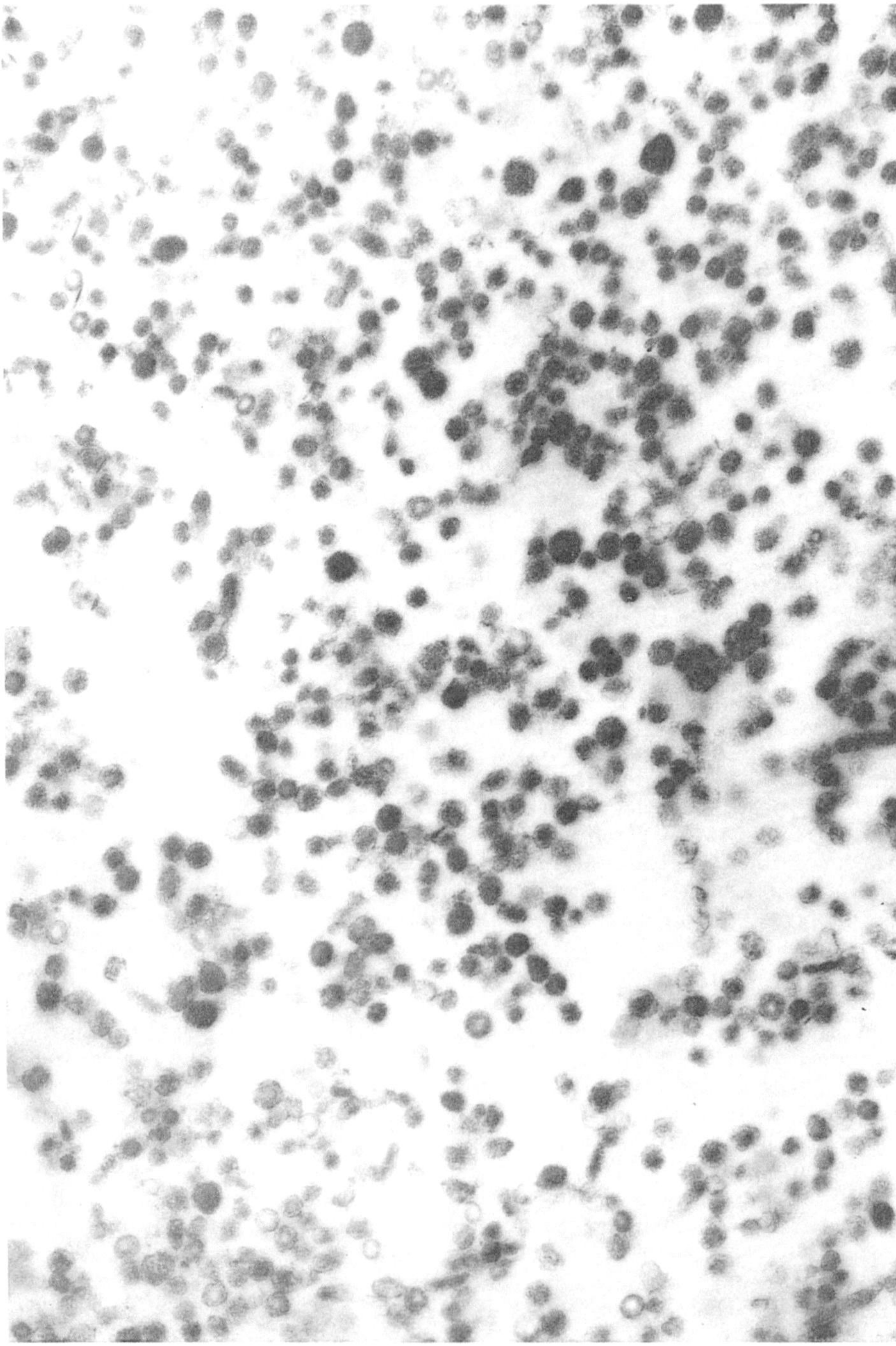

Fig. 5. Electron micrograph of neurosecretory granule fraction (× 33,030) prepared by differential centrifugation of sucrose homogenates of rabbit neurohypophysis. Reproduced with permission from BARER et al. Proc. roy. Soc. 158 B, 388—416 (1963)

of similar dimensions (100—300 mμ) and appearance to the neurosecretory granules of the nerve swellings seen by electron microscopy (LEDERIS and HELLER, 1960; WEINSTEIN, MALAMED and SACHS, 1961; SCHAPIRO and STJARNE, 1961; LABELLA et al., 1962; ISHI, YASUMASU, KOBAYASHI, OOTA, HIRANO, and TANAKA, 1962; BARER, HELLER, and LEDERIS, 1963; GINSBURG and IRELAND, 1966). The exact conditions for the preparation of neurosecretory granule fractions varies among the different groups of workers but, constantly, the highest yield of hormone activity was obtained in a fraction that sediments at centrifugal forces higher than those required from mitochondrial sedimentation but less than required for deposition of microsomes (Fig. 5). Moreover, WEINSTEIN et al. (1961) were able to distinguish the hormone bearing particles from the main mitochondrial, lysosomal and microsomal fractions by succinic dehydrogenase, glucuronidase and nucleic acid determinations. Substantial amounts of hormone activity are found in nuclear and mitochondrial fractions but these are far from homogenous and contain numerous vesicular and granular bodies that can be identified as small neural swellings or fragments of neural swellings as well as free neurosecretory granules (BARER et al., 1963). Intragranular vasopressin is protected from tryptic hydrolysis (WEINSTEIN et al., 1961) but the granular membranes can be disrupted by treatment with hot acetic acid (WEINSTEIN et al., 1961; HELLER and LEDERIS, 1962) hypotonic solution (SCHAPIRO and STJARNE, 1961; WEINSTEIN et al., 1961) or detergent (WEINSTEIN et al., 1961; BARER et al., 1963). There is some evidence that suggets that oxytocin and vasopressin may not be distributed uniformly among the population of granules and that particles may contain one or the other hormone preferentially, if not exclusively. By the use of density gradient centrifugation BARER et al. (1963) and LABELLA et al. (1962) were able to demonstrate partial separation of oxytocin-rich from vasopressin-rich granule fractions (Fig. 6). The membranes of the oxytocin particles also seem to be more fragile since BARER et al. (1963) found that treatment of the granules with octylamine liberated oxytocin more readily than vasopressin and more recently, GINSBURG and IRELAND (1966) reported an experiment in which nearly 50% of the oxytocin in a granule pellet was liberated on resuspension in an isotonic potassium phosphate buffer compared with less than 10% of the vasopressin.

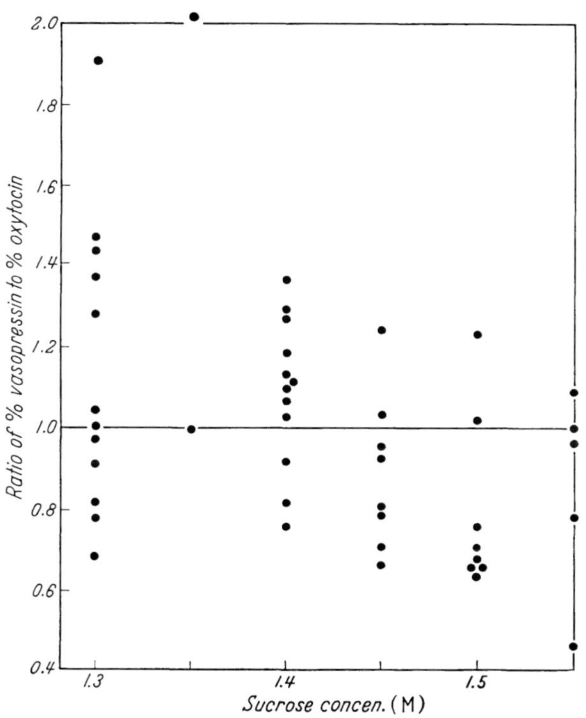

Fig. 6. Scatter diagram of the results of sucrose density gradient centrifugation of homogenates of rabbit neurohypophyses. Reproduced with permission from BARER et al. Proc. roy. Soc. 158 B, 388—416 (1963)

It is quite likely that *in situ* the separation of oxytocin and vasopressin granules might be more complete than these experiments suggest. The supernatant media of the homogenates, even under the best conditions contain oxytocin and vasopressin to the extent of about 10% or more of the content of the whole homogenate and it is feasible that some exchange of intragranular and supernatant hormone could occur in the suspension. On the other hand, *in situ*, there is the possibility that an individual neurone will contain predominantly, one or the other hormone (see p. 301) and so the conditions for exchange will be less favourable than in suspension of the particles.

Most of the biochemical investigations of the neurosecretory granule fractions were used as a means to distinguish the granules from other intracellular organelles. However, GINSBURG and IRELAND (1966) have shown that the distribution of the hormone binding protein, neurophysin, in fractions of bovine neural lobe separated by differential centrifugation from sucrose homogenates is essentially similar to the distribution of the hormones and that the neurosecretory granule fraction is richest in the carrier protein. It was estimated that neurophysin represented as much as 50% of protein in the granules soluble in 0.1 M acetic acid. GINSBURG and IRELAND (1966) were also able to obtain approximate estimates for the concentrations fo neurophysin and hormone in the intragranular space. The concentration of neurophysin in the granule water was of the order of 15—20 g/100 ml while the average hormone content (oxytocin plus vasopressin) of a single granule was 0.5—1.0 $\times 10^{-13}$ units; for each molecule of neurophysin the granules contained 1.0—1.6 molecules of peptide hormone. This is much below the maximum capacity of bovine neurophysin to bind the hormones (GINSBURG and IRELAND, 1965), and although the intracellular pH is not optimal for binding (pH 5.8; GINSBURG and IRELAND, 1964) it was concluded that the peptide hormones occur in the bound form in the granules. However, the association constant for the formation of the hormone-neurophysin complexes is such that there would be significant amounts of free hormone intragranularly in equilibrium with the bound form.

A quite substantial proportion of the hormones is found in the supernatant fraction from sucrose homogenates of neural lobes, usually quarter to half of the activity in the granule faction (BARER et al., 1963; GINSBURG and IRELAND, 1966). However, after suspension of granule pellets by homogenisation in fresh sucrose medium and recentrifugation, GINSBURG and IRELAND (1966) found that less than 10% of the hormones and protein appeared in the supernatant. GINSBURG and IRELAND (1966) also concluded that neurophysin content of the supernatant fraction was greater than could be attributed to disruption of neurosecretory granules during homogenisation, so that extra-granular hormone, like that in the granules, can exist as the free and bound forms in equilibrium. However, owing to the low association constant and the greater dilution of the hormone and neurophysin, the proportions of bound to free would be much less than in the granules. It is possible that extra-granular hormone derives from the neuronal cytoplasm and extra-neuronal spaces; BARER and LEDERIS (1966) have suggested recently that a mucopolysaccharide matrix in perivascular spaces might act as a subsidiary store of neurohypophysial hormone.

A neurosecretory granule fraction from the hypothalamo-median eminence complex of the dog has been separated by SACHS (1963a). Sedimentation of this fraction was obtained under the same conditions used for the preparation of neurosecretory granules from neurohypophysis and its vasopressin content was higher than in other fractions, both in terms of concentration and absolute amount. However, the ratio of vasopressin to protein in the hypothalamic neurosecretory particles is only about one quarter of that for neurohypophysial granules. There is no information available on the neurophysin content of these granules from hypothalamic tissue.

The occurrence of the neurohypophysial hormone in granules in the form of a labile complex is clearly important for the maintenance of the large and readily available store of hormone in the neurohypophysis. When granules are incubated at different hydrogen ion concentration within the range pH 6.2—7.4 the release of hormone increases with increasing pH, i. e. as conditions alter to favour dissociation of the hormone-neurophysin complexes (GINSBURG and IRELAND, 1966). It would appear therefore, that the granular membrane is not a barrier to the diffusion of free hormone and that the integrity of the store depends on the intragranular neurophysin. One of SACHS' (1963a) experiments suggests another role for the neurophysin in the protection of the hormones from degradation by cytoplasmic enzymes. He found that the activity of arginine vasopressin was reduced by 70—80% after incubation with a homogenate of dog hypothalamo-median eminence while there was no significant loss of vasopressin when added in the form of disrupted neurohypophysial neurosecretory particles, i. e. presumably therefore in the complex form.

3. The Nature of the Complexes Formed by Neurophysin and Neurohypophysial Hormones

Pursuing J.J. ABEL's famous 'unitary hormone' concept, MCARTHUR (1931) and later VAN DYKE, CHOW, GREEP, and ROTHEN (1941) isolated a protein fraction from posterior pituitary glands with oxytocic, vasopressor and antidiuretic activities. ROSENFELD (1940) showed that the pressor and oxytocic principles existed in the untreated press-juice of the posterior lobe of the pituitary in the form of large molecule(s), one third to one half the size of egg albumin, an observation that has been confirmed by more recent experiments (SMITH and ROSENFELD, 1961).

The protein isolated by VAN DYKE et al. (1941) was prepared under relatively mild conditions (fractional precipitation on the addition of NaCl to a concentration of 6%) and was shown to contain oxytocic and vasopressor activity in the ratio 1:1 and a high proportion of cystine. ACHER, CHAUVET, and OLIVRY (1956) and ACHER and FROMAGEOT (1957) re-examined the properties of the VAN DYKE protein and found that the oxytocin and vasopressin can be removed from the protein by dialysis in dilute acetic acid, by electro-dialysis, by trichloracetic acid precipitation of the protein and by counter current distribution. These observations suggest that the hormones are held to the protein by electrostatic forces, a conclusion reached in earlier work by HASSELBACH and PIGUET (1952) who found that oxytocin in bovine posterior pituitary extracts could be separated from protein by electrodialysis. Thus the VAN DYKE protein comprised three components that were separable quite readily; oxytocin, vasopressin and the protein moiety. The name 'neurophysin' was suggested for the protein by CHAUVET, LENCI, and ACHER (1960) who showed that the salt-precipitable complex was reformed on the addition of hormone to neurophysin. LINDNER, ELMQVIST, and PORATH (1959) while developing techniques for the purification of neurohypophysial hormones, found that by gel filtration at pH 3.0 the hormones could be separated from the protein in acetic acid homogenates of neurohypophyses.

SMITH (1963) considered that the most likely mode of combination of the hormones with neurophysin susceptible to dissociation at low pH, would be disulphide interchange between the cystine residues of the hormones and the protein. An alternative proposed by STOUFFER, HOPE, and DU VIGNEAUD (1963) and GINSBURG and IRELAND (1963, 1964) is that the complex is formed by ionic association involving the free α-amino group of a hemicystinyl residue in the peptide and carboxyl groups in the protein. STOUFFER et al. (1963) showed that desamino oxytocin (lacking the free cystinyl amino group) is not bound by bovine neurohypophysial protein while GINSBURG and IRELAND (1963, 1964) found that the pH dependence of binding of the hormones (optimum pH 5.2—5.8) was compatible only with involvement of the free cystinyl amino group of the peptides in complex formation with carboxyl groups in neurophysin.

In this connection it may be significant that a characteristic of the amino acid composition of neurophysin from both bovine and porcine sources is a high content of dicarboxylic acids as well as a high content of cystine (BLOCK and VAN DYKE, 1952; FRANKLAND, HOLLENBERG, HOPE, and SCHACHTER, 1966; GINSBURG, JAYASENA, PICKERING, and THOMAS, 1966). Neurophysin does not form complexes with other pharmacologically active peptides and bases such as catecholamines, histamine, substance P or 5-hydroxytryptamine (GINSBURG and IRELAND, 1964) and GINSBURG, JAYASENA, and THOMAS (1965) have been able to separate two components in porcine neurophysin of which one binds both oxytocin and vasopressin while the other binds oxytocin selectively (Fig. 7). It is obvious also that carboxyl groups in neurophysin do not form complexes with the ionised groups of the arginyl and lysyl residues of the vasopressins.

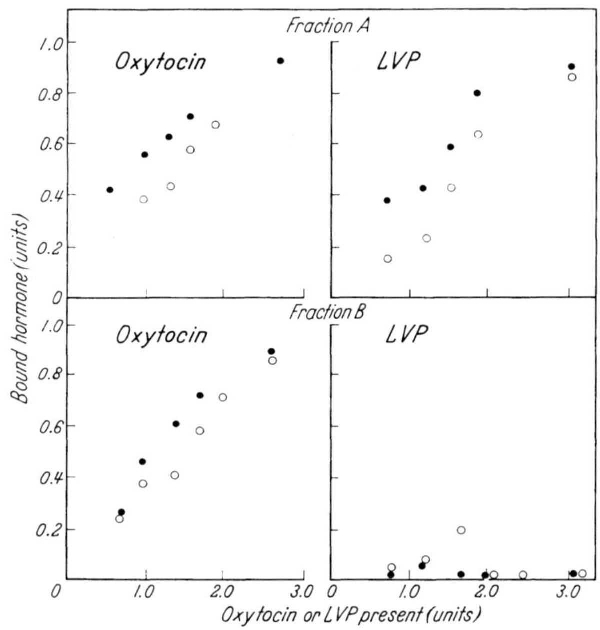

Fig. 7. Binding of oxytocin and lysine vasopressin by protein fractions from porcine neurohypophyses separated by chromatography on DEAE Sephadex. The open and closed circles distinguish results obtained with different preparations. Reproduced with permission from GINSBURG et al. J. Physiol. (Lond.) **183**, 45 (1965)

This degree of specificity is difficult to explain on the basis of the ionic association which must therefore be regarded as a primary link with specificity conferred by other forces, possibly by secondary disulphide interchange or by lipophilic interaction between other sites (GINSBURG and IRELAND, 1965).

4. Biosynthesis of Neurohypophysial Hormones

According to the BARGMANN and SCHARRER (1951) neurosecretion hypothesis the neurosecretory product is synthesised in the paraventricular and supraoptic nuclei. Morphological and endocrinological studies have provided much evidence that supports this view. Recently, SACHS and his co-workers have reported studies of vasopressin biosynthesis by incorporation of labelled amino acids and, as a result, the general outline of the original hypothesis has been confirmed, although some changes in detail have become necessary.

In the earlier experiments (SACHS, 1960) ^{35}S labelled cysteine was infused for periods of 8—36 h into a jugular vein in dogs or for 8 h into the third ventricle. The vasopressin content of the hypothalamus in the neural lobe was estimated by biological assay and then by painstaking use of chromatographic methods, assisted by the addition of unlabelled arginine vasopressin "carrier", the vasopressin was isolated. The isotopic purity of the vasopressin was established by (a) its biological activity (about 400 u/mg) (b) performic acid oxidation followed by chromatography to separate any labelled SH compounds that might have formed disulphide bridges with vasopressin and (c) in some instances the dinitrophenol derivative of oxidised vasopressin was prepared.

The essential result from these experiments was that the ratio of the specific activities of the vasopressin from the two sites $\frac{\text{hypothalamus}}{\text{neural lobe}}$ was of the order of 2—5. SACHS pointed out that, by considering the differences in the size of the pools of vasopressin in the hypothalamus and the neural lobe and on the assumption that the rate of secretion of vasopressin was 5 mu/h as estimated by SHANNON (1942), this ratio should be of the order of 400 if all the labelled vasopressin was synthesised as such in the hypothalamus.

The application to SACHS' experimental conditions (the dogs were anaesthetised with pentobarbitone) of SHANNON's (1942) value for the rate of secretion, which is an estimate of antidiuretic hormone secretion required to keep a conscious dog in normal water balance, is almost certainly in error. However, new calculations using a more realistic estimate for vasopressin secretion rate (SLOPER, 1965) gives a ratio of between 42 and 85 to 1 which is equally incompatible with the observed value between 2 and 5 to 1.

Localisation in the hypothalamic cell bodies of radioactive sulphur from the administration of labelled amino acids has been shown by many groups of workers (GAITONDE and RICHTER, 1956; MALANDRA, 1958; FORD and HIRSCHMAN, 1958; SLOPER, ARNOTT, and KING, 1960; FLAMENT-DURAND, 1961; FORD, HIRSCHMAN, RHINES, and ZIMBERG, 1961; FICQ and FLAMENT-DURAND, 1964). In most of these studies total radioactivity was measured, usually by autoradiography. It is not possible therefore to distinguish between free amino acid, amino acid incorporated in vasopressin and amino acid incorporated in protein.

SACHS (1963) also has investigated the intracellular site of vasopressin synthesis. The specific activities were measured of vasopressin isolated from subcellular particles obtained by differential centrifugation of sucrose homogenates of canine hypothalamo-median eminence complex, after infusion of (^{35}S) cysteine into the 3rd ventricle. The fraction sedimenting at 70,000 g, i.e. with sedimentation properties of neurosecretory particles (NSP) contained more vasopressin than other fractions, but the specific activity of vasopressin in the NSP fractions was equal to that in the 70,000 g supernatant and was less than in a fraction sedimented at 600 g (cell debris and nuclei). The 70,000 g supernatant was resolved into a "large granule and microsome" fraction and "cell sap" and the specific activity of vasopressin from these particles was greater than the NSP vasopressin, and even higher than in the "cell debris and nuclei" fraction. On treatment with deoxycholate the highly radioactive vasopressin was no longer sedimentable showing that it was not bound firmly to ribosomes. SACHS considered that the pool of highly active deoxycholate soluble vasopressin was not large enough or sufficiently radioactive to account for the radioactivity of the NSP fraction vasopressin. He proposed therefore that a bound and biologically inert form of vasopressin, possibly a protein, was formed on ribosomes and that the biologically active peptide was released from the inactive precursor both during the formation and the maturation of the neurosecretory particles.

More recently, the essence of this proposal has been confirmed by additional experiments of TAKABATAKE and SACHS (1964) in which evidence for *in vitro* biosynthesis of vasopressin was obtained. Labelled vasopressin was isolated from intact guinea pig hypothalamo-neurohypophysial systems that had been incubated in a tissue culture medium containing labelled amino acids. The appearance of the labelled hormone was dependent on an energy source and was inhibited by puromycin, suggesting that a protein synthesising system was involved. However, the appearance of labelled vasopressin in the system, unlike the appearance of labelled protein, was preceded by a lag period. No incorporation of labelled amino acid into vasopressin occurred when neural lobe alone was incubated, but the ability of slices of hypothalamo-median eminence complex to synthesise vasopressin was demonstrated (Fig. 8). Puromycin treatment also prevented the appearance of labelled vasopressin in *in vivo* experiments with dogs, but only if it was administered from the start of the experiment (SACHS and TAKABATAKE, 1964).

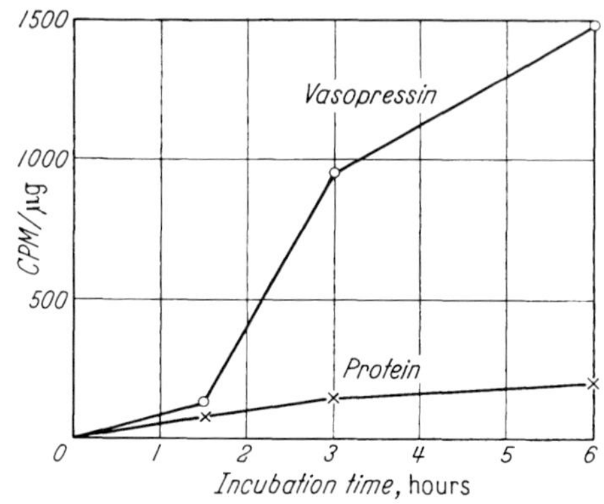

Fig. 8. Incorporation of ^{35}S cysteine into vasopressin and protein of hypothalamo-neurohypophysial tissue of guinea pigs incubated *in vitro*. Reproduced with permission from SACHS and TAKABATAKE. Endocrinology **75**, 934 (1964)

Slices of hypothalamo-median eminence tissue taken from dogs that had been infused with labelled amino acid for at least 1—5 h form labelled vasopressin *in vitro*, even if puromycin is present in the incubation mixture. Thus, the synthesis of a precursor could be prevented by puromycin but, once formed, the antibiotic did not interfere with its conversion into the active peptide.

In contrast to vasopressin, the highest specific activity of protein was found in the 70,000 g pellet from homogenates of hypothalamus from dogs in which ^{35}S cysteine had been infused into the 3rd ventricle (SACHS, 1963). When the infused labelled amino acid was ^{3}H leucine, the specific activity of the NSP protein was not conspicuously greater than in the other fractions, but it could be shown the high ^{35}S specific activity of NSP protein was not entirely due to its high content of sulphur because when expressed as counts per mg S content the specific activity remained higher than in other fractions.

It seems possible that the sulphur rich metabolically active protein of hypothalamic NSP might be the vasopressin precursor molecule and that the conversion to the biologically active peptide proceeds during the distal transport of the particles in the axons of the hypothalamo-hypophysial tract. DE ROBERTIS (1964) has suggested that alteration in the size of neurosecretory granules in different parts of the system is associated with progressive hormone synthesis during transport. The observation that the vasopressin/protein ratio is higher in neurohypophysial NSP than in hypothalamic NSP might be held to support this interpretation but could be accepted only with reservations because of the uncertain purity of the hypothalamic NSP fraction.

Neurophysin is a known component of the neurosecretory granules with a high S content. Comparison of the amino acid composition of bovine and porcine neurophysins does not show a preponderance of arginine in the former and lysine in the latter (GINSBURG et al., 1966) so it is unlikely that neurophysin has a dual role as hormone carrier and hormone precursor. One of the unique features of the neurohypophysis is the high content of free peptide of which only a small proportion is represented by the biologically active hormones (RAMCHANDRAN and WINNICK, 1957; WINNICK, WINNICK, ACHER, and FROMAGEOT, 1955). Most are rather small molecules but one of them isolated by PREDDIE and SAFFRAN (1965) has a molecular weight of the order of 8,000 and like the hormones contains a ring closed by a disulphide bridge (PREDDIE, 1965). It could be that these peptides are inactive fragments of the hormone precursor molecules or are degradative products from other proteins attacked by a hormone liberating enzyme system.

Fig 9 shows diagrammatically how SACHS and TAKABATAKE (1964) interpret their findings. Vasopressin precursor is synthesised on ribosomal RNA and is incorporated into the neurosecretory granules as these are formed possibly from the Golgi complex. They propose that some release of vasopressin from the precursor takes place during the formation of the neurosecretory granule and that the process is completed within the granule during distal transport in the axon. There are, of course, other possibilities. For example, the activation could occur outside the granules, which being rich in neurophysin would thus be able to concentrate the hormone. The answers to questions like this may be given when the precursor molecule and its activating system have been characterised and their subcellular locations determined.

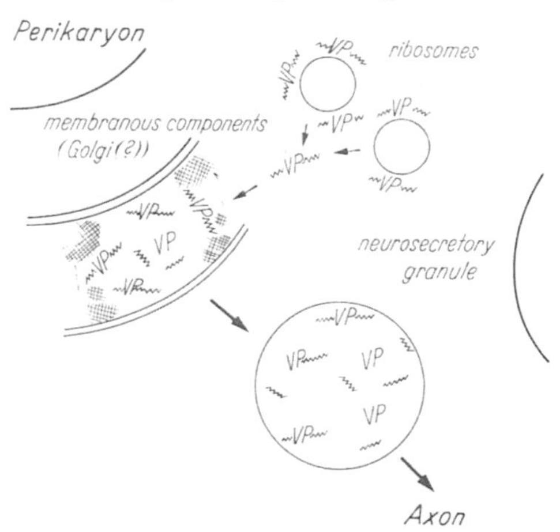

Fig. 9. A "precursor" model for vasopressin biosynthesis. VP = biologically active octopeptide. ~~ VP ~~ = precursor molecule. Reproduced with permission from SACHS and TAKABATAKE. Endocrinology **75**, 943 (1964)

There are no reports of experimental investigations of oxytocin biosynthesis but it would be surprising if, ultimately, it was shown that the mechanism did not have many features in common with that for the biosynthesis of vasopressin. The occurrence of both oxytocin and vasopressin in the hypothalamus has been demonstrated for many mammalian species (VON SCHLICHTEGROLL, 1954; VAN DYKE, ADAMSONS, and ENGEL, 1955; ADAMSONS, ENGEL, VAN DYKE, SCHMIDT-NIELSEN, and SCHMIDT-NIELSEN, 1956; LEDERIS, 1961) and the ratio of vasopressin to oxytocin in the hypothalamus usually is not different from the ratio of the two hormones in the neural lobe of the same species. However, this obscures differences in the relative amounts of the hormones in different hypothalamic areas, and where these can be separated readily by dissection, in sheep, (LEDERIS, 1961) and camel (ADAMSONS et al., 1956) it has been shown that in the supraoptic region, vasopressin is the predominant hormone while oxytocin predominates in the paraventricular region. The hypothalamus in the dog is exceptional in that while it contains substantial amounts of vasopressin, the oxytocin content is very low and might well be attributable to the intrinsic oxytocic activity of the vasopressin in the extracts (VOGT, 1953). Thus if the biosynthetic pathway for oxytocin also is by way a precursor formed in the hypothalamus, then liberation of the active oxytocin occurs more distally in the hypothalamo-hypophysial tract than the liberation of the active vasopressin. This conclusion and the differences in the relative proportions of the hormones in different regions of the hypothalamus suggest that oxytocin and vasopressin are not liberated from a common precursor and/or that the activating systems are different. The absence of vasopressin, while oxytocin is present, in the neurohypophysis of rats of the Brattleboro' strain with familial diabetes insipidus (VALTIN, SAWYER, and SOKOL, 1965) indicates the separate genetic control of the precursor synthesising and/or activating systems for the two neurohypophysial hormones. Anatomical separation of the sites of oxytocin and vasopressin synthesis also is possible. The relative concentration of each hormone in one or the other magnocellular nucleus could arise from the segregation in supraoptic region of the cell bodies of neurones in which vasopressin precursor and its activating system occurs, while the cell bodies of paraventricular region belong predominantly to neurones containing the oxytocin synthesising system.

According to OLIVECRONA (1957) and NIBBELINK (1961) placement of lesions in the paraventricular nuclei of rat and cat results in a profound fall in the oxytocin content of the neural lobe, although the antidiuretic hormone content is not changed. Since it is difficult both to destroy all the cell bodies of the paraventricular cell nucleus and to avoid retrograde degeneration of many cells in the supraoptic nucleus (OLIVECRONA, 1957) this evidence does not give unequivocal support to the proposal that the paraventricular nuclei are the main or sole sites of synthesis of oxytocin or its precursor.

SOKOL and VALTIN (1965) from studies of the morphology of the hypothalamic nuclei in relation to hereditary hypothalamic diabetes insipidus in rats point out that even in heterozygotes, that store normal amounts of oxytocin in the neural lobe, the amounts of neurosecretory material in the axons in the paraventricular nucleus is much reduced. However, the departure from normal in the appearance of the supraoptic nucleus is much more radical. This suggests that although there may not be absolute separation of the synthesis of the two hormones at the different sites in the hypothalamus there is nevertheless relative separation, and that although 'one neurone – one hormone' might be the rule the synthesis of both hormones may occur within some individual neurones.

Making the reasonable assumption that if the vasopressin content of the neurohypophysis did not vary greatly from day to day in undisturbed animals (estimated rates of secretion are of the order of 1% of the gland content of vasopressin per day), GINSBURG and BROWN (1956) pointed out that the normal rate of synthesis must equal the rate of secretion and that there were many indications that some stimuli for the release of vasopressin also increase vasopressin synthesis. When, for example, adult rats are subjected to dehydration, the concentration of antidiuretic hormone in blood rises and more hormone is excreted in urine, but the vasopressin content of the neural lobe increases during the first 48 h (AMES and VAN DYKE, 1950; DICKER and NUNN, 1957) although with dehydration of longer duration the hormone content of the gland falls. Also, in the experiments of HILD and ZETLER (1953a) when access to drinking water was restored to dogs that had been deprived of water for 14 days, the vasopressin content of the neurohypophysis increased at a rate 20—100 times faster than the normal rate of synthesis. In thus responding to secretory stimulation the neurones of the hypothalamo-neurohypophysial system seems to be acting similarly to neurones in general for, as HYDÉN (1943) has shown, if a motor or a sensory part of the central nervous system is stimulated within physiological limits, each nerve cell affected will increase its content of RNA, proteins and lipid, and enzymatic activity rises (HYDÉN and PIGON, 1960).

EDSTROM and EICHNER (1958) EDSTROM, EICHNER, and SCHOR (1961) have in fact demonstrated in rats in which vasopressin secretion was stimulated by administration of hypertonic sodium chloride solution that the amounts of RNA in the cytoplasm and the nucleus of cells in the supraoptic nucleus increases significantly, coupled with increases in the volumes of the nucleus and the nucleolus. Hypothalamo-median eminence slices from guinea pigs deprived of water for 4 days, when incubated with labelled amino acids incorporate the label into vasopressin more quickly than tissue from guinea pigs in normal water balance (TAKABATAKE and SACHS, 1964). With more severe dehydration (8 days) there is virtual loss of the ability of the hypothalamo-median eminence slices to incorporate the labelled amino acids in vasopressin. However, there was little difference in the labelling of protein in the slices from normal animals, and animals dehydrated for 4 or 8 days. It would seem thus that the formation of the specific RNA molecules required for the synthesis of proteins involved in the biosynthetic pathway for vasopressin is, in its turn, affected by the stimuli that evoke vasopressin secretion.

5. Intraaxonal Transport of Neurosecretory Material

The neurosecretion hypothesis requires the centrifugal transport of material from the cell bodies in the hypothalamus to the nerve endings in the neural lobe where most of the hormone in the system is stored. It is usually assumed that the phenomenon of proximo-distal axoplasmic flow that occurs in all neurones can account sufficiently for the process. The evidence for the existence of axoplasmic flow comes mainly from the work of WEISS and his colleagues (WEISS and HISCOE, 1948; WEISS and CAVANAUGH, 1959; WEISS, 1961). In the basic experiment a mild constriction was placed on nerve fibre by placing a tightly fitting cuff of arterial tissue around a nerve trunk. During the weeks that followed the operation the fibres developed marked asymmetry with respect to the constriction. The distal portion of the fibre shrunk to a narrower calibre, while the proximal portion was enlarged. The conclusion drawn from this type of experiment was that material synthesised in the cell body of a neurone is transported distally down the length of the axon and replenishes stores of substances, in the cytoplasm throughout the axon, that are subject to continual loss or degradation. The appearance fo the dammed-up material at the proximal side of the constriction was bead-like, or in smaller fibres the deformation resembled corkscrew-like spirals, and this would occur only if the moving mass was solid or semi-solid, but not liquid. The motive mechanism for axoplasmic flow is not known —"the movement seems to be in the nature of what in larger dimensions is effected by peristaltic waves, but this is about all that one could safely conclude at the present juncture" (WEISS, 1961).

The accumulation of cholinesterase and cholineacetylase at the proximal end of cut peripheral nerve (SAWYER, 1946; HEBB and WAITHES, 1956), the accumulation of neurosecretory material and even the regeneration of a "new" and partially functional neurohypophysis at the proximal end of a severed pituitary stalk, provide further evidence for axoplasmic flow (STUTINSKY, 1951, 1955, 1957; SLOPER and ADAMS, 1956; MOLL, 1957; BECK and DANIEL, 1961). Attempts have been made to estimate the rate of axoplasmic flow by following the appearance in the nerve fibre of radioactive labels of substances that would be incorporated into an axoplasmic component in the cell body, e.g. an amino acid into protein, or P into phosphoprotein (SAMUELS, BAJARSKY, GERARD, LIBET and BRUST, 1951; SLOPER, 1958; WEISS, 1959; SLOPER, ARNOTT, and KING, 1960; DROZ and LEBLOND, 1962).

In spite of the complexity inherent in such experiments almost all the observations suggest a rate of movement of about 1—2 mm/day. According to SLOPER (1965), taking into consideration the numbers of neurosecretory granules seen in electronmicrographs of the neural lobe and the hypothalamic cell bodies, such movement could transport vasopressin at a rate similar to the rate of secretion in the resting animal. During active restoration of the depleted store in thirsted animals vasopressin is delivered distally at a much faster rate; it is not known whether this can be accounted for by the increased synthesis of vasopressin and it may be necessary to postulate that during enhanced secretory activity in a neurosecretory neurone the rate of axoplasmic flow is increased.

a) Cellular Mechanism of Neurohypophysial Hormone Release

It is generally accepted that in the various physiological states that evoke secretion of hormone from the neurohypophysis, the response is mediated by humoral or nervous factors and do not act directly upon the store of hormone in the neurosecretory terminals of the neural lobe but through the neurosecretory cell bodies (JEWELL and VERNEY, 1957; HARRIS, 1955; ORTMANN, 1960). For example, isolated neurohypophyses do not liberate vasopressin when exposed to solution with raised osmotic pressure (DOUGLAS and POISNER, 1964) or containing acetylcholine (DOUGLAS and POISNER, 1964; DANIEL and LEDERIS, 1966) although both are effective *in vivo*, particularly when given in such a way as to reach first the anterior hypothalamus (JEWELL and VERNEY, 1957; PICKFORD, 1939, 1947; PICKFORD, and WATT 1951; ABRAHAMS and PICKFORD, 1956).

The discharge of impulses down the hypothalamo-hypophysial tract is obviously a means whereby stimuli received in the cell body can be transmitted to the nerve terminals and there affect the state of the stored hormone. It has been known for a long time that electrical stimulation of the pituitary stalk causes release of both neurohypophysial hormones in *in vivo* experiments (HATERIUS and FERGUSON, 1938; HATERIUS, 1940; FERGUSON, 1941; HARRIS, 1947, 1948; CROSS and HARRIS, 1952). More recently it has been shown, *in vitro*, that stimulation of the rat pituitary stalk (DOUGLAS and POISNER, 1964) or the passage of impulses through a suspension of guinea pig neural lobes (HALLER, SPERELAKIS, SACHS, and SHARE, 1965), cause vasopressin release into the incubation medium, and that the effect of electrical stimulation can be blocked by a local anaesthetic, tetracaine (HALLER et al., 1965). The question whether or not neurosecretory cells are neuronal not only in morphological appearance but also in conducting properties has recently been solved by several groups of workers who have made intracellular recordings from positively identified neurosecretory cells (MORITA, ISHIBASHI, and YAMASHITA, 1961; BENNETT and FOX, 1962; YAGI, BERN, and HAGEDORN, 1963) including cells of the hypothalamo-hypophysial system (KANDEL, 1962) and have established that they behave like neurones. Also, KOIZUMI, ISHIKAWA and BROOKS (1964), ISHIKAWA, KOIZUMI, and BROOKS (1966) have recorded extracellular action potentials in the pituitary stalk during stimulation of the supra-optic nuclei in cats. Thus it seems that the secretory stimulation of the neurohypophysis involves the generation of impulses in the cell body and their discharge toward the nerve terminals. Arrival of the impulses at the nerve terminals sets in motion a chain of events of which the net effect is the transfer of hormone from a compartment of the neural lobe to the circulating blood.

The number of barriers interposed between the elementary granules and the lumen of the neurohypophysial capillary is impressive. They are: (a) the limiting membrane of the neurosecretory granule, (b) the plasma membrane of the neural swelling, (c) the outer condensed layer of basement membrane, (d) the mucopolysaccharide layer of the perivascular space, (e) the inner condensed layer of the basement membrane and (f) the capillary endothelial cells or their prores. However, it is not known which compartment contains the hormone whose translocation is elicited by the arrival of impulses, nor is it known the extent to which these membranes are effective barriers to the diffusion of free hormone. Ultimately, the liberated hormone probably (though not necessarily), comes from the store in the neurosecretory granules, but the rather limited evidence suggests that the immediate effect of the secretory stimulus is upon hormone in some other compartment, possibly the extragranular hormone of the nerve swellings as proposed by THORN (1965) and GINSBURG and IRELAND (1966).

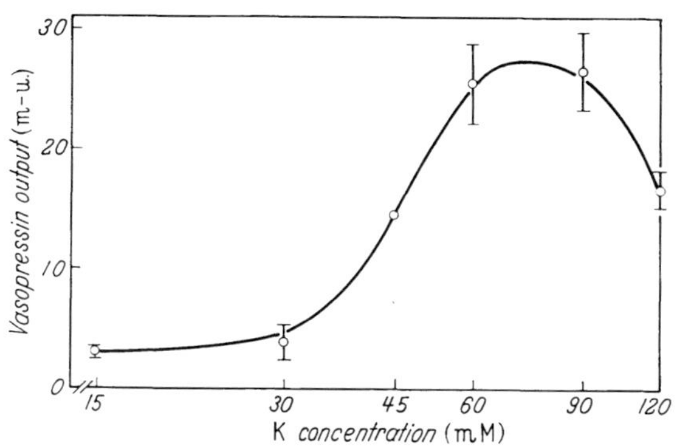

Fig. 10. Relationship between K concentration and vasopressin output from isolated incubated rat neurohypophyses. Reproduced with permission from DOUGLAS and POISNER. J. Physiol. (Lond.) **172**, 1—18 (1964)

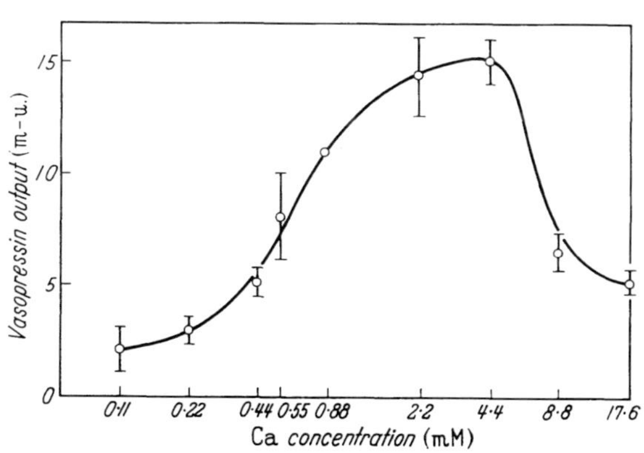

Fig. 11. Relationship between Ca concentration and vasopressin-release response to excess K (60 mM) of isolated incubated rat neurohypophyses. Reproduced with permission from DOUGLAS and POISNER. J. Physiol. (Lond.) **172**, 1—18 (1964)

In spite of the lack of knowledge on these important questions a striking advance in understanding of stimulus-secretion coupling has been achieved in recent years, mainly though the work of DOUGLAS and his colleagues, (DOUGLAS, 1963; DOUGLAS and POISNER, 1963a, 1963b; 1964a, 1964b). Rat neurohypophyses incubated *in vitro* in a modified Locke solution containing 5.2 mM K and 2.2 mM Ca, after equilibration, lose vasopressin into the medium at a fairly steady but quite low rate — about 0.1% of the gland content per 10 min. If however, the composition of the medium is changed by increasing K to 52 mM, vasopressin appearing in the medium is increased by a factor of about 10. Raising K to 30 mM has but little effect and the response was maximal at 60—90 mM (Fig. 10), and since this is similar to the relationship between K and depolarisation of muscle, it was suggested that in the media with excess K the neurohypophysial nerve terminals were depolarised.

When Ca was omitted from the incubation medium, raising K concentration no longer elicited vasopressin release, and it was shown that the effect of excess K was maximal at Ca concentrations around 2.2—4.4 mM (Fig. 11), but re-introduction of Ca free medium containing 5.6 mM K did not have a stimulant effect. Omission of Na from the medium potentiated the response to excess K and increasing the Mg concentration from 1 mM to 10—20 mM depressed the secretory response to K. DOUGLAS and POISNER (1964a) interpret these results as meaning that depolarisation, on exposure to high concentration of K, stimulates secretion by promoting the entry of Ca into the neurosecretory terminals. Confirmation of this proposal was obtained in studies of the movement of ^{45}Ca between the medium and the incubated rat hypophyses (DOUGLAS and POISNER, 1964b). It was found that on raising the K concentration from 5.6—56 mM the rate of ^{45}Ca uptake was increased 5 fold. Efflux of ^{45}Ca also was increased in the presence of excess K but only when the incubation medium contained Ca, showing that the effect of increased K was due to increased influx rather than reduced efflux of Ca. In certain respects, however, ^{45}Ca uptake did not run parallel with vasopressin release. For example, uptake in the presence of excess K was uninfluenced by the absence of Na and was inhibited only slightly by 10 mM Mg; in excess K media the release of vasopressin is much less at 8.8 mM Ca than with 2.2 mM Ca and yet the stimulation of Ca uptake by excess K is not less at the higher Ca concentration. It would seem, therefore, that while the influx of Ca into neurohypophysial cells is probably the most important factor determining the release of vasopressin, very high concentration of Ca and altered amounts of Na and Mg in the medium modify release by affecting the intracellular action of Ca and not its uptake.

The application of the hypothesis to the release of hormone from the neurohypophysis *in vivo* involves the assumption that the effect of excess K simulates the arrival of the action potentials at the nerve terminals. This assumption may be justified because the dependence on Ca concentration of vasopressin release *in vitro* is the same whether it is elicited by electrical stimulation of the stalk or by excess K in the medium (MITIKEN and DOUGLAS, 1965).

The basic observation that release of vasopressin *in vitro* from rat neurohypophyses is dependent on K and Ca concentration in the medium has been confirmed by DANIEL and LEDERIS (1963) and DICKER (1966), though, quantitatively, the effects were rather smaller than those obtained by DOUGLAS and POISNER (1964a). These workers have shown also that oxytocin release is elicited under the same conditions and in DICKER's (1966) experiments the release of oxytocin from adult rat glands under any given set of conditions was greater than the simultaneous release of vasopressin. HALLER, SACHS, SPERELAKIS, and SHARE (1965) have shown that addition of Ba to the incubation medium in which isolated guinea pig neurohypophyses are suspended increases release of vasopressin, this effect is considered not to be analogous to that of Ca but due to the increased excitability of the neuronal membrane.

A variety of metabolic inhibitors (2:4 dinitrophenol, iodoacetate, cyanide, amytal and antimycin) can prevent the release of vasopressin that normally accompanies a rise in K concentration from 5.6 mM to 56 mM (DOUGLAS, ISHIDA, and POISNER, 1965). The effect was not due to prevention of depolarisation by excess K because the inhibitors also prevented the release of vasopressin evoked by adding Ca to Ca free Locke containing 153 mM K in which rat neurohypophyses were incubated. On the assumption that the entry of Ca into the depolarised neural lobes is passive, they concluded that the metabolic inhibitors affect the process that links intracellular Ca with vasopressin extrusion. It was proposed, therefore, that the process of calcium induced secretion is tightly coupled to energy metabolism and requires the presence of an intermediate, the production of which is energy dependant. ATP might be involved as the intermediate, a role that it may play in the extrusion of hormones from chromaffin cells of the adrenal medulla (DOUGLAS, POISNER, and RUBIN, 1965). On the other hand, addition of ATP to incubated rat neurohypophyses does not increase vasopressin release (THORN, 1966) and may indeed prevent release elicited by ouabain (DICKER, 1966). Another proposal for the intracellular action of Ca that leads to neurohypophysial hormone release is that Ca promotes dissociation of the hormone-neurophysin complexes. The effect of Ca on vasopressin binding by bovine neurophysin was described first by SMITH and THORN (1965). They showed that the expected shift in the elution of arginine vasopressin when subject to gel filtration in the presence of neurophysin did not occur when $CaCl_2$ was added to the buffer to a concentration of 10 mM. GINSBURG, JAYASENA, and THOMAS (1966) confirmed and extended these observations in experiments in which binding of oxytocin and lysine vasopressin by porcine neurophysin was inhibited in the presence of Ca. The Ca concentration for inhibition of binding is extremely critical, (there is no significant inhibition of binding where the Ca concentration is 0.25×10^{-6}M while at 1.0×10^{-6}M inhibition is virtually complete) and was independent of the concentrations of hormone or neurophysin in the system, within the limits that were feasible under the condition of the experiments. It would seem therefore, that the inhibition of hormone binding by Ca is of a non-competitive nature.

Addition of Ca to suspensions of neurosecretory granules does not affect the loss of hormone from the particles (DANIEL and LEDERIS, 1963; GINSBURG and IRELAND, 1966). This is not inconsistant with the proposed action for Ca since the inhibition fraction, in the case of non-competitive enzyme inhibitors, is reduced at very high enzyme concentrations (LEYDEN-WEBB, 1963) and in the granules the neurophysin concentration is much higher than in the *in vitro* binding experiments. Nevertheless, one must conclude that if Ca affects the hormone-neurophysin complex *in situ*, it must do so in some compartment other than the neurosecretory granules.

THORN (1966) has pointed out that the stimulation of isolated rat neurohypophyses by a depolarising concentration of K in the presence of Ca affects a fraction that comprises only about 5% of the glandular vasopressin and therefore cannot be the intragranular stores. The results of cell fractionation experiments (GINSBURG and IRELAND, 1966) show that some hormone and neurophysin probably occur in an extragranular compartment. Both THORN (1965, 1966), and GINSBURG and IRELAND (1966) suggest therefore that in eliciting hormone release, Ca acts primarily by dissociating the extragranular hormone neurophysin complexes. There is the difficulty of reconciling this with the results obtained (DOUGLAS et al., 1965), using metabolic inhibitors because the effect of Ca on hormone binding elearly is not dependent on metabolic energy. Another difficulty is that Mg can prevent the release of hormone by excess Ca and yet does not influence either Ca uptake (DOUGLAS and POISNER, 1964b) or Ca inhibition of hormone binding (GINSBURG, JAYASENA, and THOMAS, 1966). Sulphydryl reagents, p-chloromercuribenzoate, salyrganic acid and N-ethyl maleimide (DOUGLAS, ISHIDA, and POISNER, 1965) or chilling the incubate to 10° or lower temperatures (DOUGLAS and ISHIDA, 1965) increase release of neurohypophysial hormones from neural lobes. These effects are not dependant on excess Ca or a depolarising concentration of K and both conditions might well affect the hormone-neurophysin association. The high content of cystine in neurophysin makes it tempting to suppose that the sulphydryl reagents interfere with the formation of disulphide bridges that might be secondary bonds between the hormones and the protein. Evidence obtained from the kinetics of the inhibition by cystine of vasopressin binding by neurophysin suggests that an allosteric transformation of the protein occurs during the binding of peptide (THOMAS and GINSBURG, 1966a). The transformation is initiated by the binding of vasopressin at one set of sites and results in the exposure of additional binding sites. At low temperatures, however, the allosteric activation of the protein is inhibited and also the binding capacity is reduced (THOMAS and GINSBURG, 1966b).

Any proposals for the cellular mechanism of hormone release must take into account the changes in the microscopic and electron microscopic appearance of the stimulated gland. The inadequate parallelism between hormone content and neurosecretory material content after acute stimulation of the neurohypophysis has been discussed (see p. 289). The characteristic changes in the electron microscopic appearance of neural lobes taken from animals in hypersecretory states is that the electron dense core of the neurosecretory granules is absent, and the number of small vesicles is increased (PALAY, 1955; BODIAN, 1963; LEDERIS, 1963; BARER, HELLER, and LEDERIS, 1963). Again, after acute stimulation of hormone release by ether anaesthesia followed by severe haemorrhage, there was complete loss of electron density of the elementary granules and yet the vasopressin and oxytocin contents of the glands were 60% and 80% respectively of the amounts in the glands of undisturbed, unanaesthetised controls (DANIEL and LEDERIS, 1966). Increased diffusablilty of the hormone from the stimulated glands was shown by enhanced liberation of hormones from the incubated, isolated neural lobes of the animals subjected to haemorrhage.

This might be consistant with the earlier observation of BARER et al. (1963) that there is a shift of hormone from the granules to the cell supernatant fraction in homogenates of neural lobes from chronically dehydrated or lactating rabbits, though it may be unwise to apply the results of chronic experiments to acute conditions. The electron density of the granules is due to the affinity of a component for heavy metal stains. It is tempting to suppose that this component is the neurophysin-hormone complex, and that the binding of heavy metal atoms is dependent on the allosteric transformation that is induced in the hormone-protein complex state. LEDERIS (1964) has pointed out that loss of electron density can be seen in neurosecretory granules throughout the course of some nerve fibres in the neurohypophysis of trout exposed to a sea-water environment. However, the conclusion that hormone release can occur from nerve fibres anywhere in the gland (i.e. whether abutting on blood vesels or not) is not acceptable because the relationship between the change in electron density and secretion is not absolute.

The ultimate fate of the neurosecretory granules is unknown. Among the numerous possibilities that have been canvassed are (a) that the small particles of the dimension of synaptic vesicles are degenerate neurosecretory granules, (b) that the contents of the granules are extruded from the nerve terminals by 'reverse pinocytosis' (c) that the neurosecretory particles penetrate into the capillaries intact (d) that when the releasing stimulus is withdrawn the particles revert to the normal electron dense appearance. While some of these are inherently more probable than others there is no positive evidence to support any one of them.

In various experimental conditions in which there is increased secretion of neurohypophysial hormones pituicytes multiply and hypertrophy (SELYE and HALL, 1943; CHAMBERS, 1945; ORTMANN, 1951; STUTINSKY, 1951, 1953; COLLIN and RACADOT, 1953; BILLENSTEIN and LEVEQUE, 1955; RENNELS and DRAGER, 1955; LEVEQUE and SMALL, 1959; DUCHEN, 1962), and there is a very close topographical relationship between pituicytes and nerve fibres which sometimes appear to be enveloped by the cytoplasm of the pituicytes (PALAY, 1957). LEVEQUE and SMALL (1959) have proposed that pituicytes may secrete a substance that acting directly on the nerves liberates neurosecretion (hormone) in a soluble form. In the light of more recent work this hypothesis seems to be unnecessary and no evidence has been offered in its support. The observations that led to its formulation remain unchallenged — the changes in pituicytes in hypersecretory states. However, these could occur as a result of hormone release (e.g. an effect of liberated hormone on the pituicytes) or some other event in the secreting gland (e.g. the increased electrical activity in the neurones).

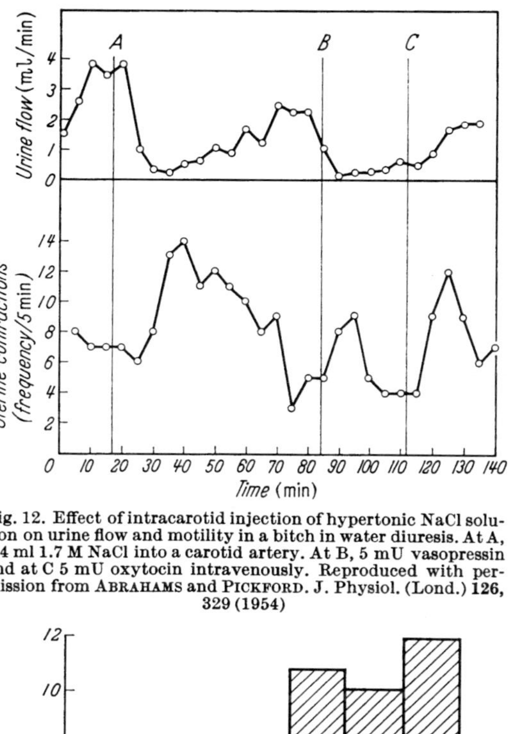

Fig. 12. Effect of intracarotid injection of hypertonic NaCl solution on urine flow and motility in a bitch in water diuresis. At A, 2.4 ml 1.7 M NaCl into a carotid artery. At B, 5 mU vasopressin and at C 5 mU oxytocin intravenously. Reproduced with permission from ABRAHAMS and PICKFORD. J. Physiol. (Lond.) **126**, 329 (1954)

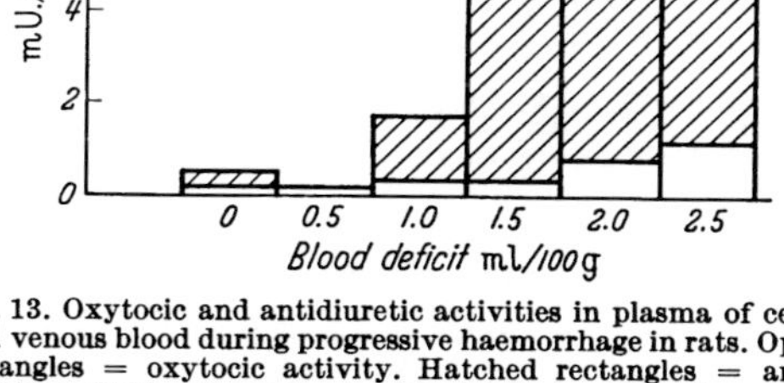

Fig. 13. Oxytocic and antidiuretic activities in plasma of cerebral venous blood during progressive haemorrhage in rats. Open rectangles = oxytocic activity. Hatched rectangles = antidiuretic activity. Reproduced with permission from GINSBURG and SMITH. Brit. J. Pharmacol. **14**, 327—333 (1959)

b) Independance of Oxytocin and Vasopressin Secretion

In the absence of any relevant evidence, it is assumed tacitly that the secretion from a given nerve terminal is related to the capacity of the neurone to synthesise one or other (or both) of the neurohypophysial hormones. The separation of the sites of synthesis of the two neurohypophysial hormones in different regions of the hypothalamus apparently is not absolute (see p. 300). It is not unexpected, therefore, that various stimuli evoke simultaneous secretion of both hormones. The proportions of oxytocin to vasopressin liberated vary with the stimulus but it is surprising that oxytocin is usually, but not invariably, secreted in the larger amounts. This is true for stimuli such as those initiated by suckling (PEETERS and COUSSENS, 1950; CROSS, 1951) where oxytocin is the mediator of a neuroendocrine reflex, for electrical stimulation of the pituitary stalk and acetylcholine administration (HARRIS, 1947, 1948; ABRAHAMS and PICKFORD, 1954) where one might expect no differentiation and even for inter-carotid injection of hypertonic salt solution (ABRAHAMS and PICKFORD, 1954) which, if it simulates dehydration would be expected, on teleological grounds, to liberate vasopressin preferentially (Fig. 12). In contrast, during severe acute haemorrhage (Fig. 13) in rats and cats, large amounts of vasopressin are liberated without equivalent amounts of oxytocin (GINSBURG and SMITH, 1959; BELESLIN, BISSETT, HALDAR, and POLAK, 1967).

With the acute stimulation of secretion, the amounts of hormone liberated are too small to have a significant effect on the hormone content of the gland or, if there is a great excess of one hormone in the secretion, on the ratio of the amounts of the hormones in the gland. In lactating rabbits the ratio of oxytocin to vasopressin released by suckling is 100 to 1 (CROSS, 1951) and yet after 5 or 10 days of lactation there is no significant change in the smounts or ratio of oxytocin to vasopressin (0.5) in the gland (BARER et al., 1963). This suggests that synthesis of oxytocin is stimulated to a rate 100 times greater than the synthesis of vasopressin giving further evidence for the independence of the synthesis of the two hormones.

Presumably the afferent pathways converging on the hypothalamic nuclei are such that they will be stimulated either together or separately. It is possible that the generation of impulse activity in a fibre may affect adjacent fibres that contain the other hormone but the rather sparse evidence suggests that with physiological stimuli this is not so. In trout exposed to sea water for 2 h there is a sharp fall in the ratio of arginine vasotocin to isotocin and yet an electron micrograph shows adjacent fibres one of which has electron dense granules and the other only 'empty' vesicles (LEDERIS, 1964).

6. Cholinergic Mechanisms and Neurohypophysial Hormone Release

Acetylcholine injected intravenously into unanaesthetised atropinised dogs causes inhibition of water diuresis that is due to liberation of vasopressin from the neurohypophysis (PICKFORD, 1939, 1947; DUKE, PICKFORD, and Watt, 1950). The effective dose of acetylcholine is smaller when injected via a carotid artery and still smaller again when given after administration of eserine (PICKFORD and and WATT, 1951). Moreover, acetylcholine in microgram quantities injected directly into the caudal cells of a supra-optic nucleus produces a marked antidiuretic effect (Fig. 14) that is absent if the neurohypophysis has been ablated previously or if the mammillary bodies are injected instead (PICKFORD, 1947; ABRAHAMS and PICKFORD, 1956). Di *iso* propyl phosphorofluoridate (DFP) injected into the supra-optic nuclei in dogs causes a profound and long lasting antidiuresis followed by a marked polyuria lasting 4—19 days (PICKFORD, 1947; DUKE, PICKFORD, and WATT, 1950). In a similar way, eserine or DFP injected into the supra-optic nuclei of dogs anaesthetised with chloralose leads to liberation of oxytocin (uterine contractions after 4—5 min; duration 45—50 min. with eserine and at least for 4 h with DFP); injection into the posterior hypothalamus or the hypothalamus lateral to the fornix is without effect (ABRAHAMS and PICKFORD, 1956). Of other parasympathomimetic drugs, Yohimbine stimulates liberation of neurohypophysial hormones (FUGO, 1944), and alteration in the electron microscopic appearance of neurohypophysis suggesting increased secretory activity has been described in rabbits treated with pilocarpine (FUJITA and HARTMANN, 1961). Addition of acetylcholine to the incubated, isolated intact hypothalamo-system of rats, even in the absence of cholinesterase inhibitor, increases the release

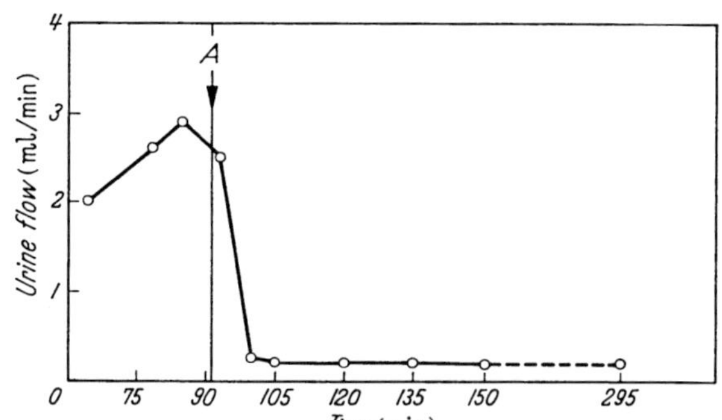

Fig. 14. The effect of hypothalamic injection of DFP on the rate of urine flow in a dog in water diuresis. At A, 120 μg DFP injected into right and left supraoptic nuclei. Reproduced with permission from DUKE, PICKFORD and WATT. J. Physiol. (Lond.) 111, 81 (1950)

of both oxytocin and vasopressin into the incubation medium (DANIEL and LEDERIS, 1966b).

These effects of acetylcholine and acetylcholinesterase inhibitors indicate that mediation at neuronal synapses in the supra-optic nucleus (the evidence for the paraventricular nucleus is sparse) is cholinergic. They suggest, also, that the post synaptic neurone bearing the cholinergic receptors might be the neurosecretory nerve of which the processes or axons and their terminals form the supra-optico hypophyseal tract and the neural lobe respectively. The distribution of cholinesterases in the hypothalamo-neurohypophysial system also is consistent with this conclusion (ABRAHAMS, KOELLE and SMART, 1957).

ABRAHAMS, KOELE, and SMART (1957) in the dog and PEPLER and PEARSE (1957) in the rat found that the region of the supraoptic and paraventricular nuclei contains both pseudocholinesterase and true cholinesterase. HOLMES (1961) investigated the distribution of cholinesterases throughout the hypothalamo-neurohypophysial system of the macaque; the supraoptic and paraventricular areas gave a consistent and strong positive reaction for both enzymes, the median eminence was negative in all preparations from the five animals studied. In the neural lobe a positive reaction occurred only around blood vessels. There are probably species differences since, HOLMES and KIERNAN (1966) reported a high content of both enzymes in the neurohypophysis of the hedgehog, and KOELLE and GEESEY (1961) found that in the neurohypophysis of the cat the nerve fibres and associated Herring bodies stain consistently for acetylcholinesterase. LEDERIS and LIVINGSTONE (1966) have shown that acetylcholinesterase is the predominant cholinesterase in the neural lobe and the anterior hypothalamus in the rabbit and the concentration of that enzyme in the former tissue is only about one half of the content in the latter.

KOELLE (1961) interprets the occurrence of cholinesterase in the neurohypophysis as an indication that acetylcholine is implicated in the release of the hormones from the neurosecretory nerve terminals. However, incubation of isolated rat neurohypophyses or of suspensions of neurosecretory granules with acetylcholine, even in the presence of cholinesterase inhibitors does not affect the rate of hormone release (DANIEL and LEDERIS, 1966b; DOUGLAS and POISNER, 1964a; DICKER, 1966). The presence at the neurone endings in the neurohypophysis of particles of the same dimensions and appearance as synaptic vesicles (PALAY, 1957; GREEN and MAXWELL, 1959; GERSCHENFELD, TRAMEZZANI and DE ROBERTIS, 1960), have been cited in support of KOELLE's hypothesis. However, the inverse relationship between the abundance of synaptic vesicles and of neurosecretory granules in a nerve terminal (LEDERIS, 1964; DANIEL and LEDERIS, 1965) suggests an alternative, hypothesis, viz. that the particles resembling synaptic vesicles are degenerate neurosecretory granules.

In the experiments of PICKFORD and her co-workers referred to earlier, dogs in which intravenous administration of acetylcholine evoked an antidiuretic response had been treated with atropine to avoid complications due to effects of acetylcholine at parasympathetic neuro-effector sites. Reflex discharge of vasopressin following stimulation of carotid sinus receptors is not blocked by atropine (CHIEN, PERIC, and USAMI, 1962). FANG, LUI , and WANG (1962) also were unable to block in dogs liberation of vasopressin after electrical stimulation of the ventromedial, supraoptic, paraventricular and medial preoptic nuclei by treatment with atropine or hyoscyamine. However, another atropine-like drug, ethybenztropine did inhibit vasopressin secretion evoked by hypothalamic stimulation. It may be questioned whether atropine and hyoscyamine reached the hypothalamus in concentration sufficient to block the release of 'intrinsic' acetylcholine in these experiments and 'extrinsic' acetylcholine in the experiments of PICKFORD and her colleagues. In later experiments, however, MILLS and WANG (1964b) obtained only slight and transient inhibition of antidiuretic hormone release following stimulation of the brain stem or ulnar or vagus nerves in animals treated with atropine or ethybenztropine, although it has been shown that atropine given systemically inhibits other activities of hypothalamic nuclei.

On the other hand there is evidence from two groups of workers that atropine inhibits release of oxytocin in response to suckling in lactating rats (GROSVENOR and TURNER, 1957; CHAUDHURY, 1961). This result should be interpreted conservatively because there was a great difference in the doses of atropine used (GROSVENOR and TURNER, 700 mg/kg subcutaneously; CHAUDHURY 10 μg intraperitoneally). It could be argued that an effect produced by a massive dose of stropine such as the larger of these might be due to an action unrelated to blockade of cholinergic receptors. Even if atropine was acting by blockade of cholinergic receptors no conclusion could be drawn as to the location of these receptors. Possibly atropine blocks transmission of a cholinergic synapse involved in the reflex a level higher than the hypothalamus. Alternatively, since most of the evidence for the failure of atropine to affect neurohypophysial secretion relates to vasopressin it may be that the characteristics of receptor on the oxytocin secreting neurone differ from those on the vasopressin secreting neurone.

The effectiveness of nicotine as a stimulator of neurohypophysial hormone secretion suggests an analogy with a peripheral autonomic ganglion(WALKER, 1957). However, there is no reason to believe that nicotine (or acetylcholine except when injected into the hypothalamus) does not act partly or even principally at levels in the brain higher than the hypothalamus. The observations of BISSET and WALKER (1953, 1957) and SUPEK and EISEN (1953) that ganglion blocking drugs do not block the antidiuretic effect or prevent the rise in circulating antidiuretic activity brought about by nicotine administration is, again, of questionable significance since it is unlikely that the quarternary bases would penetrate the blood brain barrier. CHAUDHURY (1961) how ever, has reported that pentolinium inhibits oxytocin release in response to suckling in lactating rats.

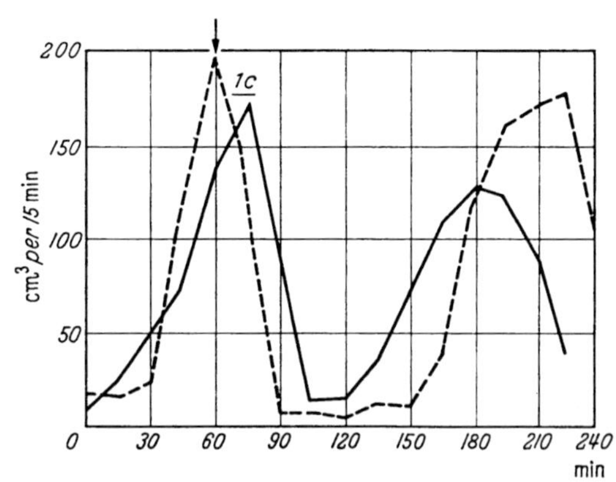

Fig. 15. Effect of intravenous nicotine (0.5 mg) and smoking one cigarette on the diuresis of a water loaded human subject. Nicotine injection (at arrow) broken line. Cigarette (at 1 c) solid line. Reproduced with permission from BURN, TRUELOVE and BURN. Brit. med. J. 1, 403—406 (1945)

The stimulant action of acetylcholine, which has already been discussed in some detail, can be defined as nicotinic in the sense that it is not abolished by atropine (PICKFORD, 1939, 1947). Nicotine itself was shown by MOTZFELDT as long ago as 1917 to produce an antidiuretic effect on rabbits. BURN, TRUELOVE, and BURN (1945) showed that the subcutaneous injection of 0.25 mg of nicotine inhibited a water diuresis in intact but not in hypophysectomised rats (Fig. 15). In human beings water diuresis was completely inhibited by 0.5 and 1.0 mg nicotine injected intravenously; the smoking of cigarettes had a similar effect (see also WALKER, 1949; CHALMERS, LEWIS, and PAWAN, 1951). Increased antidiuretic activity in the urine after smoking has been demonstrated by TAYLOR and WALKER (1951). A 'nicotine test' as an aid in the diagnosis of diabetes insipidus has been developed (CATES and GARROD, 1951; LEWIS and CHALMERS, 1951) and BISSET and WALKER, 1957 have shown in rats that nicotine raises both the antidiuretic and the oxytocic potency of the blood.

To sum up, there is a cholinergic mechanism at hypothalamic synapses involved in vasopressin secretion but the evidence for a similar mechanism in the pathway for impulses causing oxytocin secretion is incomplete. At present it is not possible to draw any conclusion as to the pharmacological characteristics of the cholinergic receptors.

7. Adrenergic Mechanisms and Neurohypophysial Hormone Release

O'CONNOR and VERNEY (1942, 1945) reported that antidiuretic effects were evoked in dogs by emotional stress brought about through weak faradic stimulation of subcutaneous tissue. In some animals the effects were of short duration and after section of the splanchnic nerves or abdominal sympathectomy the character of the response was changed to a more prolonged antidiuresis similar to that obtained by injection of posterior pituitary extract. The suggestion that the brief antidiuresis was due to adrenomedullary secretion which at the same time prevented release of vasopressin was confirmed by the demonstration that in sympathectomised dogs 15 μg of adrenaline, injected 30 sec before emotional stress, inhibited the antidiuresis. The antidiuretic action of acetylcholine in dogs (and presumably therefore the release of vasopressin) is usually but not invariably prevented by adrenaline given 5—35 sec previously (DUKE and PICKFORD, 1951), and the increase in antidiuretic activity of blood brought about by morphine is prevented by treatment with adrenaline and noradrenaline (GIERE and EVERSOLE, 1954). Changes in ultrastructure in the neurohypophysis of animals treated with adrenaline (FUJITA and HARTMANN, 1961) and the accumulation of neurosecretory substances also point to the inhibition of neurohypophysial secretion (KIVALO and ARKO, 1957).

The role of adrenaline in the emotional inhibition of the milk-ejection reflex initiated by suckling is complicated because adrenaline prevents the action of oxytocin on the mammary gland possibly by local vasoconstriction, (LINZELL, 1955; PEETERS, SIERENS, and SILVER, 1952). However, CROSS (1955a, b) showed

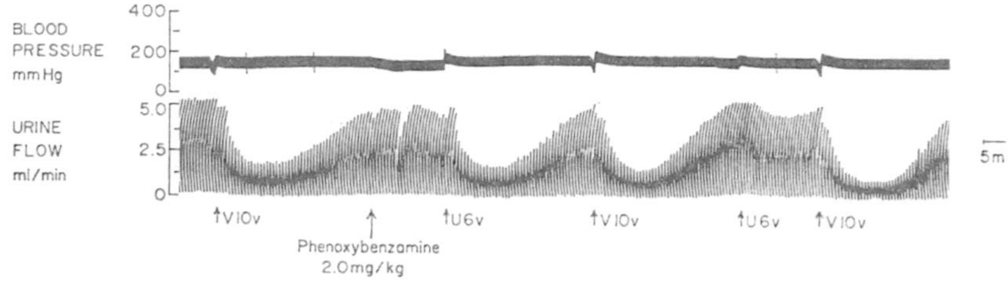

Fig. 16. Effect of Phenoxybenzamine on antidiuretic responses to stimulation of a vagus (V) and ulnar nerve (U). Note blockade of response to ulnar nerve stimulation 58 min after injection of phenoxybenzamine, while response to vagal stimulation is unaffected. Reproduced with permission from MILLS and WANG. Amer J. Physiol. 207, 1405—1416 (1965)

that in lactating rabbits in which the suckling reflex was inhibited by placing the animals under forcible restraint, after injection of oxytocin more milk was removed than during suckling alone. He concluded therefore that there was a degree of central inhibition of oxytocin release. CHAUDHURY (1961) also concluded that adrenaline and noradrenaline act centrally to inhibit oxytocin release during suckling.

While small amounts of adrenaline may thus by a central action inhibit neurohypophysial hormone release in response to suckling, nociceptive stimuli and administration of acetylcholine or morphine, there is evidence also that in higher doses, adrenaline and noradrenaline may themselves cause hormone release (DEARBORN and LASAGNA, 1952). Experiments with adrenergic blocking agents also suggest the pathway for secretory stimuli in the hypothalamus involves an adrenergic synapse. FANG, LIU, and WANG (1962) have shown the adrenergic blocking agent, phenoxybenzamine, blocked antidiuretic responses following stimulation at many points in the hypothalamus, and MILLS and WANG (1964) showed that phenoxybenzamine and dihydroergotamine blocked the antidiuretic responses to ulnar nerve stimulation (Fig. 16).

The highest concentrations of noradrenaline in the central nervous system are found in the hypothalamus (VOGT, 1954) and CALRSSON, FALCK, and HILLARP (1962) have shown that the periventricular, paraventricular and especially the supra-optic nuclei are innervated by adrenergic fibres. Furthermore, (^{3}H) noradrenaline easily crosses the blood brain barrier and is taken up preferentially in the hypothalamus in the cat (WEIL-MALHERBE, WHITBY, and AXELROD, 1961).

Thus although action at the level of the hypothalamus is possible, no evidence has been reported as to the sites and pathways of the stimulant and inhibiting effects of catecholamines and neurohypophysial hormone secretion.

8. Pathways of Secretion

According to SCHARRER and SCHARRER (1954) most if not all fibres of the supraoptic hypophysial tract end around blood vessels; the relationship between nerve terminals and blood vessels is displayed particularly well in the opossum (BODIAN, 1951). It is generally assumed, therefore, that the hormones are secreted mainly into the blood. Nevertheless, processes of neurosecretory cells have been observed to reach the third ventricle (BARGMANN, 1953), and TALANTI and KIVALO (1961) have reported that in the camel large amounts of material stainable with chrome-haematoxylin or aldehyde fuchsin are found in the ependyma of the infundibular recess, in the interstices of the ependymal cells and within the third ventricle. In ultrastructural studies dendrites have been observed to end between ependymal cells and axon terminals to abut on to flattened ependymal cells that intervene between the terminals and the ventricular lumen (NISHIOKA, BERN, and MEWALDT, 1964; E. SCHARRER, 1965).

The detection of neurohypophysial hormone activities in the CSF was reported and was denied in much early work in which the assay methods used would be regarded today as inadequate. VOGT (1953) could not detect oxytocin or vasopressin in dog CSF while HELLER and SAIFI (1966) have detected vasopressin in rat CSF. Since the antidiuretic activity of CSF is raised when large amounts of vasopressin is injected intravascularly, it cannot be stated whether the vasopressin found in CSF had reached there via the blood or by direct secretion from the neurosecretory neurones.

The main pathway of secretion is almost certainly into the blood. Surprisingly little attention has been paid to the state of the neurohypophysial circulation in relation to hormone release, no doubt because the technical difficulties are formidable. Quite large amounts of histamine are present in the neural lobe (HARRIS, JACOBSOHN, and KAHLSON, 1952; ADAM, 1961) and it could possibly have a role in the regulation of local blood flow in the neural lobe. BODIAN (1963) has indeed suggested that the mast cells in the neural lobe of the opossum might, by releasing histamine, facilitate the passage of neurosecretory material (hormone) into vascular spaces. It is possible also, that some of the neurones of the system are concerned with vasomotor control rather than (or as well as) neurosecretion (LEDERIS, 1966). If the state of the neurohypophysial circulation is a factor in hormone release, it is important to realise that vascular effects cannot influence hormone release in experiments with isolated, incubated neural lobes.

9. Secretory Stimuli

A wide variety of conditions and manipulations have been proposed as stimuli for the release of neurohypophysial hormones, but the evidence is not always convincing. Evidence obtained by estimation of hormone concentration in blood is less equivocable than that yielded by other types of experiment. The amounts are so small, however, that the experiments demand the most sensitive and difficult assay methods and the use of large animals, not normally found in laboratories, so as to provide sufficient blood without, at the same time, evoking hormone release by its withdrawal. Methods for the extraction of and concentration of the hormone in body fluids have been much improved, and methods are available for characterisation of the activity in the extracts chemically, enzymatically and chromatographically, as well as biologically. A much favoured procedure consists in showing that a given stimulus produces effects in the animal that can be matched by administration of exogenous hormone (Fig. 12). This method has been successful in the hands of experienced workers particularly when — in the case of vasopressin antidiuresis — it is accompanied by renal clearance studies, and when the experiments are repeated in animals in which neurohypophysial function has been eliminated surgically.

10. Increased Osmotic Pressure of Plasma

The proposal that changes in plasma osmotic pressure determines the release of antidiuretic hormone was made first by CHAMBERS, MELVILLE, HARE, and HARE (1945) when they showed that intravenous injection of very large amounts of NaCl in hypertonic solution causes greater increases in urine volume in dogs with diabetes insipidus than in normal control animals. It is upon the work of VERNEY (1946, 1947) however, that the proposal is securely based. The critical experiment by VERNEY is illustrated in Fig. 17. Hypertonic solution injected into the carotid artery of a conscious dog produced inhibition of water diuresis although the same dose given intravenously had no effect. The time course of the effects (slow onset and long duration) were characteristic of those produced by injection of neurohypophysial extracts and were greatly reduced in size in dogs from which the neurohypophysis had been removed. Sustained infusion of hypertonic NaCl solution into a common carotid at a rate that would increase the osmotic pressure of the blood by only 1.8% also inhibited water diuresis to an extent that could be matched in extent, onset, duration and offset by an infusion of 0.07 mU/min of posterior pituitary extract. Injections of NaCl, Na_2SO_4 and dextrose into a carotid artery in amounts and concentrations that produced the same rise in osmotic pressure of the blood released the same amount of antidiuretic hormone. Within the range of increase of osmotic pressure in carotid blood studies (1.77—5.05%) the hormone release estimated by matching the antidiuresis with infusion of posterior pituitary extract was directly related to the increase in osmotic pressure.

O'CONNOR (1950) also has studied the relationship between hormone secretion and the magnitude of the osmotic stimulus. In his experiments the hypertonic solutions were given orally and intravenously. The rate of hormone secretion was taken as 10 times the rate at which antidiuretic activity appeared in the urine during the period of osmotic stimulation; this factor was established in experi-

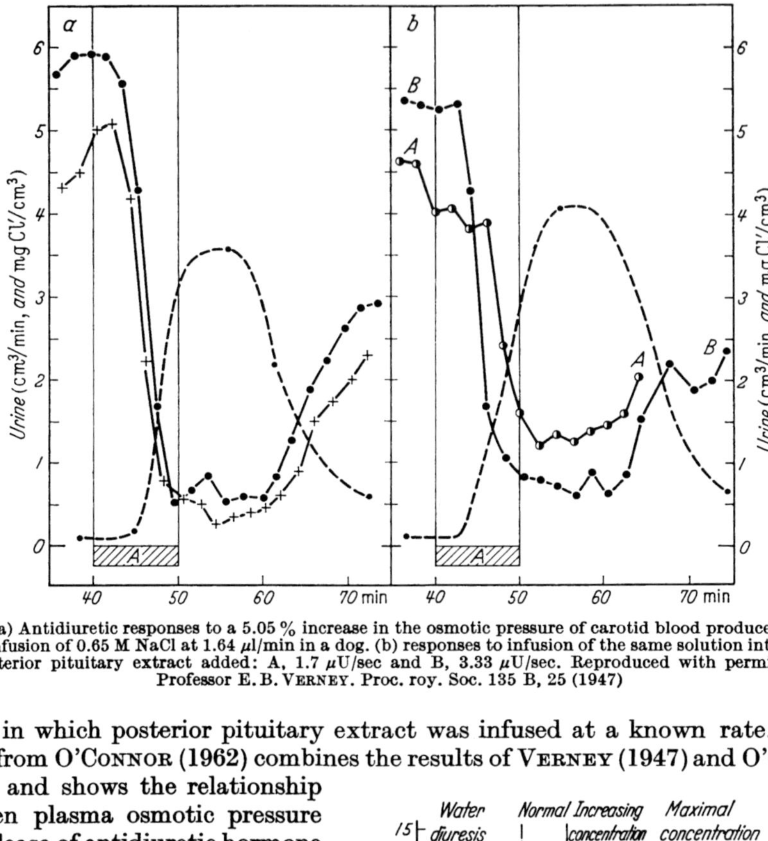

Fig. 17. (a) Antidiuretic responses to a 5.05 % increase in the osmotic pressure of carotid blood produced by intracarotid infusion of 0.65 M NaCl at 1.64 μl/min in a dog. (b) responses to infusion of the same solution intravenously with posterior pituitary extract added: A, 1.7 μU/sec and B, 3.33 μU/sec. Reproduced with permission from Professor E. B. VERNEY. Proc. roy. Soc. 135 B, 25 (1947)

ments in which posterior pituitary extract was infused at a known rate. Fig. 18 taken from O'CONNOR (1962) combines the results of VERNEY (1947) and O'CONNOR (1950) and shows the relationship between plasma osmotic pressure and release of antidiuretic hormone in the dog. It would seem paradoxical that antidiuretic hormone secretion increases very sharply with increase in osmotic pressure when the rate is such that maximum urinary concentration is already reached. As O'CONNOR (1962) points out a curve of this type is often found when response is plotted against stimulus and can usually be ascribed to the recruitment of an increasing number of units where stimulation thresholds are randomly distributed. Urea and (when infused slowly) dextrose did not inhibit water diuresis. VERNEY (1947) therefore suggested the presence of receptors that were responsive to an

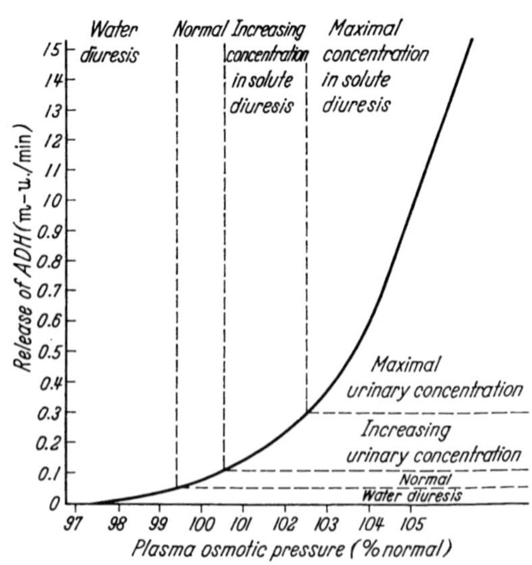

Fig. 18. The effect of changes in plasma osmotic pressure on the rate of release of antidiuretic hormone from the neurohypophysis. Reproduced with permission from Dr. W. J. O'CONNOR. Renal Function (1960)

increase in the osmotic pressure of the blood except where the excess solute in blood was not osmotically active at the receptor (i.e. the receptor membrane was permeable to the substance as in the case of urea and, to a lesser extent, dextrose). VERNEY gave the name 'osmoreceptors' to the sensitive structures.

Release of neurohypophysial hormones following an intracarotid injection of a hypertonic solution has been demonstrated not only in dogs (VERNEY, 1947; AMES, MOORE, and VAN DYKE, 1950; ABRAHAMS and PICKFORD, 1954; ZUIDEMA, CLARK, and MINTON, 1956; ZUIDEMA and CLARK, 1957) but also in goats (ANDERSSON, 1951b) and rabbits (HOLLAND et al., 1959).

ZUIDEMA et al. (1956, 1957) carried out their experiments in dogs lightly anaesthetised with chloralose and so were able to show that conditioned antidiuretic responses to irritation and pain following intra-arterial injection of hypertonic solution were not responsible for the effects. However, unlike VERNEY, they did not find any differences in the antidiuretic effects of equimolar hypertonic solutions of NaCl, Na_2SO_4, sucrose, glucose or urea. Antidiuretic activity assayed in the urine from the dogs after injection of the hypertonic solution also was independent of the solute.

In the rat ITOH (1954a) reported a decrease in the antidiuretic hormone content of the posterior lobe after the intravenous injection of NaCl or 20% glucose solution but not after 10% urea solution. LLOYD (1957) found a loss of antidiuretic activity in the posterior pituitary gland when rats were given hypertonic salt solution very rapidly (so rapidly that a number had convulsions) FRIEDMAN, HINKE, and FRIEDMAN (1956) injected hypertonic solutions of NaCl into a common carotid of unanaesthetised rats and found an antidiuretic action of 2% and 1.5% solutions. No effect was seen on injection into a femoral artery, and intra-carotid injection had no effect in hypophysectomised animals. DICKER and NUNN (1958) using the same technique, injected a 3% NaCl solution into the common carotid of unanaesthetised rats and obtained similar results. In contrast, GINSBURG and BROWN (1957) found that the injection of hypertonic NaCl solution into an internal carotid of unanaesthetised rats failed to inhibit the urine flow even though the animal responded to small doses of vasopressin. Since GINSBURG and BROWN's experiments differ from those of FRIEDMAN et al (1956) and DICKER and NUNN (1958) essentially only in that the latter injected not into the internal but into the common carotid, the discrepancy in the results may have been due to a different distribution of the hypertonic solutions in the cephalic circulation. Alternatively, it is possible that carotid sinus receptors (see p. 330) were affected in one set of experiments but not in others.

The anatomical site of the osmoreceptors in the dog was investigated by JEWELL and VERNEY (1957) by testing the effect of intracarotid injections after ligation of vessels in the cerebral blood supply. Antidiuresis resulted only when the hypertonic solutions reached a region in the anterior hypothalamus which included the supraoptic nuclei. One of the dogs in which the cell population of the paraventricular nuclei had been drastically reduced responded normally to the osmotic stimulus which is consistent with more recent evidence on the relative separation of vasopressin and oxytocin neurones. The term osmoreceptor implies the occurrence of structures that are specifically adapted to respond to changes of osmotic pressure in the *milieu interieur* and that are functionally linked with the neurohypophysis. JEWELL (1954) has described vesiculated structures in the supraoptic neurones that might be the osmoreceptors and much additional evidence is consistent with the location of the osmoreceptors in the proximity of the supraoptic nuclei. For example, antidiuretic hormone secretion in cats is not affected by central denervation of the hypothalamus or decerebration (WOODS and BARD, 1960; BARD and MACHT, 1958) while intracarotid injection of hypertonic NaCl solution evokes vasopressin release after section between the mesencephalon and the diencephalon (HOLLAND, CROSS, and SAWYER, 1959). However, it is quite clear that intracarotid injection of hypertonic solution affects many modalities in the brain apart from antidiuretic hormone secretion. One of these has been referred to already — the secretion of oxytocin in response to intracarotid injection of hypertonic NaCl solution. This important observation of ABRAHAMS and PICKFORD (1954) was made on conscious bitches prepared so that uterine contractions and urine flow could be recorded simultaneously. When the neurohypophysis was stimulated by sudden intracarotid injection of hypertonic NaCl solution the resultant increased uterine activity and antidiuresis were compared with the effects produced by intravenous injection of oxytocin and vasopressin (Fig. 12). In order to match the effects on both uterus and kidney produced by osmotic stimulation it was necessary to give vasopressin together with 10—20 times as much oxytocin. The conclusion that the osmotic stimulus released much more oxytocin than vasopressin seems inescapable, and, indeed, the disparity might be even greater than the experiment suggests, because the pituitary preparation used (Pitressin) almost certainly comprised lysine vasopressin which is a much less potent antidiuretic agent in dogs than the endogenous canine hormone, arginine vasopressin. The liberation of oxytocin by intracarotid injection of hypertonic solution has been shown also in the goat (ANDERSSON, 1951) and rabbit (HOLLAND, CROSS, and SAWYER, 1959; SIDDIQI and WALKER, 1959).

The evidence for oxytocin secretion in response to osmotic stimulation in man is less consistent. According to HENDRICKS, HELFAND, and CALDEYRO-BARCIA (1959) intravenous injection of 400 ml of 5% NaCl increases uterine activity in pregnant women. This observation has not been confirmed by THEOBALD (1959) or DICKER (1959) and GAITAN, COBA, and MIZRACHI (1964) could not show any release of oxytocin (uterine stimulation or increased intramammary pressure) in pregnant or puerpural women, although marked antidiuretic responses were demonstrated.

The effects of hypertonic solution are extremely complex and in the sense that every cell is an osmometer it would be unrealistic to expect that osmotic stimulation would affect only one system. READ and VICK (1961) have stressed the cholinergic like effects of hypertonic solutions; WAYNER, GRIMSLEY, KAHAN, and STOLLER (1963) have described marked facilitation of monosynaptic reflex discharge in rats after intracarotid injection of hypertonic saline, and in rabbits there is central sympathetic stimulation (HOLLAND, SUNDSTEN, and SAWYER, 1958). Intra-arterial injection of hypertonic solution also elicits reflex circulatory effects producing hypertension, tachycardia and tachypnoea (LASSER, SCHOENFELD, ALLEN, and FRIEDBERG, 1960). It is to be expected, therefore, that the effects of intracarotid injection of hypertonic solutions on electrical activity of the brain will be very complex and that not all of them will be functionally significant for the release of antidiuretic hormone.

Electrical responses after intravascular injection of hypertonic solution have been recorded from many parts of the brain; VON EULER (1953) described slow d.c. shifts when recording from the preoptic and supraoptic regions in the cat; SAWYER and GERNANDT (1956) after intracarotid injections of salt solutions into rabbits, obtained a triphasic response in the subcortical electro-encephalogram (EEG) which was not seen in the supraoptic nucleus but was detected in adjacent areas, and FULLER and SAWYER (1956) made similar observations in cats and rabbits. CLEMENTE, SUTIN, and SILVERSTONE (1957) also in cats, found a region in the medulla oblongata that gave a reproducible electrical response to intravenous injections of hypertonic solutions; SUNDSTEN and SAWYER (1956) in the dog have reported EEG changes in the olfactory bulb after intracarotid injections of hypertonic salt or sugar solutions. The most consistent changes in electrical activity which HOLLAND, CROSS, and SAWYER (1959) saw after the injection of hypertonic salt solutions into unanaesthetised rabbits consisted of high amplitude fast activity in the lateral preoptic area and the deep portion of the olfactory tubercle. These findings help little in establishing the site of specific osmoreceptors, and reports in some of these investigations that the intravascular injections were followed by liberation of neurohypophysial hormone are only of limited value in this context; absence of hormone release after a region responded electrically to osmotic stimuli would obviously eliminate such a site as being involved in transmitting secretory impulses to the posterior pituitary, but the occurrence of a neurohypophysial response does not necessarily establish a causal connection between the electrical phenomena and hormone release. The results of experiments by SUNDSTEN and SAWYER (1960, 1961) substantiate that viewpoint. They showed by ablating the olfactory tubercles that the EEG response in that region is not essential to the osmotic stimulation of the neurohypophysial hormone secretion. In fact the only essential region was that which included the supraoptic nuclei and an islet of tissue connecting them to the posterior pituitary. This applied to oxytocin as well as vasopressin secretion and the remarkable result was obtained that even when the paraventricular nuclei were excluded, oxytocin secretion was not inhibited. The problem is further complicated by a study of CROSS and GREEN (1959) who recorded the activity of single neurones in rabbits and found not only that many neurones in the vicinity of the supraoptic and paraventricular nuclei responded to osmotic stimuli but also that supraoptic neurones were generally accelerated while the paraventricular neurones were inhibited. Results agreeing with those of CROSS and GREEN (1959) have been obtained in more recent experiments with cats by BROOKS, USHIYAMI, and LANGE (1962) and by KOIZUMI, ISHIKAWA, and BROOKS (1964).

The secretion of vasopressin is probably most important physiologically for its antidiuretic function in the control of water balance and particular attention has been paid to its role in water conservation during dehydration. The inability to concentrate urine in animals with impaired neurohypophysial function as a result of surgery or because of a genetic defect, the depletion of vasopressin (and oxytocin) in the neurohypophysis of severly dehydrated animals (AMES and VAN DYKE, 1950; HILD and ZETLER, 1953a; DICKER and NUNN, 1957; KRECEK and HELLER, 1962) the large stores of vasopressin in the neurohypophysis of animals from a desert environment (AMES and VAN DYKE, 1950) the increase in plasma antidiuretic activity in dehydrated human subjects (BUCHBORN, 1957; BARATZ, DOIG, and ADATTO, 1960) and rats (LITTLE and RADFORD, 1964) and the excretion of an antidiuretic substance in the urine of dehydrated rats (GILMAN and GOODMAN, 1939) provides a formidable body of evidence for the water conserving role of the increased secretion of antidiuretic hormone during dehydration. Finally one may add that the increases in blood osmotic pressure of about 2% shown by VERNEY (1947) to be sufficient to elicit antidiuretic hormone release are of a similar order to the increase after the first day of water withdrawal in man (RUBINI, WOLF, and MORONEY, 1956) and dog (WOLF and EDDY, 1957). From the point of view of normal physiology, the osmotic pressure of the blood in the resting subject in water balance seems to be sufficient to allow some secretion of antidiuretic hormone. The inhibition of the resting secretion of antidiutetic hormone by decrease in plasma osmotic pressure (see Fig. 18), following ingestion of water and the resultant diuresis is probably a more familiar example of the role of osmoreceptor mechanism in water balance.

As might be expected, overhydration by continuous administration of water by intra-oesophageal tube to dogs (ANDERSSON and JEWELL, 1957) or by giving water or dextrose solution to rats (ORTMANN, 1951) increases the amount of neurosecretory material throughout the hypothalamo-neurohypophysial system and increases the abundance of neurosecretory particles in the nerve terminals. There are no reports on the hormone content of neurohypophyses from over-hydrated animals.

11. Milk-Ejection Reflex

The observation that milk-ejection could be evoked by injection of posterior pituitary extracts was reported first as long ago as 1910 (OTT and SCOTT, 1910). It was not until 1930 that TURNER and SLAUGHTER suggested that the pituitary might be involved in a neuroendocrine reflex regulating milk-ejection. They wrote that "one of the normal functions of the pituitary gland, which is so clearly connected to the nervous system, is to regulate the discharging phase of milk-secretion. If this were the case, the nerve paths would lead to the pituitary gland, causing the discharge of the hormone which would, in turn, bring about the well-known change in the gland". After the lapse of a decade, ELY and PETERSON (1941) showed that motor denervation of half of a cow's udder did not affect the milk-ejection from that half during subsequent lactation indicating that the control of milk-ejection was independent of secreto-motor innervation and PETERSON and LUDWICK (1942) showed that blood taken from a cow immediately after milking evoked an immediate flow of milk if perfused through an isolated udder, while blood from an unstimulated cow was without effect. The failure of litters to obtain milk by suckling from hypophysectomised mothers in which lactation was maintained by treatment with anterior pituitary extracts (GOMEZ, 1939; HARRIS and JACOBSOHN, 1952) indicated the involvement of a factor from the posterior pituitary in the process that COWIE, FOLLEY, CROSS, HARRIS, JACOBSOHN, and RICHARDSON (1951), the milk-ejection reflex.

Both vasopressin and oxytocin are liberated during suckling or mammary stimulation but the posterior pituitary factor mainly involved is oxytocin which when tested on the rabbit mammary gland is 5 times more potent than arginine vasopressin (BOISSONAS, BERDE, and KONZETT, 1961) and is liberated during suckling in amounts greater than vasopressin by 100 times in the rabbit (CROSS, 1951) and by 30 times in the dog (PICKFORD, 1960).

The amounts of vasopressin liberated during suckling or mammary stimulation are nevertheless sufficient to cause inhibition of urine flow in the mother, provided sufficient water is given to establish water diuresis (PEETERS, COUSSENS, and SIERENS, 1949; PEETERS and COUSSSENS, 1950; CROSS, 1951; KALLIALA and KARVONEN, 1951; THEOBALD, 1959; PICKFORD, 1960). Diabetes insipidus in women is said to regress during lactation (SCHEER, RAISZ, and LLOYD, 1959; ALEXANDER and DOWNS, 1957), but this must be a more complicated phenomenon than merely stimulation of vasopressin release.

The amounts of oxytocin liberated during suckling have been estimated by various indirect methods in which the effects of suckling are compared with effects of known amounts of oxytocin, on intramammary pressure, milk volume or uterine activity. The various estimates are as follows: — rat, 20—100 mu, (GROSVENOR and TURNER, 1957); rabbit, 20—50 mu (CROSS, 1951; CROSS and HARRIS, 1952; CROSS and VAN DYKE, 1953; FUCHS and WAGNER, 1963); goat,

1000 mu (COWIE, 1952); sow, 250—500 mu (BRAUDE and MITCHELL, 1950; WHITTLESTONE, 1954); cow, 1000 mu (PEETERS, STORMORKEN, and VANSCHOUBROEK, 1960); dog, 15—20 mu (PICKFORD, 1960); women, 10 mu (BELLER, KRUMHOLZ, and ZEININGER, 1955; THEOBALD, 1959).

There are conflicting reports on the effect of suckling on the hormone content of the neurohypophysis. The amount of hormone liberated at any single milk let-down is relatively small in relation to the storage and synthetic capacities of the neurohypophysis. Nevertheless, some authors have reported a selective fall in oxytocin content in the glands of lactating animals (DICKER and TYLER, 1953; ACHER and FROMAGEOT, 1957) while other authors have detected no change (WHITTLESTONE, BASSETT, and TURNER, 1952; MACAULEY, 1952; BARER et al., 1963). Often it is not clear what time interval elapsed between suckling and sacrifice of the animals, and clearly this could be an important factor. Possibly more important is the demonstration by HELLER and LEDERIS (1959) that a considerable proportion of oxytocin (but not vasopressin) in the neurohypophyses of lactating rats dissolves in acetone which is used frequently to dessicate pituitaries before extraction of the hormones. This may well be due to the shift of oxytocin from neurosecretory granules to cell cytoplasm that occurs in lactating rabbits (BARER et al., 1963).

It could not be assumed from the demonstration by PETERSON and LUDWICK (1942) that the substance in the blood taken from cows during milking which evoked milk-ejection from an isolated udder was oxytocin, since many naturally occurring substances may produce contraction of mammary myo-epithelium (see LINZELL, 1955). Until recently, conclusive evidence that the oxytocin concentration in blood is raised following the milking stimulus has been lacking. Thus, HAWKER (1958) and HAWKER, WALMSLEY, ROBERTS, BLACKSHAW, and DOWNES (1961) found no increase in the oxytocin content in blood during suckling in lactating women. In cows, HAWKER and ROBERTS (1957) found as much oxytocin in blood just before as during milking, although in goats they did observe an increase during the milking process, as did FITZPATRICK (1961) in ewes. The control levels of oxytocic activity in the experiments of HAWKER and his colleagues are very much higher than found by other workers using improved bioassay and extraction procedures (FITZPATRICK, 1961; KNAGGS, 1963; FOLLEY and KNAGGS, 1964, 1965, 1966), and the substance detected in their experiments appears to be quite distinct from the neurohypophysial peptides.

In the experiments of FOLLEY and KNAGGS (1964, 1965, 1966) on cows, goats and sows, greatest care was taken to accustom the animals to the experimental procedure, and so to avoid stimuli that might have been due to unfamiliar circumstances, and well-validated methods for extraction and assay of oxytocin were used, backed by chromatographic evidence for the identity of the substance in the blood extracts and oxytocin. In cows milked by machine the application of the teat cups evoked a transient appearance of oxytocin in jugular vein blood followed in some cases by a second spurt of oxytocin during the milking process. The sows were suckled by their litters during the collection of serial samples of external jugular blood, and again a transient rise in oxytocin in blood was observed just before the milk-ejection phase. In contrast, the goats were milked by hand and provided that they were milked carefully, normal milk yields could be obtained without release of oxytocin, although in a minority of animals oxytocin was detected in blood collected during milking (Fig. 19). This result agrees with other experiments that have shown that deafferentation of the udder in goats and sheep does not prevent normal milk yield, and thus, that although oxytocin release may occur during suckling in these animals, it is not essential for milk let-down (Denamur and Martinet, 1959a; Denamur, 1965).

It is often difficult to distinguish between a conditioned response and the milk-ejection that arises from the stimulation of afferents in the mammary gland. Thus it is well known that milk-ejection can occur in cows at milking-time before any

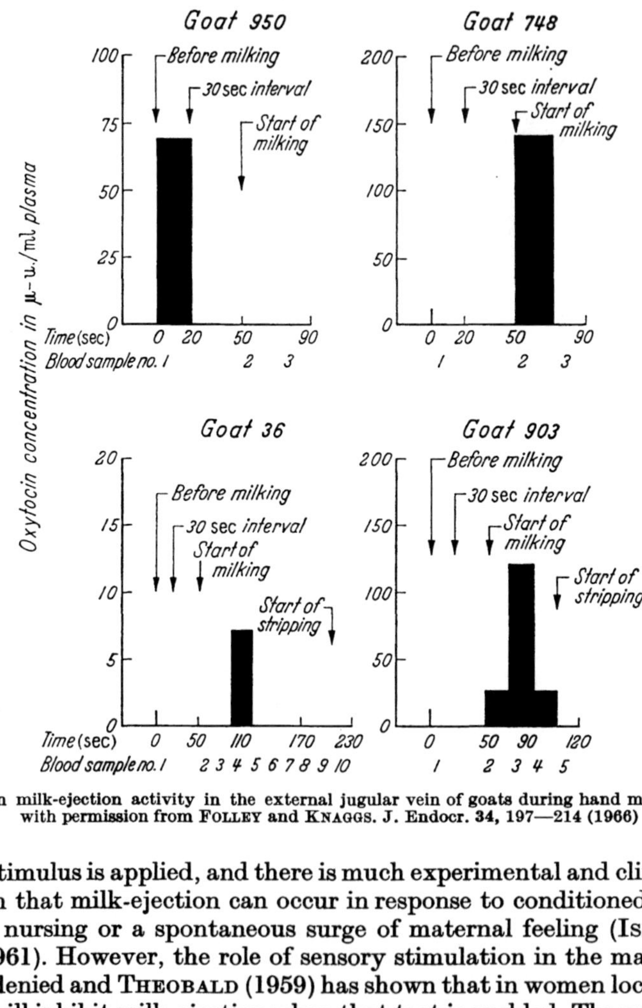

Fig. 19. Oxytocin milk-ejection activity in the external jugular vein of goats during hand milking. Reproduced with permission from Folley and Knaggs. J. Endocr. 34, 197—214 (1966)

mammary stimulus is applied, and there is much experimental and clinical evidence from women that milk-ejection can occur in response to conditioned stimuli associated with nursing or a spontaneous surge of maternal feeling (Isbister, 1954; Newton, 1961). However, the role of sensory stimulation in the mammary gland is not to be denied and Theobald (1959) has shown that in women local anaesthesia of the teat will inhibit milk-ejection when that teat is suckled. The process of milking or suckling involves stimulation of a variety of tactile and thermal modalities in the mammary gland and it is not surprising, perhaps, that electrical stimulation of the teat has not led to easily reproducible results (Denamur and Martinet, 1959a).

The afferent pathway from teat to neurohypophysis has been studied by observation of lactational performance after section or hemi-section of the spinal cord and the placement of lesions in the brain. Eayers and Baddeley (1956) carried out experiments in rats sectioning six pairs of dorsal roots between L_2 and T_7 and the bilateral sectioning of various tracts in the spinal cord. Similar experiments in goats have been reported by Denamur and Martinet (1959b). In both species, hemisection of the spinal cord suppresses the ejection reflex if the mammary stimulation is ipsilateral although stimulation of the contralateral side will cause milk-ejection from all glands and thus the main ascending pathways do not appear to be crossed.

12. Stimulation of Female Genitalia

It is well known that contractile activity of the uterus increases following stretching or other mechanical stimulation of the uterus, cervix, vagina or vulva. Although such responses might easily be the result of purely local reflexes, HATERIUS and FERGUSON (1938) and FERGUSON (1941) showed that the increase in contractions of a uterine horn following stretching of the cervix or the contralateral horn or vagina was abolished by mid-spinal section or by electrolytic destruction of the pituitary stalk. Milk-ejection effects following mechanical stimulation of the genital tract have been reported by ANDERSSON (1951), VAN DENMARK and HAYS (1951) and USUELLI, PIANA, and CURTO (1952) and has been used as a means of inducing let-down of milk by tribal Hottentots (FITZPATRICK, 1966).

The most conclusive work in this field has come from DEBACKERE and PEETERS (1960a, b) and DEBACKERE, PEETERS, and TUYTTENS (1961). In experiments in cows DEBACKERE and PEETERS (1960a) showed that inflation of a balloon in the vagina to pressures of 50—200 mm. Hg caused milk-ejection and antidiuresis although comparable distention in the rectum was without effect. Cervical stimulation also caused milk-ejection but only in about half of the experiments, whereas vaginal distention was always effective. This is contrary to the observations of VAN DENMARK and HAYS (1953) that the greatest responses were obtained with stimulation of the external os of the cervix.

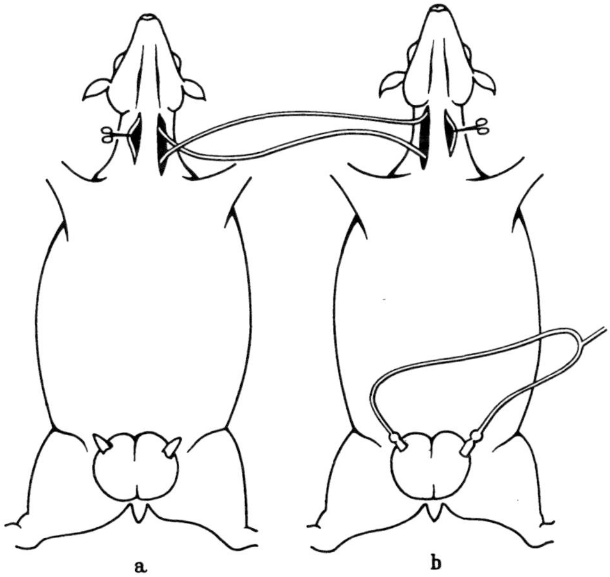

Fig. 20. Cross-circulation experiment on lactating ewes. One jugular vein of A was joined with one jugular vein of B. The other jugular veins were clamped. The vagina in A was distended and the intramammary pressure recorded in B. Reproduced with permission from DEBACKERE, PEETERS and TUYTTENS. J. Endocr. 22, 321—334 (1961)

DEBACKERE, PEETERS, and TUYTTENS (1961) described ingenious cross-circulation of experiments in ewes that are illustrated in Fig. 20. The circulations of the two ewes are connected by crossing jugular veins so that the jugular outflow in each animal passed into the venous and returns to the heart in the other. Vaginal stimulation in one ewe resulted in milk-ejection, not in the stimulated ewe but in the other, and the roles of the two ewes could be reversed. It follows that the agent responsible for the mammary response is blood borne and enters the circulation in the head, and thus, almost certainly, is oxytocin.

Increased uterine activity associated with mating has been observed in many species and has been attributed to release of oxytocin. Milk-ejection during coitus has been reported in women (PICKLES, 1953; HARRIS and PICKLES, 1953), in mares (HAMMOND, 1936) and in cows (VAN DENMARK and HAYS, 1953) and antidiureses have been reported in female rats (ERANKO, FRIBERG, and KARVONEN, 1953) and in women (FRIBERG, 1953). HAWKER, ROBERTS, and WALMSLEY (1959) examined the oxytocic activity in extracts of blood taken from ewes at the time of copulation. The interpretation of these experiments was hampered by the presence in their extracts of an oxytocic substance apart from oxytocin. Nevertheless, in one of the five ewes the increase in oxytocin content (10 mu/ml to 160 mu/ml) was sufficiently large to be detected even against the background of the non-specific oxytocic substance. Using improved methods of extraction and assay by milk-ejection

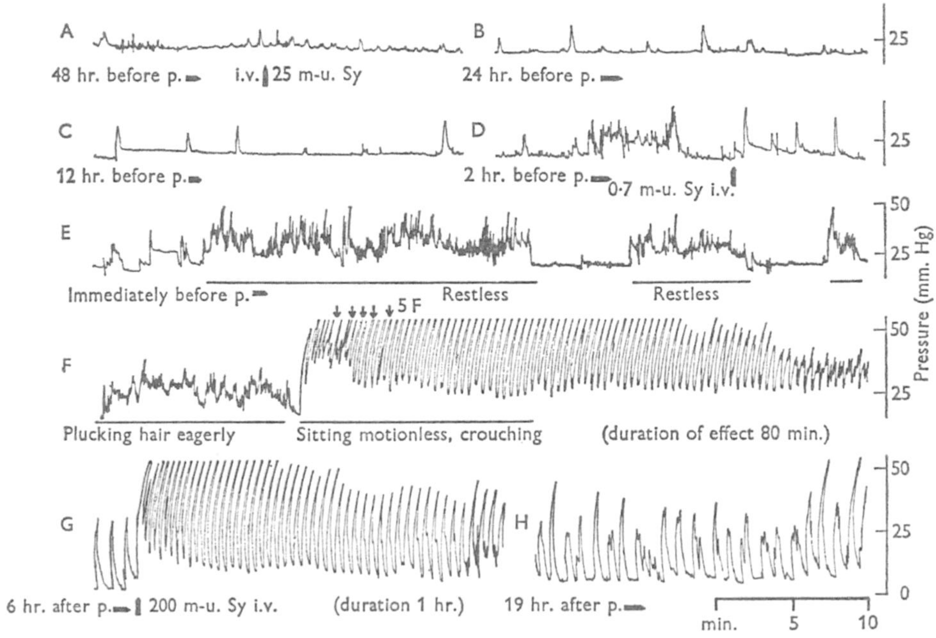

Fig. 21. Motility of uterine horn of a conscious unrestrained perturient rabbit. Recording by intra-uterine balloon in a horn from which the foetuses had been removed — the foetuses in the other horn were left *in situ*. Reproduced with permission from Dr. A. R. FUCHS. J. Endocr. 30, 217—224 (1964)

WALMSLEY (1963) carried out further experiments in four mares at mating. In one animal, in which no oxytocin could be detected in blood before coitus, measurable quantities appeared in the blood 1—4 min after the beginning of coitus. The amount was sufficiently great to allow chromatographic investigation and the properties of the milk-ejecting activity were consistent with it being oxytocin.

It should not be assumed that the release of neurohypophysial hormones during coitus in females is necessarily the result of genital stimulation. In the emotional and psychological context of mating it is difficult to isolate the causal relationships of events and as HARRIS (1955) has pointed out, the release of hormone might be evoked by a compliment by the husband as well as by specific physical contact.

Milk-ejection is commonly observed during parturition in domesticated ani mals including sows, mares and cows; GUNTHER (1948) reported that expulsion of milk in a parturient lactating woman was synchronous with labour pains and that these effects could be simulated by injection of posterior pituitary extract. Similar observations have been made in women in whom the mammary gland ducts have been cannulated (SICA-BLANCO, MENDEZ-BAUER, SALA, CABOT, and CALDEYRO-BARCIA, 1959) and CROSS (1958) has recorded milk-ejection in rabbits precisely coinciding with the delivery of the litter. FUCHS (1964) has recorded movements of uterine horn in rabbits during the final 48 h of pregnancy. The foetuses were removed from one horn and replaced by an intra-uterine balloon. Only minor changes in uterine activity were noted until a few minutes before the birth of the litter (Fig. 21), when, with very sudden onset, powerful rhythmic contractions of the uterus started during which the litter was born. Using similar techniques

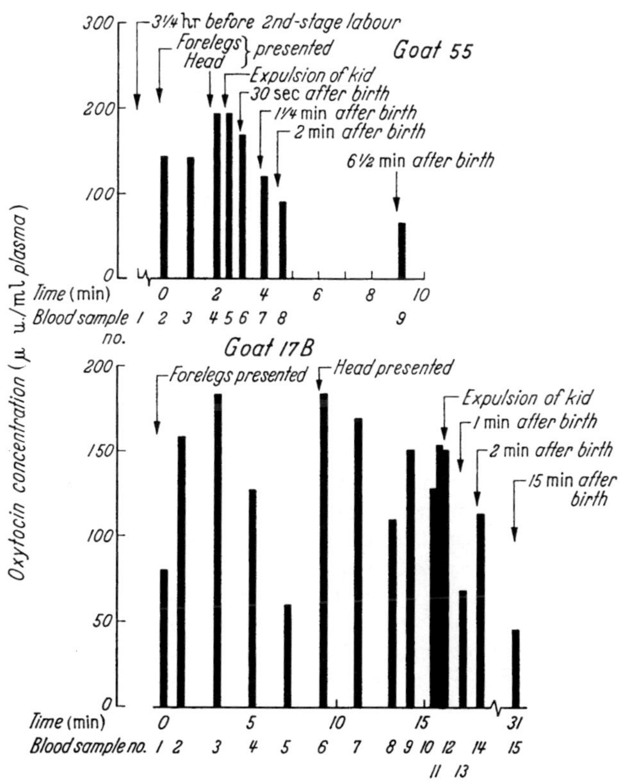

Fig. 22. Oxytocin levels in jugular vein blood of goats during parturition. Reproduced with permission from FOLLEY and KNAGGS. J. Endocr. 33, 301—315 (1965)

FUCHS (1966) also has shown that by giving rabbits a continuous infusion of alcohol, an inhibitor of neurohypophysial hormone secretion (see p. 322), the onset of labour can be prevented although effective uterine contractions can be elicited by administration of oxytocin.

HAWKER and ROBERTSON (1958) were the first to attempt to measure oxytocin levels in blood taken from women in labour. Unfortunately a large part of the oxytocic activity in their extracts was due to another substance that could be distinguished from oxytocin, since it was not inactivated by thioglycollate treatment and its presence has confused the interpretation of their results. In 1961, CALDEYRO-BARCIA showed that blood from women during labour contained measurable amounts of milk-ejecting activity and FITZPATRICK (1961) found that very low levels of oxytocin in jugular blood of sheep in late pregnancy were markedly increased immediately before and during labour and during the delivery of the placenta.

In more recent work oxytocin has been assayed in jugular blood of parturient horses, cows and goats (FITZPATRICK and WALMSLEY, 1962, 1965; FOLLEY and KNAGGS, 1964, 1965). In these domestic animal species the increase in blood oxytocin was detected only during the expulsive stage of labour and only much lower amounts or none, were detected during the stage of cervical dilatation (Fig. 22). These results indicate that the maximum rate of secretion of oxytocin occurs during the passage of the foetus through the vagina and cervix, particularly when the head emerges from the vulva and levels up to 1 mu/ml in jugular blood are reached. It is possible, therefore, that the liberation of oxytocin could be triggered by the stretching of these tissues as suggested by FERGUSON (1941). Since oxytocin levels in the first stage of labour are usually much lower than the highest values the massive discharge of oxytocin does not initiate labour but is, more probably, a result of it; that does not exclude the possibility that labour might be precipitated by an earlier, but smaller, discharge of oxytocin. Similar observations have been made in parturient women by COCH, BROVETTO, CABOT, FIELITZ, and CALDEYRO-BARCIA (1965) who were able to overcome the special difficulty of the occurrence of oxytocinase in the blood of pregnant women. Milk-ejection activity was measured in both internal jugular and peripheral vein blood and since the concentration in the former was six to nine times greater than in the latter it follows that the active substance was secreted at some site in the head, i.e. probably the neurohypophysis.

The effects of extirpation of the pituitary gland on the efficiency of parturition has been the subject of many investigations, but, before 1938, the results were extremely variable. It would seem that the reason for the variation lay in the inadequate techniques of hypophysectomy and the resultant regeneration of a functional neurohypophysis (see p. 281). FISHER, MAGOUN, and RANSON (1938) by placing lesions in the anterior hypothalamus in cats caused degeneration of the hypothalamo-neurohypophysial system distal to the lesion with resultant loss of oxytocin and vasopressin from the gland and thereby produced permanent diabetes insipidus. Lesions were placed in seven pregnant cats and at term all showed severe dystocia and only one successfully delivered and reared a litter. Similar results have been obtained in experiments with guinea pigs (DEY, FISHER, and RANSOM, 1941; ASDELL, 1946). In man, neurohypophysial deficiency of an extent sufficient to cause severe diabetes insipidus is compatible with normal labour (DANDY, 1940; HENDRICKS, 1954; ALEXANDER and DOWNS, 1957; LITTLE, SMITH, JESSIMAN, SELENKOV, VAN'T HOFF, ELGIN, and MOORE, 1958). However, diabetes insipidus is a symptom of deficient vasopressin secretion — oxytocin secretion need not necessarily be impaired, and NIBBELINK (1961) has shown that lesions in the paraventricular regions in cats may cause severe dystocia and prolongation of labour without concurrent diabetes insipidus.

Lesions placed in the hypothalamic preoptic region in the fowl interfere with egg laying (RALPH, 1959). Stalk section and neurohypophysectomy are apparently without effect (SHIRLEY and NALBANDOV, 1956) but since the operations would leave the median eminence intact the possibility of a neurohypophysial factor in egg laying was not excluded. TANAKA and NAKAJO (1962) have shown that there is a very pronounced fall in the arginine vasotocin content of posterior pituitaries in fowls killed 5 min after oviposition. More than 50 % of the vasotocin is lost and recovery to control levels is complete 6 h later; there is only a very small fall in oxytocin content. Since arginine vasotocin is a much more potent stimulator of oviduct contraction than the other naturally occurring neurohypophysial peptides, the results suggest that oviposition is controlled by a neuroendocrine reflex involving the avian neurohypophysis.

13. Stimulation of Male Genitalia

Although there is no known physiological function for oxytocin in male animals, the store of oxytocin in the neurohypophysis is not really less in male than in female animals. It is clear also that stimulation of the neurohypophysis in male animals liberates oxytocin as well as vasopressin, because, for example, dehydration causes a fall in the amounts of both hormones in the neurohypophysis. However, the method of detecting oxytocin release by observing the activity of a target organ e.g. mammary gland and uterus, is not available in experiments with male animals and this difficulty has been overcome by DEBACKERE, PEETERS, and TUYTTENS (1961) by the employment of cross-circulation techniques. The circulations of a ram and a lactating ewe were connected by attaching the distal end of a severed jugular vein in each animal to the central stump in the other, so that the male animal received the jugular blood of the female and *vice versa*. The seminal vesicles and ampullae of the male animal were stimulated manually, *per rectum*. A milk-ejection response followed that was clearly similar to that produced by intravenous injection of oxytocin and the effect could be matched by 50—100 mu. It is possible that release of oxytocin in the male might occur during coitus but no experimental test for this possibility has been reported. However, there is evidence for vasopressin release during coitus in male human subjects. FRIBERG (1953) reported antidiuresis following coitus and FITZPATRICK (1966) has been able to show more clearly that the effect is consistent with vasopressin secretion since the fall in volume is accompanied by an increase in the concentration of electrolytes in urine.

14. Haemorrhage and Changes in Blood Volume

In 1938, RYDIN and VERNEY showed that in conscious water loaded dogs the removal of small volumes of blood from an artery (5—10 ml, sufficient to lower blood pressure by 10 mm-Hg) brought about a marked inhibition of urine flow. Since the response was not affected by denervation of the kidneys or section of the splanchnic nerves they concluded that it "was humorally determined and that the humoral agent was not adrenaline." In contrast, O'CONNOR (1962) was able to remolve similar volumes of blood in unanaesthetised dogs without producing inhibition of urine flow, and in man, LEWIS (1953) withdrew as much as 1,200 ml of blood by venesection without affecting water diuresis. The sympathetic nervous system was intact in the experiments of O'CONNOR and of LEWIS, and the blood was withdrawn from a vein rather than an artery; in spite of this difference between the experiments and those of RYDEN and VERNEY (1938) it seems possible in view of the very small amounts of blood removed, that the results of the latter were due to emotional stress. A role of emotional stress in the effect of blood withdrawal on vasopressin secretion in unanaesthetised human subjects was shown clearly by the experiments of NOBLE and TAYLOR (1953). They found that subjects who fainted after physical (venesection) or emotional (venesection before withdrawal of blood) stresses excreted increased amounts of an antidiuretic substance in the urine and that there was no correlation between the amount of blood withdrawn and the occurrence of fainting. Brun, Knudsen, and Raaschou (1945a, b) also showed that fainting, produced by seating a water-loaded subject so that blood accumulated in the dependent legs, caused inhibition of urine flow of which the time course and the change in urinary composition were similar to those of antidiuretic effects produced by posterior pituitary extract.

Although the results obtained with conscious subjects and animals are thus variable and apparently not directly related to the extent of haemorrhage, experiments in anaesthetised animals have established clearly an effect of blood withdrawal on vasopressin secretion. The difference between the results in conscious and anaesthetised animals might be due to a variety of factors. For example, anaesthetic depression of central pathways mediating an inhibiting influence on neurohypophysial secretion; impairment of sympathetic tone and cardiovascular reflexes leading to an earlier and more precipituous fall in blood pressure in anaesthetised animals (Ginsburg and Brown, unpublished observation); the larger proportion of the total blood volume withdrawn in experiments with anaesthetised animals.

Ginsburg and Heller (1953a) were first to show that the antidiuretic activity of blood taken from rats anaesthetised with ether rose as the volume of blood withdrawn increased. The concentration of antidiuretic activity in external jugular blood was about 5 times that in arterial blood, indicating that the substance entered the circulation from the head. In subsequent experiments carried out under similar conditions Ginsburg and Brown (1956, 1957) showed that the substance was inactivated by treatment with thioglycollate and did not appear in the blood of neurohypophysectomised rats subjected to haemorrhage. Similar observations have been made by de Wied (1960). The discharge of a pressor substance into the circulation of dogs subjected to massive haemorrhage also has been shown by Weinstein, Berne, and Sachs (1960) who demonstrated that it had some of the chemical and chromatographic properties of vasopressin. The amounts of vasopressin found in blood after severe haemorrhage are remarkably high and samples obtained at the maximum blood deficits contain several milliunits of vasopressin per ml. Increased antidiuretic activity in blood of dogs after haemorrhage has also been reported by Baratz and Ingraham (1960) and by Jahn, Stephan, and Stahl (1960).

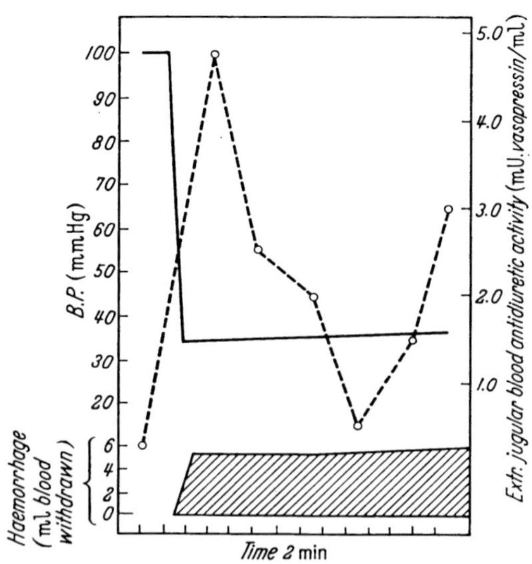

Fig. 23. Effect of rapid haemorrhage on blood pressure and antidiuretic activity in external jugular blood of a rat anaesthetised with urethane. Reproduced with permission from Ginsburg and Brown. Brit. J. Pharmacol. 11, 236 (1956)

When blood was withdrawn from anaesthetised rats in steps of 0.5 ml/100 g at 4 min intervals, Ginsburg and Brown (1956, 1957) found that the increase in antidiuretic activity in external jugular blood often occurred in two distinct phases. The first pronounced rise in antidiuretic activity coincided with the sharp fall in blood pressure and the second rise occurred after the blood pressure had been less than 50 mm Hg (and usually less than 40 mm Hg) for 15 min. When blood was withdrawn rapidly so as to lower the blood pressure to 33—37 mm Hg within 1 min, the biphasic nature of the response was seen more clearly. 4 min after the removal of blood the antidiuretic activity was 25 times greater than in the control blood sample; 12 min later it had fallen almost to the control level to be followed by another rise in the succeeding 8 min (see Fig. 23). WEINSTEIN et al. (1960) in dogs also have shown that the raised vasopressin concentration in blood after rapid haemorrhage are not sustained but they did not observe the second rise, possibly because blood pressure was lowered only to 50 mm Hg.

Unlike many other stimuli to the neurohypophysis, the secretion elicited by haemorrhage is predominantly vasopressin with little or no oxytocin. GINSBURG and SMITH (1959) withdrew up to 3.0 ml of blood/100 g body weight from anaesthetised rats and estimated antidiuretic and oxytocic activity in the same samples. They found that in blood taken when the deficit was 1.5 ml blood/100 g body weight the antidiuretic activity was about 30 times higher than in the initial samples while the oxytocic activity had hardly increased. This result has been confirmed recently by BELESLIN et al. (1957) in cats. These findings agree with the results of CHAUDHURY and WALKER (1958) who were unable to detect a release of oxytocin in rabbits from which about one third of the total blood volume had been withdrawn.

A wide variety of procedures (less drastic than but including haemorrhage) change the distribution of blood within the vascular system and those that increase the intrathoracic blood volume also initiate a diuresis of dilute urine while decrease in intrathoracic blood volume is associated with oliguria. It is claimed that these effects on water balance are mediated by increase or decrease in antidiuretic hormone secretion and that the effects of 'volume' changes may transcend the influence of concurrent changes in plasma osmotic pressure (see GAUER and HENRY, 1963). This is true, certainly, for haemorrhage itself since BARATZ and INGRAHAM (1960) have shown convincingly that the release of vasopressin is not mediated by changes in plasma osmotic pressure. Contraction of the extracellular fluid in dogs by 15% (estimated from the change in haematocrit) following intraperitoneal injection of hypertonic glucose is associated with an increase of antidiuretic activity in plasma of the order of 10—20 times; although there is a rise in plasma osmolarity due to absorbed glucose, intravenous injection of glucose in amounts giving the same increase in serum osmolarity has a much smaller and delayed affect upon plasma antidiuretic activity (SHARE, 1961). It is concluded therefore, that the stimulation of vasopressin secretion is the result of the changing extracellular fluid volume rather than changes in plasma osmotic pressure or systemic blood pressure. Antidiuresis of 'quiet standing' can be prevented by alcohol administration (PEARCE and NEWMAN, 1954) suggesting that it, also, is due to stimulation of neurohypophysial secretion independently of changes in osmotic pressure or arterial blood pressure, although changes in the distribution of blood in the vascular system could be involved.

The situation is balanced with more subtlety when the expansion of volume is coupled with increased plasma osmotic pressure as in the experiments of BLOMBERT, GERBRANDY, MOLHUYSEN, DE VRIES, and BORST (1951) who showed that the first effect on urine flow of an intravenous infusion of slightly hypertonic solutions into recumbent human subjects was a diuresis of hypotonic urine similar to that produced by simple water loading. Also, WELT and his associates (WELT and ORLOFF, 1951; PETERSDORF and WELT, 1953) have shown that expansion of plasma volume by infusion of iso-oncotic albumin solution induces diuresis which they assume to be due to inhibition of antidiuretic hormone secretion. More direct evidence has been obtained by SHARE (1962) who showed that circulating antidiuretic hormone was reduced by 50% after infusion of isotonic dextran.

Negative pressure breathing has been employed extensively as a means of increasing the intrathoracic blood volume at the expense of the extrathoracic circulation. In men and dogs breathing under reduced pressure, hypotonic diuresis of non-osmotic origin ensues (GAUER, HENRY, SIEKER, and WENDT, 1954; SURTSHIN, HOLTZENBEIN, and WHITE, 1955; HULET and SMITH, 1959; BOYLAN and ANTKOWIAK, 1959; BARATZ and INGRAHAM, 1960). A similar polyuria is produced by breathing gas mixtures of low O_2 and high CO_2 concentration, voluntary overbreathing or breathing through the resistance valves used to administer gas mixtures (BARBOUR, BULL, HUGHES-JONES, EVANS, and LOGOTHETOPOULOS, 1953; LOVE, RODDIE, ROSENWEIG, and SHANKS, 1957; CURRIE and ULLMAN, 1961). Positive pressure breathing, which is somewhat more stressing, reduces intrathoracic blood volume and inhibits water diuresis even if moderate positive pressures are used (DRURY, HENRY, and GOODMAN, 1947). The location of the sensitive parts of the central circulation has been investigated by placing obstructions of snares, or particles, or inflated balloons at strategic positions in the thoracic blood vessels. Partial occlusion of the pulmonary circulation at the level of the pulmonary capillaries or at the opening of the pulmonary veins at the left atrium caused only a slight decrease in urine volume while obstruction of the mitral orifice leading to engorgement of the left atrium caused diuresis (HENRY, GAUER, and REEVES, 1956; BAISSET and MONTASTRUC, 1959). According to ELIAHOU, CLARKE, and BULL (1960) the significant parameter of atrial receptor stimulation is not so much the absolute length but rather that the receptors respond mainly to pulsatile stretch. LEDSOME, LINDEN, and O'CONNOR (1961) also have reported experiments in dogs in which distention of the left atrium, in most cases, caused a moderate increase in urine flow. However, they deny that the effect could be due to inhibition of antidiuretic hormone secretion because the urine flow rate could not be reduced by administration of vasopressin. This is not in agreement with results of other observers who have found that the diuresis induced by negative pressure breathing in man and dogs resembles water diuresis in that it is inhibited by vasopressin and in other respects (SURTSHIN et al., 1955; MURDAUGH, SIEKER, and MANFREDI, 1959; BOYLAN and ANTKOWIAK, 1959). However, O'CONNOR (1962) has pointed out that the amounts of vasopressin required to inhibit the diuresis are approximately ten times greater than those required to inhibit diuresis induced by water ingestion, and he suggests that the larger amounts may produce their effects by an action on the renal circulation rather than on tubular reabsorption of water. On the other hand, BARATZ and INGRAHAM (1960) have shown that positive pressure breathing leads to a significant increase in plasma antidiuretic activity, and BAISSET and MONTASTRUC (1959) have observed a fall in circulating antidiuretic activity following balloon distention of the left atrium.

The afferent pathway for the impulses from the volume receptors of the atrium is located in vagal fibres since the diuretic responses to negative pressure breathing or to left atrial distention caused by obstruction are abolished by cooling the vagus nerve to 8—10°. Removal of 50 ml blood/kg body weight from a dog reduces vagal afferent traffic while there is a marked increase during atrial distention, though the increase during negative pressure breathing is not so pronounced (HENRY and PEARCE, 1956).

It would seem therefore that the impulses in the vagal afferents impinge upon a central mechanism for the *inhibition* of antidiuretic hormone secretion. The same conclusion follows from the results of experiments by SHARE and LEVY (1962), who showed that occlusion of the carotid arteries increases circulating vasopressin only if the vagi had been severed; carotid occlusion in animals in which the carotid sinus had been denervated did not affect plasma antidiuretic activity, even if the vagi were divided. CLARK and ROCHA E SILVA jr. (1966) found that carotid occlusion in vagotomised cats does not raise plasma oxytocin concentration although antidiuretic activity is increased. They confirm the finding of SHARE and LEVY (1962) that carotid sinus denervation prevents the increase in circulating vasopressin.

An interesting paradox is that while these experiments show the occurrence of vagal afferent inhibitory activity, the observations of long-standing (CHANG, CHIA, HSU, and LIM, 1937, 1938; CHAN, LIM, LU, WANG, and WANG, 1938) that electrical stimulation of the central end of a severed vagus nerve results in release of both oxytocin and vasopressin has been confirmed in recent work (MILLS and WANG, 1964; DYBALL, 1966, 1967).

These results suggest that the vagally innervated and carotid sinus receptors act in a manner analogous to their function as baroreceptors in the regulation of arterial blood pressure, viz. that inhibitory impulses from the carotid sinus are decreased by carotid occlusion but this is effective in increasing vasopressin secretion only if the inhibitory activity of vagal afferents is prevented. A similar interpretation follows from more recent experiments (SHARE and LEVY, 1966b) in which it was shown that when the perfusion of the carotid sinuses in unanaesthetised, vagotomised dogs was changed from pulsatile to steady, without change in mean pressure, the antidiuretic activity in plasma increased by more than 150%. It is concluded that decreased pulsatile stretching of carotid sinus receptors decreases the discharge of impulses in the afferent fibres that exert an inhibitory influence on vasopressin secretion. The possible contribution of chemoreceptor stimulation to vasopressin secretion during carotid occlusion (or haemorrhage) was investigated by assay of circulating antidiuretic activity during perfusion of a carotid sinus with deoxygenated blood (SHARE and LEVY, 1966a). Small but significant increases in antidiuretic activity were observed only if the mean arterial blood pressure was prevented from rising by allowing the blood volume to fall. These circumstances are so equivocal that the role of chemoreceptor stimulation is, at best, a small one. Essentially similar results have been obtained in dogs by USAMI, PERIC, and CHIEN (1962) and CHIEN, PERIC, and USAMI (1962) who showed also that occlusion of the external or internal carotids above the bifurcation was ineffective. Thus, in addition to the vagal afferents from the left atrium another group of receptors in the carotid sinuses also are involved in regulating antidiuretic hormone secretion. PERLMUTT (1963) has studied the effect of brief occlusion of the common carotids on urine flow in water diuresis. The character of the antidiuresis that resulted (hyper-osmotic urine and decrease a free water clearances) are consistent with the release of antidiuretic hormone. Unlike the results of SHARE and LEVY (1962), PERLMUTT (1963) found that occlusion above the thyrocarotid junction did not affect antidiuretic hormone secretion (as indicated by antidiuresis). The differences between the conditions of the two sets of experiments should be stressed; it is possible that an increase of vasopressin secretion sufficient to inhibit water diuresis might not be detected when plasma levels of antidiuretic activity of non-diuretic dogs are measured, and also the brief occlusion of the carotids in PERLMUTT's (1963) experiments contrasts with the longer duration of the occlusion in the experiments of SHARE and LEVY (1962). MAZER, ALLEGRINI, and LEMAIRE (1962a, b) also have found that hypotension in the carotid arteries evokes an antidiuresis.

15. Anaesthetics and Anaesthesia

The observation that inhibition of water diuresis occurs during or after anaesthesia with ether or chloroform was first made in the early years of this century

(THOMPSON, 1905; FREY, 1907). In 1932, HELLER and SMIRK showed that water retention caused by the anaesthetics could not be attributed to impaired water absorption in the gastro-intestinal tract. Since then similar observations have been recorded with other anaesthetics such as cyclopropane (CRAIG et al., 1945; MILES and DE WARDENER, 1952), halothane (BLACKMORE et al., 1960) and barbiturates (DE BODO and PRESCOTT, 1945). Obviously, the possibility of increased vasopressin secretion from the hypothalamic-neurohypophysial system under the influence of the anaesthetic agents should be taken into account as one of the factors involved. The experiments of DE BODO and PRESCOTT (1945) showing that in dogs with permanent diabetes insipidus produced by the destruction of the neurohypophysis, barbiturates failed to cause antidiuresis supported this point of view.

Additional evidence now provided by assay of antidiuretic activity in blood, shows that in rats anaesthetised with ether, pentobarbitone or urethane blood contained higher concentrations of vasopressin than in conscious animals (AMES and VAN DYKE, 1952; GINSBURG and HELLER, 1953; DICKER, 1953; GINSBURG and BROWN, 1956; CHAUDHURY and WALKER, 1958 and HELLER, 1960). The observations that concentrations of the antidiuretic activity in venous blood draining the cerebral circulation were higher than in arterial blood (GINSBURG and HELLER, 1953), that antidiuretic activity was not detectable in blood from anaesthetised, neurohypophysectomised animals (AMES and VAN DYKE, 1952; GINSBURG and BROWN, 1956) and that loss of the activity occurred after treatment with thioglycollate (GINSBURG and BROWN, 1956) provides evidence for the neurohypophysial origin of the antidiuretic substance. It has been shown also that ether anaesthesia in rabbits also increases the oxytocic activity of blood (CHAUDHURY and WALKER, 1958).

Study of the role of vasopressin in anaesthetic-induced antidiuresis is complicated by the difficulty of assessing the depth of anaesthesia by objective criteria. Cardiovascular changes during anaesthesia also make difficult the interpretation of renal function changes; moreover, increased secretion of vasopressin might well be secondary to the abrupt fall in blood pressure as inhibition of central control of vasomotion supervenes (GINSBURG and BROWN, 1956). The route of administration and secondary characteristics of the anaesthetic agent also are likely to be important. It is hardly surprising that an animal anaesthetised by ether vapour should have disturbed renal function attributable to increased antidiuretic hormone secretion. "Emotional stress" and painful irritation of mucus membranes are, under these circumstances, the most likely causes of stimulation of the neurohypophysial system, which, then, would be due to the events during induction of anaesthesia rather than the anaesthesia *per se*. In support of this interpretation, KIVALO (1966) has shown that a low dose of thiopentone given before exposure to ether apparently alleviates the emotional disturbances and lessens the antidiuresis. Similar results have been obtained in clinical experiments in man (APRAHAMIAN et al., 1959; MORRIS et al., 1959).

It is quite clear that stimulation of the neurohypophysial system, whether indirectly or not, is a property of only some anaesthetic agents and is not an invariable accompaniment to the state of anaesthesia. Thus, DE BODO and PRESCOTT (1945) found in dogs that phenobarbitone and amylobarbitone caused antidiuresis in some dogs only. Other barbiturates, particularly those with a short duration of action, e.g. thiopentone and Inaktin (5-ethyl-5(1 methyl prophyl)-2-thiobarbitone), may be used to anaesthetise animals without impairment of water diuresis and have been employed in antidiuretic assays. The latter may have an inhibiting effect on neurohypophysial secretion (WIRZ, 1956).

Ethanol is used widely as anaesthetic in rats in antidiuretic assays and its capacity to promote water diuresis (EGGLETON, 1942) is well established. VAN DYKE and AMES (1951) and DICKER (1953) have shown that secretion of vasopressin in response to an osmotic stimulus (intracarotid injection of hypertonic NaCl solution) is inhibited by ethanol anaesthesia. The stimulus to antidiuretic hormone secretion in rats given by heart puncture and by injection of acetylcholine in dogs are inhibited by ethanol anaesthesia. Ethanol also inhibits oxytocin release in response to suckling stimulus in women (FUCHS and WAGNER, 1963a) rabbit (FUCHS and WAGNER, 1963b) and rat (CHAUDHURY, 1961). FUCHS (1966) has shown that with blood ethanol levels of 0.25—0.35 ml per 100 g in parturient rabbits, the onset of labour is delayed and that uterine contractions typical of normal labour were absent which she attributes the effect of ethanol to central inhibition of reflex release of oxytocin. On the other hand ethanol does not suppress stimulation of antidiuretic hormone secretion in other circumstances. For example, GINSBURG and BROWN (1956) showed in rats that ethanol had no effect on haemorrhage induced release of oxytocin and vasopressin.

16. Morphine and Related Substances

Many analgesics of the morphine type, including pethidine, have been shown to inhibit water diuresis. Evidence for the release of antidiuretic hormone by morphine is provided by the observations that the antidiuretic effect cannot be produced in neurohypophysectomised animals (DE BODO, 1944) and that there is an increase in the antidiuretic activity of urine (GIARMAN, MATTIE, and STEPHENSON, 1953) and of blood (GIERE and EVERSOLE, 1954; HELLER, 1960). Nalorphine also is antidiuretic in rats but it has been possible to demonstrate nevertheless an antagonism between nalorphine and morphine (SCHNIEDEN and BLACKMORE, 1953). On the other hand MILLS and WANG (1964) suggest that the cardiovascular effects of pethidine and morphine might be partly responsible for the antidiuretic responses. This may, indeed, be true in their own experiments, which were performed in dogs anaesthetised with chloralose but is probably not applicable generally. After the immediate antidiuretic effect of vascular origin had passed off, MILLS and WANG found that the analgesics blocked release of antidiuretic hormone by electrical stimulation in the medulla or of the ulnar nerve while the release brought about by central vagal stimulation was unaffected. They conclude, therefore, that the analgesics inhibit vasopressin secretion by acting in two ways, (a) by inhibiting responses to nociceptive stimulation and (b) by an action at a site rostral to the mid brain.

17. Tranquillisers

Experimental workers studying antidiuretic responses are constantly impressed and frustrated by the apparent lability of antidiuretic hormone release in response to minor stresses, brought about by handling and other stimuli that fall far short of causing pain. It is not surprising therefore that drugs that block behavioural manifestations of conditioned avoidance responses will also block antidiuretic effects of minor acute stress. Thus, DE WIED and JINKS (1958) have shown that chlorpromazine prevents the antidiuretic effect of electrical stimuli applied to the feet in rats, while it does not affect the antidiureses produced by nicotine or histamine administration. (It should be noted that there is no *a priori* reason to assume than an antidiuretic response to intraperitoneal histamine in rats is mediated by antidiuretic hormone.) Methyl pentynol (DICKER, 1958) and perphanazine (HUNTER, KALANT, and OGILVIE, 1959) also have an inhibitory effect on antidiuretic hormone secretion. It is interesting to note that non-stressing stimuli also are blocked by chlorpromazine. CHAUDHURY (1961) found that oxytocin release in response to suckling stimuli, assessed by weight gain in nursed rats, was inhibited in mothers treated with chlorpromazine.

18. Environmental Temperature

Heller and Smirk (1932) in rabbits and Weiner (1945) in man showed that the diuretic response to water administration decreased at high environmental temperatures even when extrarenal losses were compensated. Hellmann and Weiner (1953) found an increase in the excretion of an antidiuretic substance in the urine of human subjects after exposure to heat. Itoh (1954b) reported subsequently that the antidiuretic activity of the serum rose and the antidiuretic hormone content of the posterior pituitary gland diminished when rats were subjected to high temperatures for 50—120 min. On re-investigation of the effects of short-term exposure of rats, sheep and man to high temperatures, Robinson and Macfarlane (1956) and Macfarlane and Robinson (1957) confirmed the rise in plasma antidiuretic activity but concluded that there was no direct stimulation of receptors in the skin or hypothalamus by heat, for the increase in plasma antidiuretic activity occurred $1^1/_2$—3 h after the rise of the skin temperature and was accompanied by an increase in plasma protein concentration and plasma osmotic pressure. They suggested therefore that the increased release of antidiuretic hormone was due to loss of water.

19. Emotion

Klisiecki, Pickford, Rothschild, and Verney (1933) observed a marked fall in the rate of urine flow in a dog when the animal was shown a cat. Similar inhibitory effects were seen by Rydin and Verney (1938) when dogs were frightened by sounding a motor-car horn. In other experiments (O'Connor and Verney, 1942, 1945) stress was produced by weak faradic stimulation of subcutaneous tissues. Three different responses were found in intact conscious dogs with an established water diuresis: 1. an immediate short inhibition with a return to a diuretic rate of flow within 10 min; 2. an inhibition of slow onset continuing much longer and returning to the previous diuretic level 30—60 min later; 3. a combination of these two responses. Removal of the posterior lobe abolished or markedly diminished the slow and prolonged antidiuresis (O'Connor and Verney, 1942). Denervation of both kidneys and adrenals eliminated the immediate shortlasting inhibition but a slow prolonged inhibition always occurred. O'Connor and Verney (1945) reported also that an intravenous injection of adrenaline given to such dogs 30 sec before the faradic stimulus, abolished the prolonged antidiuretic effect. Verney (1947) suggested, therefore, that adrenaline interfered with the release of antidiuretic hormone by an action on the central nervous system. The problem was further investigated by Dempster and Joekes (1955) who, in dogs, had found (Dempster and Joekes, 1953) that a kidney transplanted to the neck responded to a faradic stimulus in a manner indistinguishable from a normal kidney; that is to say, it produced an immediate decrease in urine flow and then a prolonged inhibition with a slow return to diuretic volumes. Intravenously injected adrenaline (15—80 μg per animal) caused an immediate inhibition of diuresis lasting 5—6 min, almost identical with that seen by Pickford and Watt (1951b) in normal dogs.

It seems therefore that the rapid inhibition of urine flow after faradic stimulation is due to a release of adrenaline and that it may be followed by a longer lasting antidiuretic response caused by an increased secretion of antidiuretic hormone. However, Dempster and Joekes (1955) in the auto-transplanted kidney were unable to confirm the prevention of the slow component of an emotional antidiuresis by previously injected adrenaline.

CHALMERS and LEWIS (1951) observed marked antidiuresis in a subject who was about to experience a painful experimental procedure. Absence of any demonstrable changes of the glomerular filtration rate and a rise in urinary chloride concentration suggested that the antidiuretic effect was due to the release of antidiuretic hormone. More investigations in man and in other species are desirable to establish the importance of the emotional release of antidiuretic hormone in ordinary life.

20. Nociceptive Stimuli

The inhibition of water diuresis in fainting subjects suggested vagal stimulation as one of the causes for an increased release of antidiuretic hormone. ANDERSSON and LARSON (1954) therefore investigated whether vomiting, which might be regarded as a mild vaso-vagal attack, had an influence on the water diuresis of conscious dogs. They found that emesis produced by either apomorphine or copper sulphate produced marked decreases in urine flow. However, 2 mg of atropine given subcutaneously 40 min before the apomorphine did not abolish the antidiuretic effect. TAYLOR, HUNTER, and JOHNSON (1957) found that laboratory induced motion sickness was consistently accompanied by an inhibition of water diuresis of the vasopressin type.

KELSALL (1949) showed that water diuresis in man can be inhibited by a period of pain produced by exercising the forearm muscles after arrest of the circulation in them. Since 1. changes in pulse rate and blood pressure subsided before the inhibition of diuresis was fully established, 2. the concentration of chloride in the urine increased, 3. the excretion of endogenous creatinine remained unchanged (KELSALL, 1951), 4. intravenous injections of adenosine triphosphate in doses which lowered the systemic blood pressure by about 10 mm Hg had no antidiuretic action (see however, DEXTER, STONER, and GREEN, 1954), 5. the antidiuretic effect of ischaemic pain could be closely paralleled by small doses of Pituitrin, KELSALL suggested that the antidiuretic effects observed were predominantly due to the release of antidiuretic hormone. CHALMERS and LEWIS (1951) produced an inhibition of water diuresis by ischaemic pain in 3 out of 6 subjects. The chloride concentration in the urine increased markedly when the diuresis was inhibited, again suggesting that the antidiuresis was due to stimulation of the neurohypophysis.

21. Neurohypophysial Function in Immaturity

New born animals (HELLER, 1949) and infants (HANSEN and SMITH, 1952; BARNETT and VESTERDAL, 1953) are unable to concentrate urine to the same extent as adults. It has been suggested that apart from the functional immaturity of the kidneys that incomplete development of the biosynthetic, storage and release mechanism for neurohypophysial hormones might also contribute. The appearance of neurosecretory material in the immature neurohypophysis has been the subject of many light microscopy investigations (SCHARRER, 1954; RODECK and CAESAR, 1956; RODECK, 1958; AMOROSO, HARRISON, HARRISON-MATTHEWS, ROWLANDS, BOURNE, and SLOPER, 1958; BARGMANN, 1949; DAWSON, 1953; BERNISCHKE and MCKAY, 1953). At birth the neurosecretory material is scanty in those species which are also immature by other criteria. Even after the 4th to 6th post-natal day in the rat it appears only as very fine dust-like particles which aggregate as the animal matures. BARER and LEDERIS (1966) have described the ultrastructure of the neurohypophysis of 5 day old rabbits. They have the impression that the relative abundance of pituicytes is rather greater than in adults and the neural swellings contain particles resembling elementary granules but very few of these have dense cores. Glycogen particles that are seen only very rarely in adult glands are very obvious in the neural swellings in the immature animals. Several investigators haven shown that the vasopressin content of the neurohypophysis is very low (HELLER, 1947; HELLER and ZAIMIS, 1949; DICKER and TYLER, 1953; ACHER, CHAUVET and OLIVRY, 1956b; HELLER and LEDERIS, 1959; KŘEČEK, DLOUHÁ, and KŘEČEKOVA, 1961; MIKULAS and DLOUHÁ, 1962) not only in absolute amounts but also when related to body weight or pituitary weight (mu/mg/wet weight of gland). During the first week of post-natal life the concentration of vasopressin in the neurohypophysis of rats is less than $^1/_9$th of that in adult animals; the ratio for human infants is of the order of $^1/_3$, while in 1 day old guinea pigs the vasopressin concentration in neurohypophysis is 60% of that in adults. HELLER and LEDERIS (1959) point out that using that criterion as an index of the maturity of the hypothalamo-neurohypophysial system the order rat, human, guinea pig parallels the overall maturity at birth as judged by other criteria.

The neurohypophysis of rats 10—20 days after birth contains less than 50 mu of antidiuretic activity per 100 g body weight (KRECEK and J. HELLER, 1962). This is somewhat discrepant in the light of the vasopressor activities of 150—200 mu/100 g body weight obtained in 14 days old rats by HELLER and LEDERIS (1959) who showed also that the active pressor substance could not be distinguished from vasopressin by chromatographic methods.

According to MIKULAS and DLOUHA (1962) the amounts of antidiuretic activity in the neurohypophysis in rats increasie sharply during the 4th post-natal week, coinciding with the end of the weaning period. At the same time an increase in plasma antidiuretic activity can be elicited by osmotic stimulation (KRECEK and J. HELLER, 1962). In human infants the response to osmotic stimulation (increased plasma antidiuretic activity) is not apparent until after the 3rd post-natal month. In younger infants the urine contains appreciable amounts of antidiuretic activity which do not appear to depend on the state of hydration (DICKER and EGGLETON, 1960). It seems unlikely therefore that the secretion of vasopressin in the neurohypophysis, at that stage, is dependent on the osmoreceptor stimulation as in adults, and this is consistent with post-natal maturation of magnocellular hypothalamic nuclei (AUER, 1951, RODECK, 1958). Immaturity thus involves both the afferent and efferent limbs of the neuroendocrine reflex and even the action of antidiuretic hormone, which does not affect the neonatal kidney. It is possible that the hyper-hydration of infants subsisting on a milk diet might be at the root of the immaturity at the hypothalamic and renal levels.

The oxytocin content of neurohypophysis of immature rats also is very low and according to DICKER and TYLER (1953) and ACHER et al. (1956b) the ratio of vasopressin to oxytocin shortly after birth may be as high as 7 or 8 but reaches unity in the third post-natal week. HELLER and LEDERIS (1959) have shown that this observation can be repeated only if the neurohypophyses are dehydrated before extraction by treatment with acetone; if the glands are extracted without acetone dehydration, the relative excess of vasopressin in the first post-natal week disappears or is reduced. The reason appears to be that a large proportion of the oxytocin in glands of new born rats is eluted by the acetone used for dessication, while such losses of oxytocin amount to only about 3% from glands of adult rats. The explanation for these results may lie in the observations of BARER et al. (1963) that over 60% of the oxytocin in sucrose homogenates of 5 day old rabbit neurohypophysis is not sedimented by ultracentrifugation compared with 20% in glands from adult animals, whereas the unsedimented vasopressin is not very different in adult and young animals. There is thus a higher proportion of oxytocin free (in the sense that it is not incorporated in sedimentable particles) in the neurohypophysis of young rabbits and it could be this fraction or a proportion of it that is eluted by acetone. According to Dicker (1966), however, the rate of loss of vasopressin from incubated neurohypophyses of new born (1—2 day) rats is rather greater than the rate of loss of oxytocin although the reverse is the case with glands from adult rats.

22. The State of Circulating Neurohypophysial Hormones

Neurohypophysial hormones in blood can be recovered quantitatively from plasma and thus penetration into erythrocytes is negligible. This has been shown for vasopressin added to rat (Heller and Zaidi, 1957), dog (Bocanegra and Lauson, 1961) and human blood (Ginsburg, 1960); vasopressin released endogenously in blood also is confined to plasma (Bocanegra and Lauson, 1961). Similar observations have been made with the recovery of oxytocin added to rat (Ginsburg and Smith, 1959), sheep (Fitzpatrick, 1961), and goat (Folley and Knaggs, 1966) blood. Vasopressin is remarkably stable in blood or plasma (Ginsburg and Heller, 1953; Heller and Zaidi, 1957); the loss of activity of vasopressin stored in plasma is no greater than in phosphate buffer (Adamson, Engel, and van Dyke, 1958). It is thus unlikely that inactivation of circulating hormone by factors in blood plays a significant role in the metabolism of oxytocin and vasopressin, with the possible exception of the case of some primates during pregnancy, when a circulating oxytocinase is present. The apparent exclusion of the peptides from the red cells raises the question of how the concentration gradients between the cells and the plasma are maintained since some diffusion of free hormone into the cells might be expected. Circulating vasopressin does not penetrate extravascular spaces (apart from organs of preferential uptake) and the restriction of the apparent volume of distribution to the plasma volume (Ginsburg and Heller, 1953b; Lauson, 1960; Czaczkes, Kleeman, and Koenig, 1964; Czaczkes and Kleeman, 1964) also means that the free diffusion of neurohypophysial peptides in blood is somehow restricted. The most obvious way in which this could be achieved would be by the association of the peptides with plasma protein but the evidence for this is conflicting and contradictory.

In experiments with human plasma Heller and Lederis (1957) compared the dialysis rates of oxytocin and vasopressin added to plasma or to isotonic Krebs-Eggleston phosphate saline buffer. Dialysis of the hormones from the plasma was shown to be slower than from the buffer, whereas there as no difference in the dialysis rates for inulin, suggesting therefore that the peptides were bound to a plasma protein fraction. Dingman (1958) tested the antidiuretic activities of human plasma protein fractions separated by Cohn's procedure: only the combined fractions II and III contained antidiuretic activity. These experiments do not satisfactorily identify the fraction containing the putative binding protein since the affinities could alter in the conditions used for protein fractionation and the possibility of co-precipitation is not excluded. Hipsley and McKellar (1960) found that by adding plasma from non-pregnant human subjects (male or female) to pregnancy plasma, the inactivation of vasopressin by the latter can be prevented; they attribute the protection of vasopressin to binding by protein in the non-pregnancy plasma.

In contrast to these observations, Czaczkes et al. (1964) were unable to detect any binding of vasopressin in human plasma by dialysis or ultrafiltration experiments. It is difficult to see what is the essential difference between these experiments and those of Heller and Lederis (1957). Czaczkes et al. (1964) used the much lower concentration of endogenous vasopressin in human plasma, while Heller and Lederis (1957) added large amounts of exogenous hormone, but this might have led one to expect a difference in the opposite direction, i.e. a failure to detectbinding in the presence of an overwhelming excess of vasopressin.

The most extensive evidence for neurohypophysial hormone binding to plasma protein comes from the work of THORN and his colleagues, using rat serum (THORN and SILVER, 1957; THORN, 1959a; SMITH and THORN, 1965). When serum of blood taken from rats (in ether anaesthesia) 1 min after intracarotid injection of hypertonic NaCl solution was subjected to ultrafiltration all of the antidiuretic activity was retained by a filter of which the pore size was such that only substances of molecular weight greater than 70,000 would be retained (THORN and SILVER, 1957).

Adequate evidence that the antidiuretic activity was due to vasopressin was obtained by the specificity of inactivation by proteolytic enzymes and by thioglycollate inactivation. In dialysis experiments, only some of the activity was found in the diffusate when dialysed against 20 volumes of water, whereas on dialysis against 0.2 N acetic acid no retention of the antidiuretic activity was observed. The rat serum was also subjected to electrophoresis on starch blocks for 41—48 min at 4° C (barbital buffer, pH 8.6, ionic strength 0.1) and it was found that all of the detectable activity migrated with the β-globulin fraction. Subsequently THORN (1959) added purified 8-arginine-vasopressin and synthetic oxytocin to serum that had been obtained from rats anaesthetised with ethanol and therefore without detectable endogenous antidiuretic activity. On electrophoresis, the oxytocic and antidiuretic activities were found, once again, in the β-globulin region; when eluted, the activities were further shown not to be ultrafiltrable. Evidence for vasopressin binding by rat serum protein was obtained by yet another method, gel filtration, by SMITH and THORN (1965). The movement of arginine vasopressin through a column equilibrated with a 1:1 mixture of rat serum and sodium acetate buffer was faster than when the rat serum was omitted. However, CZACZKES and KLEEMAN (1964) could find no difference between the concentrations of antidiuretic activity of the diffusates and retentates when rat serum was subjected to ultrafiltration or equilibrium dialysis. Since they found that the volume of distribution of vasopressin was approximately equal to the plasma volume and that the concentration of vasopressin in lymph was less than $^1/_{200}$ of the concentration in plasma, they suggested that the hormone might be bound *in vivo* although this could not be demonstrated *in vitro*.

The results of experiments on the binding of vasopressin to plasma protein in dogs is equally contradictory. BOCANEGRA and LAUSON (1961) found that 25% of the antidiuretic hormone in plasma obtained from animals in fatal haemorrhage (300 units per ml) was not ultrafiltrable. CZACZKES and KLEEMAN (1964) who, by taking not more than 40 ml from each dog, used much lower concentrations of the endogenous hormone (3—6 μu/ml) but did not find any difference in the concentration of vasopressin in diffusate and retentate; BROOK and SHARE (1966) also were unable to demonstrate binding of vasopressin to plasma protein in dogs· However, HARVEY, JONES, and LEE (1967) showed that at three different concentrations of arginine vasopressin in dog plasma (30, 100 and 290 μu/ml) 24—75% of the hormone was bound, the proportion bound decreasing with increasing hormone concentration.

There are some similarities in the properties of the hormone binding protein fraction of rat serum and those of pituitary neurophysin. For example, the dissociation of the complexes at low pH (THORN and SILVER, 1957; GINSBURG and IRELAND, 1964) and in the presence of Ca (SMITH and THORN, 1965; GINSBURG, JAYASENA and THOMAS, 1966). Indeed, GINSBURG and JAYASENA (1967) have extracted a protein fraction from pig serum that has chromatographic properties similar to neurophysin; are bound oxytocin and vasopressin and the binding is inhibited by

Ca; and that cross-reacts with neurophysin antibody. Nevertheless, there are some difficulties that should be resolved before the identity of the hormone binding protein of serum and neurophysin can be established. For example, the apparent molecular weight of the rat serum protein is greater than 70,000; the molecular weight of rat neurophysin is not known, but in other species it is 30,000 or less (VAN DYKE et al., 1941; ACHER, 1958; GINSBURG and IRELAND, 1965). However, LAUSON (1960) points out that is conceivable that neurophysin in plasma might become bound to another protein and thus the effective size would be increased. Other difficulties are that vasopressin and oxytocin are bound by the plasma protein at pH 8.6 (THORN and SILVER, 1957; THORN, 1959) while binding of the hormones by neurophysin is much reduced at pH 7.4 (GINSBURG and IRELAND, 1964). The association constants are very low and the complexes dissociate on dilution so that at the concentrations that obtain in plasma, binding might be negligible. It is possible that these difficulties might be resolved and thus that the hormone binding proteins in plasma might indeed be of neurohypophysial origin, though the occurrence of neurophysin-like proteins in kidney, uterus and mammary gland (GINSBURG and JAYASENA, 1967) would leave the interpretation problematical.

The antidiuretic activity in urine of dehydrated rats and after osmotic stimulation does not dialyse (GILMAN and GOODMAN, 1937; THORN, 1959b) and the activity in the urine of kangaroo rats (adapted to life in a desert environment) also is nondialysable (AMES and VAN DYKE, 1950). Oxytocic activity in rat urine is not dialysable, but the identity of the active substances with oxytocin is not established (AUJARD, CZANYI, and LE BRETON, 1954). AMES, MOORE, and VAN DYKE (1950) in experiments in dogs showed that the antidiuretic activity appeared in urine after intracarotid injection of hypertonic NaCl solution was not freely dialysable and was sedimented by ultracentrifugation. They were able to exclude the possibility that the macromolecule to which the activity was bound was present normally in urine as follows: Urine was first collected from a dog in water balance and the animal was then injected with hypertonic NaCl solution into a carotid artery. The antidiuretic activity in urine secreted subsequently was only partially dialysable. The "free" fraction was added to the urine collected prior to osmotic stimulation, and when the mixture was ultracentrifuged no evidence of sedimentation of the activity was obtained. It would seem, therefore, that the macromolecule appeared in urine when endogenous vasopressin is released; whether it comes from the neurohypophysis or is released from the kidney as a result of the action of vasopressin is not known. If the former is correct it would strengthen the evidence for the occurrence of neurohypophysial neurophysins in the circulation and would have important implications for the mechanism of hormone release. However many difficulties remain, not least the observation by THORN (1959a) that the vasopressin and oxytocin binding plasma protein fraction is present in rats in which neurohypophysial hormone secretion had been suppressed by ethanol treatment. It would be possible to account for this if it was shown that the proteins persist longer in the circulation than do the hormones.

23. The Clearance of Circulating Neurohypophysial Hormones

The investigation of the metabolic fate of peptide hormones is beset by the difficulty of differentiating the products of hormone metabolism from those of the metabolism of other proteins and peptides. As radioactive labelled hormones become available, better understanding of the catabolic pathways could be achieved and indeed a start has been made in the experiments of AROSKAR, CHAN, STOUFFER, SCHNEIDER, MURTI, and DU VIGNEAUD (1964) using oxytocin labelled with tritium through its leucine residue. These showed, for example, that the radioactivity excreted in urine after injection of the labelled oxytocin comprised oxytocin itself and two metabolic products that contained the label, which were not identified. Otherwise, present knowledge of the fate of neurohypophysial hormones has been gained by determination of the residual biological activity either after incubation of the hormones with tissue homogenates, cell fractions or slices *in vitro* or in body fluids or tissue extracts after injection of the hormone *in vivo*.

The capability to inactive oxytocin and vasopressin rapidly *in vitro* has been demonstrated with homogenates of kidney (DICKER and GREENBAUM, 1956; HELLER and ZAIDI, 1957; CHAUDHURY and WALKER, 1959) liver (HELLER and URBAN, 1935; BIRNIE, 1953) spleen, duodenum (CHRISTLIEB, 1940), brain (HOOPER, 1962), placenta (WERLE and MAIER, 1954; HAWKER, 1956), mammary gland (WERLE and MAIER, 1954) and myometrium from pregnant and pseudo-pregnant (SAWYER, 1954) and non-pregnant rats (AUDRIAN and CLAUSER, 1960). Inactivation by skeletal muscle homogenates is slow (SAWYER, 1954). However, the occurrence of an enzyme system which inactivates neurohypophysial peptides in a disorganised homogenate does not necessarily indicate that the tissue is involved in the metabolism of the hormones. For example, proteases of the alimentary tract inactivate oxytocin and vasopressin in accordance with their known specificities but they are not concerned in the metabolism of the hormones *in vivo*. In simple homogenates tissue barriers to the permeation of the hormones are removed and these as SMITH (1962) has shown, are important factors limiting the rate of inactivation of vasopressin in rat kidney slices. In interpreting results obtained with homogenates the possibility must be born in mind that enzymes may have been activated after disruption of the cell or subcellular particles and these may have no bearing on similar activities in the intact cell (HELLER, 1957; SMITH and SACHS, 1961).

After intravenous injection of neurohypophysial hormones, the biological activity disappears very rapidly from the circulation as first shown by HELLER and URBAN (1935) for the antidiuretic activity and by JONES and SCHLAPP (1936) for the pressor and oxytocic activities of posterior pituitary extract. Measurement of the rates at which the hormones disappear from the circulation has proved to be one of the more powerful methods for investigating the problem of the fate of neurohypophysial hormones. Two experimental situations have been used: after a single intravenous injection of the hormone (or the cessation of constant infusion of hormone) and during the steady state reached by constant intravenous infusion.

In the former case the following equations apply:

$$P = P_0 e^{-C/_V t} \text{ and } \ln (P/P_0) = -\frac{C}{V} t$$

where P = plasma concentration of hormone at time t after injection or cessation of infusion, P_0 = plasma concentrations of hormone at t_0 (time of injection or cessation of infusion), V = the virtual distribution space of the hormone, C = total clearance (= volume of distribution space of hormone cleared of hormone in unit time).

Where the relationship between t and P can be shown to follow an exponential course C is constant and the value of V can be obtained by extrapolation of the semi-logarithmic plot of plasma concentration against time to t_0. Thus, C can be obtained if P and P_0 are known. In some respects the ratio $\frac{C}{V}$, the fractional clearance, is preferable because consideration of the magnitude of V is not involved.

Alternatively these results can be expressed as half-lives given by $\log_e \frac{2V}{C}$.

The assumption of a single exponential function is not necessary and the overall clearance can be the resultant of several rate processes. Where it has been possible to follow the disappearance from the circulation over a wide range of plasma concentration it is clear that more than one exponential function is involved. For example, in man, Schroder and Rott (1959) find antidiuretic hormone concentrations in plasma withdrawn later than 30 min after injection of vasopressin deviate from the single exponential function established during the period immediately preceded by the injection of vasopressin: and in the disappearance of radioactivity from the circulation in human subjects given ^{131}I labelled arginine vasopressin two exponential functions could be discerned (Silver et al., 1961). More recently it has been shown in rats, dogs and man (Czaczkes and Kleeman, 1964) that the rate constant depends to some extent on the plasma concentration, the clearance being *slower* at *lower* plasma concentrations.

With vasopressin, most investigators have reached the conclusion that the virtual distribution space in humans, rats and dogs is, at the first approximation, equal to the plasma volume (Ginsburg and Heller, 1953b; Lauson and Bocanegra, 1961; Czaczkes and Kleeman, 1964; Smith and Thorn, 1965). This conclusion is based on constant infusion experiments and on the evidence from single injection experiments that the extrapolated concentration of vasopressin at t_o is approximately equivalent to that obtained by dilution of the amount injected in the plasma volume. Perhaps more convincingly, Czaczkes and Kleeman (1964) showed that the ratio of concentration of antidiuretic activity in blood plasma and lymph withdrawn simultaneously was greater than 200. On the other hand, Share (1962) concluded that the distribution space of vasopressin was appreciably greater than the plasma volume on the basis of the extrapolated concentration at t_o. Further evidence for virtual restriction of vasopressin within the confines of the vascular compartment in rats is given by the good agreement of estimates of C when these have been obtained by single injections or continuous infusion methods (Ginsburg, 1957); since the latter does not require the assumption of a value for V (see p. 339) it follows that assumptions required in the former method are not seriously in error. The binding of vasopressin to plasma proteins (which is inhibited by Ca) is possibly important for the containment of vasopressin in the circulation in rats; Smith and Thorn (1965) have shown in hypercalcaemic rats that the apparent volume distribution of arginine vasopressin obtained by extrapolation to t_o is three times greater than in control animals, in which it is approximately equal to the plasma volume. Another major factor is the efficiency of the preferential removal of vasopressin from the circulation by liver and kidney; the diffusion into extravascular spaces being so much slower, substantial error will not be introduced by ignoring it. On the other hand, penetration of oxytocin into extravascular compartments in the rat (Ginsburg and Smith, 1959) is of sufficient magnitude to invalidate calculations which require the assumption of the plasma volume as the volume of distribution. After an intravenous injection of oxytocin in rats deprived of organs for preferential uptake of the hormone, oxytocic activity of plasma falls rapidly during the first 8—10 min after injection; thereafter a steady state is established at a concentration of oxytocin corresponding to a volume of distribution equal to about 40% of the total body water. Observations of the distribution of radioactivity after the injection of tritium labelled oxytocin are consistent with these findings. Aroskar et al. (1964) in their experiments with tritium labelled oxytocin found that radioactivity in skeletal muscle and in cerebral cortex indicating generalised penetration of oxytocin and/or its metabolites into extravascular spaces.

In the single injection method the extrapolate of plasma concentration to t_0 can be used to obtain a value for V only if the equilibration of the injected hormone in its volume of distribution is sufficiently rapid to be considered practically instantaneous. This clearly is not so, even where penetration beyond the plasma volume is negligible, though errors due to inadequate mixing may be offset by careful choice of the conditions of the timing of the injection. Precautions of this kind are probably of no avail when applied to oxytocin, where equilibration in the ultimate volume of distribution even in steady state conditions in rats, is probably not nearly complete until at least 20 min after intravenous injection (GINSBURG and SMITH, 1959) and if, as in some investigations the blood samples are taken from a vein rather than an artery, the diffusion of oxytocin into the extravascular compartment in the vascular bed drained by the vein will bias the results. However, it should be recalled that in response to suckling stimuli and in labour, oxytocin is released in spurts (FITZPATRICK, 1961; FOLLEY and KNAGGS, 1965, 1966) that would be simulated by quick injections, and if the aim of the investigations is to discover how long the target organ could be under the influence of released endogenous hormone the theoretical objections must be set aside (KNAGGS, 1967).

In the alternative method of assessing clearance rates, the hormone is infused continuously (at a rate I) and the change in plasma concentration is defined by the differential equation: —

$$\frac{VdP}{d\,t} = I - CP;$$

when a steady state supervenes $\frac{dP}{d\,t} = O$ and thus

$$C = \frac{I}{P} \text{ (Lauson, 1960).}$$

This gives a value for C (in terms of proportion of distribution space cleared of hormone in unit time) without requiring any assumptions about the magnitude of distribution space. GINSBURG (1957) using the constant infusion method in rats obtained a mean value of 3.4 ml plasma/100 g/min which compared well with 2.7 ml plasma/100 g/min in single injection experiments in which the range of plasma concentration was approximately the same (0.2—3.2 mU/ml). The mean value for C calculated from the data of the constant infusion experiments of CZACZKES and KLEEMAN (1964) is 1.02 ml/min compared with 1.03 ml/min from single injection experiments at the same plasma levels (around 2.0 μU/ml) and the comparison with the earlier results of GINSBURG (1957) brings out the point that clearance is reduced at lower plasma concentrations. Values of C for dogs calculated from constant infusion experiments of CZACZKES and KLEEMAN (1964) also show the direct proportionality between plasma concentration and volume cleared.

Attempts have been made to obtain estimates for some of the clearance parameters by analysis of the onset and offset of antidiuretic and oxytocic responses after injection or infusion of neurohypophysial hormones (CALDEYRO-BARCIA, SICA-BLANCO, POSEIRO, GONZALEZ-PANIZZA, MENDEZ-BAUER, FIELITZ, ALVAREZ, POSE, and HENDRICKS, 1957; LAUSON, 1960). This involves the assumption that the magnitude of the responses at each instant reflects in an unvarying way, the concentration of hormone in the arterial plasma (LAUSON, 1960). It is clear, however, that this assumption is not valid. For example, antidiuresis in a rat usually is not maximal until 1—2 min after intravenous injection of vasopressin and the response continues at near maximum intensity for several minutes; in the interval between injection and the beginning of the offset of the response, the vasopressin concentration in plasma would have fallen by more than an order of magnitude.

Furthermore, the duration of the antidiuretic action of lysine vasopressin in rats is much shorter than that of arginine vasopressin (SAWYER, CHAN, and VAN DYKE, 1962) and yet the half life in the circulation of the former is greater than that for the latter hormone (GINSBURG, 1960; SAWYER, 1963). This shows clearly that the duration of the antidiuretic response is determined by some intra-renal process in addition to the concentration of hormone in blood. BURN and GREWAL (1951) attempted a mathematical description of the relationship between onset and duration and offset of antidiuretic responses with the dose of vasopressin in man. The lag to onset is inversely related to dose and they assumed that it represents the time required for the kidney to take up from the circulating blood sufficient vasopressin to evoke a detectable change in urine flow.

Table 1. *Estimates of half life for neurohypophysial hormones and some of their analogues*

Peptide	Species	Plasma concentration (mU/μl)	½-life (min)	Reference
Oxytocin	rat		1.65	GINSBURG and SMITH (1959)
	rabbit		3.3	CHAUDHURY and WALKER (1959)
	cat		8.5	JONES and SCHLAPP (1936)
	man		2.7	GONZALEZ-PANIZZA et al. (1961)
Arginine⁸-vasopressin	rat	0.2—6	0.85	GINSBURG and HELLER (1953b)
	rat	3—6	0.7	GINSBURG (1957)
	rat	0.05—3	1.1	GINSBURG (1960)
	rat	not given	0.9	SAWYER (1963)
	rat	0.008—0.05	1.5	CZACZKES and KLEEMAN (1964)
	rat	0.002—0.008	2.0	CZACZKES and KLEEMAN (1964)
	rat	0.0015—0.004	3.4	CZACZKES and KLEEMAN (1964)
	dog	0.01—2	5.4	LAUSON and BOCANEGRA (1961)
	dog	0.19	5.0	SHARE (1962)
	dog	0.01—0.04	5.0	CZACZKES and KLEEMAN (1964)
	dog	0.0004—0.01	7.5	CZACZKES and KLEEMAN (1964)
	dog*		5.0	SILVER et al. (1961)
	rhesus monkey		3.4	CHAUDHURY et al. (1961)
	man		7.8	SCHRÖDER and ROTT (1959)
	man*		4.2	SILVER et al. (1961)
	man**		10—13	CZACZKES and KLEEMAN (1964)
	man***		40	CZACZKES, KLEEMAN, KOENIG (1964)
Lys⁸-vasopressin	rat		1.7	GINSBURG (1960)
	rat		1.9	SAWYER (1963)
Phe³-oxyt.	rat		1.3	SMITH and GINSBURG (1961)
Val³-oxyt.	rat		3.7	SMITH and GINSBURG (1961)

Footnotes: * tritiated arginine-vasopressin
** normal dehydrated, or d. insipidus
*** normal overhydrated

Table 1 shows some of the published estimates of half life for neurohypophysial hormones and some of their analogues, obtained by assay of the activity in blood. There are two difficulties that lie in the way of facile comparison of the values given. Firstly, in some early experiments commercial preparation of vasopressin might have come from either bovine or porcine posterior pituitaries and thus may have contained arginine^8-vasopressin or lysine^8-vasopressin or a mixture of both. The half life for lysine-vasopressin in rats is $1^1/_2$—2 times longer than that for arginine vasopressin (GINSBURG, 1960; SAWYER, 1963); since the values obtained with arginine vasopressin agree well with those observed in work using vasopressin of uncertain composition (GINSBURG and HELLER, 1953b; GINSBURG, 1957) it seems likely that, in fact, the preparations used consisted of arginine vasopressin mainly. The second difficulty arises from the suggestion that the clearance rate of vasopressin varies with plasma concentration (there is no evidence so far for a similar dependence of the clearance on plasma concentration for any other neurohypophysial peptide) and where appropriate the range of vasopressin plasma concentration is given. CZACZKES and KLEEMAN (1964) suggest that the enhanced clearance of vasopressin at higher plasma concentrations might be due to an inductive effect on the enzyme systems involved in hormone inactivation. It is difficult to accept this suggestion because the lines on the semi-logarithmic plot of plasma concentration against time fit the points at zero time so that the "induction" would have to be effective instantaneously (Fig. 24). The finding cannot be due to the saturation of a "fast" transfer process at high plasma concentrations or the inhibitory effect of a vasopressin metabolite because the clearance rate at low plasma levels does not depend on whether or not they are at the tail-end of an experiment in which a relatively large dose of vasopressin was given. For the same reason, re-entry into the circulation of vasopressin from a small extravascular pool, established at high plasma concentration, is probably excluded.

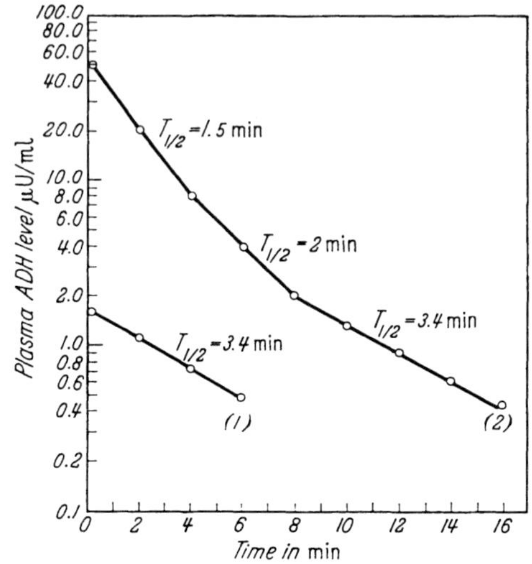

Fig. 24. Disappearance of arginine vasopressin from the plasma of rats after intravenous injection. 1. 5 μU injected, 2. 150 μU injected. Reproduced with permission from CZACZKES and KLEEMAN. J. clin. Invest. **43**, 1641 (1964)

It may be that changes in the distribution of blood flow within the kidney brought about by vasopressin (KRAMER, THURAU, and DEETJEN, 1960; FOURMAN and KENNEDY, 1966) might have an important influence on the clearance of the hormone in that organ. It is possible also that the slowing of clearance at very low plasma concentrations may not be as significant as the results suggest, because it could be influenced by very small amounts of endogenous vasopressin secretion. CZACZKES, KLEEMAN, and KOENIG (1964) suggest also that the clearance of vasopressin in normal man might also be affected by the state of body hydration. The half life of arginine vasopressin in plasma ranged from 10 min after 3 days of water deprivation to 40 min after 3 days of sustained overhydration.

24. Sites of Preferential Uptake from the Circulation

In intact animals, the clearance of the peptides is the resultant of the rate of equilibration within the distribution space and the preferential uptake by specific organs of the body. The experiments of GINSBURG and HELLER (1953c) in which the effect of removal or partial isolation from the circulation of kidneys and organs of the splanchnic vascular area on the vasopressin clearance rates in rats showed these to be the main sites of preferential uptake from the circulation (Fig. 25). The disappearance of antidiuretic activity from the circulation in acutely nephrectomised animals in which the mesenteric and hepatic arteries were tied was so slow as to be accounted for by the residual blood flow through the liver via haemorrhoidal-portal anastomases, without involving any other organ or tissue.

In experiments on similar lines by GINSBURG and SMITH (1959) with oxytocin (except that the portal vein also was tied) the clearance of oxytocin continued at a rate only about half that in intact animals during the first seven minutes after injection (Fig. 26). Thereafter the concentration of oxytocin in plasma was more or less constant

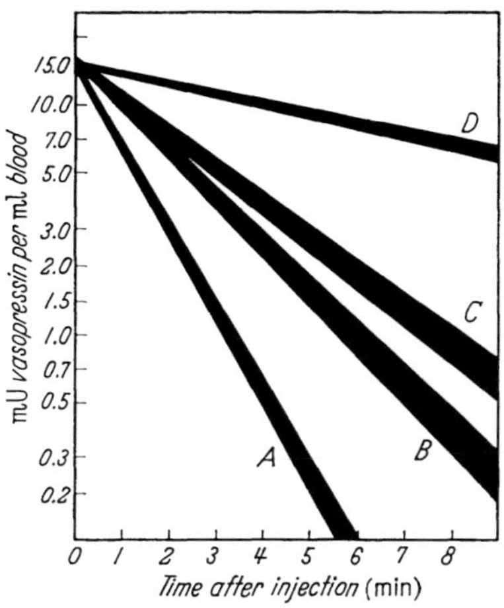

Fig. 25. Disappearance of vasopressin from the circulation following the intravenous injection of 100 mU/100 g in anaesthetised rats. A, intact rats, B, rats with coeliac and mesenteric arteries tied; C, nephrectomised rats; D, nephrectomised rats with coeliac and mesenteric arteries tied. Reproduced with permission from GINSBURG and HELLER. J. Endocr. 9, 283—291 (1953b)

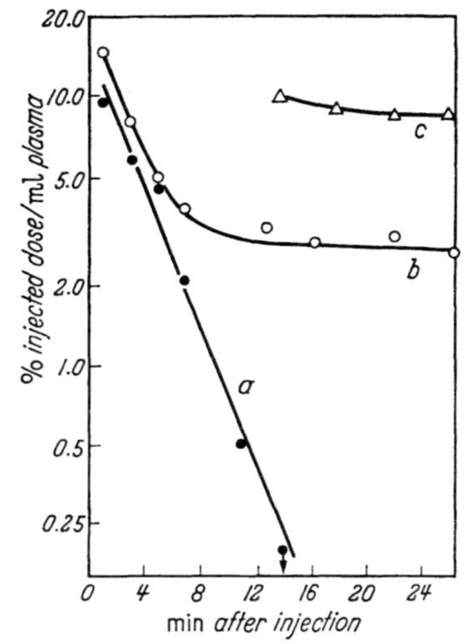

Fig. 26. Concentrations of oxytocin in arterial plasma following intravenous injection of 200 mU/100 g oxytocin in male rats. A, nephrectomised rats; B, nephrectomised rats without splanchnic circulation; C, concentration of inulin in arterial blood of rats as in B after intravenous injection of 40 μg inulin/100 g. Reproduced with permission from GINSBURG and SMITH. Brit. J. Pharmacol. 14, 327 (1959)

for the remaining period of observation (20 min) thus showing that after removal of the kidneys and the exclusion of the circulation from the splanchnic vascular area in male and non-lactating female rats no organ or tissue remained in which substantial amounts of oxytocin were removed preferentially from the circulation and rapidly destroyed or inactivated. It was suggested that the fall in plasma oxytocin concentration in the first 7 min was due to equilibration of oxytocin into a distribution space which is intermediate in size between total body water and extracellular fluid volume. If, however, the experiments were repeated in lactating rats the clearance of oxytocin continued without inflexion of the semi-logarithmic plot showing that these animals possessed a subsidiary site of oxytocin clearance, presumably the actively lactating mammary gland. Small amounts of oxytocin are found in milk of goats and cows after injection of large amounts of oxytocin (NODDLE, 1962). Investigations using tritiated oxytocin (AROSKAR et al., 1964) are essentially in agreement with the results of the experiments in which disappearance of oxytocic activity from the circulation was followed. 20 min after intravenous injection of oxytocin the concentrations of radioactivity in kidney, liver, adrenal and pituitary were higher than in blood; taking into account the relative bulk of these organs it is clear that the liver and kidney make the greater contributions to oxytocin clearance. Other organs (including skeletal muscle) contained some radioactivity but usually not in significantly higher concentration than in blood, giving confirmation of the widespread penetration of oxytocin in body water. In contrast LAUSON (1960) states that muscle removes little or no vasopressin from the circulation in dogs, which is accord with the generally agreed conclusion that vasopressin does not penetrate rapidly into the extravascular compartments in general.

The main sites of uptake of the synthetic oxytocin analogues, phenylalanine^3- and valine^3-oxytocin also are in the kidneys and organs of splanchnic vascular area but the clearance of the valine analogue is very much slower than that of oxytocin or the phenylalanine derivative (SMITH and GINSBURG, 1961). This is due not only to slower uptake by the kidney and liver but also to slower penetration into extravascular spaces. It is remarkable that the process that determines the transfer of these peptides from the circulation, whether it is a protein binding phenomenon or the surmounting of a permeability barrier, should be sufficiently specific to distinguish between oxytocin and its valine^3-analogue which differ from each other only by a single methylene group in a side-chain.

25. Clearance by the Kidneys

It has long been known that after injection of vasopressin or of undifferentiated posterior pituitary extract, antidiuretic activity is found in urine.

After a single injection of vasopressin in rats, about 5—10% of the amount injected is excreted in urine (GINSBURG and HELLER, 1953b; HELLER and ZAIDI, 1957; SMITH and THORN, 1965) and that the bulk of it is excreted within the first 3 min (HELLER and ZAIDI, 1957). This is not surprising because of the speed with which the concentration of vasopressin in blood falls. However, it does suggest that the vasopressin appearing in urine largely represents a fraction that is not concerned in the antidiuretic response of the kidney, which with the high doses used by HELLER and ZAIDI (1957) would persist for a considerable period. The same point is made, more strikingly in an experiment of AROSKAR et al. (1964) with labelled oxytocin in which it is clear that the bulk of the oxytocin excreted is found in urine even before the prolonged antidiuresis starts.

During continuous intravenous infusion of large amounts of vasopressin in water-loaded rats the rate of urinary excretion might amount to more than 30% of the infusion rate (GINSBURG, 1957). In hydrated dogs, THORN and SMITH (1965) report that about 12% of the amount of vasopressin in a single intravenous injection appears in the urine and that this value is independent of the amount injected (within the range 4—50 mU/kg). O'CONNOR (1950) infused vasopressin into conscious water-loaded dogs and also found that the urinary excretion rate was about 12% of the infusion rate and was independent of the amount infused (0.3 to 2.5 mU/min). On the other hand, LAUSON, BOCANEGRA, and BEUZEVILLE (1965) found that anaesthetised, non-hydrated dogs, infused with large amounts of vasopressin (371—511 mU/min) excreted antidiuretic activity at rates between 25% and 50% of the infusion rate and similar results have been reported by HARVEY, JONES, and LEE (1967). Urinary excretion of oxytocic activity after injection of oxytocin also occurs (DALE, 1909; LAUSON, 1935; GONZALEZ-PANIZZA et al., 1961; AROSKAR et al., 1964) but no extensive quantitative studies have been carried out.

The evidence for the suggestion that the antidiuretic activity found in urine after the injection of vasopressin is not vasopressin but a biologically active metabolic product from the peptide (DICKER and GREENBAUM, 1956) cannot be sustained (GINSBURG, HELLER, and ZAIDI, 1956). Many of the properties of vasopressin have been demonstrated in the urinary antidiuretic substance e.g. it is inactivated by thioglycollate, trypsin and carboxypeptidase, it is resistant to treatment with pepsin and carboxypeptidase (AMES, MOORE, and VAN DYKE, 1950; THORN, 1959) and the activity in human urine is indistinguishable from arginine vasopressin in the time course and dose regression of the antidiuretic response and in its chromatographic properties (MAYER, 1960). TOWBIN and FERRELL (1963) also report good agreement between antidiuretic activity and radioactivity in their experiments on renal excretion of tritiated vasopressin in dogs suggesting not only that the active substance in urine is indeed vasopressin but also that biologically active metabolites are not excreted to a significant extent. That is not to say that the antidiuretic activity as it occurs in urine is vasopressin in the free state; evidence for the binding of vasopressin by a macromolecule in urine has been discussed previously (see p. 338).

The contribution by the kidneys to the overall clearance of vasopressin has been estimated by the difference between intact and nephrectomised rats in the rate of disappearance of antidiuretic activity after intravenous injection of a single large dose of vasopressin (GINSBURG and HELLER, 1953b) (Fig. 25). It was concluded that more than 50% of the total clearance was attributable to the kidneys. This estimate was confirmed by DICKER (1954) who measured the persistence of antidiuretic activity in the circulation after cessation of sustained infusion of vasopressin in intact and nephrectomised rats. In experiments similar to those of GINSBURG and HELLER (1953b), but with smaller doses of vasopressin, CRAWFORD and PINKHAM (1954) found a somewhat greater retardation of vasopressin clearance in nephrectomised animals, suggesting that more than 70% of the amount injected was cleared by the kidneys. Under the conditions of these experiments (anaesthetised rats given large doses of vasopressin) the estimates for the volume of plasma cleared of vasopressin by the kidneys in unit time is of the same order ($>$ 70%) of the renal plasma flow indicating very efficient extraction of vasopressin in the kidneys. Since vasopressin removed from the blood by the kidneys exceeds the amount excreted in urine in rats, it would appear that the greater part of vasopressin in the kidneys is inactivated or fixed in renal cells. HELLER and ZAIDI (1957) estimated antidiuretic activity in extracts of kidney from rats that had been killed at short time intervals after the intravenous injection of a large doses of vasopressin. Three min after injection about $^1/_9$th of the amount that would have been taken up by the kidneys was in urine (in bladder and ureters plus renal pelves) while the antidiuretic activity of the kidneys themselves was equivalent to less than $^1/_{100}$th of the amount that would have been cleared from the renal arterial blood. SAWYER (1963) infused vasopressin into rats and estimated the rate of plasma clearance that accounted for the antidiuretic activity appearing in the urine, i.e. the urinary clearance, taking no account of vasopressin inactivation in the kidneys. The urinary clearance of arginine vasopressin represents only $^1/_7$th of the total clearance while that of lysine vasopressin accounts for $^1/_3$rd of the total clearance. Thus the longer half-life of lysine vasopressin is not attributable to a lower rate of excretion in urine but to slower inactivation in the kidneys and possibly other organs. With kidney slice preparations *in vitro*, SMITH (1962) has shown that lysine vasopressin is inactivated more slowly than arginine vasopressin.

The observation that the urinary clearance of vasopressin in rats exceeded the inulin clearance by about 25% led to the suggestion (GINSBURG, 1957) that some of the vasopressin excreted in urine might have been transported by a tubular secretory mechanism. The extent to which urinary clearance of vasopressin exceeded the glomerular filtration rate is rather small and may not be beyond the limits of experimental error; indeed, SAWYER (1963) finds that the urinary clearance of arginine vasopressin in rats is 15% less than the inulin clearance. This does not exclude the involvement tubular processes — the approximate correspondence of urinary clearance and GFR could be fortuitous.

In these calculations it is assumed that all vasopressin in plasma is freely filterable at the glomerulus although there is abundant, though contradictory evidence that this is not so (see p. 336). Furthermore, vasopressin in urine may represent only a proportion of the amount cleared by the kidneys, the remainder being inactivated in renal tissue.

In dogs the process of renal extraction of vasopressin appears to be less efficient than in rats but it is not clear whether the quantitative difference is a reflection of a qualitative difference in the renal handling of vasopressin in the two species. Estimates of the renal extraction of vasopressin in dogs have been obtained by LAUSON, BOCANEGRA, and BEUZEVILLE (1965) and by HARVEY, JONES, and LEE (1967). Comparison of the antidiuretic effects in the right kidney of short infusions of vasopressin given either via a peripheral vein and via the left renal artery was used to estimate renal extraction of vasopressin in conscious dogs, at "physiological" concentration of vasopressin; under these conditions the renal extraction was 25% and thus the renal clearance was approximately equal to the glomerular filtration rate (LAUSON et al., 1965). In experiments in which the antidiuretic activity was measured in urine and in plasma from renal vein and arterial blood of anaesthetised dogs during sustained infusion of vasopressin at high rates, it was found that 20% of the vasopressin in renal arterial blood is extracted during a passage through the kidney, which is equivalent to about 60% of the glomerular filtration rate (LAUSON et al., 1965). Since the mean *urinary* clearance was of approximately the same order as the *renal* clearance, LAUSON et al. (1965) concluded that in the non-hydrated anaesthetised dogs virtually all the vasopressin extracted from the blood by the kidneys was excreted unchanged. However, the variability of these results and the fact that in 3 out of 5 animals the urinary clearance quite substantially exceeded the renal clearance (urinary C/renal C = 1.5, 1.7 and 2.6) makes this conclusion doubtful. On ther other hand, they suggest that in water-loaded animals only $^1/_4$ of the vasopressin extracted by the kidneys is excreted, the remainder being inactivated. The constancy of the proportion of vasopressin excreted in urine of dogs injected with doses of vasopressin ranging from 4—50 mU/kg (THORN and SMITH, 1965) has ben interpreted as showing that antidiuretic hormone in the dog is excreted mainly by glomerular filtration. However, as these authors point out, this conclusion would follow from their observations only if it is assumed that the range of doses of vasopressin used covered the conditions of both saturation and unsaturation of a hypothetical tubular process.

In contrast, HARVEY et al. (1967) in similar experiments also in anaesthetised non-hydrated dogs, but at much lower concentrations of vasopressin, found that the amount of vasopressin in urine was always less than the amount extracted. Apart from a single experiment, the urinary clearance exceeded the amount that could be filtered even assuming that all the vasopressin in plasma was free. They suggest that the urinary clearance of vasopressin is determined by a combination of glomerular filtration, tubular extraction and secretion, and inactivation. In their view, the hormone that passes into the nephron via the glomerulus is excreted unchanged without reabsorption, but that at low plasma concentration the amount filtered may be low because of binding by plasma protein.

I^{131}-labelled vasopressin is taken up by tubular cells particularly in the distal convolutions and the collecting ducts (DARMADY, DURANDT, MATTHEWS, and STRANNACH, 1960), and inactivation of vasopressin occurs in the "tubular" fraction, rather than the "glomerular" fraction (HELLER and ZAIDI, 1957). HARVEY et al. (1967) suggest therefore that vasopressin is taken up via the non-luminal surface of the tubular cells, where it both exerts its effect and is inactivated; a similar conclusion was reached by SKADHAUGE (1964). The experiments of LAUSON et al. (1965) in anaesthetised non-hydrated dogs were carried out after a 3 h period of sustained infusion of vasopressin at very high rates (371—511 mU/min i.e. the dogs received about 80 units of vasopressin) and it is conceivable that receptor sites were saturated.

One form of fixation of vasopressin in renal cells seems to involve an -SH protein. Treatment of hypophysectomised rats with vasopressin causes a reduction in the titrable protein-bound SH groups in the convoluted portions of the proximal and distal tubules (CAFRUNY, CARHART, and FARAH, 1957). FONG, SILVER, CHRISTMAN, and SCHWARZ (1960) attributed this effect, at least as far as the distal tubules are concerned, to the formation of disulphide bridges which they considered to be the bond between hormone and active receptor.

This conclusion must now be regarded as doubtful in view of the biological activity of desthio derivatives of vasopressin. It may well be valid in a modified form, because experiments of ZEDECK, MELLETT, and CAFRUNY (1966) have shown that alkylating agents block the antidiuretic action of vasopressin, an effect they consider could be due to alkylation of SH groups of a receptor. Recent experiments have shown that extracts of porcine and guinea pig kidney contain protein similar to neurohypophysial neurophysin (GINSBURG and JAYASENA, 1967) which although it binds lysine vasopressin does not form complexes with oxytocin. The kidney protein cannot be distinguished from the neurohypophysial protein chromatographically or immunochemically and apparently has the same binding characteristics, the complex formation being inhibited in the presence of low concentration of Ca and no binding of desamino analogues of vasopressin can be demonstrated. Since these analogues are nevertheless very potent antidiuretic agents, it follows that the protein cannot be regarded as an active receptor system, though it may play a role as an "uptake" or "silent" receptor.

Calcium is implicated in many aspects of the action of vasopressin on its target organ. The action of vasopressin of increasing water permeability of cell membranes of the toad bladder (BENTLEY, 1959; PETERSEN and EDELMAN, 1964) and in the kidney of *Necturus* (WHITTEMBURY, SUGINO, and SOLOMON, 1960) is diminished by raising the concentration of Ca: hypercalcaemia lowers the capacity of the kidneys to reabsorb free water in dogs (BECK, LEVITIN, and EPSTEIN, 1959) and causes polyuria in man (LEVITT, HALPERN, POLINEROS, SWEET, and GRIBETZ, 1958) and monkeys (FREEDMAN, MOULTON, and SPENCER, 1958). Also inactivation of vasopressin by kidney slices is prevented by Ca (SMITH, 1963; THORN and WILLUMSEN, 1963) and the antidiuretic action of vasopressin is accompanied by an increase in the urinary output of Ca (THORN, 1961; DICKER and EGGLETON, 1961; NIELSEN, 1964). The correlation of these interactions between Ca and vasopressin in the kidney is obscure but there is the fascinating possibility that one or more of them might involve the inhibition by Ca of binding of vasopressin to kidney neurophysin — the target organ thus exhibiting the same reaction that might occur when the hormones are released from the neurohypophysis (see p. 306). Hypercalcaemia also increases the proportion of a dose vasopressin that is excreted in urine (SMITH and THORN, 1965). It is not clear whether this is due to an effect of Ca on the kidney or whether it is a result of the inhibition of Ca binding to plasma protein and hence more extensive penetration of vasopressin into body fluid compartments and longer persistance in the blood.

26. Clearance by the Liver

The clearance of antidiuretic activity from the circulation of anaesthetised rats injected with a large dose of vasopressin is reduced in animals in which the coeliac and mesenteric arteries are tied (GINSBURG and HELLER, 1953b). No clearance of vasopressin could be demonstrated in the mesenteric circulation in experiments in which a large dose of vasopressin was injected into the superior mesenteric artery and the antidiuretic activity in portal vein blood was estimated (GINSBURG, 1957). This seems to be true also for endogenous antidiuretic hormone at lower plasma concentrations, there being no difference in the vasopressin concentrations in arterial and portal plasmas (GINSBURG, 1957).

From the extent of the reduction of the clearance of vasopressin when the mesenteric circulation was occluded it was suggested that the extraction of vasopressin by the liver was very efficient and that under the conditions of these experiments, the hepatic contribution to vasopressin clearance was only slightly less than the contribution of the kidneys (GINSBURG and HELLER, 1953b). Other evidence in general agreement with this is that antidiuretic effects of vasopressin injected into the spleen in rats and rabbits are smaller than after intramuscular or subcutaneous injection (EVERSOLE, BIRNIE, and GAUNT, 1949; MOLLER-CHRISTENSON, 1951) and pressor responses to intraportal injection of vasopressin in rats are matched by less than half the dose given intravenously (GINSBURG, 1957; SCHNIEDEN, 1962). In contrast, the hepatic clearance of much smaller doses of vasopressin (50 or 100 μU) estimated by the comparison of antidiuretic effects from intraportal and intravenous injections, suggests a very small hepatic extraction ratio (BEUZEVILLE and LAUSON, 1964; LAUSON, 1965) perhaps no greater than 10 or 15%.

It is suggested that the essential difference between these experiments and the others quoted above lies in the plasma concentration of vasopressin, at low plasma concentration the hepatic extraction ratio being less than at high plasma concentration of vasopressin. This falls in line with the observations of CZACZKES and KLEEMAN (1964) that the total clearance also is greater at high plasma concentrations. These conclusions have been confirmed in studies of antidiuretic hormone inactivation by isolated perfused rat liver (LITTLE, KLEVAY, RADFORD, and McGANDY, 1966). The extraction ratio in single passage experiments ranged from 0.24 at concentrations of 15—25 μU/ml plasma to 0.63 at 1,000—5,000 μU/ml. It is suggested that the mechanism whereby the hepatic extraction of vasopressin increases at high plasma concentrations could involve an alteration in the distribution of hepatic blood flow; if vasopressin constricted blood vessels in a route that by-passed inactivating sites, the total hepatic clearance would be enhanced with higher doses. Acute haemorrhage is possibly the only circumstance known in which the concentration of endogenous vasopressin rises to levels where the hepatic clearance of vasopressin is enhanced. USAMI and CHIEN (1963) investigated the effect of haemorrhage on the hepatic clearance of vasopressin by comparison of the antidiuretic activities of plasma from hepatic vein and femoral artery blood. The hepatic extraction ratio was found to be in the range 0.21—0.24 and was not dependent on the extent of the haemorrhage (11—41% of blood volume). In fact, there was a fall in the contribution of the liver to total clearance of vasopressin arising from the fall in hepatic blood flow after haemorrhage.

The hepatic clearance of vasopressin in dogs also has been estimated by comparison of the antidiuretic responses to vasopressin given via a splenic vein or a peripheral vein (MATHÉ and ALTMAN, 1954; LAUSON, 1953; LAUSON and BOCANEGRA, 1961; LAUSON et al., 1965). In the earlier experiments there was no convincing difference in the antidiuretic responses to the same doses given by the different routes but with very careful studies, LAUSON et al. (1965) conclude that the mean hepatic portal extraction ratio was 15%. The difference between the antidiuretic responses is indeed slight, and it is not to detract from the considerable achievement of its demonstration to say that the mean value must be subject to considerable error. The hepatic extraction of vasopressin in conscious dogs is thus slightly less efficient than renal extraction (25%).

Arrest of the circulation in the splanchnic vascular area also retards the disappearance of oxytocin from the circulation in rats and rabbits (GINSBURG and SMITH, 1959; CHAUDHURY and WALKER, 1959) but the effect is not as pronounced as that of bilateral nephrectomy. Substantial amounts of radioactivity are found in liver after injection of tritiated oxytocin but the concentration is less than in kidney (AROSKAR et al., 1964). MANUNTA and MARONGUI (1961) have shown extraction of oxytocin by the liver in sheep by comparing the effects on intramammary pressure of oxytocin injections given into a jugular vein or the portal vein. A much smaller response was obtained with oxytocin given intraportally and it would appear that only about 20% of the dose given reached the general circulation.

27. Pregnancy Serum Oxytocinase

Inactivation of oxytocin *in vitro* by serum from pregnant women was shown first by VON FEKETE (1930); it was found later that human pregnancy serum also destroyed the pressor (SCHOCKHAERT and LAMBILLON, 1935; WERLE and KALVELAGE, 1941; WOODBURY, AHLQUIST, ABREU, TORPIN, and WATSON, 1964) and antidiuretic (DIECKMANN, EGENOLF, MORLEY, and POTTINGER, 1950) activities of vasopressin. The enzymatic nature of the process was established in 1941 by WERLE and his co-workers and TUPPY and NESVADBA (1957) showed that the enzyme split the pentapeptide ring of oxytocin between cystine and tyrosine thus acting as a cystine aminopeptidase. The structural requirements for substrate are fulfilled also by vasopressin so that the vasopressin-inactivating activity of human pregnancy plasma need not be ascribed to another enzyme. Oxytocinase activity in plasma can be assayed by inactivation of oxytocin or by the hydrolysis of a synthetic substrate L-cystine di-β-naphthylamide and the results with these methods are generally in agreement (MÜLLER-HARTBERG, NESVADBA, and TUPPY, 1959); some discrepancies occur that may be due to the presence of other enzymes in plasma that hydrolyse the synthetic substrate (TUPPY, 1960).

Significant amounts of oxytocinase can be detected in plasma as early as 8 weeks after conception (PAGE, 1946) and the activity increases throughout the course of pregnancy (WERLE, HEVELKE, and BUTHMANN, 1941). Since plasma oxytocinase occurs in pregnancy only in women and some anthropoid apes (CALDEYRO-BARCIA and POSEIRO, 1958) and is absent from plasma of pregnant rats (SAWYER, 1954), rabbits, dogs and rhesus monkeys (DICKER and WHYLEY, 1961) its occurrence is not likely to be of crucial physiological significance. HILTON and JOHNSON (1959) and DICKER and TYLER (1956) reported a sharp decline in plasma oxytocinase activity during the first stage of labour, suggesting that this might be a factor determining the onset of labour. Later investigations failed to substantiate this observation (DICKER and WHYLEY, 1959) and most observers agree that after parturition the concentration of the enzyme in plasma decreases slowly and reaches the non-pregnant level about 3 weeks *post partum*.

The importance of plasma oxytocinase is limited because (a) at the very low substrate concentration provided by the amounts of oxytocin in plasma, the reaction velocity would be infinitesimally small and (b) the efficiency of the clearance of the peptide from the circulation by penetration into extravascular spaces and by preferential uptake by kidneys and liver limits the exposure of the hormone the the enzyme in plasma.

28. Disordered Metabolism of Vasopressin and Disease

The hypothesis that the cause of the disordered water metabolism lay in the impaired metabolism of antidiuretic hormone by the diseased liver (Ralli et al., 1945) followed from the association of water retention in liver disease with the occurrence of antidiuretic activity in the urine (Ralli, Robson, Clarke, and Hoagland, 1945; van Dyke, Ames, and Plough, 1950; Hall, Frame, and Drill, 1949). This hypothesis has not, however, been substantiated by more recent investigations (White, Rubin, and Leiter, 1951, 1953; Bernstein, Weston, Ross, Grossman, Hanenson, and Leiter, 1953; Hanenson, Goluboff, Grossman, Weston, and Leiter, 1956; White, 1958) showing that the duration of the antidiuretic response to administered vasopressin or to endogenous antidiuretic hormone released by nicotine administration in patients with hepatic cirrhosis or congestive heart failure is not longer than in normal subjects. Also it has been shown by Chaudhury, Chuttani, and Ramalingswami (1961) that in monkeys with liver damage induced by protein deficiency and/or carbon tetrachloride, the clearance of vasopressin from the circulation is not lower than in normal animals. Perhaps it is as well to indicate here, that the relationship between the duration of the antidiuretic response and the rate of clearance of vasopressin from the circulation is most likely a complex one in that, although a prolongation of the response in patients with liver disease was not established, it does not necessarily follow that the metabolism of the antidiuretic hormone was undisturbed. The experiments with monkeys, too, are not above criticism, since it has not been shown whether the contribution of the liver to vasopressin clearance is so great that the half-life would be increased by its exclusion.

Schnieden (1962) obtained results, in contrast to those of Chaudhury et al. (1961), showing reduced vasopressin clearance by the liver in rats with nutritional hypoproteinaemia or with liver damage induced by carbon tetrachloride treatment; there was no evidence of the difference seen in normal animals between intravenous and intraportal equipressor doses of vasopressin. *In vitro* studies, too, have produced conflicting results in that reduction of the inactivation of vasopressin by homogenates of livers of rats and mice damaged by carbon tetrachloride or protein deficiency has been demonstrated (Gopalan, 1950; Birnie, Blackmore, and Heller, 1952; Birnie, 1953) while Miller and Townsend (1954) did not find any difference between homogenates of normal and cirrhotic human liver. Thus, indirect evidence for impaired metabolism of vasopressin as a cause of the disordered water balance in liver disease is highly equivocal. The most direct experiments in which the concentrations of vasopressin were estimated in internal jugular blood and in blood from a peripheral vein of patients with ascites due to liver cirrhosis (Lee, 1960; Lee and Kerr, 1963) led to the conclusion that while excess vasopressin might, in some patients, contribute to water retention it was not the primary cause nor even an essential factor.

It has been reported that in some patients with diabetes insipidus the duration of the antidiuretic response to vasopressin is shorter than in normal subjects (Hankiss, Keszthelyi, and Siro, 1961). This observation certainly falls into line with the finding of Czaczkes and Kleeman (1964) that the half-life of vasopressin injected in diabetes insipidus patients is very much shorter than in normal subjects given a water load. However, the suggestion of Hankiss et al. (1961) that the cause of the disorder lies in increased inactivation of the antidiuretic hormone cannot be sustained because the accelerated clearance is associated with a degree of dehydration and can be induced in normal subjects (see Table 1). Also, the hypothesis depends on an unproven assumption of a simple relationship between rate of inactivation and duration of response. The patients responded promptly to administered vasopressin and if their output of antidiuretic hormone was not deficient it is difficult to see how, when fluids were withdrawn, they could have been so severely dehydrated that diabetes insipidus was diagnosed.

The homeostatic mechanism, at least for osmotic control by antidiuretic hormone, is mediated through feed-back from the electrolyte concentration in extracellular fluid and not directly by the concentration of the hormone in blood. It follows therefore that changes in the capacity to inactivate the hormone are unlikely to provoke disorders in water metabolism provided that hormone release mechanisms and target organ function are unimpaired.

29. Inappropriate Secretion of Vasopressin

The first description of a patient with carcinoma of the bronchus associated with hyponatraemia and an usually high rate of sodium excretion was given by WINKLER and CRANKSHAW (1938). Two similar patients were studied by SCHWARZ, BENNETT, CURELOP, and BARTTER (1957) and they noted that despite the expansion of the extracellular fluid volume and the hypotonicity of the plasma, the urine was hypertonic. The parallelism of this situation with that of normal subjects given large doses of vasopressin led to the suggestion that there was, in the patients, inappropriate secretion of vasopressin. Since then the condition has been recognised with increasing frequency and up to the end of 1965 more than 30 cases had been studied and reported (BARRACLOUGH, JONES, and LEE, 1966). Usually the evidence for inappropriate vasopressin secretion has rested on the production of hypertonic urine in the presence of normal glomerular filtration rate and adequate solute excretion. More direct evidence has been provided by the demonstration of increased amounts of antidiuretic activity in urine (ALEXANDER and FILBIN, 1962; THORN and TRANSBOL, 1963; SOUSA, BERDE, and MACH, 1965; RUCH, 1966) and raised concentration of vasopressin in plasma (LEE, JONES, and BARRACLOUGH, 1964; BOWER, MASON, and FORSHAM, 1964; BARRACLOUGH et al., 1966).

The presence of an antidiuretic substance in the tumour was first shown by AMATRUDA, MULROW, GALLAGHER, and SAWYER (1963) and later by LEE et al. (1964) and BOWER et al. (1964). It has been shown by BERDE (1965) that when the material from tumours was subjected to antidiuretic, vasopressor and milk-ejection tests the potency ratios corresponded to those for arginine vasopressin.

The concentration of activity in the tumour is very much higher than in plasma and it is unlikely that the hormone was synthesised in the neurohypophysis and subsequently trapped in the tumour. Indeed, in the patient of BOWER et al. (1964) there was evidence of functional atrophy of the posterior pituitary. It would appear that the tumour cells are endowed with the capacity to synthesise vasopressin and it is of interest that it has shown recently that neoplasms may synthesise a variety of other hormonal substances (LIDDLE, ISLAND, NEY, NICHOLSON, and SHIMIZA, 1963; GREENBERG, DIVERTIE, and WOOLNER, 1964; LIPSETT, ODELL, ROSENBERG, and WALDMANN, 1964). There is no *a priori* reason to assume that the synthetic pathway in the tumour cell is different from that in the neurone of the supra-optico-neurohypophysial system and thus it would involve the formation of a protein precursor and a degradative activating step. On the other hand, release of the hormone from the tumour seems to be unrestrained and unrelated to physiological requirements, exceptionally large amounts of antidiuretic activity being found in urine. It would seem therefore that the mechanism for storage and release of vasopressin is lacking, possibly implying that the tumor cell lacks neurophysin and the equivalent of neurosecretory granules.

References

Abrahams, V. C., G. B. Koelle, and P. Smart: Histochemical demonstrations of cholinesterases in the hypothalamus of the dog. J. Physiol. (Lond.) **139**, 137—144 (1957).

—, and M. Pickford: Simultaneous observations on the rate of urine flow and spontaneous uterine movements in the dog and their relationship to posterior lobe activity. J. Physiol. (Lond.) **126**, 320—346 (1954).

— — Observations on a central antagonism between adrenaline and acetylcholine. J. Physiol. (Lond.) **131**, 712—718 (1956a).

— — The effect of anti-cholinesterases injected into the supraoptic nuclei of chloralosed dogs on the release of the oxytocic factor of the posterior pituitary. J. Physiol. (Lond.) **133**, 330—333 (1956b).

Acher, R.: Etat naturel des principles oxytocique et vasopressique de la neurohypophyse. In: Neurosecretion, 2nd Int. Symposium, pp. 71—78. Ed. by W. Bargmann, G. Hanstrom, and E. Scharrer. Berlin-Heidelberg-New York: Springer 1958.

—, J. Chauvet, et G. Olivry: Sur l'existence eventuelle d'une hormone unique neurohypophysaire. Relation entre l'ocytocine, la vasopressine et la proteine de van Dyke extraites de la neurohypophyse du boeuf. Biochim. biophys. Acta (Amst.) **22**, 421—427 (1956a).

— — — Variations des teneurs en activites ocytocique et vasopressique de la neurohypophyse du rat au cours de la croissance et de la reproduction. Biochim. biophys. Acta (Amst.) **22**, 428—433 (1956b).

—, and C. Fromageot: The relationship of oxytocin and vasopressin to active proteins of posterior pituitary origin. In: The Neurohypophysis. Ed. by H. Heller. London: Butterworths 1957.

Adam, H. M.: Histamine in the central nervous system. In: Regional Neurochemistry. Ed. by S. E. Kety and J. Elkes. London: Pergamon Press 1961.

Adams, W. M., and J. C. Sloper: The hypothalamic elaboration of the posterior pituitary principles in man, the rat and dog. Histochemical evidence derived from performic acid-alcian blue reaction for cystine. J. Endocr. **13**, 221—228 (1956).

Adamsons, K., S. L. Engel, and H. B. van Dyke: Stability of neurohypophysial hormones. Endocrinology **63**, 679—687 (1958).

— — —, B. Schmidt-Nielsen, and K. Schmidt-Nielsen: The distribution of oxytocin and vasopressin (antidiuretic hormone) in the neurohypophysis of the camel. Endocrinology **58**, 272—278 (1956).

Alexander, C. S., and J. F. Downs: Diabetes insipidus complicating pregnancy. Obstet. and Gynec. **10**, 682—683 (1957).

—, and D. M. Filbin: Extraction and bioassay of antidiuretic hormone (ADH) from human urine by a new method. J. Lab. clin. Med. **60**, 855 (1962).

Amatruda, J. J., P. J. Mulrow, J. C. Gallagher, and W. H. Sawyer: Carcinoma of the lung with inappropriate antidiuresis. Demonstration of antidiuretic-hormone-like activity in tumour extract. New Engl. J. Med. **269**, 544—549 (1963).

Ames, R. G., and H. B. van Dyke: Antidiuretic hormone in the serum or plasma of rats. Endocrinology **50**, 350—360 (1952).

— — Antidiuretic hormone in the urine and pituitary of the kangaroo rat. Proc. Soc. exp. Biol. (N.Y.) **75**, 417—420 (1950).

—, D. H. Moore, and H. B. van Dyke: The excretion of posterior pituitary antidiuretic hormone in urine and its detection in blood. Endocrinology **46**, 215—227 (1950).

Amoroso, E. C., R. J. Harrison, L. Harrison-Matthews, I. W. Rowlands, C. H. Bourne, and J. C. Sloper: Cited in Sloper (1958).

Andersson, B.: Some observations on the neuro-humoral regulation of milk-ejection. Acta physiol. scand. **23**, 1—7 (1951).

—, and P. A. Jewell: The effect of long periods of continuous hydration on the neurosecretory material in the hypothalamus. J. Endocr. **15**, 332—338 (1957).

—, and S. Larson: Inhibitory effects of emesis on water diuresis in the dog. Acta physiol. scand. **32**, 19—27 (1954).

Aprahamian, H. A., J. L. Vanderveen, J. P. Bunker, A. J. Murphy, and J. D. Crawford: The influence of general anaesthetics on water and solute excretion in man. Ann. Surg. **150**, 122—130 (1959).

Aroskar, J. P., W. Chan, J. E. Stouffer, C. H. Schneider, V. V. S. Murti, and V. du Vigneaud: Renal secretion and tissue distribution of radioactivity after administration of tritium labelled oxytocin to rats. Endocrinology **14**, 226—232 (1964).

Asdell, S. A.: Patterns of mammalian reproduction. Ithaca, New York: Cornstalk 1946.

Audrian, L., et H. Clauser: Mecanisme de l'inactivation de l'ocytocine par le tissu uterin. Biochim. biophys. Acta (Amst.) **38**, 494—501 (1960).

AUER, J.: Postnatal differentiation in the hypothalamus of the hamster. J. Neurol. (Brux.) **95**, 17—41) 1951).
AUJARD, L., E. CSANYI, et C. LE BRETON: Recherches sur l'activite oxytocique des urines. Arch. Sci. physiol. **9**, 71—82 (1954).
BAISSET, A., et P. MONTASTRUC: Modification de la diurese apres distention de l'orciette gauche. Pathol. Biol. Semaine Hop. **7**, 1691 (1959).
BARATZ, R.A., A. DOIG, and I.J. ADATTO: Plasma antidiuretic activity and free water clearance following osmoreceptor and neurohypophysial stimulation in human subjects. J. clin. Invest. **39**, 1539—1545 (1960).
—, and R.C. INGRAHAM: Renal haemodynamics and antidiuretic hormone release associated with volume regulation. Amer. J. Physiol. **198**, 565—570 (1960).
BARBOUR, A., G.M. BULL, N.C. HUGHES-JONES, B.M. EVANS, and J. LOGOTHETOPOULOS: The effect of breathing 5—7% carbon dioxide on the urine flow and mineral excretion. Clin. Sci. **12**, 1—13 (1953).
BARD, P., and M.B. MACHT: Neurological basis of behaviour. Ciba Foundation Symposium, p. 55 (1958).
BARER, R., H. HELLER, and K. LEDERIS: The isolation, identification and properties of the hormonal granules of the neurohypophysis. Proc. roy. Soc. B **158**, 388—416 (1963).
—, and K. LEDERIS: Ultrastructure of the rabbit neurohypophysis with special reference to the release of the hormones. Z. Zellforsch. **75**, 201—239 (1966).
BARGMANN, W.: Über die neurosekretorische Verknüpfung von Hypothalamus und Neurohypophyse. Z. Zellforsch. **34**, 610—634 (1949).
— Zwischenhirn und Neurohypophyse; eine neue Vorstellung über die funktionelle Bedeutung der Hinterlappen. Med. Mschr. **5**, 466—470 (1951).
— Über das Zwischenhirn-Hypophysensystem von Fischen. Z. Zellforsch. **39**, 275—298 (1953).
—, u. A. KNOOP: Elektronenmikroskopische Beobachtungen an der Neurohypophyse. Z. Zellforsch. **46**, 242—251 (1957).
—, and E. SCHARRER: The site of origin of hormones of the posterior pituitary. Amer. Sci. **39**, 255—259 (1951).
BARNETT, H.L., and J. VESTERDAL: The physiologic and clinical significance of immaturity of kidney function in young infants. J. Pediat. **42**, 99—119 (1953).
BARNETT, R.J.: Histochemical demonstration of disulfide groups in the neurohypophysis under normal and experimental conditions. Endocrinology **55**, 484—501 (1954).
—, and A.M. SELIGMAN: Histochemical demonstrations of protein-bound sulphydryl groups. Science **116**, 323—327 (1952).
BARRACLOUGH, M.A., J.J. JONES, and J. LEE: Production of vasopressin by anaplastic oat cell carcinoma of the bronchus. Clin. Sci. **31**, 135—144 (1966).
BECK, E., and P.M. DANIEL: Degeneration and regeneration in the hypothalamus. In: Cytology of nervous tissue; Proceedings,Anatomical Society, pp. 60—63. London: Taylor and Francis 1961.
—, H. LEVITIN, and F.H. EPSTEIN: Effect of intravenous infusion of calcium on renal concentrating ability. Amer. J. Physiol. **197**, 1118—1120 (1959).
BELESLIN, D., G.W. BISSETT, J. HALDAR, and R.L. POLAK: The release of vasopressin without oxytocin in response to haemorrhage. Proc. roy. Soc. B **166**, 443—458 (1967).
BELLER, F.K., K.H. KRUMHOLZ u. K. ZEININGER: Vergleichende Oxytocin-Bestimmungen, gemessen durch die Lactogenen der Milchdrüse (milk ejection). Acta endocr. (Kbh.) **29**, 1—8 (1958).
BENNETT, M.V.L., and S. FOX: Electrophysiology of the caudal neurosecretory cells in the skate and fluke. Gen. Cong. Endocrinol. **2**, 77—95 (1962).
BENTLEY, P.J.: The effects of ionic changes on water transfer across the isolated urinary bladder of the toad, *Bufo marinus*. J. Endocr. **18**, 327—333 (1959).
BERDE, B.: Les analogues synthetiques des hormones neurohypophysaires. Sont-il une clef de l'etude des troubles de l'hormonogenese de ce systeme. Extrait de les troubles congenitaux de l'hormonogenese. Rapports de la VIIIe reunion des endocrinologistes de langue francaise (1965).
BERN, H.A.: The secretory neurone as a doubly specialised cell. In: The general physiology of cell specialization, pp. 349—366. Ed. by D. MAZIA and A. TYLER. New York: Mc Graw-Hill 1963.
—, R.S. NISHIOKA, and I.R. HAGEDOORN: Association of elementary granules with the Golgi complex. J. Ultrastruct. Res. **5**, 311—320 (1962).
BERNISCHKE, K., and D.B. MCKAY: The antidiuretic hormone in fetus and infant. Obstet. and Gynec. **1**, 638—649 (1953).
BERNSTEIN, S.H., R.E. WESTON, G. ROSS, J. GROSSMAN, I.B. HANENSON, and L. LEITER: Studies in intravenous water diuresis and nicotine and pitressin antidiuresis in normal subjects and patients with liver disease. J. clin. Invest. **32**, 422—427 (1953).

BEUZEVILLE, C.F., and H.D. LAUSON: The question of vasopressin removal by rat liver. Fed. Proc. **23**, 150 (1964).
BILLENSTEIN, D.C., and J.F LEVEQUE: The reorganisation of the neurohypophyseal stalk following hypophysectomy in the rat. Endocrinology **56**, 704—717 (1955).
BIRNIE, J.H.: The inactivation of posterior pituitary antidiuretic activity by liver extracts. Endocrinology **52**, 33—38 (1953).
—, E.K. BLACKMORE, and H. HELLER: Changes in water diuresis and vasopressin inactivation in mice fed on protein deficient diets. Experientia (Basel) **8**, 20 (1952).
BISSETT, G.W., and J.M. WALKER: The effect of hexamethonium on the antidiuretic action of nicotine in the rat. Abstr. Comm. XIX Int. Physiol. Congr. 215 (1953).
— — The effects of nicotine, hexamethonium and ethanol on the secretion of the antidiuretic and oxytocic hormones of the rat. Brit. J. Pharmacol. **12**, 461 (1957).
BLACKMORE, W.P., K.W. ERMIN, O.F. WIEGAND, and R. LIPSEY: Renal and cardiovascular effects of halothane. Anaesthesiology **21**, 489—495 (1960).
BLOCK, R.J., and H.B. VAN DYKE: Amino acids in posterior pituitary protein. Arch. Biochem. **36**, 1—4 (1952).
BLOMBERT, G., J. GERBRANDY, J.A. MOLHUYSEN, L.A. DE VRIES, and J.G.G. BORST: Diuretic effect of isotonic saline solution compared to that of water. Lancet **1951 II** 1011—1015.
BOCANEGRA, M., and H.D. LAUSON: Ultrafiltrability of endogenous antidiuretic hormone from the plasma of dogs. Amer. J. Physiol. **200**, 486—492 (1961).
BODIAN, D.: Nerve endings, neurosecretory substance and lobular organisation of the neurohypophysis. Bull. Johns Hopk. Hosp. **89**, 354—376 (1951).
— Cytological aspects of neurosecretion in opossum neurohypophysis. Bull. Johns Hopk. Hosp. **113**, 57—93 (1963).
BODO, R.C. DE: Antidiuretic action of morphine and its mechanism. J. Pharmacol. **82**, 74—85 (1944).
—, and K.T. PRESCOTT: The antidiuretic action of barbiturates (phenobarbital, amytal, pentobarbital) and the mechanism involved in this action. J. Pharmacol. **85**, 222—233 (1945).
BOISSONNAS, R.A., B. BERDE, and H. KONZETT: In: Oxytocin, p. 247. Ed. by R. CALDEYRO-BARCIA and H. HELLER. Oxford: Pergamon Press 1961.
BOWER, B.F., D.M. MASON, and P.H. FORSHAM: Bronchogenic carcinoma with inappropriate antidiuretic activity in plasma and tumor. New Engl. J. Med. **271**, 934—938 (1964).
BOYLAN, J.W., and D.E. ANTKOWIAK: Mechanisms of diuresis during negative pressure breathing. J. appl. Physiol. **14**, 116—120 (1959).
BRAUDE, R., and K.G. MITCHELL: Let down of milk in the sow. Nature (Lond.) **165**, 937 (1950).
BRIGHTMAN, M.W.: Neurosecretion and milk-ejection in the mouse. Anat. Rec. **121**, 268 (1955).
BROOK, A.H., and L. SHARE: On the question of protein binding and the diffusability of circulating antidiuretic hormone in the dog. Endocrinology **78**, 785—799 (1966).
BROOKS, C.MC, J. USHIYAMI, and G. LANGE: Reactions of neurones in or near supra-optic nucleus. Amer. J. Physiol. **202**, 487—490 (1962).
BRUN, C., E.O.E. KNUDSEN, and F. RAASCHOU: Post-syncopal oliguria. Acta med. scand. **122**, 381—395 (1945a).
— — — On the cause of post-syncopal oliguria. Acta med. scand. **122**, 486—489 (1945b).
BUCHBORN, E.: Antidiuretic hormone and serum osmolarity in liver cirrhosis. Lancet **1957 I**, 1201.
BUCY, P.C.: In: The hypophysis cerebri in cytology and cellular pathology of the nervous system, p. 712. Ed. by W. PENFIELD. New York: P.B. Hoeber 1932.
BURN, G.P., and R.S. GREWAL: The antidiuretic response to and excretion of pituitary (posterior lobe) extract in man, with reference to the action of nicotine. Brit. J. Pharmacol. **6**, 471—482 (1951).
BURN, J.H., L.H. TRUELOVE, and S. BURN: The antidiuretic action of nicotine and smoking. Brit. med. J. **1945 I**, 403—406.
CAFRUNY, E.J., E. CARHART, and A. FARAH: Effect of hypophysectomy and hormones on sulphydryl concentrations in rat kidney cells. Endocrinology **61**, 143—147 (1957).
CALDEYRO-BARCIA, R.: Factors controlling the actions of the pregnant human uterus. In: Physiology of prematurity, pp. 11—17. Ed. by M. KOWLESSAR. New York: Josiah Macy 1961.
—, and J.J. POSEIRO: Oxytocin and contractility of the pregnant human uterus. Ann. N.Y. Acad. Sci. **75**, 813—830 (1958).
—, Y. SICA-BLANCO, J.J. POSEIRO, V. GONZALEZ-PANIZZA, C. MENDEZ-BAUER, C. FIELITZ, H. ALVAREZ, S.V. POSE, and C.M. HENDRICKS: A quantitative study of synthetic oxytocin on the pregnant human uterus. J. Pharmacol. **12**, 18 (1957).
CARLSSON, A., B. FALCK, and N.A. HILLARP: Cellular localisation of brain monoamine. Acta Physiol. Scand., Suppl. **196**, 1—28 (1962).

Cates, J. E., and O. Garrod: The effect of nicotine on urinary flow in diabetes insipidus. Clin. Sci. **10**, 145—160 (1951).
Chalmers, T. M., and A. A. G. Lewis: Stimulation of the supraoptic-hypophysial system in man. Clin. Sci. **10**, 127—135 (1951).
— —, and G. L. S. Pawan: The effects of posterior pituitary extracts on the renal excretion of sodium and chloride in man. J. Physiol. (Lond.) **112**, 238—242 (1951).
Chambers, G. H., E. V. Melville, R. S. Hare, and K. Hare: Regulation of the release of pituitrin by changes in the osmotic pressure of plasma. Amer. J. Physiol. **144**, 311—320 (1945).
Chang, H. C., K. F. Chia, G. H. Hsu, and R. K. S. Lim: A vagus-post-pituitary reflex. I. Pressor component. Chin. J. Physiol. **12**, 309—326 (1937).
— — —, and R. K. S. Lim: Humoral transmission at central synapses. II. Central vagus transmission after hypophysectomy in the dog. Chin. J. Physiol. **13**, 13—32 (1938).
—, R. K. S. Lim, V. M. Lu, C. C. Wang, and K. J. Wang: A vago-post-pituitary reflex. III. Oxytocic component. Chin. J. Physiol. **13**, 269—284 (1938).
Chaudhury, R. R.: Release of oxytocin in unanaesthetised rats. Brit. J. Pharmacol. **17**, 297 to 304 (1961).
—, H. K. Chuttani, and V. Ramlingswami: The antidiuretic hormone and liver damage. Clin. Sci. **21**, 199—203 (1961).
—, and J. M. Walker: The release of neurohypophysial hormones in the rabbit by anaesthetics and by haemorrhage. J. Physiol. (Lond.) **143**, 16 p. (1958).
— — The fate of injected oxytocin in the rabbit. J. Endocr. **19**, 189—192 (1959).
Chauvet, J., M. T. Lenci, et R. Acher: L'ocytocine et la vasopressine du mouton. Reconstitution d'un complexe hormonal actif. Biochim. biophys. Acta (Amst.) **38**, 266—272 (1960).
Chien, S., B. Peric, and S. Usami: Reflex nature of release of antidiuretic hormone upon common carotid occlusion in vagotomised dogs. Proc. Soc. exp. Biol. (N.Y.) **111**, 193—196 (1962).
Christlieb, M.: Über den Abbau von Oxytocin und Vasopressin *in vitro*. Arch. Exp. Pathol. Pharmakol. **194**, 44—51 (1940).
Clark, B. J., and M. Rocha e Silva jr.: Independent release of vasopressin by carotid occlusion. J. Physiol. (Lond.) **186**, 142—143 (1966).
Clemente, C. D., J. Sutin, and J. T. Silverstone: Changes in electrical activity of the medulla on the intravenous injections of hypertonic solutions. Amer. J. Physiol. **188**, 193—198 (1957).
Coch, J. A. J. Brovetto, H. M. Cabot, C. A. Fielitz, and R. Caldeyro-Barcia: Oxytocin-equivalent activity in the plasma of women in labour and during the puerperium. Amer. J. Obstet. Gynec. **91**, 10—17 (1965).
Collin, R., et J. Racadot: La chute du taux de la substance gomari-positive neurohypophysaire dans la postpartum chez le cobaye. Ann. Endocr. (Paris) **14**, 546 (1953).
Cowie, A. T., S. J. Folley, B. A. Cross, G. W. Harris, D. Jacobsohn, and K. C. Richardson: Terminology for use in lactational physiology. Nature (Lond.) **168**, 421 (1951).
— Quoted in Folley (1952).
Craig, F. N., F. E. Visscher, and C. R. Houck: Renal function in dogs under ether or cyclopropane anaesthesia. Amer. J. Physiol. **143**, 108—118 (1945).
Crawford, J. P., and B. Pinkham: The removal of circulating antidiuretic hormone by the body. Endocrinology **55**, 699—700 (1954).
Cross, B. A.: Suckling antidiuresis in rabbits. J. Physiol. (Lond.) **114**, 447—453 (1951).
— The hypothalamus and the mechanism of sympathetico-adrenal inhibition of milk-ejection. J. Endocr. **12**, 15—28 (1955a).
— Neurohumoral mechanisms in the emotional inhibition of milk-ejection. J. Endocr. **12**, 29—37 (1955b).
— On the mechanism of labour in the rabbit. J. Endocr. **16**, 261—271 (1958).
— and H. B. van Dyke: The effects of highly purified posterior pituitary principles on the lactating mammary gland of the rabbit. J. Endocr. **9**, 232—235 (1953).
—, and J. D. Green: Activity of single neurones in the hypothalamus. Effect of osmotic and other stimuli. J. Physiol. (Lond.) **148**, 554—569 (1959).
—, and G. W. Harris: The role of the neurohypophysis in the milk-ejection reflex. J. Endocr. **8**, 148—161 (1952).
Currie, J. C. M., and E. Ullman: Polyuria during experimental modifications of breathing. J. Physiol. (Lond.) **155**, 438—455 (1961).
Czaczkes, J. W., and C. R. Kleeman: The effect of various states of hydration and the plasma concentration on the turnover of antidiuretic hormone in mammals. J. clin. Invest. **43**, 1649—1658 (1964).
— —, and M. Koenig: Physiologic studies of antidiuretic hormone by its direct measurement in human plasma. J. clin. Invest. **43**, 1625—1648 (1964).
Dale, H. H.: The action of extracts of the pituitary body. Biochem. J. **4**, 427—447 (1909).

DANDY, W.E.: Section of the human hypophysial stalk. J. Amer. med. Ass. **114**, 312—314 (1946).
DANIEL, A.R., and K. LEDERIS: Hormone release from the neurohypophysis *in vitro*. Gen. Comp. Endocrinol. **3**, 693—694 (1963).
— — Effect of ether anaesthesis and haemorrhage on hormone storage and ultrastructure of the rat neurohypophysis. J. Endocr. **34**, 91—104 (1966).
— — Effects of acetylcholine on the release of neurohypophysial hormones *in vitro*. J. Endocr. **34**, X—XI (1966b).
DARMADY, E.M., J. DURANDT, E.R. MATTHEWS, and F. STRANNACH: Location of I^{131}pitressin in the kidney by autoradiography. Clin. Sci. **19**, 229—236 (1960).
DAWSON, A.B.: The early appearance of secretion in the neurohypophysis and hypothalamic nuclei of the rat. Anat. Rec. **117**, 620 (1953).
DEARBORN, E.H., and L. LASAGNA: The antidiuretic action of epinephrine and novepinephrine. J. Pharmacol. **106**, 122—128 (1952).
DEBACKÈRE, M., and G. PEETERS: The influence of vaginal distention on milk-ejection and diuresis in the lactating cow. Arch. Int. Pharmacodyn. **123**, 402—471 (1960a).
— — Le mechanism de l'ejection du lait par distention vaginale chez le mouton. Arch. Int. Pharmacodyn. **126**, 486—488 (1960b).
— —, and M. TUYTTENS: Reflex release of an oxytocic hormone by stimulation of genital organs in male and female sheep studied by a crosscirculation technique. J. Endocr. **22**, 321—334 (1961).
DEMPSTER, W.J., and A.M. JOEKES: Diuresis and antidiuresis in the auto-transplanted kidney in dogs. Quart. J. exp. Physiol. **38**, 11—24 (1953).
— — Emotional antidiuresis in the auto-transplanted kidney. J. Physiol. (Lond.) **128**, 122 to 130 (1955).
DENAMUR, R.: The hypothalamo-neurohypophysial system and the milk-ejection reflex. Dairy Sci. Abstr. **27**, 193—224 and 263—280 (1965).
—, et J. MARTINET: Énervation de la mammelle et lactation chez la brebis et la chevre. C.R. Acad. Sci. (Paris) **148**, 833—836 (1954).
— — Les stimulus nerveux mammaires sont-ils necessaires a l'entretien de la lactation chez la chevre. C.R. Acad. Sci. (Paris) **248**, 860—862 (1959a).
— — Entretien de la lactation chez la chevre apres section de la moelle epinière et sympathectomie lombaire. C.R. Acad. Sci. (Paris) **248**, 743—746 (1959b).
DENMARK, M.R. VAN, and R.L. HAYS: Effect of stimulation of the reproductive organs of the cow on the release of an oxytocin-like substance. Endocrinology **52**, 634—637 (1953).
— — Stimulatory action of breeding on the release of oxytocin as measured by intramammary pressure. J. Dairy Sci. **34**, 496—497 (1951).
DEXTER, D., H.B. STONER, and H.N. GREEN: The release of posterior pituitary antidiuretic hormone by adenosinetriphosphate. J. Endocr. **11**, 141—159 (1954).
DEY, F.L., C. FISHER, and S.W. RANSON: Disturbances in pregnancy and labour in guinea pigs with hypothalamic lesions. Amer. J. Obstet. Gynec. **42**, 459—466 (1941).
DICKER, S.E.: A method for the assay of very small amounts of antidiuretic activity with a note on the antidiuretic titre of rat's blood. J. Physiol. (Lond.) **122**, 149—157 (1953).
— The fate of antidiuretic activity of pitressin in rats. J. Physiol. (Lond.) **124**, 464—475 (1954).
— The effect of methylpentynol on ethanol and on water metabolism in rats. J. Physiol. (Lond.) **144**, 138—147 (1958).
— Possible independence of oxytocin and vasopressin secretion in the human being. J. Physiol. (Lond.) **147**, 25 (1959).
— Release of vasopressin and oxytocin from isolated pituitary glands of adult and newborn rats. J. Physiol. (Lond.) **185**, 429—444 (1966).
—, and M.G. EGGLETON: Hyaluronidase and antidiuretic activity in urine of man. J. Physiol. (Lond.) **154**, 378—384 (1960).
— — Renal excretion of hyaluronidase and calcium in man during the antidiuretic action of vasopressin and some analogues. J. Physiol. (Lond.) **157**, 351—362 (1961).
—, and A.L. GREENBAUM: Inactivation of antidiuretic activity of vasopressin by the kidneys and the liver of rats. J. Physiol. (Lond.) **126**, 116—123 (1956).
—, and J. NUNN: The role of antidiuretic hormone during water deprivation in rats. J. Physiol. (Lond.) **136**, 235 (1957).
— — Antidiuresis in adult and old rats. J. Physiol. (Lond.) **141**, 332—336 (1958).
—, and C. TYLER: Vasopressor and oxytocic activities of the pituitary gland of rats, guinea pigs and cats and of human foetuses. J. Physiol. (Lond.) **121**, 206 (1953).
— — Inactivation of oxytocin and vasopressin by blood of pregnant women. J. Obstet. Gynaec. Brit. Emp. **63**, 690—696 (1956).
—, and G.A. WHYLEY: Inactivation of oxytocin by plasma of pregnant women. J. Obstet. Gynaec. Brit. Emp. **66**, 605—609 (1959).

DICKER, S.E., and G.A. WHYLEY: In: Release and metabolism of the neurohypophysial hormones. Quoted by S.E. DICKER. J. Pharm. Pharmacol. **13**, 449—469 (1961).
DIECKMANN, S.B., G.F. EGENOLF, B. MORLEY, and R.E. POTTINGER: The inactivation of the antidiuretic hormone of the posterior pituitary gland by blood from pregnant patients. Amer. J. Obstet. Gynec. **60**, 1043—1050 (1950).
DINGMAN, J.F.: Hypothalamus and the endocrine control of sodium and water metabolism in man. Amer. J. med. Sci. **235**, 79—99 (1958).
DOUGLAS, W.W.: A possible mechanism of neurosecretion. Release of vasopressin by depolarization and its dependence on calcium. Nature (Lond.) **197**, 81—82 (1963).
—, and A. ISHIDA: The stimulant effect of cold on vasopressin release from neurohypophysis *in vitro*. J. Physiol. (Lond.) **179**, 185—191 (1965).
— —, and A.M. POISNER: The effect of metabolic inhibitors on the release of vasopressin from the isolated neurohypophysis. J. Physiol. (Lond.) **181**, 753—759 (1965).
—, and A.M. POISNER: Release of vasopressin from the rat's neurohypophysis *in vitro*. J. Physiol. (Lond.) **167**, 55—56 (1963a).
— — On the intimate mechanism of vasopressin secretion. Stimulus secretion coupling in the isolated neurohypophysis. Biochem. Pharmacol. **12**, 225 (1963b).
— — Stimulus-secretion coupling in a neurosecretory organ. The role of calcium in the release of vasopressin from the neurohypophysis. J. Physiol. (Lond.) **172**, 1—18 (1964).
— — Calcium movement in the neurohypophysis of the rat and its relation to the release of vasopressin. J. Physiol. (Lond.) **172**, 19—30 (1964a).
— —, and R.P. RUBIN: Efflux of adenine nucleotides from perfused adrenal glands exposed to nicotine and other chromaffin cell stimulants. J. Physiol. (Lond.) **179**, 130—137 (1965).
DRAGER, G.A., and E.C. RENNELS: The independent behaviour of Gomori-positive neurosecretion and the oxytocic hormone in the rat neurohypophysis. Anat. Rec. **121**, 287 (1955).
DROZ, B., and C.P. LEBLOND: Migration of proteins along axons of the sciatic nerve. Science **137**, 1047—1048 (1962).
DRURY, D.R., J.P. HENRY, and J. GOODMAN: The effects of continuous pressure breathing on kidney function. J. clin. Invest. **26**, 945 (1947).
DUCHEN, L.W.: Effects of ingestion of hypertonic saline on pituitary gland. A morphological study of pars intermedia and posterior lobe. J. Endocr. **25**, 161—168 (1962).
DUKE, H.N., and M. PICKFORD: Observations on the action of acetylcholine and adrenaline on the hypothalamus. J. Physiol. (Lond.) **114**, 325—332 (1951).
— —, and J.A. WATT: The immediate and delayed effects of di-isopropyl-fluorophosphate injected into the supraoptic nuclei of dogs. J. Physiol. (Lond.) **111**, 81—88 (1950).
DYBALL, R.E.J.: Stimuli for the release of antidiuretic hormone. J. Physiol. (Lond.) **186**, 99—100 (1966).
— Personal communication (1967).
DYKE, H.B. VAN: Die Verteilung der wirksamen Stoffe der Hypophyse auf die verschiedenen Teile derselben. Arch. Exp. Pathol. Pharmakol. **114**, 261—274 (1926).
—, K. ADAMSON jr., and S.L. ENGEL: Aspects of the biochemistry and physiology of the neurohypophyseal hormones. Recent Progr. Hormone Res. **11**, 1—35 (1955).
—, R.G. AMES, and I.C. PLOUGH: The excretion of antidiuretic hormone in the urine of patients with cirrhosis of the liver. Trans. Ass. Amer. Phycns **63**, 35—38 (1950).
— — Alcohol diuresis. Acta endocr. (Kbh.) **7**, 110—121 (1951).
—, B.F. CHOW, H.O. GREEP, and A. ROTHEN: The isolation of a protein from the pars neuralis of the ox pituitary with constant oxytocic, pressor and diuresis-inhibiting effects. J. Pharmacol. (Kyoto) **74**, 190—209 (1941).
EAYERS, J.J., and R.M. BADDELEY: Neural pathways in lactation. J. Anat. (Lond.) **90**, 161 to 171 (1956).
EDSTROM, J.E., and D. EICHNER: Relationship between nucleolar volume and cell body content of ribonucleic acid in supraoptic neurones. Nature (Lond.) **181**, 619 (1958).
— —, and M. SCHOR: Quantitative ribonucleic acid measurements in functional studies of nucleus supraopticus. In: Regional neurochemistry. Ed. by S.E. KETY and J. ELKES. Oxford: Pergamon Press 1961.
EGGLETON, M.G.: The diuretic action of alcohol in man. J. Physiol. (Lond.) **101**, 172—191 (1942).
ELIAHOU, H.E., S.D. CLARKE, and G.M. BULL: Atrial pulsation during acute distention and its possible significance in the regulation of blood volume. Clin. Sci. **19**, 377 (1960).
ELY, F., and W.E. PETERSON: Factors involved in the ejection of milk. J. Dairy Sci. **24**, 211—223 (1941).
ERANKO, O., O. FRIBERG, and M.J. KARVONEN: The effect of the act of copulation on water diuresis in the rat. Acta endocr. (Kbh.) **12**, 197—200 (1953).
EULER, C. v.: A preliminary note on slow hypothalamic "osmopotentials". Acta physiol. scand. **29**, 133—136 (1953).

EVERSOLE, W. J., J. H. BIRNIE, and R. GAUNT: Inactivation of posterior pituitary antidiuretic hormone by the liver. Endocrinology **45**, 378—382 (1949).
FANG, H. S., H. M. LUI, and S. C. WANG: Liberation of antidiuretic hormone following hypothalamic stimulation in the dog. Amer. J. Physiol. **202**, 212—216 (1962).
FEKETE, K. v.: Beiträge zur Physiologie der Gravidität. Endokrinologie **7**, 364—369 (1930).
FERGUSON, J. K. W.: A study of the motility of the intact uterus at term. Surg. Gynec. Obstet. **73**, 359—366 (1941).
FICQ, A., and J. FLAMENT-DURAND: Autoradiography in endocrine research. In: Techniques in endocrine research, pp. 73—85. Ed. by P. ECKSTEIN and F. KNOWLES (1964).
FISHER, C., W. R. INGRAM, and S. W. RANSON: Diabetes insipidus and the neurohormonal control of water balance. Ann. Arbor, Michigan: Edwards Bros. Inc. 1938.
—, H. W. MAGOUN, and S. W. RANSON: Dystocia in diabetes insipidus. The relation of pituitary oxytocin to parturition. Amer. J. Obstet. Gynec. **36**, 1—9 (1938).
FITZPATRICK, R. J.: The estimation of small amounts of oxytocin in blood. In: Oxytocin, pp. 358—379. Ed. by R. CALDEYRO-BARCIA and H. HELLER. Oxford: Pergamon Press 1961.
— The posterior pituitary gland and the female reproductive tract. In: The pituitary gland, Vol. 3, pp. 453—504. Ed. by G. W. HARRIS and B. T. DONOVAN. London: Butterworths 1966.
—, and C. F. WALMSLEY: The concentration of oxytocin in bovine blood during parturition. J. Physiol. (Lond.) **163**, 13—14 (1962).
— — The release of oxytocin during parturition. In: Advances in oxytocin. Ed. by J. PINKERTON. Oxford: Pergamon Press 1965.
FLAMENT-DURAND, J.: Etude des relations hypothalamo-hypophysaire a l'aide de radioisotopes marques au soufre 35. C.R. Acad. Sci. (Paris) **252**, 3487—3489 (1961).
FOLLENIUS, E.: Etude comparative de la cytologie fine au noyau preoptiques (NPO) et du noyau lateral du tuber (NLT) chez la truite (Salmo irideus Gibb) et chez la perche (Perca fluviatilis) comparison des deux types de neurosecretion. Gen. comp. Endocr. **3**, 66—89 (1963).
FOLLEY, S. J.: Aspects of pituitary-mammary gland relationships. Recent Progr. Hormone Res. **7**, 107—133 (1952).
— and G. S. KNAGGS: Observations on oxytocin release in ruminants. J. Reprod. Fertil. **8**, 265—266 (1964).
— — Levels of oxytocin in the jugular vein blood of goats during parturition. J. Endocr. **33**, 301—315 (1965).
— — Milk-ejection activity (oxytocin) in the external jugular vein blood of the cow, goat and sow, in relation to the stimulus of milking or suckling. J. Endocr. **34**, 197—214 (1966).
FONG, C. J. O., L. SILVER, D. R. CHRISTMAN, and T. L. SCHWARZ: On the mechanism of action of the antidiuretic hormone (vasopressin). Proc. nat. Acad. Sci. (Wash.) **46**, 1273—1277 (1960).
FORD, D. H., and A. HIRSCHMAN: The localisation of S^{35}labelled l-cystine in the central nervous system of rat. Anat. Rec. **130**, 302 (1958).
— —, R. RHINES, and S. ZIMBERG: The rate of uptake and radioautographic localisation of S^{35} in the central nervous system, pituitary and skeletal muscle of horned male rats after the injection of S^{35} cystine. Exp. Neurol. **4**, 444—459 (1961).
FOURMAN, J., and G. C. KENNEDY: An effect of antidiuretic hormone on the flow of blood through the vasa recta of the rat kidney. J. Endocr. **35**, 173—176 (1966).
FRANKLAND, B. J. B., M. D. HOLLENBERG, D. B. HOPE, and B. A. SCHACHTER: Dissociation of oxytocin and vasopressin from their carrier protein by chromatography on Sephadex G 25. Brit. J. Pharmacol. **26**, 502—510 (1966).
FREEDMAN, P., R. MOULTON, and A. G. SPENCER: The effect of intravenous calcium gluconate on the renal excretion of water and electrolytes. Clin. Sci. **17**, 247—263 (1958).
FREY, E.: Die Hinderung der Wasserdiurese durch die Narkose. Pflügers Arch. ges. Physiol. **120**, 66—92 (1907).
FRIBERG, O.: The antidiuretic effect of coitus in human subjects. Acta endocr. (Kbh.) **12**, 193—196 (1953).
FRIEDMAN, S. M., A. M. HINKE, and C. L. FRIEDMAN: Neurohypophysial responsiveness in the normal and senescent rat. J. Geront. **1956 II**, 286—291.
FUCHS, A. R.: Oxytocin and the onset of labour in rabbits. J. Endocr. **30**, 217—224 (1964).
— Inhibitory effect of alcohol on oxytocin release in rabbit parturition. J. Endocr. **35**, 125—134 (1966).
—, and G. WAGNER: Effect of alcohol on release of oxytocin. Nature (Lond.) **198**, 92—94 (1963a).
— — The effect of alcohol on release of oxytocin in rabbits. Acta endocr. (Kbh.) **44**, 593—605 (1963b).
FUGO, N. W.: The antidiuretic action of Yohimbine. Endocrinology **34**, 143—148 (1944).

Fujita, H., and J.F. Hartmann: Electron microscopy in normal, adrenalin-treated and pilocarpine-treated rabbits. Z. Zellforsch. **54**, 734—763 (1961).
Fuller, G.R., and C.H. Sawyer: Electroencephalographic changes in the cat associated with antidiuretic response to intracarotid injection of hypertonic solutions. Fed. Proc. **15**, 69—70 (1956).
Gaitan, E., E. Coba, and M. Mizrachi: Evidence for the differential secretion of oxytocin and vasopressin in man. J. clin. Invest. **43**, 2310—2322 (1964).
Gaitonde, M.K., and D. Richter: The metabolic activity of the proteins of the brain. Proc. roy. Soc. B **45**, 83—99 (1956).
Gauer, O.H., and J.P. Henry: Circulatory basis of fluid volume control. Physiol. Rev. **43**, 423—481 (1963).
— —, O.H. Sieker, and W.E. Wendt: The effect of negative pressure breathing on urine flow. J. clin. Invest. **33**, 287 (1954).
Gerschenfeld, H.M., J.M. Tramezzani, and E. de Robertis: Ultrastructure and function in neurohypophysis of the toad. Endocrinology **66**, 741—762 (1960).
Gersh, I.: Structure and function of the parachymatous glandular cells in the neurohypophysis of the rat. Amer. J. Anat. **64**, 467—443 (1939).
Giarman, M.J., L.R. Mattie, and W.F. Stephenson: Studies on the antidiuretic action of morphine. Science **117**, 225—226 (1953).
Giere, F.A., and W.J. Eversole: Effects of adrenal medullary hormones on antidiuretic substances in blood serum. Science **120**, 395—396 (1954).
Ginsburg, M.: The clearance of vasopressin from the splanchnic vascular area and the kidneys. J. Endocr. **16**, 217—226 (1957).
— Unpublished observations (1960).
—, and L.M. Brown: Effect of anaesthetics and haemorrhage on the release of neurohypophysial antidiuretic hormone. Brit. J. Pharmacol. **14**, 327—333 (1956).
— — The effects of haemorrhage and plasma hypertoxicity on the neurohypophysis. In: The neurohypophysis. Ed. by H. Heller. London: Butterworths 1957.
—, and H. Heller: Antidiuretic activity in blood obtained from various parts of the cardiovascular system. J. Endocr. **9**, 274—282 (1953a).
— — The clearance of injected vasopressin from the circulation and its fate in the body. J. Endocr. **9**, 283—291 (1953b).
— —, and S.M.A. Zaidi: Re-appraisal of the evidence for the metabolic conversion of vasopressin into a less active metabolite. Nature (Lond.) **178**, 803—804 (1956).
—, and M. Ireland: The hormone binding protein of the neurohypophysis. J. Physiol. (Lond.) **169**, 15 (1963).
— — Binding of vasopressin and oxytocin to protein in extracts of bovine and rabbit neurohypophyses. J. Endocr. **30**, 131—145 (1964a).
— — Unpublished observations (1964b).
— — The preparation of bovine neurohypophysis and the estimation of its maximum capacity to bind oxytocin and arginine vasopressin. J. Endocr. **32**, 187—198 (1965a).
— — Unpublished observations (1965b).
— — The role of neurophysin in the transport and release of neurohypophysial hormones. J. Endocr. **35**, 289—298 (1966).
—, K. Jayasena, B.J. Pickering, and P.J. Thomas: Unpublished observations (1966).
— — Unpublished observations (1967).
— —, and P.J. Thomas: Preparation and properties of porcine neurophysin and the influence of calcium on the hormone-neurophysin complex. J. Physiol. (Lond.) **184**, 387—401 (1966a).
— — — Subfractions from porcine neurophysin with different hormone binding properties. J. Physiol. (Lond.) **183**, 45—46 (1966b).
—, and M.W. Smith: The fate of oxytocin in male and female rats. Brit. J. Pharmacol. **14**, 327—333 (1959).
Gomez, E.T.: Relations of the posterior hypophysis in the maintenance of lactation in hypophysectomised rats. J. Dairy Sci. **22**, 488 (1939).
Gomori, G.: Observations with differential stains on human islets of Langerhans. Amer. J. Path. **17**, 395—406 (1941).
Gonzalez-Panizza, V.M., Y. Sica-Blanco, and C.J. Mendez-Bauer: Fate of injected oxytocin in the pregnant women near term. In: Oxytocin. Ed. by R. Caldeyro-Barcia and H. Heller. London: Pergamon Press 1961.
Gopalan, C.: Antidiuretic factor in the urine of patients with nutritional oedema. Lancet **1950 I**, 304—306.
Green, J.D., and V.L. van Breeman: Electron microscopy of pituitary and observations on neurosecretion. Amer. J. Anat. **97**, 177—227 (1955).

GREEN, J.D., and D.J. MAXWELL: The comparative anatomy of the hypophysis and observations on the mechanism of neurosecretion. In: Comparative endocrinology, pp. 368—392. Ed. by A. GORBMAN. New York: Wiley 1959.

GREENBERG, E., M.B. DIVERTIE, and L.B. WOOLNER: A review of unusual systemic manifestations associated with carcinoma. Amer. J. Med. **36**, 106—120 (1964).

GROOT, J. DE, and J.E. HARTFIELD: Quantitative changes in rat pituitary neurosecretory material in altered adrenocortical function. Acta neuroveg. (Wien) **22**, 177—183 (1960).

GROSVENOR, C.E., and C.W. TURNER: Evidence for adrenergic and cholinergic components in milk let-down reflex in lactating rats. Proc. Soc. exp. Biol. (N.Y.) **95**, 719—722 (1957).

GUNTHER, M.: The posterior pituitary and labour. Brit. med. J. **1948 I**, 567.

HALL, C.A., B. FRAME, and V.A. DRILL: Renal excretion of water and antidiuretic substances in patients with hepatic cirrhosis and rats with dietary liver injury. Endocrinology **44**, 76—82 (1949).

HALLER, E.W., N. SPERELAKIS, H. SACHS, and L. SHORE: Release of vasopressin from guinea pig posterior pituitary. Amer. J. Physiol. **209**, 79—83 (1965).

HAMMOND, J.: The physiology of milk and butterfat secretion. Vet. Rec. **48**, 519—535 (1936).

HANENSON, T.B., B. GOLUBOFF, J. GROSSMAN, R.E. WESTON, and L. LEITER: Studies on water excretion following intravenous hydration and the administration of pitressin or nicotine in congestive heart failure. Circulation **13**, 242—251 (1956).

HANKISS, J., M. KESZTHELYI, and B. SIRO: A new type of diabetes insipidus due to hormone inactivation. Its incidence in clinical material. Amer. J. med. Sci. **242**, 605—611 (1961).

HANSEN, J.D.L., and L.A. SMITH: The effects of witholding fluid intake in the immediate post-natal period. Amer. J. Dis. Child. **84**, 477—478 (1952).

HARRIS, G.W.: The innervation and action of the neurohypophysis. An investigation using the method of remote control stimulation. Phil. Trans. B **232**, 385—441 (1947).

— The excretion of an antidiuretic substance by the kidney after electrical stimulation of the neurohypophysis in the unanaesthetised rabbit. J. Physiol. (Lond.) **107**, 430—435 (1948).

— Neural Control of the Pituitary Gland. London: Arnold 1955.

—, and D. JACOBSOHN: Functional grafts of the anterior pituitary gland. Proc. roy. Soc. B **149**, 263—276 (1952).

— —, and G. KAHLSON: In: Ciba Colloquia on Endocrinology, Vol. 4, p. 186. London: J. and A. Churchill (1952.

—, and V.R. PICKLES: Reflex stimulation of the neurohypophysis (posterior pituitary gland) and the nature of posterior pituitary hormones. Nature (Lond.) **172**, 1049 (1953).

HARVEY, NANCY, J.J. JONES, and J. LEE: The renal clearance and plasma binding of vasopressin in the dog. J. Endocr. **38**, 163—172 (1967).

HASSELBACH, C.H., et A.R. PIGUET: Nature et purification partielle de l'ocytocine sur les hormones hypophysaires. 1. Helv. Clin. Acta **35**, 2131 (1952).

HATERIUS, H.O., and J.K.W. FERGUSON: Evidence for the hormonal nature of the oxytocic principle of the neurohypophysis. Amer. J. Physiol. **124**, 314—321 (1938).

— Evidence of pituitary involvement in the experimental control of water diuresis. Amer. J. Physiol. **128**, 506—513 (1940).

HAWKER, R.W.: Inactivation of antidiuretic hormone and oxytocin during pregnancy. Quart. J. exp. Physiol. **41**, 301—308 (1956).

— Oxytocin in lactating and non-lactating women. J. clin. Endocr. **18**, 54—60 (1958).

—, and V.S. ROBERTS: Oxytocin in lactating cows and goats. Brit. vet. J. **113**, 459—464 (1957).

— —, and C.F. WALMSLEY: Oxytocin and oxytocic substance in blood extracts before and during copulation in in sheep. Endocrinology **64**, 309—310 (1959).

—, and P.H. ROBERTSON: Some properties of an oxytocic substance found in blood extracts. Endocrinology **63**, 242—249 (1958).

—, C.F. WALMSLEY, V.S. ROBERTS, J.K. BLACKSHAW, and J.C. DOWNES: Oxytocic activity in blood of parturient and lactating women. J. Clin. Endocrin. **21**, 985—995 (1961).

HEBB, C.O., and G.M.H. WAITHES: Choline acetylase in antero- and retrograde degeneration of a cholinergic nerve. J. Physiol. (Lond.) **132**, 667—671 (1956).

HELLER, H.: Antidiuretic hormone in pituitary glands of new-born rats. J. Physiol. (Lond.) **106**, 28—32 (1947).

— The effects of dehydration on adult and new-born rats. J. Physiol. (Lond.) **108**, 303—314 (1949).

— The state and concentration of the neurohypophysial hormones in blood. Ciba Found. Coll. Endocr. **11**, 609—630 (1957).

—, and K. LEDERIS: Cited by H. HELLER (1957).

— — Maturation of the hypothalamo-neurohypophysial system. J. Physiol. (Lond.) **147**, 299—314 (1959).

— — Characteristics of isolated neurosecretory vesicles from mammalian neural lobes. Mem. Soc. Endocrinol. **12**, 35—50 (1962).

HELLER, H., and A.Q. SAIFI: Unpublished observations (1966).
—, and F.H. SMIRK: The influence of binding on animal, of its body temperature and of external losses of water upon diuresis. J. Physiol. (Lond.) **76**, 23—38 (1932a).
— — Studies concerning the alimentary absorption of water and tissue hydration in relation to diuresis. IV. The influence of anaesthetics and hypnotics on the absorption and excretion of water. J. Physiol. (Lond.) **76**, 292—302 (1932b).
—, and F.F. URBAN: The fate of antidiuretic principle of post-pituitary extracts *in vivo* and *in vitro*. J. Physiol. (Lond.) **85**, 502—518 (1935).
—, and S.M.A. ZAIDI: The metabolism of exogenous and endogenous antidiuretic hormone in the liver and kidney *in vivo*. Brit. J. Pharmacol. **12**, 284—292 (1957).
—, and E.J. ZAIMIS: The antidiuretic and oxytocic hormones in the posterior pituitary glands of new-born infants and adults. J. Physiol. (Lond.) **109**, 162—169 (1949).
HELLER, J.: The physiology of the antidiuretic hormone. IV. The effect of certain anaesthetics on the antidiuretic activity of rat blood plasma. Physiol. bohemoslov. **9**, 283—288 (1960).
HELLMAN, K., and J.S. WEINER: Antidiuretic substances in urine following exposure to high temperatures. J. appl. Physiol. **6**, 194—198 (1953).
HENDRICKS, C.H.: The neurohypophysis in pregnancy. Obstet. gynec. Surv. **9**, 323—341 (1954).
—, T. HELFAND, and R. CALDEYRO-BARCIA: Amer. J. Obstet. Gynec. **77**, 387 (1959).
HENRY, J.P., O.H. GAUER, and J.L. REEVES: Evidence of the atrial location of receptors influencing urine flow. Circulat. Res. **4**, 85 (1956).
—, and J.W. PEARCE: The possible role of cardiac stretch receptors in the induction of changes in urine flow. J. Physiol. (Lond.) **131**, 572 (1956).
HILD, W.: Experimentell-morphologische Untersuchung über das Verhalten der „Neurosekretonischen Bahn" nach Hypophysenstieldurchschneidung bei Eingriffen in den Wasserhaushalt und Belastung der Osmoregulation. Virchows Arch. path. Anat. **319**, 526—546 (1951).
—, and G. ZETLER: Über das Vorkommen der Hypophysenhinterlappenhormone im Zwischenhirn. Arch. Exp. Pathol. Pharmakol. **213**, 139—153 (1951).
— — Über die Funktion des Neurosekrets im Zwischenhirnneurohypophysensystem als Trägersubstanz für Vasopressin, Adiuretin und Oxytocin. Z. ges. exp. Med. **120**, 236—243 (1953a).
— — Experimenteller Beweis für die Entstehung der sog. Hyperphysenhinterlappenwirkstoffe im Hypothalamus. Pflügers Arch. ges. Physiol. **257**, 169—201 (1953b).
HILTON, J.G., and R.F. JOHNSON: Changes in blood oxytocinase during parturition. Amer. J. Obstet. Gynec. **78**, 479—482 (1959).
HIPSLEY, E.H., and J.W. MCKELLAR: Vasopressin binding capacity of plasma. J. Endocr. **19**, 345—352 (1960).
HOLLAND, R.C., B.A. CROSS, and C.H. SAWYER: E.E.G. correlates of osmotic activation of the neurohypophysial milk-ejection mechanism. Amer. J. Physiol. **196**, 796—802 (1959).
—, J.W. SUNDSTEN, and C.H. SAWYER: Anat. Rev. **130**, 316 (1958).
HOLMES, R.L.: Phosphatase and cholinesterase in the hypothalamo-hypophysial system in the monkey. J. Endocr. **23**, 63—67 (1961).
—, and J.A. KIERNAN: The fine structure of the infundibular process of hedgehog. Z. Zellforsch. **61**, 894—912 (1964).
HOOPER, K.C.: The catabolism of some physiologically active polypeptides by homogenate of dog hypothalamus. Biochem. J. **83**, 511—517 (1962).
HOPE, D.B., and M.D. HOLLENBERG: Isolation of a new hormone-binding protein from the posterior lobes of bovine pituitary glands. Biochem. J. **99**, 5—6 p. (1966).
HOWE, A., and P.A. JEWELL: Effects of water deprivation upon the neurosecretory material of the desert rat (Meriones meriones) compared with the laboratory rat. J. Endocr. **18**, 118—123 (1959).
—, and A.G.E. PEARCE: A histochemical investigation of neurosecretory substance in the rat. J. Histochem. Cytochem. **4**, 561—569 (1956).
HULET, W.H., and H.W. SMITH: Negative pressure respiration, water diuresis and natriuresis in normotensive, hypertensive and prehydrated normotensive subjects. J. clin. Invest. **38**, 1972—1980 (1959).
HUNTER, J., M. KALANT, and J.C. OGILVIE: A simple method for the assay of small amounts of antidiuretic hormone. Canad. J. Biochem. **37**, 1218—1225 (1959).
HYDEN, H.: Protein metabolism in the nerve cell during growth and function. Acta physiol. scand. **6**, suppl. **17**, 1—136 (1943).
—, and A. PIGON: A cytophysiological study of the functional relationship between oligodendroglial cells and nerve cells of Deiter's nucleus. J. Neurochem. **6**, 57—72 (1960).
ISBISTER, C.: A clinical study of the draught reflex in human lactation. Arch. Dis. Childh. **29**, 66 (1954).
ISHI, S., I. YASUMASU, H. KOBAYASHI, Y. OOTA, T. HIRANO, and A. TANAKA: Isolation of neurosecretory granules and nerve endings from bovine posterior lobe. Annotationes Zool. Japon. **35**, 121—127 (1962).

ISHIKAMA, T., K. KOIZUMI, and C.M. BROOKS: Electrical activity recorded in pituitary stalk of the cat. Amer. J. Physiol. **210**, 427—431 (1966).

ITOH, S.: The release of antidiuretic hormone from the posterior pituitary body on exposure to heat. Jap. J. Physiol. **4**, 185—190 (1945).

— Mammalian antidiuretic hormone. Sogo Igaku **11**, 395 (1954).

JAHN, H., F. STEPHAN, and J. STAHL: Diuretic activity in blood and urine after bleeding in the dog. Arch. Sci. physiol. **14**, 421—433 (1960).

JEWELL, P.A.: The occurrence of vesiculated neurones in the hypothalamus of the dog. J. Physiol. (Lond.) **121**, 167—181 (1953).

—, and E.B. VERNEY: An experimental attempt to determine the site of the neurohypophysial and osmoreceptors in the dog. Phil. Trans. B **240**, 197—324 (1957).

JONES, A.M., and W. SCHLAPP: The action and fate of injected posterior pituitary extracts in the decapitated cat. J. Physiol. (Lond.) **87**, 144—157 (1936).

KALLIALA, H., and M.J. KARVONEN: Antidiuresis during suckling in women. Ann. Med. exp. Fenn. **29**, 233—241 (1951).

KANDEL, E.R.: Spike and synaptic potentials in hypothalamic neuroendocrine cells. Fed. Proc. **21**, 361 (1962).

KELSALL, A.R.: The inhibition of water diuresis in man by ischaemic muscle pain. J. Physiol. (Lond.) **109**, 150—161 (1949).

— The urinary excretion of adrenaline during inhibition of water diuresis in man by ischaemic muscle pain. J. Physiol. (Lond.) **112**, 54—58 (1951).

KIVALO, E., and H. ARKO: The effect of noradrenaline and acetylcholine on water diuresis and neurosecretory substance of the rat. Ann. Med. exp. Fenn. **35**, 398—403 (1957).

KIVALO, I.: Effect of some anaesthetic agents on diuresis and hypothalamo-hypophysial neurosecretion in the rat. Ann. J. Med. exp. Biol. Fenn., Suppl. 5, **44**, 1—60 (1966).

KLISIECKI, A., M. PICKFORD, P. ROTHSCHILD, and E.B. VERNEY: The absorption and excretion of water by the mammal. Proc. roy. Soc. B **112**, 496—547 (1933).

KNAGGS, G.S.: Blood oxytocin levels in the cow during milking and in the parturienr goat. J. Endocr. **26**, XXIV—XXV (1963).

— Biological half-life of intravenously injected oxytocin in the sow. J. Endocr. **37**, 229—230 (1967).

KNOWLES, F.G.W.: In: 2nd Int. Symposium on neurosecretion. Ed. by W. BARGMANN, B. HAUSTRON, and E. SCHARRER. Berlin-Göttingen-Heidelberg: Springer 1958.

KOELLE, G.B.: A proposed dual neurohumoral role of acetylcholine; its function at the pre- and postsynaptic sites. Nature (Lond.) **190**, 208—211 (1961).

—, and C. GEESEY: Localisation of acetylcholine-esterase in the neurohypophysis and its functional implications. Proc. Soc. exp. Biol. (N.Y.) **100**, 625—628 (1961).

KOIZUMI, K., T. ISHIKAWA, and C. MCC. BROOKS: Control of activity of neurons in the supraoptic nucleus. J. Neurophysiol. **27**, 878—892 (1964).

KOVACS, K., D. BACHRACH, A. JAKOBOVITS, E. HORVATH u. B. KORPASSY: Hypothalamohypophyseale Beziehungen der Flüssigkeitsentziehung bei Ratten. Endokrinologie **31**, 17—29 17—29 (1954).

KRAMER, K., K. THURAU u. P. DEETJEN: Hämodynamik des Nierenmarks. 1. Capillare Passagezeit, Blutvolumen, Durchblutung, Gewebshämatokrit und O_2-Verbrauch des Nierenmarks *in situ*. Pflügers Arch. ges. Physiol. **270**, 251—269 (1960).

KRECEK, J., H. DLOUHA, and J. KRECKOVA: Cited by KRECEK and HELLER (1962).

—, and J. HELLER: Neurohypophysis and the regulation of water and electrolyte metabolism in infant mammals. Proc. XXII Int. Congr. Physiol. Sci., Vol. 1, pp. 53—69 (1962).

LABELLA, F.S., G. BEAULIEU, and R.J. REIFFENSTEIN: Evidence for the existence of separate vasopressin and oxytocin-containing granules in the neurohypophysis. Nature (Lond.) **193**, 172—173 (1962).

LARSON, E.: Tolerance and fate of the pressor principle of posterior pituitary extract in anaesthetised animals. J. Pharmacol. (Kyoto) **62**, 346—361 (1935).

LASSER, R.P., M.R. SCHOENFELD, D.F. ALLEN, and C.K. FRIEDBERG: Reflex circulatory effects elicited by hypertonic and hypotonic solutions injected into femoral and bracheal arteries of the dog. Circulat. Res. **8**, 913—919 (1960).

LAUSON, H.D.: Unpublished experiments. Cited by LAUSON (1960).

— Vasopressin and oxytocin in the plasma of man and other mammals. In: Hormones and human plasma, pp. 225—293. Ed. by H.N. ANTONIADES. Boston: Little, Brown and Co. 1960.

— Antidiuretic hormone. Fed. Proc. **24**, 731—736 (1965).

—, and M. BOCANEGRA: Clarance of exogenous vasopressin from plasma in dogs. Amer. J. Physiol. **200**, 493—497 (1961).

— —, and C.F. BEUZEVILLE: Hepatic and renal clearance of vasopressin from plasma of dogs. Amer. J. Physiol. **209**, 199—214 (1965).

LEDERIS, K.: Vasopressin and oxytocin in the mammalian hypothalamus. Gen. Comp. Endocr. **1**, 80—89 (1961).

— Ultrastructure of the hypothalamo-neurohypophysial system in teleost fishes and isolation of the hormone containing granules from the neurohypophysis. Z. Zellforsch. **58**, 192—213 (1962).

— Hormonal and ultrastructural changes in the hypothalamo-neurohypophysial system following osmotic stimulation. Gen. Comp. Endocr. **3**, 714—715 (1963).

— Fine structure and hormone content of the hypothalamo-neurohypophysial system of the rainbow trout (Salmo irideus) exposed to sea water. Gen. Comp. Endocr. **4**, 638—661 (1964).

— An electron microscopical study of the human neurohypophysis. Z. Zellforsch. **65**, 847 to 868 (1965).

— Personal communication (1966).

—, and H. HELLER: Intracellular storage of vasopressin and oxytocin in the posterior pituitary lobe. Acta endocr. (Kbh.), Suppl. **51**, 115—116 (1960).

—, and A. LIVINGSTONE: Acetylcholinesterase content of rabbit neurohypophyses. J. Physiol. (Lond.) **186**, 37—38 (1966).

LEDSOME, J.R., R.J. LINDEN, and W.J. O'CONNOR: The mechanism by which distention of the left atrium produces diuresis. J. Physiol. (Lond.) **159**, 86—90 (1961).

LEE, J.: Antidiuretic activity in the blood and urine in cirrhosis of the liver. Acta endocrin. (Kbh.), Suppl. **51**, 129—130 (1960).

—, J.J. JONES, and M.A. BARRACLOUGH: Inappropriate secretion of vasopressin. Lancet **1964 II**, 792—793.

—, and D.N.S. KERR: The concentrations of vasopressin in the blood in patients with hepatic cirrhosis. Clin. Sci. **28**, 375—384 (1963).

LEVEQUE, J.E., and M. SMALL: The relationship of the pituicyte to the posterior lobe hormones. Endocrinology **65**, 909—915 (1959).

LEVITT, M.F., M.H. HALPERN, D.P. POLIMEROS, A.Y. SWEET, and D. GRIBETZ: The effect of abrupt changes in plasma calcium concentration on renal function and electrolyte excretion in man and monkey. J. clin. Invest. **37**, 294—305 (1958).

LEWIS, A.A.G.: The control of the renal excretion of water. Ann. roy. Coll. Surg. Engl. **13**, 36—54 (1953).

—, and T.M. CHALMERS: A nicotine test for the investigation of diabetes insipidus. Clin. Sci. **167**, 137—144 (1951).

LEYDEN-WEBB, J.: Metabolic Inhibitors. New York: Academic Press 1963.

LIDDLE, G.W., D.P. ISLAND, R.L. NEY, W.E. NICHOLSON, and N. SHIMIZA: Non-pituitary neoplasm and Cushing's syndrome. Arch. Inst. Med. **111**, 471—475 (1963).

LINDNER, E.B., A. ELMQUIST, and J. PORATH: Gel filtration as a method of purification of protein bound peptides exemplified by oxytocin and vasopressin. Nature (Lond.) **184**, 1565 (1959).

LINZELL, J.L.: Some observations on the contractile tissue of the mammary glands. J. Physiol. (Lond.) **130**, 257—267 (1955).

— Some observations on the contractile tissue of the mammary gland. J. Physiol. (Lond.) **130**, 257—267 (1955).

LIPSETT, M.B., W.D. ODELL, L.E. ROSENBERG, and T.A. WALDMANN: Humoral syndromes associated with non-endocrine tumours. Ann. intern. Med. **61**, 733—756 (1964).

LITTLE, J.B., L.M. KLEVAY, E.P. RADFORD, and R.B. MCGANDY: Antidiuretic hormone inactivation by isolated perfused rat liver. Amer. J. Physiol. **211**, 786—792 (1966).

—, and E.P. RADFORD: Circulating antidiuretic hormone in rats. Effects of dietary electrolytes and protein. Amer. J. Physiol. **207**, 821—825 (1964).

—, V.W. SMITH, A.G. JESSIMAN, H. SELENKOW, W. VAN'T HOFF, J.M. ELGIN, and F.D. MOORE: Hypophysectomy during pregnancy in a patient with cancer of the breast. A case report with hormone studies. J. clin. Endocr. **18**, 425—443 (1958).

LLOYD, C.W.: In: The neurohypophysis. Ed. by H. HELLER. London: Butterworths 1957.

LOVE, A.H., R.A. RODDIE, J. ROSENSWEIG, and R.C. SHANKS: The effect of pressure changes in the respiral air on the renal excretion of water and electrolytes. Clin. Sci. **16**, 281—296 (1957).

MACARTHUR, C.G.: A new posterior pituitary preparation. Science **73**, 448 (1931).

MACAULEY, M.: Quoted in FOLLEY (1952).

MACFARLANE, W.V., and K.W. ROBINSON: Seasonal changes in plasma antidiuretic activity produced by standard heat stimulus. J. Physiol. (Lond.) **135**, 1—11 (1957).

MALANDRA, B.: Etude preliminaire du systeme neurosecretaire diencephalique neurohypophysaire par S^{35}. In: Proc. 2nd Int. Symposium on Neurosecretion. Berlin-Göttingen-Heidelberg: Springer 1958.

MANUNTA, G., e A. MARONGUI: Inattivazione dell'oxitocina *in vivo* negli ovini. Boll. Soc. ital. Biol. sper. **37**, 510—512 (1961).

MATHE, G., et J. ALTMAN: Contribution experimentale a l'etude de l'inactivation hepatique de la pitressin. Presse med. **62**, 983—985 (1954).
MAYER, F.S.: Identification of the antidiuretic substance in human urine. Acta endocr. (Kbh.) **35**, 568—574 (1960).
MAZER, A., J. ALLEGRINI, et R. LEMAIRE: Localisation des zones vaso-sensibles carotidiens responsable de la secretion de l'hormone antidiuretique chez le chien. C.R. Soc. Biol. (Paris) **156**, 718—721 (1962a).
— — — Influence des hypotensions moderees sur le reflex antidiuretique a prend depas carotidien. C.R. Soc. Biol. (Paris) **156**, 730—732 (1962b).
MIKULAS, I., and H. DLOUHA: Cited by KRECEK and HELLER (1962).
MILES, B.E., and H.E. DE WARDENER: Renal vasoconstriction produced by ether and cyclopropane anaesthesia. J. Physiol. (Lond.) **118**, 140—144 (1952).
MILLER, G.E., and C.E. TOWNSEND: The *in vitro* inactivation of Pitressin by normal and cirrhotic human liver. J. clin. Invest. **33**, 549—553 (1954).
MILLS, E., and S.C. WANG: Liberation of antidiuretic hormone; pharmacologic blockade of ascending pathways. Amer. J. Physiol. **207**, 1405—1410 (1964).
MITIKEN, J.M., and W.W. DOUGLAS: Effect of Ca^{++} and other ions on vasopressin release from rat neurohypophysis stimulated electrically *in vitro*. Nature (Lond.) **207**, 302 (1965).
MOLL, J.: Regeneration of the supraoptico-hypophyseal tracts in the hypophysectomised rat. Z. Zellforsch. **46**, 686—709 (1957).
MOLLER-CHRISTENSON, E.: Investigations on the inactivation of vasopressin in the liver. Acta endocr. (Kbh.) **6**, 153—160 (1951).
MONACI, M., et P. NOCENTINI: La 'neuricrinie' hypothalamo-hypophysaire au cours du choc et de l'hyperthermie generalisee controllee. Anesthesie **12**, 3—17 (1955).
MOREL, F.: Quelques aspects de la regulation endocrienne de l'equilibre hydroaineral enregistres chez le rat a l'aide du radio sodium Na^{24}. Bull. Biol. France Belg., Suppl. **39**, 1—110 (1955).
MORITA, H., T. ISHIBASHI, and S. YAMASHITA: Synaptic transmission in neurosecretory cells. Nature (Lond.) **191**, 183 (1961).
MORRIS, G.C., A.S. KEATS, J.H. MOYER, and M.E. DE BAKEY: Renal function during anaesthesia for cardiovascular surgery. Anaesthesiology **20**, 608—612 (1959).
MOSES, A.M., T.F. LEVEQUE, M. GIAMBATISTA, and C.W. LLOYD: Dissociation between the content of vasopressin and neurosecretory material in the rat neurohypophysis. J. Endocr. **26**, 273—278 (1963).
MOTZFELDT, K.: Experimental studies on the relation of the pituitary body to renal function. J. exp. Med. **25**, 153—188 (1917).
MÜLLER-HARTBERG, W., H. NESVADBA, and H. TUPPY: Arch. Gynaecol. **191**, 442. Quoted by H. TUPPY. In: Polypeptides which affect smooth muscles and blood vessels. Ed. by M. SCHACHTER. Oxford: Pergamon Press 1959.
MURAKAMI, M.: Neurosekretorische Zellen im Hypothalamus der Maus. Z. Zellforsch. **56**, 277—299 (1962).
MURDAUGH, H.V., H.O. SIEKER, and F. MANFREDI: Effects of altered intrathoracic pressure on renal hemodynamics, electrolyte excretion and water clearance. J. clin. Invest. **38**, 834 (1959).
NEWTON, M.: Human lactation. Chapter 7. In: Milk; the mammary gland and its secretion. Ed. by S.K. KON and A.T. COWIE. London: Academic Press 1961.
NIBBELINK, D.W.: Paraventricular nuclei, neurohypophysis and parturition. Amer. J. Physiol. **200**, 1229—1232 (1961).
NIELSEN, B.: Correlation between antidiuretic hormone effect and the renal excretion of calcium and magnesium in man. Acta endocr. (Kbh.) **45**, 151—160 (1964).
NISHIOKA, R.S., H.A. BERN, and L.R. MEWALDT: Ultrastructural aspects of the neurohypophysis of the white-crowned sparrow *Zonotrichia leucophrys gambeii*, with special reference to the relation of neurosecretory axons to ependyma in the pars nervosa. Gen. Comp. Endocrinol. **4**, 304—313 (1964).
NOBLE, R.L., and N.B.G. TAYLOR: Antidiuretic substances in human urine after haemorrhage, fainting, dehydration and acceleration. J. Physiol. (Lond.) **122**, 220—237 (1953).
NOODLE, B.: Metabolism of oxytocin in the mammary gland. Proc. Int. Union Physiol. XXII Int. Congr. Leiden, Abstr. Comm. No. 523 (1962).
O'CONNOR, W.J.: The role of the neurohypophysis of the dog in determining urinary changes and the antidiuretic activity of urine following administration of sodium chloride. Quart. J. exp. Physiol. **36**, 21—48 (1950).
— Renal Function. London: Edward Arnold 1962.
—, and E.B. VERNEY: The effect of removal of the posterior lobe of the pituitary on the inhibition of water diuresis by emotional stress. Quart. J. exp. Physiol. **31**, 393—408 (1942).
— — The effect of increased activity of the sympathetic system in the inhibition of water diuresis by emotional stress. Quart. J. exp. Physiol. **33**, 77—90 (1945).

OLIVECRONA, H.: Paraventricular nucleus and pituitary gland. Acta physiol. scand. **40**, Suppl. 136 (1957).

OOTA, Y., and H. KOBAYASHI: Fine structure of the median eminence and pars nervosa of the pigeon. Annotationes Zool. Japon. **35**, 128—138 (1962).

ORTMANN, R.: Über experimentelle Veränderungen der Morphologie des Hypophysen-Zwischenhirnsystems und die Beziehung der sog. „Gomori-Substanz" zum Adiuretin. Z. Zellforsch. **36**, 92—140 (1951).

OTT, I., and J.C. SCOTT: The action of infundibulin upon the mammary secretion. Proc. Soc. exp. Biol. (N.Y.) **8**, 48—49 (1910).

PAGE,, E.W. The value of plasma pitocinase determination in obstetrics. Amer. J. Obstet. Gynec. **52**, 1014—1021 (1946).

PALAY, S.L.: An electron microscope study of the neurohypophysis in normal, hydrated and dehydrated rats. Anat. Rec. **121**, 348 (1955).

— The fine structure of the neurohypophysis. In: Ultrastructure and cellular chemistry of neural tissue, pp. 31—49. Ed. by H. WAELSCH. New York: Hoeber 1957.

— The fine structure of secretory neurones in the preoptic nucleus of the goldfish (Carassius auratus). Anat. Rec. **138**, 417—443 (1960).

PARDOE, A.V., and M. WEATHERALL: Intracellular localization of oxytocic and vasopressor substances in pituitary glands of rats. J. Physiol. (Lond.) **127**, 201—212 (1955).

PEARCE, M.L., and E.V. NEWMAN: Some postural adjustments of salt and water excretion. J. clin. Invest. **33**, 1089 (1954).

PEETERS, G., and R. COUSSENS: The influence of the milking acts on the diuresis of the lactating cow. **84**, 209—220 (1950).

— —, and G. SIERENS: Physiology of the nerves to the bovine mammary gland. Arch. Int. Pharmacodyn. **79**, 75—82 (1949).

—, G. SIERENS, and M. SILVER: The exclusion of milk in the isolated perfused udder of the cow. Arch. int. Pharmacodyn. **88**, 413—424 (1952).

—, H. STORMORKEN, and F. VANSCHOUBROEK: The effect of different stimuli on milk-ejection and diuresis in the lactating cow. J. Endocr. **20**, 163—172 (1960).

PEPLER, W.J., and A.G.E. PEARSE: The histochemistry of the esterase of rat brains with special reference to those of the hypothalamic nuclei. J. Neurochem. **1**, 193—202 (1957).

PERLMUTT, J.H.: Reflex antidiuresis after occlusion of common carotid arteries in hydrated dogs. Amer. J. Physiol. **204**, 197—201 (1963).

PETERS, J.P.: Body water. Springfield: C.C. Thomas 1935.

PETERSDORF, R.G., and L.G. WELT: The effect of an infusion of hyperoncotic albumin on the excretion of water and solutes. J. clin. Invest. **32**, 283—291 (1953).

PETERSEN, M.J., and I.S. EDELMAN: Calcium inhibition of the action of vasopressin on the urinary bladder of the toad. J. clin. Invest. **43**, 583—594 (1964).

PETERSON, W.E., and T.M. LUDWICK: The humoral nature of the factor causing the let-down of milk. Fed. Proc. **1**, 66—67 (1942).

PICKFORD, M.: The inhibitory effect of acetylcholine on diuresis in the dog and its pituitary transmission. J. Physiol. (Lond.) **95**, 226—238 (1939).

— The action of acetylcholine on the supraoptic nucleus of the chloralosed dog. J. Physiol. (Lond.) **106**, 264—270 (1947).

— The release of oxytocin and vasopressin in polypeptides which affect smooth muscles and blood vessels, pp. 42—47. Ed. by M. SCHACHTER. Oxford: Pergamon Press 1960.

—, and J.A. WATT: A comparison of the effects of intravenous and intracarotid injections of acetylcholine in the dog. J. Physiol. (Lond.) **114**, 333—335 (1951a).

— — Comparison of the action of adrenaline and nor-adrenaline on the kidney. Quart. J. exp. Physiol. **36**, 205—212 (1951b).

PICKLES, V.R.: Blood flow estimations as indices of mammary activity. J. Obstet. Gynaec. Brit. Cwlth **60**, 301—311 (1953).

PREDDIE, E.C.: Structure of a large polypeptide of bovine posterior pituitary tissue. J. biol. Chem. **240**, 4194—4203 (1965).

—, and M. SAFFRAN: Isolation of a large polypeptide from bovine posterior pituitary powder. J. biol. Chem. **240**, 4189—4193 (1965).

RALLI, E.P., J.S. ROBSON, D. CLARKE, and C.L. HOAGLAND: Factors influencing ascites in patients with cirrhosis of the liver. J. clin. Invest. **24**, 316—325 (1945).

RALPH, C.L.: Some effects of hypothalamic lesions on gonadotrophin release in the hen. Anat. Rec. **134**, 411—421 (1959).

RAMCHANDRAN, L.K., and T. WINNICK: Peptides of neuro-intermediate lob of hog pituitary gland. Biochim. biophys. Acta (Amst.) **23**, 533—540 (1957).

RASMUSSEN, A.T.: Innervation of the hypophysis. Endocrinology **23**, 263—278 (1938).

READ, R.C., and J.A. VICK: Cholinergic-like effects of hypertonic solution. Amer. J. Physiol. **200**, 233 (1961).

RENNELS, E.G.: Effects of lactation on the neurohypophysis of the rat. Tex. Rep. Biol. Med. **16**, 219—231 (1958).

—, and G.V. DRAGER: Relationship of pituicytes to neurosecretion. Anat. Rec. **122**, 193—203 (1955).

RINNE, V.K.: Neurosecretory material around the hypophysial portal vessels in the median eminence of the rat. Studies on its histological and histochemical properties and functional significance. Acta endocr. (Kbh.) **35**, Suppl. 57, 1—108 (1960).

ROBERTIS, E. DE: Histophysiology of synapses and neurosecretion. Oxford: Pergamon Press 1964.

ROBINSON, K.W., and M.V. MACFARLANE: The influence of environmental temperature on the level of plasma antidiuretic substances in the rat. Aust. J. biol. Sci. **9**, 130—138 (1957).

RODECK, H.: Neurosekretion und Wasserhaushalt bei Neugeborenen und Säuglingen. Beih. Arch. Kinderheilk. **36**, 1—62 (1958).

— Zusammenhänge zwischen Neurosekret und den sogenannten Hypophysenhinterlappenhormonen. III. Mitt. Untersuchungen zur farbtechnischen Darstellung von synthetischem Oxytocin. Z. ges. exp. Med. **132**, 122—135 (1959a).

— Zusammenhänge zwischen Neurosekret und den sogenannten Hypophysenhinterlappenhormonen. IV. Mitt. Untersuchungen an schwefelhaltigen Aminsoäuren. Z. ges. exp. Med. **132**, 225—235 (1959b).

—, u. R. CAESAR: Zur Entwicklung des neurosekretorischen Systems bei Saugern und Mensch und der Regulationsmechanismen des Wasserhautshaltes. Z. Zellforsch. **44**, 666—691 (1956).

ROSENFELD, M.: The native hormones of the posterior pituitary gland; the pressor and oxytocic principles. Bull. Johns Hopk. Hosp. **66**, 398—403 (1940).

ROTHBALLER, A.B.: Changes in rat neurohypophysis induced by painful stimuli with particular reference to neurosecretory material. Anat. Rec. **115**, 21—41 (1953).

RUBINI, M.E., A.V. WOLF, and W.V. MORONEY: Effects of sea water on the metabolism of men without food or sufficient water. Research report WRAIR, 190-56. Cited from WOLF. THIRST. Springfield: C.C. Thomas 1958.

RUCH, W.: Estimation of antidiuretic hormone in the urine of healthy subjects and patients with inappropriate secretion of vasopressin (Schwartz-Bartter Syndrome). Acta endocr. (Kbh.) **54**, 113—121 (1967).

RYDIN, A., and E.B. VERNEY: The inhibition of water diuresis by emotional stress and muscular exercise. Quart. J. exp. Physiol. **27**, 343—374 (1938).

SACHS, H.: Vasopressin biosynthesis. I. *In vivo* studies. J. Neurochem. **5**, 297—303 (1960).

— Studies in the intracellular distribution of vasopressin. J. Neurochem. **10**, 289—297 (1963a).

— Vasopressin biosynthesis. II. Incorporation of ^{35}S cysteine into vasopressin and protein associated with cell fractions. J. Neurochem. **10**, 299—311 (1963b).

—, and Y. TAKABATAKE: Evidence for a precursor in vasopressin biosynthesis. Endocrinology **75**, 943—948 (1964).

SAMUELS, A.J., L.L. BAJARSKY, R.W. GERARD, B. LIBET, and M. BRUST: Distribution, exchange and migration of phosphate compounds in the nervous system. Amer. J. Physiol. **164**, 1—15 (1951).

SATO, G.: Über die Beziehung des Diabetes insipidus zum Hypophysenhinterlappen und zum Tuber cinereum. Arch. Exp. Pathol. Pharmakol. **131**, 45—69 (1928).

SAWYER, C.H.: Cholinesterases in degenerating and regenerating peripheral nerves. Amer. J. Physiol. **146**, 266—253 (1946).

—, and B.E. GERNANDT: Effects of intracarotid and intravenous injections of hypertonic solution on electrical activity of the rabbit brain. Amer. J. Physiol. **185**, 209—216 (1956).

SAWYER, W.H.: Inactivation of oxytocin by homogenates of uteri and other tissues from normal and pregnant rats. Proc. Soc. exp. Biol. (N.Y.) **87**, 463—465 (1954).

— Neurohypophysial peptides and water excretion in the vertebrates. Mem. Soc. Endocrinol. No. 13, 45—48 (1963).

—, W.Y. CHAN, and H.B. VAN DYKE: Antidiuretic responses to neurohypophysial hormones and some of their analogues in dogs and rats. Endocrinology **71**, 536—540 (1962).

—, H. VALTIN, and A.W. SOKOL: Neurohypophysial principles in rats with familial diabetes insipidus (Brattleboro' strain). Endocrinology **74**, 153—155 (1964).

SCHAPIRO, S., and L. STJARNE: Evidence for the granular localization of the posterior pituitary hormones. Nature (Lond.) **189**, 669 (1961).

SCHARRER, B.: The role of neurosecretion in neuroendocrine integration. In: Comparative endocrinology, pp. 134—148. Ed. by A. GORBMAN. New York: Wiley 1959.

SCHARRER, E.: The final common path in neuroendocrine integration. Arch. Anat. micr. Morph. exp. **54**, 359—370 (1965).

— The maturation of the hypothalamic-hypophyseal neurosecretory system in the dog. Anat. Rec. **118**, 437 (1954).

SCHARRER, E., and S. BROWN: Electron-microscopic studies of neurosecretory cells in lumbricus terrestris. Mem. Soc. Endocrinol. No. 12, 103—108 (1962).
—, and B. SCHARRER: Secretory cells within the hypothalamus. Res. Publ. Ass. nerv. ment. Dis. XX, 170—194 (1940).
— — Neurosecretion. In: Handbuch der mikroskopischen Anatomie des Menschen. Ed. by W. BARGMANN, Vol. VI, part 5. Berlin-Göttingen-Heidelberg: Springer 1954.
SCHEER, R., L.G. RAISZ, and C.W. LLOYD: Change in diabetes insipidus during pregnancy and lactation. J. clin. Endocr. **19**, 805—811 (1959).
SCHIEBLER, T.H.: Zur Histochemie des neurosekretonischen hypothalamisch-neurohypophysären Systems. Arch. Anat. **13**, 233—255 (1951).
— Die chemischen Eigenschaften der neurosekretonischen Substanz in Hypothalamus und Neurohypophyse. Exp. Cell Res. **3**, 249—250 (1952a).
— Cytochemische und elektronenmikroskopische Untersuchungen an granularen Fraktionen der Neurohypophyse des Rindes. Z. Zellforsch. **36**, 563—576 (1952b).
SCHLICHTEGROLL, A. v.: Vasopressorische und oxytosische Wirkung in Hypothalamus und Hypophysenhinterlappenextrakten. Naturwissenschaften **41**, 188—189 (1954).
SCHNIEDEN, H.: Comparison between the effects of intravenous and intraportal vasopressin in normal rats, malnourished rats, and rats treated with carbon tetrachloride. J. Endocr. **24**, 397—402 (1962).
—, and E.K. BLACKMORE: The effect of nalorphine on the antidiuretic action of morphine in rat and man. Brit. J. Pharmacol. **10**, 45—50 (1955).
SCHOCKHAERT, J.A., et J. LAMBILLON: Sur la presence d'une substance antagoniste de la vasopressine dans le serum des femmes enceintes. C.R. Soc. Biol. (Paris) **119**, 1194—1197 (1935).
SCHRODER, R., and D. ROTT: Über die Bestimmung und das Verhalten von ADH im menschlichen Plasma. Klin. Wschr. **37**, 1175—1181 (1959).
SCHWARTZ, W.B., W. BENNET, S. CURELOP, and F.C. BARTTER: Syndrome of renal sodium loss and hyponatremia probably resulting from inappropriate secretion of antidiuretic hormone. Amer. J. Med. **23**, 529—542 (1957).
SELYE, H., and E.C. HALL: Further studies concerning the action of sodium chloride on the pituitary. Anat. Rec. **86**, 579—583 (1943).
SHANNON, J.A.: Control of the renal excretion of water; rate of liberation of posterior pituitary antidiuretic hormone in the dog. J. exp. Med. **76**, 387—399 (1942).
SHARE, L.: Acute reduction in extracellular fluid volume and the concentration of antidiuretic hormone in blood. Endocrinology **69**, 925—933 (1961).
— Vascular volume and blood level of antidiuretic hormone. Amer. J. Physiol. **202**, 791 (1962).
— Effects of carotid occlusion and left atrial distention on concentration of ADH in blood. Amer. J. Physiol. **208**, 219—223 (1965).
—, and M.N. LEVY: Cardiovascular receptors and blood titre of antidiuretic hormone. Amer. J. Physiol. **203**, 425—428 (1962).
— — Effect of carotid chemoreceptor stimulation in plasma antidiuretic hormone titre. Amer. J. Physiol. **210**, 157—161 (1966a).
— — Carotid sinus pulse pressure as a determinent of plasma antidiuretic hormone activity. Amer. J. Physiol. **211**, 721—724 (1966b).
SHIRLEY, H.V., and A.V. NALBANDOV: Effects of neurohypophysectomy in domestic chickens. Endocrinology **58**, 477—483 (1956).
SICA-BLANCO, Y., C. MENDEZ-BAUER, N. SALA, H.M. CABOT, e R. CALDEYRO-BARCIA: Neuro metudo para el Estudio de la functionalidad mammaria en la mujer. Arch. Ginec. Obstet. **17**, 63—72 (1959).
SIDDIQI, S., and J.M. WALKER: Oxytocin activity of blood applied directly to the "superfused" uterus of the rat. J. Physiol. (Lond.) **149**, 12 p. (1959).
SILVER, L., I.E. SCHWARTZ, C.T.O. FONG, A.F. DEBONS, and L.K. DAHL: Disappearance of plasma radioactivity after injection of H^3 or I^{131} labelled arginine vasopressin. J. appl. Physiol. **16**, 1097—1099 (1961).
SKADHAUGE, E.: Effects of unilateral infusion of arginine vasotocin into the portal circulation of the avian kidney. Acta endocr. (Kbh.) **47**, 321—330 (1964).
SLOPER, J.C.: Histochemical observations on the neurohypophysis in dog and cat with reference to the relationship between neurosecretory material and posterior lobe hormone. J. Anat. (Lond.) **88**, 576 (1954).
— Hypothalamic neurosecretion in the dog and cat with particular reference to the identification of neurosecretory material with posterior lobe hormone. J. Anat. (Lond.) **89**, 301—316 (1955).
— Hypothalamo-neurohypophysial secretion. Int. Rev. Cytol. **7**, 337—389 (1958).

SLOPER, J.C.: The experimental and cytopathological investigation of neurosecretion in the hypothalamus and pituitary. In: The pituitary gland, vol. II, pp. 131—239. Ed. by G.W. HARRIS and B.T. DONOVAN: Oxford: Butterworths 1965.
—, and C.W.M. ADAMS: The hypothalamic elaboration of posterior pituitary principle in man; evidence derived from hypophysectomy. J. Path. Bact. **72**, 587—602 (1956).
—, P.J. ARNOTT, and B.C. KING: Sulphur metabolism in the pituitary gland and hypothalamus of the rat; a study of radioisotope uptake after the injection of ^{35}S dl cysteine, methionine and sodium sulphate. J. Endocr. **20**, 9 (1960).
—, and R.G. BATESON: Ultrastructure of neurosecretory cells in the supraoptic nucleus of the dog and rat. J. Endocr. **31**, 139—150 (1965).
SMITH, M.W.: The effect of hyaluronidase and cortisol on the inactivation of vasopressin by rat kidney slices. J. Endocr. **24**, 415—424 (1962).
— The effect of calcium on the inactivation of vasopressin by rat kidney slices. J. Physiol. (Lond.) **166**, 22—23 (1963).
—, and M. GINSBURG: The fate of synthetic oxytocin analogues in the rat. Brit. J. Pharmacol. **16**, 244—252 (1961).
—, and H. SACHS: Inactivation of arginine vasopressin by rat kidney slices. Biochem. J. **69**, 663—669 (1961).
—, and N.A. THORN: The effects of calcium on protein-binding and metabolism of arginine vasopressin in rats. J. Endocr. **32**, 141—151 (1965).
SMITH, R.E., and M. ROSENFELD: Chromatographic study of the native oxytocin hormone of the neurohypophysis. J. Pharmacol. (Kyoto) **136**, 1 (1961).
SMITH, S.W.: Neurohypophyseal hormones. Discussion. In: Advances in neuroendocrinology, pp. 86—89. Ed. by A.V. NALBANDOV. Urbana: University of Illinois Press 1963.
SOKOL, H.W., and H. VALTIN: Morphology of the neurosecretory system in rats homozygous and heterozygous for hypothalamic diabetes insipidus (Brattleboro' strain). Endocrinology **77**, 692—700 (1965).
SOUSA, R.C. DE, B. BERDE, et R.S. MACH: Syndrome de secretion inappropriee d'hormone antidiuretique (syndrome de Schwartz-Bartter). Secretion intrahumorale de l'arginine vasopressine ou d'analogues des vasopressines. Ann. Endocr. (Paris) **25**, 756—763 (1965).
STOUFFER, J.E., D.B. HOPE, and V. DU VIGNEAUD: Neurophysin, oxytocin and desamino-oxytocin. In: Perspectives in biology, pp. 75—80. Ed. by C.F. CORI, V.G. FOGLIA, L.F. LELOIR, and S. OCHOA. Amsterdam: Elsevier Publ. Co. 1963.
STUTINSKY, F.: Sur l'origine de la substance Gomori-positive du complexe hypothalamo-hypophysaire. C.R. Soc. Biol. (Paris) **145**, 367—373 (1951).
— Effects de l'hypophysectomie totale ou partielle sur la neurosecretion hypothalamique du rat. C.R. Ass. Anat. 42ieme Reunion (1955).
— Recherches experimentales sur la complexe hypothalamo-neurohypophysaire. Arch. Anat. micr. Morph. exp. **46**, 93—158 (1957).
SUNDSTEN, J.W., and C.H. SAWYER: Electroencephalographic evidence of osmosensitive elements in olfactory bulb of dog brain. Proc. Soc. exp. Biol. (N.Y.) **101**, 524—527 (1956).
— — Osmotic activation of the neurohypophysial milk-ejection reflex in rabbits with "diencephalic glands". Fed. Proc. **19**, 293, No. 7 (1960).
— — Osmotic activation of neurohypophysial hormone release in rabbits with hypothalamic islands. Exp. Neurol. **4**, 548—561 (1961).
SUPEK, Z., and V. EISEN: The action of nervous depressants on the antidiuretic and chloruretic effect of nicotine. Arch. int. Pharmacodyn. **93**, 75—82 (1953).
SURTSHIN, A.J., A.J. HOLTZENBEIN, and H.L. WHITE: Some effects of negative pressure breathing on urine excretion. Amer. J. Physiol. **180**, 612 (1955).
TAKABATAKE, Y., and H. SACHS: Vasopressin biosynthesis. III. *In vitro* studies. Endocrinology **75**, 934—942 (1964).
TALANTI, S., and E. KIVALO: The infundibular recess in the brain of *Camelus dromedarius* with particular reference to neurosecretory pathways into the third ventricle. Experientia (Basel) **17**, 470 (1961).
TANAKA, K., and S. NAKAJO: Participation of neurohypophysial hormone in oviposition in the hen. Endocrinology **70**, 453—458 (1962).
TAYLOR, N.B.G., J. HUNTER, and W.H. JOHNSON: Antidiuresis as a measurement of laboratory induced motion sickness. Canad. J. Biochem. **35**, 1017—1027 (1957).
—, and J.M. WALKER: Antidiuretic substances in human urine after smoking. J. Physiol. (Lond.) **113**, 312—418 (1951).
THEOBALD, G.W.: The separate release of oxytocin and ADH. J. Physiol. (Lond.) **149**, 443 to 461 (1959).
THOMAS, P.J., and M. GINSBURG: Inhibition by l cystine of the binding of lysine^8-vasopressin by porcine neurophysin. Biochem. J. **100**, 9C (1966a).
— — Unpublished observations (1966b).

THOMPSON, W. H.: Preliminary note on renal activity during anaesthesis. Brit. med. J. **1905 I**, 649—650.
THORN, N. A.: Binding *in vitro* of highly purified arginine vasopressin and synthetic oxytocin to rat serum globulin. Acta endocr. (Kbh.) **30**, 472—476 (1959a).
— Some properties of antidiuretic material in the urine of rats. Acta endocr. (Kbh.) **32**, 128 to 133 (1959b).
— Correlation between antidiuretic hormone effect and changes in renal excretion of calcium in rats and dogs. Acta endocr. (Kbh.) **38**, 563—570 (1961).
— Role of calcium in the release of vasopressin and oxytocin from posterior pituitary protein. Acta endocr. (Kbh.) **50**, 357—364 (1965).
— *In vitro* studies of the release mechanism for vasopressin in rats. Acta endocr. (Kbh.) **53**, 644—654 (1966).
—, and L. SILVER: Chemical form of circulating antidiuretic hormone in rats. J. exp. Med. **105**, 575—583 (1957).
—, and M. W. SMITH: Renal excretion of synthetic arginine vasopressin injected in dogs. Acta endocr. (Kbh.) **49**, 388—392 (1965).
—, and I. TRANSBOK: Hyponatremia and bronchogenic carcinoma associated with renal excretion of large amounts of antidiuretic material. Amer. J. Med. **35**, 257—268 (1963).
—, and N. B. S. WILLUMSEN: Inhibitory action of calcium on the inactivation of antidiuretic hormone by rat kidney slices. Acta endocr. (Kbh.) **44**, 563—569 (1963).
TOWBIN, E. J., and C. B. FERRELL: Stop-flow study of renal excretion of tritiated vasopressin. J. clin. Invest. **42**, 987 (1963).
TUPPY, H.: Enzymic inactivation and degradation of oxytocin and vasopressin. In: Polypeptides which stimulate smooth muscle and blood vessels. Ed. by M. SCHACHTER. London: Pergamon Press 1960.
—, u. H. NESVADBA: Über die Aminopeptidaseaktivität des Schwangerenserums und ihre Beziehung zu dessen Vermögen, Oxytocin zu inaktivieren. Mh. Chem. **88**, 977—988 (1957).
TURNER, C. W., and I. S. SLAUGHTER: The physiological effect of pituitary extract (posterior lobe) on the lactating mammary gland. J. Dairy Sci. **13**, 8—24 (1930).
USAMI, S., and S. CHIEN: Role of hepatic blood flow in regulating the concentration of antidiuretic hormone after haemorrhage. Proc. Soc. exp. Biol. (N.Y.) **113**, 606—609 (1963).
—, B. PERIC, and S. CHIEN: Release of antidiuretic hormone due to common carotid occlusion and its relation with vagus nerve. Proc. Soc. exp. Biol. (N.Y.) **111**, 189—193 (1962a).
USUELLI, F., G. PIANA, e G. M. CURTO: Sui momenti secretori e sulle modalito d'azione dell'Ossitocina durante il parto. Bull. Soc. Ital. Biol. Sper. **28**, 1677—1679 (1952).
VALTIN, H., W. H. SAWYER, and H. W. SOKOL: Neurohypophysial principles in rats homozygous and heterozygous for hypothalamic diabetes insipidus (Brattleboro strain). Endocrinology **71**, 701—706 (1965).
VERNEY, E. B.: Absorption and excretion of water. The antidiuretic hormone. Lancet **1946 II**, 739—744 and 781—783 (1946).
— The antidiuretic hormone and the factors which determine its release. Proc. roy. Soc. B **135**, 25—106 (1947).
VOGT, M.: Vasopressor, antidiuretic and oxytocic activities of extracts of the dogs' hypothalamus. Brit. J. Pharmacol. **8**, 193—196 (1953).
— The concentration of sympathin in different parts of the central nervous system under normal conditions and after the administration of dugs. J. Physiol. (Lond.) **123**, 451—481 (1954).
WAELSCH, H., and A. LAJTHA: Protein metabolism in the nervous system. Physiol. Rev. 709 to 736 (1961).
WAGNER, M. J., D. GRIMSLEY, S. KAHAN, and W. STOLLER: Effects of intracarotid injection of hypertonic saline on spinal reflex excitability. Nature (Lond.) **197**, 390—391 (1963).
WALKER, J. M.: The effect of smoking on antidiuresis in men. Quart. J. Med. **18**, 51—55 (1949).
— Release of vasopressin and oxytocin in response to drugs. In: The neurohypophysis, pp. 221—229. Ed. by H. HELLER. London: Butterworths 1957.
WALMSLEY, C. F.: The concentration of oxytocin in blood in relation to reproduction. Thesis: University of Bristol 1963.
WEIL-MALHERBE, H., L. G. WHITBY, and J. AXELROD: Blood-brain barrier for catecholamines in different regions of the brain. In: Regional neurochemistry, p. 284. Ed. by S. S. KETY and J. ELKES. Oxford: Pergamon Press 1961.
WEINER, J. S.: The diuretic response of men working in hot and humid conditions. J. Physiol. (Lond.) **103**, 36—37 (1945).
WEINSTEIN, H., R. M. BERNE, and H. SACHS: Vasopressin in blood. Effect of haemorrhage. Endocrinology **66**, 712—718 (1960).
—, S. MALAMUD, and H. SACHS: Isolation of vasopressin-containing granules from the neurohypophysis of the dog. Biochim. biophys. Acta (Amst.) **50**, 386—389 (1961).

WEISS, P.: Evidence by isotope tracers of perpetual replacement of mature nerve fibres from their cell body. Science **129**, 1290 (1959).
— The concept of perpetual neuronal growths and proximo-distal substance convection. In: Regional neurochemistry. Ed. by S.E. KETY and J. ELKES. Oxford: Pergamon Press 1961.
—, and M.W. CAVANAUGH: Further evidence of perpetual growth of nerve fibres. Recovery of fibre diameter after the released of prolonged constrictions. J. Exp. Zool. **142**, 461—473 (1959).
—, and H.B. HISCOE: Experiments on the mechanism of nerve growth. J. Exp. Zool. **107**, 315—395 (1948).
WELT, L.G., and J. ORLOFF: The effects of an increase in plasma volume on the metabolism and excretion of water and electrolytes in normal subjects. J. clin. Invest. **30**, 751—752 (1951).
WERLE, E., A. HEVELKE u. K. BUTHMAN: Zur Kenntnis des oxytocin-abbauenden Prinzips des Blutes. Biochem. Z. **309**, 270 (1941).
—, u. A. KALVELAGE: Über die Vasopressin inaktivierende Kraft des Blutes von Schwangeren und die Natur des inaktivierenden Prinzips. Biochem. Z. **308**, 405—412 (1941).
—, u. L. MAIER: Über den Abbau von Oxytocin und Vasopressin durch Milchdrüsenextrakte der Kuh. Naturwissenschaften **41**, 380 (1954).
WHITE, A.G.: Clinical implication of antidiuretic hormone activity. Arch. intern. Med. **102**, 685—689 (1958).
—, G. RUBIN, and L. LEITER: Studies in edema. III. The effect of pitressin on the renal excretion of water and electrolytes in patients with and without liver disease. J. clin. Invest. **30**, 1287—1297 (1951).
— — — Studies in edema. IV. Water retention and the antidiuretic hormone in hepatic and cardiac disease. J. clin. Invest. **32**, 931—939 (1953).
WHITTEMBURY, G., N. SUGINO, and A.K. SOLOMON: Effect of antidiuretic hormone and calcium on the equivalent pore radius of kidney slices from *Necturus*. Nature (Lond.) **187**, 699—701 (1960).
WHITTLESTONE, W.G.: J. Dairy Res. **21**, 19 (1954).
—, E.G. BASSETT, and C.W. TURNER: Phylogenetic study of milk "let down" hormone. Proc. Soc. exp. Biol. (N.Y.) **80**, 191 (1952).
WIED, D. DE: A simple automatic and sensitive method for the assay of antidiuretic hormone with notes on the antidiuretic potency of plasma under different experimental conditions. Acta physiol. pharmacol. neerl. **9**, 69 (1960).
—, and R. JINKS: Effect of chlorpromazine on antidiuretic response to noxious stimuli. Proc. Soc. exp. Biol. (N.Y.) **99**, 44—45 (1958).
WINKLER, A.W., and O.F. CRANKSHAW: Chloride depletion in conditions other than Addison's disease. J. clin. Invest. **17**, 1—6 (1938).
WINNICK, T., R.E. WINNICK, R. ACHER, and C. FROMAGEOT: Amino-acids and peptides of posterior pituitary and hypothalamus tissues. Biochim. biophys. Acta (Amst.) **18**, 488 to 494 (1955).
WIRZ, H.: Der osmotische Druck in den corticalen Tubuli der Rattennieren. Helv. physiol. pharmacol. Acta **14**, 353—362 (1956).
WOLF, A.V., and H.A. EDDY: Effect of hydropenia and the ingestion of tap water and artificial sea waters in the fasting dog. Research report WRAIR. 90-57. Cited from A.V. WOLF. THIRST. Springfield: C.C. Thomas 1957.
WOODBURY, R.A., R.R. AHLQUIST, B. ABREU, R. TORPIN, and W.G. WATSON: The inactivation of pitocin and pitressin by human pregnancy blood. J. Pharmacol. (Kyoto) **86**, 359—365 (1946).
WOODS, J.W., and P. BARD: Antidiuretic hormone secretion in the cat with a centrally denervated hypothalamus. Acta Endocr. **35** (suppl. **51**), 113 (1960).
YAGI, K., H.A. BERN, and T.R. HAGEDORN: Action potentials of neurosecretory neurons in the leech *Theromyzon rude*. Gen. Comp. Endocrinol. **3**, I, 490—495 (1963).
ZEDECK, M.S., L.B. MELETT, and E.J. CAFRUNY: The diuretic effects of Cyclophosphamide and nor-nitrogen mustard. Relationship to antidiuretic hormone. J. Pharmacol. **153**, 550—561 (1966).
ZUIDEMA, G.D., and N.P. CLARK: Central localization of the osmotic control centre. Amer. J. Physiol. **188**, 616—618 (1957).
— —, and M.F. MINTON: Osmotic regulation of body fluids. Amer. J. Physiol. **187**, 85—88 (1956).

The Influence of the Neurohypophysial Hormones and Similar Polypeptides on the Kidneys

NIELS A. THORN

Introduction

Several aspects concerning the subject of the present section have been dealt with in a number of previous reviews (BERDE, 1963; DICKER, 1961, 1964; HELLER, 1951, 1955, 1957; LIPSETT, SCHWARTZ and THORN, 1961; NIELSEN, 1964; PICKFORD, 1966; SAWYER, 1961a, b, c, 1963, 1966; SCHWARTZ and LIVINGSTON, 1964; RUDINGER, 1964a, b; THORN, 1958, 1960a; THORP, 1962; USSING *et al.*, 1960).

In the present chapter the main emphasis will be placed on a physiological, biochemical and pharmacological analysis of the problems involved. In order to save space, reference will sometimes be made to the previous reviews for details concerning certain aspects.

It is generally agreed that vasopressin plays a crucial role in the concentrating mechanism of the kidneys by increasing the permeability to water of the distal part of the nephron. Vasopressin changes the distribution of the pressure fall within the nephron. There is little evidence for striking direct effects on renal transport of sodium and potassium, but vasopressin does bring about a slight increase in the rate of excretion of calcium (and magnesium). In addition, vasopressin may affect the function of certain blood vessels in the kidney. Vasopressin has a general vasopressor effect, but the concentrations needed far exceed physiological ones. Some of the analogues of vasopressin have very weak general vasopressor effects and thus act nearly specifically on the kidneys.

As for oxytocin, the substance in large doses can produce an antidiuretic effect. This is hardly physiological, but it is of interest in the therapeutic use of oxytocin. Its effects on electrolyte transport in the kidney seem to be small. It may affect the function of some of the renal vessels, possibly in conjunction with vasopressin.

I. The Concentrating-Diluting Mechanism of the Mammalian Kidney

The main features of the concentrating-diluting mechanism of the kidney have been elucidated over the past 15 years. The result has been that we have now a fairly clear picture of the regulation of the concentration of water in the body fluids. However, new findings keep turning up, requiring modifications of the original models. This is not the place for a thorough discussion of the details of this mechanism. Instead, reference will be made to a number of comprehensive reviews on the subject (BERLINER *et al.*, 1958; BERLINER and BENNETT, 1967; CHINARD, 1964; FORSTER, 1965; GIEBISCH, 1962; GOTTSCHALK, 1964; THORN, 1958; ULLRICH and MARSH, 1963; KRUHØFFER in USSING *et al.*, 1960; WIRZ, 1961).

Here, a very short summary of the most important aspects of the mechanism will be given, supplemented with a few remarks on some points which need special emphasis.

The basic process underlying the concentrating mechanism of the kidney is a very active reabsorption of sodium taking place in the ascending limb of the loop of Henle and the distal convoluted tubules. The suggestion (THORN, 1960a) that the whole ascending limb is involved has recently received experimental support (JAMISON *et al.*, 1967). By means of this mechanism (arranged as an active countercurrent system) and a low permeability to water of the ascending limb a hypertonicity is created in the medulla of the kidney. To allow the mechanism to act properly, some additional factors work. The vessels are arranged in a hair-pin like structure, which — with relatively low blood flow — allows the maintenance of a passive countercurrent mechanism that prevents washing out of the hypertonicity. Also, a special recirculation goes on for urea and sodium, and the permeabilities of the tubules are "arranged" in a way which allows urea to be excreted in such a manner that it generally does not compromise the sodium pump in its work of concentrating the urine.

The permeability of the distal convoluted tubules and the collecting tubules to water and a number of solutes is of great importance for the concentration of the urine. The main action of the antidiuretic hormone is to regulate this permeability to water. Very small amounts of substance are needed to give this effect. VERNEY (1954) made a calculation of the number of molecules of vasopressin present in each receptor cell in the distal convoluted tubules when the substance exerted its action. Using various assumptions it could be calculated that there were some 500 molecules present per cell.

It should be remembered that there seems to be a species difference in the degree to which the distal convoluted tubules can be influenced by vasopressin. In dogs and monkeys this tubular section seems to be little affected (CLAPP and ROBINSON, 1966; BERLINER and BENNETT, 1967).

It is very often stated that the main point of attack of vasopressin is the medullary part of the collecting tubules. It is true that the concentration of the urine, in the sense of the increase in osmolality over that of the plasma takes place in this segment. Essential for the efficiency of this mechanism, however, is the development of isotonicity from hypotonicity and the simultaneous reduction of urine volume which takes place in the distal convoluted tubules in rats and in the cortical collecting tubules in dogs (CLAPP and ROBINSON, 1966) during antidiuresis. In terms of quantity of water transported this seems to outweigh the transport taking place in the medullary collecting tubules during the influence of vasopressin. By means of the concentrating-diluting mechanism of the kidneys the osmolality of the urine may be varied over a very wide range (in man from some 60 mosm/kg to some 1400 mosm/kg) for references see THORN (1960a). Whereas it may be said in general that antidiuretic hormone increases urine concentration over that present before the administration or release of hormone, the degree of antidiuresis depends on a great number of factors, some of which have been outlined above.

It must be stated that hypertonic urine may be excreted presumably in the total absence of vasopressin (see e.g. VALTIN, 1966b) and, on the other hand that a hypotonic urine can be excreted despite the presence of adequate amounts of vasopressin (see e.g. CLAPP and ROBINSON, 1966; McDONALD and DE WARDENER, 1965). It must also be remembered that under certain circumstances (after loading with hypertonic saline) vasopressin may have a diuretic action (see e.g. KOBINGER, 1964; SCHRÖDER *et al.*, 1961; WITTE *et al.*, 1961; see also DALE, 1957).

The degree of concentration of the urine will depend on a number of factors among which are the capacity of the sodium pumps involved, the rate of flow of blood in the vascular loops and of preurine entering the distal convoluted tubules and the collecting tubules together with tubular fluid concentrations and composition of solutes. This latter may also depend on the food taken (e.g. EPSTEIN *et al.*,

1957; MERONEY *et al.*, 1958). Since so many variables must be considered in the quantitative assessment of renal concentrating capacity, it is very difficult to express the maximum concentrating capacity of the kidneys. So e.g. max. negative free water clearance is measured under very artificial conditions. The varying passive contribution of urea to the osmolality of the urine makes the max. U/P osmolar ratio difficult to interpret.

One of the most recent modifications of the countercurrent model is that of LEVER (1965) in which it is suggested that the cells of the loop of Henle take no essential part in the formation of the countercurrent pattern, which is instead suggested to be established by a pressure effect. This hypothesis seems unlikely for different reasons. It has e.g. been well established that the concentrating mechanism is abolished in the cyanide poisoned or the cooled kidney (LUNDSGAARD, 1935; BICKFORD and WINTON, 1937; see also HERMS and MALVIN, 1963).

NIESEL and RÖSKENBLECK (1965) have worked out several models of countercurrent systems based on permeability differences in the tubular membranes. (For criticism see JAMIESON *et al.*, 1967.)

In the original countercurrent hypothesis of WIRZ and others there were some obscure points which have now been clarified. It has been demonstrated that also the fluid in the loop of Henle is hypertonic (GOTTSCHALK and MYLLE, 1959; see also GOTTSCHALK *et al.*, 1963, and SAKAI *et al.*, 1966) and the contents of the vascular loops equally so (ULLRICH *et al.*, 1961).

It has now been well established that also the medullary tissue in water diuresis is hypertonic, although only to a small degree, and that there is a solute gradient from cortex towards the papillary tip (Rats: SCHMIDT-NIELSEN, 1958; BRAY, 1960; SAIKIA, 1965a. Rabbits: CRAWFORD *et al.*, 1957. Dogs: ULLRICH and JARAUSCH, 1956; LEVITIN *et al.*, 1962; WHITE and ROLF, 1965).

There may be several causes for the fact that this osmolality is very much lower than that found in antidiuresis:

1. an increased medullary blood flow.

2. a decrease in the capacity of the sodium pump in the ascending limb or in the proximal convoluted tubule (CLAPP and ROBINSON, 1966). This might be caused by a decrease in aldosterone secretion.

3. an increased load of fluid to the distal part of the nephron would give a high rate of autonomous back diffusion of water (KIIL and AUKLAND, 1960).

The main part of the hypertonicity of the medulla is produced by electrolytes and urea, but amino acids and other as yet undefined substances contribute to a small extent (ROBINSON *et al.*, 1966).

Very recently it has been demonstrated (CLAPP and ROBINSON, 1966) that the dog differs from rodents by always having hypotonicity over the entire length of the lumen in the distal convoluted tubules.

MARSH (1966) recently claimed that a hypoosmotic reabsorption is responsible for the final phase in the development of hypertonicity of the urine in the papillary collecting ducts. The basis for the hypothesis was a demonstration of the establishment of a (rather small) increase in osmolality in drops placed in the collecting ducts of isolated papillae kept in a medium of the same composition. The assumption was made that there was no osmotic gradient between collecting duct tubular fluid and surrounding tissue, but this was not experimentally tested. More reliable results might have been obtained with isolated collecting tubules. Further evidence seems necessary before one can accept the existence of hypoosmotic reabsorption in the collecting ducts.

Much ignorance still prevails over the role of the renal circulation in the different physiological mechanisms. One reason for this fact is the small size of the medullary blood flow and the great difficulties encountered in measuring it under different circumstances (see p. 379).

Considerable controversy still exists regarding the renal transport processes for urea in the mammal. It has been known for long that urea increases the concentrating capacity of the kidney. Creatinine does not possess this property (MERTZ, 1965). It is often stated that urea contributes to the concentrating mechanism of the kidney. It is true that a considerable part of the medullary hypertonicity is due to urea. If, however, as many authors conclude, urea is treated completely passively by the human kidney, urea cannot contribute "actively" to the concentrating mechanism. However, urea has exquisite qualities as an excretory product, due to its high diffusibility in some sections of the nephron and low permeability in others. By means of the arrangement of the vessels in a countercurrent system and a high permeability to urea in the distal part of the nephron or solvent drag effect there, urea can be excreted without any marked extra work by the cells which are involved in the mechanism of concentration of the urine.

GARDNER and MAFFLY (1964) have suggested that the effect of urea on the concentrating capacity of the kidney might be that urea prevents some water from following sodium in the ascending limb and thus prevents dilution of the papilla, since the detained water is reabsorbed in the cortex before the pre-urine returns to the papilla.

In the collecting tubules a similar process might have much less effect due to a higher permeability to water and urea.

The overall effects of such processes would depend on a number of factors, among which one should emphasize the differential permeability to urea and water in the different segments of the nephron, and the influence of urea concentration on the degree of equilibrium reached (EDELMAN *et al.*, 1966) as well as the possibility of the existence in the mammal of active transport of urea such as has been suggested by various authors (e.g. SCHMIDT-NIELSEN, 1958; LASSITER *et al.*, 1966; CLAPP, 1966; ULLRICH *et al.*, 1967).

II. Comments on some of the Methods Employed in Studies of the Effects of Neurohypophysial Hormones on the Kidneys

In the following section the principles of some methods employed in studies of the effects of neurohypophyseal hormones on the kidneys will be briefly outlined together with some comments on the pitfalls of the methods and their limitations.

A. Hormone Preparation

In the use of hormone preparations some problems have been encountered: LITTLE and RADFORD (1964) described considerable variations in the potency of commercially available Pitressin ampoules. One explanation of this finding is the use of preparations which consist of two chemically different hormones, arginine^8- and lysine^8-vasopressin (HOLLANDER *et al.*, 1957; RAISZ *et al.*, 1958; SCHEER *et al.*, 1959). This inspired NIELSEN (1960) to suggest that an International Standard for Lysine-vasopressin should be established (see also BERDE and CERLETTI, 1961). Recently an International Collaborative Assay has been carried out to compare Arginine^8- and Lysine^8-vasopressin, and an International Standard for Lysine^8-vasopressin may now be established. The preparation proposed is an acetone-dried powder of hog posterior pituitary gland.

Impurities may introduce inaccuracies due to change of the potency per unit weight of the preparation, but this may also be due to an interference with the response.

The interference of substances used for preservation of the hormones should naturally be excluded (see e.g. GRANTHAM and BURG, 1966).

The stability of hormone preparations when they are kept at a pH around 3 and cooled, seems to be high, and the ratio between antidiuretic and pressor potencies seems to remain constant (ADAMSONS *et al.*, 1958; NIELSEN, 1964).

B. State of the Experimental Animal

Hydration with Water, Saline or Hyperosmotic Fluids

It has been an essential feature in many experiments on the effect of vasopressin on kidney function that animals or persons in a water diuresis have been studied, and water diuresis and antidiuresis have then been compared. This is necessary, since in the normal animal hydration has to be induced for depressing the endogenous secretion of vasopressin. Water diuresis has often been established by producing a 5—10% overhydration of the experimental subject. This can be done either by using trained animals or employing anesthetics which do not release vasopressin (Inactin e.g. in rats ULLRICH *et al.*, 1964, and dogs FANG *et al.*, 1962, Thiopental in dogs WHITE and ROLF, 1965). Often, however, care has not been taken to eliminate or reduce dead space errors from the urinary tract when studies of the dynamic or acute phases of changes have been made (see e.g. the study of CHAN, 1965). Such dead space errors are probably greater during hydration. In severe overhydration several parameters of kidney function show marked changes (PERLMUTT, 1962).

The fact that vasopressin administered during a water diuresis can only produce a concentration of the urine that is a fraction of the effect called forth by dehydration can be due to a number of factors. A reduced osmolarity of the medulla (which has been demonstrated, see p. 374) is one possibility. Another possible reason might be that during water diuresis there would be a reduced permeability to water of the proximal convoluted tubules.

It is obvious that in studying physiological mechanisms use of the extremes in experimental situations often helps in obtaining clear-cut results. It should be kept in mind, however, that a state with an overhydration equivalent to 8% of the body weight (a considerable expansion of body water volume) is somewhat artificial. Heavy hydration produces definite changes in the ultrastructure of the rat kidney (GLIMSTEDT *et al.*, 1954; ROBSON, 1963), and possibly increases in renal blood flow (see p. 379). Also, it would not seem to be correct to assume that the concentration of vasopressin in the plasma oscillates around 0, now with secretion and now with inhibition of secretion. At least in the rat it seems that the animal has always some degree of antidiuresis (RADFORD, 1959).

It would seem that many studies might gain in value as bases for drawing conclusions on physiological conditions if they had been carried out with a smaller degree of hydration. Provided that the suppression of endogenous hormone is effective and the elimination is unchanged (see e.g. MILLER *et al.*, 1967), this might be a better base line situation.

It has often been assumed that a severe overhydration completely prevents the release of vasopressin, also during experimental procedures. However, such procedures often do not bring about a complete suppression of the release of vasopressin. This is e.g. the case for the studies of AUKLAND and KJEKSHUS (1966) and BERLINER *et al.* (1958). It should, however, also be remembered that saline infusion can considerably modify renal conditions and the responsiveness to vasopressin (McDonald and de Wardener, 1965; Shuster *et al.*, 1966; Friedler and Earley, 1966).

In several studies on the mechanism of action an osmotic diuresis has been employed (e.g. Foulkes, 1966; Gottschalk *et al.*, 1965). It should be remembered that such a condition is rather artificial (see e.g. Lilien and Spitzer, 1964, and Appelboom *et al.*, 1965).

C. Use of Animals with Diabetes Insipidus

When vasopressin is not secreted, a state of diabetes insipidus develops. This condition can be reversed by injecting vasopressin (Motzfeldt, 1917; Fisher, Ingram, and Ranson, 1938). (In rabbits severe diabetes insipidus cannot be induced experimentally; Cross and Harris, 1952.) In experiments with animals with diabetes insipidus one has the advantage that the overhydration which has to be used in normal animals to suppress release of endogenous vasopressin is absent. This has as a consequence that all the secondary reactions in the body on these severe water loads are absent.

Experimental diabetes insipidus (d.i.) has most often been produced by electrolytic hypothalamic lesions (see e.g. Kennedy, 1960). This produces d.i. of a much higher severity than hypophysectomy (Alexander, 1958).

In many studies it has been tacitly assumed that an animal with diabetes insipidus is not able to release vasopressin so that effects of injections can safely be assumed to be caused exclusively by the substance injected. It should, however, be remembered that no ideal experimental diabetes insipidus exists. Sloper (1960) and Moll and de Wied (1962) and others have demonstrated that after hypophysectomy a release center can be reestablished which functions to some extent as a normal release center. It seems possible that after hypothalamic lesions and development of diabetes insipidus, a severe signal may release hormone from possible regenerated neurons, the function of which is not normally much utilized. There is a need for better methods of establishing diabetes insipidus. Here, possibilities that might be tried would be the selective destruction of the neurons by chemical substances analogous to the alloxan effect on the pancreas or development of specific antibodies to the hormone-producing cells in analogy with immunosympathectomy.

In some cases diabetes insipidus animals have been used in the acute phase after the operation (Ullrich *et al.*, 1964; Gertz *et al.*, 1964). This may yield better results probably partly due to the fact that deficiencies of adenohypophyseal functions have not developed in these animals as yet. They seem to tolerate operation better. Valtin and coworkers (see Valtin, 1967) have discovered a strain of rats with a herediatary hypothalamic diabetes insipidus. This strain would seem to offer certain advantages in experiments on the effects of vasopressin. The rats seem to have only a small disturbance of adenohypophysial function (Galton *et al.*, 1966; McCann *et al.*, 1966). In conjunction with Bauman's findings (1965) (see p. 399) it is of interest that their medullary sodium concentration is not different from that of normal rats. It seems that Valtin's rats have a defect in the synthesis of vasopressin that may be absolute, but it is very difficult to prove that not the slightest release of antidiuretically active peptide may occur under certain circumstances (see p. 402). Valtin's rats have recently been used for bioassay of vasopressin (Sawyer and Valtin, 1967; Vierling *et al.*, 1967). They are more sensitive than normal rats. Possibly they stand the operating procedures less well than normal rats.

D. Interpretation of Data Obtained with the Techniques of Micropuncture, Microperfusion etc.

During the past decade a great many experiments have been performed on kidney function using the techniques of micropuncture, microperfusion and various modifications of these procedures. It must be remembered that even if these techniques have given valuable information, possible errors from a great many factors keep turning up. Also, the experimental conditions have often been somewhat artificial. In a number of studies the composition of distal tubular urine has been compared with that of final urine. This procedure may cause errors, since by micropuncture only the superficial tubules can be punctured. Their composition may not be representative of all distal tubules. Caution should therefore be used in drawing conclusions concerning conditions in vivo from such experiments. In this connection it may be stated that it is only during recent years that methods have been developed for studying renal functions in unanesthetized, undisturbed rats (see e.g. KLEINMAN *et al.*, 1965; MALVIN and FUSCO, 1967).

III. Possible Effects of Neurohypophysial Hormones on Kidney Vessels

Vasopressin does not act on the ureter (ABRAHAMS and PICKFORD, 1956) or on the mammalian bladder (LEVINSKY and BERLINER, 1959), so the present and the following section will only deal with its effects on the nephron "membranes" and kidney vessels.

A. Possible Effects of Vasopressin on Renal Vessels

It seems safe to state that an action on vessels is not essential for the action of vasopressin on the kidney. This point is supported by the fact that the hormone acts on isolated renal collecting tubules (see p. 402), from the fact that the doses necessary to give a general vascular effect are very much higher than those necessary for an antidiuretic effect and finally from the fact that there is no fixed correlation between antidiuretic potency and vascular potency (THORN, 1959e).

In anaesthetized cats and rabbits arginine-vasopressin, lysine-vasopressin and phenylalanine^{2}-lysine^{8}-vasopressin in fairly large doses cause an increase of the renal blood flow (measured with an electromagnetic flowmeter) and a large diuresis (BARER, 1963). This is an effect similar to the original effects reported to be characteristic of vasopressin (see also DALE, 1957).

It seems generally accepted that vasopressin has no striking effect on the glomerular filtration rate (for references see THORN, 1958; BROOKS and PICKFORD, 1958; PICKFORD, 1966; see also PERLMUTT, 1961). It must be remembered in this connection, however, that glomerular filtration rate can only be measured with an accuracy of some 5—10%. In addition to previous arguments against action on glomerular vessels one might perhaps add the findings (CHAUDHURY and WALKER, 1959) that vasopressin is not inactivated by isolated glomeruli. If site of action is identical with site of inactivation, this finding would support the above hypothesis. It should, however, also be mentioned that certain experimental data may be interpreted as showing that vasopressin *does* affect glomerular vessels. This is the case with the finding by SELLWOOD and VERNEY (1955). They showed that when water was given orally to dogs, a rise in inulin clearance ensued which was earlier in onset than the diuresis. This might be due to a decrease in vasopressin effect on glomerular vessels. BOJESEN (1955) discussed whether vasopressin might cause its effect through a vascular action on the glomerular vessels.

If this were so, one should, however, expect a decrease in the rate of excretion of sodium after vasopressin. This has not been found. Otherwise one would have to assume the existence of compensatory reactions in other parts of the nephron. Such reactions have not been described as yet.

The renal medullary blood flow is of considerable importance for the concentrating capacity of the kidney (see e.g. THURAU and DEETJEN, 1962; ABBRECHT and MALVIN, 1961). There are several indications that the medullary blood flow is carried by special systems of vessels and that it may be subjected to a special regulation (see e.g. NISSEN, 1966). There is disagreement on the question whether vasopressin affects medullary blood flow.

Medullary blood flow can be measured by many techniques against practically all of which severe criticism may be raised. One of the essential problems in the interpretation of results is the uncertainties concerning the reference volume of the tissue (see AUKLAND, 1967).

KRAMER's group has mainly employed a photo-electric dye dilution technique. With this technique THURAU *et al.* (1960) demonstrated that in dogs in a water diuresis there was an increase of medullary blood flow which might be as high as about 70%. Administration of vasopressin had the effect that medullary blood flow very gradually returned to normal. In the studies of VALTIN (1966a) no change in the medullary and papillary sodium concentration (mmoles per kg. dry solid) was seen when rats with hereditary hypothalamic diabetes insipidus were treated for 3 days with vasopressin. This seems to go against the hypothesis that vasopressin should decrease a *normal* medullary blood flow (see also THURAU, 1964).

AUKLAND (see AUKLAND and BERLINER, 1964) has developed a technique employing desaturation of the outer medulla for hydrogen gas. Using this method he did not find any striking decrease of medullary blood flow by vasopressin (AUKLAND 1967). The same has been the case in the studies of GRÄNGSJÖ and PERSSON (personal communication) using removal of heat. In the technique of KRAMER and his group the blood flow in a rather large area is measured. The technique of WOLGAST (1966) in which β-sensitive semiconductor needle detectors are employed should provide the possibility of measuring blood flow in very small areas. FOURMAN and MOFFAT (1963) in an abstract described the finding of a much lower medullary blood flow in dehydrated rats than in hydrated animals. FOURMAN and KENNEDY (1966) compared the intensity of staining of the vasa recta by thioflavine S in the renal medulla of normal and d.i. rats in water diuresis and after dehydration. Intense staining was found in normal, hydrated rats. No staining was found in normal rats in endogenous or exogenous antidiuresis. Diabetes insipidus rats, however, showed intense staining, also in dehydration. The results indicated to the authors that vasopressin acts partly by decreasing medullary blood flow. Apparently they assumed that changes in staining were solely an indicator of changes in blood flow, that differences in medullary osmolality did not interfere with the staining, and that difference in staining could be quantitated with reasonable accuracy. LEVITIN *et al.* (1962) showed that the uptake into the renal medulla of radioactive sodium injected i.v. was retarded during antidiuresis as compared to the diuresis state. These data were consistent with the hypothesis that vasopressin slows the blood flow in the medulla. They might, however, also be explained by an increased reabsorption of sodium in the loop of Henle. Large doses of vasopressin are possibly able to increase blood flow through the vasa recta (TRUETA *et al.*, 1947; see also BOBA and POWERS, 1966).

Since it is so difficult to measure medullary blood flow by methods available at present, it seems safe to conclude that it is nearly impossible to exclude variations in this factor as causes of changes in concentrating capacity and as causes of part of the effect of vasopressin on urine concentration. It should be remembered that a decreasing effect of vasopressin on medullary blood flow might have other causes than a vasoconstrictive effect on the vessels. Thus the concentration of the blood subsequent to entry into the kidney medulla might slow down the blood flow (see also CARONE *et al.*, 1967).

B. Possible Effects of Oxytocin on Renal Vessels

Conflicting results have been found regarding the effects of oxytocin on glomerular filtration rate and renal plasma flow. One group of investigators (BROOKS and PICKFORD, 1958; ALI, 1958; HORSTER, KUSCHINSKY and PETERS, 1959) found an increase of these parameters. This was not found by CHAN and SAWYER (1961) (see also HEIDENREICH *et al.*, 1960). All these experiments were done on dogs. In man, variable results concerning effects on GFR and RPF have been found by MERTZ (1960) and by CROSS *et al.* (1960). No effects were found in the studies of ABDUL-KARIM and ASSALI (1961) or by SAUNDERS and MUNSICK (1966).

PICKFORD in her review (1966) advocated that there is an antagonistic effect of vasopressin and oxytocin on some renal blood vessels, so that vasopressin constricts these vessels whereas they are dilated by oxytocin. In agreement with such a hypothesis is the suggestion of LEVKOFF *et al.* (1954) that oxytocin maintains a certain degree of renal vasodilation (see also DEMUNBRUN *et al.*, 1954). It might also be in agreement with the explanation of some experiments of EZRIN *et al.* (1962) that oxytocin plays a physiological role for the regulation of the diurnal cycle of glomerular filtration rate.

In connection with the discussion of possible vascular effects of vasopressin and oxytocin on the kidney it is of interest that POISNER (1964) found an interaction of oxytocin and vasopressin with β-adrenergic receptors in the kidney. Pronethalol, a beta blocking agent, decreased the antidiuretic action of vasopressin and oxytocin somewhat. The mechanism is obscure. It might involve interference with adenyl cyclase (see p. 406).

Stilboestrol treatment may sensitize renal vessels to vasopressin and oxytocin (DEIS *et al.*, 1963).

IV. Effects of Vasopressin on the Intratubular Pressure in the Different Sections of the Nephron

WIRZ (1956) and GOTTSCHALK and MYLLE (1956, 1957) have shown that in rats under steady state conditions the pressure in the proximal convoluted tubules is some 15 mm Hg. In the distal convoluted tubules it is about 10 mm Hg during a moderate water diuresis (see also THURAU and WOBER, 1962). During antidiuresis the pressure in the distal convoluted tubules was equal to the pelvic pressure (about 1 mm Hg) whereas the pressure in the proximal convoluted tubules was not changed much. Although no studies seem to have been made on pressure changes during the transition phase from water diuresis to antidiuresis, this would seem to mean that the main pressure fall through the tubules takes place in the collecting tubules during a water diuresis, but in the Henle loop during antidiuresis, or that on transition from a water diuresis to an antidiuresis a pressure fall is introduced in the Henle loop. This is a very interesting finding, the mechanism of which is unknown. It might be speculated that a collapse induced on the loop of Henle in some way might play a part, possibly by an increase in the interstitial pressure. It is unknown whether this change of the distribution of the pressure fall within the nephron has any connection with the morphological differences found by SABOUR *et al.* (1964) in the descending limb of the Henle loop in rats during water diuresis and antidiuresis, respectively. It should be remembered in this connection that these changes have not been found to be specific for these structures by other investigators (see p. 391).

V. Effects of Neurohypophysial Hormones on Renal Transport Processes

A. Studies of Transition from Water Diuresis to Antidiuresis

A few reports have appeared, in which changes during the transition phase from water diuresis to antidiuresis have been studied. Such experiments are those of WHITE and ROLF (1965) and of JAENIKE (1963, 1964) in dogs and those of THOMAS (1964) in man. To the author's knowledge no experiments of this type have been done in rats.

WHITE and ROLF (1965) followed the acute changes occurring in urine and papillary osmolality after vasopressin injection in dogs. In animals with a hydration of about 6%, papillary osmolality was about 400 mosm/kg. Injection of vasopressin rapidly increased urine osmolality to that of the papilla, but about 6 min passed until the papillary osmolality rose. JAENIKE (1963) found that the increase in urea concentration in the urine came some time after the increase in the concentration of nonurea solutes. This was interpreted to show back diffusion of urea under the influence of vasopressin.

THOMAS (1964) found that during the decline in urine flow, the increments in osmolality and urea concentrations (and U/P ratios) relative to those in the preceding diuretic periods were smaller than those in creatinine and non-urea solute concentrations (and U/P ratios). Also, ammonium excretion relative to that of creatinine or nonurea solute fell. The data would seem to be compatible with changes in the permeability of the collecting tubules to urea and ammonium acutely induced by vasopressin. This might explain the lag found by FREY *et al.* (1960) between max. antidiuresis and max. urine osmolality after vasopressin.

B. Antidiuretic Effect of Arginine^8- and Lysine^8-Vasopressins

There is a qualitative difference between the antidiuretic response to arginine- and lysine-vasopressin in the rat, dog and man (VAN DYKE *et al.*, 1956; THORN, 1957a, 1959; NIELSEN, 1958; ALI, 1958; SAWYER, 1958; BERDE and CERLETTI, 1961; DICKER and EGGLETON, 1961; SAWYER *et al.*, 1962). The maximal antidiuretic effect of arginine-vasopressin lasts longer than that of lysine-vasopressin. This difference is not seen in the pig (MUNSICK *et al.*, 1958).

The difference between the qualitative response to arginine- and lysine-vasopressin may be due to differences in all of the processes taking place after injection of the hormones to their elimination and the end of the effect. Some of these possibilities have been tried. Half-life determinations of the activity in the plasma have been performed using different techniques against which objections may be raised. The half-life determination from the disappearance of activity from the circulation requires injection of large doses. Half-life estimations from decay of biological response are difficult to interpret since the duration of response is not necessarily related to the clearance rate (GINSBURG in RUDINGER, 1964). It has been shown that the half-life of arginine-vasopressin determined from disappearance of biological activity from the circulation is shorter than that of lysine-vasopressin (see GINSBURG in RUDINGER, 1964). It is in agreement with this fact that THORN and SCHWARTZ (1967) have shown that a larger percentage of a large dose of lys-vasopressin is excreted in the urine.

MILLER *et al.* (1967), however, determined in man the half-life in the plasma of arginine[8]- and lysine[8]-vasopressin from the response after administration of low submaximal doses. They found that AVP had a half-life of 24 min whereas LVP had a half-life of 14 min. There is not either complete agreement on the existence of a difference in the rate of inactivation of arginine- and lysine-vasopressin in the kidney and liver. THORN and WILLUMSEN (1963) did not find any marked difference, but SMITH (1962) found a small difference in the rate of inactivation of the two vasopressins in kidney slice experiments.

MILLER *et al.* (1965) in an abstract described experiments on the effects of arginine[8]- and lysine[8]-vasopressin in humans. According to their results the affinity of the two hormones to the receptors was similar, whereas the longer action of arginine-vasopressin could be ascribed to a difference in the rates of turnover of the two hormones in the circulation. In a recent paper (MILLER *et al.*, 1967) they suggested that there is a more rapid turnover of lysine[8]-vasopressin in the circulation or at the receptors.

It has not as yet been tested how the two hormones act on an isolated kidney preparation. This should be studied, since here a good deal of the variables from the intact organism have been eliminated.

The effects of the hormone on the different parameters of kidney function have been discussed on p. 400. VOGEL *et al.* (1966) studied the effects of arginine-vasopressin on stop-flow patterns and clearances in normal and diabetes insipidus rats.

C. Effects of Long-Term Administration of Natural Vasopressins

Repeated injections of short or long lasting preparations of hormone have been employed, especially to study the characteristics of the syndrome of constant overproduction of vasopressin. When free intake of water is allowed under such circumstances a syndrome evolves, now known to be typical for the state of inappropriate secretion of vasopressin (see p. 386).

D. Possible Interference of Oxytocin with the Antidiuretic Effects of Vasopressin

Previously, a depression of the antidiuretic effect of vasopressin by oxytocin has been reported. VORHERR and FRIEDBERG (1960) and VORHERR (1964) did not find this effect in rat or man. Urine flow and sodium excretion did not respond as markedly in pregnant as in non-pregnant women. SAWYER and VALTIN (1965), however, using ratios of oxytocin to vasopressin that were intermediate in relation to those employed by VORHERR, did find an inhibition of the antidiuretic effect of vasopressin by oxytocin.

E. Effects of Oxytocin on the Diuresis

The antidiuretic potency of oxytocin is small as compared to vasopressin. In large doses, however, oxytocin has marked effects on the diuresis. In the rat and dog it characteristically has a two-phasic effect, first an antidiuresis, then a diuresis (FRASER, 1937, 1942; CHAN, 1965; for more references see PICKFORD, 1966; and KRAMAR *et al.*, 1966). SAUNDERS and MUNSICK (1966) have recently published a careful study on the antidiuretic effect of oxytocin in man (see also THOMSON, 1960, and DOUGLAS, 1965). In the experiments of SAUNDERS and MUNSICK in women post partum 100 or more rat oxytocic milliunits of oxytocin invariably caused antidiuresis. Glomerular filtration rate or renal plasma flow were not affected. This antidiuretic effect of large doses of oxytocin can produce water intoxication when it is administered in large volumes of infusion fluid (for references see SAUNDERS and MUNSICK, 1966; SELF, 1966; and SILVA and ALLAN, 1966).

ABDUL-KARIM and ASSALI (1961) found that oxytocin given to humans as an infusion caused a marked antidiuresis which was a direct effect on the kidneys. Single injections had no effect. Denervation of the kidneys does not affect the renal responses to vasopressin and oxytocin in dogs (DEIS *et al.*, 1963).

F. Effects of Neurohypophysial Hormone Peptides on the Renal Excretion of Sodium and Potassium

The possible effects of vasopressin on sodium transport in the kidney tubules have been widely debated. Many authors have suggested that vasopressin increases sodium excretion. On the other hand some reports have appeared which have been interpreted to show that the hormone increases the reabsorption of sodium e.g. in the proximal convoluted tubules (see p. 400). Such a process would be analogous to the effect of vasopressin in amphibian membranes, where it seems well established that vasopressin increases inward transport of sodium.

Since there is little evidence that vasopressin causes any decrease in renal sodium excretion, it seems necessary to assume compensatory reactions, if any major increase occurs in the proximal reabsorption.

The papers on effect of neurohypophysial hormones on the renal excretion of electrolytes often show conflicting results, especially for vasopressin. Whereas some authors have found no effect of this hormone on these processes, others have found an increasing effect, both on sodium, potassium and chloride excretion, and it has even been suggested that the effect on chloride excretion could be used as an index of response in bioassays for vasopressin (HAM and LANDIS, 1942; ANSELMINO *et al.*, 1932; RALLI *et al.*, 1950). BRUN *et al.* (1945) thought that the fact that a certain substance increased the rate of chloride excretion supported the hypothesis that it was identical with vasopressin. GAUNT *et al.* put forth the hypothesis that an antagonism between a saluretic neurohypophysial hormone (possibly vasopressin) and adrenocortical hormone was of significance for the control of renal sodium excretion (see GAUNT *et al.*, 1957). It has been suggested that the persistence of such a natriuretic factor from the neurohypophysis in adrenocortical insufficiency might be of importance for the development of this condition (ROEMMELT *et al.*, 1949). The significance of such a possible mechanism seems rather limited since there are no major deficiencies in electrolyte metabolism in diabetes insipidus (EARLE *et al.*, 1951).

A number of difficulties are involved in the interpretation of studies on the effect of neurohypophysial hormones on renal electrolyte transport.

1. The preparations used have — with a few exceptions — been of a poorly defined character, often partially purified extracts with activities of both vasopressin and oxytocin have been employed. Such preparations may also contain a histaminlike substance (SWINGLE *et al.*, 1956). The preparation Pitressin has often consisted of a mixture of arginine- and lysine-vasopressin in a poorly defined ratio (see p. 375).

2. The doses used have varied considerably and have often been supramaximal in terms of an antidiuretic effect. In large doses vasopressin has effects on vessels. Such effects on the blood pressure or on renal vessels might explain some of the results.

3. Very often the hormones have not been injected i.v. As discussed elsewhere (see p. 410) this may cause considerable error.

4. The periods over which the urine has been collected have varied considerably, and often delay time, dead space errors and the possibility of effects on the kidney pelvis have been neglected.

5. Very often the status of the water and salt metabolism of the experimental animals or the persons on which the substances have been injected have not been well defined or controlled and the base-line periods have been too short.

6. Sometimes the effects of injections and infusions have been uncritically compared. Sometimes infusions of hormone preparations have been carried on for such a long time that the water retention induced — by various regulatory mechanisms — may have caused an increase of the renal excretion of sodium.

7. It has sometimes been assumed that conclusions on the sodium excretion can be inferred from changes in the chloride excretion.

8. Very often species differences exist, see e.g. effects of oxytocin on diuresis and electrolyte excretion.

In the following section the effects on sodium and potassium excretion of several preparations which are purified extracts will be described. This might seem of less interest now as several commercial preparations are available which contain synthetic hormones, that may be considered to be of a considerable higher purity than the extract preparations. However, extract preparations are still used extensively, so knowledge of their pharmacological properties in this respect retains its interest.

After this section there will be a discussion of the effects of highly purified preparations or synthetic preparations.

1. Effects of Extracts Containing Both Vasopressin and Oxytocin

SAWYER (1952) injected subcutaneously more than 1 mU/100 g rat of Pituitrin to rats to which water, 0.05% NaCl solution or Ringer solution had been given. He found an increased renal excretion of Na and K. HAM (1943) injected Pituitrin in the same doses intraperitoneally and found an increased excretion rate for chloride. In the experiments of DICKER and HELLER (1946) Pituitrin in doses of 3 mU/100 g rat caused an increased chloride excretion and an increased GFR. HELLER and STEPHENSON (1950) gave Pituitrin (3 mU per 100 g rat) to rats on a standard diet and found a slightly increased excretion of K and Cl. JACOBSON and KELLOGG (1956) gave Pituitrin to rats which received an infusion of saline. Doses of 1—100 mU i.v. gave a chloruresis.

In dogs O'CONNOR (1950) did not find any increase of chloride excretion after infusion of doses of 0.25 mU/min. SHANNON (1942) in his hydrated dogs found an increased rate of excretion of sodium and chloride (Infusions of less than 20 mU per hour of "Pituitary Liquid USP Armour").

In man DANIEL and HÖGLER (1927) using antidiuretic doses of Pituitrin i.v. or subcutaneously could not provoke any increase in the 6 hour excretion of Na, K or Cl. ROBERT (1932) found no effect on the chloride excretion when he injected "Hypophysin" to normal persons who were hydrated. LAVIETES *et al.* (1935) found no change in the 24 hour excretion of Na or Cl when they gave antidiuretic doses of Pituitrin to two patients with diabetes insipidus. SMITH and MACKAY (1936) gave "Pituitrin surgical" 0.5 ml daily to a normal man and found an increased excretion of sodium for the first two days. BARCLAY *et al.* (1949) in hydrated medical students found an increased excretion of chloride after Pituitrin i.m. (1,2 mU). CHALMERS *et al.* (1951) found that i.v. injections of single doses of 100 to 200 oxytocic mU of the posterior pituitary lobe extract (BDH) did not change the excretion of Na^+ or Cl^-.

2. Effects of Vasopressin-rich Extracts

In the experiments of DICKER and HELLER (1946) in rats Pitressin had neither effect on the GFR nor on the excretion of chloride. HELLER and STEPHENSON (1950) using 3 mU of Pitressin per 100 g rat found a decreased excretion of sodium and chloride, but an increased rate of excretion of potassium. SAWYER (1952) used doses of Pitressin above 10 mU per 100 g rat subcut. and found an increased renal excretion of Na and K. JACOBSON and KELLOGG (1956) injected i.v. 1—100 mU of Pitressin to rats which received an isotonic saline infusion. A moderate chloriuresis ensued. SCHRÖDER *et al.* (1961) found that doses of 100 μU of Pitressin increased renal excretion of sodium in hydrated rats. In rats which had received 0.9% NaCl solution, KOBINGER (1964) found that Pitressin (100 mU/rat, i.p.) increased renal sodium and potassium excretion.

In dogs SARTORIUS and ROBERTS (1949) using 8 mU per kg of Pitressin found an increased excretion of sodium. HARE *et al.* (1944) found no change in the excretion of chloride after injection of Pitressin to dogs with diabetes insipidus, whether they were normally hydrated or after infusion of 2.5% NaCl. ANSLOW and WESSON (1955) found natriuresis and kaliuresis after Pitressin infusion (15—20 mU/h) to hydrated dogs. BARGER *et al.* (1958) injected Pitressin into the renal artery of dogs and found no change in the excretion of sodium. CHAN and SAWYER (1961) found that Pitressin injected in large doses caused an increased sodium excretion in both hydrated and dehydrated dogs. The effects on potassium excretion were inconcistent. Infusion of Pitressin also caused a transient natriuresis in hydrated dogs (CHAN and SAWYER, 1962). These results seem to differ from those of PERLMUTT (1961). KÜHN and PEETERS (1965) studied the effects of an infused arginine-vasopressin preparation in physiological doses on sodium, potassium and chloride excretion in ewes. A significant increase in K excretion was found both in high and low diuresis. Na and Cl excretion was increased in the low diuresis state (see also KINNE *et al.*, 1961; CROSS *et al.*, 1963, GANS, 1964; and KÜHN and PEETERS, 1967). MACFARLANE *et al.* (1967) have demonstrated that Pitressin causes an increase in the renal excretion of potassium in Merino sheep, even if the animals had been depleted of potassium prior to the injection.

In hydrated humans ROBERT (1932) found no effect on chloride excretion after injection of "Tonephin" in antidiuretic doses. MANCHESTER (1932) found a considerable increase in the rate of excretion of Na (not K) in two boys after subcutaneous injection of Pitressin. LITTLE *et al.* (1947) gave 10 units of Pitressin to hydrated persons and found an increased excretion of chloride. SINCLAIR-SMITH *et al.* (1950) found no change in the excretion of Na and Cl after 40—100 mU of Pitressin to hydrated persons. GRASER (1950) found a considerable increase in the chloride excretion in young diabetics. MURPHY (1950) used i.v. injection of 1 mU per kg of Pitressin but found no change in the chloride excretion in persons who were normally hydrated or after i.v. saline. WHITE, RUBIN, and LEITER (1951) injected 0,57 mU/kg (Pitressin). No effect was seen on Na, Cl or K excretion in hydrated persons.

In normal subjects on a constant diet posterior pituitary extracts did not affect the 24-hour sodium output (BLACK and THOMSON, 1951). ASSALI *et al.* (1960) injected or infused Pitressin to pregnant women and to these same women after delivery. During pregnancy the output of sodium and chloride fell, after delivery electrolyte excretion increased. Different results were found by TORRES *et al.* (1966). BRODEHL *et al.* (1965) studied the effect of Pitressin and synthetic Lys^8-vasopressin in three patients with nephrogenic diabetes insipidus. The patients were on a low sodium diet. Vasopressin produced a prompt increase of the freewater clearance and a delayed increase of sodium clearance. It was suggested that vasopressin normally has this effect in addition to the effect on water permeability. The effect of Tonephin on renal electrolyte excretion during infusion of glucose was studied by SCHRÖDER *et al.* (1966).

The effect of long term administration of vasopressin-rich extracts has been studied by several investigators. LEAF *et al.* (1953) injected Pitressin tannate in oil (1 unit every 12 hours) to 10 persons, partly normal, partly with insufficiency of the posterior pituitary lobe or of the whole pituitary. When the intake of fluid was high, there was an increased rate of excretion of sodium and chloride (in spite of a low plasma concentration). This was not found when the intake of fluid was low. The increased rate of excretion was ascribed to a homeostatic mechanism, different from the vasopressin system, see also JONES *et al.* (1963). WESTON *et al.* (1953) found similar results. A clinical syndrome, due to inappropriate secretion of vasopressin has been associated with similar findings (for a survey see BOWER and GORDON, 1965; and BARTTER and SCHWARTZ, 1967). Recently, KAYE (1966) has suggested that the hyponatremia typical for this condition is not due to a renal loss of sodium, but it is due to a redistribution of sodium within the body. In dogs the reactions to long term administration of Pitressin show some differences from those found in man. Among other things, there is here also an increase in the excretion of potassium (LEVINSKY *et al.*, 1959).

3. *Effects of Extracts Rich in Oxytocin*

FRASER (1937) found an increased excretion of chloride in non-hydrated rats which received subcutaneously 0.005—0.1 U of "Postlobin O". DICKER and HELLER (1946) found that 3 mU/100 g of Pitocin to hydrated rats gave an increased excretion of chloride. HELLER and STEPHENSON (1950) gave the same dose of Pitocin subcutaneously to rats on a standard diet. Whereas there was no change in the rate of excretion of sodium, there was a decrease in chloride excretion, an increase in potassium excretion. SAWYER (1952) demonstrated that Pitocin in doses above 10 mU subcut. to rats given 0.05 N NaCl gave an increased excretion of Na and K. BRUNNER *et al.* (1956) injected 31 and 125 mU of Orasthin Hoechst subcutaneously to rats and found an increased excretion of Na and Cl, but no change in K. JACOBSON and KELLOGG (1956) found a chloriuresis when they injected 10—100 mU of Pitocin to rats in a steady state diuresis after infusion of isotonic saline. This result was also seen after hypertonic fluid.

In dogs FRASER (1942) found an increased rate of excretion of chloride after Pitocin. In two experiments ANSLOW and WESSON (1955) infused 26 mU/h to hydrated dogs. No effect on the electrolyte excretion was seen.

ROBERT (1932), CHALMERS *et al.* (1951) and GRASER (1950) found no increase in the excretion of Na or Cl after Pitocin in man. BRUNNER *et al.* (1956) found that 25—100 mU of Orasthin/kg subcut. gave a decreased rate of excretion of Cl and K. The persons were hydrated.

4. *Effects of Highly Purified Arginine- and Lysine-Vasopressin on Renal Excretion of Sodium and Potassium*

Rather few experiments have been done with these preparations. In hydrated rats THORN (1959c) found that doses of highly purified arginine-vasopressin up to 1080 micropressor units did not cause any increase in the renal excretion of sodium or potassium. Nor had highly purified lysine-vasopressin in doses up to 2160 micropressor units any effect.

BROOKS and PICKFORD (1958) studied the effects of highly purified arginine-vasopressin on renal excretion of sodium and potassium in dogs. ALI (1958) made similar experiments, but in addition he also studied the effects of highly purified lysine-vasopressin. Arginine-vasopressin given in supramaximal antidiuretic doses to dogs in a water diuresis often caused an increased rate of excretion of sodium and potassium. Submaximal doses of arginine-vasopressin had little effect on potassium excretion, lysine-vasopressin in such doses usually caused an increased rate of excretion. Arginine- and lysine-vasopressin in supramaximal antidiuretic doses to only lightly hydrated dogs had no effect on sodium or potassium excretion. Neither had they any effect when given to dogs in antidiuresis (see also ALI *et al.*, 1958).

FREY *et al.* (1960) studied the effect of "chemically pure" vasopressin preparations after i.v. injection to hydrated persons (1×10^{-4} I.U./kg). The rate of excretion of Na, K and Cl decreased.

5. *Effects of Synthetic Vasopressins on Renal Excretion of Na and K*

BARNAFI *et al.* (1962) found that synthetic Arg^8- and Lys^8-vasopressin injected subcutaneously increased renal excretion of Na and K in rats loaded with a solution of NaCl and KCl. The urine was collected over fairly long periods. CHAN (1965) found a slight natriuretic and kaliuretic effect of synthetic Lys^8-vasopressin in hydrated rats. ATHERTON *et al.* (1967) found a transient natriuresis in hydrated rats after injection or infusion of synthetic lysine-vasopressin.

6. *Effects of Highly Purified Oxytocin on Renal Excretion of Sodium and Potassium*

To the author's knowledge all experiments with this substance have been done in dogs. BROOKS and PICKFORD (1958) found that highly purified oxytocin given to dogs in an antidiuresis or to dogs in a water diuresis with vasopressin simultaneously administered caused an increased rate of excretion of sodium and potassium. The fact that oxytocin alone increased renal plasma flow, but that vasopressin and oxytocin together had no effect on this parameter would seem to suggest that the effect was extrarenal.

7. *Effects of Synthetic Oxytocin on Renal Excretion of Sodium and Potassium*

CROXATTO and LABARCA (1958) found that synthetic oxytocin increased renal excretion of sodium in rats. This was also found when renal carbonic anhydrase had been completely inhibited. In the studies of ROSAS *et al.* (1962) rats loaded with a solution of NaCl and KCl were injected subcutaneously with synthetic oxytocin (2.5 and 5 mU). Renal excretion of sodium and potassium increased somewhat (see also BARNAFI *et al.*, 1960). In the studies of CHAN (1965) similar results were found.

Syntocinon in high doses produced an increased rate of excretion of sodium in both hydrated and dehydrated dogs (CHAN and SAWYER, 1961; see also HORSTER *et al.*, 1959). In low doses it only produces natriuresis during antidiuresis (CHAN and SAWYER, 1962).

MERTZ (1960) and THOMSON (1960) found inconsistent changes in renal functions after injection of large doses of synthetic oxytocin in humans. CROSS *et al.* (1960) found no change in renal excretion of Na, K and Cl after infusion to humans.

8. *Comments on the Results of Studies of the Effects of Neurohypophysial Hormones on the Renal Excretion of Sodium and Potassium*

From the results of the many studies discussed, it is apparent that no striking effects on sodium, potassium or chloride excretion is characteristic of the hormones. The most reproducible effect seems to be a chloruretic and natriuretic effect of oxytocin preparations at least in rats and dogs. The mechanism of the effect has only been studied little (see discussion in USSING *et al.*, 1960, p. 354). BARNAFI *et al.* (1960) found that suitable doses of synthetic lysine-vasopressin were able to counteract the effect of aldosterone on sodium retention in rats. It is characteristic that all the results reviewed have been obtained by very simple methods and classical methods of renal physiology. There is a need for experiments with better defined experimental states of the animals and taking into account all the facts outlined on p. 383. Studies using micropuncture techniques — as they have been applied for aldosterone (WIEDERHOLT *et al.*, 1966) will be awaited with interest. — The effects of long term administration are clearcut, although the mechanism of the increased sodium excretion has not been elucidated. ROSAS *et al.* (1962) and BARNAFI *et al.* (1962) showed that substances which inactivated the antidiuretic effect of vasopressin and the uterotonic effect of oxytocin affected the changes in electrolyte excretion which were found in these experiments in a similar manner (see also p. 387).

G. Effect of Vasopressin on Renal Excretion of Calcium

THORN (1960b, 1961) found that antidiuretic doses of vasopressin and of oxytocin caused an increase in the rate of excretion of Ca which was small, but consistent and was well correlated in magnitude and duration with the antidiuretic response. A few scattered clinical observations had previously shown that vasopressin increases renal calcium excretion (ALBRIGHT and BARTTER, 1950; HELLMAN *et al.*, 1962). The observations of THORN in rats and dogs were confirmed in normal humans by DICKER and EGGLETON (1961) and by NIELSEN (1964). In women with breast cancer GARDNER *et al.* (1962) did not find any consistent changes in 12 hour urinary calcium excretion after administration of very large doses of a vasopressin preparation. The long collection periods may have obscured effects occuring in direct conjunction with the administration of hormone.

In hydrated ewes KÜHN (1966) found a decrease in renal excretion of calcium after infusion of arginine- or lysine-vasopressin in low concentrations. The employment of a rather short-base-line period and a low concentration of hormone in the infusion fluid (with ensuing very gradual onset of effect) makes the results difficult to interprete.

A discussion of the increased renal excretion of calcium in relation to the mechanism of action of the hormones is found on p. 405.

H. Effect of Vasopressin on Renal Excretion of Magnesium

NIELSEN (1964) demonstrated that commercial preparations of arginine- and lysine-vasopressin caused an increase in the renal excretion of magnesium in hydrated humans. The increase was well correlated with the antidiuresis and was also found following stimulation of release of endogenous vasopressin. It was of an order of about 10 microequivalents of magnesium per minute, comparable to the simultaneous increase in the rate of calcium excretion.

J. Effect of Vasopressin on Renal Transport of Urea

As previously mentioned there is a great controversy regarding the nature of the mammalian tubular transport processes for urea. Especially it seems not quite established whether active transport of urea exists (or whether it becomes of importance only under some circumstances).

Similarly, there is considerable disagreement on the question whether vasopressin affects renal handling of urea. This is also so for the possible effects of vasopressin on transport of urea and analogues of it in the amphibian membranes (see e.g. CAPEK *et al.*, 1966). The findings of JAENIKE (1963) and THOMAS (1964) have been described previously in conjunction with studies of the transition phase from water diuresis to antidiuresis (see p. 381).

In rabbits FOULKES (1966) using the technique of isotopic equilibration (with urine flow maintained by mannitol) found that vasopressin increased the back transport of urea over the nephron. However, the transport of thiourea was not affected. In conscious sheep in an osmotic diuresis CROSS *et al.* (1966a) found that vasopressin decreased urea clearance without altering glomerular filtration rate. The data were interpreted to suggest that vasopressin increases the permeability of the tubular cell membranes to urea.

GARDNER and MAFFLY (1964) using perfusion of collecting tubules in the isolated medullary pyramid of the rodent kidney demonstrated an increased transport of urea from tubular lumen to the interstitial tissue when the animals had been exposed to vasopressin. However, micropuncture studies on proximal and distal convoluted tubules (CAPEK *et al.*, 1966) and studies on isolated pieces of cortical tubules (GRANTHAM and BURG, 1966) have not shown any increased permeability of the tubules to urea under the influence of vasopressin. The findings of a positive effect of vasopressin by other authors (see also JAENIKE, 1961) made CAPEK *et al.* suggest that such findings might have been due to solvent drag effects on urea movement (see also APPELBOOM *et al.*, 1965). It should be remembered that increased permeability to urea might occur on vasopressin administration, but only in some sections of the tubules, e.g. in medullary collecting ducts.

K. Effect of Vasopressin on Renal Excretion of Ammonium

Studies done by THOMAS (1964) in man seem to show that vasopressin increases the permeability to ammonium in the distal part of the nephron. SAIKIA (1965a) found a considerable concentration gradient for ammonium towards the papillary tip of rats (for dogs see ROBINSON and OWEN, 1965).

L. Miscellaneous

SAWYER and VALTIN (1965) found that extracts of pituitaries from rats with hereditary hypothalamic diabetes insipidus caused a natriuresis. This was presumably due to the oxytocin present or to an unknown analogue possibly produced in these rats.

CORT *et al.* (1966) suggested that the natriuresis found after carotid occlusion was due to an oxytocin-like substance.

PENA and MALVIN (1962) found that 20 units of Pitressin (a very large dose) increased the permeability of proximal and distal tubules in dogs to d-arabinose. They used the stop-flow method with mannitol as an osmotic diuretic (see p. 377).

DAVEY and LOCKETT (1960) have shown that aldosterone has no effect on the isolated cat kidney, unless an oxytocin-like substance from the hypophysis is present in the perfusing blood (see also LEES and LOCKETT, 1964). In later studies it was suggested that this substance was not vasopressin or oxytocin (LOCKETT and DE LIMA, 1961), but was very likely growth hormone (LOCKETT and ROBERTS, 1963).

VI. Effects of Neurohypophysial Hormones on Histological Structures in the Kidneys

The main questions which have been asked in histological examinations of the kidneys under the influence of neurohypophysial hormones, have been whether changes could be found in the structures where the hormones have been shown to act by physiological experiments, or at other places. Such changes might then reveal details of the mechanism of action, e.g. whether the increased water transport across the epithelium occurs between the cells, whether any section of the epithelial cells are detached (as e.g. suggested by GINETZINSKY and others (see p. 407), whether e.g. pinocytotic transport could be detected after administration of the hormones or whether any explanation could be found for the changes in the "distribution" of the pressure fall within the nephron induced by vasopressin (see p. 380).

In recent years a number of electron microscopic studies have been published, but it seems safe to state, that as yet no clear picture of the effects of the neurohypophysial hormones on the kidneys has emerged from any of the histological studies.

Whereas several studies have been made on the ultrastructure of the frog skin (e.g. OTTOSON *et al.*, 1953) under conditions where it transports sodium and water, there seems to have been done little work on comparisons between the ultrastructure of this tissue before and after addition of neurohypophysial hormones.

Several extensive studies using electron microscopy have been employed on the problem of the effects of neurohypophysial hormones on the morphological features of the toad bladder (POY and BENTLEY, 1960; PEACHEY and RASMUSSEN, 1961; CARASSO *et al.*, 1962). CARASSO *et al.* (1966) suggested that the ultrastructural changes in the toad bladder seen after oxytocin were secondary to water transport. The other studies have shown that the cell plasma and interstitial spaces swell. However, they disagree in one important aspect: CARASSO *et al.* (1962) found an increased number of vesicles in membranes treated with hormone, indicating to them that the hormone might stimulate pinocytosis. This was not found in the studies of POY and BENTLEY or PEACHEY and RASMUSSEN. It remains for the future to establish whether this discrepancy has been due to differences in the preparation of the tissue.

It seems essential to raise a word of caution when dealing with interpretation of the structural changes found in such a complicated organ as the kidney during antidiuresis. As also pointed out by THOENES (1961) and GLOOR and NEIDITSCH-HALFF (1965) the fixing fluids generally used are isotonic with blood. This means that during fixation, rapid movements of water may be expected when tissues are fixed in a state where there is considerable hypertonicity, respectively only weak hypertonicity in the medulla. It would seem that the media would have to have their tonicity adapted to the one present in sections to be prepared. Also, it seems that in several studies too much time has been allowed for the tissue to develop changes before the fixation becomes effective. It has been demonstrated by HANSSEN (1960) that extensive changes develop in the proximal tubulus when the tissue is fixed in the classical ways. It would seem indicated to try the use of more rapid fixation methods, such as injection by micropuncture of fixation fluid or retrograde injection from the pelvis. Perfusion with glutaraldehyde gave good preparations of proximal convoluted tubules (ERICSSON, 1966; see also GRIFFITH *et al.*, 1967).

It is striking that no marked differences of similar nature as those found in the toad bladder have been described between the state of water diuresis and antidiuresis in the structures which are considered to be the place where the major part of the action of vasopressin occurs (the distal convoluted tubules and the collecting tubules). It is also striking that it appears that no special emphasis has been put on examining the question whether the hormones increase water transport between the cells, such as occurs in the gall bladder (DIAMOND and TORMEY, 1966) or through them and whether they act by stimulating pinocytosis. The most marked changes from antidiuresis to water diuresis seem to have been found in the descending part of Henle's loop and the interstitial cells of the medulla. SABOUR *et al.* (1964) stated that the main difference between the electronmicroscopical picture of dehydrated and water-loaded rats was the presence in the hydrated animals of marked thickening and fibrillary changes of the basement membrane of the pars recta of the proximal tubule and the descending limb of the loop of Henle. These changes were reversed by dehydration or administration of Pitressin. It is very difficult to find any connection between these findings and the action of vasopressin, since the hormone is generally not considered to act on the permeability of these structures (see p. 400) and since in the rat the urine is normally always more concentrated than the plasma, so that water diuresis is a very unusual situation for a rat (RADFORD, 1959). On p. 380 the phenomenon was mentioned that during hydration a pressure fall has been shown to occur over the collecting tubule, but that this pressure fall "moves to" the Henle loop during antidiuresis. Whether this fact has any connection with the morphological findings just cited is unknown. It might be that the thickening of the Henle loop present during hydration stabilizes this wall. It should, however, still be remembered that not all anatomists have found those thickenings specifically located in the Henle loop (see below). Also, it should be remembered that ROBSON (1963) stated that the structure was unaltered when vasopressin was given to hydrated rats, i.e. the alterations are not acutely reversible. This would agree with the assumption of ROBSON that they are due to the hydration and not to the lack of vasopressin.

SABOUR *et al.* also found that in rats which had received large water loads, there was seen *a lateral separation of collecting* tubule cells in addition to a vacuolization, whereas dehydrated rats did not show such changes. The authors speculated that the findings might be consistent with a large reabsorption of water in the collecting ducts during a water diuresis as suggested by KIIL and AUKLAND (see p. 401). GLIMSTEDT *et al.* (1954) found a nuclear oedema in collecting tubule cells of hydrated rats. Recently OSVALDO and LATTA (1966a) have published results of electron-microscopic studies of the thin limbs of the loop of Henle. They comment on the findings of SABOUR *et al.* and state that in their studies thickening of the basement membranes were seen not only in the descending limb of the loop of Henle, but also in several other structures in the medulla. In addition they made the comment that the supposedly passive descending limb has a more complex structure than the supposedly active ascending limb in the loop of Henle.

GLOOR and NEIDITSCH-HALFF (1965) who described the ultrastructure of the *interstitial cells* of the kidney medulla in rats cite findings by MUEHRKE and co-workers and also relate findings by themselves showing a swelling of these cells during antidiuresis and a shrinking during diuresis.

BULGER *et al.* (1966) have published the finding of changes in the structure of the endoplasmic reticulum of interstitial cells in the rat kidney papilla during severe dehydration. Cylindrical bodies occured confluent with membranes of the endoplasmic reticulum. These cylinders might represent a morphological expression of altered ergoplasmic function possibly related to the production of concentrated urine (if they are not artefacts produced during fixation, or due to the very severe dehydration) (see also OSVALDO and LATTA, 1966b).

On the basis of caryometric measurements BUCHER and GRANDJEAN (1961) suggested that vasopressin may have an effect on the proximal convoluted tubules (mice). It seems peculiar, however, that so long latency periods as were reported should exist.

For a discussion of the histological findings which have been made and discussed in conjunction with the hypothesis of GINETZINSKY that vasopressin releases hyaluronidase in the kidney, the reader is referred to the symposium paper by DICKER (1964) (see also p. 407) and to the papers by HANCOX and KOMENDER (1963) and SABOUR *et al.* (1964).

Very few electron microscopic studies seem to have been carried out on kidneys in which the concentrating mechanism and the effects of the hormone have been compromised. The only one seems to be that of ROBSON (1963) in potassium depletion, in which changes similar to those found in hydration were noted. No studies on kidneys subjected to interference with calcium or kidneys of patients with vasopressin-resistant diabetes insipidus seem to have been carried out.

VII. Effects of Neurohypophysial Hormones on the Chemical Composition of the Kidneys

A number of studies have been performed in which the effect of vasopressin injected or infused i.v. has been studied on the composition of the different parts of the kidney (concentration and content of water, sodium, urea and other solutes). In another group of experiments these parameters have been compared in animals in endogenous antidiuresis and water diuresis. For the majority of such studies most of the points are valid which were outlined on p. 383 in relation to the very different effects which have been reported by various investigators on the renal excretion of sodium and potassium caused by neurohypophysial hormones.

Most often animals in a state of considerable overhydration have been used, and generally rather small effects have been found. Doses and methods of administration have varied widely. It seems possible that some of the results in which there were changes in the medullary concentration of sodium might have been due to vascular effects only appearing when very large doses are given. More useful information might be obtained from studies on animals in which vasopressin is given during only slight hydration.

Studies of changes in the chemical composition of the kidneys are complicated to interpret for many reasons. The general problem of reference point is very difficult. GARDNER (1966) recently demonstrated significant variations in the contents of rat kidney papillae solids. This stresses the caution that must be used when employing dry weight as a reference substance.

The different parts of the kidney perform widely different functions. The papilla plays the most important part for the final step in the concentrating process. In studies of the papilla e.g. changes in composition are difficult to interpret due to the many compartments that exist, the composition of which may differ widely. In water diuresis, the content of the collecting tubules will be very hypotonic, whereas the extracellular and intracellular fluids differ from that. Some studies seem to indicate that variations introduced by these factors are of a fairly low magnitude. According to BRAY (1960) the volume of urine in segments of the papilla of dogs is only about 5%. This agrees with the findings of APPELBOOM *et al.* (1965). According to LEVITIN *et al.* (1962) there is no difference between the histologically measured interstitial area during antidiuresis and water diuresis.

It has been mentioned on p. 374 that medullary hypertonicity is still present during a water diuresis but that it is much reduced. It is unknown whether this is an effect of the lack of vasopressin or an effect of other changes induced by water diuresis, e.g. a change in the efficiency of the sodium pump or the medullar blood flow (see p. 374).

Most of the studies done have been made in a steady state whereas few have been done during transition from water diuresis to antidiuresis. A study of the latter kind was performed by WHITE and ROLF (1965) in dogs. It would seem to be interesting to do experiments of a similar nature in rats (in this species papillary osmolarity may be rather high during hydration). See also p. 381.

SAIKIA (1965b) analysed the composition of kidney tissue in hydrated rats before and 30 min after i.v. injections of Lys^8-vasopressin. He did not find any great change in the osmolality of the papilla. It may be, however, that the dose of Lys^8-vasopressin he used has been too small to give an effect. ZAIN-UL-ABEDIN (1965) using higher doses stated to have found a considerable increase in the osmolality of papillary tissue, although not an increase which reached anything near the osmolality present in hydropenia. CROSS and SHERRINGTON (1965) found that vasopressin caused a decrease in the papillary water content of hydrated rats. This agrees with the findings by YUNIBHAND and HELD (1965).

There seems to be no contradiction in the fact that vasopressin increases the water content of isolated kidney slices in rats (THORN and WILLUMSEN, 1963; although HANDLER and ORLOFF, 1963, did not find it in rabbit medulla) and perfused isolated kidney papillae (GARDNER and MAFFLY, 1964), whereas it decreases the water content of intact kidney papillae, as measured when they are removed during antidiuresis produced by hormone (see references above). Slices and isolated papillae are systems where the countercurrent mechanisms are no longer functioning.

A decrease in the water content of the papilla would be expected if vasopressin increases the permeability to water of the distal convoluted tubules, and if this effect is responsible for the major part of the increased water reabsorption. Even if the permeability to water in the collecting tubules is increased by the action of the hormone, the load of preurine may be so greatly decreased that a smaller quantity of water is reabsorbed in the collecting tubules during antidiuresis than during water diuresis (see p. 401).

LEVITIN *et al.* (1962), PERLMUTT (1962) and RUIZ-GUINAZU *et al.* (1964) have shown that in steady state experiments vasopressin increases the osmolarity of the papilla in hydrated dogs.

There is a considerable disagreement in the reports on the sodium concentration in the kidney medulla in water diuresis versus dehydration (or influence of vasopressin). SAIKIA (1965a) found a difference in hamsters. In rats in a rather moderate water diuresis there was a small and doubtful reduction of sodium in the medulla. YUNIBHAND and HELD (1965) found that dehydration changed sodium concentration in rat renal medulla only to a small extent. KOBINGER (1964) reported a reduction of the papillary sodium concentration of rats in severe water diuresis compared with rats dehydrated for 36 hours. GARDNER (1966) found hydration in rats to be associated with a significant reduction in papillary sodium content. CROSS (1964) studied rat renal medullary concentrations of Na and K during osmotic diuresis and after vasopressin. Varying results were found depending on the loading solution. CROSS and SHERRINGTON (1965) found results which seemed to demonstrate that vasopressin causes an accumulation of sodium in the papilla of rats.

In the studies of BAER *et al.* (1962) rats with diabetes insipidus had a sodium concentration in the interstitial fluid which was no different from controls. VALTIN (1966a) found that the medullary and papillary concentration of sodium (mmoles per 100 g dry solids) was not greater in normal rats than in diabetes insipidus rats drinking ad lib. Nor were the contents increased in diabetes insipidus rats after 3 days of vasopressin administration or after 28 days (VALTIN, 1967). MALVIN and FUSCO (1966) found a correlation between urinary osmolality in diabetes insipidus rats and the Na ratio: papilla/cortex during steady state conditions.

LEVITIN *et al.* (1962) and PERLMUTT (1962) found that in hydrated dogs there was a reduction in the contents of sodium per unit dry solids in the kidney medulla. JAENIKE (1963) found results which seemed to disagree with this concept.

LEVITIN *et al.* (1962) seem to have shown that vasopressin increases the papillary sequestration of radiosodium when administered to dogs in a water diuresis.

PHILIPPSON (1964) confirmed earlier findings of ULLRICH and PEHLING (see also ULLRICH, 1959) that there is during antidiuresis in the kidney medulla a considerably higher concentration of glycerylphosphorylcholine and glycerylphosphorylethanolamine than in a water diuresis. The possible functional significance of these results is unknown.

JACOBSEN *et al.* (1964) found that the hexosamine content in the papillae of rats was high in diuresis, but low in antidiuresis. This was taken as support for the hypothesis of GINETZINSKY (see p. 407).

CROSS *et al.* (1966b) found a very varying uptake of ^{131}J labelled albumin in the renal papilla of rats after vasopressin.

VIII. Effects of Neurohypophysial Hormones on the Kidney of Birds

Phylogenetically birds are the first vertebrates to possess a kidney which is capable of producing a concentrated urine (BENTLEY, 1963). The concentrating power of the kidney is limited, however. The domestic chicken can maximally concentrate the urine to a concentration about twice that of blood (KORR, 1939; DICKER and HASLAM, 1966; SKADHAUGE and SCHMIDT-NIELSEN, 1967a). Certain birds, however, such as the Savannah sparrow and the zebra finch can produce a urine of a much higher osmolality.

In recent years a considerable amount of work has been done on the countercurrent system in the kidney of birds (POULSON, 1965; VOGEL, 1963, 1965; DICKER *et al.*, 1966) and on other mechanisms by which the fowl may conserve water (reduction of glomerular filtration rate, reabsorption of water through intestinal sections). It has been clarified that the relative contribution of urea to the hypertonicity in the renal medulla seems to be considerably smaller in birds than in mammals (SKADHAUGE and SCHMIDT-NIELSEN, 1967b).

It seems well established that the antidiuretic hormone of chickens is arginine-vasotocin (MUNSICK, 1964).

The antidiuretic effect of arginine-vasotocin in the chicken seems to be caused mainly by a tubular effect (SKADHAUGE, 1964b; DANTZLER, 1966). It appears that the hormone has not to be filtered to have an effect, or in other words that it acts on the cells from the blood side (SKADHAUGE, 1964). This is an analogy with the relations in the toad bladder and the frog skin and kidney of rats (see p. 403).

Some studies have been done using neurohypophysial peptides which are not physiological in the fowl. HOLMES and ADAMS (1963) when using very large doses of Pitressin and Pitocin found an antidiuretic effect of both preparations, but only Pitocin increased renal excretion of sodium.

VOGEL *et al.* (1965) found a slight antidiuretic effect of Hypophysin in turkeys.

IX. Effects of Artifical Hormone Analogues on the Kidneys

For analyses of the significance of the different functional groups in the molecules for the antidiuretic effect the reader is refered to previous reviews (BOISSONNAS *et al.*, 1961; KONZETT, 1963; SCHWARTZ and LIVINGSTON, 1964; RUDINGER, 1964a; BERDE and BOISSONNAS, 1966) and the other sections of this book.

Recently the significance of the carboxamido groups for the biological activities has been studied (BRANDA and DU VIGNEAUD, 1966). Such analogues of oxytocin have very little antidiuretic effect.

The configuration of the basic amino acid at position 8 seems to be more important for the pressor than for the antidiuretic component of the hormonal effect (ZAORAL *et al.*, 1966; SAWYER *et al.*, 1962).

Although some principles in correlation between chemical structure and biological effect have been established by these studies, it is still hard to predict effects of structural changes on biological activity, see e.g. BERDE and CERLETTI (1964), STÜRMER *et al.* (1965).

Several problems are encountered in studies of the effects of artificial analogues of the neurohypophysial hormones on the kidneys. Since derivatives of lysine-vasopressin are much more easily synthetized than those of arginine-vasopressin, the course of the work has generally been to synthetize lysine-vasopressin analogues with the prospect of following up possible leads with arginine-analogues (RUDINGER, 1964a).

Several aspects are of interest in the development of such artificial analogues. Especially the specific potencies, the qualitative response to the substances (duration of response) and the development of antagonists. It is possible to develop substances with a higher potency than the naturally occuring hormones. It is possible to develop hormones with a more rational potency relation between antidiuretic effect and pressor effect than the naturally occurring hormones. Such compounds may have a smaller potency per mol of the effect selected than the naturally occurring hormones. This, however, may be of less significance, since larger doses may be used. Further it may be of interest to develop substances with a protracted effect.

It is a very difficult problem to express the antidiuretic potencies of such compounds, since the biological standardization versus a certain hormone peptide has no meaning in the usual sense, if their qualitative responses are different. For a further discussion of these problems see p. 416. For these reasons the potencies and potency ratios given below should be taken with a grain of salt.

When such compounds have been synthetized one should try to clarify the reasons why they have the specific qualities. Here, differences in each of the separate partial processes in the fate of the hormone come into question, but also transformation of hormonogens to hormones is a possibility (see e.g. RYCHLIK in RUDINGER, 1964a, and BERÁNKOVÁ-KSANDROVÁ *et al.*, 1966). Very little work has been done along these lines.

Deamino-oxytocin has a higher antidiuretic (15 IU/mg) and a lower pressor activity (1 IU/mg) than oxytocin (HOPE *et al.*, 1962).

$Asp(NH_2)^4$-lysine-vasopressin has an antidiuretic potency of about 700 IU/mg. The pressor potency is slightly lower than that of lysine-vasopressin (ZAORAL *et al.*, 1963a).

Deamino-arginine-vasopressin has an antidiuretic potency of 1300 IU/mg, but a pressor potency of some 370 IU/mg (HUGUENIN *et al.*, 1965). It is more potent antidiuretic substance than any of the other neurohypophysial hormone peptides.

$Deamino^1$-Phe^2-Arg^8-vasopressin has a rat antidiuretic potency of 800 IU/mg. Since the pressor potency is 29 IU/mg, the antidiuretic/pressor ratio is 28/1 (STÜRMER *et al.*, 1965). For other deamino –/– analogues see ZAORAL *et al.* (1967b).

D-Arg^8- and D-Lys^8-vasopressin have a higher a.d./pressor ratio than the natural compounds (antidiuretic potency: 114 IU/mg, pressor potency: 4 IU/mg) (ZAORAL *et al.*, 1966, 1967a). D-Dab^8-vasopressin has similar activities (ZAORAL and SORM, 1966). $Tyr(Me)^2$-lysine-vasopressin showed an even greater ratio of antidiuretic to pressor activity (40), but the ratio varied considerably between species (see also ZAORAL *et al.*, 1965). This was in contrast to the findings for D-Dab^8-vasopressin.

Some of the artificial analogues have qualitative effects which are similar to those of arginine-vasopressin. Thus, the antidiuretic effect of Deamino-lysine-vasopressin lasts longer than that of lysine-vasopressin and is stronger. Its pressor effect is smaller (CHAN, 1965). The reason for these qualities is unknown. CHAN suggested that this compound should be used in the treatment of diabetes insipidus. The antidiuretic effect of Deamino-^{1}-Phe^2-Arg^8-vasopressin is qualitatively similar to that of arginine-vasopressin (STÜRMER *et al.*, 1965).

Other analogues have qualitative effects which are more similar to those of lysine-vasopressin. Phe[2]-vasopressin has an antidiuretic effect which is qualitatively similar to that of lysine-vasopressin, but 2.4 times weaker (BERDE *et al.*, 1961; see also GUHL, 1961). However, NIELSEN (1965) found that in rats the analogue had a potency that was 3 times stronger than that of Lys-vasopressin. He ascribed this difference to a difference in the strain of rats. The citrulline[8] analogues of vasopressin and oxytocin have a qualitative antidiuretic effect similar to that of Lys[8]-vasopressin (VAN DYKE *et al.*, 1963). D-Dab[8]-vasopressin shows the same characteristics (ZAORAL and SORM, 1966).

Gly.cys[1]-lysine-vasopressin and Gly.cys[1]Tyr(Me)[2]-lysine-vasopressin have an antidiuretic effect which is considerably more prolonged than that of lysine-vasopressin (ZAORAL *et al.*, 1963b) (see also RYCHLIK in RUDINGER, 1964a, and KASAFIREK *et al.*, 1966).

Whereas Acetyl[1]-Arg[8]-vasopressin seems to function as an antagonist to the pressor action of arginine-vasopressin (STUDER and CASH, 1963) nothing is known of antagonists to the antidiuretic action of vasopressin (still see oxytocin p. 382).

Some analogues have a diuretic action (Valyl- and leucyl-analogues of oxytocin; BERDE *et al.*, 1957).

Since no clear-cut results have been obtained concerning the question about effects of the naturally occurring neurohypophysial hormones on renal excretion of Na and K, it is impossible to try to analyse for relations between structural changes and changes in effect on electrolyte excretion. CHAN (1965) studied the effects of deamino analogues of Lys-vasopressin and oxytocin on renal excretion of sodium and potassium. He found a very slight increase of sodium and potassium excretion after the vasopressins, but a large increase after oxytocins. However, several facts may invalidate his conclusion. First, only 10 min were used as the base line period and secondly, no measures were taken to decrease urinary tract dead space.

CHAN and SAWYER (1961) found that arginine-vasotocin and Leu[8]-vasopressin caused an increase in the renal excretion of sodium in dogs. The effect caused by the latter was brief.

Val[3]-oxytocin in doses which caused submaximal antidiuresis increased the renal excretion of sodium and potassium in hydrated rats and dogs (THORN, 1960). The same was the case for Phe[2]-oxytocin (THORN and MILEWSKI, 1959).

In the studies of BARNAFI *et al.* (1962) in rats, Phe[2]-Lys-vasopressin increased renal excretion of Na and K in rats loaded with solutions of these ions. His[2]-Lys-vasopressin had no effect. ROSAS *et al.* (1962) injected (subcutaneously) synthetic oxytocin, Val[3]-oxytocin and Phe[2]-Tyr[3]-oxytocin in doses which were equivalent in uterotonic effect to rats loaded with a solution of NaCl and KCl. All these substances increased the renal excretion of Na and K, but Phe[2]-Tyr[3]-oxytocin had only weak effects. Inactivation of the uterotonic activity gave similar reductions in the effects on electrolyte excretion. THOMSON (1960) found that Phe[3]-oxytocin had no effect on renal electrolyte excretion in man.

It would seem pertinent to examine the question whether analogues which are stronger antidiuretic agents than the naturally occurring hormones, also increase renal excretion of calcium to a larger extent (see p. 388).

X. Factors Influencing the Responsiveness of the Kidneys to Neurohypophysial Hormones

A number of factors influence the responsiveness of the kidneys to vasopressin. Some of them (high Ca, pH, the disease nephrogenic diabetes insipidus) seem directly to interfere with the action of vasopressin on the kidneys, possibly by decreasing the rate of entry of the hormone to the receptor sites, possibly directly interfering with the interaction between the hormone and the "receptors". A great number of factors cause derangements in the processes which form the background on which the permeability changes cause the increase in the urine concentration.

A. Effects of Calcium, pH and Nephrogenic Diabetes Insipidus

It has been demonstrated that the effect of posterior pituitary peptide hormones on various in vitro preparations of amphibian membranes can be inhibited by high concentrations of calcium (see e.g. PETERSEN and EDELMAN, 1964).

Recently this effect has also been demonstrated by micropuncture experiments on segments of the kidney tubules where vasopressin acts (the distal convoluted tubules) LASSITER *et al.* (1965). No experiments seem to have been made on the collecting tubules. This would be of interest in connection with the possible difference in the mechanism of the increased water permeability found in the different sections of the distal part of the nephron after vasopressin (see p. 405). The effect of calcium may be due to several mechanisms. One would be a direct antagonism between vasopressin and calcium, another a decrease of the permeability to hormone, or it might be due to a combination of these facts. For a discussion of the role of calcium in the biochemical mechanism of action of vasopressin the reader is referred to p. 405.

The effect of *pH* on the action of different neurohypophysial polypeptides has been studied thoroughly in reference to peptide effects on the toad bladder and the uterus. One aim has been to establish values of pH for the hypothetical receptor groups. Some of the difficulties involved in such interpretations have been stressed recently by GULYASSY and EDELMAN (1965).

A lack of clarity exists concerning the problem of the effect of pH on the action of neurohypophysial peptides on the kidney. In some cases opposite effects have been reported by different groups of investigators but often the experimental conditions have been so different that this might explain the discrepancies. Thus CZACZKES *et al.* (1961) have described in man that infusion of bicarbonate solution diminished the response to fairly small doses of Pitressin. On the other hand, CURTIS and DE WARDENER (1963) stated that they could not find this effect. However, they used smaller doses, and inspection of their data seems to show that in some cases there was actually an effect. ULLMANN *et al.* (1965) reported that in dogs excreting a dilute urine and infused with alkaline solutions, the renal tubules showed a decreased responsiveness to exogenous vasopressin, whereas the tubular sensitivity to vasopressin was enhanced during the administration of an acid solution. GOODMAN and LEVITIN (1965) used dogs in an osmotic diuresis. In those experiments, no change in the $T^{C}_{H_2O}$ accompanied alkalization of the urine. In rats, alkali loading induced an acute and reversible decrease in the maximum concentrating ability, expressed as maximum urine osmolality.

It would appear that more work needs to be done on the problem including the use of different species and a wider range of hydration and doses. Even if in some cases there seems to have been an effect of pH on the concentrating mechanism, the mechanism of action remains obscure.

A number of references on the disease nephrogenic diabetes insipidus are found in the recent paper by BERLYNE *et al.* (1965) (see also SCHOEN, 1960; CUTLER *et al.*, 1962, and DARMADY *et al.*, 1964). LINDEMAN *et al.* (1961) concluded from their experiments that cortisol does not alter the sensitivity of the renal tubules to vasopressin. A similar conclusion was drawn from studies on diabetes insipidus rats (see VALTIN, 1967).

B. Effects of Other Factors

DE WARDENER (1960), ROBSON (1963), BUCHBORN (1964), BLACK (1965), EPSTEIN (1966), SCHWARTZ and RELMAN (1967) have summarized many causes for interference with the concentrating mechanism of the kidneys. In some of these cases it has been established that the interference with the concentrating mechanism is due to changes in renal medullary osmotic gradients or other factors not involving the direct reactivity to vasopressin. In other cases such direct interferences do occur, but on the whole the detailed mechanism of these disturbances is still little elucidated.

Some authors have reported a decrease in the concentrating capacity with age, but others have found results which disagree with these findings (VAN EPS *et al.*, 1966). There is much literature on decreased concentrating capacity in the newborn (see e.g. HELLER, 1958, and DLOUHA *et al.*, 1965).

Prolonged exposure of rats to dehydration produces a refractiveness to vasopressin in the recovery phase which is due to a decreased ability to form a medullary solute gradient (WELLER, 1965). Fasting decreases the max. urinary osmolality obtained after vasopressin (BAUMANN *et al.*, 1964; MORRISON *et al.*, 1967). After acute renal failure a reduced renal concentrating ability may persist for a long period (WARD *et al.*, 1966).

Overhydration, maintained for several days reduces the sensitivity of the kidney to vasopressin (DE WARDENER and HERXHEIMER, 1957; EPSTEIN, KLEEMAN and HENDRIKX, 1957; LEVINSKY, DAVIDSON and BERLINER, 1959; JAENIKE and WATERHOUSE, 1961; YOON and HONG, 1961). The reason is probably a decreased osmolality of the renal medulla. HAYS and LEAF (1961) in toads found results suggesting that hydration caused changes in the sensitivity of bladder cells to vasopressin. Such reports for kidney cells do not seem to exist. It has been reported several times in clinical studies that ureteral blockade causes a decrease in the concentrating ability of the kidneys (for references see JAENIKE and BRAY, 1960; see also MEES, 1960; for chronic obstruction see BERLYNE and MACKEN, 1962). This phenomenon has been studied in more detail by JAENIKE and BRAY and especially by SELKURT (1963). SELKURT found that ureteral blockade caused an increase in total renal blood flow accompanied by a decrease in the extraction of paraaminohippurate. This combination would fit well with an increased perfusion of vascular circuits of the A-v communicating type involving the medulla. How this change comes about, however, is unclear (see p. 379).

It is also known (see e.g. STEINESS and LUNDING, 1966) that acute relief of urinary tract obstruction may be followed by a severe vasopressin-resistant polyuria, probably most often due to an inhibition of proximal tubular sodium reabsorption.

Besides interfering directly with the responsiveness of the tubules to vasopressin, hypercalcemia may disturb the establishing of hypertonicity in the medulla (see e.g. SCHWARTZ and RELMAN, 1967).

A voluminous literature — full of disagreements — exists on the effect of potassium depletion on the concentrating mechanism of the kidneys. For a recent review the reader is referred to SCHWARTZ and RELMAN (1967). Many techniques for studying kidney function have been used in attempts at clarifying this phenomenon (classical clearance techniques: BRUNNER and SELDIN, 1966; electron microscopy: ROBSON, 1963; micropuncture: BANK and AYNEDJIAN, 1964; GOTT-

SCHALK *et al.*, 1965). A recent one has been the employment of the method of tubular microinjection with a study of transit times (JONES *et al.*, 1965). It appears from the studies of GOTTSCHALK and his group that, in the rat, potassium depletion causes a disturbance of the countercurrent system. The explanations of the effect of potassium depletion discussed have been such a derangement (caused by decreased delivery of solute or a deficiency of the sodium pump; see e.g. BUCKALEW *et al.*, 1967) and alternatively, a defect in the permeability of the collecting tubules. Whereas the permeability of the collecting tubules seems normal in the rat in potassium depletion, in other species it seems to be affected (see discussion in the paper by JONES *et al.*, 1965). GARDNER (1966) in a careful study found no change in papillary sodium content in kaliopenic rats. FINN *et al.* (1966) demonstrated that in the toad bladder a decrease in cell potassium was necessary to provoke the effect of K lack.

Patients with diabetes insipidus are unable to concentrate their urine to the same extent as normal persons when given vasopressin (ALEXANDER and FILBIN, 1959).

Long-term consumption of phenacetin in rats decreases the concentrating capacity (ANGERWALL *et al.*, 1964; see also NUSYNOWITZ *et al.*, 1967). Removal of one kidney causes a decrease in the medullary hypertonicity of the other (BOYLAN and ASSHAUER, 1962). Papillectomy reduces the response of the animal to vasopressin (MARSHALL *et al.*, 1963). Renal venous occlusion reduces the concentrating ability (SELKURT *et al.*, 1964). BAUMAN (1965) has published findings which seem to support the hypothesis that anterior pituitary hormones are essential for maintaining the concentration gradient within the kidneys which is the basis for action of ADH.

CRABBÉ (1962) showed that injection of aldosterone increased the concentrating capacity of the human kidney, presumably due to a stimulation of sodium reabsorption in the ascending limb of the loop of Henle. The mechanism may be that the hormone increases the passive permeability of the urinary side of the cells to sodium (CRABBÉ and DE WEER, 1965; see also GUINNEBAULT, 1962; KESSLER *et al.*, 1964, and WIEDERHOLT *et al.*, 1966).

SIGLER *et al.* (1965) found that in adrenalectomized rats renal concentrating ability was decreased as was the sodium concentration at the papillary tip. The possibility that aldosterone acts on medullary blood flow should be kept in mind, however.

Mercaptomerin decreases the sodium concentration of the medulla (AIKAWA and PILLIOD, 1959; see also AU and RAISZ, 1960, and DOW and IRVINE, 1967) as do digitalis glycosides (KUPFER and KOSOVSKY, 1962). Sodium depletion (BAKER *et al.*, 1961) or an acute reduction in sodium excretion (GOODMAN *et al.*, 1964) cause a reduction in the concentrating capacity of the kidneys.

SCHRÖDER (1966) found that angiotensin increased urinary concentration when it was infused to hydrated normal persons who received an infusion of vasopressin. The effect was explained to be due to alterations in the intrarenal hemodynamics and increased distal reabsorption of sodium and water.

WESTON *et al.* (1956) reported a decreased response to Pitressin-tannate-in oil in patients with hyperthyroidism. The mechanism was not elucidated (see also GLATTE *et al.*, 1965).

GOLDBLATT *et al.* (1967) reported that ethyleneimine reduces the renal action of vasopressin in diabetes insipidus dogs. It has been suggested that dexamethasone inhibits the renal action of vasopressin (CHABRIA and GAITONDE, 1966). Other drugs have been claimed to potentiate the action (e.g. MARTIN *et al.*, 1964).

XI. Localization of the Site of Action of Neurohypophysial Hormones on the Subdivisions of the Mammalian Nephron

It has been generally agreed for a long time that the major site of action of vasopressin is the distal part of the nephron. This conclusion was originally based on the apparent equality of the volume of water not reabsorbed in the proximal tubules and the volume excreted in diabetes insipidus (see USSING *et al.*, 1960, p. 344). During diabetes insipidus approximately 20% of the filtered urine is excreted in the bladder. Since some $^2/_3$ of the preurine has been demonstrated always to be reabsorbed in the proximal tubules (obligatory water reabsorption) the rest (under influence of vasopressin) was named the facultative water reabsorption. (For the distal back diffusion of water which is independent of vasopressin see p. 401.)

On the following pages there will be discussion each section of the nephron where evidence exists that the neurohypophyseal hormones exert an action on it. The possibility that the hormone might affect glomerular filtration rate has been discussed on p. 378).

A. Proximal Convoluted Tubules

As mentioned elsewhere (p. 391) there are a few histological studies which might seem to suggest an action of vasopressin on the proximal convoluted tubules. The evidence seems frail, however. An action on proximal convoluted tubules might be suggested by the finding of a water diuresis above 30 ml per minute in patients treated with cortisone (ROSENBAUM *et al.*, 1952). This might be explained in other ways, however (RAISZ *et al.*, 1957).

Micropuncture studies in rats (GERTZ *et al.*, 1964; ULLRICH *et al.*, 1964) and dogs (CLAPP *et al.*, 1963) agree that vasopressin has no effect on the permeability to water in the proximal convoluted tubules. There is some evidence that it may stimulate sodium reabsorption in the proximal convoluted tubules of rats (GOTTSCHALK, cited by GERTZ *et al.*, 1964) and in dogs (CLAPP *et al.*, 1963). The evidence was the finding of a higher tubular fluid to plasma ratio for inulin in antidiuresis than in water diuresis, whereas the glomerular filtration rate seemed to be similar. As CLAPP *et al.* point out themselves, these findings should be confirmed by single nephron perfusion experiments. If vasopressin does increase sodium reabsorption in the prox. convoluted tubules, there must be a compensatory decrease elsewhere, unless the increased reabsorption of sodium is rather small. It was pointed out by LEVITIN *et al.* (1962) that the total amount of sodium that would need to be reabsorbed to increase medullary sodium concentration to the values of antidiuresis was only small (this assumes that there was no spill-over). Very few reports (e.g. the abstract of FREY *et al.*, 1960), on *decrease* in the rate of sodium excretion after vasopressin in mammals seem to exist. Recently DAVIS *et al.* (1967) have found results which do not suggest that vasopressin has any significant influence on sodium transport in the proximal tubule of dogs.

B. Loop of Henle

Little physiological evidence seems to exist that the permeability of this section of the nephron is influenced by neurohypophysial hormones. However, this section of the nephron is very difficult to examine directly, so the possibility should be kept in mind. The fact that on transition from a water diuresis to an antidiuresis the essential pressure fall within the nephron goes from the collecting tubules to the Henle loop (see p. 380) would suggest an effect of the hormone directly or indirectly on the Henle loops. How this interesting effect comes about is obscure (see p. 380). Elsewhere (p. 390) the morphological differences which exist between the descending limbs when they are in a water diuresis and in an antidiuresis have been described and discussed.

An action of vasopressin on the permeability of the ascending limb of the loop of Henle might explain the finding by CLAPP and ROBINSON (1966) of a diminished osmolality of early distal tubular fluid in dogs in water diuresis, but several other explanations of this phenomenon seem possible.

DARMADY *et al.* (1960) injected ^{131}I Pitressin to rats and studied its location to the different sections of the nephron by autoradiography. Unfortunately, the delicate nature of the thin limb of the loop of Henle did not allow preparation of satisfactory autoradiograms of this section. No activity was observed over the ascending limb of the loop of Henle.

Although this may be fortuitous, it should be mentioned that Boss *et al.* (1962) found that the medullary part of the proximal convoluted tubule and the thin segment of Henle's loop both differentiate in the period when the kidney first responds in the adult manner to antidiuretic hormone.

C. Distal Convoluted Tubules

It seems generally agreed that vasopressin exerts its main action on this section and on the collecting tubules. This conclusion is drawn from stop-flow, micropuncture and many other experiments (see *e.g.* THORN, 1958, 1960). Recently CLAPP and ROBINSON (1966), however, have demonstrated in dogs that in this species the distal convoluted tubular fluid is hypotonic all through its length, even during antidiuresis. This finding might explain why rats concentrate their urine better than other species.

DARMADY *et al.* (1960) have demonstrated that after i.v. injection of ^{131}I Pitressin in very large doses the radioactivity was mainly located over the distal convoluted tubule and the upper two thirds of the collecting tubule. If this location is an indication of the site of action and only that (not special sites of excretion or inactivation) it would strengthen the concept just outlined.

D. Collecting Tubules

It has been a long-standing argument how permeable to water the distal convoluted tubules and the collecting tubules are when vasopressin is not present at the receptor sites. One group of authors has advocated the hypothesis that the permeability to water in this situation is very low (LEAF *et al.*, 1954; GRANBERG, 1963; PAPPER *et al.*, 1957). On the other hand KIIL and AUKLAND (1960) (see, however, also AUKLAND and KJEKSHUS, 1966 for a different formulation) have suggested that segments of the collecting tubules are "freely permeable" to water in water diuresis. Conclusions of a similar nature have been reached by others (DEL GRECO and DE WARDENER, 1956; BERLINER and DAVIDSON, 1957; KLEEMAN *et al.*, 1957; see also CUTLER *et al.*, 1962; HILGER *et al.*, 1958; ABBRECHT and MALVIN, 1960; GRANTHAM and BURG, 1966). Diffusion of water out of the lumen of the collecting tubules has been assumed to occur in the stop flow experiments of JAENIKE and BERLINER (1960) as in the multiple tracer microinjection studies of MOREL *et al.* (1965) in diabetes insipidus rats. It might explain the results of MARSH (1966). Criticism may, however, be raised against the techniques employed in such studies. For example in the studies of BERLINER and DAVIDSON or those of KLEEMAN *et al.* and CUTLER *et al.* there was no proof that vasopressin release was completely lacking, and in the experiments of GRANTHAM and BURG the isolated kidney tubulus may not have been functioning completely normally (e.g. they were kept at room temperature).

The question of the degree of permeability to water in the distal part of the nephron in complete absence of antidiuretic neurohypophyseal polypeptides is difficult to solve. The main problem is to prepare an animal in which there is certainty that no such substance can influence the permeability. It would seem that one of the best experimental procedures possible would be that of employing an isolated kidney preparation in which the glomerular filtration rate could then be lowered. (It is admitted that an isolated kidney preparation does not function as well as an intact one (SCHRÖDER *et al.*, 1965; BAHLMANN *et al.*, 1967). This has actually been done in the experiments of ROSENFELD *et al.* (1959) on isolated rabbit kidneys. Here they found that a reduction of the glomerular filtration rate caused an increase of the creatinine U/P ratio. However, other experiments on collecting tubule permeability to water in the absence of vasopressin have given different results. Using diabetes insipidus rats in the acute phase after the operation GERTZ *et al.* (1964) found evidence against water reabsorption in the collecting tubules during strong water diuresis. The basis for the conclusion was, however, an extrapolation on the basis of tubular fluid/plasma ratios for Inulin that showed considerable dispersion. It may be added that ULLRICH and RUMRICH, according to GERTZ *et al.* (1964) infused very hypotonic solutions into the distal convoluted tubules of diabetes insipidus rats and found no change in osmolality after the solution had moved 1 mm in the tubule.

If the observed differences are not due to a difference between species, it would indicate that even with the best available experimental preparations, conflicting results are found.

The fact that a certain degree of permeability to water exists in all situations does not mean that vasopressin cannot increase this permeability. There is ample evidence that the hormone can increase the permeability of (distal convoluted tubules and) collecting ducts. This evidence derives from experiments on: 1. isolated collecting tubules (GRANTHAM and BURG, 1966), 2. isolated kidney papillae (GARDNER and MAFFLY, 1964), 3. preparations of isolated kidneys (e.g. ROSENFELD *et al.*, 1959), 4. experiments on intact animals (ULLRICH *et al.*, 1964; GOTTSCHALK *et al.*, 1965; AUKLAND and KJEKSHUS, 1966) and findings in diseased humans (CARONE and EPSTEIN, 1960). It would seem to be reasonable to state that these tubules are somewhat permeable to water even in a water diuresis, allowing what might be called the vasopressin independent back diffusion of water or the autonomous concentration of the urine. However, their permeability to water can be increased considerably when they are under the influence of vasopressin. It would seem to be in agreement with this hypothesis that VALTIN (1966a) found that the urinary osmolality remained lower in dehydrated diabetes insipidus rats than in similar rats treated with vasopressin.

It would also seem to be in agreement with this hypothesis that VALTIN (1966b) has reported that dehydrated diabetes insipidus rats that appeared to have an absolute defect for synthetizing vasopressin (see p. 377) may produce a urine with an osmolality above 1000 mosm/kg. The studies of DARMADY *et al.* (1960) (see p. 401) also support this hypothesis. It is interesting that DARMADY *et al.* found that the radioactivity (due to J^{131} labelled Pitressin) which was located to the collecting tubules, was focal in character. The possible significance of this finding is unknown. It might be added here that BROWN and PETKAS (1961) found that vasopressin increased the uptake of water in medullary mitochondria, but not in mitochondria prepared from cortical tissue of dogs.

It may be that the absolute amount of water reabsorbed per unit area of tubular membrane per unit time is larger in water diuresis than in antidiuresis, since in antidiuresis, the load of solution to the collecting tubules has been so very markedly reduced by the effect of the hormone on the distal convoluted tubules (see also GERTZ *et al.*, 1964). However, the fractional reabsorption, that is the fraction of the tubular load that is reabsorbed is much larger in antidiuresis than in water diuresis.

Although these cells do not form part of the tubular walls proper, it should be remembered that several investigators have speculated (see e.g. STERNBERG *et al.*, 1956) that the interstitial cells in the medulla are the target for vasopressin. There is no physiological proof of this hypothesis. On p. 391 some of the morphological evidence for it has been discussed.

XII. Route of Entry of the Hormones to the Kidney Receptors

It seems well established, especially from the experiments of USSING and coworkers (see USSING *et al.*, 1960) and from those of LEAF and coworkers (see LEAF, 1965) that vasopressin has to be added to the "blood side" of the membrane in order to exert an effect on amphibian membranes.

There is also some evidence on this problem in the mammalian kidney. Antidiuretic material, which seems to be vasopressin, is excreted in the urine after stimulation of the release (THORN, 1959b), and after injection of vasopressin (FRANDSEN, 1967), so the luminal membranes of the tubules *are* exposed to active material (in this connection it may be mentioned that cyclic AMP [see p. 406] has been isolated from rat urine [ASHMAN *et al.*, 1963]). SKADHAUGE (1964) injected vasopressin (and India ink as a tracer) retrogradely to rats in a water diuresis. No antidiuretic effect was noticed, although fluid did reach sections of the collecting tubules which are presumably sensitive to hormone. It is true that only a limited number of collecting tubules were found to be stained on the histological examination, but the concentration of hormone in the fluids employed were very great, so it would appear that these experiments can be interpreted to support the hypothesis that also in the mammals hormone has to be "added" to the blood side.

GRANTHAM and BURG (1966) using isolated sections of collecting tubules of rats demonstrated that vasopressin was ineffective when added to the solution bathing the luminal cell surface whereas it did change the permeability to water when it was added to the solution bathing the outside of the tubule.

XIII. Localization of Possible Hormone Receptors within Tubular Cells

The autoradiographic technique used in the studies of DARMADY *et al.* (1960) on the location of ^{131}I Pitressin (after i.v. injection to rats) to the different sections of the nephron did not allow any precise localization within the cell or the basement membrane.

There do not seem to have been done any studies on the uptake into renal cells and subcellular distribution of the natural hormones. LEUSCHNER (1960), however, studied the uptake and subcellular distribution of Phe^2-Leu^8-vasopressin. He found that the major part of the intracellular hormone was localized to the cytoplasmic microsome fraction. It is naturally an essential problem in such studies that one can be sure that distribution of hormone to specific subcellular fractions has not taken place during the preparation of the cell fractions. LEUSCHNER made special efforts to be sure that this was not the case.

A few reports exist on effects of vasopressin on subcellular kidney structures. LEUSCHNER (1960) demonstrated that Phe^2-Leu^8-vasopressin protected renal mitochondria (presumably prepared from whole mouse kidney) against osmotic swelling. The possible role of this effect in the mechanism of action is unknown. In the paper of BROWN and PETKAS (1961) it was demonstrated that Lys[8]-vasopressin in a high concentration increased the water uptake of dog kidney mitochondria. That this might have something to do with its physiological effect was indicated by the fact that only mitochondria prepared from the renal medulla were responsive, not mitochondria prepared from kidney cortex, liver or pituitary. GREENBAUM and DICKER (1963a) found similar effects on kidney mitochondria with arginine-vasopressin in concentrations similar to the physiological ones. However, they did find a positive effect of the hormones on mitochondria from rat liver also. In Aplodontia rufa (an animal unresponsive to vasopressin) kidney mitochondria were unaffected by vasopressin (GREENBAUM and DICKER, 1963b).

It has become a generally used model to speak of lumen-near and blood-near "membranes" of the cells in the kidney tubules and to dissolve effects on permeability of the cell layer in terms of effects on one or the other of these "membranes". MOREL, MYLLE, and GOTTSCHALK (1965) from a number of assumptions and an analysis of data obtained by tracer microinjection studies in rats drew the conclusion that vasopressin increases the diffusion permeability to water of the luminal surface of the cellular membranes in the distal convolutions and/or collecting ducts. The use of an osmotic diuretic to keep up urine flow removes conditions somewhat from being physiological. The "membrane" localization of the hypothetical pores in the distal part of the nephron has not been established.

XIV. Biochemical Mechanism of Action of Neurohypophysial Hormones on the Kidneys

Most of the work that has been done on the biochemical mechanism of action of vasopressin has been performed on amphibian membranes. Since the present section deals with the kidney, and since the effects on the amphibian membranes have been described otherwhere in this volume, the author will restrict himself mainly to giving a discussion of the limited information available on biochemical mechanism of action in the kidneys.

On p. 413 a discussion is found on the disagreement that exists in the literature whether Michaelis-Menten kinetics are valid for the effect of vasopressin on free water clearance by the kidneys.

A. Are the Different Biological Effects of a Neurohypophysial Hormone Due to the Same Configuration in the Molecule?

It has been a standing discussion whether the groups in the molecule which are responsible for the antidiuretic effect are identical with the ones which are involved in the pressure effect. That this may not be the case was suggested by some experiments by DICKER and GREENBAUM (1958), but their findings were not supported by the results of the experiments of BARNAFI *et al.* (1962). However, the fact that some synthetic analogues have a pressor activity which is more than 200 times higher than their antidiuretic activity would have to be considered in this connection.

B. Hypothesis About Chemical Bond Between Receptors and Hormone Through SS Bridges

A binding process, where a chemical bond was established between the SS group of the hormone molecule and a similar group in a receptor has been thought to be involved in the biochemical mechanism of action of vasopressin (and oxytocin) (see SCHWARTZ *et al.* in RUDINGER, 1964a). The synthesis by RUDINGER and

JOST (1964) of an analogue of oxytocin which has an S atom replaced by a carbon atom and which was still rather active, seems to have shown that a double SS bond between hormone and receptor cannot be critical for hormone activity (see also SCHWARTZ *et al.*, 1964; JOST and RUDINGER, 1967).

C. Does Vasopressin Mainly Affect Diffusion Permeability to Water or Bulk Transport of Water Through "Pores" in the Distal part of the Nephron?

For a recent discussion of transport of water across cell membranes (existence of water filled channels, "pores" etc.) the reader is referred to DICK (1966). USSING and coworkers (see USSING *et al.*, 1960) and LEAF (1965) have formulated the hypothesis that vasopressin acts on amphibian membranes not so much by increasing diffusion permeability to water, but mainly by causing an expansion of the diameter of "pores" thus allowing a much higher "bulk" flow of water induced by the osmotic gradient present. DAINTY and HOUSE (1966) suggested that the reason why vasopressin does not significantly affect diffusion permeability to water is that there are regions in the isolated frog skin that are not stirred well. It would seem to the present reviewer, however, that this objection would not be valid for toad bladder, since such regions would be of a considerably smaller size in the very thin bladder wall. DAINTY and HOUSE stated that whereas a body of experimental data can be explained by the presence of pores in the cell membranes of the amphibian skin, further evidence for their existence is needed.

Some evidence exists that the hormone works on the distal convoluted tubules in a similar manner as suggested by USSING and coworkers for amphibian membranes, but cortical and outer medullary collecting tubules appear to behave differently. Analyses of the mechanism of the effect on papillary collecting tubules in this regard do not seem to have been performed. MOREL, MYLLE, and GOTTSCHALK (1965) stated that the osmotic permeability coefficient (as determined in the experiments of ULLRICH *et al.* (1964) when vasopressin was present, was increased very much more than the diffusion permeability coefficient determined in their own experiments on distal convoluted tubules and/or collecting ducts. However, the comparisons (besides involving two different studies) involved different sections of the distal part of the nephron. GRANTHAM and BURG (1966) claimed to have found evidence that the diffusion permeability to water in isolated cortical and outer medullary collecting tubules was increased by vasopressin to a similar degree as the osmotic permeability to water.

More work seems needed — under more physiological conditions than previously — before a clear picture of these problems can be obtained.

It would seem reasonable to state that as concerns the mechanism of action of vasopressin on the distal part of the nephron, the "pore" hypothesis is a useful working hypothesis, but it should be added that even it it is confirmed, it only explains the phenomena in "biophysical terms". The biochemical mechanism of action (how changes in pore radius come about) would still have to be elucidated.

D. Calcium

It has been known for a great number of years that hypercalcemia inhibits the action of vasopressin on the kidneys (for references see THORN, 1960a). This made THORN try the simple reasoning: If calcium can inhibit the action of vasopressin it might be possible that vasopressin acts by removing membrane-bound calcium from the cells. In experiments in rats and dogs (THORN, 1960b, 1961) it turned out that vasopressin (or oxytocin) injected in doses which gave antidiuresis produced a slight, but definite increase in the rate of excretion of calcium in the urine. This effect was well correlated with the antidiuretic effect, both as concerned the magnitude as the duration (see also p. 388).

Since about 99% of the filtered calcium is reabsorbed, and since calcium is also secreted, the increased rate of excretion might mean either an increased filtration rate, a decreased reabsorption, an increased secretion or detachment of calcium from tubular membranes.

Due to the complexity of the kidney functions and the difficulties of locating such small changes in the rate of excretion to any of the possible partial functions mentioned, it was tested in a simpler system whether hormone affected cellular calcium (Thorn and Schwartz, 1965).

In these experiments toad bladder tissue from Bufo Marinus was "loaded up" with Ca^{45} by incubation for 60 min in a toad Ringer fluid, after which washout-curves for the radioactive calcium were obtained. When hormone was added to the medium during the washout procedure, there was a sudden increase in the release of Ca^{45} to the medium. This increased release was influenced by pH changes and changes in the concentration of calcium in the medium in the same way as was affected the permeability to water by the hormone. There thus seemed to be a good correlation between effect of hormone on the permeability to water and its effect on release of Ca^{45} to the medium during the washout.

Other experiments on amphibian membranes have demonstrated that calcium can interfere with the action of vasopressin. Bentley (1959) showed that calcium inhibits the effect of Pitressin on the isolated toad bladder. Similar effect in the isolated frog skin have been noted by Gill and Nedergaard (see Gill and Bartter, 1961). A corresponding effect in the intact frog skin was found by Pigeon and Epstein (1963). Findings of a similar nature have been reported for kidney slices of Necturi by Whittembury *et al.* (1960).

The hypothesis that calcium is crucially involved in the mechanism of action of vasopressin seems to be attractive for different reasons: It has long been known that calcium is very important for the permeability to water of a number of animal membranes (e.g. Fukuda, 1936; Bozler, 1959). It has been shown by Lassiter *et al.* (1965) that calcium inhibits the permeability to water in the distal part of the nephron, but not in the more proximal parts where the hormone presumably does not act on the water permeability. It is known that calcium is crucial for the action of oxytocin on the uterus. The concentration of calcium is crucial for the inhibitory action of certain analogues of oxytocin (Rudinger, 1964b). Several hypotheses could be advanced for the biochemical mechanism of action of vasopressin-involving calcium. A displacement of calcium from crucial membrane sites might open up channels or pores and allow a more free passage of water. Displacement of calcium from pore regions might be brought about e.g. by interaction of the disulphide groups or the peptide links of the hormones with lipid constituents of the membrane (Robinson, 1966; Sanyal and Snart, 1967). Calcium induced activation of cyclic AMP might also be involved in a pore reaction.

E. Adenyl Cyclase

The group of Orloff and his coworkers have studied the possible role of adenyl cyclase as an intermediate in the mechanism of action of vasopressin (see Orloff and Handler, 1964). The starting point was the finding of Hilton *et al.* (1959) that vasopressin exerts a corticosteroid stimulating effect and that adenyl cyclase is involved in this effect. The evidence has mainly been gained from studies on the toad bladder, but some experiments have also been done on mammals. Thus it was found (Brown *et al.*, 1963, and Anderson and Brown, 1963) that high concentrations of arginine[8]-vasopressin stimulate the production of 3',5' cyclic AMP in dog kidneys. It has also been demonstrated that large concentrations of arginine[8]-vasopressin stimulate phosphorylase activity in the dog kidney (HANDLER and ORLOFF, 1963). Cyclic 3',5' AMP in high concentrations (10^{-2} M) increases the permeability to water in isolated collecting tubules when added to the blood side (GRANTHAM and BURG, 1966; see also ORLOFF and HANDLER, 1967).

The main criticism that can be raised against the hypothesis of ORLOFF *et al.* is the following:

a) The concentration of cyclic 3',5' AMP necessary for an antidiuretic effect has been very high, much higher than that which may be found in the tissues.

b) The response of the toad bladder to cyclic 3',5' AMP does not have all the characteristics of the vasopressin effect.

c) Theophyllin (which inhibits the inactivation of cyclic 3',5' AMP) is antidiuretic in the toad bladder, but diuretic in mammals.

d) It does not seem to have been shown conclusively that cyclic 3',5' AMP can cause a direct antidiuretic effect in mammals. ALEXANDER (1965) did not find any antidiuretic effect in rats or one dog. LEVINE (1966) injected cyclic 3',5' AMP to humans in a water diuresis. One of them was a patient with diabetes insipidus. As stated on p. 377 it is very difficult to secure that a diabetes insipidus is complete. It was characteristic that cyclic AMP, besides giving an antidiuretic effect, very often caused circulatory changes (see also LEVINE and VOGEL, 1966). It seems very probable that the antidiuretic effects may have been secondary to release of vasopressin from the neural lobe (see p. 377).

e) The fact that so many hormones increase the activity of adenyl cyclase would seem to caution against a hypothesis of specificity of the mechanism of action. One should be sure that it is not a secondary effect.

Even if one accepts the hypothesis that the mechanism of action of vasopressin is mediated through adenyl cyclase, the hard question remains: How does an increased formation of cyclic 3',5' AMP increase the permeability of the tubules to water?

F. Hyaluronidase

It has been the subject of a considerable debate whether hyaluronidase is involved in the mechanism of action of vasopressin. The basic hypothesis was that vasopressin acts by a liberation in the kidneys of hyaluronidase, which by depolymerization of mucopolysaccharides in the tubular membranes increases the permeability of these structures. This hypothesis has been advances by GINETZINSKY (1958) on the basis of histological findings as well as findings of an increased hyaluronidase activity of the urine during antidiuresis. For a detailed discussion of the hypothesis the reader is referred to the symposium section by DICKER (1964) and a recent paper by DICKER and FRANKLIN (1966). In the latter paper the evidence *for* a role of hyaluronidase in the mechanism of action of vasopressin have been outlined. They were that hyaluronic acid and chondroitin sulphate have been isolated and identified in the medulla and the cortex of the kidneys of three different species (see also p. 391). Hyaluronidase has been extracted from the urine of man. It is different from commercial hyaluronidase. Hyaluronidase exists in the urine during antidiuresis and is absent in urine from patients suffering from nephrogenic diabetes insipidus. DICKER and FRANKLIN were very reserved in interpreting the evidence cited as supporting GINETZINSKY's hypothesis. In the present author's opinion there still lacks crucial evidence for this hypothesis. Such evidence would e.g. be a correlation between changes in negative free water clearance and the rate of excretion of hyaluronidase in the urine, or a clear demonstration of a increase in the rate of excretion of hyaluronidase after administration of hormone. The main problem is the determination of hyaluronidase (by viscometric methods), since this among other things requires special precautions due to the influence of varying salt concentrations on the activity. It is very likely that the antidiuretic effects which have been caused by injections of hyaluronidase are due to a systemic effect and not to a direct effect on the kidneys (see e.g. ROSENFELD *et al.*, 1967).

G. Carbonic Anhydrase

KASHIWAGI (1959) studied the effect of posterior pituitary extracts (Pharm. Japon.) on the carbonic anhydrase activity extracted from cow's red blood cells. The posterior pituitary extract added in very large concentrations increased the activity of the carbonic anhydrase. From these experiments the author arrived at the conclusion that "the net mechanism of acceleration of reabsorption of water in the renal tubules by vasopressin can be ascribed to activation of this enzyme occuring in the tubule cells". Besides the part which impurities in the preparation may have played for the effect — and which is stressed by the author, it seems unwarranted to draw this conclusion without studying the possible effect of the hormone on carbonic anhydrase from the kidneys. Such studies have been performed by KURIAKI and BABA (1959) who used homogenates from rat kidneys. Pitressin given to hydrated animals in doses sufficient to suppress the water diuresis did not produce any statistically significant changes in the carbonic anhydrase activity. That carbonic anhydrase is not critically involved in the mechanism of action of vasopressin at least in the toad bladder seems to be supported by the findings of BENTLEY (1958). He showed that diamox only in very large concentrations inhibited the action of vasopressin.

H. Miscellaneous

No effects on glutaminase — 1 or on ATP-ase were found in the studies on rat kidney homogenates by KURIAKI and BABA (1959). In these same studies an uncoupling action of Pitressin was found.

XV. Methods of Assay for Antidiuretic Effects of Neurohypophysial Hormones

The blood pressure method for assay of vasopressin can be used for many purposes and has a number of advantages over the assay methods using the renal effects. Thus the preparation of the animal is easy, and the effect on the blood pressure has a duration which is about 5—10 times shorter than that of the renal effects. This has as a consequence that many more injections can be made on the same animal in each assay with the ensuing higher precision. This method thus is convenient and accurate in terms of the time spent. It should be stated, however, that antidiuretic potency of a hormone or an analogue cannot be derived directly from its pressor potency, since different peptides have a different ratio between pressor and antidiuretic effect (see p. 378).

The antidiuretic assay methods allow only few injections in each assay due to the long duration of even small effects. A submaximal effect lasts some 20—30 min in rats, 40—50 min in dogs and several hours in toads. This has tempted some workers to refrain from the well-established principle in bioassays of comparing unknown and standards in the same animal with different doses of each and repeating the standards at different times during an assay to take into account changes in sensitivity (see e.g. CZACKES *et al.*, 1964; LITTLE and RADFORD, 1964). Objection should be raised against abandoning the principles mentioned above.

Another consequence of the long duration of responses has been that several workers have employed a rather narrow dose-response curve and that many assays have been done recording the responses of very small doses which give responses that do not differ much when standard deviations are considered (e.g. DE WIED, 1960; LITTLE and RADFORD, 1964; CZACKES *et al.*, 1964). This reduces the precision of the assays. The main reasons for the overlap at the small doses would seem to be difficulties in measuring the small volume changes accurately as well as changes in the dead space of the urinary tract.

On the other hand, working in the lower dose ranges (using refined recording methods, such as e.g. a drop divider [PLISKA and RYCHLIK, 1967]) has the advantage that one saves time and that there is a smaller risk of tachyphylaxis and changes in glomerular filtration rate.

The antidiuretic assay methods have one advantage in comparison with the pressor assays: Some of them are about 500 times as sensitive as the pressor methods, and can thus be used in a number of studies where weak activities in body fluids are to be measured and where concentration procedures are impossible or difficult.

It can thus be concluded that antidiuretic assay methods are much more sensitive, but less accurate than pressor methods.

Among the general requirements for a bioassay method are: Specificity, sensitivity, reproducibility and ease of performance.

In a previous review (THORN, 1958) *a number of problems in assay methods for antidiuretic activity of vasopressin have been discussed* (see also SAWYER, 1961c). In the following section the *different assay methods* with their main characteristics *will be commented on*. The main emphasis will be put on *discussing the criticism which has been raised against and can be raised against the methods*. The author is fully aware that it is easy to criticise the methods of other workers. Such an evaluation is important, however, in order that the user can make his choice. The job must then be from the great number of assay methods described to combine the various facts which bring the assay method towards that optimum of sensitivity and precision that can be obtained with the species in question. It is the opinion of the present reviewer that the development of immunoassay methods for vasopressin and oxytocin has not yet reached the state where reliable and specific determinations can be carried out. Therefore, bioassay methods seem to be the only ones available for making such determinations.

When comparing the results obtained by different groups in antidiuretic assays it is obvious that many reasons exist for discrepancies in such results. However, in recent years some facts have been established which would seem to prevent some of these discrepancies in the future (e.g. it has become generally agreed that i.v. injections of hormone should always be used). The main variables are now the hydration solution (composition, amount) and differences in measuring the response (differences in deadspace and time over which response is measured as well as differences in index of response).

A. Hydration of the Assay Animal

The degree of hydration produced in the assay animals has varied considerably (THORN, 1958). The same has been the case with the composition of the hydration solution used. In many of the more recent assays for which a very high sensitivity has been claimed, dilute electrolyte solutions have been employed. A systematic study of the best composition of the hydration solutions is needed.

Training of the animals to the water loads seems to be an essential procedure. It has been mentioned by Thorn (1957), de Wied (1960), Dettelbach (1958) and Berde and Cerletti (1961).

B. Use of Unanaesthetized Animals

Procedures without anaesthesia have only for a few methods been used in rats (Ginsburg and Heller, 1953; Little and Radford, 1964; Leuschner, 1960). Most of the dog methods have employed unanaesthetized animals (Ames, Moore, and van Dyke, 1950; Thorn, 1959; Bocanegra and Lauson, 1961).

In use of non-anaesthetized animals or man it should be secured that no pain is caused by the injection, since this will liberate endogenous hormone (Thorn, 1958).

C. Anaesthesia

The anaesthetics used in the different assay methods are seen in Table 1. It is seen that ethanol has been very much used. The introduction of Inactin in kidney micropuncture studies paved the way for use of this substance in assays for antidiuretic hormone activity. Inactin has also been used in dogs (Fang *et al.*, 1962). One of the difficulties of ethanol anaesthesia is that the high rate of urine flows causes high rates of excretion of ethanol. Consequently, the fluid used for maintenance of hydration must contain ethanol given in an amount equivalent to the urinary loss *and* the metabolism of ethanol. The ethanol concentrations in the plasma reached in these assays is approximately 0,5% (see e.g. Pliska and Rychlik, 1967).

D. Value of Performing Operations Before Assays

There is disagreement on whether the operative procedures involved in the assay should be done some time before the assay itself. Little and Radford (1964), and de Wied (1960), as well as Ahmed *et al.* (1967) used preoperated animals, but Jones and Lee (1965) found no larger sensitivity when using pre-operated animals.

E. Route of Injection

It seems now generally agreed that assay of substances for antidiuretic effect should take place through an intravenous route. The problems involved have been discussed previously (Thorn, 1958). As an example of the difficulties encountered when one uses the subcutaneous route it can be cited that van Dyke *et al.* in 1956 found a difference in the "relative antidiuretic potency" between arginine- and lysine-vasopressin when they were injected i.v. to dogs, but not when they were injected s.c. to rats. However, when they were injected i.v. to rats, there was a similar difference between the effect of the two substances as in dogs (Thorn, 1959e).

It has recently been confirmed that the antidiuretic effect which is seen after subcutaneous injection of "physiological doses" of 5 hydroxytryptamine to rats is unspecific and indirect and probably due to afferent nerve stimuli from the site of injection (Frandsen and Nielsen, 1966).

The method of close arterial injection of assay substances has recently been introduced. By this method, the dilution and elimination of hormone before it reaches the receptors in the kidney is considerably diminished. Leuschner (1960) in his assay method in conscious rats injected into an indwelling aorta catheter. Sawyer (1966) quotes a personal communication from Holliday that he has employed a similar method.

Lauson (1965) employed an intrarenal artery catheter in dogs.

F. Transfusion Methods

MARX (1930) transfused 10—15% of the blood from non-hydrated and from hydrated dogs to assay dogs in a water diuresis. Only blood from the dehydrated dogs caused an antidiuresis. For references on use of this method in man see p. 424.

G. Registration of the Response

Some of the main problems in registration of and calculation of the response are the establishment of a stable baseline and the avoidance of dead-space errors in the registration of the diuresis. LITTLE and RADFORD (1964) have reported diuretic effects of plasma or saline injections. This will disturb the baseline. The importance of injecting the same volume of fluid each time has been stressed by GINSBURG *et al.* (1955) as well as by DICKER and GREENBAUM (1956) and ROBINSON and MACFARLANE (1957). Dead-space errors have been tackled by reducing the volume of the bladder by tying off its major part THORN (1957a), PLISKA and RYCHLIK (1967), AHMED *et al.* (1967), or by removing the bladder and establishing a cystotomy, either on the day of assay or previously (J. HELLER and STULC, 1959). Dead-space problems in the urinary bladder might e.g. be encountered in the methods of LITTLE and RADFORD (1964) and that of DE WIED (1960). Rats with diabetes insipidus have a bladder hypertrophy.

It should be remembered that even if the dead-space of the urinary tract is reduced, there remains a considerable dead-space in the pelves of the kidneys (e.g. BOJESEN, 1955) and that variations in this part of the dead-space are very difficult to control.

Various techniques have been developed for the automatic recording of the diuresis (rats: BOURA and DICKER, 1953; dogs: FANG *et al.*, 1962) or the urinary conductivity (ALBERS and BRIGHTMAN, 1959; SAWYER, 1961c). Methods for automatic recording of the rate of urine flow coupled with regulation of the delivery of hydrating solution to the animal have been described by BOURA and DICKER (1953), DE WIED (1960), BERDE and CERLETTI (1961). DYBALL *et al.* (1966) have recently stressed the value of a considerable simplification of the method of BOURA and DICKER. The principle involves only a balance, a photoelectric relay and a twin pump.

In studying the qualitative response of analogues it is important to have methods which secure a continous recording of the response. This has been done in the method of PLISKA and RYCHLIK (1967). (An improved technique for recording conductivity. A drop divider secures a very accurate registration of small changes in the diuresis.)

H. Index of Response

As indices of response changes in the rate of urine flow, changes in urine osmolality or density and changes in urine conductivity have been used. It has even been suggested to use changes in chloride ion excretion rate.

For description of some of the most accurate methods of measuring changes in these parameters the reader is referred to the following papers: Changes in diuresis and Changes in urine conductivity: PLISKA and RYCHLIK (1967); Changes in urine osmolality and Changes in urine density: THORN (1960a). Whereas changes in the diuresis and in urine conductivity can easily be recorded continously by the methods just mentioned, the changes in urine osmolality and density have to be done on fractions collected. This naturally increases very much the labor involved in making registration of the responses with short intervals.

It must be remembered that responses measured by changes in osmolarity or changes in urine conductivity or density do not show the same thing. Discrepancies between changes in diuresis and changes in urine conductivity could be due to the fact that some peptides have distinct effects on electrolyte excretion in the kidney. Discrepancies between effect on conductivity and osmolarity would be due especially to effects on handling of urea by the kidney (see p. 388), changes that would be registered in the osmolarity methods, but not in the conductivity methods.

Changes in urine osmolarity seem well correlated to changes in urine density (THORN, 1960a; MATHE and ALTMAN, 1954).

It might be discussed whether the use of ethanol anaesthesia would introduce errors due to changing concentration of ethanol in the blood and thus in the urine. However, the variations which can occur only produce negligible errors when osmolality is the index of response (THORN, 1960a).

The base line is more stable when one is measuring osmolarity or density, a fact which is explained by the relation between urine osmolarity and the diuresis (see e.g. SMITH, 1962, p. 121).

The main problems in choosing the correct way of calculating the index of response is the problem whether intensity of response or the total effect should be preferred. The total effect requires that one has recording facilities for the effect as a function of time. This has been obtained in some of the earlier assay methods and especially in the very recent one of PLISKA and RYCHLIK (1967).

Evaluations of differences in results with intensity and total response are described in the papers of THORN (1959e) and PLISKA and KREJČÍ (1966).

The main source of error in using maximum intensity of the antidiuretic effect is the possibility of inaccurate recording of the change in the rate of urine flow due among other things to a dead-space effect of a large bladder — if that has not been excluded from the urinary tract — or a dead-space effect from the kidney pelves.

On the other hand, a continous recording of urine osmolarity or conductivity (PLISKA and RYCHLIK, 1967) might yield a better picture of the intensity of the response.

It would appear that back diffusion of solutes through the bladder wall (LEVINSKY and BERLINER, 1959) only occurs during so very low urine flows that they are not present during ordinary assays.

The time during which the antidiuresis has been used for registering the antidiuretic effect has varied somewhat. Often 20 min have been used, but also 10, and in some dog methods 30 min.

The interest in the time course of the antidiuretic effect has been increased considerably since the discovery of different relations here for arginine- and lysine-vasopressin. THORN (1959e) discussed different results obtained with different indices of response and different analogues. This has had as a consequence that the procedure of measuring antidiuresis for 20 min after injection previously used much has become less common, and that in many assays the total deviation is measured of the diuresis from the base line flow, either continously or in small fractions.

SAWYER (1958) described how the relative antidiuretic potency of arginine-vasopressin in relation to lysine-vasopressin was dependent on the index of response used (he tried the maximal intensity of the effect, the effect for a 10 min period and the effect over longer periods).

GINSBURG and HELLER (1953) claimed that percentage antidiuresis (two 20 min periods) gave a more reliable dose-response curve than maximal intensity of antidiuresis.

It can be stated that no index of response is specific for vasopressin. The main effect of vasopressin is an increase of permeability to water with no major change in solute excretion rate. This means that there is an antidiuretic effect combined with an increase in urinary osmolality. Decreases in diuresis without change in urinary osmolality have been reported, as a consequence of decrease of glomerular filtration rate, by some authors (see p. 401) and some substances can produce changes in the rate of solute excretion without any change in diuresis. It is obvious that a true effect of vasopressin involves a simultaneous reduction of urine flow and an increased urine osmolality. These two effects can be combined in the free-water clearance. This requires a measurement of plasma osmolality, which is possible in dogs, but not very easily practicable in rats (unless one uses a microdetermination of the osmolality). Therefore, in rats it seems preferable to measure diuresis and urine osmolality (or density or conductivity).

J. Dose-Response Relation

Assay method for vasopressin have generally shown a fairly well fitting straight line relation between log dose and the different indices of response which have been used. Other correlations have also been tried, however. Thus HOLLANDER *et al.* (1957) studied the relation between changes in free water clearance and Pitressin infused in doses of 0.5—15 mU per hour in man. This represents a fairly small dose-response range. The data would fit three simple equations for a curvelinear relation. They fit excellently in an equation relating reciprocal dose to reciprocal response. This relationship would apparently fit the hypothesis that a "pore effect" was involved in the response.

In the recent studies of MILLER *et al.* (1967), however, it was demonstrated that changes in free water clearance are not a simple function of dose of arginine-vasopressin, whereas the data fit well for lysine-vasopressin.

GAUER and TATA (1966) have described that the antidiuretic effect was a constant deficit of water per unit vasopressin within the dose-response range. In other words that when the base line rate of urine flow was high, the antidiuretic effect was short lasting, whereas it lasted longer when the base line rate of urine flow was lower.

TATA and GAUER (1966) related the antidiuretic response (total urine deficit) to dose of Tonephin (a commercial preparation of vasopressin). They did not use the conventional way of relating response to log dose but plotted log response as a function of log dose. Although there seemed to be some relation between these parameters when all results were considered together, the results in the individual assay animals varied considerably. Apparently, the method, like all other assays, has caused a good deal of trouble, since the authors conclude their discussion with the followings statement: "The initial hope of employing the method in batteries of test rats in clinical research did not materialize."

PLISKA and RYCHLIK (1967) found a linear relation between the logarithm of the dose and the ratio of the observed effect and the maximal effect. The effects were changes in urine conductivity. The slope of the function was about 0.6. This is a slope generally found for drug action in cases where one molecule of the drug is thought to react with a single receptor unit.

K. Specificity

It is obvious that to secure the specificity of a response when one is assying very small amounts of hormone, the assays should be done in duplicate, i.e. in two different animals. Thus unspecific responses due to changes in dead-space or spontaneous release of epinephrine or similar substances are not taken for responses to vasopressin, injected at the same time. An unspecific response may be detected by its uncharacteristic shape when one registers the response continually. Also, parallelism between the dose response curves employing two different doses of unknown and standard is a good sign of specificity.

Although it can be said generally that the antidiuretic assays are more specific than the pressor assays, it must be stated, that no index of response is specific for antidiuretic hormone. This means that an antidiuretic action may be caused by other substances or factors, and that it should consequently be proved when assaying e.g. body fluids, that a substance giving an antidiuretic action is vasopressin (either by inactivation procedures or by chemical identification procedures). The chemical identification procedures (chromatography and similar methods) are very difficult to use when assaying hormone in body fluids — due to the very small concentrations found.

In identification of substances as vasopressin in such cases some use has been made of the "proteolytic enzyme inactivation pattern" for arginine-vasopressin besides the employment of reduction procedures. The hormone seemed to be inactivated by trypsin and chymotrypsin but not by pepsin and pancreatic carboxypeptidase (THORN, 1957b; see also BISSET, 1962). Very recent studies by BARTH, PLISKA, and RYCHLIK (1967) seem to establish that chymotrypsin, when it is not contaminated by trypsin, does not inactivate the hormone. BOCANEGRA and LAUSON (1961) encountered trouble when they assayed enzyme treated plasma in dogs.

L. Sensitivity

One of the main problems in the bioassay procedures for vasopressin is the question of whether it is possible reliably to measure plasma concentrations of hormone in cases where these concentrations are low, normal or only slightly elevated. One of the most reliable methods of determining vasopressin activity in plasma directly seems to be that of LITTLE and RADFORD (1964). However, these authors did not find concentrations in rat plasma above 4 μU/ml (their minimum sensitivity value). The antidiuretic activity of untreated plasma was normally below this level. It may be mentioned that in what appears to be one of the most reliable extraction methods (AHMED *et al.*, 1967) the concentrations found in normal persons was between 2.5 and 10 μU/ml (see also BARATZ *et al.*, 1960, for results with a non-extraction method).

During recent years a number of reports have appeared describing assay methods with a very high sensitivity. Characteristic of some of these methods has been the use of rats in which a cystotomy has been performed before the assay. Also, a catheter to the ext. jugular vein has been inserted before the assay day. Characteristic has also been the hydration with a salt solution (see p. 409) and sometimes use of rats having a rather small body weight. The method originally suggested by J. HELLER and STULC (1959) has been used mainly by three groups: J. HELLER *et al.* (see J. HELLER and STULC, 1959), TATA and GAUER (see TATA and GAUER, 1966) and by CZACZKES and KLEEMAN (see CZACZKES *et al.*, 1964; see also GUZEK and LESNIK, 1966). The procedure of CZACZKES *et al.* was used by BOWER *et al.* (1964) in a study in which it was claimed that an abnormally high concentration of vasopressin was found in the plasma of a patient with hyponatremia and bronchogenic carcinoma.

The method of CZACZKES *et al.* was used for a number of estimations on human plasma and for various other problems. The main criticism that can be raised against that method is the use of an unconventional assay principle (see p. 408). Apparently, the sensitivity of the animal was tested at the beginning and sometimes also at the end of the assay to see whether the responses to a standard fell on the value expected from a "standard curve" made on a small number of similar rats. Thus one did not adhere to the principle of testing two doses of standard and unknown in the same animal thereby taking into account possible changes in sensitivity occurring during the assay. The base line value for urine flow of 1,35 ml per 10 min given in the typical protocol seems surprisingly stable, and the responses (per cent reduction of urine flow) shown in their Table 1 seem surprisingly reproducible.

What was considered a fairly large response was obtained with 0,5 μU, giving a reduction in the urine flow of 14% or as little as some 140 μl in 10 min, measured in a not very refined way. The occurrence of a very variable dead space in the urinary tract (see p. 411) would also seem to reduce the apparent exactness of these measurements.

The standard used by Czaczkes *et al.* seems to be well defined. This appears to be less well documented for the standards used by J. Heller and Stulc and by Tata and Gauer. Little and Radford (1964) have tried the method of J. Heller and Stulc. They were not able to reproduce the very high sensitivity claimed by these authors, and they pointed out various inconsistencies between figures and tables of their publication. Vierling *et al.* (1967) were unable to reproduce the very high sensitivity claimed in the method of Czaczkes *et al.*

Jones and Lee (1965) tried to reproduce the high sensitivities in the methods reported by J. Heller and Stulc (1959) and by Czaczkes *et al.* (1964) using rats of the Sprague-Dawley and the Wistar strain. They were unable to obtain the extreme sensitivity reported by Heller and Stulc and by Czaczkes *et al.*. The possibility of difference in sensitivity between different strains of rats exists, of course, but no systematic studies on this phenomenon seem to have been done. It is known that there are genetic differences in the diuretic response to a water load (Stewart and Spickett, 1965). For some time Kleeman and Czaczkes (personal communication, see also Miller *et al.*, 1967) have been unable to reproduce the high sensitivity reported in their papers from 1964. The results found in patients with adrenocortical insufficiency have not been confirmed in the experiments of Ahmed *et al.* (1967). The results found on difference in turnover of hormone between the hydrated and dehydrated state were not confirmed by Miller *et al.* (1967). Other results have been critizised by Brook and Share (1966). In a recent publication (Linkenbach *et al.*, 1967) using a different procedure for maintaining hydration, the sensitivity of the method of Tata and Gauer was given as 5 μU.

Little and Radford (1964) found no increase in sensitivity when the overhydration was increased from 6—10%. Low-salt, high-salt or high-protein diets had no effect either, nor did addition of electrolytes to the hydration fluid. It seems that old rats have less sensitivity than young ones (see J. Heller and Stulc, 1959; Dicker and Nunn, 1958). In conclusion it seems safe to state that the sensitivity of the various assay methods in rats seems to be roughly the same whether changes in diuresis or conductivity, osmolarity or density are used as index of response. A minimum response can generally be detected after injection of 2—5 μU of arginine-vasopressin. Close arterial injection of the assay substance may increase the sensitivity somewhat (see p. 410).

Rats with hereditary hypothalamic diabetes insipidus are about twice as sensitive as normal rats to intravenous vasopressin under conditions of ethanol anaesthesia and water loading (Valtin, 1967; Jones and Lee, 1967; see also Yamane and Kunishige, 1966). Daily pretreatment of the rats with vasopressin does not increase the sensitivity. Disadvantages in the use of these rats for bioassay are the hypertrophy of their urinary bladder (see p. 411) and possibly a higher sensitivity to the anaesthesia. It has recently been demonstrated (Forsling *et al.*, 1967) that a background infusion of arginine- or lysine-vasopressin enhances the antidiuretic effect of single i. v. injections of these hormones. The mechanism is obscure.

M. Further Comments on Various Assay Methods

In Table 1 characteristics of most of the antidiuretic assay methods which have been reported are found. In addition to the criticism already stated, a few points might be mentioned. The methods of BUCHBORN (1955) on the European toad and LAUBER (1961) on the toad, Bufo Marinus, represent measurements in which the combined effects of vasopressin on water uptake and diuresis can be measured. They allow only few injections in each animal, since the duration of the response is several hours. This means that the precision must be fairly low.

The method of BUCHBORN has been critizised by HERKEN (1958) and by WIRZ (1961). It has apparently been used by GAUER *et al.* (see TATA and GAUER, 1966) but without much success.

It would seem to be fairly risky to inject as much fluid as BUCHBORN did (5% of the body weight, or about equal to the blood volume). This might explain the good correlation found with this method between serum osmolality and concentration of vasopressin activity in the serum.

The method of LAUBER *et al.* has been criticised by LITTLE and RADFORD (1964) mainly due to the large volume of plasma required to each animal with the consequent lack of precision of the assay.

In the method of ANDERSSON and PERSSON (1958) using goats there are possibilities of dead space errors. The method has a low sensitivity. An advantage is the easy method of maintenance of overhydration.

BINKLEY and CHRISTENSEN (1959) have suggested the use of increases in kidney weight in hypophysectomized rats as index of response for rather large doses of vasopressin (see also GLIMSTEDT *et al.*, 1954). This would seem to be a fairly expensive method if accurate determinations are wanted.

Tachyphylaxis after injection with short time interval in rats was found by DICKER (1953) but not by DETTELBACH (1958).

Although the dog methods have the advantage that the animals may be reused within limits and that rather large volumes of fluid may be administered, they have a number of disadvantages.

1. The training of the animals is time consuming.

2. The time required for obtaining a maximal diuresis (min urine osmolality) after water loading is long. (The elimination of endogenous vasopressin is slow.) This fact combined with the long duration of responses has probably been the cause of the fact that there is very little statistics available on the precision and accuracy of such methods.

3. The methods have a fairly low sensitivity (about 1 mU).

4. It is only possible to use the same animal about twice weekly.

5. There is a risk of development of hypersensitivity when repeated injections of impure solutions containing polypeptides are done. THORN (1960a; reactions to rat plasma), DINGMAN (1958; reactions to human plasma), BOCANEGRA and LAUSON (1961; reactions to plasma which had been under the influence of proteolytic enzymes).

N. Assays of Hormone Analogues

In evaluations of specific activities of analogues of vasopressin and oxytocin a number of problems arise. The analogues may have a different qualitative effect on the kidneys. This may be due to differences in all the processes involved from

Table 1. *Main points of assay methods for antidiuretic hormone activity.*

Reference	Animal	Hydration	Maintenance of hydration	Anaesthesia	Route of injection	Index of response	Sensitivity	Precision	Standard
BUCHBORN (1955)	toad Bufo bufo	8 h in water; 0.5 ml water/10 g in dorsal lymph sac	—	none	dorsal lymph sac.	weight change in 2 h after inj.	0.01 mU/10g	$\lambda = 0.228$	highly-purified vasopressin
LAUBER (1961)	Bufo Mar.	In water over night	—	—	same	same 3 h after	0.005 mU	—	Pitressin
GIBBS (1930) GLAUBACH and MOLITOR (1932)	mouse (2 groups of 4)	water; 1 ml intraperit./mouse	—	none	subcut.	urinevol. for 3 h	—	—	Pitressin
NELSON and WOODS (1934)	mouse (group)	water; 5% of body wt. intraperit.	—	none	intra-perit. or subcut.	urinevol. for 3 h	20 mU/10 g	—	Pituitrin "O"
HELLER and BLACKMORE (1952)	mouse (group)	water; 3 times 5 ml/100 g	—	none	i. v. (max. 0.05 ml/10 g mouse	% water excreted	0.01 mU/10g	S/b = 0.26	Pitressin
BURN (1931)	rat (4 groups of 4)	water; 5% of body weight	—	none	subcut.	time to max. rate of water excretion	4.0 mU	average variation 12%	Pituitary extract (Parke, Davis & Co.)
GILMAN and GOODMAN (1937)	rat (groups of 4)	as Burn with priming water gavage (2.5% of body weight) 3 hours before	—	none	subcut.	time to excretion of 50% of water load	5.0 mU/rat	—	Pituitrin
ROBINSON and FARR (1940)	rat (10 groups of 2)	water; 2.5 ml/100 g + 5 ml/100 g	—	none	intra-perit.	time for excretion of 2.5% of body wt.	—	—	No standard
HAM and LANDIS (1942) HAM (1943)	rat (3 groups of 6)	0.2% NaCl 2.5 ml/100 g + 5 ml/100 g	—	none	intra-perit.	urinevol. for 3 h Chloride-excretion	0.5 mU 0.1 mU	—	Pituitrin
JEFFERS et al. (1942)	rat	water; 8% of body weight	—	ethanol	i. v.	change in rate of urine flow	0.02 mU	$\lambda = 0.249 \pm 0.04$	Pitressin

Table 1. Cont. a)

Reference	Animal	Hydration	Maintenance of hydration	Anaesthesia	Route of injection	Index of response	Sensitivity	Precision	Standard
Ralli et al. (1950)	rat (group)	Burn's procedure	—	none	subcut.	time to excretion of 50% ingested H_2O. μEq Cl/min.	2.0 mU 10.0 mU	—	Pitressin
Birnie et al. (1950)	rat (group)	water; 3 gavages of 3 ml/100 cm^2 at hourly intervals	—	none	intra-perit.	% water excreted 90 min. after inj.	—	—	Pitressin
Leaf and Mamby (1952)	(hypophy-sect.) rat (group)	water; 8% hydration	—	none	intra-perit.	change in urine water conc.	—	—	—
Stein et al. (1952)	rat (4 groups)	0.2% NaCl; 5 ml twice with 1 hour interval	—	none	intra-perit.	reciprocal of urine vol at 60 min. divided by urine vol. at 20 min.	0.1 mU	$\lambda = 0.329$	Pitressin
Ginsburg and Heller (1953)	rat	water; 6—9% of body weight maintained	+	none	i. v.	% fall in urine vol.	0.05–0.2 mU	Percentage error −41–+38	Pitressin
Dicker (1953)	rat	water; + 12% ethanol 8% of body wt.	+	ethanol	i. v.	change in rate of urine flow	3.5 μU/100 g	—	Pitressin
Crawford and Pinkham (1954)	rat (groups of 6)	water; 1 load of 350 ml/m^2; 3 loads of 250 ml/m^2	—	none	intra-perit.	% change in urine water conc.	0.1 mU	$\lambda = 0.13$	Pitressin
Thorn (1957a)	rat	As Dicker	+	ethanol	i. v.	change in urine density	8 μU/100 g Pitressin 2 μU/100 g Arg.-vasopr.	$\lambda = 0.144$	Pitressin. Arg.-vasopressin
McCreary et al. (1957)	rat (groups of 2)	water; 5% of body wt. twice, 1 hour interval	—	—	subcut.	urine vol. excreted in 3 hours	—	—	Pitressin

Table 1. Cont. b)

Reference	Animal	Hydration	Maintenance of hydration	Anaesthesia	Route of injection	Index of response	Sensitivity	Precision	Standard
DETTELBACH (1958)	rat	12% ethanol; 5% of body wt. + 2% ethanol; 5% of body wt.	+	ethanol	i. v.	change in rate of urine flow	2 μU	$\lambda = 0.232$	Pitressin
ALBERS and BRIGHTMAN (1959)	rat	as DICKER	—	ethanol i. p.	i. v.	Cumulative conductivity change	—	—	Pitressin
BARATZ and INGRAHAM (1959)	rat	as DICKER	+	ethanol	i. v.	percentage change in urine spec. gravity, as N. A. THORN, 1957a)	<30 μU	—	Pitressin
HUNTER et al. (1959)	rat	0.05% NaCl 8% of body wt.	+	perphenazine	i. v.	change in rate of urine flow, time also considered	25 μU	$\lambda = 0.143$	Pitressin
J. HELLER and STULC (1959)	rat	12% ethanol 3% of body wt. 2 ×	—	ethanol	i. v.	change in rate of urine flow	1.25 μU	$\lambda = 0.016$	Pitressin
DE WIED	rat	2% ethanol in 0.2% NaCl 5 ml also 12% ethanol	+	ethanol	i. v.	change in rate of urine flow	5 μU	$\lambda = 0.184$	Pitressin
LEUSCHNER (1960)	rat	0.2% NaCl 5% of body wt.	—	none	i. a.	percentage antidiuresis	10 μU/100 g	$\lambda = 0.113$	Tonephin
SAWYER (1961e)	rat	1.5% ethanol 0.05% NaCl 8% of body wt.	+	Inactin i. p.	i. v.	percentage antidiuresis. Conductivity also considered	—	—	—
BERDE and CERLETTI (1961)	rat	H_2O 5% of body wt. 12% ethanol 5% of body wt.	+	ethanol	i. v.	change in rate of urine flow	appr. 5 μU Lys-V	see paper	Synth Lys-V Internat. Stand.
LEE (1961)	rat	10% ethanol 5% of body wt. + H_2O, 3% of body wt.	+	ethanol	i. v.	percentage antidiuresis	7 μU	—	Pitressin

Table 1. Cont. c)

Reference	Animal	Hydration	Maintenance of hydration	Anaesthesia	Route of injection	Index of response	Sensitivity	Precision	Standard
SHARE (1961) YOSHIDA et al. (1963)	rat	H_2O 5% of body wt. 12% ethanol 5% of body wt.	+	ethanol	i. v.	cumulative conductivity change	< 20 μU	λ = 0.135	USP Post. Pit. Ref. Stand.
HEINTZ et al. (1964)	rat	H_2O 5% of body wt. 12% ethanol 5—9% of body wt.	+ (with. 0.4% NaCl.	ethanol	i. v.	percentage antidiuresis	0.1 μU	—	Synth. Lys.-Vasopressin
LITTLE and RADFORD (1964)	rat	12.5% ethanol 7% of body wt. H_2O, 3% of body wt.	+	ethanol	i. v.	cumulative antidiuresis over 10 min	2—3 μU	—	USP Post. Pit. Ref. Stand.
CZACZKES et al. (1964)	rat	12% ethanol 2×3% of body wt. + app. 2% of body wt.	+	ethanol	i. v.	percentage antidiuresis	0.25 μU	—	Synth. Arg-vasopressin
TATA and GAUER (1966)	rat	12% ethanol 2×3% of body wt. H_2O, 2% of body wt.	+	ethanol	i. v.	urine deficit during antidiuresis	0.25 μU	—	Tonephin
DYBALL et al. (1966)	rat		+			change in urine mass	—	—	—
PLISKA and RYCHLIK (1967)	rat	1% ethanol 8—10% of body wt.	+	ethanol pendiomide	i. v.	change in diuresis and urine conductivity	5 μU	—	Arg-vasopressin Lys-vasopressin
AHMED et al. (1967)	rat	10% ethanol 5% of body wt. 5% ethanol 5% of body wt.	+	ethanol	i. v.	percentage antidiuresis	2 μU	λ = 0.08	USP Post. Pit. Ref. Stand.
VIERLING et al. (1967)	(hered.) hypothal d. i. rat	12% ethanol 5.7% of body wt.	+	ethanol	i. v.	percentage antidiuresis	0.75 μU/100 g	—	USP Post. Pit. Ref. Stand.

Table 1. Cont. d)

Reference	Animal	Hydration	Maintenance of hydration	Anaesthesia	Route of injection	Index of response	Sensitivity	Precision	Standard
ANSELMINO et al. (1932)	rabbit	water; 90 cc by stomach tube	—	none	subcut.	change in rate of urine flow; change in NaCl excreted $2^1/_2$ hours after injection	—	—	Pituigan (Henning)
WALKER (1939)	rabbit	1 ml paraldehyde, water 100 ml + 50 ml/kg repeated	+	paralde-hyde	i. v.	change in rate of urine flow	0.2–0.5 mU/rabbit	—	Pituitrin
FUGO and ARAGON (1947) LINDQUIST and ROWE (1949)	rabbit	water; 5% of body wt. + 0.9% NaCl; 50 ml + 20% glucose; 25 ml i. v.	—	morphine + urethane	i. v.	change in rate of urine flow	0.2–0.3 mU/rabbit	—	Pitressin
KESTRANEK, MOLITOR and PICK (1925)	dog	water orally 250 ml/dog	—	none	subcut.	urine vol. in $1^1/_2$ hr. after inj.	—	—	Vögtlin's standard prep.
THEOBALD (1934)	dog	water; 250 ml/dog	—	chlora-lose	i. v.	change in rate of urine flow	—	—	Infundin (Burroughs, Wellcome & Co.)
SAMAAN (1935)	dog	water; 20—25 ml/kg repeated	+	none	i. v.	change in rate of urine flow	—	differences of 20% in dosage may be detected	Post. pit. (Burroughs, Wellcome & Co.)
HARE, HICKEY and HARE (1941)	D. I. dog	creatinine in water; 5 gm in 100 ml/dog	—	none	i. v.	creatinine U/P	0.25 mU/dog	—	Pitressin
HICKEY, HARE and HARE (1941)	D. I. dog	creatinine in water; 5 gm in 100 ml/dog	—	none	i. v.	area of curve plotting creatinine U/P against time	0.25 mU/dog	—	Pitressin

Table 1. Cont. e)

Reference	Animal	Hydration	Maintenance of hydration	Anaesthesia	Route of injection	Index of response	Sensitivity	Precision	Standard
HARE, MELVILLE, CHAMBERS and HARE (1945)	D. I. dog	creatinine in water; 5 gm in 100 ml/dog	—	none	i. v.	per cent. change in creatinine U/P	0.25 mU/dog	—	Pitressin
AMES, MOORE and v. DYKE (1950)	n. or D.I. dog	water; 8%	+	none	i. v.	change in rate of urine flow	0.25 mU	0.25 mU dist. from 0.5; 0.75 mU dist. from 0.5 or 1.0	Pitressin
BOCANEGRA and LAUSON (1961), LAUSON (1965)	dog	water	+	none	i. v. i. a.	cumulated antidiureses	—	—	All-beef Pitressin
FANG et al. (1962)	dog	0.45% NaCl by infusion	+	Chloralose or Inactin + ethanol	i. v.	Decrease in urine flow	—	—	Pitressin
MUNSICK et al. (1958)	„Miniature" pig	H_2O, appr. 5% of body wt.	+	none	i. v.	Percentage decrease in urine volume	—	—	Arginine-vasopressin. Synth. Lys-vasopressin
ANDERSSON and PERSSON (1958)	goat	water; 20%	+	none	i. v.	change in rate of urine flow	2 mU	—	Pitressin

injection of the substance to its effects on the receptors. The problems involved in assaying analogues have been discussed by NIELSEN (1964) and more recently by PLISKA *et al.* (PLISKA and RYCHLIK, 1967; PLISKA and KREJČÍ, 1966). The magnitude of the problems can be illustrated by the fact quoted by PLISKA and KREJČÍ (1966) that the antidiuretic activity of asparagine^4-lysine^8-vasopressin was found to be 600—800 U/mg by ZAORAL *et al.* but only 24 U/mg by BOISSONNAS *et al.* It was suggested that the cause of this difference was non-parallelism in the log dose response curves for the analogue and Lys^8-vasopressin.

The differences may play a part not only on the antidiuretic effect but also on possible effects on solute excretion. Thereby there might be differences in potency when comparing methods in which the index of response is urine volume or conductivity/osmolaritiy. Differences in strains of assay animals were found in the study of NIELSEN (1965) as compared with that of BERDE *et al.* (1961) on the relative antidiuresis potency of Phe^2-Lys^8-vasopressin and Lys^8-vasopressin.

O. Determination of the "Relative Antidiuretic Potency"

Determination of the so-called "relative antidiuretic potency" of different polypeptide preparations has been undertaken in some cases. It should, however, be remembered that this concept has certain limitations. This potency will be dependent on the index of response used. Also, however, the reference value, the pressor potency which is presumed to be identical may have been determined e.g. by different methods, where the relative pressor potency of the two substances need not be identical (NIELSEN, 1960).

It is obvious that one kind of antidiuretic units cannot be compared uncritically with others. There is, at least in some cases a difference in potency (effect per unit weight) between different analogues in the same animal and for the same peptide when it is assayed in different species.

This means that a proper indication of the antidiuretic potency of a preparation should include the species on which it has been determined, recording procedure and detailed description of the index of response.

P. Clinical Use of Assays for Antidiuretic Hormone Activity

1. Single Injection Assays

The main clinical situations in which determination of the antidiuretic activity of extracts of organs or of body fluids are of interest (possibly also after extraction, concentration, purification etc.) would seem to be the cases in which an inappropriate secretion of vasopressin occurs (see BARTTER and SCHWARTZ, 1967). This involves primarily cases of bronchogenic carcinoma (for a survey see BOWER and GORDON, 1965) in which vasopressin-like substances can be produced (BERDE, 1965), released to the blood (BOWER *et al.*, 1964) and excreted in the urine (THORN and TRANSBØL, 1963; RUCH, 1967).

Inappropriate secretion of vasopressin has also been reported in a number of cerebral diseases (GOLDBERG, 1963) as well as in acute intermittent porphyria (NIELSEN and THORN, 1965; CORNIL *et al.*, 1965), digitoxin intoxication (FOËX and KORALNIK, 1966), adrenocortical insufficiency (AHMED *et al.*, 1967) and postoperatively (see e.g. DEUTSCH *et al.*, 1966). It is common to all the studies on these problems that the criticisms raised against the assay methods outlined previously is also valid for assay methods employed here.

2. Transfusion Assays

Although this procedure would seem to have only limited application in the cases mentioned, one should here call attention to a principle which has been used in some studies in man (for dogs see p. 411), the method of transfusion assay, when only small concentrations of vasopressin are present in the blood. The transfusion can be given to the same person when he has been hydrated or to another, hydrated person. This method has e.g. been used by BRUN *et al.* (1945), BARNETT, FORMAN, and LAUSON (1952), and by EPSTEIN *et al.* (1961).

XVI. Pharmacological Application of Effects of Neurohypophysial Hormones on the Kidneys

Use of Synthetic Vasopressin Preparations in the Treatment of Diabetes Insipidus

The synthesis of neurohypophysial hormone peptides and analogues of them has introduced new possibilities in the treatment of diabetes insipidus due to vasopressin deficiency. Synthetic Lys^8-vasopressin has several advantages in comparison with the purified extracts previously used. It can be administered in a nasal spray instead of by injection and allergic reactions do not seem to occur. For descriptions of the clinical use of this preparation, the reader is referred to the paper by GOODMAN (1966) (which has a number of references; see also BARLTROP, (1963), DINGMAN and HAUGER-KLEVENE (1964), and RALLISON and TYLER (1967).

References

ABBRECHT, P. H., and R. L. MALVIN: Flow rate of urine as a determinant of renal countercurrent multiplier system. Amer. J. Physiol. **199**, 919—922 (1960).

— — Effects of GFR and renal plasma flow on urine osmolarity. Amer. J. Physiol. **201**, 754—758 (1961).

ABDUL-KARIM, R., and N. S. ASSALI: Renal function in human pregnancy. V. Effects of oxytocin on renal hemodynamics and water and electrolyte excretion. J. Lab. clin. Med. **57**, 522—532 (1961).

ABRAHAMS, C. V., and M. PICKFORD: The effect of 5-hydroxytryptamine on the urethra and on the blood pressure of dogs, and of adrenaline, noradrenaline and posterior pituitary extract on the urethra. Brit. J. Pharmacol. **11**, 44—49 (1956).

ADAMSONS, K. jr., S. L. ENGEL, and H. B. VAN DYKE: The stability of natural and synthetic neurohypophysial hormones in vitro. Endocrinology **63**, 679—681 (1958).

AHMED, A. B. J., B. C. GEORGE, C. GONZALES-AUVERT, and J. F. DINGMAN: Increased plasma arginine vasopressin in clinical adrenocortical insufficiency and its inhibition by glucosteroids. J. clin. Invest. **46**, 111—123 (1967).

AIKAWA, J. K., and J. P. PILLIOD: Changes in renal tissue composition induced in rabbits by various intravenous doses of mercaptomerin sodium. Proc. Soc. exp. Biol. (N.Y.) **101**, 61—66 (1959).

ALBERS, R. W., and M. W. BRIGHTMAN: A major component of neurohypophysial tissue associated with antidiuretic activity. J. Neurochem. **3**, 269—276 (1959).

ALBRIGHT, F., and F. C. BARTTER: The effects of anterior pituitary adrenocorticotropic hormone (ACTH) on bone metabolism. Transactions of the 2nd Conf. on Metabolic Interrelations. New York: J. Macy Found. 1950.

ALEXANDER, C.: The effect of 3',5'-cyclic AMP and other nucleotides on urine flow and hemodynamics in the rat. J. clin. Invest. **44**, 1025 (1965).

ALEXANDER, C. S.: Production of diabetes insipidus in the rat. Proc. Soc. exp. Biol. (N.Y.) **99**, 142—146 (1958).

—, and D. M. FILBIN: Failure of vasopressin to produce normal urine concentration in patients with diabetes insipidus. J. Lab. clin. Med. **54**, 566—571 (1959).

ALI, M. N.: A comparison of some activities of arginine vasopressin and lysine vasopressin on kidney function in conscious dogs. Brit. J. Pharmacol. **13**, 131—137 (1958).

—, R. B. CROSS, and M. PICKFORD: Electrolyte excretion in diuretic and non-diuretic dogs. J. Physiol. (Lond.) **41**, 177—182 (1958).

AMES, R. G., D. H. MOORE, and H. B. VAN DYKE: The excretion of posterior pituitary antidiuretic hormone in the urine and its detection in the blood. Endocrinology **46**, 215—227 (1950).

ANDERSON, W.A., and E. BROWN: The influence of arginine vasopressin on the production of adenosine 3',5'-monophosphate by adenyl cyclase from the kidney. Biochim. biophys. Acta (Amst.) **67**, 674—676 (1963).

ANDERSSON, B., and N. PERSSON: Intravenous assay of antidiuretic hormone using the goat. Acta physiol. scand. **42**, 257—261 (1958).

ANGERVALL, L., L. LEHMANN, and U. BENGTSSON: The renal concentrating capacity in albino rats after long-term consumption of phenacetin, napa and acetylsalicylic acid. Acta med. scand. **175**, 155—160 (1964).

ANSELMINO, K.J., F. HOFFMANN, and W.P. KENNEDY: The relation of hyperfunction of the posterior lobe of the hypophysis to ecclampsia and nephropathy of pregnancy. Edinb. med. J. **39**, 376—388 (1932).

ANSLOW, W.P., and L.G. WESSON jr.: Some effects of pressor-antidiuretic and oxytocic fractions of posterior pituitary extract on sodium, chloride, potassium and ammonium excretion in the dog. Amer. J. Physiol. **182**, 561—566 (1955).

APPELBOOM, J.W., W.A. BRODSKY, and W.N. SCOTT: Effect of osmotic diuresis on intrarenal solutes in diabetes indipidus and hydropenia. Amer. J. Physiol. **208**, 38—45 (1965).

ASHMAN, D.F., R. LIPTON, M. MELICOW, and T.D. PROCE: Isolation of adenosine 3',5'-monophosphate and guanosine 3',5'-monophosphate from rat urine. Biochem. biophys. Res. Com. **11**, 330 (1963).

ASSALI, N.S., W.J. DIGNAM, and L. LONGO: Renal function in human pregnancy. III. Effects of antidiuretic hormone (ADH) on renal hemodynamics and water and electrolyte excretion near term and post partum. J. clin. Endocr. **20**, 581—592 (1960).

ATHERTON, J.C., M.A. HAI, and S. THOMAS: Transient saluresis due to lysine-vasopressin administration in the conscious water diuretic rat. J. Physiol. (Lond.) 190, 30—31 P (1967).

AU, W.Y.W., and L.G. RAISZ: Studies on the renal concentrating mechanism. V. Effect of diuretic agents. J. clin. Invest. **39**, 1302—1311 (1960).

AUKLAND, K.: Studies of renal circulation with inert gas. Measurements in tissue. Proc. 3rd Congr. Nephrol. Washington 1966.

—, and R.W. BERLINER: Renal medullary countercurrent system studied with hydrogen gas. Circulat. Res. **15**, 430—442 (1962).

—, and J. KJEKSHUS: Tubular salt and water transport in hydrated dogs studied with pushflow technique. Amer. J. Physiol. **210**, 971—979 (1966).

BAER, J.E., A.V. BROOKS, R.M. NOLL, and K.B. BEYER: Effect of hydrochlorothiazide on renal electrolyte gradient in glucose diuresis and experimental diabetes insipidus. J. Pharmacol. exp. Ther. **137**, 319—323 (1962).

BAHLMANN, J., J.G. GIEBISCH, B. OCHWADT, and W. SCHOEPPE: Micropuncture study of isolated perfused rat kidney. Amer. J. Physiol. **212**, 77—82 (1967).

BAKER, G.P., H. LEVITIN, and F.H. EPSTEIN: Sodium depletion and renal conservation of water. J. clin. Invest. **40**, 867—873 (1961).

BANK, N., and H.S. AYNEDJIAN: A micropuncture study of the renal concentrating defect of potassium depletion. Amer. J. Physiol. **206**, 1347—1354 (1964).

BARATZ, R.A., A. DOIG, and I.J. ADATTO: Plasma antidiuretic activity and free water clearance following osmoreceptor and neurohypophyseal stimulation in human subjects. J. clin. Invest. **39**, 1539—1545 (1960).

—, and R.C. INGRAHAM: Sensitive bioassay method for measuring antidiuretic hormone in mammalian plasma. Proc. Soc. exp. Biol. (N.Y.) **100**, 296—299 (1959).

BARCLAY, J.A., R.F. CRAMPTON, and D.M. MATTHEWS: Henle's loop and the sodium content of the medullae of mammalian kidneys. J. Physiol. (Lond.) **147**, 48 P (1959).

BARER, G.R.: The action of vasopressin, a vasopressin analogue (PLV_2) oxytocin, angiotensin, bradykinin and theophylline ethylene diamine on renal blood flow in the anaesthetized cat. J. Physiol. (Lond.) **169**, 62—72 (1963).

BARGER, A.C., R.D. BERLIN, and J.F. TULENKO: Infusion of aldosterone, 9-fluorohydrocortisone and antidiuretic hormone into the renal artery of normal and adrenalectomized, unanesthetized dogs. Effect on electrolyte and water excretion. Endocrinology **62**, 804—815 (1958).

BARLTROP, D.: Diabetes insipidus treated with synthetic lysine vasopressin. Lancet **1963**, 176—278.

BARNAFI, L., R. ROSAS, M. DE LA LASTRA, and H. CROXATTO: Influence of oxytocin and vasopressin on sodium-retaining activity of aldosterone in the rat. Amer. J. Physiol. **198**, 255—259 (1960).

— —, T. PEREDA, and H. CROXATTO: Effect of vasopressin structural modifications on rat renal excretion of Na, K and water. Amer. J. Physiol. **202**, 593—596 (1962).

BARNETT, H.L., C.W. FORMAN, and H.D. LAUSON: The nephrotic syndrome in children. Advanc. Pediat. **5**, 53—128 (1952).

Barth, T., W. Pliska, and I. Rychlik: Chymotryptic and tryptic cleavage of oxytocin and vasopressin. Collection Czech. Chem. Commun. **32**, 1058—1063 (1967).
Bartter, F. C., and W. B. Schwartz: The syndrome of inappropriate secretion of antidiuretic hormone. Amer. J. Med. **42**, 790—806 (1967).
Bauman, J. W.: Effect of hypophysectomy on the renal concentrating ability of the rat. Endocrinology **77**, 496—500 (1965).
—, C. Guyot-Jeannin, and J. Dobrowolski: Nutritional state and urine concentrating ability in the rat. J. Endocrin. **30**, 147—148 (1964).
Bentley, P. J.: The effects of neurohypophyseal extracts on water transfer across the wall of the isolated urine bladder of the toad, bufo marinus. J. Endocr. **17**, 201—209 (1958).
— The effects of ionic changes on water transfer across the isolated urinary bladder of the toad bufo marinus. J. Endocr. **18**, 327—333 (1959).
— Neurohypophysial function in amphibians, reptiles and birds. Symp. Zool. Soc. London **9**, 141—152 (1963).
Beránková-Ksandrová, Z., G. W. Bisset, K. Jost, I. Krejčí, V. Pliska, J. Rudinger, I. Rychlik, and F. Sorm: Synthetic analogues of oxytocin acting as hormonogens. Brit. J. Pharmacol. **26**, 615—632 (1966).
Berde, B.: Pharmacologie des hormones neurohypophysaires. Paris: Masson & Cie 1963.
— Les analogues synthetique des hormones neurohypophysaires sont-ils une clef de l'etude des troubles de l'hormonogenese de ce systeme? Rapport de la VIIIe reunion des endocrinologistes de langue française, p. 33—49 (1965).
—, and R. A. Boissonnas: Synthetic analogues and homologues of the posterior pituitary gland. In: The pituitary gland. Ed. by G. W. Harris and B. T. Donovan. London: Butterworths 1966.
—, u. A. Cerletti: Über die antidiuretische Wirkung von synthetischem Lysin-Vasopressin. Helv. physiol. pharmacol. Acta **19**, 135—150 (1961).
— — Medizinische und biologische Aspekte von pharmakologischen Arbeiten mit synthetischen Peptiden von neurohypophysärem Typus. Klin. Wschr. **42**, 1159—1165 (1964).
—, W. Doepfner, and H. Konzett: Some pharmacological actions of four synthetic analogues of oxytocin. Brit. J. Pharmacol. **12**, 209—214 (1957).
—, H. Weidmann, u. A. Cerletti: Über Phenylalanin²-Lysin-Vasopressin. Helv. physiol. pharmacol. Acta **19**, 285—302 (1961).
Berliner, R. W., and C. M. Bennett: Concentration of urine in the mammalian kidney. Amer. J. Med. **42**, 777—789 (1967).
—, and D. G. Davidson: Production of hypertonic urine in the absence of pituitary antidiuretic hormone. J. clin. Invest. **36**, 1416—1427 (1957).
—, N. Levinsky, D. G. Davidson, and M. Eden: Dilution and concentration of the urine and the action of antidiuretic hormone. Amer. J. Med. **24**, 730—744 (1958).
Berlyne, G. M., and A. Macken: On the mechanism of renal inability to produce a concentrated urine in chronic hydronephrosis. Clin. Sci. **22**, 315—324 (1962).
—, S. Nilwarangkur, K. Janabi, and M. Cooper: Nocturnal nephrogenic diabetes insipidus. Quart. J. Med. **34**, 463—479 (1965).
Bickford, R. G., and F. R. Winton: The influence of temperature on the isolated kidney of the dog. J. Physiol. (Lond.) **89**, 198—219 (1937).
Binkley, F., and G. M. Christensen: An effect of vasopressin on renal weight. Endocrinology **64**, 307—308 (1959).
Birnie, J. H., W. J. Eversole, W. R. Boss, C. M. Osborn, and R. Gaunt: An antidiuretic substance in the blood of normal and adrenalectomized rats. Endocrinology **47**, 1—12 (1950).
Bisset, G. W.: Effect of tyrosinase preparations on oxytocin, vasopressin and bradykinin. Brit. J. Pharmacol. **18**, 405—420 (1962).
Black, D. A. K.: Renal rete mirabile. Lancet **1965**, 1141—1152.
—, and A. E. Thomson: Day-to-day changes in sodium and water output with and without posterior pituitary extract. Clin Sci. **10**, 511—520 (1951).
Boba, A., and S. R. Powers: Mannitol-vasopressin in the splenectomized dog. J. surg. Res. **6**, 265—273 (1966).
Bocanegra, M., and H. D. Lauson: Ultrafilterability of endogenous antidiuretic hormone from plasma of dogs. Amer. J. Physiol. **200**, 486—493 (1961).
Boissonnas, R. A., St. Guttman, B. Berde, and H. Konzett: Relationship between the chemical structures and the biological properties of the posterior pituitary hormones and their synthetic analogues. Experientia (Basel) **17**, 377—391 (1961).
Bojesen, E.: Den tubulære saltvandsresorption. København: Christtreus 1955.
Boss, J. M. N., H. Dlouha, M. Kraus, and J. Krecek: The development of the kidney in young rats. J. Physiol. (Lond.) **161**, 51—52 P (1962).

BOURA, A., and S. E. DICKER: An apparatus for the maintenance of a constant water load and the recording of urine flow in rats. J. Physiol. (Lond.) **122**, 144—148 (1953).
BOWER, B. F., and G. S. GORDON: Hormonal effects of nonendocrine tumors. Ann. Rev. Med. **16**, 83—118 (1965).
—, D. M. MASON, and P. H. FORSHAM: Bronchogenic carcinoma with inappropriate antidiuretic activity in plasma and tumor. New Engl. J. Med. **271**, 934—938 (1964).
BOYLAN, J. W., and E. ASSHAUER: Depletion and restoration of the medullary osmotic gradient in the dog kidney. Pflügers Arch. ges. Physiol. **276**, 99—116 (1962).
BOZLER, E.: Osmotic effects and diffusion of nonelectrolytes in muscle. Amer. J. Physiol. **197**, 505—510 (1959).
BRANDA, L. A., and V. DU VIGNEAUD: Synthesis and pharmacological properties of 9-decarboxamido-oxytocin. J. med. pharm. Chem. **9**, 169—172 (1966).
BRAY, G. A.: Distribution of urea, thiourea-C^{14} and sucrose-C^{14} in dog kidney during antidiuresis. Amer. J. Physiol. **199**, 1211—1214 (1960).
— Freezing point depression of rat kidney slices during water diuresis and antidiuresis. Amer. J. Physiol. **199**, 915—918 (1960).
BRODEHL, J. A., K. GELLISSEN, u. W. HAGGE: Die Wirkung des Vasopressins beim Diabetes Insipidus Renalis. Klin. Wschr. **43**, 72—78 (1965).
BROOK, A. H., and L. SHARE: On the question of protein binding and the diffusibility of circulating antidiuretic hormone in the dog. Endocrinology **78**, 779—785 (1966).
BROOKS, F. P., and M. PICKFORD: The effect of posterior pituitary hormones on the excretion of electrolytes in dogs. J. Physiol. (Lond.) **142**, 468—493 (1958).
BROWN, E., D. L. CLARKE, V. ROUX, and G. H. SHERMAN: The stimulation of adenosine 3',5'-monophosphate production by antidiuretic factors. J. biol. Chem. **238**, PC 852—PC 853 (1963).
BROWN, J. H. U., and A. A. PETKAS: The behavior of kidney mitochondria under the influence of ADH. Endocrinology **69**, 182—183 (1961).
BRUN, C., E. O. E. KNUDSEN, and F. RAASCHOU: On the cause of postsyncopal oliguria. Acta med. scand. **122**, 486—500 (1945).
BRUNNER, F. P., and D. W. SELDIN: The mechanism of the urinary concentrating defect in potassium dificient rats. Pflügers Arch. ges. Physiol. **290**, 202—210 (1966).
BRUNNER, H., G. KUSCHINSKY, O. MÜNCHOW, u. G. PETERS: Der Einfluß von Oxytocin auf Diurese und Salzausscheidung bei Ratte und Mensch. Klin. Wschr. **34**, 451—452 (1956).
BUCHBORN, E.: Ein quantitativer biologischer Adiuretin-(Vasopressin-)Nachweis an der Kröte. Z. ges. exp. Med. **125**, 614—625 (1955).
— Klinische Pathophysiologie der Harnkonzentrierung. Schweiz. med. Wschr. **94**, 1273—1283 (1964).
BUCHER, O. VON, u. PH. GRANDJEAN: Zur Frage der Angriffspunkte des antidiuretischen Hormons in der Niere. Z. Biol. **113**, 67—76 (1961).
BUCKALEW, V. M., M. A. RAMIREZ, and M. GOLDBERG: Free water reabsorption during solute diuresis in normal and potassium depleted rats. Amer. J. Physiol. **212**, 381—386 (1967).
BULGER, R. E., L. D. GRIFFITH, and B. F. TRUMP: Endoplasmic reticulum in rat renal interstitial cells. Molecular rearrangement after water deprivation. Science **151**, 83—86 (1966).
BURN, H.: Estimation of the antidiuretic potency of pituitary (posterior lobe) extract. Quart. J. exp. Biol. (N.Y.) **4**, 517—529 (1931).
CAPEK, K., G. FUCHS, G. RUMRICH, u. K. J. ULLRICH: Harnstoffpermeabilität der corticalen Tubulusabschnitte von Ratten in Antidiurese und Wasserdiurese. Pflügers Arch. ges. Physiol. **290**, 237—249 (1966).
CARASSO, N., P. FAVARD, J. BOURGUET, et S. JARD: Role du flux net d'eau dans les modifications ultrastructurales de la vessie de grenouille stimulée par l'oxytocine. J. Microsc. **5**, 519—522 (1966).
— —, and J. VALERIEN: Variations des ultrastructure dans les cellules epitheliales de la vessie du crapaud apres stimulation par l'hormone neurohypophysaires. J. Microscopie **1**, 143—158 (1962).
CARONE, F. A., and F. H. EPSTEIN: Nephrogenic diabetes insipidus caused by amyloid disease. Amer. J. Med. **29**, 539—544 (1960).
—, B. A. EVERETT, N. J. BLONDEEL, and M. GOLDBERG: Renal localization of albumin and its function in the concentrating mechanism. Amer. J. Physiol. **212**, 387 (1967—393).
CHABRIA, N. L., and B. B. GAITONDE: Effect of dexamethasone on urine output and electrolyte excretion in rats. Arch. int. Pharmacodyn. **162**, 364—370 (1966).
CHALMERS, T. M., A. A. G. LEWIS, and G. L. S. PAWAN: The effect of posterior pituitary extracts on the renal excretion of sodium and chloride in man. J. Physiol. (Lond.) **112**, 238—242 (1951).

Chan, W. Y.: Effects of neurohypophysial hormones and their deamino analogues on renal excretion of Na, K and water in rats. Endocrinology **77**, 1097—1104 (1965).
—, and H. Sawyer: Saluretic actions of neurohypophysial peptides in conscious dogs. Amer. J. Physiol. **201**, 799—803 (1961).
—, and W. H. Sawyer: Natriuresis in conscious dogs during arginine vasopressin infusion and after oxytocin injection. Proc. Soc. exp. Biol. (N.Y.) **110**, 697—699 (1962).
Chaudhury, R. R., and J. M. Walker: The fate of injected oxytocin in the rabbit. J. Endocr. **19**, 189—192 (1959).
Chinard, F. P.: Kidney, water and electrolytes. Ann. Rev. Physiol. **26**, 187—226 (1964).
Clapp, J. R.: Renal tubular reabsorption of urea in normal and protein-depleted rats. Amer. J. Physiol. **210**, 1304—1308 (1966).
—, and R. R. Robinson: Osmolality of distal tubular fluid in the dog. J. clin. Invest. **45**, 1847—1853 (1966).
—, J. F. Watson, and R. W. Berliner: Osmolality, bicarbonate concentration and water reabsorption in proximal tubule of the dog nephron. Amer. J. Physiol. **205**, 273—279 (1963).
Crabbé, J.: The role of aldosterone in the renal concentration mechanism in man. Clin. Sci. **23**, 39—46 (1962).
—, and P. de Weer: Action of aldosterone and vasopressin on the active transport by the isolated toad bladder. J. Physiol. (Lond.) **180**, 560—568 (1965).
Cornil, A., J. C. Demant, P. van Geel, et P. A. Bastenie: Syndrome de Schwartz Bartter au cours d'une porphyrie aigue intermittente. Acta clin. belg. **20**, 286—299 (1965).
Cort, J. H., J. Rudinger, B. Lichardus, and J. Hagemann: Effects of oxytocin antagonists on the saluresis accompanying carotid occlusion. Amer. J. Physiol. **210**, 162—168 (1966).
Crawford, R. F., A. Paresi, P. Meara, and M. L. Terry: Urine composition and renal tissue electrolytes. Amer. J. Dis. Child. **94**, 512—513 (1957).
—, and B. Pinkham: An assay method for antidiuretic hormone based on a more specific response index. Endocrinology **55**, 521—529 (1954).
Cross, B. A., and G. W. Harris: The role of the neurohypophysis in the milk-ejection reflex. J. Endocr. **8**, 148—161 (1952).
Cross, R. B.: The effects of osmotic diuresis and vasopressin upon the distribution of sodium, potassium and urea in the rat kidney. Aust. J. exp. Biol. med. Sci. **42**, 523—538 (1964).
—, S. E. Dicker, A. H. Kitchin, S. Lloyd, and M. Pickford: The effect of oxytocin on urinary excretion of water and electrolytes in man. J. Physiol. (Lond.) **153**, 553—561 (1960).
—, E. Lee, and W. M. Thornton: The effect of vasopressin on urea excretion by the sheep. J. Physiol. (Lond.) **187**, 34—35 (1966a).
—, and L. A. Sherrington: The effect of vasopressin on water distribution in the rat kidney. Aust. J. exp. Biol. med. Sci. **43**, 505—510 (1965).
— —, and W. M. Thornton: The effect of vasopressin upon the distribution of serum albumin in the rat kidney. Aust. J. exp. Biol. med. Sci. **44**, 137—142 (1966b).
—, W. M. Thornton, and E. D. Twedell: The effect of vasopressin on water and electrolyte excretion by the sheep. Aust. J. exp. Biol. med. Sci. **41**, 629—636 (1963).
Croxatto, H., u. E. Labarca: Die Wirkung von synthetischem Oxytocin (Syntocinon) und Acetazolamid auf die Ausscheidung von Wasser, Natrium und Kalium. Experientia (Basel) **14**, 339—341 (1958).
Curtis, J. R., and H. E. de Wardener: Effect of urine pH on the changes in urine concentration produced by vasopressin. Clin. Sci. **24**, 159—166 (1963).
Cutler, R. E., C. R. Kleemann, M. H. Maxwell, and J. T. Dowling: Physiologic studies in nephrogenic diabetes insipidus. J. clin. Endocr. **22**, 827—838 (1962).
Czaczkes, J. W., M. Eliakim, and T. D. Ullman: Diminished antidiuretic response to pitressin in diabetes insipidus during the infusion of sodium bicarbonate solution. J. Lab. clin. Med. **57**, 938—945 (1961).
—, C. R. Kleeman, and M. Koenig: Physiologic studies of antidiuretic hormone by its direct measurement in human plasma. J. clin. Invest. **43**, 1625—1640 (1964).
Dainty, J., and C. R. House: An examination of the evidence for membrane pores in frog skin. J. Physiol. (Lond.) **185**, 172—241 (1966).
Dale, H.: Evidence concerning the endocrine function of the neurohypophysis and its nervous control. In: The Neurohypophysis. Ed. by H. Heller. London: Butterworths 1957.
Dalton, A. J., and F. Haguenau: Ultrastructure of the kidney. New York: Academic Press (1967).
Daniel, J., u. F. Högler: Über die Diuresehemmung durch Pituitrinum infundibulare (infundibulin). Wien. Arch. inn. Med. **13**, 481—508 (1927).
Dantzler, W. H.: Renal response of chickens to infusion of hyperosmotic sodium chloride solution. Amer. J. Physiol. **210**, 640—646 (1966).

DARMADY, E.M., and J. DURANT, E.R. MATTHEWS, and F. STRANACK: Location of ^{131}J Pitressin in the kidney by autoradiography. Clin. Sci. **19**, 229—241 (1960).
—, J. OFFER, J. PRINCE, and F. STANACK: The proximal convoluted tubule in the renal handling of water. Lancet **1964**, 1254—1257.
DAVEY, M.J., and M.F. LOCKETT: Actions and interactions of aldosterone, monoacetate and neurohypophysial hormones on the isolated cat kidney. J. Physiol. (Lond.) **152**, 206—219 (1960).
DAVID, M.A., u. K. KOVACS: Die Wirkung der Oestronbehandlung auf die antidiuretische Aktivität des Vasopressins. Endokrinologie **46**, 217—223 (1964).
DAVIS, B.B., F.G. KNOX and R.W. BERLINER: The effect of vasopressin on proximal tubule sodium reabsorption in the dog. Amer. J. Physiol. **212**, 1361—1364 (1967).
DE BODO, K.C., and K.F. PRESCOTT: The antidiuretic action of barbiturates (phenobarbital, amytal, Pentobarbital) and the mechanism involved in this action. J. Pharmacol. exp. Ther. **85**, 222—233 (1945).
DEIS, R.P., S. LLOYD, and M. PICKFORD: The effects of stilboestrol and progesterone and of renal denervation on the response of the kidney to vasopressin and oxytocin. J. Physiol. (Lond.) **165**, 348—357 (1963).
DEL GRECO, F., and H.E. DE WARDENER: The effect on urine osmolarity of a transient reduction in glomerular filtration rate and solute output during a water diuresis. J. Physiol. (Lond.) **131**, 307—316 (1956).
DEMUNBRUN, T.W., A.D. KELLER, A.H. LEVKOFF, and R.M. PUSSER, jr.: Pitocin restoration of renal hemodynamics to pre-neurohypophysectomy levels. Amer. J. Physiol. **179**, 429—438 (1954).
DETTELBACH, H.R.: A method for assaying small amounts of antidiuretic substances with notes on some properties of vasopressin. Amer. J. Physiol. **192**, 379—386 (1958).
DEUTSCH, S., M. GOLDBERG, and R.D. DRIPPS: Postperative hyponatremia with the inappropriate release of antidiuretic hormone. Anesthesiology **27**, 250—256 (1966).
DE WARDENER, H.E.: Polyuria. J. chron. Dis. **2**, 199—212 (1960).
—, and A. HERXHEIMER: The effect of a high water intake on the kidney's ability to concentrate the urine in man. J. Physiol. (Lond.) **139**, 42—52 (1957).
DE WIED, D.: A simple automatic and sensitive method for the assay of antidiuretic hormone with notes on the antidiuretic potency of plasma under different experimental conditions. Acta physiol. pharmacol. neerl. **9**, 69—81 (1960).
DIAMOND, J.M., and J. McD. TORMEY: The role of long extracellular channels in fluid transport across epithelia. Nature (Lond.) **210**, 817—820 (1966).
DICK, D.A.T.: Cell water. London: Butterworth 1966.
DICKER, S.E.: A method for the assay of very small amounts of antidiuretic activity with a note on the antidiuretic titre of rat's blood. J. Physiol. (Lond.) **122**, 149—157 (1953).
— Release and metabolism of neurohypophyseal hormones. J. Pharm. Pharmacol. **13**, 449—469 (1961).
— The mechanism of action of oxytocin and vasopressin and their analogues on the kidney of mammals. In: Oxytocin, vasopressin and structual analogues. Ed. by J. RUDINGER. Pergamon Press, Czech. Medical Press 1964.
—, M.C. EGGLETON, and J. HASLAM: The effects of urea and hydrochlorothiazide on the renal functions of rat and domestic fowl. J. Physiol. (Lond.) **187**, 247—255 (1966).
—, and M.G. EGGLETON: Renal excretion of hyaluronidase and calcium in man during the antidiuretic action of vasopressin and some analogues. J. Physiol. (Lond.) **157**, 351—362 (1961).
—, and C.S. FRANKLIN: The isolation of hyaluronic acid and chondroitin sulphate from kidneys and their reaction with urinary hyaluronidase. J. Physiol. (Lond.) **186**, 110—120 (1966).
—, and A.L. GREENBAUM: The destruction of the antidiuretic activity of vasopressin by -SH active compounds. J. Physiol. (Lond.) **141**, 107—116 (1938).
—, and J. HASLAM: Water diuresis in the domestic fowl. J. Physiol. (Lond.) **183**, 225—235 (1966).
—, and H. HELLER: The renal action of posterior pituitary extract and its fractions as analyzed by clearance experiments on rats. J. Physiol. (Lond.) **104**, 353—360 (1946).
—, and J. NUNN: Antidiuresis in adult and old rats. J. Physiol. (Lond.) **141**, 332—336 (1958).
DINGMAN, J.F.: Hypothalamus and the endocrine control of sodium and water metabolism in man. Amer. J. med. Sci. **235**, 79—99 (1958).
—, and J.H. HAUGER-KLEVENE: Treatment of diabetes insipidus: synthetic vasopressin nasal solution. J. clin. Endocr. **24**, 550—553 (1964).
DLOUHA, H., J. KRECEK, M. KRAUS, and V. PLISKA: Sensitivity of rats to vasopressin in the weaning period. Physiol. bohemoslov. **14**, 217—224 (1965).
DOUGLAS, C.P.: Oxytocin and antidiuresis in pregnancy at term. Clin. Sci. **28**, 39—42 (1965).

Dow, J., and R. O. H. Irvine: The effect of diuretics on cortico-medullary gradients of sodium and urea in rat kidney. Nephron **4**, 25—31 (1967).

Dyball, R. E. J., G. J. Lane, and R. G. Morris: A simplified automatic device for the performance of antidiuretic assays. J. Physiol. (Lond.) **186**, 43P—44P (1966).

Earle, D. P. jr., R. C. de Bodo, I. L. Schwartz, S. J. Farber, M. Kurtz, and J. Greenberg: Effect of hypophysectomy on electrolyte and water metabolism in the dog. Proc. Soc. exp. Biol. (N.Y.) **76**, 608—612 (1951).

Edelmann, C. M., H. L. Barnett, and H. Stark: Effect of urea on concentration of urinary nonurea solute in premature infants. J. appl. Physiol. **21**, 1021—1025 (1966).

Epstein, F. H.: Disorders of renal concentrating ability. Yale J. Biol. Med. **39**, 186—190 (1966).

—, C. R. Kleeman, and A. Hendrikx: The influence of bodily hydration on the renal concentrating process. J. clin. Invest. **36**, 629—634 (1957).

—, H. Levitin, G. Glaser, and P. Lavietes: Cerebral hyponatremia New. Engl. J. Med. **265**, 513—518 (1961).

Ericsson, J. L. E.: Glutaraldehyd perfusion of the kidney for preservation of proximal tubules with patent lumens. J. Microscopie **5**, 97—100 (1966).

Ezrin, C., L. Loach, and T. F. Nicholson: Diuretic effect of oxytocin in a patient with reversed diurnal rhythm of water and electrolyte excretion. Canad. med. Ass. J. **87**, 673—675 (1962).

Fang, H. S., H. M. Liu, and S. C. Wang: Liberation of antidiuretic hormone following hypothalamic stimulation in the dog. Amer. J. Physiol. **202**, 212—216 (1962).

Finn, A. L., J. S. Handler, and J. Orloff: Relation between toad bladder potassium content and permeability response to vasopressin. Amer. J. Physiol. **210**, 1279—1285 (1966).

Fisher, C., W. R. Ingram, and S. W. Ranson: Diabetes insipidus and the vaso-humoral control of water balance. Ann. Arbor. J. W. Edwards (1938).

Foëx, P., and O. Koralnik: Sécrétion inadéquate d'hormone antidiuretique lors d'une intoxication digitalique massive. Schweiz. med. Wschr. **96**, 1750—1751 (1966).

Forsling, M. L., J. J. Jones, and J. Lee: A change of sensitivity to neurohypophysial hormones induced by their intravenous infusion in the rat. J. Physiol (Lond.) **191**, 127P (1967).

Forster, R. P.: Kidney, water and electrolytes. Ann. Rev. Physiol. **27**, 183—232 (1965).

Foulkes, E. C.: The action of pitressin on solute permeability of the rabbit nephron in vivo. J. gen. Physiol. **50**, 1—8 (1966).

Fourmann, J., and G. C. Kennedy: An effect of antidiuretic hormone on the flow of blood through the vasa recta of the rat kidney. J. Endocr. **35**, 173—176 (1966).

—, and D. B. Moffat: The effect of water intake on the efferent arterioles of the juxtamedullary glomeruli. 2nd Int. Congr. Nephrology Prague 1963. Excerpta med. Int. Congr. Series **78**, 627—629.

Frandsen, P.: The specific pressor and antidiuretic activity in rat urine after infusion of lysine-vasopressin. Acta pharmacol. (Kbh.) **25**, 197—200 (1967).

—, and Aa. Theil Nielsen: The antidiuretic effect of 5-hydroxytryptamine in the rat after subcutaneous injection of "physiological doses". Acta pharmacol. (Kbh.) **24**, 50—54 (1966).

Fraser, A. M.: The diuretic action of the oxytocic hormone of the pituitary and its effect on the assay of pituitary extracts. J. Pharmacol. exp. Ther. **60**, 89—95 (1937).

— The action of the oxytocic hormone of the pituitary gland on urine secretion. J. Physiol. (Lond.) **101**, 236—251 (1942).

Frey, J., L. Kerp, u. W. Reichardt: Antidiurese und Zunahme der Harnkonzentration nach i.v. Vasopressin-Gabe beim Menschen. Pflügers Arch. ges. Physiol. **272**, 80—81 (1960).

Friedler, R. M., and L. E. Earley: Reduced renal concentrating capacity during isotonic saline loading. Proc. Soc. exp. Biol. (N.Y.) **121**, 352—357 (1966).

Fugo, N. W., and G. T. Aragon: The utilization of an old technique for a sensitive antidiuretic assay. Fed. Proc. **6**, 330—331 (1947).

Fukuda, T. R.: Tonic antagonism in the water permeability of sea urchin eggs. J. cell. comp. Physiol. **7**, 301—311 (1936).

Galton, V. A., H. Valtin, and D. G. Johnson: Thyroid function in the absence of vasopressin. Endocrinology **78**, 1224—1228 (1966).

Gans, J. H.: Vasopressin-induced saluresis in sheep. Amer. J. vet. Res. **25**, 918—923 (1964).

Gardner, B., G. S. Gordan, and J. Witt: Urinary calcium excretion of women with breast cancer during post-hypophysectomy polyuria, spontaneous interphase and vasopressin-induced antidiuresis. Proc. Soc. exp. Biol. (N.Y.) **109**, 71—75 (1962).

Gardner, K. D., and R. H. Maffly: An in vitro demonstration of increased collecting tubular permeability to urea in the presence of vasopressin. J. clin. Invest. **43**, 1968—1975 (1964).

Gardner, K. D. jr.: Dry weight as a point of reference in studies of renal papillary composition. Amer. J. Physiol. **211**, 1031—1035 (1966).

Gauer, O. H., and P. S. Tata: Vasopressin studies in the rat. II. The amount of water reabsorbed by the rat kidney after single i.v. injection of vasopressin: The vasopressin water equivalent. Pflügers Arch. Physiol. **290**, 286—293 (1966).

GAUNT, R., C.W. LLOYD, and J.J. CHART: The adrenal-neurohypophysial interrelationship. In: The Neurohypophysis, p. 233. Ed. by H. HELLER. London: Butterworths 1957.

GERTZ, K.H., G.C. KENNEDY u. K.J. ULLRICH: Mikropunktionsuntersuchungen über die Flüssigkeitsruckresorption aus den einzelnen Tubulusabschnitten bei Wasserdiurese (diabetes insipidus). Pflügers Arch. ges. Physiol. **278**, 513—519 (1964).

GIBBS, O.S.: A practical test for the antidiuretic action of pituitary. J. Pharmacol. exp. Ther. **40**, 129—137 (1930).

GIEBISCH, G.: Kidney, water and electrolyte metabolism. Ann. Rev. Physiol. **24**, 357—420 (1962).

GILL, J.R., jr., and F.C. BARTER: On the impairment of renal concentrating ability in prolonged hypercalcemia and hypercalciuria in man. J. clin. Invest. **40**, 716—722 (1961).

GILMAN, A., and L. GOODMAN: The secretory response of the posterior pituitary to the need for water conservation. J. Physiol. (Lond.) **90**, 113—124 (1937).

GINETZINSKY, A.G.: Role of hyaluronidase in the re-absorption of water in renal tubulus. The mechanism of action of the antidiuretic hormone. Nature (Lond.) **182**, 1218—1219 (1958).

GINSBURG, M., and H. HELLER: The antidiuretic assay of vasopressin by intravenous injection into unanaesthetized rats. J. Endocr. **9**, 267—273 (1953).

— —, and H. SCHNIEDEN: Unpublished observations. In: The hormonal control of water and salt-electrolyte metabolism with special reference to higher vertebrates. Ed. by H. HELLER. Mem. Soc. Endocr. **5**, 35 (1955).

GLATTE, H., R.E. CUTLER, and J.T. DOWLING: Studies of the renal concentrating defect in thyrotoxicosis. J. clin. Invest. **44**, 1050 (1965).

GLAUBACH, S., u. H. MOLITOR: Vergleich der Auswertungsmethoden von Gesamtextrakten des Hypophysenhinterlappens am isolierten Meerschweinchenuterus und an der Diuresehemmung von Hunden, Ratten und Mäusen. Arch. exp. Pathol. Pharmakol. **166**, 243—264 (1932).

GLIMSTEDT, G., N. JOUSSON, and H.R. ROSSMAN: The collecting tubules of the kidney in the rat at water overloading. Kungl. Fysiogr. Sällsk i Lunds Forh. **24**, 1—9 (1954).

GLOOR, F., u. L.A. NEIDITSCH-HALFF: Die interstitiellen Zellen des Nierenmarkes der Ratte. Z. Zellforsch. **66**, 488—495 (1965).

GOLDBERG, M.: Hyponatremia and the inappropriate secretion of antidiuretic hormone. Amer. J. Med. **35**, 293—298 (1963).

GOLDBLATT, E.L., M.L. KAUKER, R.S. HARE, and K. HARE: Effects of ethyleneimine on renal action of vasopressin. Proc. Soc. exp. Biol. (N.Y.) **123**, 845—847 (1967).

GOODMAN, B., A. COHEN, M.F. LEWITT, and M. KAHN: Renal concentration in the normal dog. Effect of an acute reduction in salt excretion. Amer. J. Physiol. **206**, 1123—1128 (1964).

GOODMANN, A., and H. LEVITIN: Effect of urinary pH on the renal concentrating mechanism. Amer. J. Physiol. **208**, 847—851 (1965).

GOODMANN, R.: Diabetes insipidus. A two-year study with lysine^8-vasopressin. Curr. ther. Res. **8**, 56—60 (1966).

GOTTSCHALK, C.W.: Osmotic concentration and dilution of the urine. Amer. J. Med. **36**, 670—685 (1964).

—, W.E. LASSITER, M. MYLLE, K.J. ULLRICH, B. SCHMIDT-NIELSEN, R. O'DELL, and G. PEHLING: Micropuncture study of composition of loop of Henle fluid in desert rodents. Amer. J. Physiol. **204**, 532—535 (1963).

—, F. MOREL, and M. MYLLE: Tracer microinjection studies of renal tubular permeability. Amer. J. Physiol. **209**, 173—178 (1965).

—, and M. MYLLE: Micropuncture study of pressures in proximal tubules and peritubular capillaries of the rat kidney and their relation to ureteral and renal venous pressures. Amer. J. Physiol. **185**, 430—439 (1956).

— — Micropuncture study of pressures in proximal and distal tubules and peritubular capillaries of the rat kidney during osmotic diuresis. Amer. J. Physiol. **189**, 323—328 (1957).

— — Micropuncture study of the mammalian urinary concentrating mechanism. Evidence for the countercurrent hypothesis. Amer. J. Physiol. **196**, 927—936 (1959).

— —, N.F. JONES, R.W. WINTERS, and L.G. WELT: Osmolality of renal tubular fluids in potassium-depleted rodents. Clin. Sci. **29**, 249—260 (1965).

GRANBERG, P.-O.: Effect of acute hypoxia on renal haemodynamics and water diuresis in man. Stockholm: Svenska Tryckeriaktiebolaget 1963.

GRANTHAM, J.J., and M.B. BURG: Effect of vasopressin and cyclic AMP on permeability of isolated collecting tubules. Amer. J. Physiol. **211**, 255—259 (1966).

GRASER, F.: Die Beeinflussung der Chlorurese durch Oxytocin und Vasopressin beim diabetes insipidus. Klin. Wschr. **28**, 551—552 (1950).

GREEN, H.H., A.R. HARRINGTON, and H. VALTIN: Impaired water diuresis in rats with hereditary hypothalamic diabetes insipidus (DI) after adrenalectomy. 3rd Int. Congr. Nephrology, Washington, D.C., Abstr. II, p. 202 (1966).

GREENBAUM, A.L., and S.E. DICKER: The effects of mammalian posterior lobe hormones on the swelling of liver and kidney mitochondria in the rat and the dog. Biochim. biophys. Acta (Amst.) **74**, 519—524 (1963a).

— — The swelling of mitochondria from the liver and kidney of a primitive rodent. Biochem. biophys. Res. Commun. **12**, 402—404 (1963b).

GRIFFITH, L.D., R.E. BULGER, and B.F. TRUMP: The ultrastructure of the functioning kidney. Lab. Invest. **16**, 220—246 (1967).

GUHL, U.: Die antidiuretische und pressorische Wirksamkeit von Arginin[8]-Vasopressin, Lysin[8]-Vasopressin und Phenylalanin[2]-Lysin[8]-Vasopressin beim Menschen. Schweiz. med. Wschr. **91**, 798—805 (1961).

GUINNEBAULT, M.: Mise en Evidence du Role de l'Aldosterone dans le Mecanisme de Concentration de l'Urine. Rev. Franc. d'Etudes Cliniques et Biol. **7**, 920—926 (1962).

GULYASSY, P.F., and I.S. EDELMAN: Hydrogenion dependence of the antidiuretic action of vasopressin, oxytocin and deaminooxytocin. Biochim. biophys. Acta (Amst.) **102**, 185—197 (1965).

GUZEK, J.W., and H. LESNIK: Antidiuretic activity of the hypothalamus, neurohypophysis and blood plasma in various states of water metabolism in the guinea pig. Bulletin de l'Academie Polonaise des Sciences **14**, 723—726 (1966).

HAM, G.C.: Reproducible diuresis and chloruresis for bioassay of antidiuretic activity. Proc. Soc. exp. Biol. (N.Y.) **53**, 210—213 (1943).

—, and E.M. LANDIS: A comparison of pituitrin with antidiuretic substance found in human urine and placenta. J. clin. Invest. **21**, 455—470 (1942).

HANCOX, N.M., and J. KOMENDER: Quantitative and qualitative changes in the "dark" cells of the renal collecting tubules in rats deprived of water. Quart. J. exp. Physiol. **48**, 346—354 (1963).

HANDLER, J.S., and J. ORLOFF: Activation of phosphorylase in toad bladder and mammalian kidney by antidiuretic hormone. Amer. J. Physiol. **205**, 298—302 (1963).

HANSSEN, O.E.: Early post mortem renal changes studied in mice with one kidney exteriorized. II. The functional and the early post mortem morphology of the kidney. Acta path. microbiol. scand. **49**, 297—320 (1960).

HARE, K., R.C. HICKEY, and R.S. HARE: The renal excretion of an antidiuretic substance in the dog. Amer. J. Physiol. **134**, 240—244 (1941).

—, E.V. MELVILLE, G.H. CHAMBERS, and R.S. HARE: The assay of antidiuretic material in blood and urine. Endocrinology **36**, 323—331 (1945).

HARE, R.S., K. HARE, and D.M. PHILIPS: The renal excretion of chloride by the normal and by the diabetes insipidus dog. Amer. J. Physiol. **140**, 334—348 (1944).

HAYS, R.M., and A. LEAF: The problem of clinical vasopressin resistance. In vitro studies. Ann. intern. Med. **54**, 700—709 (1961).

HEIDENREICH, O., Y. KOOK, V. LING u. H. MENZEL: Der Einfluß von Oxytocin auf die Nierendurchblutung und die Größe des Glomerulusfiltrats bei normalen und total hypophysectomierten Hunden. Arch. exp. Pathol. Pharmakol. **239**, 328—335 (1960).

HEINTZ, R., E.F. DREWS, G. DREWS u. H. BRASS: Untersuchungen über den Gehalt des menschlichen Plasmas an antidiuretischem Hormon mit einer verbesserten Methode zum Hormonnachweis. Klin. Wschr. **42**, 771—776 (1964).

HELLER, H.: Antidiuretic substances. J. Pharm. Pharmacol. **3**, 609—630 (1951).

— The active principles of the neurohypophysis. J. Pharm. Pharmacol. **7**, 225—247 (1955).

— (Ed.): The Neurohypophysis. London: Butterworths 1957.

— Die Hypophysenhinterlappen- und Nebennierenrindenhormone während der ersten Lebenszeit im Zusammenhang mit der Regulation des Wasserhaushaltes. Mschr. Kinderheilk. **106**, 81—87 (1958).

—, and K.E. BLACKMORE: The assay of small amounts of antidiuretic activity by intravenous injection into mice. J. Endocr. **8**, 224—228 (1952).

—, and R.P. STEPHENSON: Effect of posterior pituitary extract and its fractions on renal electrolyte excretion. Nature (Lond.) **165**, 189 (1950).

HELLER, J., and J. STULC: Physiology of the antidiuretic hormone. I. A simple titration method. Physiol. bohemoslov. **8**, 558—564 (1959).

HELLMAN, E.S., D.P. TSCHUDY, and F.C. BARTTER: Abnormal electrolyte and water metabolism in acute intermittent porphyria. The transient inappropriate secretion of antidiuretic hormone. Amer. J. Med. **32**, 734—747 (1962).

HERKEN, H.: Schlußwort zu der Veröffentlichung von E. BUCHBORN: Vasopressin und Ödementstehung. Dtsch. med. Wschr. **48**, 2137 (1958).

HERMS, W., and R.L. MALVIN: Effect of metabolic inhibitors on urine osmolality and electrolyte excretion. Amer. J. Physiol. **204**, 1065—1070 (1963).

HICKEY, R.C., K. HARE, and R.S. HARE: Some cytological and hormonal changes in the posterior lobe of the rat's pituitary after water deprivation and stalk section. Anat. Rec. **81**, 319—322 (1941).

HILGER, H.H., J.D. KLÜMPER u. K.J. ULLRICH: Wasserrückresorption und Ionentransport durch die Sammelrohrzellen der Säugetierniere. Pflügers Arch. ges. Physiol. **267**, 218—237 (1958).
HILTON, J.G., L.F. SCIAN, C.D. WESTERMANN, and O.R. KRUERI: Direct stimulation of adrenocortical secretion by synthetic vasopressin in dogs. Proc. Soc. exp. Biol. (N.Y.) **100**, 523—525 (1959).
HOLLANDER, W. jr., T.F. WILLIAMS, C.C. FORDHAM, and L.G. WELT: III. A study of the quantitative relationship between antidiuretic hormone (vasopressin) and the renal tubular reabsorption of water. J. clin. Invest. **36**, 1059—1071 (1957).
HOLMES, W.N., and B.M. ADAMS: Effects of adrenocortical and neurohypophysial hormones on the renal excretory pattern in the water loaded duck. Endocrinology **73**, 5—10 (1963).
HOPE, D.B., V.V.S. MURTI, and V. DU VIGNEAUD: A highly potent analogue of oxytocin, desamino-oxytocin. J. biol. Chem. **237**, 1563—1567 (1962).
HORSTER, F.A., G. KUSCHINSKY u. G. PETERS: Die diuretische Wirkung von Oxytocin beim Hund. Arch. exp. Pathol. Pharmakol. **237**, 241—246 (1959).
HUGUENIN, R.L., E. STÜRMER, R.A. BOISSONNAS, and B. BERDE: Desamino-arginine-vasopressin. An analogue of arginine-vasopressin with high antidiuretic activity. Experientia (Basel) **21**, 68 (1965).
HUNTER, J., H. KALANT, and J.C. OGILVIE: A simple method for the assay of small amounts of antidiuretic hormone. Canad. J. Biochem. **37**, 1215—1225 (1959).
JACOBSEN, A., A. GRIECO, and S.J. FARBER: Hexosamine analysis of renal papillae in diuretic and antidiuretic rats. Proc. Soc. exp. Biol. (N.Y.) **115**, 1153—1156 (1964).
JACOBSON, H.N., and R.H. KELLOGG: Isotonic NaCl diuresis in rats. Antidiuresis and chloruresis produced by posterior pituitary extracts. Amer. J. Physiol. **184**, 376—389 (1956).
JAENIKE, J.H.: The relative rates of urea and water permeation in the distal nephron of the intact kidney. J. clin. Invest. **43**, 45—55 (1964).
JAENIKE, J.R.: The influence of vasopressin on the permeability of the mammalian collecting duct to urea. J. clin. Invest. **40**, 144—151 (1961).
— Acute effects of the administration of vasopressin during water diuresis in the dog. J. clin. Invest. **42**, 161—170 (1963).
—, and R.W. BERLINER: A study of distal renal tubular functions by a modified stop flow technique. J. clin. Invest. **39**, 481—490 (1960).
—, and G.A. BRAY: Effects of acute transitory urinary obstruction in the dog. Amer. J. Physiol. **199**, 1219—1222 (1960).
—, and C. WATERHOUSE: The renal response to sustained administration of vasopressin and water in man. J. clin. Endocr. **21**, 231—243 (1961).
JAMISON, R.L., C.M. BENNETT, and R.W. BERLINER: Counter current multiplication by the thin loops of Henle. Amer. J. Physiol. **212**, 357—366 (1967).
JEFFERS, W.A., M.A. LIVEZEY, and J.H. AUSTIN: A method for demonstrating an antidiuretic action of minute amounts of pitressin, statistical analysis of results. Proc. Soc. exp. Biol. (N.Y.) **50**, 184—188 (1942).
JONES, J.J., and J. LEE: The value of the pre-operated rat in the bioassay of vasopressin. J. Endocr. **33**, 329—330 (1965).
— — The value of rats with hereditary hypothalamic diabetes insipidus for the bioassay of vasopressin. J. Endocr. **37**, 335—344 (1967).
JONES, N.F., M.A. BARRACLOUGH, and I.H. MILLS: The mechanism of increased sodium excretion during water loading with 2.5% Dextrose and vasopressin. Clin. Sci. **25**, 449—457 (1963).
—, M. MYLLE, and C.W. GOTTSCHALK: Renal tubular microinjection studies in normal and potassium-depleted rats. Clin. Sci. **29**, 261—275 (1965).
JOST, K., and J. RUDINGER: Amino acids and peptides. LXIX. Synthesis of two biologically active analogues of deamino-oxytocin not containing a disulphide bond. Collection Czech. Chem. Commun. **32**, 1229—1241 (1967).
KASAFIREK, E., V. RABEK, J. RUDINGER, and F. SORM: Amino acids and peptides. LXVI. Synthesis of ten extended-chain analogues of lysine-vasopressin. Collection Czech. Chem. Commun. **31**, 4581—4591 (1966).
KASHIWAGI, R.: Mechanism of the antidiuretic effect of vasopressin. Nature (Lond.) **184**, 991 (1959).
KAYE, M.: An investigation into the cause of hyponatremia in the syndrome of inappropriate secretion of antidiuretic hormone. Amer. J. Med. **41**, 910—926 (1966).
KENNEDY, G.C.: The effect of adrenal steroids upon the secretion of hypotonic urine by the rat. J. Endocr. **20**, 365—374 (1960).
KESSLER, E., R.L. ALLEN, jr., D. KIRMAN, and H. STRAUSS: Effect of aldosterone and cortisol on sodium and water content of the rat kidney. Amer. J. Physiol. **207**, 109—112 (1964).
KESTRANEK, W.H., H. MOLITOR u. E.P. PICK: Über die Wirkungsstärke von Hypophysenextrakten, gemessen an ihren antidiuretischen Eigenschaften. Biochem. Z. **164**, 34—43 (1925).

Kiil, F., and K. Aukland: Renal tubular localization of water and sodium reabsorption in antidiuresis and water diuresis. Scand. J. clin. Lab. Invest. **12**, 277—289 (1960).

Kinne, R., W. V. Macfarlane, and O. E. Budtz-Olsen: Hormones and electrolytic excretion in sheep. Nature (Lond.) **192**, 1084—1085 (1961).

Kleeman, C. R., M. H. Maxwell, and R. Rockney: Production of hypertonic urine in humans in the probable absence of antidiuretic hormone (ADH). Proc. Soc. exp. Biol. (N.Y.) **96**, 189—191 (1957).

Kleinman, L. I., E. P. Radford jr., and G. Torelli: Urea and inulin clearances in undisturbed, unanesthetized rats. Amer. J. Physiol. **208**, 578—584 (1965).

Kobinger, W.: Die Wirkung von Vasopressin auf die Konzentrationsgradienten von Natrium und Harnstoff im Nierengewebe bei verschiedenen Diuresezuständen. Naunyn-Schmiedebergs Arch. exp. Path. Pharmak. **246**, 538—551 (1964).

Konzett, H.: Synthetische Analoge von Hypophysen-Hinterlappen-Hormonen. Arch. exp. Pathol. Pharmakol. **245**, 153—166 (1963).

Korr, J. H.: The osmotic function of the chicken kidney. J. cell. comp. Physiol. **13**, 175—193 (1939).

Kramar, J., E. H. Grinell, and W. M. Duff: Studies on the renal activity of oxytocin. Amer. J. med. Sci. **252**, 331—340 (1966).

Kupfer, S., and J. D. Kosovsky: The effects of intrarenal arterial injection of digitalis glycosides on urinary concentration. Fed. Proc. **21**, 435—437 (1962).

Kuriaki, K., et N. Baba: Effets de la vasopressine et de la serotonine sur l'anhydrase carbonique, la glutaminase-I, l'atpase et la phosphorylation oxydative dans le rein de rat. C.R. Soc. Biol. (Paris) **153**, 1638—1640 (1959).

Kühn, E.: Influence de l'antidiurese obtenu par infusion de l'arginine-vasopressine (AVP) de la lysine-vasopressine (LVP) et de l'ocytocine sur l'excretion du calcium chez la brebis. Arch. int. Pharmacodyn. **160**, 480—484 (1966).

—, et G. Peeters: Influence de l'arginine-vasopressin sur l'excretion d'electrolytes chez le mouton. Arch. int. Pharmacodyn. **155**, 455—458 (1965).

— — Influence de la secretion par voie reflexe des hormones post hypophysaires sur l'excretion du potassium chez la chevre. Arch. int. Pharmacodyn. **166**, 214—215 (1967).

Lassiter, W. E., A. Frick, G. Rumrich, and K. J. Ullrich: Influence of ionic calcium on the water permeability of proximal and distal tubules in the rat kidney. Pflügers Arch. ges. Physiol. **285**, 90—95 (1965).

—, M. Mylle, and C. W. Gottschalk: Micropuncture study of urea transport in rat renal medulla. Amer. J. Physiol. **210**, 965—970 (1966).

Lauber, J. K.: A bio-assay and histochemical study of antidiuretic hormone in adrenalectomized rats. Amer. J. Physiol. **200**, 898—900 (1961).

Lauson, H. D.: Antidiuretic hormone. Fed. Proc. **24**, 731—736 (1965).

Lavietes, P. H., L. M. d'Esopo, and H. E. Harrison: The water and base balance of the body. J. clin. Invest. **14**, 251—265 (1935).

Leaf, A.: Transepithelial transport and its hormonal control in toad bladder. Ergebn. Physiol. **56**, 216—263 (1965).

—, F. C. Bartter, R. F. Santos, and O. Wrong: Evidence in man that urinary electrolyte loss induced by pitressin is a function of water retention. J. clin. Invest. **32**, 868—878 (1953).

—, W. S. Kerr, O. Wrong, and J. Y. Chatillon: Effect of graded compression of the renal artery on water and solute excretion. Amer. J. Physiol. **179**, 191—208 (1954).

—, and A. R. Mamby: The normal antidiuretic mechanism in man and dog, its regulation by extracellular fluid tonicity. J. clin. Invest. **31**, 54—59 (1952).

Lee, J.: Neurohypophysial hormones and fluid balance in hepatic cirrhosis. Thesis: London 1960.

Lees, F., and M. F. Lockett: The influence of hypophysectomy and of adrenalectomy on the urinary changes induced by oxytocin in rats. J. Physiol. (Lond.) **17**, 403—410 (1964).

Leuschner, F.: Untersuchungen über die Wirkung des Vasopressins und analoger Polypeptide auf die Niere. Z. Vitamin-, Hormon- u. Fermentforsch. **11**, 98—158 (1960).

Lever, A. F.: The vasa recta and countercurrent multiplication. Acta med. scand. Suppl. **434**, 33 pp. (1965).

Levine, R., and J. A. Vogel: Cardiovascular and metabolic effects of cyclic adenosine 3',5'-monophosphate in unanesthetized dogs. J. Pharmacol. exp. Ther. **151**, 262—272 (1966).

Levine, R. A.: The antidiuretic action of adenosine 3',5'-monophosphate (3',5'-AMP) in man. J. clin. Invest. **45**, 1039 (1966).

Levinsky, N. G., and R. W. Berliner: Changes in composition of the urine in ureter and bladder at low urine flows. Amer. J. Physiol. **196**, 549—553 (1959).

—, D. G. Davidson, and R. W. Berliner: Changes in urine concentration during prolonged administration of vasopressin and water. Amer. J. Physiol. **196**, 451—456 (1959).

LEVITIN, H., A. GOODMAN, G. PIGEON, and F.H. EPSTEIN: Composition of renal medulla during water diuresis. J. clin. Invest. **41**, 1145—1152 (1962).

LEVKOFF, A.H., T.W. DEMUNBRUN, and A.D. KELLER: Disparity between fluid intake and renal concentrating capacity in dogs with diabetes insipidus. Amer. J. Physiol. **176**, 25—32 (1954).

LILIEN, O.M., and R. SPITZER: The countercurrent system and osmotic diuresis. J. Urol. (Baltimore) **92**, 9—16 (1964).

LINDEMANN, R.D., H.C. VON BUREN, and L.G. RAISZ: Effect of steroids on water diuresis and vasopressin sensitivity. J. clin. Invest. **40**, 152—158 (1961).

LINDQUIST, K.M., and L.W. ROWE: The antidiuretic activity of the posterior pituitary and its quantitative evaluation. J. Amer. pharm. Ass. **38**, 227—232 (1949).

LINKENBACH, H.J., P. ECKERT u. O.H. GAUER: Nachweis eines diuretischen Faktors im menschlichen Serum während der durch Expansion des intrathorakalen Blutvolumens ausgelösten Diurese. Pflügers Arch. ges. Physiol. **293**, 107—114 (1967).

LIPSETT, M.B., I.L. SCHWARTZ, and N.A. THORN: Hormonal control of sodium, potassium, chloride and water metabolism. Mineral Metab. **1** B, 473—549. New York: Academic Press 1961.

LITTLE, J.B., and E.P. RADFORD: Bio-assay for antidiuretic activity in blood of undisturbed rats. J. appl. Physiol. **19**, 179—186 (1964).

LITTLE, J.M., S.L. WALLACE, E.C. WHATLEY, and G.A. ANDERSON: Effect of pitressin on the urinary excretion of chloride and water in the human. Amer. J. Physiol. **151**, 174—185 (1947).

LOCKETT, M.F., and T. LIMA: The failure of neurohypophyseal hormones to prevent excessive loss of sodium from isolated cat kidneys perfused with blood drawn from headless donors. Arch. Int. Physiol. Biochim. **69**, 327—328 (1961).

—, and E.N. ROBERTS: Some actions of growth hormone on the perfused cat kidney. J. Physiol. (Lond.) **169**, 879—888 (1963).

LUNDSGAARD, E.: The effect of phloridzin on the isolated kidney and isolated liver. Scand. Arch. Physiol. **72**, 265—270 (1935).

MACFARLANE, W.V., R. KINNE, C.M. WOHNSLEY, B.D. SIEBERT, and D. PETER: Vasopressin and the increase of water and electrolyte excretion by sheep, cattle and camels. Nature (Lond.) **214**, 979—981 (1967).

MALVIN, R.L., and M.M. FUSCO: Alteration in the countercurrent gradient by lesion in the median eminence. Nature (Lond.) **212**, 1591—1592 (1966).

— — Renal function in unanesthetized normal and diabetes insipidus rats. J. appl. Physiol. **22**, 380—382 (1967).

MANCHESTER, R.C.: Influence of posterior pituitary extracts on mineral and water exchange in children. Proc. Soc. exp. Biol. (N.Y.) **29**, 717—719 (1932).

MARSH, D.J.: Hypo-osmotic reabsorption due to active salt transport in perfused collecting ducts of the rat renal medulla. Nature (Lond.) **210**, 1179—1180 (1966).

MARSHALL, S., T.B. MILLER, and A.E. FARAH: Effect of renal papillectomy on ability of the hamster to concentrate urine. Amer. J. Physiol. **204**, 363—368 (1963).

MARTIN, G.J., J.N. MOSS, and R.D. SMYTH: Vasopressin potentiation and stimulation by bromelain. Arch. int. Pharmacodyn. **152**, 445—449 (1964).

MARX, H.: Zur Theorie der Diurese. Klin. Wschr. **9**, 2384 (1930).

MATHÉ, G., et J. ALTMANN: Contribution expérimentale a l'étude de l'inactivation hépatique de la pitressine. Presse méd. **62**, 983—985 (1954).

MCCANN, S.M., J. ANTUNES-RODRIGUES, R. NALLAR, and H. VALTIN: Pituitary-Adrenal function in the absence of vasopressin. Endocrinology **79**, 1058—1064 (1966).

MCCREARY, A.B., J.Q. ADAMS, and R.R. OVERMAN: A bioassay technique for plasma antidiuretic activity. J. Lab. clin. Med. **49**, 626—629 (1957).

MCDONALD, S.J., and H.E. DE WARDENER: Some observations on the production of a hypo-osmotic urine during the administration of 0.9% saline and vasopressin in the dog. Clin. Sci. **28**, 445—459 (1965).

MEES, E.J.D.: Reversible water losing state, caused by incomplete ureteric obstruction. Acta med. scand. **168**, 193—197 (1960).

MERONEY, W.H., M.E. RUBINI, and W.B. BLYTHE: The effect of antecedent diet on urine concentrating ability. Ann. intern. Med. **48**, 562—573 (1958).

MERTZ, D.P.: Über die akute Wirkung von synthetischem Oxytocin auf die Nierenhämodynamik und renale Elektrolytausscheidung beim Menschen. Naunyn-Schmiedebergs Arch. exp. Path. Pharmak. **239**, 410—424 (1960).

— Zur Frage einer Beteiligung von Nichtelektrolyten (Harnstoff, Kreatinin) am Vorgang der Harnkonzentrierung beim Menschen. Klin. Wschr. **43**, 661—673 (1965).

Miller, L., L. Fisch, and C. R. Kleeman: Comparative potency of the antidiuretic hormones lysine[8]- and arginine[8]-vasopressin in humans. J. clin. Invest. **44**, 1075—1076 (1965).
— — — Relative potency of arginine[8]-vasopressin and lysine[8]-vasopressin in humans. J. Lab. clin. Med. **69**, 270—291 (1967).
Moll, J., and D. de Wied: Observations on the hypothalamo-posthypophyseal system of the posterior lobectomized rat. Gen. comp. Endocr. **2**, 215—228 (1962).
Morel, F., M. Mylle, and C. W. Gottschalk: Tracer microinjection studies of effect of ADH on renal tubular diffusion of water. Amer. J. Physiol. **209**, 179—187 (1965).
Morrison, S. D., C. Mackay, E. Hurlbrink, J. K. Wier, M. S. Nick, and F. K. Miller: The water exchange and polyuria of rats deprived of food. Quart. J. exp. Physiol. **52**, 51—67 (1967).
Motzfeldt, K.: Experimental studies on the relation of the pituitary body to renal function. J. exp. Med. **25**, 153—188 (1917).
Munsick, R. A.: Neurohypophysial hormones of chickens and turkeys. Endocrinology **75**, 104—112 (1964).
—, W. H. Sawyer, and H. B. van Dyke: The antidiuretic potency of arginine- and lysine-vasopressin in the pig with observations on porcine renal function. Endocrinology **63**, 688—693 (1958).
Murphy, R. J. F.: Studies on the mechanisms of saline diuresis. J. clin. Invest. **29**, 836 (1950).
Nelson, E. E., and G. G. Woods: The diuretic-antidiuretic activity of posterior pituitary extracts. J. Pharmacol. exp. Ther. **50**, 241—253 (1934).
Nielsen, Aa, Th.: A note on the relative antidiuretic potency of beef and hog vasopressin. Acta endocr. (Kbh.) **29**, 561—564 (1958).
— Dissimilarity between arginine and lysine vasopressin in rat pressor assays. Acta endocr. (Kbh.) **35**, 299—311 (1960).
— Hypofysebaglapshormoner. København: Kandrup & Wunsch Bogtrykkeri 1964 [Thesis in Danish, with summary in English].
— On the antidiuretic activity of Phe[2]-Lys[8]-vasopressin in the rat. Acta endocr. (Kbh.) **49**, 312—319 (1965).
Nielsen, B.: Correlation between antidiuretic hormone effect and the renal excretion of magnesium and calcium in man. Acta endocr. (Kbh.) **45**, 151—160 (1964).
—, and N. A. Thorn: Transient excess urinary excretion of antidiuretic material in acute intermittent porphyria with hyponatremia and hypomagnesiemia. Amer. J. Med. **38**, 345—358 (1965).
Niesel, W., u. H. Röskenbleck: Konzentrierung von Lösungen unterschiedlicher Zusammensetzung durch alleinige Gegenstromdiffusion und Gegenstromosmose als möglicher Mechanismus der Harnkonzentrierung. Pflügers Arch. ges. Physiol. **283**, 230—241 (1965).
Nissen, O. I.: The filtration fractions of plasma supplying the superficial and deep venous drainage area of the cat kidney. Acta physiol. scand. **68**, 275—285 (1966).
Nusynowitz, M. L., L. G. Wegienka, B. F. Bower, and P. H. Forsham: Effect on vasopressin action of analgesic drugs in vitro Amer. J. Med. Sci **252**, 424—428 (1966).
O'Connor, W. J.: The role of the neurohypophysis of the dog in determining urinary changes and the antidiuretic activity of the urine following the administration of sodium chloride or urea. Quart. J. exp. Physiol. **36**, 21—48 (1950).
Orloff, J., and J. S. Handler: The cellular mode of action of antidiuretic hormone. Amer. J. Med. **36**, 686—697 (1964).
— — The role of adenosine 3'. 5'-phosphate in the action of antidiuretic hormone. Amer. J. Med. **42**, 757—768 (1967).
Osvaldo, L., and H. Latta: The thin limbs of the loop of Henle. J. Ultrastruct. Res. **15**, 144—168 (1966a).
— — Interstitial cells of the renal medulla. J. Ultrastruct. Res. **15**, 589—613 (1966b).
Ottoson, D., F. Sjøstrand, S. Stenström, and G. Svaetichin: Microelectrode studies on the E.M.F. of the frog skin related to electron microscopy of the dermo-epidermal junction. Acta physiol. scand. 29 suppl. **106**, 611—624 (1953).
Papper, S., L. Saxon, M. B. Burg, H. W. Seifer, and J. D. Rosenbaum: The effect of morphine sulfate upon the renal excretion of water and solute in man. J. Lab. clin. Med. **50**, 692—704 (1957).
Peachey, L., and H. Rasmussen: Structure of the toad urinary bladder as related to its physiology. J. biophys. biochem. Cytol. **10**, 529—553 (1961).
Pena, J. C., and R. L. Malvin: Transcellular diffusion of non-electrolytes across the renal tubular epithelium. J. gen. Physiol. **45**, 643—649 (1962).
Perlmutt, J. H.: Renal activity of vasopressin in anesthetized dogs. Amer. J. Physiol. **200**, 400—404 (1961).
— Influence of hydration on renal function and medullary sodium during vasopressin infusion. Amer. J. Physiol. **202**, 1098—1104 (1962).

PETERSEN, M.J., and I.S. EDELMANN: Calcium inhibition of the action of vasopressin on the urinary bladder of the toad. J. clin. Invest. **43**, 583—594 (1964).

PHILIPPSON, CHR.: Der Gehalt an Glycerylphosphorylcholin und Glycerylphosphoryläthanolamin von Nierenmark und Nierenrinde hochreiner Wistarratten während forcierter Wasserdiurese und extrem langer Durst-Antidiurese. Pflügers Arch. ges. Physiol. **280**, 30—37 (1964).

PICKFORD, M.: Neurohypophysis and kidney function. In: The pituitary gland, Vol. 3. Ed. by G.W. HARRIS and B.T. DONOVAN. London: Butterworths 1966.

PIGEON, G., and H. EPSTEIN: Water uptake in the intact frog. Amer. J. Physiol. **204**, 217—221 (1963).

PLISKA, V., and I. KREJČÍ: The dose-response relation of the antidiuretic and vasopressor activities of ^{4}-asparagine^{8}lysine-vasopressin. Arch. int. Pharmacodyn. **161**, 289—297 (1966).

—, and I. RYCHLIK: Determination of antidiuretic activity in the rat for structural analogues of the neurohypophysial hormones. Acta endocr. (Kbh.) **54**, 129—140 (1967).

POISNER, A.M.: Interaction of oxytocin and vasopressin with β-adrenergic receptors in the kidney. Nature (Lond.) **201**, 199—200 (1964).

POULSON, T.L.: Countercurrent multipliers in avian kidneys. Science **148**, 389—391 (1965).

POY, R.F.K.P., and P.J. BENTLEY: Fine structure of the epithelial cells of the toad urinary bladder. Exp. Cell. Res. **20**, 235—237 (1960).

RABASA, S.L., and F. BERGMAN: A method to measure the renal sensitivity to ADH in the rat. Acta physiol. lat.-amer. **14**, 89—93 (1964).

RADFORD, E.P.: Factors modifying water metabolism in rats fed dry diets. Amer. J. Physiol. **196**, 1098—1108 (1959).

RAISZ, L.G., W.F. MCNEELY, L. SAXON: Studies on the renal concentrating mechanism. J. Lab. clin. Med. **52**, 437—445 (1958).

— — —, and J.D. ROSENBAUM: The effects of cortisone and hydrocortisone on water diuresis and renal function in man. J. clin. Invest. **36**, 767—779 (1957).

RALLI, E.P., L.G. RAISZ, S.H. LESLIE, M.E. DUMM, and B. LAKEN: Evidence for more than one antidiuretic substance in pitressin. Amer. J. Physiol. **163**, 141—147 (1950).

RALLISON, M.L., and F.H. TYLER: Treatment of diabetes insipidus in children with lysine^8-vasopressin. J. Pediat. **70**, 122—125 (1967).

ROBERT, F.: Über die Einwirkung von Hypophysin und seine Fraktionen auf den Wassersalzstoffwechsel. Arch. exp. Pathol. Pharmakol. **164**, 367—371 (1932).

ROBINSON, J.D.: Interaction between protein sulphydryl groups and lipid double bonds in biological membranes. Nature (Lond.) **212**, 199—200 (1966).

ROBINSON, J.H., jr., and L.E. FARR: Relation between clinical oedema and excretion of antidiuretic substance in the urine. Ann. intern. Med. **14**, 42—54 (1940).

ROBINSON, K.W., and W.V. MACFARLANE: Plasma antidiuretic activity of marsupials during exposure to heat. Endocrinology **60**, 679—680 (1957).

ROBINSON, R.R., and E.E. OWEN: Intrarenal distribution of ammonia during diuresis and antidiuresis. Amer. J. Physiol. **208**, 1129—1134 (1965).

— —, and B. SCHMIDT-NIELSEN: Intra-renal distribution of free amino acids in antidiuretic ruminants. Comp. Biochem. Physiol. **19**, 187—195 (1966).

ROBSON, J.S.: Factors affecting renal concentrating ability. Electron-microscopic study of the kidney during antidiuresis, diuresis and potassium depletion. In: Hormones and the Kidney. Ed. by P.C. WILLIAMS. Mem. Soc. Endocr. No. 13, p. 105—119. New York: Academic Press 1963.

ROEMMELT, J.C., O.W. SARTORIUS, and R.F. PITTS: Excretion and reabsorption of sodium and water in the adrenalectomized dog. Amer. J. Physiol. **159**, 124—136 (1949).

ROSAS, R., L. BARNAFI, T. PEREDA, and H. CROXATTO: Effect of oxytocin structural changes on rat renal excretion of Na, K and water. Amer. J. Physiol. **202**, 901—904 (1962).

ROSENBAUM, J.D., R.K. DAVIS, and B.C. FERGUSON: The influence of cortisone on water diuresis in man. J. clin. Invest. **30**, 668 (1951).

ROSENFELD, J.B., K. HIRATA, A.N. BREST, and J.H. MOYER: Effect of large doses of hyaluronidase upon urine concentration in dogs. Israel. J. Med. Sci. **3**, 119—130 (1967).

ROSENFELD, S., A.L. SELLERS, and J. KATZ: Development of an isolated perfused mammalian kidney. Amer. J. Physiol. **196**, 1155—1159 (1959).

RUCH, W.: Estimation of antidiuretic hormone in the urine of healthy subjects and patients with inappropriate secretion of vasopressin (Schwartz-Bartter syndrome). Acta endocr. (Kbh.) **54**, 113—121 (1967).

RUDINGER, J.: Synthetic analogues of oxytocin with inhibitor activity or protracted action. Excerpta Med. Int. Congr. Ser. No. 83, p. 1202—1206. London 1964.

— (Ed.) Oxytocin, vasopressin and their structural analogues. Proc. 2nd Int. Pharmacol. Meeting, Praha, Aug. 1963. Oxford: Pergamon Press; Praha: Czech. Med. Press 1964a.

RUDINGER, J., and K. JOST: A biologically active analogue of oxytocin not containing a disulfide group. Experientia (Basel) **20**, 570 (1964).
RUIZ-GUINAZU, A., E. E. ARRIZURIETA, and L. YELINEK: Electrolyte, water and urea concent in dog kidneys in different states of diuresis. Amer. J. Physiol. **206**, 725—730 (1964).
SABOUR, M. S., M. K. MAC DONALD, A. T. LAMBIE, and J. S. ROBSON: The electron microscopic appearance of the kidney in hydrated and dehydrated rats. Quart. J. exp. Physiol. **49**, 162—170 (1964).
SAIKIA, T. C. Composition of the renal cortex and medulla of rats during water diuresis and antidiuresis. Quart. J. exp. Physiol. **50**, 146—157 (1965a).
— The acute effect of vasopressin upon the composition of the rat renal cortex and medulla. Quart. J. exp. Physiol. **50**, 158—168 (1965b).
SAKAI, F., M. TADOKORO, and J. YAMAGUCHI: Osmolality of loop of Henle fluid in golden hamster. Jap. J. Pharmacol. **16**, 492 (1966).
SAMAAN, A.: The effect of pituitary (posterior lobe) extract upon the urinary flow in non-anaesthetized dogs. J. Physiol. (Lond.) **85**, 37—46 (1935).
SANYAL, N. N., and R. S. SNART: Absorption of octapeptide hormones on to lipid monolayers. Nature (Lond.) **1**, 798—799 (1967).
SARTORIUS, O. W., and K. ROBERTS: The effects of pitressin and desoxycorticosterone in low dosage on the excretion of sodium, potassium and water by the normal dog. Endocrinology **45**, 273—283 (1949).
SAUNDERS, W. G., and R. A. MUNSICK: Antidiuretic potency of oxytocin in women post partum. Amer. J. Obstet. Gynec. **95**, 5—11 (1966).
SAWYER, W. H.: Posterior pituitary extracts and excretion of electrolytes by the rat. Amer. J. Physiol. **169**, 583—587 (1952).
— Differences in the antidiuretic response of rats to the intravenous administration of lysine and arginine vasopressin. Endocrinology **63**, 694—698 (1958).
— Comparative physiology and pharmacology of the neurohypophysis. Rec. Progr. Horm. Res. **17**, 437—465 (1961a).
— Neurohypophysial hormones. Pharmacol. Rev. **13**, 225—277 (1961b).
— Biological assays for oxytocin and vasopressin. Meth. med. Res. **9**, 210—219 (1961c).
— Neurohypophyseal peptides and water excretion in the vertebrates. In: Hormones and the kidney. Ed. by P. C. WILLIAMS. Mem. Soc. Endocr. No. 13. London: Academic Press 1963.
— Biological assays for neurohypophysial principles in tissues and blood. In: The pituitary gland. Ed. by G. W. HARRIS and B. T. DONOVAN. London: Butterworths 1966.
—, W. Y. CHAN, and H. B. VAN DYKE: Antidiuretic responses to neurohypophysial hormones and some of their synthetic analogues in dogs and rats. Endocrinology **71**, 536—540 (1962).
—, and H. VALTIN: Inhibition of vasopressin antidiuresis by extracts of pituitaries from rats with hereditary hypothalamic diabetes insipidus and by oxytocin. Endocrinology **76**, 999—1001 (1965).
— — Antidiuretic responses of rats with hereditary hypothalamic diabetes insipidus to vasopressin, oxytocin and nicotine. Endocrinology **80**, 207—210 (1967).
SCHEER, R. L., L. G. RAISZAND, and C. W. LLOYD: Changes in diabetes insipidus during pregnancy and lactation. J. clin. Endocr. **19**, 805—811 (1959).
SCHMIDT-NIELSEN, B.: Urea excretion in mammals. Physiol. Rev. **38**, 139—168 (1958).
SCHOEN, E. J.: Renal diabetes insipidus. Pediatrics **26**, 808—816 (1960).
SCHRÖDER, R.: Herstellung und Funktion eines isolierten Nierenpräparates vom Hund. Pflügers Arch. ges. Physiol. **286**, 189—198 (1965).
— Die Wirkung einer Angiotensininfusion auf die Harnkonzentration des Menschen unter maximaler ADH-Wirkung. Pflügers Arch. ges. Physiol. **290**, 193—201 (1966).
—, H.J. BUSCHMANN u. K. EHRENTAHL: Die Wirkung von Tonephin auf die renale Elektrolyt- und Harnstoffausscheidung bei Infusion von Glucose und Sterofundin. Klin. Wschr. **44**, 943—951 (1966).
—, G. MEYER-BURGDORFF, D. ROTT u. O. BRAHMS: Vergleichende Untersuchungen über die Wirkung von ADH, Hypertensin und Renin auf renale Wasser- und Elektrolytausscheidung der Ratte. Arch. exp. Pathol. Pharmakol. **240**, 285—312 (1961).
SCHWARTZ, I. L., and L. M. LIVINGSTON: Cellular and molecular aspects of the antidiuretic action of vasopressin and related peptides. Vitamins and Hormones **22**, 261—358 (1964).
—, H. RASMUSSEN, and J. RUDINGER: Activity of neurohypophysial hormone analogues lacking a disulfide bridge. Proc. nat. Acad. Sci. (Wash.) **52**, 1044—1045 (1964).
SCHWARTZ, W. B., and A. S. RELMAN: Effects of electrolyte disorders on renal structure and function. New Engl. J. Med. **276**, 383—389 (1967).
SCHWARZ, W., u. J. WOLFF: Veränderungen am Hauptstück und peritubulären Kapillaren der Rattenniere nach Hypophysectomie. Z. Zellforsch. **71**, 441—454 (1966).
SELF, J.: Water intoxication induced by oxytocin administration. Amer. J. med. Sci. **252**, 573—574 (1966).

SELKURT, E.E.: Effect of ureteral blockade on renal blood flow and urinary concentrating ability. Amer. J. Physiol. **205**, 286—292 (1963).

—, M.J. ELPERS, and J. WOMACK: Effects of renal venous occlusion on renal haemodynamies and concentrating ability. Amer. J. Physiol. **207**, 989—997 (1964).

SELLWOOD, R.V., and E.B. VERNEY: The effect of water and of isotonic saline administration on the renal plasma and glomerular filtrate flows in the dog with incidental observations on these flows of compression of the carotid arteries. Phil. Trans. B. **238**, 361—396 (1955).

SHANNON, J.A.: The control of the renal excretion of water. J.exp.Med. **76**, 387—399 (1942).

SHARE, L.: Acute reduction in extracellular fluid volume and the concentration of antidiuretic hormone in blood. Endocrinology **69**, 925—933 (1961).

SHUSTER, A., E.A. ALEXANDER, R.C. LALONE, and N.G. LEVINSKY: Renal blood flow, sodium excretion and concentrating ability during saline infusion. Amer. J. Physiol. **211**, 1181—1186 (1966).

SIGLER, M.H., J.N. FORREST, and J.R. ELKINGTON: Renal concentrating ability in the adrenalectomized rat. Clin. Sci. **28**, 29—37 (1965).

SILVA, P., and M.S. ALLAN: Water intoxication due to high doses of synthetic oxytocin. Obstet, and Gynec. **27**, 517—520 (1966).

SINCLAIR-SMITH, B.C., J. SISSON, A.A. KATTUS, A. GENECIN, C. MONGE, W. MCKEEVER, and E.V. NEWMAN: The effects of posterior pituitary extract and smoking on water, sodium and chloride excretion in normal subjects and in patients with congestive cardiac failures. Bull. Johns Hopk. Hosp. **87**, 221—234 (1950).

SKADHAUGE, E.: Effects of retrograde injections of vasopressin into the upper urinary tract of hydrated rats. Proc. Soc. exp. Biol. (N.Y.) **117**, 807—810 (1964a).

— Effects of unilateral infusion of arginine-vasopressin into the portal circulation of the avian kidney. Acta endocr. (Kbh.) **47**, 321—330 (1964b).

—, and B. SCHMIDT-NIELSEN: Renal function in domestic fowl. Amer. J. Physiol. **212**, 793—798 (1967a).

— — The renal medullary electrolyte and urea gradient in chickens and turkeys. Amer. J. Physiol. **212**, 1313—1318 (1967b).

SLOPER, J.C.: The presence of a posterior pituitary-like structure in the hypothalamus after hypophysectomy. Acta endocr. suppl. **51**, 101 (1960).

SMITH, F.M., and E.M. MACKAY: Influence of posterior pituitary extracts on sodium balance in normal subjects and patients with diabetes insipidus. Proc. Soc. exp. Biol. (N.Y.) **34**, 116—119 (1936).

SMITH, H.W. Principles of renal physiology. New York: Oxford University Press 1962.

SMITH, M.W.: The effect of hyaluronidase and cortisol on the inactivation of vasopressin by rat kidney slices. J. Endocrin. **24**, 415—425 (1962).

STEIN, M., R. JINKS, and I.A. MIRSKY: The bioassay of pitressin and antidiuretic substances in blood and urine. Endocrinology **51**, 492—501 (1952).

STEINESS, I., and M. LUNDING: Pronounced polyuria and natriuresis following surgical relief of urinary tract obstruction. Acta med. scand. **180**, 159—166 (1966).

STERNBERG, W.H., E. FARBER, and C.E. DUNLAP: Histochemical localization of specific oxidative enzymes. J. Histochem. Cytochem. **4**, 266—283 (1956).

STEWART, J., and S.G. SPICKETT: Genetic variation in diuretic responses to water loads: Definition of some parameters of diuretic response and initial results of selection for these parameters. J. Endocr. **33**, 417—428 (1965).

STUDER, R.O., and W.D. CASH: Synthesis of ^{1}acetyl^{8}-arginine-vasopressin and a study of its effects in the rat pressor assay. J. biol. Chem. **238**, 657—659 (1963).

STÜRMER, E., R.L. HUGUENIN, R.A. BOISSONNAS, and B. BERDE: Deamino^{1}-phenylalanine^{2}-arginine^{8}-vasopressin: A peptide with highly selective antidiuretic activity. Experientia (Basel) **21**, 583 (1965).

SWINGLE, W.W., L.J. BRANNICK, S.J. LE BRIE, and A.F. PARLOW: A histaminelike component of commercial pitressin. Proc. Soc. exp. Biol. (N.Y.) **91**, 223—226 (1956).

TATA, P.S., and O.H. GAUER: Vasopressin studies in the rat. I. A sensitive bioassay for exogenous vasopressin. Pflügers Arch. ges. Physiol. **290**, 279—285 (1966).

THEOBALD, G.W.: The allerged relation of hyperfunction of the posterior lobe of the hypophysis to eclampsia and the nephropathy of pregnancy. Clin. Sci. **1**, 225—239 (1934).

THOENES, W.: Die Mikromorphologie des Nephron in ihrer Beziehung zur Funktion II. Klin. Wschr. **39**, 827—839 (1961).

THOMAS, S.: Washout and re-accumulation of urea during diuresis and antidiuresis. In: Hormones and the kidney. Ed. by P.C. WILLIAMS. Mem. Soc. Endocr. No. 13. New York: Academic Press 1963.

— Solute excretion in man during changing urine flow occurring spontaneously and induced by vasopressin injection. J. clin. Invest. **43**, 1—10 (1964).

Thomson, W.B.: The effect of oxytocin and vasopressin and of phenylalanin[3]-oxytocin on the urinary excretion of water and electrolytes in man. J. Physiol. (Lond.) **150**, 284—294 (1960).
Thorn, N.A.: A densimetric method for assay of small amounts of antidiuretic hormone. J. exp. Med. **105**, 585—590 (1957a).
— Mammalian antidiuretic hormone. Physiol. Rev. **38**, 169—191 (1958).
— Binding in vitro of highly-purified arginine-vasopressin and synthetic oxytocin to rat serum globulin. Acta endocr. (Kbh.) **30**, 472—476 (1959a).
— Some chemical properties of antidiuretic material in the urine of rats. Acta endocr. (Kbh.) **32**, 128—133 (1959b).
— Effect of highly purified arginine- and lysine-vasopressin on urinary excretion of sodium and potassium in hydrated rats. Acta endocr. (Kbh.) **32**, 123—128 (1959c).
— Effects of arginine-, lysine-, and leucine-vasopressin on urinary osmolality and rate of urine flow in hydrated rats and dogs. Acta endocr. (Kbh.) **32**, 134—141 (1959e).
— Antidiuretiske hormoner og deres Analoge. Thesis. København: Danish Science Press 1960a.
— An effect of antidiuretic hormone on renal excretion of calcium in dogs. Dan. med. Bull. **7**, 109—112 (1960b).
— Effect of valyl[3]-oxytocin on renal excretion of sodium and potassium in hydrated rats and dogs. Dan. med. Bull. **7**, 113—115 (1960c).
— Correlation between antidiuretic hormone effect and changes in renal excretion of calcium in rats and dogs. Acta endocr. (Kbh.) **38**, 563—570 (1961).
—, and B. Milewski: Effect of leucine-vasopressin (phenyl-alanine-oxytocin) on renal excretion of sodium and potassium in hydrated rats and dogs. Proc. Soc. exp. Biol. (N.Y.) **100**, 267—269 (1959d).
—, and I.L. Schwartz: Effect of antidiuretic hormone on washout curves of radioactive calcium from isolated toad bladder tissue. Gen. comp. Endocr. **5**, 710 (1965).
— — Renal excretion of natural lysine-vasopressin injected into rats (unpublished).
—, and L. Silver: Chemical form of circulating antidiuretic hormone in rats. J. exp. Med. **105**, 575—583 (1957b).
—, and I. Transbøl: Hyponatremia and bronchogenic carcinoma associated with renal excretion of large amounts of antidiuretic material. Amer. J. Med. **35**, 257—268 (1963).
—, and N.B.S. Willumsen: Inactivation of arginine- and lysine-vasopressin by slices from different zones of the rat kidney and by rat liver slices. Acta endocr. (Kbh.) **44**, 545—562 (1963).
Thorp, R.H.: Posterior pituitary hormones. In: Methods in hormone research. Vol. 2, Bioassay, pp. 495—516. Ed. by R.J. Dorfman. New York: Academic Press 1962.
Thurau, K.: Renal hemodynamics. Amer. J. Med. **36**, 698—719 (1964).
—, u. P. Deetjen: Bedeutung der Hämodynamik des Nierenmarkes für die Harnkonzentrierung. Pflügers Arch. ges. Physiol. **274**, 567—580 (1962).
— — u. P. Kramer: Hämodynamik des Nierenmarks. II. Wechselbeziehung zwischen vasculärem Gegenstromsystem bei arteriellen Drucksteigerungen. Wasserdiurese und osmotischer Diurese. Pflügers Arch. ges. Physiol. **270**, 270—285 (1960).
—, u. E. Wober: Zur Lokalisation der autoregulativen Widerstandsänderungen in der Niere. Pflügers Arch. ges. Physiol. **274**, 553—566 (1962).
Torres, C., L. Schewitz, and V.E. Pollach: The effect of small amount of antidiuretic hormone on sodium and urate excretion in pregnancy. Amer. J. Obstet. Gynec. **94**, 546—558 (1966).
Trueta, J., A.E. Barclay, P.M. Daniel, K.J. Franklin, and M.M.L. Pritchard: Studies of the renal circulation. Oxford: Blackwell 1947.
Ullmann, T.D., W.J. Czackes, and J. Menczel: Modification of the antidiuretic effect of vasopressin by acid and alkaline loads. J. clin. Invest. **44**, 754—764 (1965).
Ullrich, K.J.: Das Nierenmark, Struktur, Stoffwechsel und Funktion. Ergebn. Physiol. **50**, 433—489 (1959).
—, u. K.H. Jarausch: Untersuchungen zum Problem der Harnkonzentrierung und Verdünnung. Über die Verteilung der Elektrolyte (Na, K, Ca, Mg, Cl, anorg. Phosphat), Harnstoff, Aminosäuren und exogenem Kreatinin im Rinde und Mark der Hundeniere bei verschiedenen Diuresezuständen. Pflügers Arch. ges. Physiol. **262**, 537—550 (1956).
—, and J. Marsh: Kidney, water and electrolyte metabolism. Ann. Rev. Physiol. **25**, 91—142 (1963).
—, G. Pehling, A. Ruiz-Guinazu u. Espinar-Lafuente: Veränderung des Blutes bei der Passage durch das vasculäre Gegenstromsystem im Nierenmark. Pflügers Arch. ges. Physiol. **274**, 64—65 (1961).

ULLRICH, K. J., G. RUMRICH u. G. FUCHS: Wasserpermeabilität und transtubulärer Wasserfluß corticaler Nephronabschnitte bei verschiedenen Diuresezuständen. Pflügers Arch. ges. Physiol. **280**, 99—119 (1964).
— —, and B. SCHMIDT-NIELSEN: Urea transport in the collecting duct of rats on normal and low protein diet. Pflügers Arch. ges. Physiol. **295**, 147—156 (1967).
USSING, H.H., P. KRUHØFFER, J. HESS THAYSEN, and N.A. THORN: The alkali metal ions in biology. Handbuch d. exper. Pharmacol., Ergänzungswerk Bd. 13. Berlin-Göttingen-Heidelberg: Springer 1960.
VALTIN, H.: Sequestration of urea and nonurea solutes in renal tissues of rats with hereditary hypothalamic diabetes insipidus. Effect of vasopressin and dehydration on the countercurrent mechanism. J. clin. Invest. **45**, 337—345 (1966a).
— Effect of dehydration on urinary concentration in the absence of vasopressin. J. clin. Invest. **45**, 1082 (1966b).
— Hereditary hypothalamic diabetes insipidus in rats (a useful experimental model). Amer. J. Med. **42**, 814—827 (1967).
VAN DYKE, H.B., S.L. ENGEL, and K. ADAMSON, jr.: Comparison of pharmacological effect of lysine and arginine vasopressin. Proc. Soc. exp. Biol. (N.Y.) **91**, 484—486 (1956).
—, W.H. SAWYER, and N.I.A. OVERWEG: Pharmacologic activities of the [8]-citrulline-analogues of oxytocin and vasopressin. Endocrinology **73**, 637—639 (1963).
VAN EPS, S.W.S., C.CH.T.H. ROMENY-WACHTER, H. SCHOUTEN, and A.M. STRUYKER BOUDIER: Renal concentration test in a tropical climate. Clin. chim. Acta **14**, 637—644 (1966).
VERNEY, E.B.: Water diuresis. Irish J. med. Sci. **6**, 377—402 (1954).
VIERLING, A.F., J. B. LITTLE, and E.P. RADFORD: Antidiuretic hormone bioassay in rats with heriditary hypothalamic diabetes insipidus (Brattleboro strain). Endocrinology **80**, 211—220 (1967).
VOGEL, G.: Daten zur Physiologie der Harnbereitung beim Truthuhn. Pflügers Arch. ges. Physiol. **278**, 32—43 (1963).
—, I. STOECKERT, W. KRÜGER, I. DOBBERSTEIN u. R. WINKLER: Vergleichende Stop-Flow-Untersuchungen an Nieren mit geringem und wenig ausgebildetem System Henlescher Schleifen. Pflügers Arch. ges. Physiol. **238**, 160—170 (1965a).
— — — u. I. DOBBERSTEIN: Harn und Harnbereitung bei terrestrisch lebenden Vögeln. Untersuchungen am Truthuhn (Meleagris pavo L.). Zbl. Vet.-Med. **12**, 132—160 (1965b).
— — u. R. WINKLER: Clearance und Stop-Flow-Untersuchungen an intakten und diabetes-insipidus-Ratten in Wasser- und osmotischer Diurese ohne und mit Zufuhr exogenen Vasopressins. Acta endocr. (Kbh.) **52**, 239—254 (1966).
VORHERR, H.: Über die Wirkung von synthetischem Oxytocin auf die Wasserdiurese der Ratte. Z. ges. exp. Med. **133**, 602—608 (1960).
— Zur Frage des Oxytocin-Vasopressin-Antagonismus an der Diurese bei Mensch und Tier. Klin. Wschr. **42**, 198—201 (1964).
WALKER, A.M.: Experiments upon the relation between pituitary gland and water diuresis. Amer. J. Physiol. **127**, 519—540 (1939).
WARD, E.E., P. RICHARDS, and O.H. WRONG: Urine concentration after acute renal failure. Nephron **3**, 289—294 (1966).
WELLER, C.P.: On the mechanism of the refractoriness to ADH induced by water deprivation in the rat. Acta physiol. lat.-amer. **15**, 411—416 (1965).
WESTON, R.E., I.B. HANENSON, J. GROSSMAN, G.A. BERDASCO, and M. WOLFMAN: Natriuresis and chloruresis following pitressin-induced water retention in non-edematous patients: Evidence of homeostatic mechanism regulating body fluid volume. J. clin. Invest. **32**, 611—618 (1953).
—, H.B. HOROWITZ, J. GROSSMAN, I.B. HANENSON, and L. LEITER: Decreased antidiuretic response to betahypophamine in hyperthyroidism. J. clin. Endocr. **16**, 322—337 (1956).
WHITE, A.G., G. RUBIN, and L. LEITER: Studies in oedema. III. The effect of pitressin on the renal excretion of water and electrolytes in patients with and without liver disease. J. clin. Invest. **30**, 1287—1297 (1951).
WHITE, H.L., and D. ROLF: Urine and papilla concentrations during transition from hypotonic to hypertonic urine. Amer. J. Physiol. **208**, 397—400 (1965).
WHITTEMBURY, G., N. SUGINO, and A.K. SOLOMON: Effect of antidiuretic hormone and calcium on the equivalent pore radius of kidney slices from necturus. Nature (Lond.) **187**, 699—701 (1960).
WIEDERHOLT, M.H. STOLTE, J.P. BRECHT u. K. HIERHOLZER: Mikropunktionsuntersuchungen über den Einfluß von Aldosteron, Cortison und Dexamethason auf die renale Natriumresorption adrenalektomierter Ratten. Pflügers Arch. ges. Physiol. **292**, 316—333 (1966).
WIRZ, H.: Die Druckverhältnisse in der normalen Niere. Schweiz. med. Wschr. **86**, 377—382 (1956).
— Kidney, water and electrolyte metabolism. Ann. Rev. Physiol. **23**, 577—606 (1961).

Witte, E., H. Reineck u. O. H. Gauer: Antidiurese and Diurese nach kleinen Tonephingaben bei der Ratte abhängig vom oralen NaCl-Angebot. Pflügers Arch. ges. Physiol. **274**, 262—271 (1961).

Wolgast, M.: Regional renal blood flow measured with P^{32}-labelled red cells and beta-sensitive semiconductor detectors. Acta physiol. scand. **68**, suppl. **277**, 223 (1966).

Yamsane, Y., and K. Kunishige: Bioassay of ADH on experimental diabetes insipidus rats with a study on the ADH level in normal human plasma. Jap. Circulat. J. (Enh.) **30**, 1381—1386 (1966).

Yoon, M. C., and S. K. Hong: Effect of prolonged bodily hydration on the renal concentrating operation. J. appl. Physiol. **16**, 815—818 (1961).

Yoshida, S., K. Motohashi, H. Ibayashi, and S. Okinaka: Method for the assay of antidiuretic hormone in plasma with a note on the antidiuretic titer of human plasma. J. Lab. clin. Med. **62**, 279—285 (1963).

Yunibhand, P., u. U. Held: Der Einfluß der zunehmenden Hydropenie auf Nierenmark, Serum und Urin bei Albinoratten. Helv. physiol. pharmakol. Acta **23**, 139—144 (1965).

Zain-ul-Abedin, M.: Effect of a single large vasopressin injection upon the chemical composition of kidney. J. Physiol. (Lond.) **181**, 67p—68p (1965).

Zaoral, M., E. Kasafirek, J. Rudinger, and F. Sorm: Amino acids and peptides. LI. Synthesis of 2-O-Methyltyrosine- and 2-O-Ethyltyrosine-lysine-vasopressin. Collection Czech. Chem. Commun. **30**, 1809—1873 (1965).

—, J. Kolc, and F. Sorm: Synthesis of D-arg⁸- and D-lys⁸-vasopressin. Collection Czech. Chem. Commun. **31**, 382—383 (1966).

— — — Amino acids and peptides LXX. Synthesis of D-Arg⁸- and D-lys⁸-vasopressin. Collection Czech. Chem. Commun. **32**, 1242—1249 (1967a).

— — — Amino acids and peptides LXXI. Synthesis of 1-deamino-8-D-aminobutyrine-vasopressin, 1-deamino-8-D-lysine-vasopressin, and 1-deamino-8-D-argine-vasopressin. Collection Czech. Chem. Commun. **32**, 1250—1257 (1967b).

—, V. Pliska, K. Rezabek, and F. Sorm: Synthesis of a highly effective analogue of lysine-vasopressin. Collection Czech. Chem. Commun. **28**, 746—747 (1963a).

— — —, and F. Sorm: Synthesis of two lysine-vasopressin analogues with protracted hormonal activity. Collection Czech. Chem. Commun. **28**, 747—749 (1963b).

—, and F. Sorm: Amino acids and peptides. LX. Synthesis of D-DAB⁸-vasopressin. Collection Czech. Chem. Commun. **31**, 310—314 (1966).

The Effect of Neurohypophysial Hormones and Similar Polypeptides on the Uterus and other Extravascular Smooth Muscle Tissue*

ROBERT A. MUNSICK

I. Introduction

In this review attention will be principally directed to the effects of neurohypophysial hormones and their analogues on the smooth muscle of the uterine portion of the oviduct. The effects on other nonvascular smooth muscle will be considered at less length. Because of the wide scope of the subject, certain areas will be discussed cursorily, and the interested reader will be referred when possible to review articles or specific papers which deal in depth with that particular subject area. The literature of the past 20 years is covered in some depth, especially as it relates to the neurohypophysial hormones and analogues directly. However, in areas of background information, e.g., the physiology of uterine contractions, review articles will be cited principally. The author has endeavored to make the text readable rather than have it a mere citation of the literature.

All of the diverse ramifications of this subject can not be considered in a publication of less than textbook size. Therefore, very little attention will be devoted to the clinical applications of these polypeptide drugs. Those interested in reading detailed accounts of the history of the use of oxytocin in obstetric practice and of the general pharmacology and clinical application of oxytocin are referred to the recent review articles of SOGOLOW (1966) and MUNSICK (1965a), respectively, and to textbooks of pharmacology and obstetrics.

In reviewing this subject, the author has attempted to present the data in an orderly, logical sequence, beginning with a succinct review of the physiology of uterine contractions, proceeding to the mechanism by which neurohypophysial hormones cause their oxytocic action, considering some aspects of the techniques involved in uterine biological assays, and then devoting attention to specific areas of interest which relate to the above considerations.

II. Uterine Contractility and Responses to Neurohypophysial Hormones and Analogues

A. Physiology of Uterine Contractions

The general field of uterine physiology will not be considered; it has been considered *in extenso* elsewhere, e.g., REYNOLDS (1965). Likewise, the overall field of smooth muscle physiology has been extensively reviewed (see CSAPO, 1960; and BOHR, 1964). BOHR's extensive review of electrolytes and smooth muscle contraction is highly relevant to many aspects of the points which follow and is recommended reading.

---

* Some of the author's cited unpublished data were supported by Research Grant HD-290651 from the National Institutes of Health.

Uterine smooth muscle cells, like most other visceral nonstriated muscle cells, are close-packed and admixed with variable amounts of connective tissue. In some if not all species of mammalian uteri, there is an autonomic nervous system innervation of the tissues, and the tissue has an abundant supply of catecholamines (WURTMAN, CHU, and AXELROD, 1963).

Each muscle cell has an electrically charged cell membrane, with membrane and cellular enzyme systems which contribute to the maintenance or restoration of this charge, and specific intracellular contractile proteins, which, when activated, combine to form the protein material which is directly responsible for the smooth muscle contraction. All of the biochemical details of the interactions of these proteins, what proteins are actually present in the cells and which are artifacts caused by chemical methods of extraction are subjects which are currently receiving much investigation. A recent discussion of the contractile protein, actomyosin, and others, such as the meromyosins, tropomyosin, etc., can be found in articles by NEEDHAM and WILLIAMS (1959), CSAPO (1960), and CARSTEN (1965).

Individual smooth muscle cell membranes in the inactive, resting state are more permeable to K^+ than to Na^+ and the intracellular concentration of K^+ is higher and of Na^+ is lower than in the extracellular fluid. Na^+ is actively pumped out of the cell and therefore the cell is electrically charged, positive outside and negative inside, i. e., the cell membrane potential is negative. Upon activation of the cell membrane, it becomes permeable to Na^+, net flow of Na^+ becomes inwards, and this region of the cell becomes more electropositive. In the adjacent, inactive part of the cell membrane, the charges are opposite. Therefore, a flow of current is established. The impulse or action potential continues along the membrane, while, in its wake, the charge is being restored by the pumping mechanism. With restoration of charge, Na^+ permeability diminishes, and the continuously active sodium pump restores the process to the original, resting state. Having swept down the cell, the action potential must then spread to adjoining cells if the entire tissue is to respond with a synchronous contraction. It is uncertain how depolarization spreads from cell to cell — it may be through membrane apposition, through interconnecting holes in the membranes, membrane fusion, or other as yet unproved mechanisms. Acetylcholine applied to rat uterine smooth muscle cells causes membrane depolarization, action potentials and contraction of the muscle (MARSHALL, 1962).

It is generally agreed that propagated action potentials are responsible for ultimate smooth muscle contractions. These contractions are of short duration and can occur spontaneously or as a result of stimulation with a dilute concentration of neurohypophysial hormone. A second type of contraction, in which a sustained, tonic shortening occurs in the absence of spike potentials, is known as contracture. JUNG (1961) has explained that low doses of oxytocin affect the first type of contractile system — the "tetanic system" — by slightly lowering threshold and membrane potential and thus favoring spread of the excitation waves and the frequency of contractions. Large doses, on the other hand, cause depolarization of the membrane, thus excluding the "tetanic system", and activate the "tonic system" leading to maintained contraction, or "contracture". JUNG (1961) believes that "contracture" is caused by altered permeability of the membrane to K^+. If action potentials are not propagated from cell to cell to involve the entire muscle, contractions will not be maximal and may not even be measurable.

Effects of Sex Steroids

Estrogen and progestagens have a profound influence on uterine smooth muscle physiology. MARSHALL (1959) found that uteri from spayed rats have resting membrane potentials of about —35 mV. Estrogen treatment caused a marked rise in resting membrane potential to about —57 mV, and estrogen plus progesterone caused a further rise to about —64 mV. Also measuring from single myometrial cells, JUNG (1965) has found that *high* doses of estradiol can raise the resting membrane potential to —75 mV, and that the addition of progesterone causes no further increase in the potential.

Estrogen treatment causes uterine muscle to contract spontaneously and regularly. The contractions are large and are initiated by action potentials. The action potentials are propagated over the entire muscle and are synchronized from cell to cell. In uterine muscle from rats treated with estrogen and progesterone contractions are weak and irregular, action potential discharges vary from cell to cell, and conduction block is evident.

Progesterone elevates the resting membrane potential and seems to produce a conduction block. It has been suggested that progesterone may also block uterine smooth muscle directly at the cell membrane — so-called depolarization block (CSAPO, 1961). In a series of experiments, CSAPO (1961) and his colleagues have pursued the effects of progesterone on both *in vitro* and *in vivo* systems. Most investigators agree that progesterone dominated uteri from at least some species do exhibit block. Ascertions that the progesterone block is in part caused by progesterone hyperpolarization of the membrane are not well founded, however, for, as mentioned earlier, JUNG (1965) has found that the membrane can be brought to highest potentials by estrogen without progesterone. Such uteri do not exhibit block. Hence, the high potential is not responsible, *per se*, for block. JUNG (1965) does not challenge the existence of progesterone block; rather, he confirms it. He has provided evidence that the rate of climb of the action potential upstroke is affected by progesterone. Because the rising phase of the action potential is related to influx of Na^+, JUNG (1965) argues that at least part of the progesterone blocking effect is due to a block of the Na^+ carrier mechanism.

In general, oxytocin causes depolarization of estrogen dominated mammalian uteri with a subsequent contractile response. As pointed out by MARSHALL (1962), "Evidently the action of oxytocin is not depolarization or repolarization *per se*, but oxytocin brings the membrane potential into the range most suited for activity." More will be said later concerning the mechanism of action of oxytocin. It should be emphasized, however, that the manner by which oxytocin affects the membrane electrophysiologic phenomena is not yet known.

In progesterone dominated rat and rabbit uteri (naturally dominated, as in pregnancy, or in estrogen plus progesterone treated castrated animals) the resting membrane potential is elevated and there is a depolarization block, as we have previously mentioned. Oxytocin, at least in usual, low, oxytocic concentrations, is ineffectual in depolarizing the membrane or in producing a contractile response. This observation and many others have lead several investigators (e. g., CSAPO, 1956, 1961; MARSHALL, 1962; JUNG, 1961) to enlarge on the original work of KNAUS (1927, 1928, 1934) and to postulate that the gravid uterus is refractory to oxytocin because of the "progesterone block." This controversial subject will be treated in greater detail later.

Progesterone and estrogens are not the only sex steroids which affect uterine response to oxytocin. They are, however, the principal and most important ones.

B. Mechanism of Oxytocic Action of Neurohypophysial Hormones

We have already referred to the fact that oxytocin acts on smooth muscle, at least in part, by affecting the electrophysiologic status of the myometrial membrane. In the following section an attempt will be made to answer the following questions: How does oxytocin affect the membrane potential? Are there other effects or mechanisms by which the neurohypophysial hormones cause uterine smooth muscle to shorten?

1. *Membrane Phenomena*

First, what evidence is there that oxytocin does affect the membrane potential? In multiple, confirmed experiments it has been shown that the estrogen dominated smooth muscle cell responds to oxytocin with a slight, but definite depolarization of the cell membrane. Concomitantly, the frequency and duration of spike discharges are increased. These events, accompanied by myometrial contraction, occur even at very low concentrations of oxytocin (MARSHALL, 1962). With a large dose of oxytocin the membrane is profoundly depolarized and sustained contracture occurs, accompanied by a cessation of spike discharges. MARSHALL (1962) has pointed out that these effects resemble those which occur when similar tissue is exposed to acetylcholine and other myometrial stimulants such as histamine and 5-hydroxytryptamine.

CSAPO (1961), JUNG (1961), and MARSHALL (1962) have performed numerous other experiments relevant to the effects of oxytocin on the myometrial cell membrane. In a K^+ free solution oxytocin causes minimal depolarization of the parturient rat uterus and no action potentials occur. Raising the K^+ concentration to 15 mM/L causes intensification of the normal effects of oxytocin. In the parturient rabbit uterus, raising extracellular K^+ to 120 mM/L causes membrane depolarization and nearly nullifies the electrical and oxytocic effects of oxytocin. Nevertheless, an electrical stimulus still causes maximal contractions (CSAPO, 1961; CSAPO, in MARSHALL, 1963b, p. 21).

Varying the Na^+ concentration of the extracellular fluid, MARSHALL (1963a), found that an increase of Na^+ augments the effects of oxytocin — membrane depolarization is intensified and contractions are increased. Using sucrose to increase the osmotic pressure equivalently, and keeping all ions at normal concentrations MARSHALL could not duplicate the findings which occurred with increased Na^+. She concluded, therefore, that the observed effect was due to Na^+, and was not simply an osmotic effect. Ca^{++}-rich solutions produce augmentative effects similar to Na^+-rich solutions. Conversely, Na^+-free and Ca^{++}-free solutions abolish the oxytocin effects. MARSHALL (1963a) has also studied the effects of Na^+-deficient solutions, i. e., 35.8 mM/L, on parturient rat uteri. She has shown that the consequent decreased frequency in spike potentials and diminution in the individual action potentials with diminution of the rate of rise of the upstroke velocity of each action potential is partially rectified by the addition of oxytocin. It was also found that Ca^{++} enrichment enhanced and Ca^{++} depletion inhibited this restorative action of oxytocin in Na^+ depleted solutions. MARSHALL (1963b, p. 63) has suggested that oxytocin may act by mobilizing Ca^{++}, and possibly other ions, "to act as inward current carriers during the upstroke of the action potential."

It is certainly fair to say that Ca^{++} plays an important part in membrane phenomena and in the mechanism by which oxytocin affects the membrane. Likewise, Ca^{++} probably plays some part in determining the difference between estrogen and progesterone dominated uteri. It has been shown, for example, that diminution of extracellular Ca^{++} affects the estrogen dominated more rapidly and intensely than the progesterone dominated rat uterus (GOTO and CSAPO, 1960; BERGER and MARSHALL, 1961). With estrogen domination, deprivation of Ca^{++} quickly leads to membrane depolarization and generation of trains of action potentials, followed by further decline in membrane potential to about —20 mV.

Here, action potentials cease and muscular relaxation occurs. In contrast, progesterone dominated muscle remains refractory to lowered Ca^{++} for over an hour.

From the above studies it has been suggested that oxytocin acts by liberating Ca^{++} from the membrane and that the demonstrable difference in oxytocin responses between estrogen and progesterone dominated uterine muscle may be accounted for by supposing that progesterone causes far tighter binding of Ca^{++} than does estrogen (Goto and Csapo, 1960; Berger and Marshall, 1961). It has also been found that monovalent cations are less firmly bound when uteri are progesterone dominated (Kao, 1961). However, Evans, Schild and Thesleff (1958) found that in the totally depolarized membrane, with complete abolition of action potentials, caused by applying an isotonic K^+ solution, a contractile response to large doses of oxytocin could still be evoked. Despite the artificiality of the conditions and the abnormality of the contractions, this finding certainly leads one to wonder if the action of oxytocin may not be at several biochemical levels (Jung, 1965), or at a level which has not yet been explored.

2. Other Findings

An important point which needs emphasis is the fact that oxytocin is not a direct myometrial stimulant. Although several of the indirect experiments listed earlier would seem to make this point clear, the ones performed by Csapo and his colleagues (see Csapo, 1961), in which potentially contractile isolated uterine actomyosin-ATP systems failed to contract in response to oxytocin, appeared to finalize the issue. It is tempting, therefore, to assume that oxytocin, and perhaps most oxytocic agents, such as acetylcholine, histamine and 5-hydroxytryptamine, act solely *via* the cell membrane to influence ionic permeability and contractility. The experiment by Schild's group, described above, is discomfiting for those who are prepared to accept this hypothesis totally. Also disturbing is the study of Kumar, Wagatsuma, and Barnes (1965a) in which glycerine-extracted rabbit psoas muscle fibers developed significantly greater tension in response to ATP with than without a relatively small amount of oxytocin (1 mU/ml). An explanation for this finding is not apparent. Another intracellular effect of oxytocin has been demonstrated by Leonard and Crandall (1963), who noted an increase in the ratio of active to total phosphorylase in estrogen treated rat uteri after exposure to oxytocin or epinephrine.

This finding need not necessarily indicate a direct, non-membranous, intracellular effect of oxytocin, however. The change in phosphorylase activity may result from the contraction, the alteration in ionic milieu or other factors initiated at the membrane by oxytocin.

3′, 5′-cyclic AMP has been studied in many of the biologic systems which are affected by, among other agents, the neurohypophysial hormones. To the author's knowledge this system has not been studied in the uterus. When it is it will be surprising if activation of 3′,5′ AMP is not demonstrated and held to be responsible for the action of oxytocin, for it seems that in most other systems studied such has been the case. Far more refined studies would be required, however, to adduce the manner by which this activation occurs, where in the cell it occurs, and what transpires after its occurrence.

C. Receptor Theory

There must be rather specific receptor sites for the neurohypophysial hormones in uterine smooth muscles. Most of the limited studies on this issue have not taken into account the several events which occur between introducing hormone and measuring contractile response. Indeed, it is probable that in our present state of ignorance concerning the entire gamut of events which leads to contraction, an unequivocal model of receptors cannot be synthesized.

It can be speculated, however, that the receptor sites are located somewhere in or on the cell membrane, and that the neurohypophysial peptides are bound with variable affinity to the receptor site. Binding and activation may very well be two entirely different phenomena, however. Hence, an analogue with no indigenous oxytocic activity (no receptor activation) also might have no inhibitory properties (no receptor binding). Another analogue without activity might act as an inhibitor (positive receptor binding) of active peptides. Utilizing carbamylated and acetylated analogues of oxytocin, DEREK G. SMYTH (personal communication) has prepared N-carbamyl-O-carbamyloxytocin, N-carbamyl-O-acetyloxytocin and N-acetyl-O-acetyloxytocin. All three of these compounds lack intrinsic oxytocic activity and show inhibitory activity. SMYTH is currently formulating a theory of binding and receptor activation by utilizing these and other similar analogues with and without substitutions on the N^1-position, the hydroxyl group of the Tyr^2 and with utilization of substituted De-$Amino^1$-analogues.

The possibility that uterine receptor sites contain reactive disulfide groups was entertained and evaluated by BENTLEY (1964), after MARTIN and SCHILD (1962, 1965), showed that thioglycollic acid inhibits the response of rat uteri to oxytocin and SCHWARTZ *et al.* (1960) showed that N-ethylmaleimide (NEM), a sulphydryl group blocking compound, inhibited vasopressin-induced increased water permeability of the toad bladder. BENTLEY found that reduced and oxidized glutathione reversibly and competitively inhibited the contractile action of oxytocin on isolated rat uteri. 1 mM NEM irreversibly blocked the oxytocic response to oxytocin and acetylcholine, but so many profound effects on the uterus occurred (prevents relaxation and causes increased uterine swelling) that it is impossible, now, to be certain of the exact mechanism by which its inhibition occurred. The above findings may indicate that SH and S—S groups are present at receptor sites, but it is also possible that sites and phenomena other than receptors have been influenced by these substances. For example, MARSHALL and MILLER (1964) have shown that dinitrophenol (DNP), which probably uncouples reactions between phosphorylation and electron transfer, and monoiodoacetic acid (IAA), an inhibitor of glycolysis, both inhibit the contractile response of rat uteri to oxytocin. Studying both contraction and membrane potential, they found that DNP depolarized the membrane and reversibly blocked oxytocin. IAA, on the other hand, did not affect the membrane potential, but irreversibly blocked responses to oxytocin. DANIEL (1964) has provided detailed studies of the effects of various enzyme inhibitors on ion transport and on the phenomenon of contracture in uterine muscle of rats, rabbits and cats.

What would a similar study show for the effects of NEM and the glutathiones? Is the oxytocin receptor site inextricably associated with membrane electrophysiologic phenomena? How specific are these sites? We know some of the questions but few of the answers.

D. Oxytocic Assay Methods

Hill, quoted by CSAPO (1960, p. 229), has made the following poignant comment concerning the utilization of smooth muscle for pharmacologic studies of drugs: "The mechanical response of active muscle is easy to record; indeed too easy, for very inadequate methods have been used and the older physiological literature is burdened with results of experiments which depended more on the properties of levers than on those of muscle." This acerb statement has much to recommend it, and it is hoped that the situation will improve in the future.

Nevertheless, the pharmacologist with his crowbar approach has contributed sizeably to our knowledge of both the pharmacology and physiology of the oxytocic action of the neurohypophysial hormones and analogues. Indeed, using isotonic levers, a smoked drum, a kymograph and a simple bath, DALE (1906) serendipidously discovered the oxytocic action of posterior lobe extracts and later proffered the first assay for the neurohypophysial hormones (DALE and LAIDLAW, 1912).

1. Isolated Rat Uterus

Many modifications of oxytocic assays exist and some are more suitable than others in various situations. However, the assay which is most commonly used is based upon the one described by HOLTON (1948). This assay has so many intrinsic advantages over others that a description of it will follow. Other methods will then be discussed at less length.

Isolated uteri from virgin guinea-pigs were initially utilized for oxytocic assays. These animals were expensive and difficult to obtain in suitable numbers. BEAUVILLAIN (1943) first advocated the use of rat uteri, but his paper went unnoticed. It remained for HOLTON (1948) to popularize not only the use of rat uteri, but the bath solution, the exact details of recording, of conducting the assay and of performing the statistical analysis of the results by the method of SCHILD (1942).

First, let us consider the test animal. Most investigators use young rats. No differences in responses to the neurohypophysial hormones or analogues have been demonstrated for different strains. More dependable and sensitive uteri are obtained if estrous rats are chosen or if the animals are treated with an estrogen preparation (GADDUM, 1953; MUNSICK and JERONIMUS, 1965). Recently, FOLLETT and BENTLEY (1964) have shown that three daily injections of 0.1 mg diethylstilbestrol increase sensitivity even more than a single injection. The animal is killed and a uterine horn is quickly excised, immersed in a suitable solution (*vide infra*), fastened within a bath chamber, and fixed to a lever for isotonic recording or to a strain gauge for isometric recordings. Despite numerous, stentorian objections to the use of isotonic methods for recording contractions of smooth muscle, either isotonic or isometric measurements are entirely suitable for this type of assay (MUNSICK and JERONIMUS, 1965). HOLTON recommended that the uterus be counter-weighted by a 3 g load.

In the oxygenated solution the uterus is allowed to equilibrate at about 32° C for a short time. 30 min will usually suffice. Now the assay can be started. In a fixed dose ratio the Standard (usually International or USP Posterior Pituitary Reference Standard or an accurately assayed preparation of oxytocin) and unknown are injected into the bath at exact 3 min intervals in random order, forming groups of four injections. For further details the reader is strongly urged to read HOLTON's work, for her advice is sound and explicit, and her paper is truly a classic.

When a suitable number of groups of graded responses has been obtained, the data are subjected to SCHILD's (1942) method of analyzing variances and fiducial limits of potency of the unknown. Often numerous assays on one unknown must be combined. We have recently reviewed some of the statistical methods which are useful for combining potencies and determining the significance of differences in potencies and potency ratios (MUNSICK and JERONIMUS, 1965).

a) Bath Solution: In this biological assay several points need special emphasis. First, the bath solution is extraordinarily important, for what might appear to be extremely minor, inconsequential differences between one variety of eponomized salt water and another can profoundly influence the reliability of the uterine preparation, the magnitude of responses, and the potency estimates of different neurohypophysial peptides. The last point will be considered in detail under "Influence of Ions."

The salt concentrations of some solutions which have been advocated for *in vitro* assays of the posterior lobe hormones are shown in Table 1. Note that the majority of listed solutions have essentially identical amounts of Na^+, K^+, HCO_3^- and glucose. The amounts of $CaCl_2$ and $MgCl_2$ vary considerably, however. In van Dyke-Hastings solution (VAN DYKE and HASTINGS, 1928) the ionic composition is considerably different, for it contains both high bicarbonate and phosphate buffers. This plasma surrogate has advantages over many others, for it is well buffered at

Table 1. *Comparison of various physiologic salt solutions. All values mM/L, unless otherwise noted. Bicarbonate concentration computed from added $NaHCO_3$*

Na^+	K^+	HCO_3^-	$H_2PO_4^-$ $HPO_4^=$	Ca^{++}	Mg^{++}	Glucose	pH	Remarks	Ref.
160	5.6	6.0	0	2.2	0	5.55	Variable	(See Text re. pH)	1
160	5.6	6.0	0	2.2	0.052	2.78	Variable	(See Text re. pH)	2
160	5.6	6.0	0	2.2	0.026	2.78	Variable	(See Text re. pH)	3
160	5.6	6.0	0	1.1	0.026	1.39	Variable	(See Text re. pH)	4
160	5.6	6.0	0	0.54	0.052	2.78	Variable	(See Text re. pH)	5
160	5.6	6.0	0	0.54	0	2.78	Variable	(See Text re. pH)	6
144	2.7	7.1	0.36	1.8	1.1	5.55	7.88 / 8.00	(According to VAN DYKE and HASTINGS, 1928)	7
144	6.2	30	1.0	0.53	1.0	—	7.4	(Gassed with CO_2 in O_2)	8
144	6.2	30	1.0	0.53	0 or 0.50	2.78	7.4	(Gassed with CO_2 in O_2)	9

References. 1: DALE and LAIDLAW (1912); 2: BURN and DALE (1922); 3: *Brit. Pharmacopoeia* (1948); 4: *Brit. Pharmacopoeia* (1963); 5: *Beauvillain* (1943); 6: GADDUM *et al.* (1949); 7: TYRODE (1910); 8: VAN DYKE and HASTINGS (1928); 9: MUNSICK (1960), Modification of VAN DYKE and HASTINGS (1928).

pH 7.4 when gassed with approximately 5% CO_2 in O_2, and its ionic composition more nearly approximates that of plasma. Addition of sodium phenosulfonphthalein in a dilute concentration allows the experienced assayist to monitor pH constantly by observing the color of the solution (VAN DYKE and HASTINGS, 1928; MUNSICK, 1960). Beauvillain solution (BEAUVILLAIN, 1943), which is the one basic to most others listed, reached the undesirable pH's of 6.8, 8.3 and 7.9 after $1^1/_2$ hours of gassing with 5% CO_2 in O_2, gassing with air, or not gassing a solution in an unstoppered volumetric flask, respectively (MUNSICK, 1960).

Because there is much confusion concerning what solutions have been recommended by various authors several recommended solutions are shown in Table 1. HOLTON (1948) advocated use of "de Jalon solution," referring to the publication of GARCIA DE JALON, BAYO BAYO and GARCIA de JALON (1945). However, these investigators had used BEAUVILLAIN (1943) solution unless uteri became hyperactive. In that case, they reduced the Ca^{++} concentration by 80% and added Ca^{++} just prior to injecting the next dose of drug. In the next publication of this group (GARCIA DE JALON and GARCIA DE JALON, 1945) they stated that they used a solution of Locke, and in it, according to their table, were 3.8 mM Ca^{++} and 3.2 mM K^+. Finally, GARCIA DE JALON (1947) did publish results of experiments in which guinea-pig uteri could be made more suitable for assays by employing a high Mg^{++} solution. The basic solution used here was stated to have contained

2.2 mM Ca^{++} but was otherwise identical to Beauvillain solution. The author is uncertain, therefore, of what "de Jalon's solution" is and which variant HOLTON recommended. Because of these discrepancies and others, the author urges present and future investigators not to use eponyms for solutions unless they convey a clear meaning and the references to them are easily obtainable in most libraries. The composition of the fluid, even though documented by reference, might always best be elaborated to obviate future confusion. At the risk of seeming dogmatic and pleonastic, the author again wishes to emphasize that it would be highly desirable if one solution were agreed upon for the *in vitro* oxytocic assays of neurohypophysial hormones and analogues. As of now, results have been obtained in a spate of different solutions which have contained variable amounts of Ca^{++} and Mg^{++}, have varied greatly in pH, and have often been unspecified. Consequently, these results should not be compared with one another. The three solutions used most frequently have been: 1. the modification (MUNSICK, 1960) of the one of VAN DYKE and HASTINGS (1928), using O or 0.5 mM/L Mg^{++}; 2. the one of GADDUM (1949) and 3. the one of DE JALON. Because of the confusion concerning the last solution (*vide supra*), the author strongly recommends choosing between the first two. Gaddum's is poorly buffered and when gassed with air will have a high pH. For these reasons and the ones previously mentioned, the author chooses and recommends van Dyke-Hastings solution for further work.

b) Temperature: The temperature of the bath solution is very important. HOLTON (1948) advised 32° C for the rat uterus assay. She stated that higher temperatures cause increased spontaneous activity and sensitivity and that lower temperatures decrease spontaneous contractions and responsiveness. Excellent, precise control of temperature is requisite to accurate assays, for periodic fluctuations of as little as 0.5° C are assiciated with perceptible alterations of responses. HAMBURGER (1946), using guinea-pig uteri, studied quantitative aspects of the responses to oxytocin as they are influenced by temperature. A 14% change in contraction height was observed for each 1° C change on either side of the curve whose maximal value was observed to be 32° C.

c) Superfusion: For assays of minute amounts of neurohypophysial peptides the Holton (1948) method, even when modified by serially injecting diethylstilbestrol to increase sensitivity (FOLLETT and BENTLEY, 1964), may be too insensitive. GADDUM (1953) has devised a technique of superfusion in which the bath solution trickles over the uterus, which is suspended in air. The test drug is added to the solution as it runs over the preparation. This method has been found to be quite acceptable, and effective doses of oxytocin in the order of 0.02 mU can be assayed. Seldom can doses of less than 0.5 mU be assayed by the classic Holton method, using a 10 ml bath chamber.

2. Other Methods

In many respects the above types of assay leave much to be desired. The conditions established bear little or no resemblance to those extant in the living animal and are therefore extremely artificial and "unphysiologic". Factors which differ so remarkably from *in vivo* conditions are: low temperature, low Ca^{++} and other ionic concentrations in the plasma surrogate, direct delivery of the drug to muscle, by-passing the uterine vasculature (if a drug alters uterine hemodynamics it may not reach the uterus in a concentration or manner similar to the situation *in vivo*), presence of hormonal states not necessarily resembling those *in vivo*, and the fact that the drug is flushed out of the bath as soon as the first contraction has attained its maximal value. *In situ* the prolonged action of the drug on a series of contractions is usually measured. Hence, the *in vitro* method already described does not give information on the effects of a drug on contractile rhythmicity, frequency, amplitude or uterine tonus.

SANDBERG *et al.* (1959) have developed methods of evaluating each of the above parameters but the methods have lacked acceptance because each parameter is measured separately and the methods are complex. BÖSCH and KÄSER (1956) used the difference between the plain metric measurements of the surface area of the changed and baseline activities. Their method is somewhat cumbersome and involved and it has not been received with enthusiasm. STYLES and SULLIVAN (1962) have utilized modern electronic methods to integrate muscle tension. From the output voltage of a transducer a servo recorder traces the curve of uterine activity and an electronic integrator shows the product of time and tension. BERDE and SAAMELI (1966) are currently utilizing similar techniques for *in situ* preparations. Such ingenious applications of modern electronic equipment may soon allow us to evaluate oxytocic drugs in greater depth and in more realistic terms than has hitherto been possible.

Until recently, inadequate methods existed for measuring the oxytocic potency of drugs on the uterus *in situ.* Much greater emphasis has been directed toward this problem, especially in pregnant women, since CALDEYRO-BARCIA and his colleagues showed that intra-amniotic pressure recording could be performed with relative safety and convenience. Previously, most *in situ* measurements had been performed on nonpregnant animals utilizing isotonic measurements from the horn of a uterus, isometric recordings from a portion of a horn or pressure recordings from within the horn or uterus by mean of balloons. This is not to say that pregnant experimental animals have not been used for assays. Several assays have been developed which give satisfactory results. Balloon techniques, in which pressure changes are transmitted to a recorder, are quite popular. These can be used in pregnant rabbits, for example, with the balloon replacing one of the fetuses or being inserted between them (FUCHS, 1964; MENDES, 1960). When successfully fixed to the uterine wall, the animal can be allowed to recover from anesthesia.

Another assay method, which by design has the appeal of duplicating a common clinical use of oxytocic drugs, is the measurement of the ability of drugs to induce labor in experimental animals. Rabbits have been successfully used in such a system for quantitative assays of the neurohypophysial hormones and analogues (BERDE and CERLETTI, 1958). Thismethod has two serious short-comings, however: 1. the necessity of waiting exactly 30 days post-conception and 2. the large number of test animals required. FLÜCKINGER (cited in BERDE and SAAMELI, 1966) and SCHOFIELD (1964) have shown that this method can not, unfortunately, be applied to mice or guinea-pigs, respectively.

For the *clinical* use of oxytocic drugs, information is desired which will reflect the drug's potency in women, not rats, rabbits or other mammalian species. What's more, it is usually desirable that the woman be near term, in labor, or postpartum. Presently, several methods are being used to record contractions under the above circumstances. Small balloons can be inserted into the nongravid or gravid uterus prior to or during labor (MOIR, 1936; CSAPO and PINTO-DANTAS, 1966), fine plastic catheters can be introduced transabdominally *via* a needle directly into the amniotic cavity (ALVAREZ and CALDEYRO-BARCIA, 1950; CALDEYRO-BARCIA and SERENO, 1961; HENDRICKS, 1966) or in the myometrium or endometrium as an "open catheter" technique (HENDRICKS and MOAWAD, 1965). Contractions can also be recorded by external tokography and used for assays (MYERSCOUGH and SCHILD, 1955, 1958). A more detailed review of the uses of different methods of *in situ* assays, with many considerations of their relative advantages and disadvantages has recently been reported by BERDE and SAAMELI (1966).

In separate chapters of this volume STÜRMER and FITZPATRICK, and BENTLEY have considered in detail the general areas of bioassays and specific assays for neurohypophysial hormones in body fluids, respectively.

E. Influence of Anesthetic Agents and Other Drugs

The effect of various anesthetic agents on the uterus is not usually relevant to *in vitro* assays of the neurohypophysial hormones. Generally, the uterus is removed after the animal has been killed by decapitation or stunned by a blow on the head. Even if an anesthetic agent is used, any effects are probably nullified by the prolonged submersion in and frequent changes of the bath solution.

If, however, an anesthetic or other agent, such as a preservative, is introduced as an additive with the neurohypophysial preparation to be tested, interference or modification of the response might possibly ensue. Thus, BUENO-MONTANO *et al.* (1966) have confirmed some previous findings and added new ones in showing that the spontaneous contractions of isolated human pregnant and non-pregnant myometrial strips are inhibited by chlorobutanol, ethanol, sodium acetate, phenol and propylene glycol. Effective inhibitory concentrations of each drug are shown in Table 2. The tabulated results have been estimated by the author from the original

Table 2. *Minimal dose at which inhibition of spontaneous contractions of isolated human myometrial strips was demonstrated (μg/ml of bath solution)* (after BUENO-MONTANO *et al.*, 1966)

Preservative	Non-Pregnant	Pregnant	Remarks
Chlorobutanol . . .	0.2	0.2—2.0	Complete inhibition at 20 μg/ml
Ethanol	20—200	2.0—20	Decreased frequency and tone. Still motile at 200 μg/ml
Sodium acetate . .	ca. 1.0	0.01	Decreased frequency. Still motile at 10 μg/ml
Phenol	2.0—20.0	2.0—20.0	Decreased tone and Frequency. Still motile at 20 μg/ml
Propylene glycol . .	10.0—100.0	1.0—10.0	Decreased tone and Frequency. Still motile at 1000 μg/ml

paper. In undiluted Syntocinon (Sandoz Pharmaceuticals) and many other commercial preparations of oxytocin, concentrations of chlorobutanol, ethanol, and sodium acetate are 5,000 μg/ml, 5,000 μg/ml and 1,000 μg/ml, respectively. For oxytocic assays of oxytocin and other *potent* neurohypophysial hormones and analogues less than 10 mU is usually introduced into a 10 ml bath. Therefore, the concentrations in the bath of the above preservatives would be 0.5, 0.5 and 0.1 μg/ml, or less, respectively. It is unlikely that these concentrations would influence spontaneous motility even additively. Their possible influence on drug-induced responses is conjectural, but would likely be small or absent. On the other hand, the oxytocic potencies of analogues stored with identical preservatives and with far less activity than oxytocin might be greatly diminished. Likewise, a preparation with low intrinsic sensitivity to which large doses of neurohypophysial peptides are administered, could be affected by the preservatives.

The possible effects of chlorobutanol and ethanol on uteri of intact animals must also occasionally be considered. While observing the effects of gigantic doses of oxytocin on the rat kidney, BYROM and PRATT (1958) found that the chlorobutanol anesthetized the animals. Hence, they were forced to purify the commercial oxytocin in order to obtain valid results. A.-R. FUCHS (1966), in the course of her excellent, extensive studies on the initiation of labor, has found that ethanol inhibits the onset of labor in rabbits. For inhibition to occur ethanol concentrations of 2,500—3,500 μg/ml blood were required. If rabbit uteri resemble those of women, the data of BUENO-MONTANO *et al.* (1966) suggest that the inhibition of labor observed by FUCHS may have been caused in part at least by direct ethanol-induced myometrial depression rather than to blockade of oxytocin release from the neurohypophysis. Although FUCHS reported that a direct depressive effect had been excluded, the published evidence she presents for this exclusion is not, in the author's opinion at least, totally convincing.

BUENO-MONTANO (1966) has studied the effects of numerous other drugs on the contractility of isolated uteri of numerous mammalian species. In Table 3, some of his findings are summarized. The effects of these drugs on oxytocin-induced contractions were not studied. BERDE and SAAMELI (see Table 4 of BERDE and SAAMELI, 1966) have shown that several drugs can inhibit the contractile response to oxytocin in isolated estrous rat uteri. Those with greatest potency are isoprenaline and epinephrine. Contrary to once popular opinion, succinylcholine has been shown to relax hypertonic parturient human uteri *in situ* (ALVER *et al.*, 1962).

Table 3. *Effects of some drugs on the motility of isolated uteri from several species* (after BUENO-MONTANO, 1966)

	Homo	Monkey	Sheep	Dog	Rabbit	Mouse
Oxytocin	Increased	Increased	Increased	Increased	Increased	Increased
Sparteine	Increased	Increased	Increased	Increased	Increased	Increased
Mg^{++}	Decreased	Decreased	Decreased	Decreased	Decreased	Decreased
Ether	Decreased	Decreased	Decreased	Decreased	Decreased	Decreased
N_2O	Decreased	Decreased	Decreased	Decreased	Decreased	Decreased
Isoxuprine	Decreased	Decreased	Decreased	Decreased	Increased	Decreased
Morphine	No Effect	No Effect	No Effect or Increased	No Effect	Decreased	Decreased
Cyclopropane	Decreased	Decreased	Increased	Increased	Increased	Decreased

FEINSTEIN (1966) has shown that two local anesthetic drugs. tetracaine and procaine, abolish depolarized rat uterine contractile responses to calcium. Using Ca^{45} to follow Ca^{++} movement, he concluded that the local anesthetic drugs antagonize the uterine response by inhibiting the entry of Ca^{++} into or through the myometrial cell membrane.

Volatile anesthetic drugs such as diethyl ether and halothane and gases such as cyclopropane are known to depress uterine tonus and contractility *in situ* when deep surgical anesthesia is obtained with them. Diethyl ether inhibition has been especially well studied (VASICKA and KRETCHMER, 1961). Recently, KUMAR, WAGATSUMA and BARNES (1965b) have shown that ether causes hyperpolarization of the membrane potential of human uterine myometrium. Hence, hyperpolarization and stabilization of the membrane potential probably account in part, at least, for the inhibitory effect of ether.

Rather than digress at length on the effects of various non-neurohypophysial substances on the uterus, suffice it to say that investigations in which anesthetics and other drugs are used should be viewed with these factors kept clearly in mind. Use of unanesthetized animals will usually give data which more closely resemble those which occur naturally, provided that the animal is not uncomfortable at the time of the experiment.

F. Effects of Ionic Changes on Uterine Responses to Neurohypophysial Hormones and Analogues

Mention has already been made of several alterations of uterine behavior and electrical phenomena which follow profound changes in the Ca^{++}, K^+ and Na^+ concentrations of the bath solution. In this section, attention will be directed predominantly toward the effects of specific ionic alterations on the responses of uteri to posterior pituitary extracts and specific hormones or analogues. The thorough study of VAN DYKE and HASTINGS (1928) is recommended to the interested reader for background in this area of research. In their study, submaximal isotonic contractions of virgin guinea-pig uteri were recorded and responses to stimulation with whole posterior lobe extract of unstated source were compared. The bath solution was devised by them (van Dyke-Hastings solution), and has already been described in detail (see Table 1).

1. Sodium

VAN DYKE and HASTINGS (1928) found that diminished Na^+ caused decreased responses and *vice versa*. It will be recalled that MARSHALL (1963a) elicited similar findings with rat uteri.

2. Potassium

With small changes of K^+ concentration, changes of responses to posterior pituitary extract were found to resemble qualitatively those to Na^+ (VAN DYKE and HASTINGS, 1928). These findings have been confirmed repeatedly.

3. Calcium

Responses to posterior lobe extracts parallel the Ca^{++} concentration. Total removal of Ca^{++} eliminates responses entirely (KOCHMANN, 1921; BURN and DALE, 1922; VAN DYKE and HASTINGS, 1928). These findings have been repeatedly confirmed, both for whole extracts and for oxytocin. Because so much has already been written in this section on the effects of Ca^{++}, no repetition seems necessary here. BOHR's (1964) review is especially complete concerning Ca^{++} and smooth muscle.

4. Magnesium

Magnesium has received considerable attention by pharmacologists and physiologists. Unfortunately, many observations have been at variance with one another, probably because results from different species of animals and from *in vitro* and *in vivo* investigations have been compared. The ionic composition of the bath solutions, both in regard to Mg^{++} and to other ions, have not been identical, and methods of performing experiments and interpreting results have varied. The findings which will be reviewed are the salient ones which have been published since 1928.

VAN DYKE and HASTINGS (1928) used their own solution with 1.0 mM Mg^{++} and found that decreasing or markedly increasing Mg^{++} concentration caused diminution of uterine responses to whole posterior lobe extracts. They concluded that the 1.0 mM concentration was approximately optimal, but they apparently did not test at a concentration of 2.0 mM.

GENELL (1938) used isolated rat uteri in Tyrode's solution (TYRODE, 1910). Using no Mg^{++} and adding $MgCl_2$, he found that Mg^{++} concentration from 0.53 to 10.5 mM potentiated responses to Pitocin. Concentrations above 10.5 mM inhibited responses. Maximal augmentation occurred at about 5.3 mM. At this concentration responses were increased 5—10 fold. GENELL reported that Mg^{++} augmentation also occurred in uteri from mice, dogs, guinea-pigs, cows and women.

Using guinea-pig uteri in van Dyke-Hastings solution, FRASER (1939) was the first investigator to examine the effect of Mg^{++} on both oxytocin and vasopressin. He used impure commercial preparations of oxytocin and vasopressin (Postlobin-O and Postlobin-V, respectively). FRASER found that the ratio of oxytocic activity of Postlobin-O/Postlobin-V (the pressor fraction expressed in pressor units, the oxytocic fraction in oxytocic units) varied with Mg^{++} as follows: 0.0 Mg^{++} — 0.05, 1.0 mM Mg^{++} — 0.2, 2.6 mM Mg^{++} — 0.4, 5.3 mM Mg^{++} — 0.67, and 10.5 — 21.0 mM Mg^{++} — 1.0. In other words, at the high Mg^{++} concentrations of 10—20 mM, the vasopressin and oxytocin preparations were equiactive. Maximal responses to Postlobin-V occurred at 5.3 mM Mg^{++}; higher Mg^{++} caused diminution of the response. Some potentiation to Mg^{++} was observed at 0.2 mM Mg^{++} for Postlobin-V. A 0.1 mM Mg^{++} solution caused some potentiation for Postlobin-O and maximal responses were observed at 0.53—1.1 mM. Higher Mg^{++} concentrations caused a diminution of responses to Postlobin-O.

STEWART (1949), also utilized guinea-pig uteri but obtained results which did not entirely agree with those of FRASER. Increasing Mg^{++} from 0.026 mM to 0.16 mM did not influence contractile responses to Pitressin or Pitocin. Increasing Mg^{++} to 0.26 through 0.53 mM caused definite enhancement of contractions to both Pitressin and Pitocin, however. Pitressin responses were augmented more than Pitocin responses. Further increase to 1.1 mM through 5.3 mM caused further, fairly equal enhancement of the two, but concentrations above 10.5 mM caused more enhancement of Pitocin than Pitressin.

In nonpregnant cows, FITZPATRICK (1956) showed that elevation of serum Mg^{++} to about three times the normal value caused increased responses to Pitressin, but not to Pitocin.

ABARBANEL (1945) performed an excellent study which revealed the potent spasmolytic effect of Mg^{++} in pregnant women. Intravenous doses of 2 ml of 50 % or 10 ml of 20 % magnesium sulfate solution were found to be highly efficatious in overcoming and preventing uterine contracture caused by Pituitrin, Pitocin, Pitressin and other oxytocic drugs. In this report some of the previous clinical observations concerning magnesium were discussed in detail. PRITCHARD (1955) opined that doses of $MgSO_4$ used for the treatment of eclampsia do not affect contractions significantly. Recently, HUTCHINSON *et al.* (1964) restudied the effect of magnesium on pregnant human uterine contractions. Administration of 4.0 g of $MgSO_4$ failed to produce potentiation of oxytocin induced uterine contractions, but did augment the contractions produced by Val^3-oxytocin. KUMAR, ZOURLAS, and BARNES (1963), on the other hand, have clearly demonstrated that a marked increase in serum Mg^{++} does diminish the human uterine response to oxytocin.

MUNSICK (1960) and MUNSICK and JERONIMUS (1965) have obtained precise *in vitro* data for the oxytocic potencies of several neurohypophysial hormones and analogues. These results will be presented below. Suffice it to say at this juncture that the *potencies* of almost all analogues and hormones, except for oxytocin, are greater with 0.5 mM Mg^{++} than without Mg^{++}. BENTLEY (1965) has provided further data on Mg^{++} potentiation, which will also be discussed in more detail below.

Contrasting the heights of contractions of rat uteri in response to oxytocin and other neurohypophysial peptides with 0.5 mM or no Mg^{++}, we have found that Mg^{++} inevitably augments contractions (MUNSICK, 1960; MUNSICK and JERONIMUS, 1965). However, BENTLEY (1965), using quantitative data rather than impressions, has found that the contractile heights of rat uterine responses to oxytocin are not significantly altered by 0.5 mM Mg^{++}. He did find that contractions in response to Val^3-oxytocin are significantly augmented by the presence of 0.5 mM Mg^{++}. Using Val^3-oxytocin, BENTLEY (1965) also showed that 0.1 mM Mg^{++} caused minimal or no increase in responses compared with no magnesium, and that 1.0 mM Mg^{++} caused less potentiation than 0.5 mM Mg^{++}. Hence, *for*

Val³-oxytocin, a concentration of 0.5 mM Mg^{++} seems to cause greatest potentiation. It should be emphasized, however, that contractile height and potency are two different things. The latter is a function of the first *only in comparison with the contractions caused by the Standard*. Hence, if a concentration of 1.0 mM Mg^{++} caused greater potentiation of oxytocin (the Standard) responses, than of Val^3-oxytocin responses, the potency of the Val^3-oxytocin would not be greater despite slight, further potentiation of the responses to this analogue.

In connection with Val^3-oxytocin, BERDE and SAAMELI (1959) found that its potency was approximately 2.7 times as great for human uterine muscle *in situ* as *in vitro*, and 4.7 times as potent for human uterus *in situ* as rat uterus *in vitro*. MUNSICK (1960) conjectured that the greater potency *in situ* might have reflected a magnesium effect. Although this may be part of the story, species difference probably accounts for differences, also (see Tables 6 and 9). The differences in potency between *in vitro* and *in situ* assays performed on human pregnant uteri (BERDE and SAAMELI, 1959) may also be partially accounted for by the fact that the myometrial strips used for the *in vitro* experiments were obtained from the lower uterine segment.

The manner in which Mg^{++} effects an augmentation of responses is unknown. BENTLEY (1965) has hypothesized that Mg^{++} increases the affinity of the peptide for its receptors. MUNSICK and JERONIMUS (1965) have shown that the alterations of potency of oxytocin, $De\text{-}Amino^1$-oxytocin, Arg^8-oxytocin and Arg^8-vasopressin produced by estrogen or by 0.5 mM Mg^{++} are not parallel and in some instances are in opposite directions from one another. Hence, it is unlikely that the augmentation of responses caused by estrogen and magnesium are mediated by identical mechanisms. CLEGG, HOPKINSON, and PICKLES (1963), have again shown for the guinea-pig uterus that magnesium potentiates contractions from vasopressin. Using variable Ca^{++} and Mg^{++} concentrations they have concluded that vasopressin may act at only one cellular location, whereas other oxytocic substances may act at two or more sites.

5. *Manganese*

BENTLEY (1965) also studied the influence of Mn^{++} on the potency of several neurohypophysial peptides. He found that 0.1 mM Mn^{++} was generally more effective than 0.5 mM Mg^{++} in causing potentiation of potency and that potentiation was even demonstrable at a 0.01 mM concentration. Here again it should be emphasized that potency changes are contingent upon two variables, the alterations of responses to the analogue and to the standard. It will be interesting to note the effect of Mn^{++} on the potency of oxytocin (compared to International or U.S.P. Standard, both of which contain oxytocin and Arg^8-vasopressin) and on the heights of contractions produced by individual peptides. BENTLEY (1965) has used the findings with Mn^{++} to support the theory that Mg^{++} may act to alter the steric configuration of the peptide molecule, producing a better "fit" with receptors, or that it favorably influences the binding of peptides to their receptors, or both.

6. *Phosphate*

VAN DYKE and HASTINGS (1928) showed that increasing the phosphate concentration from 0—1.0 mM caused no significant alteration of the contractions produced by posterior lobe extract. A further increase to 3.0 mM phosphate did cause potentiation. They hypothesized that at a 1.0 mM phosphate concentration Ca^{++} was bound. Lack of a decrease in response (with diminished available ionized Ca^{++}) was therefore interpreted to indicate that phosphate ions do potentiate responses *per se*.

7. *Carbon Dioxide, Bicarbonate, Carbonate and Hydronium Ions*

It is difficult to control individual variables when studying these four factors. Also, under some conditions the solubility constant for $CaCO_3$ may be exceeded, further complicating an already complex ionic milieu.

In a series of imaginative, well devised experiments VAN DYKE and HASTINGS (1928) varied the concentrations of the above ions and measured responses to posterior lobe extract. They concluded that the changes noted could be directly attributed most clearly to alterations of $CO_3^=$ ion rather than to acidity, HCO_3^- or CO_2. They did not exempt direct influences of altered pH, etc., but felt that these were of secondary importance. Their tabulated data are shown in Table 4 and reveal that increased $CO_3^=$ is regularly correlated with diminished responsiveness, whereas decreased $CO_3^=$ is associated with increased responses.

Table 4. *Effects of varying hydronium, bicarbonate, and carbonate ions and CO_2 tension on responses of isolated guinea-pig uteri to posterior pituitary extract* (after VAN DYKE and HASTINGS, 1928)

pH	HCO_3^-	CO_2 Tension	$CO_3^=$	Response
Increased	Unchanged	Decreased	Increased	Decreased
Increased	Increased	Unchanged	Increased	Decreased
Unchanged	Increased	Increased	Increased	Decreased
Increased	Decreased	Decreased	Unchanged	Unchanged
Decreased	Increased	Increased	Unchanged	Unchanged
Decreased	Unchanged	Increased	Decreased	Increased
Decreased	Decreased	Unchanged	Decreased	Increased
Unchanged	Decreased	Decreased	Decreased	Increased

This subject has been studied in detail by many others. For example, HALPERN *et al.* (1958) drew conclusions similar to those of VAN DYKE and HASTINGS, although they were apparently unaware of the earlier study. BENTLEY and DICKER (1955) studied the effects of altered pH on diestrous rat uteri immersed in the poorly buffered solution described by DE JALON, BAJO-BAYO and DE JALON (1945) (see Table 1 and previous discussion concerning electrolyte solutions). Like VAN DYKE and HASTINGS (1928) they found increased responses after the uteri were subjected to lowered pH caused by addition of dilute acetic acid solution. Although they excluded acetate as the cause and attributed the alteration to an increase in hydronium ion concentration *per se*, they did not control the concentrations of carbonate, etc., as VAN DYKE and HASTINGS did. BENTLEY and DICKER's findings have practical value, for they revealed that the 0.25% acetic acid solvent for neurohypophysial extracts must be diluted 100 or more times to avoid sensitizing the uterus. The sensitization lasts for about $^1/_2$ h even from transient exposure to the mildly acidic solution. Their study certainly serves to emphasize the importance of using a well buffered solution, such as the one of VAN DYKE and HASTINGS.

G. Influence of Peptide Structure on Oxytocic Potency

There is a spate of information concerning the potencies of various neurohypophysial hormones and analogues on the isolated rat uterus and less information concerning other uterine assay systems. Despite this wealth of information, a good working hypothesis to explain structure-activity relationships in detail has, unfortunately, yet to be tendered. Because of this and the fact that such disparate methods have been used to assay the oxytocic potencies of these peptides, a complete tabulation is unwarranted here. SAWYER (1961) has enumerated the oxytocic potencies of 41 of the neurohypophysial hormones and analogues, and BERDE and BOISSONNAS (1966) have tabulated the oxytocic potencies of numerous additional analogues. They have discussed at length the specific changes in potency which occur with modification of structure. In separate chapters of this text BOISSONNAS and GUTTMANN have discussed the chemistry of the neurohypophysial hormones and analogues, and BERDE and BOISSONNAS have elaborated in great detail many aspects of their pharmacology and structure-activity relationships.

Structural alterations may be analyzed in terms of 1. modification of one or more specific amino acids, 2. substitutions of one or more amino acids, 3. deletions of amino acids, 4. deletions of amide or amino groups, 5. additions to amino groups, 6. disruption of the disulfide bond, 7. substitutions of D for L-amino acids, 8. increase or decrease of the size of the ring or the side chain, and 9. other miscellaneous changes. The analogues which have been prepared so far have been synthesized for the specific purpose of delineating what parts of the molecule are responsible for particular activities. Hopefully, the day will come that such studies will allow us to describe and identify how the molecule acts upon its receptor.

For oxytocic activity, the following statements seem justified. Addition of organic radicals, including amino acids, to the N-terminal extremity of oxytocin has always resulted in a marked, albeit variable, diminution in oxytocic potency. Some of these compounds have antagonistic activity.

Deamination of oxytocin produces De-Amino^1-oxytocin, which has greater oxytocic potency than the parent hormone. Considerably more will be said in in other sections concerning this interesting compound.

Disruption of the disulfide bond results in total loss of activity, but replacement of one sulfur atom in De-Amino^1-oxytocin with methylene, retaining the ring structure, results in a compound with persistent, but decreased, activity.

Shortening the lateral peptide chain by totally eliminating it or removing only one of the three amino acids in it results in marked, but not total loss, of potency. Interestingly, deletion of one, two or all three amino acids of the side chain results in very little difference in the percentage decrease of potency. Hence, the ring structure *per se* has slight intrinsic oxytocic activity, but for marked activity, the side chain must probably be of fixed length, corresponding to the one in oxytocin.

Shortening or lengthening the size of the ring invariably markedly diminishes oxytocic potency and may produce compounds with antagonistic properties.

Substitutions of amino acids in various positions of the oxytocin molecule result in variable changes in potency. Rarely, potency is unaffected or is increased; generally, it is diminished. In our present state of knowledge the change in rat oxytocic potency is unpredictable. The only known amino acid substituted analogue with potency equal or greater than oxytocin is Cit^8-oxytocin. For the cat uterus *in situ*, Ile^8-oxytocin is more potent than oxytocin. BERDE and BOISSONNAS (1966, and this text) have elaborated in more detail on many of these structure-activity relationships, and they have analyzed the results of substitutions at many of the nine positions of oxytocin.

D-oxytocin, the enantiomer of oxytocin, has been synthesized by FLOURET and DU VIGNEAUD (1965). As one might expect, this compound is devoid of oxytocic or antagonistic activity for the rat uterus.

1. Magnesium Ratios

A pharmacological phenomenon previously mentioned, the potentiation by magnesium of the oxytocic potencies of various neurohypophysial peptides, has received considerable attention. Indeed, use of the quantitative change in potency, expressed as a ratio of potency with 0.5 mM Mg^{++} against potency without magnesium, has become one of the principle tools for investigations of natural oxytocin-like peptides.

This ratio, $\frac{\text{Potency with 0.5 mM Mg}^{++}}{\text{Potency with 0.0 mM Mg}^{++}}$, known as the $R_{Mg^{++}}$, has been determined for many of the known natural neurohypophysial principles and some analogues. A list of some $R_{Mg^{++}}$'s is presented in Table 5. It is immediately apparent that oxytocin and De-Amino¹-oxytocin are the only two substances tested whose $R_{Mg^{++}}$'s are equal to or less than unity. Values of $R_{Mg^{++}}$ will vary slightly,

Table 5. *$R_{Mg^{++}}$ for some neurohypophysial hormones and analogues. Results for isolated estrous or estrogen treated rat uteri suspended in van Dyke-Hastings solution (see table 1), unless otherwise noted*

Peptide	$R_{Mg^{++}}$	References and Remarks
oxytocin	0.97	Diethylstilbestrol Treated (MUNSICK and JERONIMUS, 1965)
	0.86	Metestrous Uteri (MUNSICK and JERONIMUS, 1965)
Ile⁸-oxytocin	1.3	MUNSICK (1966)
	1.1	BENTLEY (1965)
Arg⁸-oxytocin	2.0	Diethylstilbestrol Treated (MUNSICK and JERONIMUS, 1965)
	1.2	Metestrous Uteri (MUNSICK and JERONIMUS, 1965)
	1.9	BENTLEY (1965)
Cit⁸-oxytocin	1.5	VAN DYKE, SAWYER, and OVERWEG (1963)
Ala⁸-oxytocin	2.2	SAWYER (personal communication)
Lys⁸-oxytocin	1.9	SAWYER (personal communication)
Ser⁴-Ile⁸-oxytocin	2.9	FOLLETT and HELLER (1964)
	2.8	SAWYER and VAN DYKE (1963)
Ser⁴-oxytocin	3.1	SAWYER (personal communication)
Decarboxamido⁴-oxytocin	3.0	SAWYER (personal communication)
Val-³-oxytocin	3.6	Estrus Status unknown (MUNSICK, 1960)
	5.7	BENTLEY (1965)
Phe²-oxytocin	2.9	Estrus status unknown (MUNSICK, 1960)
Phe³-oxytocin	1.4	Estrus status unknown (MUNSICK, 1960)
De-Amino¹-oxytocin	0.88	Diethylstilbestrol treated (MUNSICK and JERONIMUS, 1965)
	1.0	Metestrous uteri (MUNSICK and JERONIMUS, 1965)
Arg⁸-vasopressin	2.3	Diethylstilbestrol (MUNSICK and JERONIMUS, 1965)
	2.2	Metestrous uteri (MUNSICK and JERONIMUS, 1965)
Lys⁸-vasopressin	2.6	Estrus status unknown (MUNSICK, 1960)
Cit⁸-vasopressin	3.4	VAN DYKE, SAWYER, and OVERWEG (1963)

depending upon the standard used in the assays. If the standard is oxytocin, then oxytocin will, of course, have an $R_{Mg^{++}}$ of 1.0. However, if the standard is whole posterior lobe extract, e.g. International or U.S.P. Posterior Pituitary Reference Standard, the situation changes. Because there is Arg⁸-vasopressin in the International or U.S.P. Standards, and because vasopressin is potentiated considerably more than oxytocin by Mg^{++}, these standards are more potent, relative to oxytocin, in the 0.5 mM Mg^{++} solution. Therefore, the least potentiated peptides, oxytocin and De-Amino¹-oxytocin, have $R_{Mg^{++}}$'s of less than unity and other analogues have comparably lower $R_{Mg^{++}}$'s than when oxytocin is used for standard. This may seem to be a point of little consequence; nevertheless, it is extremely important in instances where slight, statistical differences in potency ratios are used to differentiate one natural principle from another or to exclude the presence of a particular principle.

2. Sex Steroids and Endocrine Status

Although it has been known for many years that the endocrine status of animals can influence the relative potencies of oxytocin and vasopressin, very little quantitative information has been available until recently. In nonpregnant women, it has long been held that vasopressin has approximately equal or greater oxytocic potency than oxytocin. (see GARDINER and BRADBURY, 1940, for post-partum uteri; McLELLAN, 1940, and MOIR, 1944, for nonpregnant uterus). Opinions concerning the relative effects of oxytocin, vasopressin and other peptides on gravid human uteri have differed significantly. Some of these differences are explained in detail by CALDEYRO-BARCIA and SERENO (1961). Although there are still some dissenting opinions, the views of CALDEYRO-BARCIA and of EMBREY (1959) are now generally accepted. It appears that human uteri become rapidly more sensitive to oxytocin from the 10th to about the 20th week of gestation. After this, increase of sensitivity does continue until near term, but to a much lessened extent. Controversial aspects of these statements are discussed in detail by CALDEYRO-BARCIA and SERENO (1961), and by CALDEYRO-BARCIA and CSAPO (in: MARSHALL, 1963b, pp. 29—70). EMBREY (1959) has contributed findings not considerably different from Caldeyro's group concerning human gestational changes in sensitivity to oxytocin. He has shown, in addition, that sensitivity to Arg^8-vasopressin varies little from early pregnancy throughout gestation and into the early puerperium. CIBILS, POSEIRO, and NORIEGA-GUERRA (1961) have infused Arg^8-vasopressin at rates up to 16 mU/min without eliciting a significant change in uterine activity in pregnant women near term. At a rate of 64 mU/min activity was increased somewhat, but tonus was also markedly affected. It may be that the vasoactive properties of vasopressin influence its action *in situ*.

Although most studies of the effects of neurohypophysial hormones on the human uterus have been conducted on pregnant subjects, considerable information has been acquired concerning their effects on human uteri during the menstrual cycle. SAHAKO (1925, 1926) first showed that uteri were insensitive to posterior lobe extracts if active corpora lutea were present. He found that sensitivity returned very late in pregnancy. Early investigators, such as KNAUS (1927, 1928) and ROBSON (1933), extended these observations considerably. More recently, investigators such as MARSHALL (1962), SCHOFIELD (1957), CSAPO (1961) and CALDEYRO-BARCIA and SERENO (1961) have added more knowledge to the earlier studies and have modified some of the conclusions derived from them.

KNAUS (1927, 1928, 1930, 1933, 1934), reasoned that the human uterus might respond in a manner similar to rabbits, and administered posterior pituitary extract to women throughout the menstrual cycle. He found that oxytocic responses disappeared in the luteal phase, usually by about day 19 of a 28 day cycle. He correctly deduced that ovulation usually had occurred in midcycle. KNAUS' results were confirmed to a considerable extent by WITTENBECK (1930), but SCHULTZE (1931), and later others, found that the uterine response was greatest in the luteal phase. Recently, FUCHS (in: MARSHALL, 1963b, p. 70) has likewise failed to find receptivity of isolated human uterine strips to *oxytocin* in the follicular phase, but has found them slightly sensitive in the luteal phase. BYGDEMAN and ELIASSON (1963) have shown that isolated human myometrial strips are insensitive to oxytocin at midcycle, but that they are extremely sensitive to vasopressin. These findings are in agreement with those of MOIR (1944). DAHLE (1950) has reviewed and studied the above subject in detail and has also concluded that nonpregnant human myometrium has greater sensitivity to vasopressin than to oxytocin.

GARDINER and BRADBURY (1940) studied women postpartum and found that Pitocin and Pitressin had approximately equivalent oxytocic potencies in the sixth to ninth days of the puerperium. More recent studies by EMBREY (1959) on uteri throughout pregnancy and in the puerperium have revealed equal sensitivity to oxytocin and vasopressin in early pregnancy, followed by rather constant, fixed sensitivity to vasopressin throughout the remainder of pregnancy and in the puerperium. The sensitivity to oxytocin, on the other hand, progressively increased throughout pregnancy, becoming maximal during labor, and diminished slightly postpartum. Postpartum sensitivity was still much greater for oxytocin than vasopressin, however.

EMBREY (1959) and CALDEYRO-BARCIA and SERENO (1961) have extensively reviewed the often confusing, conflicting findings concerning the responses of human uteri to neurohypophysial hormones at various times in pregnancy, in the puerperium and during the menstrual cycle. Many of the conflicting issues can probably be attributed to manifold factors such as differences in recording techniques, comparing *in vitro* and *in situ* experiments, failing to take the hormonal status of the subject into account, using impure hormone preparations, failing to realize that commercial vasopressin preparations, such as Pitressin, may contain Arg^8, Lys^8 or both vasopressins, etc. In this reviewer's opinion it appears safe to state that during the menstrual cycle uteri are minimally if at all sensitive to oxytocin. Vasopressin — the relative potency of Arg^8 *versus* Lys^8-vasopressin is an open question — does stimulate such uteri, especially during the luteal phase. In pregnancy and the puerperium sensitivity to vasopressin probably changes very little, but the pregnant uterus early acquires greater sensitivity to oxytocin, which increases less rapidly after the 20th week until labor ensues. In the puerperium, oxytocin sensitivity decreases rapidly and becomes equivalent to vasopressin after several days. These conclusions apply for the human uterine fundus. However, they probably do not apply for the muscular tissue of the uterine isthmus or for the cervix uteri. Studies of the cervix *in situ* have revealed that it contracts in response to vasopressin, but that responses are variable to oxytocin (SCHILD, FITZPATRICK, and NIXON, 1951; BAINBRIDGE *et al.*, 1956). Isolated strips of term lower uterine segment muscle were found by RUSSELL (1943) to be more sensitive to Pitressin than Pitocin, and BACHINSKI and ALLMARK (1947) found that the same tissue responded equally well to either fraction. These points are important, for they emphasize that different areas of the uterus may respond in different ways and may have different pharmacologic sensitivites to the neurohypophysial hormones. Hence, using strips of term uterus taken at the time of Cesarean Section, the location of the excised tissue should be carefully ascertained. Because modern cesarean sections are usually performed through the lower uterine segment or cervix and it is easy to obtain tissue from the incised border, many tissues said to be uterus may actually be cervical rather than fundal. Obviously, this important area of investigation still provides fertile ground for more extensive, refined experiments.

Under conditions better controlled than those which prevail in pregnant women, some interesting quantitative data have been published showing that estrogens can not only enhance the size of uterine responses, but can also alter the relative potencies of some neurohypophysial hormones and analogues. CHAN, O'CONNELL, and POMEROY (1963) found that oxytocin is more potent in estrous and metestrous than diestrous and proestrous rats. These differences were not significant, however. $De\text{-}Amino^1$-oxytocin is most potent in metestrous rats, and potency decreases going from diestrus to proestrus and estrus where sensitivities are essentially identical. Their findings are shown in Table 6.

MUNSICK and JERONIMUS (1965) studied the effects of estrogen and magnesium on the potencies of oxytocin, $De\text{-}Amino^1$-oxytocin, Arg^8-vasopressin and Arg^8-oxytocin. Some of their results are shown in Table 7. It is apparent that estrogen, in this case diethylstilbestrol, can materially alter the potencies of some of these peptides on the rat uterus. As previously mentioned, the $R_{Mg^{++}}$ is also affected, as was shown in Table 5.

Unfortunately, a thorough study of the effects of varying Ca^{++} or progesterone on neurohypophysial hormone potency has not yet been reported. We (MUNSICK and JERONIMUS, unpublished) attempted to study the inter-relationships of Ca^{++} and estrogen on the potencies of the peptides shown in Table 7, but were unsuccessful because of the difficulties of performing classical Holton-type assays in bath

Table 6. *Potencies (USP U/Mg) of oxytocin and De-Amino¹-oxytocin on isolated rat uteri suspended in van Dyke-Hastings solution (see Table 1) without Mg^{++}, showing effect of estrous cycle.* All assays against USP Posterior Pituitary Reference Standard. (Retabulation of results of CHAN, O'CONNELL and POMEROY, 1963)

Peptide	Potency			
	Diestrus	Proestrus	Estrus	Metestrus
oxytocin	497 ± 14	483 ± 13	546 ± 18	533 ± 28
De-Amino¹-oxytocin	771 ± 36	564 ± 17	551 ± 17	899 ± 24

Table 7. *Comparison of potencies of 4 peptides, with and without Mg^{++}, showing effect of Diethylstilbestrol versus metestrus* (MUNSICK and JERONIMUS, 1965)

Peptide	0 Mg^{++}		0.5 mM Mg^{++}		
	R_{des}[1]	p	R_{des}[1]	p	
oxytocin	0.874 ± 0.010	<0.01	0.980 ± 0.008	>0.01	<0.02
De-Amino¹-oxytocin	0.893 ± 0.021	<0.01	0.781 ± 0.012	<0.01	
Arg⁸-oxytocin	0.925 ± 0.026	<0.01	1.49 ± 0.06	<0.01	
Arg⁸-vasopressin	1.00 ± 0.05	>0.5	1.06 ± 0.05	>0.1	<0.5

[1] R_{des} equals $\frac{\text{Potency, Diethylstilbestrol Treated}}{\text{Potency, Metestrus}} \pm \text{S.E.}$

p = Probability of difference of ratio from 1.0.

solutions with Ca^{++} concentrations much greater or lower than those ordinarily utilized. KREJČÍ *et al.* (1964) have stated: "The effect of calcium on the one hand and of the hormonal state of the myometrium on the other on the behavior of some of our analogues could have a common denominator; the membrane potential comes to mind because this is known to be influenced both by estrogen and by calcium."

H. Correlation Between Bioassays in Animals and in Pregnant Women

For oxytocic assays to have any meaning as they relate to the human uterus and to the clinical use of oxytocic preparations, it is obvious that the best result should agree with results obtained from human uteri *in situ*. Recent evidence has revealed that such agreement does not always exist. The manner by which the human response is measured is, of course, just as important as the method for the biological assays in animals. Thus, one could use as his standard of response in the pregnant human subject the ability of a substance to cause a certain number of contractions per minute, a certain average amplitude of contractions, a certain increase in tonus, the product of the average amplitude and frequency ("Montivedeo units," see CALDEYRO-BARCIA and SERENO, 1961), the threshold dose which causes any of the above effects, the success of induction of labor, etc. Likewise, should the assay on the human subject be conducted before term, at term, in labor or postpartum? No completely specific or satisfactory answer can be tendered for these questions. Nevertheless, the subject has desperately needed study and several recent reports have given tentative answers and relatively satisfactory methods for assaying in gravid or postpartal women. These various assay methods have recently been reviewed in detail by BERDE and SAAMELI (1966).

Assays using balloons or intra-amniotic catheters for measurements in gravid women have the disadvantages of necessitating some slight risk to the gravida and even more danger to the fetus and mother should the administered oxytocic agent cause contracture to occur. Hence, both EMBREY (1965) and SAAMELI (1960, 1964) have utilized external tokographic methods on postpartal uteri. This assay has been modified after the techniques advocated by MYERSCOUGH and SCHILD (1955, 1958). In this assay, the duration of elevated tonus is the measured response and comparisons are made between an unknown and oxytocin. EMBREY (1965) has shown that for De-Amino^1-oxytocin, at least, results obtained in this manner agree closely with those obtained in women before and during labor.

Accepting this assay method as one which gives results typifying potency in term pregnant women, what then, does a comparison with oxytocic potencies determined in other ways reveal? SAAMELI (1964) has reported the data shown in Table 8. It should be noted that the potency of oxytocin is identical in all three oxytocic assays because it was used as the Standard. Use of whole extract, contraindicated in the *in situ* assays because vasopressin may induce severe side effects, might have revealed differing values for oxytocin. Perusal of Table 8

Table 8. *Activities (U/Mg ± S.E.) of several peptides in assays commonly used for oxytocin and on the human uterus postpartum.*
Italic values are closest to the value for the assay on human uterus *in situ* (after SAAMELI, 1964)

Peptide	Rat Uterus *in Vitro*	Avian Depressor	Rabbit Milk ejection	Cat Uterus *in Situ*	Human Uterus *in Situ*
oxytocin	450	450	450	450	450
Val^3-oxytocin	59 ± 8	58 ± 4	207 ± 14	*226 ± 17*	277 ± 65
Ile^8-oxytocin	289 ± 21	498 ± 37	*328 ± 21*	563 ± 74	365 ± 70
Asp^4-oxytocin	*108 ± 29*	202 ± 12	300 ± 128	335 ± 75	150 ± 40
De-Amino^1-oxytocin	360 ± 55	710 ± 60	440 ± 45	*900 ± 130*	1030 ± 300
Ser^4-Ile^8-oxytocin	150 ± 12	*320 ± 15*	300 ± 15	250 ± 40	335 ± 95

immediately reveals that neither the rat uterus *in vitro* nor the cat uterus *in situ* assay method provides results identical to those for the human uterus *in situ*. If the differences were minor there could be few objections to using the animal data for generalizations concerning potencies in human beings. The differences are striking at times, however, and emphasize the fact that we still have no oxytocic assay using experimental animals which will accurately reflect the activity of neurohypophysial hormones and analogues on the human uterus.

The ultrapotent oxytocic analogue, De-Amino^1-oxytocin, is more potent than oxytocin not only in some of the assays in experimental animals, but also in pregnant and postpartal women. GOLUBOW, CHAN, and DU VIGNEAUD (1963) and GOLUBOW and DU VIGNEAUD (1963) have shown that De-Amino^1-oxytocin, unlike oxytocin, is resistant to inactivation by pregnancy serum oxytocinase and Leu-aminopeptidase. This finding, of course, has lead to speculation of whether or not the oxytocinase resistance of De-Amino^1-oxytocin accounts for its high potency in pregnant women. SAAMELI (1964) has considered this question. In view of the high potency of De-Amino^1-oxytocin on the cat uterus *in situ* and on the fowl blood pressure (neither the cat nor the chicken has oxytocinase) he has justifiably challenged the necessity of proposing such an explanation.

There may be a place for using De-Amino[1]-oxytocin in clinical obstetric practice. Its greater human oxytocic potency certainly does not represent enough of an advantage over oxytocin to warrant its use, for the oxytocic potency of oxytocin is inherently so great that undesirable pharmacologic side effects are almost unheard of, at least when it is used as a dilute infusion. However, at times oxytocin is ineffectual in stimulating abnormal labors or in inducing labors. Provided that the dysfunctional labor is not already hypertonic, when stimulation may be contraindicated, and that there is an indication for an oxytocic drug, then there is need for an agent other than oxytocin which would be effective. BABUNA and YENEN (1966) have shown that serum oxytocinase was elevated in 11/12 women with "primary uterine inertia." Is it possible that in cases such as these De-Amino[1]-oxytocin would be effective where oxytocin sometimes is not? An answer to this question cannot be given as yet. Many more studies. which exactly define the type of dysfunctional labor, confirm the elevation of serum oxytocinase, show minimal or no response to oxytocin and reveal a "normal" response to De-Amino[1]-oxytocin will be required before conclusions can be drawn. Nevertheless, the possibilities are intriguing.

One aspect of structure-activity relationship which has not been treated in this text concerns the analogues which inhibit the oxytocic response to oxytocin and other oxytocic peptides. This field has obvious pharmacologic and possible clinical importance and is discussed in a separate chapter by RUDINGER and KREJČÍ.

III. Non-mammalian Uterine Responses

In another part of this text, MOREL and JARD have considered the effects of neurohypophysial hormones on non-mammalian vertebrates; however, some attention should be directed to uterine responses of animals other than mammals, even though studies of this subject are few.

A. Avian Oviduct

More is known of the responses of hen (*Gallus domesticus*) uteri to neurohypophysial hormones and analogues than of other non-mammalian species. RIDDLE (1921) first showed that Pituitrin could cause premature oviposition in hens. MORASH and GIBBS (1929) and BURROWS and FRAPS (1942) found that the pressor fraction was a more potent oxytocic agent than the mammalian oxytocic fraction. McKENNEY, ESSEX, and MANN (1932) found that the uterine (shell gland) portion of the hen oviduct was far more responsive than the infundibulum or magnum, and SYKES (1955) found that the vaginal portion was quite insensitive.

In order to study the active neurohypophysial principles in chicken posterior pituitaries, we (MUNSICK, SAWYER, and VAN DYKE, 1960; MUNSICK, 1962, 1964) developed an *in vitro* hen oxytocic assay. Several unexpected findings were elicited. Hen uteri have greatest spontaneous activity at low temperatures (30 °C lowest tested) and become progressively less active as the temperature is raised. Activity ceases at about 48—50 °C without causing tissue death. Responsiveness to neurohypophysial peptides is greatest at low and least at high temperatures. Ca^{++} concentration in the van Dyke-Hastings solution with 0.5 mM Mg^{++} was 0.15 mM — higher concentrations were attended by so much spontaneous activity that assays were impossible. The assay is conducted in a manner similar to HOLTON's (1948).

Hen oxytocic potencies were obtained for several hormones and analogues provided to us by Professor DU VIGNEAUD. In studying the structure-activity relationships of several hormones and analogues we hypothesized that Arg^8 and

Ile^3 were important for optimal hen oxytocic activity. An analogue, Arg^8-oxytocin or "arginine vasotocin" (Katsoyannis and du Vigneaud, 1958), with these amino acid moieties was made available to us by Professor du Vigneaud and it proved indeed to have extremely high hen oxytocic activity. As explained by Sawyer in another chapter, this finding contributed heavily to the tentative identification of Arg^8-oxytocin in chicken posterior lobes. Recently, Munsick (1965b) has shown that De-$Amino^1$-oxytocin, more potent than oxytocin in many assay systems, has only about 25% of the activity of oxytocin on a weight basis, when the two are compared for hen oxytocic potency. The striking differences between rat and hen oxytocic potencies of several peptides are shown in Table 9.

Table 9. *Ratios of isolated rat/hen oxytocic potencies for some neurohypophysial hormones and analogues. Rat oxytocic potencies determined in van Dyke-Hastings solution (see table 1) without magnesium*

Peptide	Ratio	References
oxytocin	9.5	Munsick (1965b)
Arg^8-oxytocin	0.058	Munsick, Sawyer, and van Dyke (1960)
De-$Amino^1$-oxytocin . . .	51.	Munsick (1965b)
Ile^8-oxytocin	280.	Munsick (1966)
Arg^8-vasopressin	0.038	Munsick, Sawyer, and van Dyke (1960)
Lys^8-vasopressin	0.33	Munsick, Sawyer, and van Dyke (1960)

Although the hen oxytocic assay has great utility for studying Arg^8-oxytocin in various extracts and fractions (Munsick, Sawyer and van Dyke, 1960; Munsick, 1964, 1966) it lacks precision and is somewhat capricious. Therefore, it is not recommended as a "standard" method for assaying Arg^8-vasopressin or Arg^8-oxytocin.

B. Other Non-mammalian Oviducal Responses

Responses of turtle *(Chrysemys picta)* oviduct were also studied by Munsick, Sawyer, and van Dyke (1960). They found that this preparation, like the hen uterus, was moderately sensitive to Arg^8-vasopressin, far less sensitive to oxytocin and very sensitive to Arg^8-oxytocin. Relatively little has been published on the responses of other bird and reptilian oviducts to the neurohypophysial hormones and analogues. We (Munsick, Sawyer, and van Dyke, unpublished data) did observe scarcely discernible contractions from an amphibian *(Rana catesbiana)* oviduct in response to Arg^8-oxytocin, but the contractions were so feeble that their significance is dubious. No response was elicited from U.S.P. Standard or Arg^8-oxytocin when tested on the isolated, gravid oviduct of the Black Molly, *(Mollienisia sphenops)* (Munsick, unpublished observation), a tropical teleost fish. Using mammalian and elasmobranch neurohypophysial extracts, Perks (personal communication) could not elicit contractions from the oviducts of an elasmobranch fish. In summary, some neurohypophysial hormones and analogues are known to have potent oxytocic effects on some birds and reptiles, but there is presently no evidence that they significantly stimulate the oviducts of amphibians or fishes.

IV. Effects on Other Nonvascular Smooth Muscle

A. Uterine Adnexa

Hendricks and Moawad (1965) have reported studies on the contractility of human round ligaments in situ. They inserted open ended polyethylene catheters through needles into areas of the myometrium and the round ligaments at the time of cesarean section or laparotomy for postpartal sterilization and found that the round ligaments demonstrated rhythmic contractile activity. The contractions approximately resembled those of the uterus, but this was not always the case. Although the uteri responded predictably to intravenously administered oxytocin, the round ligament response was variable.

The response of human fallopian tubes to oxytocin has been studied by RORIE and NEWTON (1965). Using different portions of the tubes of puerperal (30—50 h postpartum) and nonpregnant, nonpuerperal women, they found that oxytocin caused a definite increase in the amplitude and frequency of contractions of the puerperal tubes, which were suspended in a 12 ml chamber in "Locke-Ringer" solution. Oxytocin caused these changes in a concentration of 8 μU/ml. The responses of nonpuerperal tubes were rather inconsistent. Unfortunately, the authors did not analyze differences in sensitivity between various areas of the tube or in various times of the menstrual cycle. The effect of vasopressin was not tested, the source and purity of the oxytocin were not stated and the composition of the bath solution was not mentioned. This extreme sensitivity to oxytocin of human fallopian tubes is extremely interesting. Hopefully, more details and information will soon be forthcoming.

B. Urinary Tract

Few studies have been performed on the smooth muscle structures of the urinary tract. The statements which follow have been taken from the texts of VAN DYKE (1936) and SOLLMAN (1957); consulting these texts will provide detailed references. The bladder is said to contract and to become sensitized to pelvic but not hypogastric nerve stimulation in response to posterior pituitary extract. According to SOLLMAN (1957, p. 520), excised ureter responds to dilute but not to concentrated extracts. VAN DYKE (1936, p. 347) reports that GRUBER found isolated pig ureters responded to posterior lobe extracts with an increase in the amplitude and rate of contractions. CALDEYRO-BARCIA (in: MARSHALL, 1936b, p. 63) has stated that large intravenous doses of oxytocin caused no alteration in the ureteral contractions of pregnant women, despite induction of marked uterine responses.

C. Gastrointestinal Tract

Both VAN DYKE and SOLLMAN state that previous investigators have found little or no contractile effect of posterior pituitary extract on the stomach of man or dogs. Vary large doses can cause hemorrhagic necrosis of the gastric wall, ulceration and bleeding (VAN DYKE, 1936, pp. 348—349).

Effects of posterior lobe hormones on the small intestine have been reviewed by VAN DYKE (1936, pp. 345—347), SOLLMAN (1957, p. 520), and, recently, by LEVY (1963). LEVY has shown that both oxytocin and vasopressin (Pitressin) have an inhibitory effect on the contractility of the isolated ileum of guinea-pigs and rabbits and of canine small intestine *in situ*. The results on the dog intestine probably can not be challenged, but those on the *in vitro* preparations can. LEVY states that oxytocin concentrations of 0.3 U/ml in the bath caused definite inhibition of spontaneous and histamine, acetylcholine and barium chloride induced contractions of rabbit ileum. The amount of Syntocinon, the oxytocin preparation he used, provides a bath concentration of 350 μg/ml of both chlorobutanol and ethanol. If these smooth muscles are inhibited by these agents in a manner similar to human uterine muscle, then the results of BUENO-MONTANO *et al.* (1966), would raise the serious question of whether or not inhibition was caused, at least in part, by the drug preservatives. Unfortunately, LEVY did not use a solvent control to test this possibility.

HIATT, GOODMAN, and BIRCHER (1966) have studied the effects of drugs on isolated segments of canine ilium (Thiry-Vella loops). In doses of 700 mU/Kg, neither Pitressin nor Pituitrin caused any contractile response when injected either intravenously or intraluminally.

In a long review article on the effects of drugs on intestinal motility, INGELFINGER (1943) postulated that in man posterior pituitary extract causes increased small and large bowel propulsive waves with decreased tone. Hence, he argued, the effect on intestinal propulsive activity is positive. The well known clinical fact that vasopressin or whole extract causes rapid defecation, mobilization of gas and intestinal cramps certainly adds weight to the above argument. Another study and review of this subject was provided by PUESTOW (1942). Absence of any subjective or objective effects on the bowel from large doses of oxytocin adds further evidence that it is vasopressin which is the active component of posterior pituitary extract. There may be species differences in responses of the large bowel to oxytocin and vasopressin. Many of the older reports, reviewed by VAN DYKE (1936, pp. 345—347) and SOLLMAN (1957, p. 520) derived conclusions which were not in agreement. However, some of the discrepancies, as pointed out by SOLLMAN (1957, p. 520), may have been caused by species differences, techniques of recording, diet, the level of the segment utilized, etc.

An extremely interesting study of the effect of neurohypophysial hormones on guinea-pig intestine has recently been published by BOTTING (1965). He used a segment of the intestine which forms the junction of the ileum, caecum and colon and found that this segment was extremely sensitive to vasopressin. Other parts of the intestine, the same part from female guinea-pigs or from males weighing greater than 400 g all were often insensitive. A strip of this portion of the intestine was placed in a physiologic saline solution at 32° C and longitudinal muscle contractions were recorded isotonically. This preparation was found to have threshold values for vasopressin of 0.001—1.0 mU/ml in the bath. In his illustrations, the author was administering doses of 0.5—5.0 mU of vasopressin and obtaining excellent, assayable responses. BOTTING found that pentolinium and hexamethonium

Table 10. *Activities of some neurohypophysial hormones and analogues on guinea-pig proximal colon. Activities compared with Lys⁸-vasopressin, the Reference standard.*
Oxytocin and Ile⁸-oxytocin administered in oxytocic unitage, all others in pressor unitage (after BOTTING, 1965)

Peptide	Activity	Peptide	Activity
oxytocin	0.05	Lys^8-oxytocin	0.5
Ile^8-oxytocin	0.1	Arg^8-vasopressin	1.0
Arg^8-oxytocin	0.5	Phe^2-Lys^8-vasopressin	2.5—3.0

inhibited the vasopressin-induced contractions and hypothesized that the contractile response may be mediated *via* autonomic nerves or nerve endings. The relative potencies of several hormones and analogues are shown in Table 10. Note that the activities are expressed in ratios, compared with Lys^8-vasopressin. They therefore do not depict absolute potency or activity. Unfortunately, the standard errors of the mean potencies and individual assays were not reported by the author.

BERDE, WEIDMANN, and CERLETTI (1961) have shown that isolated rabbit ileum responds quite readily and in a graded manner to Phe^2-Lys^8-vasopressin and Lys^8-vasopressin; furthermore Stürmer (personal communication) states that the vasopressins and some of their synthetic analogues are potent stimulants for *in situ* rabbit colon preparations.

Recently, Bauer, Gmeiner, and Winkler (1966) have studied Lys^8-vasopressin, Phe^2-Lys^8-vasopressin and oxytocin on the intestine of rabbits and cats *in situ*. For rabbits, the vasopressins caused a mild increase in motility when given in large doses. There was no clear-cut effect in cats.

Surprisingly, rabbit and cat intestine responded *in situ* to intravenous infusions of 150—1,000 mU/kg/min of oxytocin. These responses were apparently predominantly from the ileum.

van Dyke (1936, p. 347) and Sollman (1957, p. 520), both reported that posterior pituitary extract has been shown to contract the gall bladder, although there have been discrepant findings which may have been caused by species differences or drug preservatives. Recently, Homsher and Cotzias (1965) found that bile flow in rats was transiently inhibited by 300—600 mU/100 g of Pitressin given intravenously. Further study revealed that this effect was probably partially caused by a direct constrictive effect on the bile ducts.

The author has found no evidence that vasopressin or oxytocin causes constriction of the pancreatic or salivary ducts. It is worthy of note, however, that Perks, Shapiro, and Woodward (1964) have described increased water resorption from the pancreatic fluid after small doses of vasopressin. According to Sollman (1957, p. 520) canine salivary secretion is diminished by posterior pituitary injection.

D. Respiratory Tract

Sollman (1957, p. 520) reviewed early reports and concluded that bronchial muscle is unaffected by posterior pituitary extract. On the other hand, Levy (1963) found that isolated guinea-pig tracheal rings were relaxed by oxytocin and vasopressin. When the tracheal rings were made to contract maximally with histamine or acetylcholine, addition of 100—500 mU of oxytocin caused an immediate relaxation of the smooth muscle. However, a 5 ml bath was used for this large dose of oxytocin. Hence, the bath concentrations of ethanol and chlorobutanol may have been adequate to cause inhibition by themselves (see previous discussion under gastrointestinal tract).

References

Abarbanel, A. R.: The spasmolysant action of magnesium ions on the tetanically contracting human gravid uterus. Amer. J. Obstet. Gynec. **49**, 473 (1945).

Alvarez, H., and R. Caldeyro-Barcia: Contractility of the human uterus recorded by new methods. Surg. Gynec. Obstet. **91**, 1 (1950).

Alver, E. C., C. W. White, J. Weiss, and D. K. Heerdegen: An effect of succinylcholine on the uterus. Amer. J. Obstet. Gynec. **83**, 795 (1962).

Babuna, C., and E. Yenen: Further studies on serum oxytocinase in pathologic pregnancy. Amer. J. Obstet. Gynec. **94**, 868 (1966).

Bachinski, W. M., and M. G. Allmark: On the oxytocic activity of Pitocin and Pitressin on isolated segments of mammalian uteri by a graded response method. J. Amer. Pharm. Ass. **36**, 73 (1947).

Bainbridge, M. N., W. C. W. Nixon, H. O. Schild, and C. N. Smyth: Synthetic Oxytocin. Brit. Med. J. **1**, 1133 (1956).

Bauer, G., R. Gmeiner u. H. Winkler: Über die Wirkung synthetischer Polypeptide auf den Darm in situ. Arch. Int. Pharmacodyn. **159**, 373 (1966).

Beauvillain, A.: Titrage des préparations Post-hypophysaires par leur seuil d'action sur l'uterus isolé de rat adulte. C. R. Soc. Biol. (Paris) **137**, 284 (1943).

Bentley, P., and S. E. Dicker: Effects of transient changes of acidity on the isolated rat's uterus, with reference to the assay of oxytocic activity. Brit. J. Pharmacol. **10**, 424 (1955).

Bentley, P. J.: The effects of N-ethylmaleimide and glutathione on the isolated rat uterus and frog bladder with special reference to the action of oxytocin. J. Endocr. **30**, 103 (1964).

— The potentiating action of magnesium and manganese on the oxytocic effect of some oxytocin analogues. J. Endocr. **32**, 215 (1965).

BERDE, B., and R. A. BOISSONNAS: Synthetic analogues and homologues of the posterior pituitary hormones. In: The pituitary Gland, Ed. by G. W. HARRIS and B. T. DONOVAN, p. 624. London: Butterworths 1966.
—, and A. CERLETTI: Quantitative comparison of substances related to oxytocin: a new test. Acta endocr. (Kbh.) **27**, 314 (1958).
—, and K. SAAMELI: The action of the synthetic polypeptide valyl-oxytocin on the human uterus *in vitro* and *in vivo*. Acta endocr. (Kbh.) **32**, 391 (1959).
— — Evaluation of substances acting on the uterus. In: Methods in drug evaluation, p. 481. Amsterdam: North-Holland Publishing Co. 1966.
—, H. WEIDMANN u. A. CERLETTI: Über phenylalanin²-lysin-vasopressin. Helv. Physiol. Acta **19**, 285 (1961).
BERGER, E., and J. M. MARSHALL: Interactions of oxytocin, potassium and calcium in rat uterus. Amer. J. Physiol. **201**, 931 (1961).
BOHR, D. F.: Electrolytes and smooth muscle contraction. Pharmacol. Rev. **16**, 85 (1964).
BÖSCH, K., u. O. KÄSER: Die Anwendung von oxytocin in der Geburtsleitung. Schweiz. Med. Wschr. **86**, 229 (1956).
BOTTING, J. H.: An isolated preparation with a selective sensitivity to vasopressin. Brit. J. Pharmacol. **24**, 156 (1965).
British Pharmacopoeia, London, Pharmaceutical Press 1948 and 1963.
BUENO-MONTANO, M.: Species variations in contractile response of excised mammalian uterine tissue. Amer. J. Obstet. Gynec. **94**, 1062 (1966).
—, H. S. MCGAUGHEY, C. M. HARBERT, and W. N. THORNTON: Drug preservatives and uterine contractility. Amer. J. Obstet. Gynec. **94**, 1 (1966).
BURN, J. H., and H. H. DALE: On the physiological standardization of extracts of the posterior lobe of the pituitary body. Med. Res. Counc. Spec. Rep. **69**, 1 (1922).
—, D. J. FINNEY, and L. C. GOODWIN: Biological standardization, 2nd Ed. New York: Oxford University Press 1950.
BURROWS, W. H., and R. M. FRAPS: Action of vasopressin and oxytocin in causing premature oviposition by domestic fowl. Endocrinology **30**, 702 (1942).
BYGDEMAN, M., and R. ELIASSON: The effect of various oxytocin analogues on the motility of the human uterus *in vitro*. Med. exp. (Basel) **9**, 31 (1963).
BYROM, F. B., and O. E. PRATT: Oxytocin and renal cortical necrosis. Lancet **1959** I, 753.
CALDEYRO-BARCIA, R., and J. A. SERENO: The Response of the human uterus to oxytocin throughout pregnancy. In: Oxytocin, p. 177, ed. by R. CALDEYRO-BARCIA and H. HELLER. New York: Pergammon Press 1961.
CARSTEN, M. E.: A study of uterine actin. Biochemistry (Wash.) **4**, 1049 (1965).
CHAN, W. Y., M. O'CONNELL, and S. R. POMEROY: Effects of the estrous cycle on the sensitivity of rat uterus to oxytocin and desamino-oxytocin. Endocrinology **72**, 279 (1963).
CIBILS, L. A., J. J. POSEIRO, and L. NORIEGA-GUERRA: Comparison of the effects on the pregnant human uterus of highly purified natural oxytocin, pitocin, synthetic oxytocin (Syntocinon), valyl³-oxytocin and arginine-vasopressin. In: Oxyciton, p. 266 Ed. by R. CALDEYRO-BARCIA and H. HELLER. New York: Pergammon Press 1961.
CLEGG, P. C., P. HOPKINSON, and V. R. PICKLES: Some effects of calcium and magnesium ions on guinea-pig uterine muscle. J. Physiol. (London) **167**, 1 (1963).
CSAPO, A. I.: Progesterone "Block." Amer. J. Anat. **98**, 273 (1956).
— Molecular structure and function of smooth muscle. In: The structure and function of smooth muscle, Vol. I, pp. 232—264. Ed. by G. H. BOURNE. New York: Academic Press 1960.
— The effects of oxytocic substances on the excitability of the uterus. In: Oxytocin, p. 100. Ed. by R. CALDEYRO-BARCIA and H. HELLER. New York: Pergammon Press 1961.
—, and C. R. PINTO-DANTAS: The cyclic activity of the nonpregnant human uterus. A new method for recording intrauterine pressure. Fertil. and Steril. **17**, 34 (1966).
DAHLE, T.: The effect of postpituitary gland extract on the activity of the human uterus. Acta Obstet. Gynecol. Scand. **30**, Suppl. 4 (1950).
DALE, H. H.: On some physiological actions of Ergot. J. Physiol. (London) **34**, 163 (1906).
—, and P. P. LAIDLAW: A method of standardizing pituitary (infundibular) extracts. J. Pharmacol. exp. Ther. **4**, 75 (1912).
DANIEL, E. E.: The interconnection between active transport and contracture in uterine tissues. Canad. J. Physiol. Pharmacol. **42**, 453 (1964).
DYKE, H. B. VAN, and A. B. HASTINGS: The response of smooth muscle in different ionic environments. Amer. J. Physiol. **83**, 563 (1928).
— The physiology and pharmacology of the pituitary body. Chicago: Univ. of Chicago Press 1936.
—, W. H. SAWYER, and N. I. A. OVERWEG: Pharmacologic activities of the 8-Citrulline analogues of oxytocin and vasopressin. Endocrinology **73**, 637 (1963).

EMBREY, M.P.: A criterion of oxytocic activity. J. Obstet. Gynaec. Brit. Cwlth. **66**, 871 (1959).
— The action of desamino-oxytocin on the human pregnant uterus. J. Endocr. **31**, 185 (1965).
EVANS, D.H., H.O. SCHILD, and S. THESLEFF: Effects of drugs on depolarized plain muscle. J. Physiol. (London) **143**, 474 (1958).
FEINSTEIN, M.B.: Inhibition of contraction and calcium exchangeability in rat uterus by local anesthetics. J. Pharmacol. exp. Ther. **152**, 516 (1966).
FITZPATRICK, R.J.: The *in vivo* potentiation by magnesium salts of uterine responses to posterior pituitary extract in the bovine. J. Pharm. Pharmacol. **8**, 403 (1956).
FLOURET, G., and V. DU VIGNEAUD: The synthesis of D-oxytocin, the enantiomer of the posterior pituitary hormone, oxytocin. J. Amer. Chem. Soc. **87**, 3775 (1965).
FOLLETT, B.K., and P.J. BENTLEY: The bioassay of oxytocin. Increased sensitivity of the rat uterus in response to serial injections of stilbestrol. J. Endocr. **29**, 277 (1964).
—, and H. HELLER: The neurohypophysial hormones of lungfishes and amphibians. J. Physiol. (London) **172**, 92 (1964).
FRASER, A.M.: The effect of magnesium on the response of the uterus to posterior pituitary hormones. J. Pharmacol. exp. Ther. **66**, 85 (1939).
FUCHS, A.-R.: Oxytocin and the onset of labour in rabbits. J. Endocr. **30**, 217 (1964).
— The inhibitory effect of ethanol on the release of oxytocin during parturition in the rabbit. J. Endocr. **35**, 125 (1966).
GADDUM, J.H., W.S. PEART, and M. VOGT: The estimation of adrenaline and allied substances in blood. J. Physiol. (London) **108**, 467 (1949).
— The technique of superfusion. Brit. J. Pharmacol. **8**, 321 (1953).
GARCIA DE JALON, M., and P. GARCIA DE JALON: Modifications más sensibles al método de valoración de la Pituitrina en úteru aislado de cobayo. Farmacoterap. Act. **2**, 514 (1945).
GARCIA DE JALON, P.: El use de las sales de magnesio en los ensayos de los extractos de lóbulo posterior de hipófisis. Farmacoterap. Act. **4**, 177 (1947).
—, J. BAYO BAYO, and M. GARCIA DE JALON: Sensible y nuevo método de valoración de adrenalina en útero aislado de rata. Farmacoterap. Act. **2**, 313 (1945).
GARDINER, S., and J.T. BRADBURY: Responses of the human post-partum uterus to posterior pituitary extracts. Amer. J. Obstet. Gynec. **39**, 1 (1940).
GENELL, S.: Die Bedeutung des Magnesiums ions für die Motorik des überlednaden Uterus. Skand. Arch. Physiol. **80**, 124 (1938).
GOLUBOW, J., W.Y. CHAN, and V. DU VIGNEAUD: Effect of human pregnancy serum on avian depressor activities of oxytocin and desamino-oxytocin. Proc. Soc. exp. Biol. (N.Y.) **113**, 113 (1963).
—, and V. DU VIGNEAUD: Comparison of susceptibility of oxytocin and desamino-oxytocin to inactivation by leucine aminopeptidase and a-chymotrypsin. Proc. Soc. exp. Biol. (N.Y.) **112**, 218 (1963).
GOTO, M., and A. CSAPO: The effect of the ovarian steroids on the membrane potential of uterine muscle. J. gen. Physiol. **43**, 455 (1960).
HALPERN, B.N., R. BINAGHI, M. MAYER, and C. BUGNARD: The mechanism of the inhibition by carbonic acid of the smooth muscle contraction produced by histamine and oxytocin. Brit. J. Pharmacol. **14**, 19 (1959).
HAMBURGER, C.: Assay of posterior pituitary extract (oxytocin). II. Influence of the temperrature on the sensitivity of the uterine preparation. Acta pharmacol. (Kbh.) **2**, 212 (1946).
HENDRICKS, C.H.: Amniotic fluid pressure recording. Clin. Obstet. Gynec. **9**, 535 (1966).
— Inherent motility patterns and response characteristics of the nonpregnant human uterus. Amer. J. Obstet. Gynec. (To be published).
—, and A.H. MOAWAD: Round ligament *in vivo* studies in man. J. Obstet. Gynaec. Brit. Cwlth. **72**, 618 (1965).
HIATT, R.B., I. GOODMAN, and R. BIRCHER: Control of motility in Thiry-Vella ileal segments in dogs. Amer. J. Physiol. **210**, 373 (1966).
HOLTON, P.: A modification of the method of Dale and Laidlaw for standardization of posterior pituitary extract. Brit. J. Pharmacol. **3**, 328 (1948).
HOMSHER, E., and G.C. COTZIAS: Antidiuretic hormone and bile flow. Nature (Lond.) **208**, 687 (1965).
HUTCHINSON, H.T., M.M. NICHOLS, C.R. KUHN, and A. VASICKA: Effects of magnesium sulfate on uterine contractility, intrauterine fetus, and infant. Amer. J. Obstet. Gynec. **88**, 747 (1964).
INGELFINGER, F.J.: The modification of intestinal motility by drugs. New Engl. J. Med. **229**, 114 (1943).
JUNG, H.: The effect of oxytocin on the mechanism of uterine excitation. In: Oxytocin, p. 87. Ed. by R. CALDEYRO-BARCIA and H. HELLER. New York: Pergammon Press 1961.
— Zur Physiologie und Klinik der hormonalen Uterusregulation. Fortschr. Geburtsh. Gynäk. **22**, 155 (1965).

KAO, C. Y.: Contents and distributions of potassium, sodium and chloride in smooth muscle. J. Physiol. (Lond.) **201**, 717 (1961).
KATSOYANNIS, P. G., and V. DU VIGNEAUD: Arginine-vasotocin, a synthetic analogue of the posterior pituitary hormones containing the ring of oxytocin and the side chain of vasopressin. J. Biol. Chem. **233**, 1352 (1958).
KNAUS, H.: Experimentelle Untersuchungen zur Physiologie und Pharmakologie der Uterusmusculatur in der Schwangerschaft. Arch. exp. Path. Pharmak. **124**, 152 (1927).
— Experimentelle Untersuchungen zur Physiologie und Pharmakologie der Uterusmusculatur in der Schwangerschaft im Puerperim. Arch. exp. Path. Pharmak. **134**, 225 (1928).
— Zur Physiologie des Corpus Luteum. Arch. Gynäk. **141**, 395 (1930).
— Zur Technik der Registration von Bewegungen der menschlichen Gebärmutter. Zbl. Gynäk. **57**, 2658 (1933).
— Die periodische Fruchtbarkeit und Unfruchtbarkeit des Weibes. Wien: Mandrich 1934.
KOCHMAN, M.: Zur Wertbestimmung der Hypophysenpräparate und anderer Wehemittel. Hoppe-Seylers Z. physiol. Chem. **115**, 305 (1921).
KREJČÍ, I., I. POLACEK, B. KUPKOVA, and J. RUDINGER: Dose-Response analysis of the action of some oxytocin analogues on the isolated uterus: The effect of ions. In: Oxytocin, Vasopressin and Their Structural Analogues, p. 181. Ed. by J. RUDINGER. New York: MACMillan Co. 1964.
KUMAR, D., T. WAGATSUMA, and A. BARNES: Studies on the mechanism of action of ether on human myometrium. Amer. J. Obstet. Gynec. **91**, 709 (1965b).
—, P. ZOURLAS, and A. BARNES: In vitro and in vivo effects of magnesium sulfate on human uterine contractility. Amer. J. Obstet. Gynec. **86**, 1036 (1963).
— — — Potentiating effect of oxytocin on contraction of glycerine extracted psoas muscle fibre induced by adenosine triphosphate. Nature (Lond.) **206**, 1050 (1965a).
LEONARD, S. L., and M. CRANDALL: Hormonal stimulation of phosphorylase activity in the rat uterus *in vitro*. Endocrinology **73**, 807 (1963).
LEVY, B.: The intestinal inhibitory response to oxytocin, vasopressin, and bradykinin. J. Pharmcol. exp. Ther. **140**, 356 (1963).
MCKENNEY, F. D., H. E. ESSEX, and F. C. MANN: The action of certain drugs on the oviduct of the domestic fowl. J. Pharmacol. exp. Ther. **45**, 113 (1932).
MCLELLAN, A.: Response of non-pregnant human uterus to posterior pituitary extract and its fractions oxytocin and vasopressin. Lancet **1940 I**, 919.
MARSHALL, J. M.: Effects of estrogen and progesterone on single uterine muscle fibers in the rat. Amer. J. Physiol. **197**, 935 (1959).
— Regulation of activity in uterine smooth muscle. Physiol. Rev. **42**, 213 (1962).
— Behavior of uterine muscle in Na-deficient solutions; Effects of oxytocin. Amer. J. Physiol. **204**, 732 (1963a).
— (Editor): Initiation of labor. Proc. Interdisciplinary Conf. Initiation of Labor. Publ. Hlth Serv., Publ. No. 1390, U.S. Department of Health, Education and Welfare (1963b).
—, and M. D. MILLER: Effects of metabolic inhibitors in the rat uterus and on its response to oxytocin. Amer. J. Physiol. **206**, 437 (1964).
MARTIN, P. J.: The antagonism of disulphide polypeptides by thiols. Brit. J. Pharmacol. **25**, 418 (1965).
—, and H. O. SCHILD: Pharmacological antagonism of oxytocin and vasopressin by thiol compounds. J. Physiol. (Lond.) **163**, 51P (1962).
MENDES, M. L.: Accão do Palerol sobre a motilidade uterina de anímais grávidos, in vivo. Coimbra Med. **7**, 963 (1960).
MOIR, C.: The effect of posterior lobe pituitary gland fractions on the intact human uterus. J. Obstet. Gynaec. Brit. Cwlth **51**, 181 (1944).
MOIR, J. C.: Expulsive force of the uterus during labor. Lancet **230**, 414 (1936).
MORASH, R., and O. S. GIBBS: The effect of pituitary on the bird. J. Pharmacol. exp. Ther. **37**, 475 (1929).
MUNSICK, R. A.: Effect of magnesium ion on the response of the rat uterus to neurohypophysial hormones and analogues. Endocrinology **66**, 451 (1960).
— The tentative identification of the neurohypophysial principles of the domestic fowl principally by pharmacological methods. Dissertation Abstracts **23**, (1962).
— Neurohypophysial hormones in chickens and turkeys. Endocrinology **75**, 104 (1964).
— The pharmacology and clinical application of various oxytocic drugs. Amer. J. Obstet. Gynec. **93**, 442 (1965a).
— Hen oxytocic activities of Oxytocin and 1-Deamino-oxytocin. Endocrinology **76**, 161 (1965b).
— Chromatographic and pharmacologic characterization of the neurohypophysial hormones of an amphibian and a reptile. Endocrinology **78**, 591 (1966).
—, and S. C. JERONIMUS: Effects of diethylstilbestrol and magnesium on the rat oxytocic potencies of some neurohypophysial hormones and analogues. Endocrinology **76**, 90 (1965).

MUNSICK, R.A., W.H. SAWYER, and H.B. VAN DYKE: Avian neurohypophysial hormones. Pharmacological properties and tentative identification. Endocrinology **66**, 860 (1960).
MYERSCOUGH, P.R., and H.O. SCHILD: Biological assay of oxytocic drugs on the human uterus. Proc. roy. Soc. Med. **48**, 679 (1955).
— — Quantitative assays of oxytocic drugs on the human postpartum uterus. Brit. J. Pharmacol. **13**, 207 (1958).
NEEDHAM, D.M., and J.M. WILLIAMS: Some properties of uterus actomyosin and myofilaments. Biochem. J. **73**, 171 (1959).
PERKS, A.M., H. SCHAPIRO, and E.R. WOODWARD: The influence of antidiuretic hormones on pancreatic exocrine secretion. Acta endocr. (Kbh.) **45**, 340 (1964).
PRITCHARD, J.A.: The use of the magnesium ion in the management of eclamtogenic toxemias. Surg. Gynec. Obstet. **100**, 131 (1955).
PUESTOW, C.B.: Intestinal motility and postoperative distention. Experimental and clinical studies. J. Amer. med. Ass. **120**, 903 (1942).
REYNOLDS, S.R.M.: Physiology of the uterus. Revised 2nd Ed. New York: Hafner Publ. Co. 1965.
RIDDLE, O.: A simple method of obtaining premature eggs from birds. Science **54**, 664 (1921).
ROBSON, J.M.: The reactivity and activity of the rabbit's uterus during pregnancy, parturition and the puerperium. J. Physiol. (Lond.) **78**, 309 (1933).
RORIE, D.K., and M. NEWTON: Response of isolated human fallopian tube to oxytocin. A preliminary report. Fertil. and Steril. **16**, 27 (1965).
RUSSELL, C.S.: The response of isolated muscle strips from the upper and lower segments of the human full-time pregnant uterus to Pitressin and to Pitocin. J. Obstet. Gynaec. Brit. Cwlth **50**, 287 (1943).
SAAMELI, K.: Tokographische Untersuchungen am postpartalen Uterus. Geburtsh. u. Frauenheilk. **30**, 202 (1960).
— Quantitative comparison between oxytocin and four related neurohypophysial peptides on the human uterus in situ. Brit. J. Pharmacol. **23**, 176 (1964).
SAHAKO, N.: Über die Pituitrinwirkung auf den ausgeschnittenen Kaninchenuterus. Folia Jap. Pharmacol. **1**, 352 (1925).
— Über die Pituitrinwirkung auf den Kaninchenuterus in situ. Folia Jap. Pharmacol. **2**, 1 (1926).
SANDBERG, F., A. INGELMAN-SUNDBERG, L. LINDGREN, and G. RYDÉN: In vitro studies of the motility of the human uterus. IV. The effects of oxytocin, methylergometrine, dihydroergotamine and two new oxytocics on the spontaneous motility in different parts of the pregnant and non-pregnant uterus. J. Obstet. Gynaec. Brit. Cwlth **66**, 417 (1959).
SAWYER, W.H.: Neurohypophysial hormones. Pharmacol. Rev. **13**, 225 (1961).
—, and H.B. VAN DYKE: Isolation of the oxytocin-like pituitary principle of a teleost fish *(pollachius virens)* and comparison of its properties with those of synthetic 4-serine, 8-isoleucine oxytocin. Endocrinology **73**, 394 (1963).
SCHILD, H.O.: A method of conducting a biological assay on a preparation giving repeated graded responses illustrated by the estimation of histamine. J. Physiol. (Lond.) **101**, 115 (1942).
—, R.J. FITZPATRICK, and W.C.W. NIXON: Activity of the human cervix and corpus uteri. Their response to drugs in early pregnancy. Lancet **1951 I**, 250.
SCHOFIELD, B.M.: The hormonal control of myometrial function during pregnancy. J. Physiol. (Lond.) **138**, 1 (1957).
— Myometrial activity in the pregnant guinea-pig. J. Endocr. **30**, 347 (1964).
SCHULTZE, G.K.F.: Die Reaction der nichtschwangeren menschlichen Gebärmutter auf Hypophysenhinterlappenenextrakte. Zbl. Gynäk. **55**, 3042 (1931).
SCHWARTZ, I.L., H. RASMUSSEN, M.A. SCHOESSLER, H. SILVER, and T.O.F. FONG: Relation of chemical attachment to physiological action of oxytocin on the isolated uterus. Proc. nat. Acad. Sci. (Wash.) **46**, 1288 (1960).
SOGOLOW, S.R.: An historical review of the use of oxytocin prior to delivery. Obstet. gynec. Surv. **21**, 155 (1966).
SOLLMAN, T.: A manual of pharmacology and its applications to therapeutics and toxicology, 8th Ed. Philadelphia: W.R. Saunders Co. 1957.
STEWART, G.A.: An examination of factors affecting the precision of the assay of the oxytocic hormone in posterior pituitary lobe preparations. J. Pharm. Pharmacol. **1**, 436 (1949).
STYLES, P.R., and T.J. SULLIVAN: Measurement of uterine activity in vitro by integrating muscle tension. Brit. J. Pharmacol. **19**, 129 (1962).
SYKES, A.H.: The effect of adrenaline on oviduct motility and egg production in the fowl. Poult. Sci. **34**, 622 (1955).
TYRODE, M.V.: The mode of action of some purgative salts. Arch. Int. Pharmacodyn. **20**, 205 (1910).

VASICKA, A., and H. KRETCHMER: Effect of conduction and inhalation anesthesia on uterine contractions. Experimental study of the influence of anesthesia on intra-amniotic pressures. Amer. J. Obstet. Gynec. **82**, 600 (1961).
WITTENBECK, F.: Ovulationstermin und Konzeptionsfähigkeit bei der Frau. Arch. Gynäk. **142**, 446 (1930).
WURTMAN, R.J., E.W. CHU, and J. AXELROD: Relation between the oestrous cycle and the binding of catecholamines in the rat uterus. Nature (Lond.) **198**, 547 (1963).

The Milk-Ejection Reflex and the Actions of Oxytocin, Vasopressin and Synthetic Analogues on the Mammary Gland

G. W. BISSET

With 7 Figures

I. Lactation and the Milk-Ejection Reflex

A. Terminology

In discussing the physiology of lactation, the following terminology introduced by FOLLEY and his co-workers (FOLLEY, 1947b, 1949; COWIE, FOLLEY, CROSS, HARRIS, JACOBSOHN, and RICHARDSON, 1951; COWIE, FOLLEY, and RICHARDSON, 1954) will be adopted. This terminology has made an important contribution to our understanding of the subject because it separates two distinct processes — α) milk secretion and β) milk removal.

Lactation

α) *Milk secretion*

(i) Synthesis of milk by the cells of the alveolar epithelium.

(ii) Passage of milk from the cytoplasm of the alveolar epithelial cells into the alveolar lumen.

β) *Milk removal*

(i) Passive withdrawal.

(ii) Milk ejection.

Milk secretion, which consists of (i) the synthesis of milk, and (ii) its passage into the alveolar lumen, is controlled by a complex of hormones (COWIE, KNAGGS, and TINDAL, 1964; COWIE and TINDAL, 1964; AVERILL, 1966) one of the most important of which is prolactin secreted by the adenohypophysis (anterior pituitary). Milk removal is divided into two components — (i) passive withdrawal from the cisterns and sinuses in the mammary gland, and (ii) an active process of milk ejection from the alveoli.

B. The Milk-Ejection Reflex

Milk ejection is controlled by a neurohormonal reflex which involves the release of oxytocin from the neurohypophysis (posterior pituitary). Suckling or milking stimulates sensory receptors in the teat, afferent nerve impulses travel by way of the spinal cord and the brain stem to reach the neurosecretory cells in the paraventricular and supraoptic nuclei in the anterior hypothalamus and stimulation of these cells causes oxytocin to be released into the circulation from nerve endings in the neurohypophysis. The action of the circulating hormone is to cause contraction of the myoepithelial cells which surround the alveoli and the finer ducts. Milk is ejected into the larger ducts, and in some species into cisterns and sinuses, from which it is obtained by the young after overcoming the resistance of the teat sphincter. Passive withdrawal refers to the removal of milk which is already present in the cisterns and sinuses by suckling or milking or simply by cannulation of the teat. The amount which can be obtained in this way varies in different species. According to DENAMUR and MARTINET (1959b) it has been estimated as 5% of the total milk content of the gland in the dog, 30% in the rabbit, 30—70% in the cow and 50—80% in the goat. CROSS (1955b) found in the rabbit that it never exceeded 15% and in 10 out of 13 experiments, it was under 5%. The milk which is still contained in the alveoli at the commencement of milking or suckling can be obtained only by active contraction of the myoepithelial cells, i. e. by milk ejection. The milk-ejection reflex is indispensable for milk removal in most but not in all species. In the goat and possibly in other ruminants, a considerable quantity of milk may overflow from the alveoli into the cisterns during the intervals between milkings and this milk can be removed by passive withdrawal (DENAMUR and MARTINET, 1959b). Moreover, vigorous massaging of the denervated mammary gland in the goat can cause discharge of milk from the alveoli (TVERSKOI, 1958), probably by mechanical stimulation of the myoepithelium as in the responses to tap stimuli described in the rabbit by CROSS (1954a) and YOKOYAMA (1956) and in the rat by GROSVENOR (1965a).

The generally accepted view is that milk ejection is controlled by a purely humoral mechanism, the release of oxytocin in response to suckling. However, Russian physiologists have advanced the theory that the final link in the milk-ejection reflex involves not only oxytocin but also the efferent nerves to the mammary gland (TSAKHAEV, 1955; PAVLOV, 1955; GOFMAN, 1955; TVERSKOI, 1955a, b; BARYSHNIKOV, 1964). Oxytocin acts on the myoepithelial cells surrounding the alveoli and smaller ducts. The efferent nerves are said to control the tonus of smooth muscle in the ducts, cisterns and teats. An increase in tonus of the ducts would inhibit, and a decrease facilitate, the action of oxytocin in ejecting milk from the alveoli. It is suggested that suckling initiates, in addition to a neurohormonal reflex involving the release of oxytocin, a purely nervous segmental reflex with a shorter latent period which causes a relaxation of tonus in the ducts. The presence in the alveolar lumen of interoceptors initiating local nervous reflexes is also postulated (ZAKS, 1955). It has been shown in the cow, sheep, goat, cat and dog that the mammary gland is supplied by sympathetic adrenergic fibres which are vasoconstrictor to blood vessels. In the cow, sheep and goat these fibres are also excitor to smooth muscle in the teat and sphincter. There is no evidence for a parasympathetic (cholinergic) innervation (PEETERS, COUSSENS, and SIERENS, 1949; PEETERS, GENIE, and COUSSENS, 1951; PEETERS, BOUCKAERT, and OYAERT, 1952; LINZELL, 1950, 1956, 1959). Adrenaline causes contraction of isolated sections cut from the walls of the large ducts, cistern and teat sphincter of the cow's udder (TVERSKOI, 1955a). The topical application of adrenaline to the living gland of the mouse, or stimulation of the nerve supply, causes a constriction of the ducts visible under the microscope (LEVITSKAYA, 1955; ZOTIKOVA, 1955). It appears, therefore that a nervous mechanism exists which could control the tonus of the duct system in the mammary gland, but its physiological significance is controversial.

The milk-ejection reflex is influenced by higher centres in the central nervous system. It can be inhibited by emotional stress (ELY and PETERSEN, 1941; WHITTLESTONE, 1951; CROSS 1953a, 1954b, 1955a, b; NEWTON and NEWTON 1948; ISBISTER, 1954; CHAUDHURY, CHAUDHURY, and LU, 1961; FUCHS and WAGNER, 1963a) and it can be conditioned both to natural (GAINES, 1915; ELY and PETERSEN, 1941; WALLER, 1943, 1947a; ISBISTER, 1954) and artificial (GOFMAN, 1955) stimuli. Apart from its intrinsic importance in the physiology of lactation the milk-ejection reflex serves as a model system for studying the pharmacology of transmission of impulses in the central nervous system.

C. The Different Functions of the Adeno- and Neurohypophysis in Controlling Milk Secretion and Milk Ejection

Milk secretion is controlled by the adenohypophysis and milk ejection by the neurohypophysis. The different functions of the two parts of the pituitary gland are well illustrated by experiments on the lactating rat. In this species little or no milk is obtained by passive withdrawal and removal of milk is almost entirely dependent on the milk-ejection reflex. GOMEZ (1939, 1940) found that "lactation" (i.e. milk secretion), which ceases immediately after complete hypophysectomy in lactating rats, was maintained for 7—10 days by injecting anterior pituitary extracts, adrenocortical extract and glucose into the mother; but although milk was present in quantities in the mammary gland and the young suckled almost continuously, they died in 2—3 days of starvation. When posterior pituitary extract was also injected into the mothers, milk ejection was restored, the young were able to obtain milk and lactation was maintained for periods of over 28 days. Experiments on functional grafts of the anterior pituitary provide a further illustration (HARRIS and JACOBSON, 1951). Pituitary glands were grafted under the median eminence in hypophysectomized rats. The adenohypophysis was revascularised by the hypophysial portal vessels and functioned normally but the neurohypophysial tissue degenerated. When these rats subsequently lactated the mammary glands were well developed and contained milk but it could not be removed by the young despite vigorous suckling. The litters survived when the milk was made available to them by injecting oxytocin into the mother. Similarly COWIE (1952) and BENSON and COWIE (1956) showed that after posterior pituitary lobectomy in lactating rats the young could be reared only if the mothers were given regular daily injections of oxytocin.

D. Oxytocin and the Control of Secretion of Prolactin

Suckling not only initiates the milk-ejection reflex; it is also a necessary stimulus for the continuance of milk secretion, as first shown by SELYE and his co-workers (SELYE, 1934; SELYE, COLLIP, and THOMSON, 1934) in experiments on lactating rats. On the 3rd day of lactation the nipples were excised from the mammary glands on one side of the body and the ducts ligated on the other side. The mothers were returned to their litters which continued to suckle the intact nipples although they could obtain no milk. Examination of the glands on both sides showed active secretion 14 days after the operation whereas in control experiments in which the litters were removed on the 3rd day of lactation, secretion ceased after 3—5 days. It was concluded that involution of the glands after weaning is due not to accumulation of secretion but to withdrawal of the suckling stimulus. Since suckling delayed involution in glands from which the nipples had been excised a humoral factor was involved in maintaining secretion. It was suggested that suckling stimulated the secretion of prolactin from the anterior pituitary in much the same way as copulation in some species stimulates the secretion of gonadotrophin. PETERSEN (1944) put forward the idea that it was the oxytocin released by suckling which constituted the stimulus for the release of prolactin. This hypothesis was developed independently by BENSON and FOLLEY (1956, 1957a, b. See also BENSON [1960] and BENSON, COWIE, and TINDAL, 1958). They showed in lactating rats that the involution of the mammary glands which normally follows removal of the litter could be greatly retarded by the injection of oxytocin thrice daily into the mothers. Oxytocin was effective only in intact and not in hypophysectomized rats and, unlike prolactin, it did not stimulate secretion when injected directly into the mammary gland through a milk duct. They concluded that oxytocin, released from nerve endings in the neurohypophysis by the milk-ejection reflex, reaches the adenohypophysis by the hypophysial portal vessels and stimulates it to release prolactin. In support of this theory, McCann, Mack, and Gale (1959) showed that injections of oxytocin retarded mammary involution in rats in which hypothalamic lesions in the supraoptico-hypophysial tract had blocked both milk secretion and milk ejection. Since the lesions must have blocked any neural control of the adenohypophysis by the hypothalamus a direct stimulant action of oxytocin on the adenohypophysis was postulated. Other workers have also confirmed that oxytocin retards mammary involution after removal of litters from lactating animals (Meites, 1959; Meites and Nicoll, 1959; Meites, Nicoll, and Talwalker, 1959; Meites, Nicoll, Talwalker, and Hopkins, 1960; Yokoyama and Ota, 1959b). Moreover, lactation can be artificially prolonged in rats for 70 days after litter withdrawal by repeated replacement with fresh litters (Nicoll and Meites, 1959) and in the sheep the mean daily milk yield is increased by regular injections of oxytocin throughout the period of lactation (Denamur and Martinet, 1961). However, although it is not disputed that oxytocin retards mammary involution several arguments have been advanced against the theory that it stimulates the release of prolactin. The fact that milk secretion was shown to occur independently of milk ejection in hypophysectomized rats with pituitary grafts (Harris and Jacobsohn, 1951), in rats after posterior pituitary lobectomy (Benson and Cowie, 1956) or lesions in a restricted part of the hypothalamus (Yokoyama and Ota, 1959a) and in rabbits after lesions in the supraoptico-hypophysial tract (Cross and Harris, 1952) suggests that oxytocin is not indispensable for the secretion of prolactin. Moreover, the secretion of prolactin continues from pituitary glands transplanted under the renal capsule (Everett, 1954), although oxytocin injected systemically increases the secretion of prolactin by such glands (Benson and Folley, 1960). Grosvenor and Turner (1958b) found that oxytocin injected into lactating rats under anaesthesia did not reduce the content of lactogenic hormone in the anterior pituitary, although a depletion could be demonstrated after normal nursing. This confirms an earlier report that posterion pituitary extract (Pituitrin) does not release lactogenic hormone (Meites and Turner, 1942). It has also been found that whereas reserpine inhibits the milk-ejection reflex it stimulates release of prolactin from the anterior pituitary (Moon and Turner, 1959). Meites and his co-workers have shown that a combination of prolactin with oxytocin is more effective than prolactin alone in retarding mammary involution (Meites, 1959; Meites and Nicoll, 1959; Meites and Hopkins, 1961). They also showed, in disagreement with Haun (1959), that oxytocin failed to initiate milk secretion in animals in which development of the mammary glands had been induced by a series of injections of oestrogens or by giving chorionic gonadotrophin to produce pseudopregnancy. (Meites, Nicoll, and Talwalker, 1959; Meites, Talwalker, and Nicoll, 1960; Meites, Nicoll, Talwalker, and Hopkins, 1960). These authors have proposed the theory that there are independent mechanisms controlling the release of oxytocin and prolactin by suckling and that oxytocin retards mammary involution not by releasing prolactin but by a direct local action on the mammary gland. The emptying of the alveoli by the action of oxytocin on the myoepithelium reduces the pressure of accumulated secretion against the epithelial cells and the blood capillaries permitting more synthesis of milk to occur under the influence of prolactin or other lactogenic hormones (Meites, Nicoll, and Talwalker, 1960). Tverskoi's work on goats supports this view (Tverskoi, 1955b).

Not only has the role of oxytocin in releasing prolactin been questioned but also the importance of an intact sensory innervation of the mammary gland. It appears to be necessary in many but not all species. INGELBRECHT (1935) showed that if rats were allowed to suckle denervated mammary glands below the level of a spinal transection they were unable to obtain milk, but when they were allowed to suckle intact glands above the level of the lesion, milk was obtained from all glands, innervated or not. This result invokes a reflex with an afferent neural and an efferent hormonal component but it is difficult to decide if the lesion affected primarily milk ejection or milk secretion. Spinal transection in lactating cats (BEYER, MENA, PACHECO, and ALCAREZ, 1962) and rats (GROSVENOR, 1964) greatly reduced the milk yield obtained by the litters and the injection of oxytocin into the mothers to ensure milk ejection failed to restore the yield; this implies a failure of milk secretion. Similarly, EAYRS and EDWARDSON (1965) showed in rats that systemic injections of oxytocin failed to maintain more than a trace of milk secretion when suckling was confined to nipples denervated by section of the sensory nerves in the intercostal spaces. On the other hand, good milk yields were obtained from lactating rabbits after spinal transection, provided that oxytocin was injected into the mothers (MENA and BEYER, 1963); this suggests that denervation of the mammary gland had abolished milk ejection without significantly impairing milk secretion. Similarly it has been clearly demonstrated that after denervation or transplantation of the mammary gland in the goat and sheep, when the milk-ejection reflex is absent, practically normal milk yields can be obtained (TVERSKOI, 1957, 1958; DENAMUR and MARTINET, 1959a, b, 1960; LINZELL, 1960, 1963). It has therefore been argued that in these species at least the secretion of prolactin is not exclusively dependent on nervous stimuli from the mammary gland and that physiological mechanisms other than that proposed by BENSON and FOLLEY are involved (DENAMUR and MARTINET (1959b). Other factors which have been suggested are a feedback mechanism and the secretion by the mammary gland of a substance stimulating the release of prolactin from the anterior pituitary (see COWIE and TINDAL, 1964). Exteroceptive or environmental stimuli may be involved; for example, GROSVENOR (1965b) has shown that if the young are returned to lactating rats after separation, but prevented from suckling by interposing a wire screen, the pituitary gland of the mothers shows the same degree of depletion of prolactin as after normal nursing. TALWALKER, RATNER, and MEITES (1963) showed that the hypothalamus contains a "prolactin inhibiting factor" or PIF which acts on the anterior pituitary to depress the synthesis or release of prolactin. Suckling can deplete the hypothalamus of PIF (RATNER and MEITES, 1964a, b; RATNER, 1966) and it has been suggested (GROSVENOR, 1965c) that the hypothalamic response to suckling in the rat is a temporary inhibition of the release of this factor. According to another theory recently proposed, the uptake of milk precursors by the actively secreting mammary gland stimulates the appetite centre or inhibits the satiety centre in the hypothalamus, and these centres have some functional association with hypothalamic control of anterior pituitary secretion (COWIE and TINDAL, 1964).

Whether or not oxytocin indirectly stimulates milk secretion by releasing prolactin, its direct action on the mammary gland is to cause the expulsion of pre-formed milk from the alveoli. It should be emphasized that the whole of the milk removed is already present in the gland when suckling or milking begins (GAINES and SANMANN, 1927; GOWEN and TOBEY, 1927; PETERSEN, PALMER, and ECKLES, 1929).

E. Reviews

Important aspects of the milk-ejection reflex are reviewed in papers by PETERSEN (1944), KAY (1949, 1955), MACAULAY (1950), FOLLEY (1947a, b, 1949,

1952, 1956), CROSS (1952b, 1953b, 1955c, 1961), COWIE and FOLLEY (1957), HARRIS (1958), LINZELL (1959), COWIE and TINDAL (1964), BARYSHNIKOV (1964), DENAMUR (1965), AVERILL (1966).

II. Evolution of the Concept of a Neurohormonal Reflex in the Control of Milk Ejection

The theory that milk ejection is brought about by a neurohormonal reflex which involves the release of oxytocin from the posterior pituitary gland was enunciated by ELY and PETERSEN in 1941. The evolution of this idea is of much historical interest.

The effect of posterior pituitary extract on the mammary gland was first reported in 1910 by OTT and SCOTT who showed that intravenous injection of the extract into a lactating goat greatly increased the outflow of milk from a cannulated teat. This they described as a galactagogue action. Within five years a similar effect was demonstrated in a number of other species including man, the cow, the cat and the dog (MACKENZIE, 1911; SCHÄFER and MACKENZIE, 1912; GAVIN, 1913; HEANEY, 1913; SCHÄFER, 1913, 1915; SIMPSON and HILL, 1915) but there were opposing views about the mechanism of action of the extract. MACKENZIE (1911) supposed that it was due to a direct stimulant action on the secretory epithelium. SCHÄFER (1915), however, produced photomicrographs showing that, after the intravenous injection of posterior pituitary extract in the cat the alveoli were distended in one gland with an intact nipple but empty in an adjacent gland in which the nipple had been excised to allow a free escape of milk. He suggested that the effect of posterior pituitary extract was to cause expulsion of milk from the gland by acting on contractile tissue in the walls of the alveoli similar to that which is present in sweat glands. This was an early adumbration of the classical work of RICHARDSON (1949) on myoepithelial tissue in the mammary gland (see Fig. 1). As further evidence against the secretory hypothesis, SCHÄFER showed that if the injection of posterior pituitary extract was repeated after the mammary gland had been emptied, it did not cause an outflow of milk unless sufficient time had elapsed to allow some secretion to accumulate in the alveoli. GAINES (1915) also recognized that posterior pituitary extract caused milk ejection and not milk secretion. The idea that a reflex involving the central nervous system governs the milk ejection produced by suckling was founded on his observation that pups were unable to obtain milk from a bitch under ether anaesthesia but that they obtained a full yield as soon as the anaesthetized bitch was given an intravenous injection of posterior pituitary extract. He produced further evidence of a reflex by showing that when one gland in a lactating goat was stimulated by the kid, a rise of pressure and an increased flow of milk occurred in the opposite gland. GAINES concluded that the reflex was initiated by sensory stimulation of the teat and that the central nervous system was involved in a reflex arc part of which was interrupted by anaesthesia. He pointed out the similarity of the responses to posterior pituitary extract and to the natural stimulus of suckling, but although it was almost implicit in his work, GAINES did not actually state that the efferent component of the reflex consisted of a discharge of posterior pituitary hormone into the blood. This final step was taken by ELY and PETERSEN (1939, 1940, 1941) who showed that the hormone involved was oxytocin. They also demonstrated the inhibitory effect of fright and of adrenaline on the milk-ejection reflex.

It should be noted that only crude extracts of the posterior pituitary gland were available to GAINES. However in 1928 KAMM, ALDRICH, GROTE, ROWE, and BUGBEE separated two active fractions from posterior pituitary extracts — the one, Alpha-hypophamine, having predominently oxytocic, and the other, Beta-hypophamine having predominently pressor, activity. Their solutions containing Alpha- and Beta-hypophamine were named oxytocin and vasopressin, respectively (Bugbee and Kamm, 1928) and the corresponding commercial preparations, Pitocin and Pitressin. These preparations were available to Ely and Petersen who investigated which of the two active fractions of posterior pituitary extract was responsible for its action on the lactating mammary gland. Their work was carried out on cows in which one half of the udder had been denervated and the other left intact. No difference was found between the rates at which the two halves of the udder ejected milk in response to milking. Therefore, the act of milk ejection was not directly under the control of the nervous system but depended on a humoral factor. Fright or the intravenous injection of adrenaline at the start of milking prevented or delayed milk ejection from both halves of the udder. The inhibitory effect of both fright and adrenaline could be counteracted by the intravenous injection of either Pitocin or Pitressin and of these two fractions, Pitocin was much the more potent. From these observations Ely and Petersen formulated their theory that sensory stimulation of the teat by suckling or milking, or stimuli associated with milking, such as the washing of the udder and the rattling of milk pails, to which the cow becomes conditioned, initiate afferent impulses which reach the central nervous system. This stimulates the pituitary to secrete oxytocin into the blood. Oxytocin is the humoral factor responsible for the increase in intraglandular pressure which squeezes the milk from the alveoli and finer ducts. At the same time, fright can cause the release of adrenaline from the adrenal medulla. It was thought that the rate of ejection of milk is determined by a balance between the opposing effects of circulating adrenaline and oxytocin.

Petersen and his co-workers demonstrated that a humoral factor capable of causing milk ejection from the mammary gland is actually released into the circulation during suckling or milking. A technique was developed for perfusing the isolated udder of the cow with warm, oxygenated blood at constant pressure and measuring the outflow of milk from a cannulated teat (Petersen, Shaw, and Visscher, 1939, 1941). Petersen and Ludwick (1942) showed that perfusion of the udder with 1 litre of blood withdrawn from a cow in which the milk-ejection reflex had been elicited, caused an outflow of milk within 15 sec. The factor producing this effect was labile since it disappeared from blood which had been left standing for 30 min. A control sample of blood had no effect on the perfused udder. Blood from a cow which had been frightened at the start of milking did not cause an outflow of milk from the perfused gland but reduced the blood flow to one quarter normal. Adrenaline and Pitressin also reduced blood flow. Pitressin was less effective than Pitocin in expelling milk from the perfused udder (Petersen, 1942). Similar results were obtained by Peeters and his co-workers who developed independently a technique for perfusing separately the two halves of the isolated bovine udder (Peeters and Massart, 1947). Although control samples of blood from a cow produced an increase in the flow of milk when perfused through one half of the udder, due to the presence of a factor which could not be identified (Peeters, Massart, and Coussens, 1947b: Peeters, Sierens, and Silver, 1952), a much greater increase was obtained when the other half was perfused with samples of jugular venous blood collected after stimulation of the teats (Peeters, Massart and Coussens, 1947a; Peeters and Massart, 1950). It was shown also that test samples of blood produced an increase in pressure in the cistern of the perfused gland similar to that obtained with Pitocin (Peeters and Massart, 1950).

Positive evidence that the humoral factor released into the blood during suckling or milking is oxytocin, has been obtained by the recent development of highly sensitive and specific methods for assaying this hormone in blood (see the chapter by Fitzpatrick and Bentley in this volume). The methods used involve extraction of the plasma with acetone or by gel filtration on Sephadex columns and assay of the extracts for oxytocic activity on the superfused rat uterus (Fitzpatrick, 1961) or for milk-ejecting activity by retrograde injection into the mammary gland of the lactating guinea-pig (Tindal and Yokoyama, 1962). With the use of these techniques, oxytocin has been identified and assayed in blood collected from ewes (Fitzpatrick, 1961) cows and sows (Knaggs, 1963; Folley and Knaggs, 1964, 1965a, 1966) during suckling or milking. In cows the presence or absence of oxytocin in the blood could be correlated with the milk yield. The application of the teat cups was the stimulus which most consistently elicited the release of oxytocin. There was no evidence in these experiments of any conditioning of oxytocin release to visual auditory or olfactory stimuli associated with the milking routine, although it is known from other work that the milk-ejection reflex can be conditioned (see p. 476). It is interesting that in the majority of experiments on goats, no oxytocin was detected in blood collected during hand milking although the milk yields were normal (Folley and Knaggs, 1964, 1965a, 1966). This may be related to the fact that in the goat the milk-ejection reflex is apparently not indispensable for milk removal (see Section I).

III. Milk-Ejection Reflex in Man

Following the work of Ely and Petersen on the cow, Waller (1943, 1947a) concluded from clinical observations that milk is ejected from the human mammary gland during suckling by a reflex which is highly susceptible to interference and conditioning. If suckling is interrupted milk can often be seen to stream for a distance of several inches from the duct orifice in the teat, showing that milk is obtained by the baby as a result of an active expulsion on the part of the mother. The fact that when the baby is put to one breast, milk is sometimes forcibly ejected from the other breast, clearly invokes a reflex mechanism. Milk ejection is accompanied by a subjective sensation of a tingling nature which is recognized in the lay term "draught." This sensation may be experienced not only during suckling, but in response to a variety of stimuli associated with preparation for nursing and in the absence of the baby (Isbister, 1954). As in cattle, therefore, the milk-ejection reflex is readily conditioned.

To test how far the theory of Ely and Petersen could be extended to the human subject, Newton and Newton (1948) attempted to inhibit milk ejection in a lactating woman by causing her emotional stress. They showed that the amount of milk obtained by the baby was reduced when the mother was distracted by exposure to cold or by emotional conflict or painful stimuli, without disturbance to the baby. A significantly greater amount of milk was produced when oxytocin was injected intramuscularly during the period of distraction.

Recognition of the fact that milk ejection involves a reflex which is easily inhibited by emotional disturbance has been of great importance in the clinical management of breast feeding and in prevention of its failure (Waller, 1947b; Newton and Newton, 1950, 1951; Robinson, 1943; Isbister, 1954).

Newton and Newton (1951) concluded that engorgement of the breast during lactation begins with retention of milk in the alveoli. The alveoli become distended and compress the neighbouring ducts; this obstructs the outflow of milk and leads to further distension of the alveoli. If this is unrelieved secondary vascular and lymphatic stasis may follow and milk secretion cease in the obstructed portion of the breast. They suggested that one of the factors causing the initial retention of milk is a failure of the milk-ejection reflex which might be caused by emotional inhibition of oxytocin release. In fact, milk retention has been successfully treated with oxytocin (Haeger and Jacobsohn, 1953).

The vascular changes which occur as a result of engorgement have been investigated experimentally in the rat by Silver (1956) and Cross and Silver (1956). The teat ducts were ligated in lactating rats on the day after parturition and the mothers were allowed to continue nursing their young. The tied glands became distended after 8 hours and engorgement was maximal after 24 hours. At this stage, if the ligatures were loosened or the teats cut, the intravenous injection of oxytocin (5—10 mU) caused milk ejection. Histologically, the alveoli were distended but surrounded by an extensive capillary network which was full of blood. After 48 hours there was no longer a response to the intravenous injection of oxytocin although the topical application of only 0.001 mU caused a localized contraction of the gland. The capillary bed was now collapsed and almost devoid of blood cells. It is relevant to note that Pickles (1953) obtained evidence of a reduction in mammary blood flow in primary engorgement of the human breast.

IV. The Neural Pathway involved in the Milk-Ejection Reflex

Milk ejection is governed by a reflex arc having neural afferent and efferent components. The afferent pathway extends from sensory nerve endings in the mammary gland to the neurosecretory cells in the supraoptic and paraventricular nuclei. The efferent pathway consists of the neurones of these two nuclei running in the hypothalamo-neurohypophysial tract. The neurohypophysis, which consists of the median eminence of the tuber cinereum, the infundibular stem and the infundibular process (Rioch, Wislocki and O'Leary, 1940) contains the nerve endings from which oxytocin is released into the circulation.

A. The Efferent Component

1. The Neurohypophysis

The role of the neurohypophysis in the milk-ejection reflex was established by the classical experiments of Cross and Harris on the effects of electrical stimulation and lesions of the supraoptico-hypophysial tract in lactating rabbits (Cross and Harris, 1950a, b; 1951, 1952; Cross, 1952b; Harris, 1958). To register milk ejection a cannula was inserted into a teat duct, partly filled with citrate solution and connected with a piston or float recorder writing on a kymograph. The ejection of milk into the cannula was recorded as a volume change. The pituitary stalk was stimulated in the unanaesthetized animal with a glass insulated platinum electrode having an exposed tip of 1 mm inserted stereotactically. Unipolar stimulation at 1 V and 50 c.p.s. for 1 min produced a milk-ejection response which had a latent period of 25 sec, reached its peak in 90 sec and subsided in 4—7 min. The volume of milk ejected from a single teat duct was 0.5—1.5 ml; the total number of teat ducts in the rabbit is 48. The response was matched by the intravenous injection of 50—200 mU posterior pituitary extract (Pituitrin), the latent period in this case being 10—15 sec. All effective stimuli were shown to have been situated within 0.5 mm of the supraoptico-hypophysial tract. Electrolytic lesions in the region of the median eminence and infundibular stem which interrupted this tract, interfered with the milk-ejection reflex. The young were unable to obtain more than 30% of the pre-operative yield of milk. At the end of suckling a considerable quantity of milk remained in the mammary gland but the injection of 50—200 mU posterior pituitary extract before suckling commenced resulted in complete emptying. In the presence of the lesions, stimulation in the region of the supraoptico-hypophysial tract failed to elicit milk ejection. Lesions in the dorsal and posterior hypothalamic and premamillary areas which did not involve the supraoptico-hypophysial tract caused no interference with milk ejection in response either to suckling or to electrical stimulation of the tract. Lesions of the median eminence and infundibular stem abolished milk ejection and the gulping phase of suckling, but not the nursing behaviour of the mother which therefore appears to be integrated at a different level in the central nervous system, probably in the cortex (CROSS, 1952a).

Electrolytic lesions of the median eminence in the rat (GALE, TALEISNICK, FRIEDMAN, and MCCANN. 1961) and radiolesions in the pituitary gland and in the region of the median eminence and pituitary stalk in the goat (GALE and LARSSON, 1963) have been shown to abolish the milk-ejection reflex. Milk ejection has been produced in the cow by electrical stimulation of the pituitary gland by means of an electrode permanently implanted through the sphenoid bone (HYNEK, BÍLEK, and LIS, 1965).

2. *The Supraoptic and Paraventricular Nuclei*

The neurohypophysis represents the final common path for neurones which originate in the supraoptic and paraventricular nuclei and converge in the infundibular region to enter the pituitary stalk. An important question which is still undecided is whether there is any differentiation of function between these two nuclei i. e. does one nucleus control the release of vasopressin in the regulation of water balance and the other the release of oxytocin in the milk-ejection reflex and possibly in parturition? There are three main approaches to this problem — the distribution of oxytocin and vasopressin in the two nuclei, the effects of lesions placed within the nuclei and finally the release of the hormones in response to discrete electrical stimulation within the anterior hypothalamus.

a) *Distribution of Hormones:* The ratio of the content of vasopressin to that of oxytocin in the supraoptic and paraventricular nuclei of fours species is shown in Table 1. This ratio is variable but in all the species examined it is higher in the

Table 1. *Vasopressin:Oxytocin (V/O) ratios in supraoptic (SON) and paraventricular (PVN) nuclei*

	V/O ratios		Ref.
	SON	PVN	
Camel	2.6	0.26	1
Sheep	3.3	0.7	2
Dog	24	15	1
Dog	18.0	9.0	2
Elephant (1 experiment)	15.4	2.7	2

References: 1. VAN DYKE, ADAMSONS, and ENGEL (1955); ADAMSONS, ENGEL, VAN DYKE, SCHMIDT-NIELSEN, and SCHMIDT-NIELSEN (1956). — 2. LEDERIS (1961, 1962).

supraoptic than in the paraventricular nuclei. In the paraventricular nuclei of the sheep and camel, the ratio is low; LEDERIS (1961) reported that in one experiment in which the paraventricular nuclei from three sheep were pooled, no vasopressin could be detected. The results suggest that in the sheep and camel the paraventricular nucleus may be concerned principally or entirely with the secretion of oxytocin.

b) *The Effects of Experimental Lesions:* The results of experimental lesions placed in one or other nucleus strongly suggest that in the cat and the rat the supraoptic nucleus is concerned mainly with the secretion of vasopressin and the paraventricular nucleus with that of oxytocin. In the rat, OLIVECRONA (1954, 1957) showed that after bilateral destruction of the paraventricular nucleus the posterior pituitary gland was depleted of oxytocin but there was little or no decrease in the content of vasopressin and the lesions did not result in a disturbance of water balance. Similar lesions have been shown to cause a decrease in the oxytocic activity of the blood in rats (DUGGAN and REED, 1958) but, as shown by the use of the thioglycollate test, only a part of this activity was due to oxytocin. In the cat, NIBBELINK (1961) found that bilateral destruction of the paraventricular nuclei caused a 90% depletion of oxytocic activity in the posterior pituitary gland. When the lesions were made in pregnant cats dystocia resulted but there was no disturbance in water balance. This is in agreement with the finding of FISHER, INGRAM, and RANSON (1938) that lesions confined to the paraventricular nuclei did not produce diabetes insipidus in cats.

In the rabbit, however, SUNSTEN and SAWYER (1961) demonstrated that in three animals with hypothalamic islands from which the paraventricular nuclei had been removed milk ejection was still obtained in response to an osmotic stimulus. This implies that, unless the milk ejection was due to the release of vasopressin (see Section X) the supraoptic nucleus in this species is concerned with the secretion of oxytocin.

c) *The Response to Electrical Stimulation:* The experiments of ANDERSSON (1951 b) and ANDERSSON and MCCANN (1955) on lactating sheep and goats suggest that each nucleus releases both hormones. Discrete points in the anterior hypothalamus were stimulated in the unanaesthetized animal. Electrodes having an uninsulated tip of 1.5 mm were inserted under x-ray control and unipolar stimulation was carried out with a modified square wave pulse of 12.5 msec duration at 0.5—1.5 V and 20 or 50 c.p.s. Stimulation in or at points adjacent to the supraoptic and paraventricular nuclei caused milk ejection as well as inhibition of water diuresis. The milk-ejection response was shown to be humorally mediated since it was observed in a denervated half of the udder and during sacral anaesthesia, and blood taken from one goat during the response caused milk ejection when injected intravenously into a second goat.

CROSS (1958a), using a similar technique to that used for stimulating the pituitary stalk, found that in oestrogenized lactating rabbits electrical stimulation of both the supraoptic and paraventricular nuclei caused milk ejection and an increase in uterine motility. This suggests that both nuclei are concerned with the release of oxytocin. HARRIS (1947) concluded that the paraventricular nucleus in the rabbit did not release vasopressin since water diuresis was not inhibited by electrical stimulation of this nucleus in the conscious animal whereas in the cat and dog, electrical stimulation of both nuclei has been reported to cause an antidiuresis (KOELLA, 1949; FANG, LIU, and WANG, 1962). These results suggest a duality of function of the two nuclei. However, their interpretation depends upon assessment of the spread of the stimulating current. Moreover, since the release of hormones was inferred from the response of the animal's own target organs possible interference from stimulation of autonomic centres must be excluded. For example, electrical stimulation in the region of the paraventricular nucleus in the rabbit causes the release of both oxytocin and catecholamines. The catecholamines, especially adrenaline, block the action of oxytocin on the mammary gland, and a milk-ejection response to stimulation of the nucleus is obtained only when the release of adrenaline is prevented by acute adrenalectomy, spinal anaesthesia or section of the spinal cord (CROSS, 1955a, 1958a, b). Antidiuresis may be caused by renal vascular changes resulting from autonomic stimulation. It must also be remembered that vasopressin possesses a considerable degree of intrinsic milk-ejecting activity and unless quantitative measurements are made of the amounts of both oxytocin and vasopressin released by stimulation, the possibility that milk ejection is a side effect of vasopressin cannot be excluded (see Section X).

A more direct approach is to assay oxytocin and vasopressin in samples of blood collected during stimulation. HAWKER, WALMSLEY, ROBERTS, and ROBERTSON (1959) found an increased concentration of oxytocin in the blood of the rat after electrical stimulation of the paraventricular nucleus. BISSET, HILTON, and POISNER (1963, 1967) attempted to define neurosecretory pathways for the release of oxytocin and vasopressin in the cat by assaying both hormones in samples of blood collected during electrical stimulation of discrete points in the anterior hypothalamus. An electrode having an uninsulated tip of < 30 μ was inserted stereotactically. The stimulus consisted of a square wave pulse of 2 msec duration at 80 c.p.s. and of sufficient voltage to give a current of 200 μA. The hormones were extracted from blood with alcohol by a simple method which gave a recovery of about 75% and the extracts were assayed for antidiuretic activity on the water loaded rat (DICKER, 1953; DETTELBACH, 1958; BISSET, 1962a) and for milk-ejecting activity on the lactating guinea-pig (BISSET, 1962a; TINDAL and YOKOYAMA, 1962). In calculating the concentration of oxytocin in a blood sample, allowance was made for the intrinsic milk-ejecting activity of the vasopressin in the sample. Stimulation of the supraoptic nucleus or the supraoptico-hypophysial tract resulted in high concentrations of vasopressin in the blood with little or no oxytocin. It was concluded that in the cat the supraoptic nucleus and its neurones are concerned principally or wholly with the release of vasopressin. Release of moderate amounts of vasopressin without detectable amounts of oxytocin was obtained on stimulation of points in the rostral part of the paraventricular nucleus and in the tractus paraventricularis cinereus of GREVING (GREVING, 1923, 1925, 1926, 1928; BARGMANN, 1949a, b). This suggests that the paraventricular nucleus also controls the release of vasopressin either directly, or indirectly through stimulation of the supraoptic nucleus. In addition to GREVING's lateral tract, a direct medial tract has been described in the dog by LAQUEUR (1954) which originates from the dorso-caudal part of the paraventricular nucleus, passes dorsal then lateral to the fornix and finally joins the fibres from the supraoptic nucleus in the proximal part of the infundibular stem. Another medial tract has been described by LARUELLE (1934) and FORD and KANTOUNIS (1957). It was found in the cat that oxytocin was released into the blood on stimulation of points in the tuberal region which corresponded in their distribution with the distal part of LAQUEUR's tract in the dog. It was suggested that, if this tract exists also in the cat and in other species, it could represent a specific neurosecretory pathway for the release of oxytocin. Evidence that the paraventricular nucleus is involved in the milk-ejection reflex in the cat has been obtained by BROOKS, ISHIKAWA, KOIZUMI, and LU (1966) who showed that suction applied to the teat induced a milk-ejection response which was correlated with an increase in unit discharge recorded with micro-electrodes from the neurones of the paraventricular nucleus.

In summary, the evidence regarding the efferent pathway for the release of oxytocin in the milk-ejection reflex is contradictory but there are indications that at least in some species this pathway may be represented by a paraventriculo-neurohypophysial system of fibres.

3. Mechanism of Release of Hormones from the Neurohypophysis

The term "neurosecretory" which is applied to the neurones of the supraoptic and paraventricular nuclei implies that these neurones have the dual function of transmitting electrical impulses and of elaborating an endocrine secretion. That they can transmit impulses like ordinary neurones has been shown by a number of investigations. CROSS and GREEN (1959) recorded action potentials of normal amplitude and wave-form, from single neurones in the two nuclei of the rabbit and showed that in response to the intracarotid injection of hypertonic saline, the rate of discharge was increased in neurones of the supraoptic nucleus and decreased in those of the paraventricular nucleus. Synaptic and action potentials and temporal summation have been demonstrated by intracellular recording from cell bodies in the caudal neurosecretory system of the eel (MORITA, ISHIBASHI, and YAMASHITA, 1961). Intracellular recording from neuroendocrine cells in the hypothalamus of the goldfish revealed that these cells had electrical membrane properties significantly different from those of salivary gland cells but similar to those of other central neurones (KANDEL, 1964).

Electrical activity has been recorded from the pituitary stalk in cats (ISHIKAWA, KOIZUMI, and BROOKS, 1966). Repetitive electrical stimulation of the supraoptic and paraventricular nuclei evoked an increase in the rate of discharge of stalk fibres. Increased activity in these fibres was also produced reflexly by the stimulus of gentle suction applied to a nipple in the mammary gland and this was accompanied by milk ejection. In other work it was shown that the same stimulus, which again caused milk ejection, increased unit discharge in the paraventricular nucleus (BROOKS, ISHIKAWA, KOIZUMI, and LU, 1966). These experiments clearly implicate the paraventricular and possibly the supraoptic nucleus in the milk-ejection reflex and suggest that it is the transmission of an electrical impulse from the cell body to the nerve ending which triggers the release of oxytocin.

How the impulse causes release is uncertain but a cholinergic mechanism has been invoked. Although FELDBERG and VOGT (1948) concluded from their studies of the distribution of choline acetylase in the central nervous system that the nerve fibres in the posterior pituitary of the dog were noncholinergic, the presence of acetylcholine itself has been demonstrated in both the hypothalamus and the neural lobe of the rabbit (LEDERIS and LIVINGSTON, 1966) and acetylcholinesterase has been found in the neurohypophysis of the ox (PASETTO, 1952) the cat (KOELLE and GEESEY, 1961) and the hedgehog (KIERNON, 1964). In the dog ABRAHAMS, KOELLE, and SMART (1957) found high concentrations of acetylcholinesterase in the cell bodies of the supraoptic and paraventricular nuclei but the enzyme could be traced along the axon for a distance of not more than 400 μ and it was not detectable in the supraoptico-hypophysial tract. The authors considered that the presence of the enzyme in the proximal part of the neurones could indicate that either the neurones themselves or presynaptic neurones impinging on the nuclei were cholinergic. They suggested that if the neurones of the supraoptic and paraventricular nuclei were cholinergic, this would represent a unique example of a neurone's own transmitter releasing its own endocrine product. A similar conclusion was reached independently by GERSCHENFELD, TRAMEZZANI, and DE ROBERTIS (1960), from electron microscopic studies of the preoptico-neurohypophysial tract in the toad. The axons in this tract contained two different types of vesicles. One type, of high electron density, containing neurosecretory granules, was present throughout the tract, the size varying from 620 Å in the hypothalamus to 1350—1500 Å in the hilum of the infundibular process and near capillaries. The second type having a mean size of 420 Å, was confined to the nerve endings and resembled the synaptic vesicles which are generally associated with the release of acetylcholine at presynaptic nerve endings (DE ROBERTIS, 1962, 1964a, b). It was suggested that the second type of vesicle in the axons of the preoptico-neurohypophysial tract contained acetylcholine or a similar mediator which was released in response to an electrical impulse and in its turn released hormone from the neurosecretory granules. This concept of double transmission is analogous to the hypothesis advanced by BURN and RAND (1959) and BURN (1963, 1965, 1966) concerning the intermediary role of acetylcholine in releasing catecholamines from adrenergic neurones. It fits into the more general concept that acetylcholine has a dual neurohumoral role (KOELLE 1961, 1962). When released by a conducted presynaptic impulse it may act at two sites: postsynaptically and at the presynaptic terminal itself to bring about release from the terminal of additional acetylcholine or of some other neurohormonal agent. However the contention that the small vesicles seen in the nerve endings of the neurohypophysis are analogous to synaptic vesicles occuring in nerve terminals in other parts of the nervous system has been challenged by the suggestion that these vesicles represent precursors or remnants of elementary granules (HOLMES and KNOWLES, 1960; LEDERIS, 1964, 1965; DANIEL and LEDERIS, 1966a).

DOUGLAS and POISNER have shown that vasopressin is released from nerve terminals in the isolated neurohypophysis of the rat by excess potassium and by electrical stimulation of the pituitary stalk (DOUGLAS, 1963; DOUGLAS and POISNER, 1962a, b; 1963, 1964a, b). They conclude that impulses from the supraoptic and paraventricular nuclei depolarize the nerve endings of the supraoptico-hypophysial tract and that this promotes Ca influx which in turn causes release of stored hormone. They suggest that Ca acts as a crucial link in the process of "stimulus secretion coupling" and that a common mechanism may underlie the release of typical secretory products of nerves, neurosecretory cells and the chromaffin cells of the adrenal medulla, all of which show a common developmental origin. DOUGLAS and POISNER limited their observations to vasopressin. However DICKER (1966) has shown that on incubation of isolated pituitary glands from rats, including lactating rats, oxytocin is released as well as vasopressin. In the presence of a sufficiently high concentration of calcium, the release of both hormones from glands of adult rats was increased by excess potassium and by ouabain. It is suggested that the function of calcium is to release oxytocin and vasopressin from binding to neurophysin (THORN, 1965; DICKER, 1966). Acetylcholine, either alone or in the presence of an anticholinesterase, does not release oxytocin or vasopressin from the isolated neurohypophysis of the rat (DOUGLAS and POISNER, 1963; DICKER, 1966). DANIEL and LEDERIS (1966b) found that neither hormone was released by acetylcholine from the isolated neural lobes of the rat, ox or hedgehog. On the other hand both hormones were released by acetylcholine if the hypothalamus of the rat was incubated with the pituitary stalk and gland attached. They concluded that acetylcholine is involved in the process of release of neurohypophysial hormones by acting on the hypothalamic nuclei but there was no evidence for a direct action on nerve endings in the neurohypophysis. It seems questionable, however, whether the external application of acetylcholine to nerve terminals in an incubation medium is comparable with the release of acetylcholine from synaptic vesicles within the terminal. In this connection BURN (1965) has suggested that the ability of mecamylamine and pempidine to block postganglionic fibres may be related to the fact that, as secondary and tertiary amines, they are able to penetrate cells, whereas other ganglion blocking agents such as hexamethonium which contain two quaternary nitrogen groups fail to block the postganglionic fibre because they do not penetrate.

B. The Synapse at the Supraoptic and Paraventricular Nuclei

1. Evidence for Cholinergic Transmission at the Synapse

CHANG, CHIA, HSU and LIM (1937a, b, c, 1938) and HUANG (1938) obtained evidence that stimulation of the central end of the vagus in the dog produced a reflex release of vasopressin from the posterior pituitary in association with a release of acetylcholine into the cerebral circulation. This work, together with the demonstration by DIKSHIT (1934, 1935) that central effects could be produced in the cat by injecting acetylcholine into the hypothalamus or cerebral ventricles, suggested to PICKFORD that acetylcholine might be the chemotransmitter of impulses at the supraoptic nucleus.

PICKFORD (1939) first showed that acetylcholine had an antidiuretic action in the conscious dog which was abolished by hypophysectomy. Intracarotid injection was more effective than intravenous (PICKFORD and WATT, 1951) and an inhibition of diuresis was obtained by direct injection of acetylcholine (PICKFORD, 1947) or diisopropylfluorophosphate (DFP) into the supraoptic nucleus (DUKE, PICKFORD, and WATT, 1950). These experiments showed that acetylcholine stimulates the supraoptic nucleus to release vasopressin. To test whether it also causes release of oxytocin, eserine (40 μg) or DFP (40—80 μg) was injected directly into the supraoptic nucleus of anaesthetized dogs treated with stilboestrol and it was shown that this resulted in a prolonged increase of spontaneous uterine activity (ABRAHAMS and PICKFORD, 1956b). A milk-ejection response similar to that obtained with 20 mU oxytocin was produced in a lactating bitch by the intracarotid injection of 200 μg acetylcholine; the same dose given intravenously was ineffective (PICKFORD, 1960). These results, supported by the demonstration of the presence of choline acetylase (FELDBERG and VOGT, 1948; FELDBERG, 1949) and acetylcholine-esterase (ABRAHAMS, KOELLE, and SMART, 1957) in the supraoptic nucleus, provide strong evidence that a cholinergic transmitter to the supraoptic neurones is indirectly responsible for the release of both oxytocin and vasopressin. The experiments of BROOKS, ISHIKAWA, KOIZUMI, and LU (1966) provide evidence for a cholinergic transmission of impulses to the paraventricular nucleus in the milk-ejection reflex. The intracarotid injection of 40—80 μg acetylcholine produced a milk-ejection response equivalent to that produced by 5 mU oxytocin and this was accompanied by an increase in the rate of discharge recorded by microelectrodes in the neurones of the paraventricular nucleus. Stimulation of the nipple by gentle intermittent suction for 1 min elicited similar responses. All neurones in the paraventricular nucleus which were reflexly excited by stimulation of the nipple were sensitive to acetylcholine.

2. The Nicotinic Action of Acetylcholine at the Synapse

The antidiuretic, oxytocic and milk-ejection responses to acetylcholine were obtained in the presence of atropine which had been given to prevent the peripheral actions of the acetylcholine. This suggests that its central action at the supraoptic and paraventricular nuclei is nicotinic, rather than muscarinic and that nicotine itself should release oxytocin and vasopressin. BURN, TRUELOVE, and BURN (1945) demonstrated an antidiuretic action of nicotine in rats, which was abolished by hypophysectomy. They found that smoking in man had the same effect. A number of investigators have since obtained further evidence for the release of vasopressin in man by smoking or by the intravenous injection of nicotine (WALKER, 1949; BURN and GREWAL, 1951; TAYLOR and WALKER, 1951; LEWIS and CHALMERS, 1951; CHALMERS and LEWIS, 1951; BERNSTEIN, WESTON, ROSS, GROSSMAN, HANENSON, and LEITER, 1953; BISSET and LEE, 1958). Nicotine has been shown to release both vasopressin and oxytocin into the blood in rats (WALKER, 1957; BISSET and WALKER, 1957; GREWAL, LU, and ALLMARK, 1962).

To test the hypothesis put forward by WALKER (1957) that the synapse at the supraoptic nucleus is similar in its pharmacological properties to that at an autonomic ganglion, BISSET and WALKER (1957) attempted to inhibit the action of nicotine at this nucleus by means of a ganglion blocking agent. However, in rats the intraperitoneal injection of hexamethonium in doses which were sufficient to block the pressor and convulsant actions of nicotine, failed to reduce its anti-diuretic action or the release of oxytocin into the blood. Previously SUPEK and EISEN (1953) had shown that the antidiuretic and chloruretic actions of nicotine in the rat were not inhibited by tetraethylammonium or pentamethonium. The negative results must be qualified by the reservation that these quaternary ammonium compounds may not have passed the blood brain barrier and therefore not have reached the supraoptic nucleus.

CHAUDHURY (1960, 1961) investigated the action of pentolinium and other drugs on the release of oxytocin in unanaesthetized lactating rats. The release of oxytocin was assessed by measuring the increase in weight after suckling of rats separated overnight from the mother. The intraperitoneal injection of pentolinium (0.1—1.0 μg) just before suckling caused partial or complete block of the milk-ejection reflex. Since the normal milk yield could be restored by injecting oxytocin (50 mU) with pentolinium (10—50 μg), this drug apparently caused a central, and not a peripheral block. The intraperitoneal injection of acetylcholine (10 μg) 2 min before pentolinium (1 μg) partly or completely prevented its blocking action. This suggests that pentolinium blocks the milk-ejection reflex by preventing cholinergic transmission at the synapse at the supraoptic or paraventricular nuclei. However it is possible that the dose of acetylcholine required to antagonize pentolinium might itself have caused milk-ejection either by releasing endogenous oxytocin or by a direct action on the mammary gland. The significance of the block caused by pentolinium in these experiments is difficult to assess because block was produced by a large variety of other substances including atropine. It was thought unlikely however, that the block could be explained simply by an emotional inhibition of the milk-ejection reflex caused by the stress of the experiment.

3. Adrenergic Transmission at the Synapse

GROSVENOR and TURNER (1957c) have invoked an adrenergic in addition to a cholinergic component in the milk-ejection reflex. This is based on the effect of adrenolytic drugs on milk ejection in rats. It was found that if ergotamine 3 mg/kg/day was administered daily to lactating rats from the 9th to 12th day post partum, the weight gain of the litters over this period was smaller than that of control groups. This was not caused by altered nursing behaviour of the mothers or to reduced secretion of milk but was apparently due to failure of the young to obtain milk on suckling (GROSVENOR, 1956a, b). In later work a quantitative method was devised (GROSVENOR and TURNER, 1957a) for assessing milk ejection in the rat which is similar in principle to that used later by CHAUDHURY. Each litter was reduced to six young shortly after birth. At 14 days the litter was separated from the mother for 10 hours, then replaced and allowed to suckle for 30 min. The criterion used to assess milk ejection was the weight of milk obtained expressed as a percentage of the body weight of the litter. The results in control experiments followed a normal distribution and were reproducible. A single injection of ergotamine tartrate (1 mg/kg) given to the mothers 10 min before suckling caused a significant reduction in the weight gain of the litters from $3.7 \pm 0.43\%$ to $0.7 \pm 0.21\%$ (GROSVENOR and TURNER, 1956). This could have been due to a central or a peripheral block of the milk-ejection reflex. It was argued that it was not due to the peripheral vasoconstrictor effect of ergotamine, which might limit access of oxytocin to the mammary gland, because on topical application of both drugs, although ergotamine caused pronounced arteriolar constriction, oxytocin still evoked alveolar contraction. However this experiment does not exclude inhibition of the effect of endogenously released oxytocin by a vasoconstrictor effect of ergotamine administered systemically. It does appear however to exclude a direct competition between the two drugs for the receptors in the myoepithelial cells. Further evidence against a peripheral block was provided by showing that when oxytocin (0.2—0.4 U/kg) was injected 8 min after ergotamine and 2 min before suckling, a normal milk yield was obtained.

In an extension of this work (GROSVENOR and TURNER, 1957c) it was found that three different ergot preparations, methylergonovine (1—2 mg/kg), Hydergine (2—4 mg/kg) and dihydroergotamine (2—4 mg/kg) inhibited the milk-ejection reflex. Since the block could be reversed by injecting oxytocin (0.2 U/kg) after the drugs and immediately before suckling, it was apparently central in origin. The greatest inhibition was seen with methylergonovine which is the least potent of the three preparations in its adrenolytic action but causes depression of the central nervous system. On the other hand, Hydergine and dihydroergotamine inhibited milk ejection without causing central depression. Inhibition was also observed 120 min after dibenamine (60—80 mg/kg) when its adrenolytic action would be expected to have reached a peak. From these results the authors concluded that the blocking action of these drugs was specifically related to their adrenolytic action and this implicates an adrenergic component in the milk-ejection reflex. Further evidence for an adrenergic component was the finding that when reserpine (0.1 mg/kg) was injected subcutaneously into lactating rats 10 or 120 min before suckling, the milk yield obtained by the litter was significantly reduced but could be restored by injecting oxytocin (0.2 U/kg) into the mother (MOON and TURNER, 1959). This suggested that reserpine had suppressed sympathetic centres normally involved in the milk-ejection reflex. On the other hand, CHAUDHURY (1960, 1961) found that reserpine in doses of 2.5—4.0 mg/kg injected intraperitoneally into lactating rats 30—60 min before suckling did not block the milk-ejection reflex but adrenaline (1 μg) and noradrenaline (1 μg) did produce a block which was partly or completely reversed by oxytocin (50 mU).

The adrenergic component postulated by GROSVENOR and TURNER must be an excitatory one. Other work on the release of vasopressin suggests an adrenergic pathway to the supraoptic or paraventricular nucleus which is inhibitory. O'CONNOR and VERNEY (1945) found that the emotional inhibition of water diuresis in dogs (RYDIN and VERNEY, 1938) could be prevented by adrenaline which apparently acted centrally by blocking the release of vasopressin. Since the stimulus of emotional stress does not cause antidiuresis after the injection of DFP into the supraoptic nucleus (DUKE, PICKFORD, and WATT, 1951) it is probably mediated by a cholinergic mechanism. These results imply an antagonism between acetylcholine and adrenaline in the transmission of impulses at the nuclei. Such an antagonism has been demonstrated by ABRAHAMS and PICKFORD (1956a) who showed that when both drugs were given by intracarotid injection in the dog, the antidiuretic response to 200 μg acetylcholine was prevented by 1—3 μg adrenaline injected not less than 8 sec and not more than 45 sec before the acetylcholine. However in previous work (DUKE and PICKFORD, 1951) adrenaline sometimes reinforced the antidiuretic action of acetylcholine. A variable effect of this kind recalls the finding that in small doses adrenaline augments, and in large doses, inhibits transmission at autonomic ganglia (BÜLBRING and BURN, 1942).

The possibility of adrenergic transmission to the supraoptic and paraventricular nuclei is underlined by the recent histochemical demonstration of high concentrations of adrenaline and noradrenaline in these nuclei (SHUTE and LEWIS, 1966). The possible role of adrenaline in mediating emotional inhibition of the milk-ejection reflex by blocking the release of oxytocin is discussed in Section II.

4. The Actions of Central Depressants at the Synapse

Inhibition of the milk-ejection reflex by anaesthetics has been shown in the dog (GAINES, 1915; PICKFORD, 1960) the rabbit (CROSS, 1955b; CROSS and HARRIS, 1952) the cat (BEYER and MENA, 1965) and the rat (GROSVENOR and TURNER, 1957b). This inhibition is not absolute. CROSS (1958b) observed that during labour in rabbits anaesthetized with pentobarbitone sodium, the delivery of the young was sometimes accompanied by milk ejection. The anaesthetic had not blocked the reflex release of oxytocin in response to distension of the uterus (see Section V). Milk ejection in response to stimulation of the nipples or uterine distension, accompanied by increased electrical activity in the neurones of the paraventricular nucleus, has been observed in cats under chloralose anaesthesia (BROOKS, ISHIKAWA, KOIZUMI, and LU, 1966). Anaesthetics may differ in their potency in inhibiting the reflex release of oxytocin. The degree of inhibition probably depends on the strength of the stimulus. The inhibition may be caused by a block in the transmission of afferent nerve impulses to the supraoptic and paraventricular nuclei, by excitation of inhibitory pathways to these nuclei or by direct depression of the neurosecretory cells.

Ethyl alcohol is known to inhibit the release of vasopressin from the neurohypophysis. The diuresis produced by alcohol has been likened to a "transient incomplete diabetes insipidus" (VAN DYKE and AMES, 1951). Alcohol inhibited the antidiuretic response to intracarotid injections of acetylcholine in the dog (VAN DYKE and AMES, 1951) and of hypertonic saline solutions in the rat (DICKER, 1954) although it did not inhibit the antidiuretic action of nicotine in man (EGGLETON, 1949) or the release of vasopressin and oxytocin by nicotine in the rat (WALKER, 1957; BISSET and WALKER, 1957). It also did not block the release of vasopressin by haemorrhage in the rat (GINSBURG and BROWN, 1956). The effect of alcohol on the milk-ejection reflex is therefore of particular interest and has been studied in the rabbit by FUCHS and WAGNER (1963b). They measured the milk yield obtained from unanaesthetized mothers by suckling and also recorded uterine activity as an index of the amount of oxytocin released. A uterine response to suckling, which was matched by the intravenous injection of 10 mU oxytocin, was blocked by ethyl alcohol 0.8 g/kg and one equivalent to 50—100 mU oxytocin by 2.0 g/kg. The amount of milk obtained by the litter on suckling was 38.3 g without alcohol, 38.2 g after 0.8 g/kg, 27.7 g after 1.2 g/kg and only 3.6 g after 2.0 g/kg. Since the milk yield could be substantially restored by injecting oxytocin into the mother the block caused by the ethyl alcohol was central and not peripheral. Moreover since the response of the uterus to 10 mg acetylcholine given intravenously was blocked by alcohol 0.8 g/kg, the inhibition caused by alcohol appeared to involve not the afferent link of the milk-ejection reflex but the synapse itself. In post partum women the uterine response to suckling was suppressed after drinking 100 ml cognac (FUCHS and WAGNER, 1963c). A central depressant closely related to ethyl alcohol, methylpentynol, when given in a dose of 50 mg/kg by intracarotid injection, inhibited the release of both pressor and oxytocic activities in response to osmotic stimulation of the neurohypophysis in rats (DICKER, 1958). It would be interesting to test the effect of this drug on the milk-ejection reflex.

C. The Afferent Component

1. Sensory Innervation of the Mammary Gland

It has been shown convincingly in the goat that if the nerves to the mammary gland are cut, the milk-ejection reflex is abolished, although milk secretion continues (TVERSKOI, 1957; DENAMUR and MARTINET, 1959a, b). It is the sensory denervation of the gland which abolishes the reflex. The demonstration that milk could be ejected from the denervated half of an udder on milking the intact half provided essential support for the theory of ELY and PETERSEN (1941) that the efferent link of the milk-ejection reflex is humoral. The contrast between an afferent neural and an efferent humoral link is strikingly illustrated in LINZELL's experiments on transplanted mammary glands in the goat (LINZELL, 1960, 1963). Milk ejection was demonstrated in the transplant when a control gland was milked but not in the control gland when a transplant was milked.

The teat contains encapsulated and unencapsulated nerve endings (CROSS, 1961; CATHCART, GAIRNS, and GARVEN, 1949) which probably serve as sensory receptors responding to tactile and thermal stimuli during suckling or milking (CROSS, 1961). The afferent pathway from these receptors to the neurosecretory cells in the diencephalon is not known in its entirety but sections of it have been traced through the spinal cord and the brain stem.

2. Spinal Cord

DENAMUR and MARTINET (1959b) and TVERSKOI (1958) showed in the goat, and MENA and BEYER (1963) in the rabbit, that the milk-ejection reflex is abolished by section of the spinal cord. EAYRS and BADDELEY (1956) traced the pathway by which suckling maintains lactation in the rat by studying the effects of limited tractotomies on milk production. Since the injection of oxytocin into the mother caused at least a temporary restoration of the milk yield when this had ceased as a result of spinal lesions, it may be assumed that the pathway revealed by their experiments includes the afferent limb of the milk-ejection reflex. This pathway was shown to pass through the dorsal roots and to run ipsilaterally in the deep part of the lateral funiculus of the cord. Failure to trace the pathway into the brain stem by MARCHI degeneration suggested that it was unmyelinated or multisynaptic or that it was not fasciculated but widely dispersed throughout the reticular formation.

3. Brain Stem

CROSS and SILVER (CROSS ,1961) have traced the afferent pathway through the brain stem by recording milk-ejection responses to localized electrical stimulation in lactating rabbits. At the level of the midbrain, positive sites for eliciting a milk-ejection response, equivalent to that produced by the intravenous injection of >2 mU oxytocin, were found in the medial lemniscus, central grey matter and reticular formation and also rostrally in the subthalamus, supramamillary area and the mamillary peduncle. It was proposed that the afferent pathway of the milk-ejection reflex in the brain stem involves both lemniscal and reticular afferent systems passing directly to the hypothalamus without thalamic relay. Electrical stimulation of the medial leminiscus rostral to the inferior olive produced milk ejection in the goat (ANDERSSON, 1951b).

BEYER and MENA (1965) have studied the effect on established lactation in the cat of placing electrolytic lesions in the brain. Although lesions at several sites outside the diencephalon were ineffective, the milk-ejection reflex was abolished by large lesions in the caudal hypothalamus involving the whole of the periventricular region at the level of the mamillary bodies but sparing the supraoptic and paraventricular nuclei. Loss of the milk-ejection reflex was attributed to interruption of the periventricular diencephalic system of fibres which is regarded as a rostral extension of the dorsal longitudinal fasciculus or bundle of SCHULTZE. This fasciculus appears to constitute an ascending system of fibres running through the mesencephalic central grey matter and joining the hypothalamus with the lower brain stem. In the rabbit electrical stimulation of the mesencephalic central grey matter elicited evoked potentials in the supraoptic and paraventricular nuclei (Beyer, Tindal, and Sawyer, 1962). The short latency of these potentials and their resistance to anoxaemia and barbiturate anaesthesia, strongly suggested that they were mediated by direct fibres.

4. Higher Centres in the Central Nervous System

Since the milk-ejection reflex can be centrally inhibited and conditioned, afferent impulses from higher centres must impinge on the supraoptic and paraventricular nuclei. Cross and Silver (Cross, 1961) applied electrical stimulation to various regions of the telencephalon in the lactating rabbit. Milk-ejection responses were recorded after stimulation of the cingulate gyrus, the septum and the fimbria of the fornix. This suggested an efferent projection from the hippocampus to the supraoptic and paraventricular nuclei. Lesions placed in the ventral hippocampal commissure did not interfere with the natural milk-ejection reflex, but it was suggested that a functional connection between the hippocampus and these nuclei might be involved in other ways, for example, conditioning of the reflex. Elecetroencephalographic recording in conscious rabbits revealed that distinct activation patterns could be elicited in the septum, hippocampus, thalamus and cortex after suckling or manual stimulation of the teats (Holland and Cross, unpublished; Quoted by Cross, 1961). The cingulate gyrus has been implicated in other work. Stimulation of this structure in the cat has been shown to elicit milk ejection (Beyer, Anguiano, and Mena, 1961) and to excite neurones in the supraoptic nucleus from which single unit activities were recorded (Brooks, Ishikawa, and Koizumi, 1963; Koizumi, Ishikawa, and Brooks, 1964). The cingulate gyrus, the septum, the hippocampus and their interconnections form the medial division of the limbic system; according to MacLean (1958) and MacLean, Ploog, and Robinson (1960) this division is concerned with functions which are in general directed towards the reproduction and preservation of the species. The limbic system is connected through the medial forebrain bundle with the hypothalamus, the central grey matter and the reticular formation of the midbrain.

The cerebral cortex has been implicated in emotional inhibition of the milk-ejection reflex (Taleisnik and Deis, 1964). Stress induced by trauma in rats caused a reduction in the weight gain of the litter on suckling. Since this could be at least partially reversed by the injection of oxytocin, the milk-ejection reflex was centrally inhibited. Topical application of 25% KCl to the cortex to induce cortical spreading depression abolished the inhibitory effect of stress on the release of oxytocin in response to suckling.

V. Milk Ejection in Response to Stimulation of the Uterus

Milk ejection in a lactating animal serves as a useful indication of the release of oxytocin during stimulation of the neurohypophysis under physiological and experimental conditions. Ferguson (1941) advanced the theory that distension of the birth canal by the foetus during parturition augments uterine contractions by causing a reflex release of oxytocin from the neurohypophysis. Coitus is also thought to result in a reflex secretion of oxytocin which, by increasing uterine activity, speeds the transport of seminal fluid from the vagina to the uterine cavity (Harris, 1947). These theories receive strong support from the fact that milk ejection has been observed during coitus in women (Pickles, 1953; Harris and Pickles, 1953; Campbell and Petersen, 1953) in cows, (Hays and Vandemark, 1953; Campbell and Petersen, 1953) and in mares (Hammond, 1936) and during parturition — coincidentally with uterine contractions in a woman

(GUNTHER, 1948) and with expulsion of the foetuses in rabbits (CROSS, 1958b). The subject has been reviewed by CROSS (1955c) and FITZPATRICK (1957).

It is thought that the release of oxytocin during coitus and parturition is elicited by a neurohormonal reflex having the same efferent link as the milk-ejection reflex. There is experimental evidence for an afferent pathway from the uterus to the supraoptic and paraventricular nuclei. Action potentials have been recorded from the peripheral ends of the uterine nerves in the rabbit in response to mechanical stimulation of the uterus (BOWER, 1959) and evoked potentials from the region of the supraoptic nucleus in the cat in response to electrical stimulation. (ABRAHAMS, LANGWORTH, and THEOBALD, 1964). Milk ejection in response to distension of the uterus in post partum cats has been shown to be associated with an increased rate of electrical discharge in the neurones of the paraventricular nucleus (BROOKS, ISHIKAWA, KOIZUMI, and LU, 1966).

There is also evidence that milk ejection elicited by mechanical stimulation of the external genitalia is mediated by a humoral mechanism. The milk-ejection response to manual stimulation of the uterus in lactating sheep and goats (ANDERSSON, 1951a) and to vaginal distension in the lactating cow (DEBACKERE and PEETERS, 1960a) is of the same magnitude in a denervated as in the intact half of the udder. HAYS and VANDEMARK (1953) showed that massage of the vulva and cervix in lactating cows caused a rise of intramammary pressure and that blood collected after, but not before, massage caused a contraction of the excised, perfused udder similar to that obtained with oxytocin. Convincing evidence for a neurohormonal reflex is provided by the cross-circulation experiments of DEBACKERE and PEETERS (1960b, c) and DEBACKERE, PEETERS, and TUYTTENS (1961). In one series of experiments, a cross-circulation through the jugular veins was established between two lactating ewes. Vaginal distension for 40 sec in one ewe elicited, after a latent period of 35—45 sec, an increase in intracisternal pressure in the udder of the second ewe. This response could be elicited repeatedly. The pressure curves obtained after vaginal distension could be imitated by injecting 20—50 mU oxytocin into the second ewe, the latent period of the response in this case being 30 sec (DEBACKERE and PEETERS, 1960b). In another series of experiments, a cross-circulation was established between a lactating ewe and a sexually mature ram. Rectal stimulation of the ampullae and seminal vesicles of the ram for 60 or 120 sec elicited, after a latent period of 30—130 sec, a rise in intramammary pressure in the ewe which could be matched by the injection of 40—100 mU oxytocin (DEBACKERE and PEETERS, 1960c). These experiments were carried out in the conscious animal. It would be interesting to know if the release of oxytocin in response to genital stimulation, like that in response to suckling, is blocked by anaesthesia and emotional stress.

In the rabbit, cat and ferret coitus induces ovulation by reflex release of gonadotrophin. It thus appears that several reproductive functions, including coitus, parturition, suckling and in some species, ovulation, involve a neurohormonal reflex acting through the neuro- or the adenohypophysis.

VI. Milk Ejection in Response to Osmotic Stimulation of the Neurohypophysis

The physiological stimulus for the release of vasopressin is an increase in the osmotic pressure of the blood (VERNEY, 1947, 1957). The question arises whether this stimulus also releases oxytocin. Milk ejection has been observed in several species in response to the intracarotid injection of hypertonic saline (Table 2). In most of the experiments shown in the table, intravenous injections of hypertonic saline or intracarotid injections of isotonic saline were given as controls and found to be ineffective. Since both neurohypophysial hormones have milk-ejecting activity (see Section X), a part or the whole of the milk-ejection response observed in these experiments could have been due to vasopressin released by osmotic stimulation. PICKFORD's experiments, however, were carried out on water-loaded

Table 2. *Milk ejection in response to intracarotid injection of hypertonic saline*

Species	Anaesthetic	Saline Solution Vol (ml)	Molarity (M)	Duration of injection (sec)	Amount of intravenous oxytocin matching response (mU)	Ref.
Goat	None	20—60	0.684—1.368	10—30	—	1
Dog	Thiopentone	3—5	1.7	?	15[1]	2
Rabbit	Ether and curare	0.5	1.7	1	1	3
		1.0	1.7	1	>10	3
Cat	Chloralose	1	1	10—15	2—3	4
Rabbit	Ether and curare a)	2—4	0.5	2—4	?	5
	Ether and curare b)	1—3	0.5	1—7	2—8	6
		0.5—3.0	1.5	1—7	3—20	6

[1] Injection of hypertonic saline matched 15 mU oxytocin in enabling pups to make maximal weight gain on suckling.

References: 1. ANDERSSON (1951a); 2. PICKFORD (1960); 3. SUNDSTEN and SAWYER (1961); 4. BROOKS, ISHIKAWA, KOIZUMI, and LU (1966); 5. HOLLAND, CROSS and SAWYER (1958); 6. HOLLAND, CROSS and SAWYER (1959a).

dogs and the antidiuresis resulting from the intracarotid injection of hypertonic saline provided a measure of the amount of vasopressin released. This was too small to account for the milk-ejection response. It was concluded that in the dog, osmotic stimulation of the neurohypophysis, in common with suckling and the intracarotid injection of acetylcholine, releases both hormones in the ratio of about 1 part of vasopressin to 30 parts of oxytocin.

Correlation of EEG patterns with milk-ejection responses in the rabbit suggested that the osmoreceptors responding to hypertonic saline might be in or close to the olfactory tubercle (HOLLAND, CROSS, and SAWYER, 1959b). However, SUNDSTEN and SAWYER (1961) showed that milk ejection was still produced by osmotic stimulation in rabbits in which, after resection of most of the brain, only a hypothalamic island containing the supraoptic nuclei remained. This suggests that the milk ejection results from direct stimulation of neurosecretory cells in the supraoptic nuclei. Further evidence in favour of this view is that barbiturate anaesthesia, which would be expected to block the transmission of impulses to the nuclei from other parts of the brain, does not abolish the milk-ejection response to hypertonic saline (ANDERSSON, 1951a; HOLLAND, CROSS, and SAWYER, 1959a; PICKFORD, 1960). An action on the nerve endings in the neurohypophysis is unlikely since hypertonic solutions do not release vasopressin from the isolated pituitary gland (DOUGLAS and POISNER, 1964a).

An examination of Table 2 suggests that the rapid injections of relatively large amounts of hypertonic saline which were required to elicit milk-ejection responses would have caused a far greater increase in the osmotic pressure of the blood than could occur under physiological conditions. For example, in the dog 3—5 ml of 1.7 M NaCl was injected. VERNEY (1947) calculated that the intracarotid injection of 2.0 ml of 1.7 M NaCl in 10 sec in the dog would raise the osmotic pressure of carotid blood by 113%. By giving intracarotid infusions of hypertonic saline over a period of 40 min it was shown that an increase of only 1.8% in the osmotic pressure of carotid blood would cause a 95% inhibition of water diuresis. Similarly CROSS and GREEN (1959) estimated that the intracarotid injection of 1.0 ml of 1.5 M NaCl in 5 sec in the rabbit would roughly double the tonicity of the blood. On the other hand, changes in the frequency of discharge of single neurones in the supraoptic and paraventricular nuclei without an observable effect on milk ejection (CROSS, 1961) could be produced by the intracarotid injection of hypertonic solutions which were estimated to increase the osmotic pressure of the blood by less than 1%.

Hypertonic saline in the concentrations used to elicit milk ejection produces widespread activation of the brain in the rabbit. This is evident from EEG recordings and pressor responses caused by stimulation of sympathetic centres. (HOLLAND, CROSS, and SAWYER, 1959b). Milk ejection may therefore result from a non-specific stimulation of the supraoptic and paraventricular nuclei. The experimental results given in Table 2 do not allow the conclusion that oxytocin is normally released with vasopressin in response to physiological increases in the osmotic pressure of the blood.

VII. Effect of Suckling on Water Diuresis in the Lactating Animal

If suckling occurs in a lactating animal during the course of a water diuresis, milk ejection is frequently accompanied by inhibition of the diuresis. This has been observed in the cow (PEETERS, COUSSENS, BOUCKAERT, and OYAERT, 1949; PEETERS and COUSSENS, 1950; PEETERS, STORMORKEN, and VANSCHOUBROEK, 1960) the rabbit (CROSS, 1950, 1951) the dog (KALLIALA, KARVONEN, and LEPPÄNEN, 1952; PICKFORD, 1960) and in women (KALLIALA and KARVONEN, 1951; THEOBALD, 1959). In the rabbit the antidiuretic response to suckling was matched by the intravenous injection of 0.4—1.0 mU vasopressin and the milk-ejection response by 50—200 mU oxytocin (CROSS, 1950, 1951). This result is often quoted as an example of the release of both hormones in a ratio of 1 part of vasopressin to 100 parts of oxytocin. However, since oxytocin has intrinsic antidiuretic activity in the rabbit equal to one hundredth of its milk-ejecting activity (BOISSONNAS, GUTTMANN, BERDE, and KONZETT, 1961) the observed antidiuresis could have been a side effect of oxytocin. This possibility was considered by CROSS. Such an explanation does not apply to the dog. In this species the estimated ratio of vasopressin to oxytocin was only 1:30 and although the milk-ejection response was matched by 15 mU oxytocin the injection of as much as 50 mU did not cause antidiuresis (PICKFORD, 1960).

THEOBALD (1959) observed that in women antidiuresis did not invariably occur in response to suckling and that when it did occur the onset was often delayed for 10—15 min after suckling commenced. Similar observations have been made in the rabbit and in cows. In well-hydrated goats, milking was accompanied only occasionally by antidiuresis although the quantity of milk withdrawn was about the same as under normal conditions (PEETERS and DEBACKERE, 1963). GAITAN, COBO, and MIZRACHI (1964) found that on 24 occasions when suckling occurred and on 11 when the mammary duct was dilated in one breast in lactating women, an increase in intramammary pressure was observed in the other breast without any antidiuresis. A possible interference by oxytocin with the renal response to vasopressin was excluded.

The occasional concurrence of milk ejection and antidiuresis has been used as an argument in favour of the theory that, even if a particular stimulus is appropriate to the release of one or other hormone, both oxytocin and vasopressin are invariably released simultaneously (HARRIS and PICKLES, 1953; PICKFORD, 1960;

DICKER, 1961). On the contrary the frequent dissociation of milk ejection and antidiuresis argues in favour of independent mechanisms of release.

VIII. The Site and Mode of Action of Oxytocin on the Mammary Gland

A. Site of Action

As early as 1915 GAINES clearly recognized that the action of posterior pituitary extract on the mammary gland was concerned not with milk secretion but with the ejection of preformed milk. The secreted milk is held up in the alveoli and smaller ducts of the mammary gland, as in the interstices of a sponge, presumably because of the viscosity of the milk and the collapsibility of the ducts. Some contractile force is obviously needed to expel the milk into the larger ducts and cisterns from which it can be passively withdrawn. That contraction of the alveoli does occur during milk ejection can be seen by comparing the histological appearances of a gland fixed while distended with milk and a gland which has been milked out (Fig. 1). However, when ELY and PETERSEN (1939, 1941) formulated their theory that milk ejection was produced by a reflex release of oxytocin there was no general agreement about the nature of the contractile mechanism within the mammary gland on which oxytocin might be supposed to act. In this sense, therefore, their theory was incomplete. Three possible sites of action of oxytocin within the mammary gland are the blood vessels, smooth muscle and myoepithelium.

1. Blood Vessels

In an exhaustive review of the literature HAMMOND (1936) came to the conclusion that stimulation of the nipple by suckling or milking produced erection in the udder similar to that which occurs through vascular engorgement in other reproductive organs on tactile stimulation and that this erection caused compression of the alveoli and ducts resulting in milk ejection. Such a theory can be disproved by showing that mechanical compression of the venous outflow from a perfused mammary gland does not cause milk ejection although this can be produced by an injection of oxytocin into the artery supplying the gland (PEETERS, SIERENS, and SILVER, 1952; LINZELL, 1950, 1952).

2. Smooth Muscle

SWANSON and TURNER (1941) claimed to have demonstrated the presence of smooth muscle elements surrounding the alveoli in the mammary gland of the cow and suggested that contraction of these elements could expel milk from the alveoli into the ducts. It now seems likely that what they observed were myoepithelial cells which could not have been distinguished from smooth muscle cells by the staining technique used in their study.

RICHARDSON (1947, 1949, 1950a, b) and LINZELL (1952) investigated the distribution of smooth muscle in the mammary gland of the goat and other species. Smooth muscle is most concentrated in association with the major blood vessels. It is found also in the teat and nipple where circular fibres act as sphincters and in the walls of the gland cistern, but there are no sphincters in the ducts. Scattered bundles of smooth muscle occur in connective tissue septa between the lobules of the gland but there are no smooth muscle fibres interspersed between the alveoli or along the course of the intralobular ducts. It is clear, therefore, from its distribution alone that smooth muscle cannot function to eject milk from the alveoli and smaller ducts.

PEETERS (1948) and PEETERS, MASSART, OYAERT, and COUSSENS (1948) showed that the muscle of the teat in the cow undergoes rhythmical contractions at the time

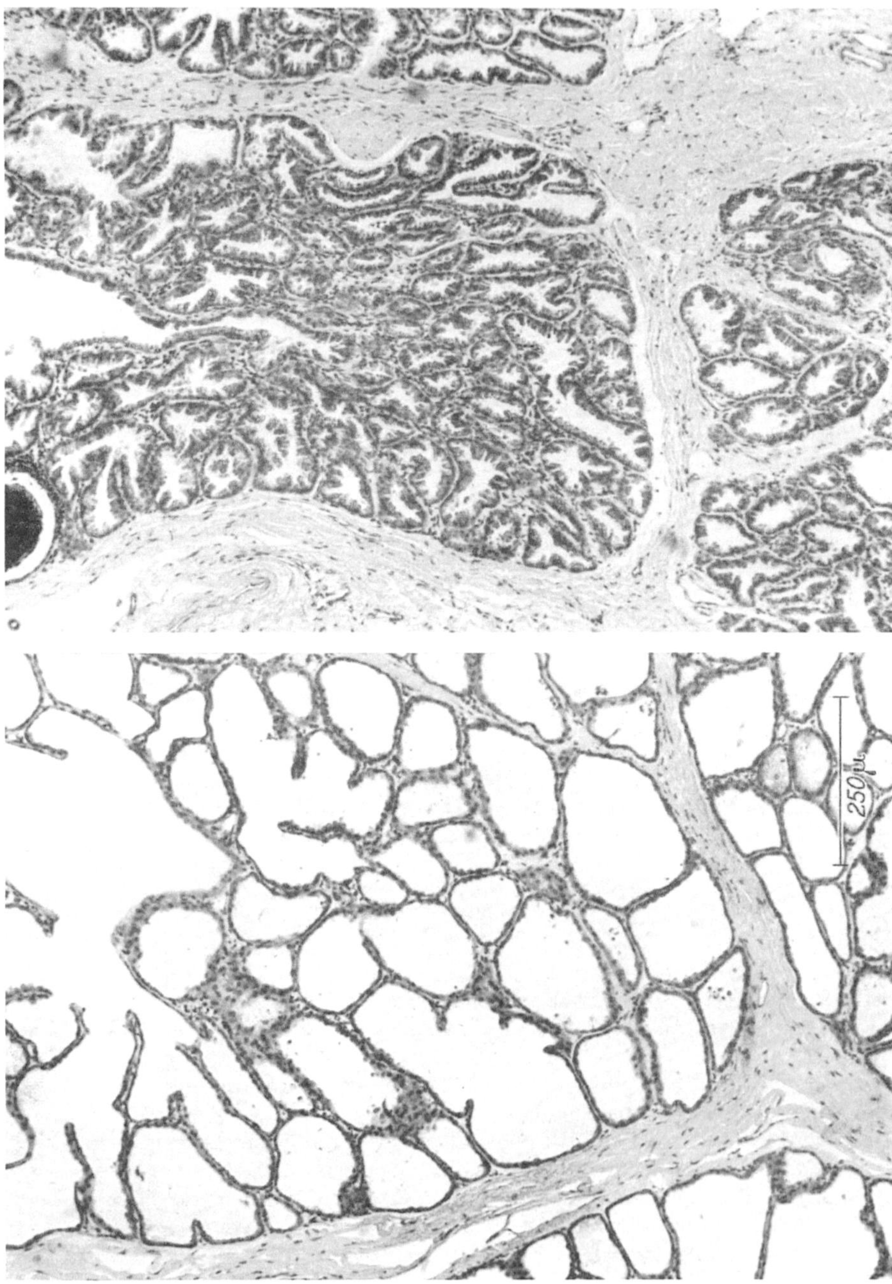

Fig. 1. (A) Part of the lobule from the left half of a goat's udder fixed while distended with milk. (B) The right half of the udder from the same goat as (A) which was milked out as completely as possible before fixation. Note the contracted lobules with collapsed alveoli and ducts lined with a thick folded epithelium. Figs. A and B are at the same magnification. From K.C. RICHARDSON, Proc. Roy. Soc. B., *136*, 30—45, (1949) (Figs. 15 and 17, plate 4). Reproduced by kind permission of the author and the Royal Society

of milk ejection and that it contracts in response to posterior pituitary extract (Pituitrin). However, TVERSKOI (1955a) found that even in high concentrations, Pituitrin had no significant effect on isolated sections cut from the large ducts, cistern and teat sphincters of the mammary gland of the cow, although they contracted in response to acetylcholine and adrenaline. Smooth muscle in these structures might therefore be under the control of the efferent nerves to the gland but not of oxytocin.

3. *Myoepithelium*

As long ago as 1894 BENDA described myoepithelial cells lying between the epithelium and the basement membrane in both sweat glands and the mammary gland and he suggested that these cells were contractile. Myoepithelium occurs also in the lachrymal glands and it was thought by BABKIN (1944) to be the only contractile tissue in salivary glands. It is now considered to be the site of action of

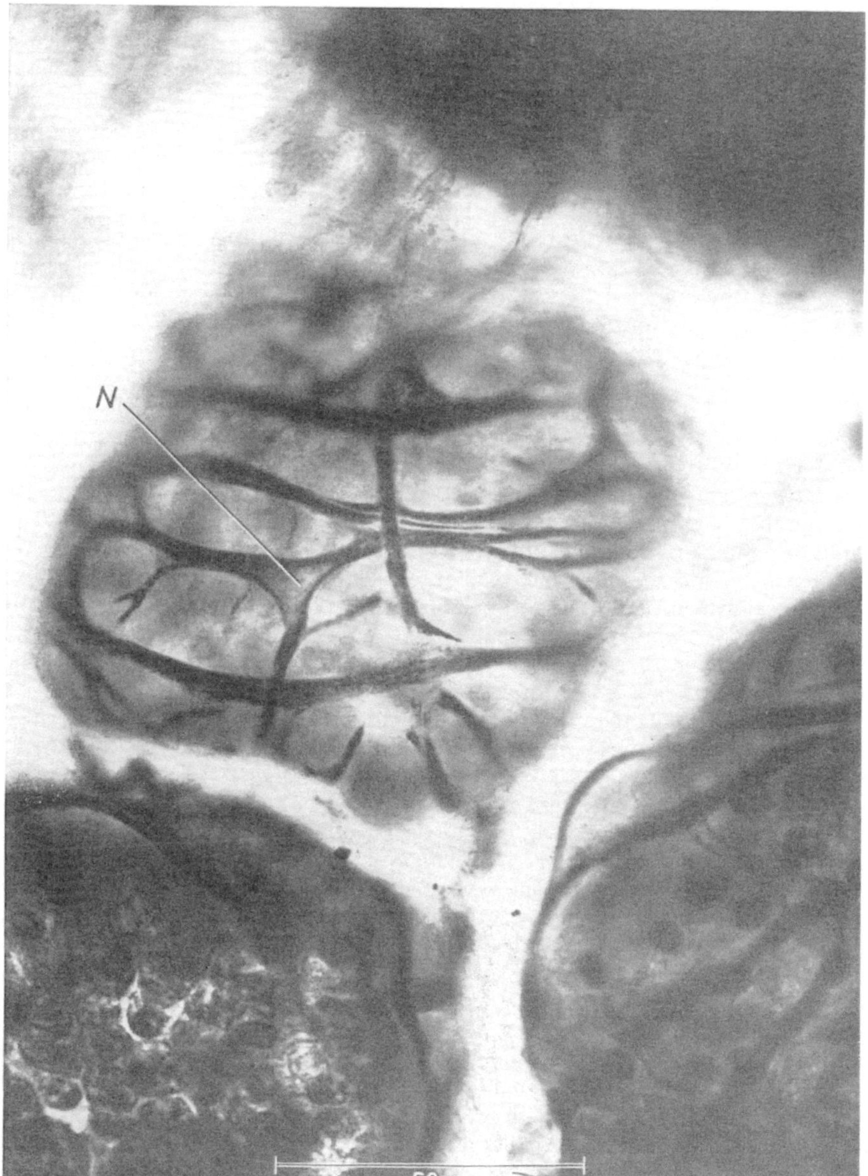

Fig. 2. Silver impregnated section of lactating mammary gland of goat. A small contracted alveolus in surface view, showing a myopethelial cell with nucleus (N) and branching processes. From K.C. RICHARDSON, Proc. Roy. Soc. B., *136*, 30—45, (1949) (Fig. 12, plate 3). Reproduced by kind permission of the author and the Royal Society

oxytocin in the mammary gland, but convincing evidence for this view was not obtained until 1947 when RICHARDSON discovered the technique of silver impregnation for selectively staining myoepithelial cells in 50— 100 μ sections of the mammary gland. According to the description given by RICHARDSON (1947, 1949, 1950a, b) for the goat, the myoepithelial cells lie inside the basement membrane, closely applied to the stromal surface of the alveoli. They may be spindle shaped or stellate with branching processess extending from the central cell body (Fig. 2) and forming an irregular network, but probably not a syncytium, over the surface of the alveoli. The cells spread in continuity over the intralobular ducts on which they are arranged spirally or longitudinally (see Fig. 3a). The myoepithelium extends to the cisterns and teat ducts. RICHARDSON observed that the processess of the myoepithelial cells were shorter and thicker over contracted alveoli (as in Fig. 1b) than over distended alveoli (as in Fig. 1a; see also Fig. 3a). Moreover, the processes were parallel to the folds of epithelium in the contracted alveoli and did not lie passively across their surface. This orientation suggested that the folds in the alveoli had been produced by an active contraction of the myoepithelial cells which embraced them. LINZELL (1952, 1959) who also used the technique of silver impregnation, independently confirmed RICHARDSON's results on goats and extended the observations to other species including man, the dog, cat, rabbit and rat. He reported that there is no visible nerve supply to the myoepithelial cells. This is consistent with the idea that milk ejection is a humoral mechanism and can be elicited reflexly in denervated or transplanted udders. He noted also that the capillaries are in close apposition to the myoepithelial cells over the alveoli and ducts, so that oxytocin reaching these cells in the blood stream might be expected to affect them almost simultaneously. DEMPSEY, BUNTING, and WISLOCKI (1947) argued against a contractile function of myoepithelial cells and suggested that they might act as a relay system for the transmission of substances from one place to another in the gland. This view was largely based on an observation that in the rat these cells showed an alkaline phosphatase activity which, while pronounced in the developing gland, was only slight in the lactating gland. However SILVER (1954) demonstrated alkaline phosphatase activity in myoepithelial cells of lactating mammary glands from rabbits, sheep and rats.

The longitudinal arrangement of the myoepithelial cells along the finer intralobular ducts which was observed by RICHARDSON, LINZELL, and SILVER is of functional significance. RICHARDSON (1947, 1950b) suggested that contraction of these cells would tend to shorten and widen the ducts and this would aid in the expulsion of milk from the alveoli. On the basis of measurements of intramammary pressure in the sow and cow, WHITTLESTONE (1950b) suggested that when the milk-ejecting hormone acts on the mammary gland it causes contraction of the myoepithelial cells surrounding both the alveoli and the smaller ducts. This results in an opening of the ducts simultaneously with an increase of pressure in the alveoli. The fall in resistance in the smaller ducts would permit a rapid flow of milk into the larger ducts and cisterns. Direct evidence in favour of this mechanism of action, which is illustrated diagramatically in Fig. 3a, has been obtained by LINZELL (1954, 1955) from experiments in which the exposed mammary glands of lactating mice, rats, guinea-pigs and rabbits were examined *in situ* under the microscope. After topical application of oxytocin and of a number of drugs which stimulate smooth muscle the alveoli were seen to contract and the milk contained within them was squeezed into the ducts (Fig. 3b). Although dilatation of the ducts was observed this could have resulted from passive distension with milk ejected from the alveoli. To avoid this possibility, further experiments were carried out on involuted glands in the mouse in which the alveoli were empty but the ducts still contained milk and were visible. The ducts were photographed with a micrometer eyepiece and the width measured at intervals of 100 μ along the length of the duct. LINZELL (1955) was able to show that the topical application of oxytocin caused a statistically significant increase in the mean width of the ducts

A

B

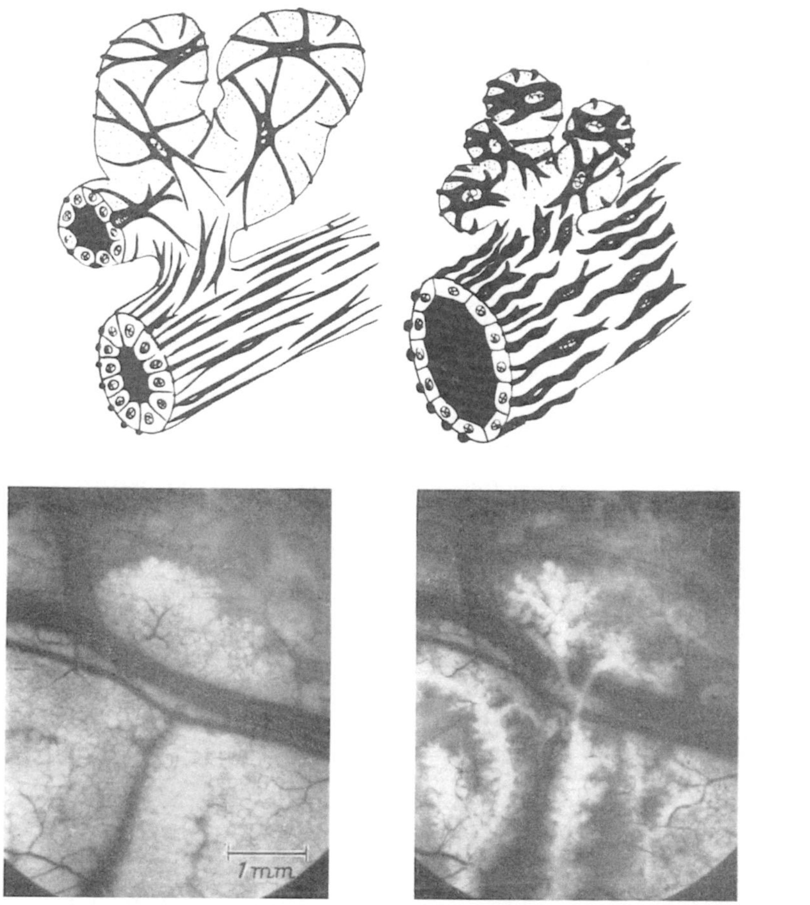

Fig. 3. (A) Disposition of myoepithelial cells (black) around alveoli and ducts. Left: myoepithelial cells relaxed, alveoli full. Right: myoepithelial cells contracted, alveoli emptied, ducts widened. (B) Milk ejection in living mammary tissue of mouse. Left: before, and Right: just after ,dropping oxytocin 0.01 mU on the surface of the tissue. Each alveolus appears as a white spot. From J. L. LINZELL, Veterinary Annual, *1961*, pp 44—53 (Recent Advances in the Physiology of the Udder — plate 13). Reproduced by kind permission of the author and the publishers, Messrs. John Wright & Sons Ltd.

which also straightened and shortened, the length decreasing by 8—10%. LEVITSKAYA (1955) has also observed contraction of the alveoli and dilatation of the ducts on topical application of oxytocin to the mammary gland of the mouse observed microscopically *in situ*.

Electron microscopy of human myoepithelial cells has provided further evidence for a contractile function. The cytoplasm was seen to contain bundles of filaments having a diameter of 40—80 Å which were identical with myofilaments in smooth muscle and so disposed that their contraction would alter the conformation of the basement membrane (LANGER and HUHN, 1958).

B. Mode of Action

A drug may stimulate smooth muscle to contract by causing excitation through an effect on the cell membrane or by a direct action on the contractile mechanism. One method of determining the mode of action is to test the effect of a drug on isolated smooth muscle in which membrane function has been temporarily suspended by calcium deficiency or by depolarization with an excess of potassium (CSAPO, 1954). This method has been applied effectively to the action of oxytocin on the uterus. It was first shown in 1960 by MÉNDEZ-BAUER, CABOT, and CALDEYRO-BARCIA that an isolated strip of mammary gland suspended in Tyrode's solution will develop contractile tension in response to oxytocin. From the evidence given in the previous section it may be assumed that the contractile tissue on which oxytocin acts in the isolated gland is the myoepithelium. Experiments have been carried out recently on the isolated mammary gland of both the rabbit and the rat, analogous to those on the rat uterus, to test the effect of depolarization on the response to oxytocin.

MOORE and ZARROW (1965) showed that when sodium was replaced by potassium in the Tyrode's solution, the response of a strip of isolated rabbit mammary gland to oxytocin although not abolished, decreased exponentially with time. The decrease was reversed in normal Tyrode's solution. When calcium was omitted from the Tyrode's solution, the strip eventually became inexcitable; the excitability was restored by adding calcium. COUTHINO and CSAPO (1959) and CSAPO (1961) had previously found that the isolated rabbit uterus depolarized by excess potassium or calcium deficiency would not respond to oxytocin although it could still be stimulated to give an almost maximal response by a strong electric field. They concluded that oxytocin and other oxytocic drugs regulate membrane function and do not directly activate the contractile mechanism of uterine smooth muscle. Similarly, MOORE, and ZARROW concluded from their results that oxytocin acts upon the membrane of the myoepithelial cells in the mammary gland.

In experiments on isolated strips of rat mammary gland, POLÁČEK, KREJČÍ, and RUDINGER (personal communication) found that as the calcium concentration in the Tyrode's solution was lowered the response to oxytocin decreased progressively and was finally abolished. The decline in response was accelerated by adding Na_2 EDTA (0.25 mM) to the solution. Strontium could substitute at least partially for calcium; when the response to oxytocin had been abolished by substituting calcium-free for normal Tyrode's solution, the addition of strontium itself caused an increase in tension of the strip and oxytocin then induced a further increase in tension which, although somewhat smaller, was similar qualitatively to that produced by the same dose of oxytocin in the original Tyrode's solution. The response of the isolated rat uterus to oxytocin is reduced or abolished by calcium deficiency (BERGER and MARSHALL, 1961; MARSHALL and CSAPO, 1961; KURIYAMA and CSAPO, 1961) and again strontium can substitute for calcium (DANIEL, SEHDEV, and ROBINSON, 1962). POLÁČEK et al. observed that when K_2SO_4-Ringer's solution was substituted for Tyrode's solution, the excess potassium itself produced a depolarization contracture of the isolated strip of rat mammary gland. This contracture occurred only in the presence of a normal concentration of calcium and the addition of strontium to calcium-free KCl-Ringer's solution caused a contracture. In all these respects, similar results have been observed with the isolated rat uterus (EVANS and SCHILD, 1957; EDMAN and SCHILD, 1961a, b, 1962; DURBIN and JENKINSON, 1961; DANIEL et al., 1962).

In contrast with the results obtained by MOORE and ZARROW with the rabbit mammary gland, POLÁČEK et al. (pers. comm.) found that when strips of rat mammary gland were suspended in K_2SO_4-Ringer's solution, the responses to oxytocin were not diminished compared with those obtained in normal Tyrode's solution. The isolated rat uterus suspended in K_2SO_4-Ringer's solution also responds to oxytocin (EVANS and SCHILD, 1957; EVANS, SCHILD, and THESLEFF, 1958; BERGER and MARSHALL, 1961; DANIEL et al., 1962). If it is assumed that the excess potassium causes complete depolarization (see BERGER and MARSHALL, 1961) it seems that in the rat at least, oxytocin can activate the contractile elements in the myoepithelium of the mammary gland as well as in the smooth muscle of the uterus without the mediation of membrane depolarization. Calcium appears to be an essential link between excitation and contraction in both polarized and depolarized rat uterine muscle; it has been suggested that drugs may activate depolarized muscle by releasing calcium bound at the cell surface or by increasing permeability to calcium ions (EDMAN and SCHILD, 1962; DANIEL et al., 1962). The same mechanism may explain the action of oxytocin on myoepithelial cells depolarized by excess potassium. It is interesting to note that the mammary gland and the uterus show the same species differences between the rat and rabbit in the effects of ions.

That oxytocin acts on the cell membrane of uterine muscle in the rat has been shown by electrophysiological techniques. JUNG (1961) found that the intravenous injection of 10 mU oxytocin produced a repetitive discharge of spike potentials recorded from the surface of the uterus *in situ* which was accompanied by a contraction. Recording with intracellular microelectrodes (KURIYAMA and CSAPO, 1961; CSAPO, 1961) or with the sucrose gap method (MARSHALL and CSAPO, 1961) has shown that oxytocin either raises or lowers the membrane potential to an optimal level, and increases the frequency of the action potential and the duration of the train of discharges. Similar methods might be used to investigate the action of oxytocin on the membrane potential and action potentials of myoepithelial cells in the lactating mammary gland although the technical difficulty would probably be considerable.

There is an interesting parallel between the mammary gland and other tissues in the effect of magnesium on the response to oxytocin and vasopressin. Magnesium has been shown to potentiate the response to oxytocin or vasopressin or to both hormones of the isolated rat uterus (MUNSICK, 1960; MUNSICK and JERONIMUS, 1965) the isolated guinea pig uterus CLEGG, HOPKINSON, and PICKLES, 1963) and isolated human umbilical veins, canine arteries and strips of rabbit mammary gland (SOMLYO, WOO, and SOMLYO, 1966). When the strips of mammary gland were suspended in a Mg free bath solution, and the increase in tension caused by oxytocin and vasopressin had reached a plateau, the addition of Mg (1.2 mM) caused a secondary increase in tension from 0.2—14 times the original response. A figure in the paper by SOMLYO et al. shows that vasopressin (400 mU/ml) failed to cause a contraction in Mg-free Tyrode's solution but a contraction did occur when Mg (1.2 mM) was added. The authors concluded that potentiation by Mg was a general property of the action of neurohypophysial hormones on contractile tissues. They suggested that a possible action of magnesium was to induce conformational changes in the membrane which led to a greater affinity of the hormones for the tissue receptors. On the other hand, POLÁČEK et al. (pers. comm.) found that magnesium, unlike strontium, was unable to restore the contractile response to oxytocin of the isolated strips of rat mammary gland suspended in Ca-free solution.

In summary the myoepithelium of the mammary gland shows many similarities to smooth muscle in its response to neurohypophysial hormones despite the difference in structure between the two tissues, and in embryological origin, the one being derived from ectoderm and the other from mesoderm. Sensitivity to oxytocin appears to be a specialized property of the myoepithelium of the mammary gland. For example it has been shown that oxytocin does not stimulate the myoepithelium of sweat glands in the cow (FINDLAY and ROBERTSHAW, 1965).

IX. Analysis of the Milk-Ejecting Activity of Oxytocin in Different Species

This section gives an analysis of the action of oxytocin on the mammary gland classified according to species and the method of investigation. The actions of a number of other drugs will be contrasted with that of oxytocin. Vasopressin and adrenaline are considered separately in later sections.

A. Observation of Milk Ejection and Measurement of Milk Yield in the Intact Animal

In some species the injection of oxytocin into the lactating animal results in a visible ejection of milk from the mammary gland. In women this provides a rapid and simple means of determining the threshold dose of oxytocin by different routes of injection. In large domestic animals such as the cow and sow it is a simple procedure to measure the total yield of milk and the rate or duration of milk ejection in response to suckling or to an injection of oxytocin.

1. Man

NICKERSON, BONSNES, DOUGLAS, CONDLIFFE, and DU VIGNEAUD (1954) found that in lactating women in the early puerperium the milk-ejection response to oxytocin could be easily recognized by the appearance of a bead of milk at the breast or by dripping or streaming of milk from the nipple. Consistent responses were obtained with 2 U oxytocin injected intramuscularly or 0.5 U intravenously; one patient responded to 0.1 U intravenously. The latent period between the completion of injection and the response was 15—60 sec by the intravenous and 40—60 sec by the intramuscular, route. The milk-ejecting activity of synthetic oxytocin was indistinguishable from that of highly purified natural oxytocin. This established the fact that milk-ejecting activity is inherent in the molecular structure of oxytocin and laid the foundation for the therapeutic application of this property of the hormone. BELLER, KRUMHOLZ, and ZEININGER (1958) observed milk-ejection responses in women to intravenous injections of only 0.01 U oxytocin.

THEOBALD (1959) observed in lactating women that suckling from one breast invariably caused milk to escape from the nipple of the other breast and that this effect could be matched within $1^1/_2$—3 min by a single intravenous injection of 5—10 mU oxytocin or by its intravenous infusion at the rate of 0.2—1 mU/min.

2. Cow

In the work on which ELY and PETERSEN (1941) based their concept of the milk-ejection reflex, cows were milked by machine and the weight of the milk yield was recorded at intervals of 15 sec. By plotting weight against time, curves were obtained showing the effect of adrenaline and of neurohypophysial hormones on the rate of milk ejection. Using a milk-flow recording apparatus WHITTLESTONE (1946, 1951) studied the characteristics of the milk-ejection curves of normal dairy cows under standard milking conditions throughout lactation. Such studies are of obvious value in applying the theory of the milk-ejection reflex to the practical problem of obtaining maximum milk yields.

Peeters, Stormorken, and Vanschoubroek (1960) measured the volumes of milk-ejected from the left forequarter after intravenous injection of 20—1000 mU oxytocin. The dose-response curve obtained by plotting log-dose against milk volume was a straight line within a wide range. In cows weighing about 450 kg, the threshold dose of oxytocin was about 20 mU.

Labouche (1957) observed that in a tropical climate, cows will deliver on milking only a small fraction ($<8\%$) of the total available milk yield, but milk ejection can be induced by the intravenous injection of oxytocin. The volume of milk ejected, expressed as a percentage of the full yield, was related to the dose of oxytocin within the two ranges of 0—0.2 U and 0.5—1.5 U. The threshold dose of oxytocin was between 0.007 and 0.04 U. The amount of milk obtained by a calf on suckling corresponded with that of an intravenous injection of 0.2 U oxytocin; this represents an estimate of the quantity of hormone normally released from the neurohypophysis by the milk-ejection reflex in the cow.

3. Sow

For experimental work the sow offers a number of advantages (Braude and Mitchell, 1950; Whittlestone, 1950a, 1952). In the cow the interpretation of milk-ejection curves is complicated by factors such as the tension in the teat sphincter, the large size of the cistern in the udder and the rate of flow of milk through the large ducts into the cistern (Whittlestone, 1952). In the sow there is no cistern and only a small pressure difference across the sphincter is required before milk will flow. After an injection of oxytocin milk trickles freely from the teat; the flow starts and stops abruptly so that the duration of flow can be measured precisely. The yield can be measured by hand or machine milking.

Braude and Mitchell (1950) gave four sows a series of daily injections of 1, 3, 5, and 10 U oxytocin intravenously over a period of 4 weeks, each sow receiving a total of six injections of each dose. The sows were hand milked. Both the yield of milk and the duration of milk flow were found to be related to the dose of oxytocin. The mean yields per udder were 41 ml for 1 U, 78 ml for 3 U, 82 ml for 5 U, and 104 ml for 10 U and the corresponding mean durations of flow 80, 131, 135 and 179 sec.

Whittlestone, Bassett, and Turner (1952) found that the threshold dose of oxytocin for eliciting milk ejection in the sow was 0.02—0.03 U intravenously. The yield produced by 1.5—2 U was comparable with that obtained during natural suckling (Smith, Whittlestone, and Allen, 1951). Whittlestone (1952) developed a quantitative method for the assay of oxytocin by its milk-ejecting activity in the sow. All glands but one were milked by machine to determine the total milk yield; the remaining gland was milked by hand to measure the duration of milk ejection. The assays were carried out one hour after natural suckling. When nine successive injections of 0.5 U oxytocin were given intravenously at intervals of 5 min the yield varied from 43—72 g and the duration declined from 34 sec for the first to 12 sec for the last injection. Duration of flow was found to be a more consistent parameter than total yield. Normally assays were carried out by giving four injections at 5 min intervals in any one experiment and adjusting the amount of the unknown to give a response equal to that of a fixed dose of standard. This method of assay was used to demonstrate milk-ejecting activity in the protein isolated from the pars nervosa of the ox by van Dyke, Chow, Greep, and Rothen (1942) and to obtain one of the first reliable estimates of the intrinsic milk-ejecting activity of vasopressin (Whittlestone, 1952).

Whittlestone and Turner (1952) observed that acetylcholine (0.2—0.3 g) and carbachol (0.1—0.2 mg) caused milk ejection on intravenous injection into the lactating sow, but the responses were not consistent and the relationship between milk yield and duration of flow was different from that observed with oxytocin. Since the latent period between injection and response was the same for acetylcholine and oxytocin it was argued that acetylcholine acted directly on the mammary gland rather than by releasing oxytocin from the neurohypophysis.

B. Measurement of the Weight Gain of Litters and Estimation of the Amount of Oxytocin Released by Suckling

The release of oxytocin in response to the natural stimulus of suckling is blocked by anaesthesia. The injection of oxytocin into the anaesthetized mother to induce milk ejection, enables the young to obtain milk on suckling. The amount obtained can be determined from the difference in weight of the litter before and after suckling or from the weight of the stomach contents. That dose of oxytocin which on intravenous injection into the anaesthetized mother allows the young to make a normal weight gain, gives an indication of the amount of hormone normally released by suckling.

1. Rat

A quantitative method has been developed in this species (Grosvenor and Turner, 1957a). The litters are reduced to six shortly after birth. When 14 days old, they are isolated from the mothers for 10 hours. At the end of this time, the stomachs are empty and the litters are replaced and allowed to suck for 30 min. After suckling, the litters are killed and the stomach contents weighed. With a series of 40 unanaesthetized lactating rats, it was found that the weight of milk obtained by the litters expressed as a percentage of the litter weight showed a normal distribution with a mean of 3.8 ± 0.19. When sodium pentobarbitone (3 mg/100 g) was injected into the mothers 10—20 min before the end of the isolation period the milk-ejection reflex was blocked. The intravenous injection of oxytocin a few minutes after nursing commenced induced milk ejection; the flow commenced after a latent period of 5—10 sec and lasted 4—5 min. Doses of 0.02, 0.05 and 0.1 U/kg produced percentage weight gains by the litters of 3.0 ± 0.82, 3.8 ± 0.20 and 5.9 ± 0.45, respectively. It was concluded that the average amount of oxytocin released on suckling is 0.05 U/kg with a range of < 0.02—0.1 U/kg (Grosvenor and Turner, 1957b). This technique has been used as an assay method for comparing the milk-ejecting activity of natural and synthetic oxytocin (Grosvenor and Turner, 1958a).

2. Dog

The intravenous injection of 15—20 mU oxytocin into bitches anaesthetized with sodium thiopentone enabled the pups to make a maximal weight gain on suckling (Pickford, 1959, 1960). The injection of 10 mU produced half the maximal weight gain or less and 5 mU no gain. In another experiment on a conscious animal which never voluntarily gave milk under observation and did not therefore require an anaesthetic to block the milk-ejection reflex, it was found that when one pup was allowed to suck one gland for at least 6 min during the first 3 weeks of lactation, an injection of 15—20 mU oxytocin into the mother permitted a maximal weight gain by the pup. During the 4th and 5th weeks of lactation, the amount of oxytocin required in the same animal was only 5 mU; this suggests that during the course of lactation, there is an increase in the sensitivity of the myoepithelial cells to oxytocin.

3. Rabbit

Cross (1955b) found that from mothers anaesthetized with sodium pentobarbitone, the young could not obtain more than 15% of the normal yield of milk: this fraction probably represents the amount that can be obtained in the rabbit by passive withdrawal. The intravenous injection of 50 mU oxytocin into the mother restored the normal yield; doses of 10 and 20 mU were insufficient. Cross obtained further evidence that the amount of oxytocin normally released in the rabbit by the milk-ejection reflex is of the order of 50 mU. In a conscious rabbit in which the restraint imposed by the experimental procedure did not cause any emotional inhibition of the milk-ejection reflex, he allowed the young to suck at some teats while he simultaneously recorded a milk-ejection response from a cannulated duct in another teat. The response to suckling was matched by the intravenous injection of 50 mU oxytocin. It is interesting to compare this finding with the following result which was also obtained in the conscious rabbit but by a different method (Fuchs and Wagner, 1963a). The release of oxytocin during natural suckling was estimated by matching the oxytocic response, recorded from an intrauterine balloon, against an intravenous injection of oxytocin. It was concluded that in the early puerperium, each young evokes the release of 0.5—1 mU oxytocin, but later, in response to suckling the entire litter 50—100 mU or at the end of the period of lactation, 250 mU may be released.

C. Registration of Milk-Ejection Responses from a Cannulated Teat Duct with Volume or Pressure Recorders

The method now used most commonly for investigating the milk-ejecting activity of pharmacologically active substances is the measurement of milk-ejection pressure from a cannulated teat duct in the mammary gland. Historically, three main stages can be traced in the development of this method. First, for their classical study of the physiology of milk ejection in the lactating rabbit, Cross and Harris (1952) had to devise a means of recording milk-ejection responses to electrical stimulation of the neurohypophysis (see Section IV A, 1). This they achieved by cannulating a teat duct and connecting the cannula with a piston recorder writing on a kymograph. The cannula, partly filled with citrate solution, was mounted vertically. In response to an intravenous injection of oxytocin, milk was ejected into the cannula and a volume change recorded. As the response subsided the milk returned to the mammary gland by virtue of the hydrostatic pressure in the cannula. With this type of preparation milk-ejection responses could be elicited repeatedly in the course of a single experiment. The second stage was the replacement of volume recorders by electronic pressure transducers which are not only highly sensitive but have the important advantage that the fluid displacement accompanying changes of pressure is extremely small. In the original method described for the rabbit by van Dyke, Adamsons, and Engel (1955) milk-ejection pressure was recorded with a Sanborn electromanometer. The principle has been extended with modifications to a number of other species. The third stage was the introduction by Fitzpatrick (1961) in the rabbit of retrograde arterial injections into the mammary gland in place of intravenous injections. The increase in sensitivity with the use of this technique has permitted the detection of minute amounts of oxytocin in body fluids.

1. Characteristics of the Milk-Ejection Response to Oxytocin

Table 3 shows some parameters of the milk-ejection responses to oxytocin observed in a number of species using pressure or volume recorders. The latent

Table 3. *Characteristics of the milk-ejection response to oxytocin measured with volume or pressure recorders from a cannulated teat duct*

Species	Reference	Method of Recording	Route of Injection	Dose of oxytocin or posterior pituitary extract (mU) Threshold	Working Range	Response Latent Period (sec)	Duration (min)
Rabbit . .	CROSS and HARRIS (1952)	Piston (volume) recorder and kymograph	IVI	5	5—200	7—15	2—7
	VAN DYKE, ADAMSONS and ENGEL (1955)	Sanborn electromanometer with high-sensitivity condenser microphone	IVI	0.5	0.5—5[1]	14—21[1]	$\not>$0.5[1]
	YOKOYAMA (1956)	Tambour and kymograph	IVI	2.5—5	2.5—100	10—30	0.6—5
	BERDE and CERLETTI (1957)	Statham strain gauge transducer and mirror galvanometer recorder	IVI	$\not>$2.5[1]	—	—	$<$1[1]
	HOLLAND, CROSS, and SAWYER (1959a)	Statham strain gauge transducer and Varian recorder	IVI	1.0	1—100	12—20	0.5—4[1]
	FITZPATRICK (1961)	Prism cell volume recorder and Ever-shed Vignoles recording voltmeter	IVI	2—10	—	—	—
			RAI	0.075—0.3 (mean 0.149)	—	ca 15[1]	—
Guinea-pig	LINZELL (1955)	Volume recorder and kymograph	IVI	1.5 (1—2)	—	—	ca 2
	BISSET (1962a, 1964)	Statham strain gauge transducer and 10″ potentiometric recorder	IVI	0.25	0.5—4	—	$<$1
			RAI[2]	0.05	0.05—0.2	—	$<$1
	TINDAL and YOKOYAMA (1962)	Statham strain gauge transducer and Grass polygraph	IVI	0.05—0.3	0.3—1.2	15	—
			RAI	0.001—0.01	0.015—0.06	5	—
Rat . .	BISSET, CLARK, HALDAR, HARRIS, LEWIS and ROCHA E SILVA (1967)	Strain gauge transducer and 10″ potentiometric recorder	IVI	0.02—0.1	0.1—0.3	—	$>$1
			RAI	0.001—0.005	0.005—0.02	4.7 $\pm$ 0.34	0.36 $\pm$ 0.015
Goat . . .	DENAMUR and MARTINET (1953)	Kymograph and ? piston recorder	IVI	0.05—0.1	0.1—10	—	1—4[1]
Sheep . .	DEBACKERE, PEETERS, and TUYTTENS (1961)	Marey tambour or piston recorder and kymograph	IVI	$\not>$15[1]	15—100	25—43	1—2[1]
Sow . . .	WHITTLESTONE (1954a, b, c)	Mercury manometer with platinum resistance and electronic recorder	IVI	50	50—600	14—29	0.25—0.75
Man . . .	SICA-BLANCO, MÉNDEZ-BAUER, SALA, CABOT, and CALDEYRO-BARCIA (1959)	Electromonometer and Sanborn Poly-Viso recorder	IVI	0.25—1	2.5—20	ca 30[1]	1[1]
	FRIEDMAN (1960)	External pressure at nipple relayed to Sanborn electromanometer	IVI	1.0	1—10	20 (mean)	0.7—1
	WIEDERMAN and STONE (1962)	Pressure transducer and Sanborn Poly-Viso recorder	IVI	2.0	2—100	20—40	1—2
	GAITAN, COBO, and MIZRACHI (1964)	Pressure transducer and Sanborn Poly-Viso recorder	IVI	0.1—2.0	0.5—40	3—30	1.3—6.2
Monkey .	BISSET and BANGHAM (unpublished)	Strain gauge transducer and 10″ potentiometric recorder	IVI	0.75	0.75—5	12—45	0.5—5
Dog . .	PICKFORD (1959, 1960)	5 ml volume recorder and kymograph	IVI	$\not>$2.5	5—25	—	—
Cat. . . .	ISHIKAWA, KOIZUMI, and BROOKS (1966)	Statham transducer and Gilson recorder	IVI	$\not>$5	5—10	—	$<$2[1]

[1] = Estimated from figures in paper. IVI = Intravenous injection
[2] = By method of TINDAL and YOKOYAMA (1962). RAI = Retrograde arterial injection

period of the response to intravenous injection of oxytocin appears to be little longer than the circulation time and with retrograde arterial injection, it is only a few seconds. The use of pressure transducers increases sensitivity and reduces the apparent duration of the responses. In routine assays with the use of transducers, injections of oxytocin can be given at intervals of only 2—3 min without inducing tachyphylaxis (BERDE and CERLETTI, 1957; TINDAL and YOKOYAMA, 1962). The threshold dose of oxytocin required to elicit a milk-ejection response in most species is very small. If body weight is taken into account, man seems to be the most sensitive species investigated. The lowest threshold dose recorded (GAITAN et al., 1964) is 0.1 mU. In a 50 kg woman this would be equivalent to about 4×10^{-12} g/kg of the pure peptide.

Several of the authors included in Table 3 have used the methods described to investigate the effect of intravenous infusions of oxytocin in the experimental animal. CROSS (1958a), using the method of CROSS and HARRIS (1952) in rabbits, found that the minimum effective rate of infusion was 6 mU/min, and this produced an oscillating or "saw-tooth" type of milk-ejection response. With rates of 12—24 mU/min, the individual contractions fused and produced a tetanic or "plateau" response. BERDE and CERLETTI (1960) described two types of response: a "tonic reaction" in which there was a maintained increase in milk-ejection pressure without significant fluctuations or a "rhythmic reaction" consisting of a series of increases of pressure at more or less regular intervals. A threshold effect was obtained with a rate of infusion of 3.3 mU/min. To match the responses produced by intravenous infusion, 1.5—8 times as much oxytocin was required by intramuscular injection and 10—100 times as much by intranasal administration. Similar patterns of response to intravenous injection of oxytocin were obtained in the rabbit by KULLANDER (1963). BERÁNKOVÁ-KSANDROVÁ, BISSET, JOŠT, KREJČÍ, PLIŠKA, RUDINGER, RYCHLÍK, and ŠORM (1966) found in the guinea-pig that the intravenous infusion of oxytocin at rates of 1—4 mU/min produced little change in the basal milk-ejection pressure but inhibited the response to small doses of oxytocin given by intravenous injection during and after the infusion (Fig. 7). In women during parturition and the puerperium, SICA-BLANCO, MÉNDEZ-BAUER, SALA, CABOT, and CALDEYRO-BARCIA (1959) observed that the intravenous infusion of oxytocin at rates of 4—8 mU/min produced a rhythmic series of increases in milk-ejection pressure which persisted until the end of the infusion. Some women responded to as little as 0.2 mU/min. Infusion at rates of 4—16 mU/min closely simulated the pattern of milk-ejection response which was recorded from one breast when the baby was suckled at the other breast.

From a therapeutic standpoint the effects of intranasal and oral administration of oxytocin to lactating women are of interest. FRIEDMAN and SACHTLEBEN (1961), using the method of FRIEDMAN (1960), found that a sublingual tablet containing 10 U oxytocin produced an increase in milk-ejection pressure in 2—10 min with the occurrence of irregular waves of contraction at intervals of 60—80 sec over a period of 20—40 min. The intranasal administration of 20 U produced a pronounced increase in pressure within 1.5—3 min which lasted only for 2 min and was followed by a period of 30 min in which the gland became refractory to oxytocin. It is probable that the dose used was excessive. WIEDERMAN and STONE (1962) found that the amount of intranasal oxytocin required to elicit an increase in milk-ejection pressure was about 200 times the intravenous dose; they obtained responses with 2 U which had a latent period of 90—130 sec and lasted for 10—15 min. In the experiments of SICA-BLANCO et al. (1959) the application for 2 sec of a nasal spray containing 40 U/ml oxytocin produced an increase in milk-ejection pressure within 1 min. This increase lasted for about

4 min and was greater than that observed after the intravenous injection of 20 mU oxytocin.

2. Contrast between the Lactating Mammary Gland and the Uterus in Situ

The response of the lactating mammary gland to oxytocin differs in several respects from that of the uterus *in situ*. The oxytocic response to an intravenous injection of oxytocin usually consists of a series of irregular contractions which can be measured quantitatively only by the use of an integrating device (BISSET, HALDAR, and LEWIN, 1966). In contrast, the response of the myoepithelial cells to oxytocin in doses within the useful range for purposes of bioassay, usually consists of a single well defined contraction with a sharp peak which permits a simple measurement of the amplitude of the response. A "multiple-response effect" in which the initial contraction is followed by a series of smaller contractions has been observed in the guinea-pig (TINDAL and YOKOYAMA, 1962) the sow (WHITTLESTONE, 1954c), the sheep (DEBACKERE, PEETERS, and TUYTTENS, 1961), man (WIEDERMAN, FREUND, and STONE, 1964), the monkey (BANGHAM and BISSET, unpublished), and the rat (BISSET, CLARK, HALDAR, HARRIS, LEWIS, and ROCHE E SILVA, 1967), but it is usually observed only after relatively large doses.

The lactating mammary gland also differs from the uterus in that it does not generally exhibit spontaneous activity, although this has been observed in conscious women (SICA-BLANCO, MÉNDEZ-BAUER, SALA, CABOT, and CALDEYRO-BARCIA, 1959; WIEDERMAN and STONE, 1962). CROSS (1958a) carried out a comparative study of uterine motility and milk-ejection pressure in the oestrogenized lactating rabbit. The threshold dose of oxytocin was the same (1—5 mU) for eliciting an increase in uterine activity or in milk-ejection pressure. The uterus exhibited continuous spontaneous activity but this did not occur in the mammary gland. This observation was in fact taken as evidence against the view (FERGUSON, 1941) that spontaneous uterine activity is due to a tonic release of oxytocin from the neurohypophysis maintained reflexly by stimuli arising from the genital tract.

A further contrast between the uterus and the mammary gland was revealed in the work of WIEDERMAN, FREUND, and STONE (1964). They measured the milk-ejection responses to oxytocin in women throughout pregnancy from the twelfth week of gestation. Although it is well known that the sensitivity of the uterus to oxytocin increases during pregnancy, these authors found no change in the threshold dose of oxytocin required to elicit milk ejection or in the slopes of the dose-response curves. In their study the threshold dose on intravenous injection was 0.25—10 mU (mean 3.6) and the latent period with threshold doses, 24—52 sec.

3. The Effect of Substances other than Oxytocin on Milk-Ejection Pressure

Table 4 shows the effects of pharmacologically active peptides and other naturally occurring substances on milk-ejection pressure in the lactating rabbit, guinea-pig and rat. The only substances other than oxytocin which have been shown to cause an increasse in milk-ejection pressure on intravenous injection are acetylcholine and substance P. On retrograde arterial injection into the mammary gland in both the guinea-pig and rat, acetylcholine, 5-hydroxytryptamine, bradykinin and angiotensin produce milk-ejection responses. For acetylcholine the threshold dose is similar in the two species, but there are large differences with other substances. The rat is about 80 times more sensitive than the guinea-pig to 5-hydroxytryptamine (base), and 10 times more sensitive to bradykinin but 10 times less sensitive to angiotensin. The most active substance is acetylcholine. However it should be noted that its threshold dose by retrograde arterial injection in the guinea-pig and rat is 10—30 ng whereas the threshold dose of oxytocin is about 10—20 pg. On a weight basis, therefore, the threshold dose of oxytocin is 1000 times smaller.

Table 4. *The effect of some pharmacologically active peptides and other naturally occurring substances on milk-ejection pressure*

Substance	Rabbit IVI µg	Guinea-pig IVI µg	Guinea-pig RAI (method of Tindal and Yokoyama, 1962) µg	Rat RAI µg
Oxytocin* . . .	+ (1.1×10^{-3})[1] = 0.5 mU	+ (2.2×10^{-3})[5] = 1.0 mU	+ ($1.1—2.2 \times 10^{-5}$)[6] = 5—10 µU	+ ($1.1—2.2 \times 10^{-5}$)[8] = 5—10 µU
Acetylcholine chloride		+ (5)[5]	+ (0.02—0.03)[6] +[7]	+ (0.01)[8]
5-hydroxytryptamine			+[7]	
Base	— (10—50)[1]			+ (0.1)[8]
Creatinine sulphate			+ (25)[6]	
Histamine . . .			+[7]	
Base	— (20—150)[1]			— (20)[8]
Acid Phosphate			+ (50)[6]	
Adenosine Triphosphate (disodium salt)			+ (100)[6]	
KCl			— (40 m-eq./l.)[7]	
Bradykinin . .	— (0.01—10)[2]	— (10)[5]	+ (1)[6]; — (3)[7]	+ (0.1)[8]
Angiotensin . .	— (0.5—500)[2]	— (25)[5]	+ (1—2)[6]; —[7]	+ (10—20)[8]
Pepsitensin . .			—[7]	
Plasma Kinin .			—[7]	
Substance P . .		+ (1.25) = 37.5 U)[5]	+ (20 U)[7]	
Anephrotensin			—[7]	
Eledoisin . . .	— (l/kg)[3]			+ (0.8)[8]
U.O.S. (unknown oxytocic substance	—[4]			

Abbreviations and signs used are:
* 1 mU is equivalent to 2.2 ng of pure oxytocin, assuming an oxytocic activity of 450 U/mg (after Boissonnas, Guttman, Berde and Konzett, 1961).
IVI = Intravenous injection; RAI = retrograde arterial injection.
\+ = Increase, — = No increase, in milk-ejection pressure; figures in parentheses give range of doses, or largest dose, tested.

References: [1] Van Dyke, Adamsons, and Engel (1955). [2] Berde and Cerletti (1961). [3] Stürmer and Berde (1963). [4] Hawker and Robertson (1958); Hawker (1961). [5] Bisset and Lewis (1962). [6] Folley and Knaggs (1965b). [7] Fitzpatrick and Walmsley (1962, 1965). [8] Bisset, Clark, Haldar, Harris, Lewis, and Rocha e Silva (1967).

The specificity of the mammary gland for oxytocin is emphasized by the fact that the potencies of oxytocin, bradykinin, angiotensin and 5-hydroxytryptamine tested on the isolated rat uterus do not differ by more than a factor of 10 (Bisset and Lewis, 1962; Bisset, Haldar, and Lewin, 1966).

D. Perfusion of the Isolated Mammary Gland

1. Cow

Using the method (see p. 481) of Petersen, Shaw, and Visscher (1939, 1941) for perfusing the isolated udder of the cow, Petersen (1942) tested a number of drugs for milk-ejecting activity. The drugs were injected into the arterial blood supplying the gland. Cannulation of the teats and collection of the venous effluent enabled the milk-ejecting activity of the drugs and their effect on blood flow to be measured simultaneously. Oxytocin (10 U), acetylcholine (4.0—100 mg), acetyl-β-methylcholine (25.0—150 mg), and histamine (0.5—10 mg) caused milk ejection from the perfused gland but only oxytocin and acetylcholine produced complete expulsion of milk. Carbamylcholine (2—8 mg) and ergonovine (0.2—0.6 mg) had no milk-ejecting activity. Oxytocin reduced blood flow by 8—20 % and histamine by 50—100 %; acetylcholine had no effect. Atropine (2—4 mg) abolished the milk ejection response to acetylcholine but did not affect the response to oxytocin. Since any milk which had collected in the large ducts and cistern during the perfusion would drain away passively through the cannulated teats, the expulsion of milk from the gland by the injection of a drug must involve an active contraction of the alveoli and this implies that the site of action of the drug is the myoepithelial cells.

In Section II it was pointed out that PEETERS and MASSART (1947) independently developed a method for perfusing bovine mammary glands which is similar in principle to that of PETERSEN et al. except that the two halves of the udder were perfused separately with no vascular connection between them. PEETERS, MASSART, and COUSSENS (1947a) found that when blood taken from a cow which had been milked was perfused through one half of the udder, it produced a milk-ejection response which was attributed to the presence in the blood of oxytocin. However a control sample of blood from a cow which had not been milked also caused milk ejection, although to a less extent, when perfused through the other half of the udder. The source of the milk-ejecting activity of normal blood was investigated by PEETERS, SIERENS, and SILVER (1952). Mechanical factors related to the expansion of the blood vessels at the onset of perfusion were excluded. The blood used was heparinized and citrated blood was less active but heparin itself (100 mg) had no milk-ejecting activity. It was concluded that some other factor was present in blood which depended for its milk-ejecting activity on the presence of calcium ions (PEETERS, MASSART, and COUSSENS, 1947b; PEETERS and MASSART, 1950), but this factor was not identified. Oxytocin was excluded because, although the injection of 10 U caused a complete expulsion of milk from the gland, there was no difference in the milk-ejecting activities of samples of blood collected from the same animal before and after death. Acetylcholine (20—100 mg) was found to cause a partial expulsion of milk but atropine, (2—4 mg) which abolished the effect of acetylcholine, did not inhibit the milk-ejecting activity of heparinized blood. Histamine (5—100 mg) reduced blood flow through the gland and had slight milk-ejecting activity. Adenosine (100 mg) had no milk-ejecting activity and adrenaline little or none. It was concluded that the milk-ejecting activity of normal heparinized blood was due to some factor such as histamine or possibly 5-hydroxytryptamine, released into the blood during its collection or perfusion. Another possible factor is bradykinin released by contact of blood with the glass or metal parts of the perfusion apparatus. In the perfusion experiments of PETERSEN and LUDWICK (1942) in which care was taken to avoid contact of blood with metal, milk-ejecting activity was not detected in control samples of blood.

PEETERS, COUSSENS, and OYAERT (1949) found that oxytocin (3 U) caused an increase in cistern pressure in the isolated perfused udder whether the initial pressure was low (10 cm H_2O) or had been raised artificially to 35 cm H_2O by filling the cistern with milk.

2. Cat and Dog

LINZELL (1950) perfused the isolated mammary glands of cats and dogs with the animal's own blood, using a constant volume pump in series with the animal and the gland. The threshold dose of oxytocin for eliciting milk ejection on intraarterial injection into the gland was 10 mU in the cat and 1 mU in the dog.

E. Direct Microscopic Examination of Mammary Tissue in Situ or in Vitro

LINZELL (1954, 1955) observed the actions of drugs applied topically to the mammary gland in the living animal. Observations were made chiefly in the mouse but also in the rat, rabbit and guinea-pig. The surface of the gland was exposed under anaesthesia by reflecting the skin and examined under a microscope using a magnification of X20—X50. The drugs were applied in a volume of 0.0002—0.1 ml from a micrometer syringe as drops at the end of a 20 gauge needle. In response to a number of drugs which cause contraction of smooth muscle, the alveoli were observed to contract and sometimes the neighbouring ducts filled with milk. The time course of the response was similar to that for smooth muscle; the latent period was 2—20 sec, the contraction lasted 2—5 sec and relaxation occurred in 0.5—5 min. LINZELL concluded from his observations that the contractile elements producing the response were the myoepithelial cells. In most experiments tests could be repeated every 5 min for 2—3 h on the same area of gland. The threshold dose of oxytocin for producing a visible contraction of the alveoli in the mouse was 1×10^{-8} to 2×10^{-4} mU. The mean of 10 observations was 3×10^{-5} mU, i. e. 0.03 μU; this is equivalent to about 1×10^{-7} μg of the pure peptide. LINZELL (1959) has calculated that the threshold dose represents about 100 molecules per alveolus. In three experiments on guinea-pigs, the threshold was 2×10^{-11}, 5×10^{-6} and 2×10^{-6} mU; it may be noted that the lowest recorded threshold for producing a milk-ejection response by retrograde arterial injection into the mammary gland in the guinea-pig and in the rat is 1×10^{-3} mU (see Table 3).

The threshold doses of other active substances applied topically to the living gland of the mouse were: for acetylcholine chloride: 0.00001—0.01 μg; pilocarpine chloride: 0.002—1.0 μg; histamine acid phosphate: 0.05—1.0 μg; barium chloride: 1—50 μg; 5-hydroxytryptamine creatinine sulphate: 1 μg. With the last substance, tachyphylaxis occurred. The action of acetylcholine was abolished by atropine. LINZELL also injected oxytocin intravenously in the mouse and detected a milk-ejection response by observing microscopically a flow of milk into the main duct; the threshold dose for eliciting this effect was 0.1—0.4 mU with a mean of 0.22 mU in nine observations. In the guinea-pig, stimulation of the spermatic nerves did not affect the response to topical application of oxytocin but it prevented the response to an intravenous injection, presumably by causing vasoconstriction in the gland. Stimulation of the cutaneous nerves to the gland had no effect on the alveoli.

LEVITSKAYA (1955), also using the method of microscopic examination of the exposed gland in the mouse, observed that the topical application of acetylcholine (2×10^{-8}) and posterior pituitary extract (Pituitrin) ("1×10^{-4} to 2×10^{-5}" — ? 0.1—0.02 mU/ml) caused contraction of the alveoli and dilatation of the ducts. Acetylcholine acted in 1—2 sec. First the alveoli contracted. The small ducts dilated and filled with milk which flowed to the main duct and beyond to the teat. When the alveoli relaxed milk flowed back into them. The entire process of contraction and relaxation lasted not more than 15 sec. Pituitrin had a similar action. It could not be determined whether the ducts actively dilated or were passively distended by expulsion of milk from the alveoli. ZOTIKOVA (1955) confirmed these results and, using cine-micrography, added the observation that electrical stimulation of the pudendal or spermatic nerves caused the appearance of sphincter-like formations in the ducts. When Pituitrin was applied after nerve stimulation the time required for expulsion of milk from the alveoli into the large duct was prolonged from 1—4 to 20—30 sec. This was taken as evidence in support of the theory that the efferent nerve supply to the mammary gland is of functional importance in the regulation of milk ejection (see Section I).

In the rat GROSVENOR and TURNER (1956) observed a response to oxytocin applied topically to the gland under a dissecting microscope. A solution containing 200 mU/ml was delivered as drops from a 24 gauge needle. The alveoli contracted in 2—4 sec and the ducts filled with milk. There was no visible effect on blood vessels. When the alveoli were distended, milk which had been squeezed into the ducts ran back into the alveoli; this process of relaxation occurred in 1—5 min.

VAN DONGEN and HAYS (1966) have introduced an *in vitro* assay method for oxytocin. Small pieces (2 mm^3) of rat mammary tissue containing milk are placed into drops (0.01 ml) of solutions containing oxytocin (1×10^{-2} to 1×10^{-10} U/ml) at 15° C and the expulsion of milk from the alveoli into the solutions is observed under a dissecting microscope. The time interval between exposure of the tissue to the solutions and the initiation of milk ejection from the alveoli is used as a quantitative parameter. Some tissues responded to 1×10^{-16} U oxytocin: 1×10^{-12} U represents the lowest threshold for quantitative purposes.

F. Measurement of Tension in Isolated Strips of Mammary Gland

It was shown by MÉNDEZ-BAUER, CABOT and CALDEYRO-BARCIA in 1960 that it was possible with the use of conventional pharmacological methods to study the mammary gland as an isolated organ preparation. They showed that if a narrow

Table 5. *Effect of oxytocin, acetylcholine, 5-hydroxytryptamine and histamine on isolated strip of mammary gland*

	Rabbit	Rabbit	Rat	Rat	Guinea-pig
Days post partum . . .	15—30	9—40		3—14	ca. 7
Resting tension of strip (mg)	50—100	1300—3400	500	160	160
Effective concentration of oxytocin (mU/ml):					
minimum	0.1	0.1	0.2—0.4	0.0005	0.025
working range	0.5—10	0.5—10		0.005—0.1	0.05—0.4
Effect of other drugs. Concentration in μg/ml of highest dose or range of doses tested:					
Acetylcholine		+ (25)		+ (1×10^{-6} to 1×10^{-5})	
5-hydroxytryptamine .		— (50)		+ (0.01—1)	
Histamine		— (125)		+ (1×10^{-5} to 1×10^{-2})	
Number of Reference . .	1	2	3	4	5

+ = Increase in tension; — = no effect.

References: 1. MÉNDEZ-BAUER, CABOT, and CALDEYRO-BARCIA (1960); 2. MOORE and ZARROW (1965); 3. SMITH (1961); 4. RYDÉN and SJÖHOLM (1962), SJÖHOLM and RYDÉN (1962); 5. BERÁNKOVÁ-KSANDROVÁ, BISSET, JOŠT, KREJČÍ, PLIŠKA, RUDINGER, RYCHLÍK, and ŠORM (1966).

strip taken from the mammary gland of a lactating rabbit was set up in an organ bath and connected with a highly sensitive strain gauge transducer, an increase in tension was recorded when oxytocin was added to the bath. This technique has been applied by other workers (see Table 5) to the rabbit and also to the rat and guinea-pig. Since smooth muscle in the mammary gland, apart from that in the teat, is insensitive to oxytocin and since the mammary tissue in the preparation of Smith (1961) consisted only of alveoli and the smaller ducts, it can be assumed that the tension in the strips is derived from contraction of the myoepithelial cells (see Section VIII, A). The increase in tension which develops in response to oxytocin is recorded isometrically and ranges from 5—15 mg in the rat to several hundred mg in the rabbit. The maximum tension is reached within 1—5 min.

Moore and Zarrow (1965) found in the rabbit that the sensitivity of isolated strips of mammary gland to oxytocin increased up to the ninth day post partum and then remained constant up to the 44th day. The optimal resting tension was 200—400 mg/mm^2 or 1300—1400 mg for the whole strip. Maximal responses were obtained within a range of temperature of 32—36° C. Below 15° C the strips were almost inactive and irreversible changes occurred above 41° C. They adopted a temperature of 32° C; that used by other workers is 37—38° C. The usual solution in the organ bath is Tyrode's but Smith (1961) used a modified Ringer's solution. Strips may be taken from the mammary gland of an animal which has been used for measuring milk-ejection pressure and can be stored at 4° C for 72 h without loss of sensitivity. Unlike the isolated rat uterus the strips of mammary gland do not show spontaneous activity.

The lowest threshold concentration of oxytocin recorded is 0.0005 mU/ml in the rat (Rydén and Sjöholm, 1962; Sjöholm and Rydén, 1962) which is equivalent with a 4 ml organ bath to 2 μU. It should be noted (Table 4) that this level of sensitivity can be attained by measuring milk-ejection pressure in the guinea-pig and rat using retrograde arterial injections (see Table 3). As an assay preparation the isolated strip has the disadvantage that an interval of 15 min may be necessary between doses. Further, Moore and Zarrow (1965) report that in some of their experiments it required 3 h to obtain a stable response to oxytocin after the resting tension had been applied. It might be possible to increase the sensitivity of the isolated strip by using the method of superfusion as applied to the rat uterus by Fitzpatrick (1961).

The table shows a striking contrast between the sensitivities of the rat and rabbit gland to acetylcholine, histamine and 5-hydroxytryptamine. With the rat strip, the minimum effective concentration for acetylcholine is the same as that for oxytocin (10^{-6} μg/ml) although acetylcholine is 1000 times less active than oxytocin on the rat mammary gland *in situ* when tested by retrograde arterial injection (Table 4). The rat strip also responds to histamine and 5-hydroxytryptamine. On the rabbit strip, these two substances are inactive and acetylcholine is active only at a concentration of 25 μg/ml. It is significant that the rabbit strip did not respond to samples of heparinized blood or plasma (Méndez-Bauer et al.) or haemolysed blood from males or non-pregnant females (Moore and Zarrow, 1965). This is in contrast with the isolated rat uterus since attempts to use this preparation for assaying oxytocin in blood extracts have been complicated by the difficulty of eliminating interfering substances (Bisset and Walker, 1954; Hawker, 1961; Bisset, 1961).

X. The Action of Vasopressin on the Mammary Gland

A. Vasopressin and the Identity of the Milk-Ejecting Hormone

Dale (1957) has given an account of the controversy which existed over the unitary and multiple hormone theories; that is, whether extracts of the posterior pituitary contained a number of active principles or a single principle with multiple pharmacological activities. The argument was partly resolved when KAMM and his co-workers (KAMM, ALDRICH, GROTE, ROWE, and BUGBEE, 1928; BUGBEE and KAMM, 1928) separated an oxytocic fraction, Pitocin, from a pressor fraction, Pitressin (see section II.). However, there was not a complete separation of activities in these two fractions since Pitocin possessed about 5% of the pressor activity of Pitressin, and Pitressin about 5% of the oxytocic activity of Pitocin. This meant either, that the fractionation was incomplete or, that there were two distinct hormones (oxytocin and vasopressin) which overlapped in their pharmacological activities.

In elaborating their theory of the milk-ejection reflex (see Section II) ELY and PETERSEN (1941) compared the milk-ejecting activities of Pitocin and Pitressin. They concluded that oxytocin was the natural hormone responsible for milk ejection and that the effect of Pitressin on the mammary gland was due to contamination with oxytocin. In the same year, however, TURNER and COOPER found that, on intravenous injection into the lactating rabbit, the mean threshold dose of Pitressin for producing a visible contraction of the mammary gland and dilatation of the duct system was 5.1 mU, compared with 1.82 mU for Pitocin and 1.04 mU for Pituitrin (whole posterior pituitary extract). The activity of Pitressin was clearly too great to be accounted for by 5 % contamination with oxytocin and they concluded that either the oxytocic and pressor fractions combined to produce the milk-ejecting activity of whole posterior pituitary extract or that a third factor specific for milk-ejection was present in variable proportions in Pitocin and Pitressin. Other workers also found that the milk-ejecting activity of Pitressin was considerably in excess of its oxytocic activity in the rabbit (CROSS and HARRIS, 1952) and in the goat (ANDERSSON, 1951c) and sow (WHITTLESTONE, 1950a). CROSS and HARRIS (1952) again suggested the possibility of a third, milk-ejecting principle in the posterior pituitary.

The problem was finally settled when the highly purified preparation of (arginine) vasopressin made by TURNER, PIERCE, and DU VIGNEAUD (1951) became available. It was shown that no leucine or isoleucine, which are present in oxytocin, could be detected in chromatograms of a hydrolysate of this preparation and that if there was any contamination with oxytocin, it could not exceed 0.7 % (POPENOE, PIERCE, DU VIGNEAUD, and VAN DYKE, 1952). When this purified vasopressin was tested for milk-ejecting activity in the rabbit (CROSS and VAN DYKE, 1953) and the sow (WHITTLESTONE, 1952) it was found to be about one fifth as potent as oxytocin. It was concluded that milk-ejecting activity, like oxytocic activity, is an intrinsic property of vasopressin. This conclusion has since been supported by the demonstration of milk-ejecting activity in synthetic vasopressin.

The fact that vasopressin has a relatively high intrinsic milk-ejecting activity recalls the question of which of the two posterior pituitary hormones is responsible for milk ejection in response to suckling. CROSS (1950, 1951, 1953b) showed that it could not be vasopressin. The antidiuretic response to suckling in water-loaded rabbits was matched by 0.5—1.0 mU vasopressin which represents only one tenth of the threshold dose of this hormone for causing milk ejection. Similarly in the water-loaded dog, PICKFORD (1960) found that the antidiuretic response to suckling was matched by 0.1—0.5 mU vasopressin and the intravenous injection of 2 mU of this hormone did not cause milk ejection. HALDAR (1966) showed that the blood of conscious rabbits contained oxytocin but no detectable vasopressin when the young obtained milk on suckling. In some experiments vasopressin was detected without oxytocin when the young failed to obtain milk. This result could be explained by the occurrence of emotional stress which would stimulate the release of vasopressin but block the milk-ejection reflex and inhibit the release of oxytocin. These results show that, although vasopressin may be released during suckling, it is the release of oxytocin which brings about milk ejection.

B. The Milk-Ejecting Activity of Vasopressin in Different Species

Table 6 shows the milk-ejecting activity of vasopressin estimated by various methods of assay in a number of species. This activity is expressed as a percentage of the milk-ejecting activity of oxytocin in the same assay, as illustrated by the following example from the data of WHITTLESTONE (1952). On intravenous injection into the sow, 2.5 U arginine-vasopressin was required to produce a milk-ejection response equivalent (in terms of milk yield and duration of milk flow) to that given by 0.5 U oxytocin[1]. Therefore, in this example, the milk-ejecting activity of arginine vasopressin is 20%.

It will be seen from the table that the milk-ejecting potency of vasopressin varies in different species and even in the same species according to the method of assay. For example, the potency of arginine-vasopressin is similar in the guinea-pig and mouse, but equal only to about one half of that of lysine-vasopressin in the guinea-pig and of arginine-vasopressin in the rabbit and sow. It appears that vasopressin has almost negligible milk-ejecting activity in lactating women. There is a striking difference between the two values given for arginine-vasopressin in the rat, one of which (13.6%) is based on retrograde arterial injection in the whole animal and the other (3.2%) on the isolated organ.

C. Importance of the Intrinsic Milk-Ejecting Activity of Vasopressin in Experimental Work

The occurrence of milk ejection in response to a stimulus to the neurohypophysis such as the intracarotid injection of hypertonic saline, cannot be taken as evidence that that stimulus has caused a release of oxytocin unless it has been proved, as in the experiments of CROSS and PICKFORD on suckling antidiuresis, that the milk ejection could not have been caused by vasopressin.

CROSS and VAN DYKE (1953) pointed out that if milk-ejecting activity is used to assay the amount of oxytocin in blood, a parallel determination of antidiuretic or pressor activity should be carried out in order to discount the intrinsic milk-ejecting activity of vasopressin. A further caution might be added that the milk-ejecting activity of vasopressin should first be determined on the same assay preparation as that used for oxytocin. The importance of carrying out parallel estimations of antidiuretic and milk-ejecting activities in the same samples of blood is exemplified by recent work in cats on the release of neurohypophysial hormones by electrical stimulation of the supraoptic nucleus (BISSET, HILTON, and POISNER, 1967), haemorrhage (BELESLIN, BISSET, HALDAR, and POLAK, 1967) and carotid occlusion (CLARK and ROCHA E SILVA, 1966). Blood samples collected during stimulation of the neurohypophysis by these procedures frequently contained milk-ejecting activity which might have been attributed to oxytocin. However, it was found that in almost all the samples this activity could be

[1] In most of the reports included in Table 6 doses are quoted in units, based on pressor bioassays in the case of vasopressin and on oxytocic or avian depressor assays in the case of oxytocin. These assays are relatively specific and refer ultimately to the International Standard for Oxytocic, Vasopressor and Antidiuretic Substances (BANGHAM and MUSSETT, 1958) which by definition contains 1 unit of oxytocic, vasopressor and antidiuretic activity in 0.5 mg. Therefore no significant inaccuracy is introduced by the fact that the hormone preparations tested by most authors were not pure chemical substances. Units disappear when activities are calculated as a percentage.

Table 6. *Estimations of milk-ejecting activity of vasopressin*

Species	Method of assay	Route of in-jection	Preparation of vasopressin	Standard for comparison	Milk-ejecting activity of vasopressin as a percentage of the milk-ejecting activity of oxytocin
Sow .	1 Milk yield.	IVI	Pitressin	Pitocin	~25
	2 Milk yield and duration of milk ejection	IVI	Purified[1] arginine vasopressin	Pitocin	20
	3 Milk-ejection pressure	IVI	Pitressin	Pitocin	~20
Rabbit	4 Cannulated teat duct and volume recorder	IVI	Purified[1] arginine vasopressin	Purified[1] oxytocin	(12.5—20) 17[4]
	5 Milk-ejection pressure	IVI	Pitressin	Pitocin	(10—50) 20
	6 Isolated strip of mammary gland		Arginine vasopressin (? synthetic)	Syntocinon	15
Goat .	7 Threshold for milk ejection	IVI	Pitressin	Pitocin	18
	8 Cannulated teat duct and volume recorder	IVI	Vasopressin (Roussel)	Oxytocin (Roussel)	~10
Guinea-pig . .	9 Cannulated teat duct and volume recorder	IVI	Purified[1] arginine vasopressin	Purified[1] oxytocin	9.1
	10 Milk-ejection pressure	IVI	Synthetic lysine vasopressin	Syntocinon	20
	11 Milk-ejection pressure	RAI	Synthetic lysine vasopressin	Pitocin	16
	12 Milk-ejection pressure	RAI	Purified[2] arginine vasopressin	PPE	9.2 ± 0.67 (= SE 5. obs)
Mouse .	13 Topical application to living gland	—	Purified[1] arginine vasopressin	Purified[1] oxytocin	11.5
	13 Milk-ejection by microscopic examination of living gland	IVI	Purified[1] arginine vasopressin	Purified[1] oxytocin	7.3
Rat . .	14 Isolated strip of mammary gland	—	Purified[3] arginine vasopressin	Syntocinon	3.2 ± 0.24 (= SE 9 obs)
	15 Milk-ejection pressure	RAI	Synthetic arginine vasopressin	PPE	13.6 ± 0.59 (= SE 8 obs)
Man .	16 Milk-ejection pressure	IVI	Pitressin	Pitocin	~1

References: 1. Whittlestone (1950a); 2. Whittlestone (1952); 3. Whittlestone (1954b); 4. Cross and van Dyke (1953); 5. Holland, Cross, and Sawyer (1959a); 6. Moore and Zarrow (1965); 7. Andersson (1951c); 8. Denamur and Martinet (1953); 9. Linzell (1955); 10. Bisset and Lewis (1962); 11. Folley and Knaggs (1965b); 12. Bisset, Hilton, and Poisner (1967), Haldar (1966); 13. Linzell (1955); 14. Smith (1961); 15. Bisset, Clark, Haldar, Harris, Lewis, and Rocha e Silva (1967); 16. Gaitan, Cobo, and Mizrachi (1964).

IVI = intravenous injection.
RAI = retrograde arterial injection.
PPE = posterior pituitary extract (3rd Int. Standard for Oxytocic, Vasopressor, and Antidiuretic Substances — Bangham and Musset, 1958). Arginine-vasopressin was assayed against this standard for antidiuretic (ADA) and milk-ejecting (MEA) activity. The values of 9.2% and 13.6% $= \frac{\text{MEA}}{\text{ADA}} \times 100$.

---

1 = prepared by Dr. V. du Vigneaud and co-workers.
2 = prepared by Dr. B.K. Follett.
3 = prepared by Dr. H. Sachs.
4 = oxytocin 5—8 times more potent than vasopressin (mean $= 6.1 \pm 0.4 =$ SE of 9 observations)

entirely accounted for by their content of vasopressin. In fact the experiments provided evidence for the release of vasopressin independently of oxytocin.

A possible complication of assaying oxytocin and vasopressin in blood is that one hormone might interfere with the assay of the other. KULLANDER (1963) showed that when vasopressin was infused into a lactating rabbit simultaneously with oxytocin in a ratio of 1:4 to 1:1, the milk-ejection response to oxytocin was inhibited. On the other hand, GAITAN, COBO, and MIZRACHI (1964) found no evidence of any interaction between the two hormones in lactating women. The intravenous infusion of vasopressin at the rate of 40 mU/min did not inhibit the milk-ejection response to an intravenous injection of 1—10 mU. oxytocin and a mixture of 50 mU oxytocin with 250 mU vasopressin produced the same response as 50 mU oxytocin alone. WHITTLESTONE (1950a, 1954b) demonstrated an additive effect of oxytocin and vasopressin in sows and it has been found that if threshold amounts of oxytocin are added to blood extracts containing a relatively high concentration of vasopressin, the milk-ejection response to the oxytocin in the mixture is not inhibited (BISSET et al., 1967; BELESLIN et al., 1967).

XI. The Interaction of Adrenaline and Oxytocin on the Mammary Gland and Emotional Inhibition of the Milk-Ejection Reflex

A. The Action of Adrenaline on the Mammary Gland

Although there have been a few isolated reports which suggest that adrenaline can stimulate contractile tissue in the mammary gland, it is a well established fact that its main action is to inhibit the milk-ejection response to oxytocin.

1. Evidence for a Stimulant Action

PETERSEN (1942) reported that adrenaline (0.05—0.2 mg) caused expulsion of milk from the isolated perfused udder of the cow, although it differed from oxytocin in producing only a partial emptying of the gland. However, PEETERS, SIERENS, and SILVER (1952) observed little or no expulsion of milk after adrenaline in their experiments on the perfused udder. BRAUDE and MITCHELL (1952) observed milk ejection in three out of seven sows after the intravenous injection of adrenaline (0.4—1 mg) but WHITTLESTONE (1954d) never observed an increase in intramammary pressure in the sow after doses of adrenaline up to 1 mg. No increase in milk-ejection pressure has been reported in the rabbit, guinea-pig, rat or dog after intravenous or retrograde arterial injections of adrenaline. Isolated strips of mammary gland from the rat respond to adrenaline (1×10^{-5} to 1×10^{-4} μg/ml) and to noradrenaline (1×10^{-5} μg/ml) with an increase in tension (RYDÉN and SJÖHOLM, 1962) but no such response was obtained from strips of rabbit gland with concentrations of adrenaline as high as 30 μg/ml (CHAN, 1965) or 100 μg/ml. (MOORE and ZARROW, 1965). Ejection of milk or increase in tension of the isolated strip in response to adrenaline may be due to an action on some contractile tissue other than myoepithelium, since no contraction of the alveoli is visible under the microscope when adrenaline is applied topically to the living gland of the mouse in concentrations sufficient to cause pronounced vasoconstriction (LINZELL, 1955; LEVITSKAYA, 1955).

2. Inhibitory Action in Different Species

Since ELY and PETERSEN (1941) demonstrated in the cow that the intravenous injection of adrenaline (1—4 mg) at the beginning of milking slowed down the rate of ejection of milk, the inhibitory effect of adrenaline on the response of the mammary gland to oxytocin has been extensively investigated in a number of species.

a) *Cow:* Adrenaline has been shown to inhibit the action of oxytocin on the isolated perfused udder. The previous injection of adrenaline (0.05 mg) retarded the expulsion of milk caused by oxytocin (5—10 U). Since the total quantity of milk expelled was not reduced, the inhibitory effect of adrenaline was thought to be due to vasoconstriction in the gland (PEETERS, SIERENS, and SILVER, 1951).

b) *Sow:* BRAUDE and MITCHELL (1952) found that the milk yield in response to an intravenous injection of oxytocin (1 U) was reduced by the simultaneous injection of adrenaline (0.4 mg) intravenously. The injection of 1 mg adrenaline 62—90 sec before oxytocin (1 U) suppressed the milk-ejection response; 0.4 mg caused a partial inhibition. Similarly WHITTLESTONE (1954d) found that an intravenous injection of adrenaline (0.2 mg) 3 sec before oxytocin (0.5 U) prevented milk ejection. However, when the same amount of adrenaline was injected simultaneously with oxytocin and milk-ejection pressure was recorded, a definite inhibition was not seen unless the amount of oxytocin in the mixture was reduced to 0.2 U.

c) *Rabbit:* Several investigations have been made in the intact animal using the method of volume or pressure recording from a cannulated teat duct. In all cases injections were given intravenously. CROSS (1953a) showed that adrenaline (5 μg) abolished the milk-ejection response to oxytocin or posterior pituitary extract (Pituitrin) (20, 30 or 50 mU) provided that the adrenaline was injected first. In 2 min the inhibitory effect of the adrenaline had almost disappeared. When adrenaline (5 μg) was injected simultaneously with oxytocin (50 mU) the response was reduced, but not abolished. In its inhibitory effect on the milk-ejection response to oxytocin, adrenaline was $1^1/_2$—4 times more potent than noradrenaline (CROSS, 1955a, 1958a). Adrenaline (3—5 μg) also inhibited for several minutes the tonic or rhythmic response to an infusion of oxytocin at a rate of 24 mU/min (CROSS, 1958a), an effect confirmed by KULLANDER (1963). YOKOYAMA (1956) found that in two out of three experiments, adrenaline (5 μg) inhibited the milk-ejection response to posterior pituitary extract (Pituitan) (50 mU) when injected simultaneously and an inhibitory effect was still present after 130—140 sec. CHAN (1965) produced graded inhibition of the milkejection response to oxytocin (12 mU) with doses of adrenaline from 0.2 to 0.8 μg injected 10—15 sec before the oxytocin. In general, a dose ratio of 0.1 μg: 1 mU caused complete inhibition. The inhibitory effect of noradrenaline was about one half or one quarter that of adrenaline.

CHAN (1965) also demonstrated an inhibitory effect of adrenaline on the response to oxytocin of isolated strips from the mammary gland of the rabbit. Adrenaline and oxytocin were applied in the same solution. The ratio of adrenaline: oxytocin required for inhibition was much higher than *in vivo:* with a ratio of 3 μg: 1 mU the inhibition was only partial. MOORE and ZARROW (1965) observed a decrease of 42 % in the response of the isolated strip to oxytocin following exposure to adrenaline (10^{-5}).

d) *Dog:* In the unanaesthetized dog in which a cannulated teat duct was connected with a volume recorder, 0.25 μg adrenaline injected intravenously caused partial, and 0.5 and 1.0 μg complete, inhibition of the milk-ejection response to oxytocin (25 mU) injected 10 sec later (PICKFORD, 1959).

e) *Mouse:* LINZELL (1955) examined microscopically the action of adrenaline and noradrenaline applied topically to the living gland of the mouse. Oxytocin applied topically at the height of the vasoconstriction caused by the amines still elicited contraction of the alveoli. Mixtures of adrenaline and oxytocin produced vasoconstriction and alveolar contraction simultaneously. In two experiments the addition of adrenaline 0.0005 and 0.001 μg to solutions of oxytocin did not increase the threshold dose of oxytocin required to elicit alveolar contraction.

f) *Guinea-Pig and Rat:* Both adrenaline and noradrenaline have been shown to inhibit the milk-ejection response to oxytocin in the guinea-pig (Bisset, Hilton, and Poisner, 1966) and the rat (Bisset, Clark, and Lewis, 1967). Adrenaline was the more potent inhibitor. In both species solutions containing one or other amine mixed in varying proportions with oxytocin or posterior pituitary extract (PPE - see footnote to Table 6) were injected by the retrograde arterial route and milk-ejection pressure was recorded from a cannulated teat duct. In the guinea-pig, 5.5 ng adrenaline (base) inhibited the response to 200 μU PPE by 34 % whereas 10 ng noradrenaline (base) inhibited it by only 20 %. The percentage inhibition was calculated by determining from a log-dose-response curve the amount of PPE which corresponded with the response given by the mixture. In the rat the amount of adrenaline (base) which was required to reduce the response to 20 μU oxytocin by 50—75 % varied in 5 experiments from 5—20 ng. In one experiment in which a comparison was made, adrenaline was about twice as potent as noradrenaline. Adrenaline should thus be considered as a possible interfering factor when oxytocin is assayed in blood extracts by retrograde arterial injection (see Bisset, Hilton, and Poisner, 1967).

3. *Mechanism of the Inhibitory Action*

There are three possible ways in which adrenaline might inhibit the milk-ejection response to oxytocin. First, it could cause contraction of the smooth muscle of the teat sphincter or of the ducts causing a mechanical obstruction to the ejection of milk. Secondly, by causing vasoconstriction of blood vessels it could prevent the access of circulating oxytocin to its site of action in the gland. Thirdly, it could have a direct inhibitory action on the myoepithelial cells, like that on the rat uterus, opposing the contractile effect of oxytocin.

Adrenaline has been shown to cause contraction of isolated sections cut from the walls of the large ducts, cistern and teat sphincter of the cow's udder (Tverskoi, 1955a). Levitskaya (1955) observed that the topical application of adrenaline (1×10^{-5}) to the living gland of the mouse caused within 5—15 sec a contraction of the walls of the ducts. Some small ducts collapsed completely and sphincter-like formations were observed in the openings of outlet ducts. Similar observations were made by Zotikova (1955). The inhibitory effect of adrenaline on milk-ejection in the whole animal could not be explained by contraction of the teat sphincter because it still occurred when the teat was cannulated.

Experiments on the isolated perfused gland show that adrenaline is a potent vasoconstrictor of mammary blood vessels. Petersen (1942) found that 0.05 mg adrenaline caused a 50 % reduction and 0.1—0.2 mg a complete stoppage of blood flow in the perfused udder. Similar responses were obtained by Peeters, Sierens, and Silver (1952) who showed also that the vasoconstriction could be reversed by dibenamine (7 mg/kg). Using the technique of perfusing the isolated gland with the animal's own blood, Linzell (1950) found that the threshold dose of adrenaline for causing vasoconstriction on arterial injection into the gland was 0.005—0.05 μg in the cat and 0.0001—0.001 μg in the dog. Plethysmography revealed that in the intact cat, the threshold dose by intravenous injection for causing a diminution in volume of the gland was 0.01—0.1 μg. In later work (Hebb and Linzell, 1951) the blood flow through the isolated gland was greatly increased by including the animal's lungs in the perfusion circuit. This preparation was much more sensitive to adrenaline; the threshold dose for vasoconstriction on arterial injection into the gland was 10^{-7}, 10^{-6} and 10^{-4} μg for the cat, dog and goat, respectively. Generally the threshold for noradrenaline was higher than that for adrenaline but the ratio varied from 1:1 to 37.5:1. By plethysmography in the intact cat, the ratio of threshold doses was 1.25:1 to 7.5:1.

Cross (1953a, 1954a, b, 1955a, b, 1958a) has advanced a number of arguments in favour of the view that the inhibitory effect of adrenaline is due chiefly or entirely to its vasoconstrictor action. Several examples have been given of the observation that adrenaline is more effective when injected before, than simultaneously with oxytocin. This can be explained by supposing that inhibition is more pronounced if the vessels are already constricted when oxytocin is injected. The following findings argue against a direct inhibitory action of adrenaline on the myoepithelial cells: adrenaline does not inhibit the milk-ejection response to mechanical (tap) stimuli applied directly to the gland (Cross, 1954a, b, 1955a; Yokoyama, 1956) nor does it inhibit the contraction of the alveoli by oxytocin when both drugs are applied topically to the living gland of the mouse (Linzell, 1955). On the other hand adrenaline has been observed to inhibit the action of oxytocin on isolated strips of mammary gland (Moore and Zarrow, 1965; Chan, 1965). Another argument in favour of the vasoconstrictor hypothesis is that the relative potencies of adrenaline and noradrenaline are similar for vasoconstriction and for inhibition of the milk-ejection response to oxytocin. Cross and Silver (1962) have provided further evidence in favour of vasoconstriction. They measured oxygen tension (pO_2) polarographically from needle electrodes inserted into the lactating mammary gland in the rabbit; pO_2 gives a measure of capillary blood flow. The intravenous injection of adrenaline (1—5 μg) depressed pO_2 and inhibited the milk-ejection response to oxytocin injected 10—15 sec later. Full inhibition of the response occurred only if the oxytocin reached the gland at a time when pO_2 was falling rapidly. Control experiments showed that the inhibition was related not so much to the absolute level of pO_2 tension as to the blood flow.

Recently an attempt has been made to define the inhibitory effect of adrenaline on milk ejection in terms of classical α and β receptors. Vasoconstriction would be expected to involve an action on α receptors and a direct inhibitory action on the myoepithelial cells, an action on β receptors analogous to that demonstrated in the rat uterus (Levy and Tozzi, 1963). In his experiments on the inhibitory effect of intravenous adrenaline on the milk-ejection response to oxytocin in the lactating rabbit (see p. 521) Chan (1965) found that an equipressor dose of angiotensin caused no inhibition whereas isoprenaline in a dose (0.2 μg) which produced only a depressor response was as potent an inhibitor as adrenaline. Moreover adrenaline still caused inhibition after its pressor action had been reversed by the α blocking agent, phenoxybenzamine. These observations appear to exclude vasoconstriction or any other action on α receptors as the cause of the inhibition of the milk-ejection response to oxytocin. The fact that, of several sympathomimetic amines tested, isoprenaline was the most potent inhibitor of milk-ejection, suggests an action on β receptors. However, when both phenoxybenzamine and the β blocking agent pronethalol were given, adrenaline still inhibited milk ejection although its vascular effects were blocked. On the other hand, in their experiments on the lactating rat, in which adrenaline and oxytocin were given by retrograde arterial injection (see p. 522), Bisset, Clark, and Lewis (1967) did obtain evidence for an action of adrenaline on β receptors. The inhibitory effect of adrenaline (5—20 ng) on the milk-ejection response to oxytocin (20—40 μU) was not blocked by phentolamine (0.1—0.4 mg) although the pressor response to large doses of adrenaline (0.2—0.4 μg) injected intravenously was reversed. In contrast, intravenous pronethalol (1 mg) consistently blocked the inhibition caused by adrenaline which appears, therefore, to be mediated by an effect on β receptors. However it cannot be excluded at present that, under different experimental conditions, a vasoconstrictor effect involving α receptors also occurs.

B. Significance of Adrenaline in Emotional Inhibition of the Milk-Ejection Reflex

The milk-ejection reflex can be inhibited by fright or pain or emotional disturbance. This has been demonstrated experimentally in the cow (Ely and Petersen, 1941; Whittlestone, 1951), in women (Newton and Newton, 1948), in the rabbit (Cross, 1953a, 1954b, 1955a, b; Fuchs and Wagner, 1963a) and in the guinea-pig (Chaudhury, Chaudhury, and Lu, 1961). The reflex could be blocked centrally by preventing the release of oxytocin or peripherally by some mechanism interfering with the action of oxytocin on the mammary gland.

The effectiveness of adrenaline in inhibiting the milk-ejection response to oxytocin suggests that the sympathetico-adrenal system might be involved in a peripheral block of the milk-ejection reflex. The sympathetic innervation of the mammary gland has been discussed on p. 476.

Cross (1953a, 1954b, 1955a, 1958a) has demonstrated in the rabbit that the milk-ejection reflex can be blocked by the injection of adrenaline and by stimulation of the sympathetic nervous system centrally as well as peripherally. The intravenous injection of adrenaline (5—50 μg) into lactating rabbits before nursing prevented the young from obtaining more than three quarters of the normal yield of milk. The injection of not less than 5 μg intravenously also inhibited milk ejection in response to electrical stimulation of the supraoptico-hypophysial tract (Cross, 1953a). Stimulation of the dorsal, lateral and posterior parts of the hypothalamus in the rabbit produced signs of sympathetic stimulation, such as dilatation of the pupil and exophthalmos, and inhibited the milk-ejection response to posterior pituitary extract (Pituitrin) (5—100 mU) injected intravenously 10—30 sec after the end of stimulation. This inhibitory effect, which was equivalent to that produced by an intravenous injection of 1—5 μg adrenaline, was abolished by bilateral adrenalectomy. However, some inhibition was also observed in the adrenalectomized animal when oxytocin was injected during stimulation of the hypothalamus. This suggested that the inhibition involved not only the adrenal medulla but also a direct inhibitory pathway through the sympathetic innervation of the mammary gland and it was shown that stimulation of mammary sympathetic nerves also inhibited the response to oxytocin (Cross, 1954b, 1955a). Electrical stimulation in the region of the paraventricular nucleus produced signs of sympathetic activity but no milk-ejection response, presumably because of concurrent stimulation of sympathetic centres situated near this nucleus in the hypothalamus. A milk-ejection response was obtained after adrenalectomy, mid-thoracic section of the spinal cord or spinal anaesthesia (Cross, 1955a, 1958a). Stimulation of sympathetic centres in the hypothalamus was associated with inability of the young to obtain milk during suckling (Cross, 1955a).

Whether the block which occurs in the emotional inhibition of the milk-ejection reflex in the conscious animal is central or peripheral, can be determined by the effectiveness of replacement therapy with oxytocin. If the block is central the intravenous injection of an appropriate amount of oxytocin should restore normal milk ejection. Ely and Petersen (1941) and Newton and Newton (1948) were able to overcome the effect of emotional inhibition in cows and in women by injections of oxytocin, but it seems probable that the amounts injected were unphysiological and sufficiently high to counteract any peripheral block which might have been present (Cross, 1953a). On investigating this problem in rabbits,

Cross (1955b) first determined the amount of oxytocin which is normally released in this species in response to suckling (see Section 9 B). This was estimated to be 50 mU. In 35 out of 42 experiments in which does were suckled under forcible restraint, the amount of milk removed by the young was reduced by 20—100%. In 29 cases, the injection of 50 mU oxytocin restored the normal yield. This suggests that a central block of release of oxytocin had occurred. Further evidence was obtained by recording milk-ejection responses kymographically from a cannulated teat duct during suckling. Normal milk removal was associated with a reflex milk-ejection response equivalent to that produced by an intravenous injection of 50 mU oxytocin; when milk removal was incomplete there was no response or one equivalent to only 5—10 mU oxytocin. In 6 of the 35 experiments, the injection of 50 mU oxytocin did not fully restore the normal milk yield and the inhibitory effect of stress was matched by the intravenous injection of 1 μg adrenaline. Cross concluded from these experiments that, while peripheral inhibition resulting from activation of the sympathetico-adrenal system does occur, the main factor in emotional disturbance of the milk-ejection reflex is a central mechanism acting by partial or complete inhibition of oxytocin release.

The possibility that adrenaline acts centrally by blocking the release of oxytocin in a dose too small to cause peripheral inhibition appears to be excluded by the experiments of Chaudhury, Chaudhury, and Lu (1961). They showed that block of the milk-ejection reflex induced by stress in guinea-pigs could be reduced by injecting the tranquillizing drugs, reserpine, chlorpromazine and meprobamate into the mothers before suckling, but that the anti-adrenaline drugs, dibenamine and dichloroisoprenaline were without effect. This suggests that emotional inhibition of the milk-ejection reflex is mediated by non-adrenergic inhibitory pathways within the central nervous system and not by release of adrenaline from the sympathetico-adrenal system.

XII. The Action on the Mammary Gland of Synthetic Analogues of Oxytocin

The chief theoretical interest in the study of synthetic analogues of oxytocin is to discover the structural requirements for different biological activities and eventually to define the chemical nature of the tissue receptors for the hormone. Many of the analogues which have been synthesized show an almost total loss of all the biological activities of oxytocin. Of greater importance from a practical standpoint are analogues which show an alteration in the ratio of activities or act as antagonists or produce a type of pharmacological response different from that which is typical of oxytocin. Two groups of analogues are of particular interest in this context. The first contains analogues which have a selective action on the mammary gland. The second consists of a number of analogues which have been termed "synthetic hormonogens." This term was introduced by Jošt, Rudinger, and Šorm (1963b) to define analogues the main action of which is not due to the analogue itself but occurs only after its conversion into the active hormone when injected into an animal or applied to an isolated organ preparation. In general the effect of hormonogens on the mammary gland is to produce a protracted type of milk-ejection response and inhibit the action of oxytocin.

A. Analogues Having a Selective Action on the Mammary Gland

Modifications of the chemical structure of oxytocin do not necessarily affect its various biological activities equally. In general, milk-ejecting activity is less susceptible than other activities to changes in structure. For example, in most synthetic analogues the ratio of milk-ejecting to oxytocic activity is higher than in oxytocin. This applies also to the vasopressins. For lysine-vasopressin the ratio is 12 and for arginine-vasopressin, 4. Deamino-oxytocin is an exception since its activity on the rabbit mammary gland is only 400 U/mg compared with 684 U/mg on the isolated rat uterus (Hope, Murti, and du Vigneaud, 1962).

No analogue has been synthesized which has a greater milk-ejecting activity on a weight basis than oxytocin itself. However the absolute potency is of less interest than the ratio of activities. As a therapeutic agent a potentially useful analogue would be one which is more active on the mammary gland than on the

Table 7. *Analogues of oxytocin with selective milk-ejecting activity*

Analogue	Activity (U/mg) Oxytocic (OA) (isolated rat uterus)	Milk-ejecting (MEA) Rabbit	Milk-ejecting (MEA) Guinea-pig	Antidiuretic (ADA) (rat)	Ratios MEA/OA	Ratios MEA/ADA	Ref.
A. Oxytocin	450 ± 30	450 ± 30		5 ± 1	1	90	1
Ile^8-oxytocin (Mesotocin)	289 ± 21	328 ± 21		1.1 ± 0.1	1.1	298	2
Ser^4-Ile^8-oxytocin (Ichthyotocin, Isotocin)	150 ± 12	300 ± 15	—	0.18 ± 0.03	2.0	1666	3
B. Phe^2-oxytocin	32 ± 2	141 ± 21	—	~0.5	4.4	282	4
(Me) Tyr^2-oxytocin	13		61		4.7	—	5
(O-Me) Tyr^2-oxytocin	<2 (anti)	—	7	0.01	>3.5	700	5
C. Leu^3-oxytocin	6 (4.4—7.7)	—	35	1	5.8	35	6
a Ile^3-oxytocin	24	—	125	0.05	5	2500	6
Nle^3-oxytocin	4 (2.0—5.1)	—	25	0.5	6.3	50	6
Nva^3-oxytocin	7	—	85	5	12.1	17	6
D. Ala^4-oxytocin	36 ± 6	240 ± 55	—	<0.01	6.7	>24000	7
Asp (NH$_2$)^4-oxytocin	108 ± 29	300 ± 128	—	0.044 ± 0.005	2.8	6820	8
Ser^4-oxytocin	195 ± 30	255 ± 45	—	0.06 ± 0.01	1.3	4250	9
Gly^4-oxytocin	2.8 ± 0.1	17 ± 1	—	<0.005	6.1	>3400	10
	3.9 ± 1.8	50 ± 25	—	—	12.8	—	11
E. Val^8-oxytocin	200 ± 15	310 ± 20	—	0.8 ± 0.1	1.6	388	12
Gly^8-oxytocin	16 ± 1	46 ± 7	—	0.16 ± 0.03	2.9	288	13
Ala^8-oxytocin	141 ± 17	208 ± 8	—	0.08 ± 0.01	1.5	2600	14
(Ne-For-Lys)^8-oxytocin	148 ± 12	220 ± 12	—	0.3 ± 0.03	1.5	733	15
F. De-Carboxamido^4-oxytocin	72 ± 2	225 ± 7	—	~0.3	3.1	750	16
De-Amino-De-Carboxamido^4-oxytocin	93 ± 2	266 ± 2	—	~2	2.9	133	17

References: 1. Berde and Boissonnas (1966); 2. Jaquenoud and Boissonnas (1961), Berde and Konzett (1960); 3. Berde and Boissonnas (1966); 4. Jaquenoud and Boissonnas (1959), Bodanszky and du Vigneaud (1959), Konzett and Berde (1959); 5. Zhuse, Jošt, Kasafirek, and Rudinger (1967), Law and du Vigneaud (1960), Jost, Rudinger, and Šorm (1963a), Bisset (1962b, 1964); 6. Nesvadba, Honzl, and Rudinger (1963), Bisset (1962b); 7. Guttman and Boissonnas (1963); 8. Jaquenoud and Boissonnas (1962), Berde and Stürmer (1962); 9. Guttmann and Boissonnas (1963); 10. Drabarek (1964); 11. Fosker and Law (1965); 12. Jaquenoud and Boissonnas (1961), Berde, Konzett and Stürmer (1960); 13. Jaquenoud and Boissonnas (1963); 14. Jaquenoud and Boissonnas (1964), Berde and Stürmer (1964); 15. Huguenin and Boissonnas (1963); 16. du Vigneaud, Denning, Drabarek, and Chan (1964); 17. Branda, Drabarek, and du Vigneaud (1966), du Vigneaud (1965).

uterus and which has only weak antidiuretic and pressor activity. A number of analogues which meet these requirements are listed in Table 7. The action of synthetic analogues on the mammary gland is usually studied by measuring milk-ejection pressure in the cannulated teat duct of a lactating rabbit or guinea-pig, although a few observations have been made on the isolated gland. The table shows oxytocic (OA) milk-ejecting (MEA) and antidiuretic (ADA) activities and the ratios: MEA:OA and MEA:ADA. The higher these ratios, the more selective is the action of an analogue on the mammary gland.

Two naturally occurring analogues, Ile^{8}-oxytocin (Mesotocin) and Ser^{4}-Ile^{8}-oxytocin (Ichthyotocin, Isotocin) have been included in the table (part A) because it is of interest that these two hormones occurring in some amphibians and fishes are more selective than oxytocin in their action on the mammary gland.

The three analogues given in part B involve a modification of the hydroxyl group in the tyrosine residue in position 2 of oxytocin. In Phe^{2}-oxytocin (deoxy-oxytocin), the hydroxyl group has been deleted; in (Me) Tyr^{2}-oxytocin it has been replaced by a methyl, and in (O-Me) Tyr^{2}-oxytocin by a methoxyl group. These three analogues form a graded series. All show a relatively high ratio of MEA:OA. The least potent, (O-Me) Tyr^{2}-oxytocin, inhibits under certain conditions the action of oxytocin on the isolated rat uterus (Beránková, Rychlík, Jošt, Rudinger and Šorm, 1961; Rudinger and Krejčí, 1962; Bisset, 1962b, 1964; Krejčí, Poláček, Kupková, and Rudinger, 1964) but no inhibitory effect was observed in assays of milk-ejecting activity in the lactating guinea-pig. This difference could be caused by metabolic or other factors involved in the two assay systems, one of which is an isolated organ and the other a preparation *in vivo*. It does not necessarily imply a difference in the nature of the tissue receptors for oxytocin in the uterus and the mammary gland.

The conditions under which oxytocic activity is tested on the isolated rat uterus are quite artificial. In order to abolish the spontaneous activity of this preparation it is usual to lower the temperature of the organ bath and to reduce the concentration of calcium to one quarter of that normally used in physiological salt solutions. A reduction in the concentration of calcium is a factor which enhances the inhibitory effect of (O-Me) Tyr^{2}-oxytocin on the uterus. (Krejčí et al., 1964). It is significant that this analogue does not inhibit the action of oxytocin on the rat uterus *in situ* (Bisset, unpublished). On the other hand (O-Me) Tyr^{2}-oxytocin and some related analogues have been shown to cause tachyphylaxis and inhibition of the response to oxytocin when tested under suitable conditions on the isolated rat mammary gland (Poláček, Krejčí, and Rudinger, unpublished). This finding illustrates the value of testing synthetic analogues not only on the mammary gland *in situ* but also on the isolated gland.

Recently quantitative methods have been developed for assaying oxytocin on the rat uterus *in situ* (Bisset, Haldar, and Lewin, 1966) and for milk-ejecting activity in the lactating rat (Bisset, Clark, Haldar, Harris, Lewis, and Rocha e Silva, 1967). These methods permit the comparison of oxytocic and milk-ejecting activities assayed *in situ* in the same species.

Parts C—F of the table show that analogues having a selective action on the mammary gland can be produced by substitution in positions 3 (C) 4 (D) and 8 (E) of oxytocin as well as in position 2, and also by omission of the carboxamide group in position 4 or of both this group and the terminal amino group in position 1 (F). Three analogues with a particularly selective action on the mammary gland are a Ile^{3}-, Ala^{4}- and Gly^{4}-oxytocin. In all these analogues the ratio of MEA:OA is 5 or more and the ratio of MEA:ADA is so high that they can be said to be almost devoid of antidiuretic activity. These analogues therefore approach the ideal of a specific milk-ejecting hormone.

B. Synthetic Hormonogens

The analogues included in this group are Gly. Cys^{1}-, Leu. Cys^{1}-, Phe. Cys^{1}-, Pro. Cys^{1}-, Gly. Gly. Cys^{1}-, Leu. Leu Cys^{1}-, and Leu. Gly. Gly. Cys^{1}-oxytocin. Their action on the mammary gland has been investigated by BERÁNKOVÁ-KSANDROVÁ, BISSET, JOŠT, KREJČÍ, PLIŠKA, RUDINGER, RYCHLÍK, and ŠORM (1966). On intravenous injection into the lactating guinea-pig the typical effect is to cause a protracted increase in milk-ejection pressure followed by tachyphylaxis and inhibition of the response to oxytocin. Under certain experimental conditions the analogues inhibit oxytocin without themselves producing any increase in milk-ejection pressure. In all the analogues an amino-acid or a short peptide chain is

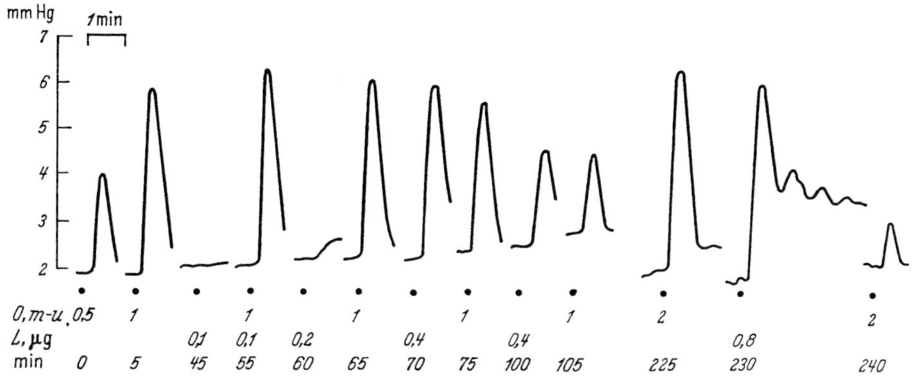

Fig. 4. Effect of Leu. Cys[1]-oxytocin (L) on milk-ejection pressure, and on its response to oxytocin (O), in the lactating guinea-pig. Intravenous injections. From BERÁNKOVÁ-KSANDROVÁ et al, Brit. J. Pharmacol., *26*, 615—632, (1966). Reproduced by kind permission of the Editorial Board.

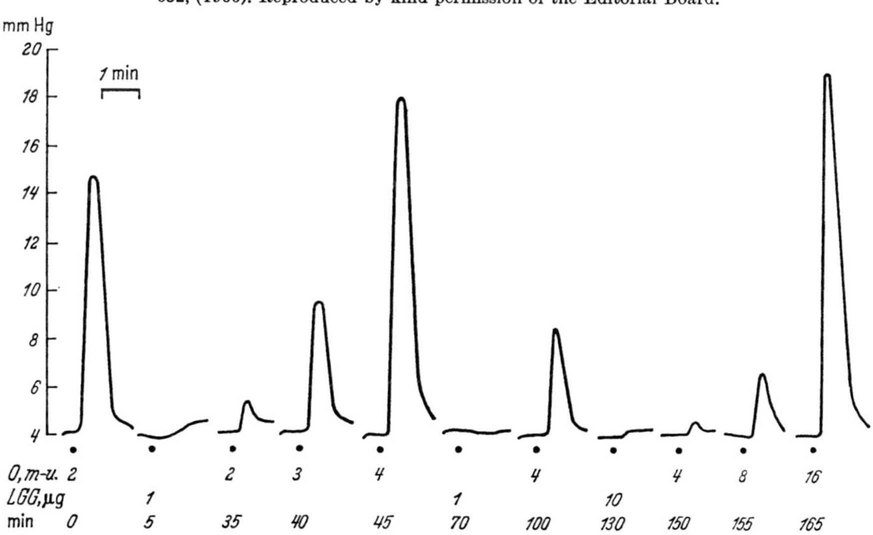

Fig. 5. Effect of Leu. Gly. Gly. Cys[1]-oxytocin (LGG) on milk-ejection pressure, and on its response to oxytocin (O), in the lactating guinea-pig. Intravenous injections. From BERÁNKOVÁ-KSANDROVÁ et al, Brit. J. Pharmacol. *26*, 615—632, (1966). Reprocuded by kind permission of the Editorial Board

attached to the terminal amino group of the hemicystine residue in position 1 of oxytocin. The substituent group is believed to be split off by aminopeptidases *in vivo* causing a continuous liberation of oxytocin. This effect is thought to explain many of the pharmacological actions of these analogues which have been termed "hormonogens."

A typical response to the intravenous injection of a hormonogen is illustrated in Fig. 4 which is taken from an experiment with Leu. Cys[1]-oxytocin on the lactating guinea-pig. The threshold dose of oxytocin for eliciting an increase in milk-ejection pressure was 0.5 mU (1.1 ng); the pressure increased in a single peak and 1 min after the injection it had practically returned to the control level. The threshold dose of the analogue was 0.2 μg. A subthreshold dose of 0.1 μg did not inhibit the response to 1 mU oxytocin injected simultaneously. The injection of 0.4 μg produced an increase in pressure similar in amplitude to that obtained with 1 mU oxytocin but of longer duration. The response to a second injection of 0.4 μg of the analogue was reduced and tachyphylaxis was accompanied by inhibition of the response to oxytocin. The injection of 0.8 μg produced an increase in pressure which persisted with fluctuations for 10 min. After this injection the response to 2 mU oxytocin was smaller than that obtained initially with 0.5 mU.

The various analogues of the hormonogen series differ in the intensity of their effects. Tachyphylaxis and inhibition of the response to oxytocin are common features, but Pro. Cys^1- and Gly. Gly. Cys^1-oxytocin are exceptional in not

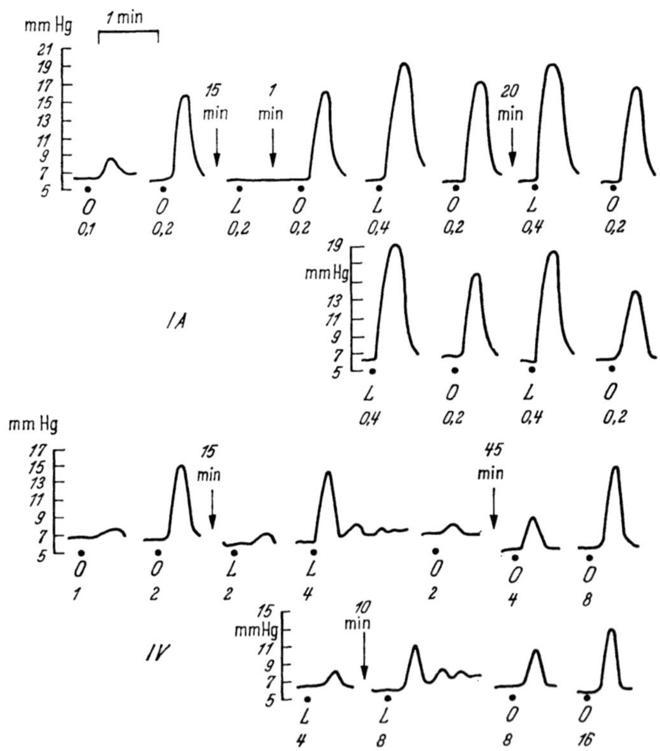

Fig. 6. Effect on milk-ejection pressure in the lactating guinea-pig of intra-arterial (IA) and intravenous (IV) injections of oxytocin (O) and Leu. Gly. Gly. Cys^1-oxytocin (L). The responses shown were obtained at intervals of 5 min except where indicated by the arrows. Doses of oxytocin in mU and of Leu. Gly. Gly. Cys^1-oxytocin in μg. From G. W. BISSET: Oxytocin, Vasopressin and their Structural Analogues, pp 21—29. Ed. by J. RUDINGER, (Proc. 2nd. Intern. Pharmacol. Meeting Vol. 10, 1964). Reproduced by permission of the publishers, Pergamon Press Limited

producing a protracted type of response. These differences probably depend on the degree of susceptibility of the analogues to aminopeptidases. A further complication in interpreting the mode of action of hormonogens is that they appear to possess an inherent milk-ejecting activity in addition to the property of liberating oxytocin. This inherent activity is most likely to be seen if the first dose injected is relatively high. If on the other hand the dose is initially low and gradually increased, an inhibitory effect may develop before the threshold for inherent activity is reached. This type of response is illustrated in Fig. 5 taken from an experiment with Leu. Gly. Gly. Cys¹-oxytocin. The analogue itself did not produce an increase in milk-ejection pressure but it strongly inhibited the response to oxytocin. The inhibition could be surmounted by an eightfold increase in the dose of oxytocin. However, in the experiment shown in Fig. 6 (IV), the same analogue produced a pattern of response similar to that given by Leu. Cys¹-oxytocin (Fig. 4) with a prolonged increase in milk-ejection pressure, tachyphylaxis and inhibition of oxytocin.

In contrast with its effect on intravenous injection, Leu. Gly. Gly. Cys¹-oxytocin did not cause tachyphylaxis or inhibition when tested by close arterial injection into the mammary gland (Fig. 6, IA) or on the isolated guinea-pig gland. The

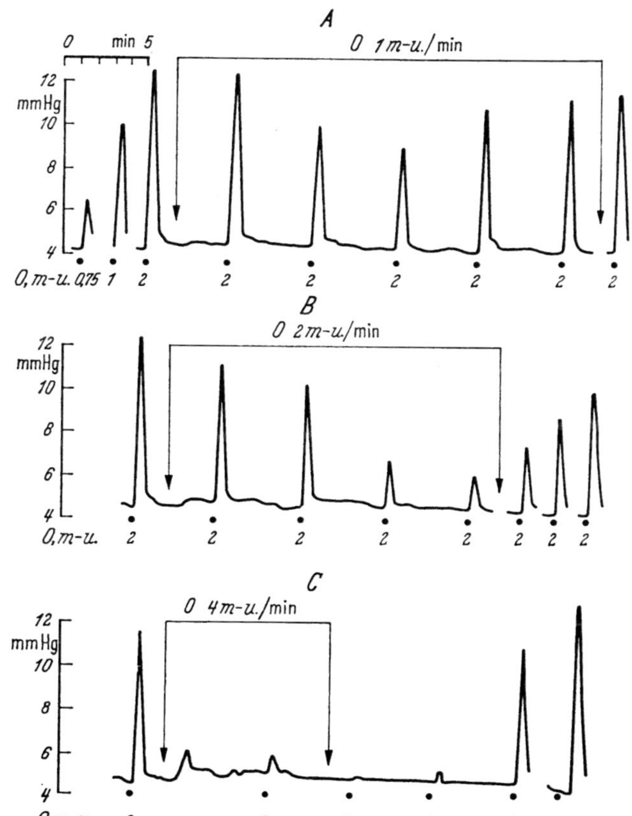

Fig. 7. Effect of intravenous infusions (between arrows) of oxytocin (O) on the response of the milk-ejection pressure to single intravenous injections of oxytocin in the lactating guinea-pig. Dots mark intravenous injections of oxytocin. In the discontinuous parts of the tracing, injections were given at intervals of 5 min. From Beránková-Ksandrová et al, Brit. J. Pharmacol., *26*, 615—632 (1966). Reproduced by kind permission of the Editorial Board

responses to the analogue were indistinguishable from those to oxytocin and the analogue had the same activity (0.5 U/mg) on the two assay systems. This probably represents inherent activity. In the experiment of Fig. 6 the dose ratio of oxytocin and the analogue was the same for the intraarterial (IA) and intravenous (IV) routes of injection. The difference in the two responses shown in Fig. 6 seems therefore to depend on the actual amount of analogue injected into the circulation and metabolised: it could be explained by supposing that only the relatively large amount which is required to produce a milk-ejection response by intravenous injection liberates enough oxytocin to elicit the pattern of response typical of a hormonogen.

Further evidence in support of the hormonogen hypothesis is provided by the results of experiments with three synthetic analogues of oxytocin, Me. Cys[1]-, Sar. Cys[1]- and D—Leu. Cys[1]-oxytocin, having substituents in the terminal NH_2 group which would not theoretically be susceptible to the action of aminopeptidases. When tested intravenously in the lactating guinea-pig, these analogues exhibited none of the effects typical of hormonogens but they did possess a small degree of milk-ejecting activity amounting to 0.3—1.0 U/mg.

An attempt was made to mimic the effect of hormonogens by infusing oxytocin intravenously into a guinea-pig at rates comparable with those at which its liberation from a hormonogen might be supposed to occur *in vivo*. An experiment of this kind is shown in Fig. 7. With a rate of infusion of 4 mU/min a small and transient increase in milk-ejection pressure occurred; this was not observed with lower rates of 1 and 2 mU/min. During the infusions at all three rates, the responses to single intravenous injections of oxytocin were inhibited. The inhibition was graded according to the rate of infusion and could be surmounted by increasing the dose of oxytocin. This result suggests that the inhibitory effect of the hormonogens as well as the protracted response and tachyphylaxis could be explained by the hypothesis of a continuous liberation of oxytocin *in vivo*.

The effects of the hormonogens are not confined to the mammary gland. du Vigneaud, Fitt, Bodanszky, and O'Connell (1960) first described a hormonogen-like effect with Gly. Cys[1]-oxytocin on chicken blood pressure. The mechanism of inhibition on various biological assay systems is discussed in the chapter by Krejčí and Rudinger in this volume.

References

Abrahams, V. C.: The effect of anticholinesterases injected into the supraoptic nuclei of chloralosed dogs on the release of the oxytocic factor of the posterior pituitary. J. Physiol. (Lond.) **133**, 330—333 (1956b).

—, G. B. Koelle, and P. Smart: Histochemical demonstration of cholinesterases in the hypothalamus of the dog. J. Physiol. (Lond.) **139**, 137—144 (1957).

—, E. P. Langworth, and G. W. Theobald: Potentials evoked in the hypothalamus and cerebral cortex by electrical stimulation of the uterus. Nature (Lond.) **203**, 654—656 (1964).

—, M. Pickford: Observations on a central antagonism between adrenaline and acetylcholine. J. Physiol. (Lond.) **131**, 712—718 (1956a).

Adamsons, K., Jr., S. L. Engel, H. V. van Dyke, B. Schmidt-Nielsen, and K. Schmidt-Nielsen: The distribution of oxytocin and vasopressin (antidiuretic hormone) in the neurophysis of the camel. Endocrinology **58**, 272—278 (1956).

Andersson, B.: Some observations on the neurohumoral regulation of milk ejection. Acta physiol. scand. **23**, 1—8 (1951a).

— The effect and localisation of electrical stimulation of certain parts of the brain stem in sheep and goats. Acta physiol. scand. **23**, 8—23 (1951b).

— Further studies on the milk-ejection mechanism in sheep and goats. Acta physiol. scand. **23**, 24—30 (1951c).

—, and S. M. McCann: Drinking, antidiuresis and milk-ejection from electrical stimulation within the hypothalamus of the goat. Acta physiol. scand. **35**, 191—201 (1955).

Averill, R. L. W.: The hypothalamus and lactation. Brit. med. Bull. **22**, 261—265 (1966).

Babkin, B. P.: Secretory mechanism of the digestive glands, p. 676. New York: Hoeber 1944.

Bangham, D. R., and G. W. Bisset, unpublished.

—, and M. V. Mussett: Third International Standard for Posterior Pituitary. Bull. Wld. Hlth Org. **19**, 325—340 (1958).

Bargmann, W.: Über die Neurosekretorische Verknüpfung von Hypothalamus und Neurohypophyse. Z. Zellforsch. Abt. Histochem. **34**, 610—634 (1949a).
— Über die Neurosekretorische Verknüpfung von Hypothalamus und Hypophyse. Klin. Wschr. **27**, 617—622 (1949b).
Baryshnikov, I.A.: Nervous control of mammary function. The reflex regulation of lactation. In: 2nd Int. Congr. Endocr., pp. 655—659, 1964.
Beleslin, D., G.W. Bisset, J. Haldar, and R.L. Polak: The release of vasopressin without oxytocin in response to haemorrhage. Proc. roy. Soc. B **166**, 443—458 (1967).
Beller, F.K., K.H. Krumholz, and K. Zeininger: Vergleichende Oxytocin-Bestimmungen. Gemessen durch den lactagogen Effect der Milchdrüse. Acta endocr. (Kbh.) **29**, 1—8 (1958).
Benda, C.: Das Verhältnis der Milchdrüse zu den Hautdrüsen. Derm. Z. **1**, 94—110 (1894).
Benson, G.K.: Pituitary-adrenal relationships in the retardation of mammary gland involution by oxytocin. J. Endocr. **20**, 91—100 (1960).
—, and A.T. Cowie: Lactation in the rat after hypophysial posterior lobectomy. J. Endocr. **14**, 54—65 (1956).
— —, and J.S. Tindal: The pituitary and the maintenance of milk secretion. Proc. roy. Soc. B. **149**, 330—336 (1958).
—, and S.J. Folley: Oxytocin as stimulator for the release of prolactin from the anterior pituitary. Nature (Lond.) **177**, 700 (1956).
— — Retardation of mammary involution in the rat by oxytocin. J. Endocr. **14**, xl (1957a).
— — The effect of oxytocin on mammary gland involution in the rat. J. Endocr. **16**, 189—202 (1957b).
— — Effects of oxytocin on the functional capacity of pituitary grafts with particular reference to prolactin secretion. In: 1st Int. Congr. Endocr., Copenhagen, Abstr. No. 578, 1147, 1960.
Beránková, Z., I. Rychlík, K. Jošt, J. Rudinger, and F. Šorm: Inhibition of the uterus-contracting effect of oxytocin by O-methyloxytocin. Coll. Czechoslov. Chem. Commun. **26**, 2673—2675 (1961).
Beránková-Ksandrová, Z., G.W. Bisset, K. Jošt, I. Krejčí, V. Pliška, J. Rudinger, I. Rychlík, and F. Šorm: Synthetic analogues of oxytocin acting as hormonogens. Brit. J. Pharmacol. **26**, 615—632 (1966).
Berde, B., and R.A. Boissonnas: Synthetic analogues and homologues of the posterior pituitary hormones. In: The pituitary gland, pp. 624—661. Ed. by G.W. Harris and B.T. Donovan. London: Butterworths 1966.
—, and A. Cerletti: Démonstration expérimentale de l'action de l'ocytocine sur la glande mammaire. Gynaecologia (Basel) **144**, 275—278 (1957).
— — Über die Wirkung pharmakologischer Oxytocindosen auf die Milchdrüse. Acta endocr. (Kbh.) **34**, 543—557 (1960).
— — Prüfung von Bradykinin and Hypertensin an der Milchdrüse. Helv. physiol. pharmacol. Acta. **19**, C7—10 (1961).
—, and H. Konzett: Isoleucyl[8]-Oxytocin, ein biologisch-hochwirksames Polypeptid. Med. exp. (Basel) **2**, 317—322 (1960).
— —, and E. Stürmer: (1960, 1962, 1964, unpublished). Cited by B. Berde, and R.A. Boissonnas. In: The pituitary gland, pp. 624—661. Ed. by G.W. Harris and B.T. Donovan. London: Butterworths 1966.
Berger, E., and J.M. Marshall: Interactions of oxytocin, potassium, and calcium in the rat uterus. Amer. J. Physiol. **201**, 931—934 (1961).
Bernstein, S.H., R.E. Weston, G. Ross, J. Grossman, I.B. Hanenson, and L. Leiter: Studies on intravenous water diuresis and nicotine and pitressin antidiuresis in normal subjects and patients with liver disease. J. clin. Invest. **32**, 422—427 (1953).
Beyer, C., and F. Mena: Blockage of milk removal in the cat by periventricular diencephalic lesions. Amer. J. Physiol. **208**, 585—588 (1965).
— —, P. Pacheco, and M. Alcarez: Effect of central nervous system lesions on lactation in the cat. Fed. Proc. **21**, 353 (1962).
—, J.S. Tindal, and C.H. Sawyer: Electrophysiological study of projections from mesencephalic central gray matter to forebrain in the rabbit. Exp. Neurol. **6**, 435—450 (1962).
Beyer, F.C., L.G. Anguiano, and F.J. Mena: Oxytocin release in response to stimulation of cingulate gyrus. Amer. J. Physiol. **200**, 625—627 (1961).
Bisset, G.W.: The assay of oxytocin and vasopressin in blood and the mechanism of inactivation of these hormones by sodium thioglycollate. In: Oxytocin, pp. 380—399. Ed. by R. Caldeyro-Barcia and H. Heller. Oxford: Pergamon Press 1961.
— Effect of tyrosinase preparations on oxytocin, vasopressin and bradykinin. Brit. J. Pharmacol. **18**, 405—420 (1962a).
— Synthetic analogues of oxytocin acting as antagonists. J. Physiol. (Lond.) **165**, 69—71 (1962b).

BISSET, G.W.: The effect on milk-ejecting activity of modifying two functional groups in oxytocin. In: Oxytocin, vasopressin and their structural analogues, 2nd Int. Pharmacological Meeting, Prague, pp. 21—29. Oxford: Pergamon Press 1964.
—, B. J. CLARK, J. HALDAR, M.C. HARRIS, G. P. LEWIS, and E. ROCHA E SILVA, Brit. J. Pharmakol. **31**, 537—549 (1967).
— —, and G.P. LEWIS: Brit. J. Pharmakol. **31**, 550—559 (1967).
—, J. HALDAR, and J.E. LEWIN: Actions of oxytocin and other biologically active peptides on the rat uterus. Mem. Soc. Endocrin. **14**, 185—198 (1966).
—, S.M. HILTON, and A.M. POISNER: Parallel assays of vasopressin and oxytocin in blood on localized electrical stimulation of the hypothalamus. J. Physiol. (Lond.) **169**, 40—41 (1963).
— — — Hypothalamic pathways for independent release of vasopressin and oxytocin. Proc. roy. Soc. B **166**, 422—442 (1967).
—, and J. LEE: Antidiuretic activity in the blood after stimulation of the neurohypophysis in man. Lancet **2**, 715—719 (1958).
—, and G.P. LEWIS: A spectrum of pharmacological activity in some biologically active peptides. Brit. J. Pharmacol. **19**, 168—182 (1962).
—, and J.M. WALKER: Assay of oxytocin in blood. J. Physiol. (Lond.) **126**, 588—595 (1954).
— — The effects of nicotine, hexamethonium and ethanol on the secretion of the antidiuretic and oxytocic hormones of the rat. Brit. J. Pharmacol. **12**, 461—467 (1957).
BODANSZKY, M., and V. DU VIGNEAUD: Synthesis of a biologically active analog of oxytocin, with phenylalanine replacing tyrosine. J. Amer. chem. Soc. **81**, 1258 (1959).
BOISSONNAS, R.A., ST. GUTTMANN, B. BERDE, and H. KONZETT: Relationships between the chemical structures and the biological properties of the posterior pituitary hormones and their synthetic analogues. Experientia (Basel) **17**, 377—432 (1961).
BOWER, E.A.: Action potentials from uterine sensory nerves. J. Physiol. (Lond.) **148**, 2P (1959).
BRANDA, L.A., S. DRABAREK, and V. DU VIGNEAUD: The synthesis and pharmacological properties of deamino-4-decarboxamido-oxytocin (1-β-mercaptopropionic acid-4-α-aminobutyric acid-oxytocin). J. biol. Chem. **241**, 2572—2575 (1966).
BRAUDE, R., and K.G. MITCHELL: "Let-down" of milk in the sow. Nature (Lond.) **165**, 937 (1950).
— — Observations on the relationship between oxytocin and adrenaline in milk ejection in the sow. J. Endocr. **8**, 238—241 (1952).
BROOKS, C.McC., T. ISHIKAWA, and K. KOIZUMI: Control of activity in supraoptic nucleus neurons. Physiologist **6**, 147 (1963).
— — —, and H.-H. LU: Activity of neurones in the paraventricular nucleus of the hypothalamus and its control. J. Physiol. (Lond.) **182**, 217—231 (1966).
BÜLBRING, E., and J.H. BURN: An action of adrenaline on transmission in sympathetic ganglia which may play a part in shock. J. Physiol. (Lond.) **101**, 289—303 (1942).
BUGBEE, E.P., and O. KAMM: Recent progress in the investigation of the posterior lobe of the pituitary gland. Endocrinology **12**, 671—679 (1928).
BURN, G.P., and R.S. GREWAL: The antidiuretic response to and excretion of pituitary (posterior lobe) extract in man, with reference to the action of nicotine. Brit. J. Pharmacol. **6**, 471—482 (1951).
BURN, J.H.: The concept of double transmission. In: The autonomic nervous system, p. 111. Oxford: Blackwell Scientific Publications 1963.
— Current concepts about adrenergic transmission. J. med. Sci. **11**, 3—18 (1965).
— Adrenergic transmission. Pharmacol. Rev. **18**, Part 1, 459—470 (1966).
—, and M.J. RAND: Sympathetic postganglionic mechanism. Nature (Lond.) **184**, 163—165 (1959).
—, L.H. TRUELOVE, and I. BURN: Antidiuretic action of nicotine and of smoking. Brit med. J. **1**, 403—406 (1945).
CAMPBELL, B., and W.E. PETERSEN: Milk "let-down" and the orgasm in the human female. Human Biol. **25**, 165—168 (1953).
CATHCART, E.P., F.W. GAIRNS, and H.S.D. GARVEN: The innervation of the human quiescent nipple, with notes on pigmentation, erection and hyperneury. Trans. roy. Soc. Edinb. **51**, 699—718 (1949).
CHALMERS, T.M., and A.A.G. LEWIS: Stimulation of the supraoptico-hypophysial system in man. Clin. Sci. **10**, 127—135 (1951).
CHAN, W.Y. Mechanism of epinephrine inhibition of the milk-ejecting response to oxytocin. J. Pharmacol. exp. Ther. **147**, 48—53 (1965).
CHANG, H.C., K.F. CHIA, C.H. HSU, and R.K.S. LIM: Humoral transmission of nerve impulses at central synapses. I. Sinus and vagus afferent nerves. Chin. J. Physiol. **12**, 1—35 (1937a).
— — —, and R.K.S. LIM: Vagus — post-pituitary reflex. I. Pressor component. Chin. J. Physiol. **12**, 309—326 (1937b).

Chang, H. C., K. F. Chia, C. H. Hsu, and R. K. S. Lim: Reflex secretion of the posterior pituitary elicited through the vagus. J. Physiol. (Lond.) **90**, 87—89 (1937c).
— — — — Humoral transmission of nerve impulses at central synapses. II. Central vagus transmission after hypophysectomy in the dog. Chin. J. Physiol. **13**, 13—32 (1938).
Chaudhury, R. R.: The release of oxytocin in unanaesthetized lactating rats. In: 1st Int. Congress of Endocrinology, Copenhagen 1960, p. 123.
— Release of oxytocin in unanaesthetized lactating rats. Brit. J. Pharmacol. **17**, 297—304 (1961).
—, M. R. Chaudhury, and F. C. Lu: Stress-induced block of milk ejection. Brit. J. Pharmacol. **17**, 305—309 (1961).
Clark, B. J., and M. Rocha e Silva, jr.: Independent release of vasopressin by carotid occlusion. J. Physiol. (Lond.) **186**, 142—143 (1966).
Clegg, P. C., P. Hopkinson, and V. R. Pickles: Some effects of calcium and magnesium ions on guinea-pig uterine muscle. J. Physiol. (Lond.) **167**, 1—17 (1963).
Couthino, E. M., and A. Csapo: The effect of oxytocics on the "ca-deficient" uterus. J. gen. Physiol. **43**, 13—27 (1959).
Cowie, A. T.: Unpublished work, quoted by S. J. Folley. Recent Progr. Hormone Res. **7**, 107, (1952).
—, and S. J. Folley: Neurohypophysial hormones and the mammary gland. In: The neurohypophysis, pp. 183—201. Ed. by H. Heller. London: Butterworths 1957.
— —, B. A. Cross, G. W. Harris, D. Jacobsohn, and K. C. Richardson: Terminology for use in lactational physiology. Nature (Lond.) **168**, 421 (1951).
— —, and K. C. Richardson: Terminology in lactational physiology. Lancet **2**, 601—602 (1954).
—, G. S. Knaggs, and J. S. Tindal: Complete restoration of lactation in the goat after hypophysectomy. J. Endocr. **28**, 267—279 (1964).
—, and J. S. Tindal: Some aspects of the neuro-endocrine control of lactation. In: Proc. 2nd Int. Congr. Endocr., pp. 646—654, 1964.
Cross, B. A.: Suckling antidiuresis in rabbits. Nature (Lond.) **166**, 612—613 (1950).
— Suckling antidiuresis in rabbits. J. Physiol. (Lond.) **114**, 447 (1951).
— Nursing behaviour and the milk-ejection reflex in rabbits. J. Endocr. **8**, XIII (1952a).
— Milk ejection and neurohypophysial function. Endocrinology **9**, IX (1952b).
— Sympathetico-adrenal inhibition of the neurohypophysial milk-ejection mechanism. J. Endocr. **9**, 7—18 (1953a).
— Milk ejection and neurohypophysial function. J. Endocr. **9**, IX (1953b).
— Milk ejection resulting from mechanical stimulation of mammary myoepithelium in the rabbit. Nature (Lond.) **173**, 450—451 (1954a).
— The hypothalamus and the mechanism of sympathetico-adrenal inhibition of milk-ejection. J. Endocr. **11**, IV (1954b).
— The hypothalamus and the mechanism of sympathetico-adrenal inhibition of milk-ejection. J. Endocr. **12**, 15—28 (1955a).
— Neurohormonal mechanisms in emotional inhibition of milk-ejection. J. Endocr. **12**, 29—37 (1955b).
— The posterior pituitary gland in relation to reproduction and lactation. J. Endocr. **11**, 151—155 (1955c).
— The motility and reactivity of the oestrogenized rabbit uterus *in vivo*; with comparative observations on milk-ejection. J. Endocr. **16**, 237—260 (1958a).
— On the mechanism of labour in the rabbit. J. Endocr. **16**, 261—276 (1958b).
— Neural control of oxytocin secretion. In: Oxytocin, pp. 24—47. Ed. by R. Caldeyro-Barcia and H. Heller. Oxford: Pergamon Press 1961.
—, and H. B. van Dyke: The effects of highly purified posterior pituitary principles on the lactating mammary gland of the rabbit. J. Endocr. **9**, 232—235 (1953).
—, and J. D. Green: Activity of single neurones in the hypothalamus. Effect of osmotic and other stimuli. J. Physiol. (Lond.) **148**, 554—569 (1959).
—, and G. W. Harris: Milk-ejection following electrical stimulation of the pituitary stalk in rabbits. Nature (Lond.) **166**, 994—995 (1950a).
— — Milk ejection following electrical stimulation of the pituitary stalk in rabbits. Colloq. int. Cent. nat. Rech. Sci. (Paris) No. 32, 157 (1950b).
— — The neurohypophysis and "let-down" of milk. J. Physiol. (Lond.) **113**, 35 P (1951).
— — The role of the neurohypophysis in the milk-ejection reflex. J. Endocr. **8**, 148—161 (1952).
—, and I. A. Silver: Milk-ejection and mammary engorgement. Proc. roy. Soc. Med. **49**, 978—979 (1956).

CROSS, B.A., and I.A. SILVER: Mammary oxygen tension and the milk-ejection mechanism. J. Endocr. **23**, 375—384 (1962).
— — (Unpublished). Cited by B.A. CROSS. In: Oxytocin, pp. 24—47. Ed. by R. CALDEYRO-BARCIA and H. HELLER. Oxford: Pergamon Press 1961.
CSAPO, A.: A link between "models" and living muscle. Nature (Lond.) **173**, 1019—1021 (1954).
— The effects of oxytocic substances on the excitability of the uterus. In: Oxytocin, pp. 100 to 123. Ed. by R. CALDEYRO-BARCIA and H. HELLER. London: Pergamon Press 1961.
DALE, H.: Evidence concerning the endocrine function of the neurohypophysis and its nervous control. In: The neurohypophysis, pp. 1—9. Ed. by H. HELLER. London: Butterworths 1957.
DANIEL, A.R., and K. LEDERIS: Effects of ether anaesthesia and haemorrhage on hormone storage and ultrastructure of the rat neurohypophysis. J. Endocr. **34**, 91—104 (1966a).
— — Effects of acetylcholine on the release of neurohypophysial hormones *in vitro*. J. Endocr. **34**, X—XI (1966b).
DANIEL, E.E., H. SEHDEV, and K. ROBINSON: Mechanisms for activation of smooth muscle. Physiol. Rev. Suppl. **5**, 228—260 (1962).
DEBACKERE, M., and G. PEETERS: The influence of vaginal distension on milk ejection and diuresis in the lactating cow. Arch. int. Pharmacodyn. **123**, 462—471 (1960a).
— — Milk ejection studied by means of a crossed-circulation technique on sheep. Naturwissenschaften **47**, 189 (1960b).
— — Release of hormone induced by massage of the seminal vesicles and ampullae in the ram. Naturwissenschaften **47**, 329 (1960c).
— — and N. TUYTTENS: Reflex release of an oxytocic hormone by stimulation of genital organs in male and female sheep studied by a cross-circulation technique. J. Endocr. **22**, 321—334 (1961).
DEMPSEY, E.W., H. BUNTING, and G.B. WISLOCKI: Observations on the chemical cytology of the mammary gland. Amer. J. Anat. **81**, 309—333 (1947).
DENAMUR, R.: The hypothalamo-neurohypophysial system and the milk-ejection reflex. Dairy Sci. Abstr. **27**, 193—224, 263—280 (1965).
—, and J. MARTINET: Sensibilité de la glande mammaire de la chèvre aux hormones posthypophysaires. C.R. Soc. Biol. (Paris) **147**, 1217—1220 (1953).
— — Les stimulus nerveux mammaires sont-ils necessaires a l'entretien de la lactation chez la Chèvre. C.R. Acad. Sci. (Paris) **248**, 743—745; 860—862 (1959a).
— — Le rôle du système nerveux de la glande mammaire dans l'entretien de la lactation. Arch. Sci. Physiol. **13**, 271—352 (1959b).
— — Physiological mechanisms concerned in the maintenance of lactation in the goat and sheep. Nature (Lond.) **185**, 252—253 (1960).
— — Action de l'oxytocine sur la sécrétion du lait de brebis. Ann. Endocr. (Paris) **22**, 777 to 781 (1961).
DETTELBACH, H.R.: A method for assaying small amounts of antidiuretic substance with notes on some properties of vasopressin. Amer. J. Physiol. **192**, 379—386 (1958).
DICKER, S.E.: A method for the assay of very small amounts of antidiuretic activity with a note on the antidiuretic titre of rat's blood. J. Physiol. (Lond.) **122**, 149—157 (1953).
— The fate of the antidiuretic activity of Pitressin in rats. J. Physiol. (Lond.) **124**, 464—475 (1954).
— The effects of methylpentynol on ethanol drinking and on water metabolism in rats. J. Physiol. (Lond.) **144**, 138—147 (1958).
— Release and metabolism of the neurohypophysial hormones. J. Pharm. Pharmacol. **13**, 449—469 (1961).
— Release of vasopressin and oxytocin from isolated pituitary glands of adult and newborn rats. J. Physiol. (Lond.) **185**, 429—444 (1966).
DIKSHIT, B.B.: The production of cardiac irregularities by excitation of the hypothalamic centres. J. Physiol. (Lond.) **81**, 382—394 (1934).
— Action of acetylcholine on the "sleep centre." J. Physiol. (Lond.) **83**, 42 P (1935).
VAN DONGEN, C.G., and R.L. HAYS: A sensitive in vitro assay for oxytocin. Endocrinology **78**, 1—6 (1966).
DOUGLAS, W.W.: A possible mechanism of neurosecretion. Release of vasopressin by depolarization and its dependence on calcium. Nature (Lond.) **197**, 81—82 (1963).
—, and A.M. POISNER: On the mode of action of acetylcholine in evoking adrenal medullary secretion. Increased uptake of calcium during the secretory response. J. Physiol. (Lond.) **162**, 385—392 (1962a).
— — Importance of calcium for acetylcholine-evoked salivary secretion. Nature (Lond.) **196**, 379—380 (1962b).
— — Release of vasopressin from the rat's neurohypophysis in vitro. J. Physiol. (Lond.) **167**, 55 P (1963).

DOUGLAS, W.W., and A.M. POISNER: Stimulus-secretion coupling in a neurosecretory organ. Therole of calcium on the release of vasopressin from the neurohypophysis. J. Physiol. (Lond.) **172**, 1—18 (1964a).
— — Calcium movement in the neurohypophysis of the rat and its relation to the release of vasopressin. J. Physiol. (Lond.) **172**, 19—30 (1964b).
DRABAREK, S.: Analogs of oxytocin containing glycine in place of tyrosine, isoleucine, or glutamine. J. Amer. chem. Soc. **86**, 4477—4481 (1964).
DUGGAN, A.W., and G.W. REED: Hypothalamus and oxytocin. Nature (Lond.) **181**, 1278 to 1279 (1958).
DUKE, H.N., and M. PICKFORD: Observations on the action of acetylcholine and adrenaline on the hypothalamus. J. Physiol. (Lond.) **114**, 325—332 (1951).
— —, and J.A. WATT: The immediate and delayed effects of diisopropylfluorophosphate injected into the supraoptic nuclei of dogs. J. Physiol. (Lond.) **111**, 81—88 (1950).
— — — Antidiuretic action of morphine. Its site and mode of action in the hypothalamus of the dog. Quart. J. exp. Physiol. **36**, 149—158 (1951).
DURBIN, R.P., and D.H. JENKINSON: The calcium dependence of tension development in depolarized smooth muscle. J. Physiol. (Lond.) **157**, 90—96 (1961).
VAN DYKE, H.B., K. ADAMSONS, jr., and S.L. ENGEL: Aspects of the biochemistry and physiology of the neurohypophyseal hormones. Recent Progr. Hormone Res. **11**, 1—35 (1955).
—, and R.G. AMES: Alcohol diuresis. Acta endocr. (Kbh.) **7**, 110—121 (1951).
—, B.F. CHOW, R.O. GREEP, and A. ROTHEN: The isolation of a protein from the pars neuralis of the ox pituitary with constant oxytocic, pressor and diuresis inhibiting activities. J. Pharmacol. exp. Ther. **74**, 190—209 (1942).
EAYRS, J.T., and R.M. BADDELEY: Neural pathways in lactation. J. Anat. (Lond.) **90**, 161 to 171 (1956).
—, and J.A. EDWARDSON: Neuroendocrine interactions in the maintenance of lactation. Acta endocr. (Kbh.) Suppl. **100**, 154 (1965).
EDMAN, K.A.P., and H.O. SCHILD: Interactions of acetylcholine, adrenaline and magnesium with calcium in the contraction of depolarized rat uterus. J. Physiol. (Lond.) **155**, 10—11 (1961a).
— — Interaction of acetylcholine, calcium and depolarization in the contraction of smooth muscle. Nature (Lond.) **190**, 350—353 (1961b).
— — The need for calcium in the contractile responses induced by acetylcholine and potassium in the rat uterus. J. Physiol. (Lond.) **161**, 424—441 (1962).
EGGLETON, M.G.: The effect of nicotine on the diuresis induced by ethyl alcohol. J. Physiol. (Lond.) **108**, 482—490 (1949).
ELY, F., and W.E. PETERSEN: Factors involved in the ejection of milk. In: Report of Proceedings of the 32nd Annual Meeting; American Society of Animal Production, p. 80, 1939.
— — The ejection of milk from the mammary gland. J. Dairy Sci. **23**, 536—537 (1940).
— — Factors involved in the ejection of milk. J. Dairy Sci. **24**, 211—223 (1941).
EVANS, D.H.L., and H.O. SCHILD: Mechanism of contraction of smooth muscle by drugs. Nature (Lond.) **180**, 341—342 (1957).
— —, and S. THESLEFF: Effects of drugs on depolarized plain muscle. J. Physiol. (Lond.) **143**, 474—485 (1958).
EVERETT, J.W.: Luteotrophic function of autografts of the rat hypophysis. Endocrinology **54**, 685—690 (1954).
FANG, H.S., H.M. LIU, and S.C. WANG: Liberation of antidiuretic hormone following hypothalamic stimulation in the dog. Amer. J. Physiol. **202**, 212—216 (1962).
FELDBERG, W.: The role of acetylcholine in the central nervous system. Brit. med. Bull. **6**, 312—321 (1949).
—, and M. VOGT: Acetylcholine synthesis in different regions of the central nervous system. J. Physiol. (Lond.) **107**, 372—381 (1948).
FERGUSON, J.K.W.: Study of motility of intact uterus at term. Surg. Gynec. Obstet. **73**, 359—366 (1941).
FINDLAY, J.D., and D. ROBERTSHAW: The role of the sympatho-adrenal system in the control of sweating in the ox (*Bos taurus*). J. Physiol. (Lond.) **179**, 285—297 (1965).
FISHER, C., W.R. INGRAM, and S.W. RANSON: Diabetes insipidus. Michigan: Edwards Bros. Inc. 1938.
FITZPATRICK, R.J.: On oxytocin and uterine function. In: The neurohypophysis. Ed. by H. HELLER. London: Butterworths 1957.
— The estimation of small amounts of oxytocin in blood. In: Oxytocin, pp. 358—379. Ed. by R. CALDEYRO-BARCIA and H. HELLER. Oxford: Pergamon Press 1961.
—, and C.F. WALMSLEY: The concentration of oxytocin in bovine blood during parturition. J. Physiol. (Lond.) **163**, 13P (1962).
— — The release of oxytocin during parturition. In: Advances in Oxytocin Research. Ed. by J.H.M. PINKERTON, pp. 51—73. London: Pergamon Press 1965.

FOLLEY, S.J.: Endocrine control of the mammary gland. Brit. med. Bull. **5**, 135—141 (1947a).
— The nervous system and lactation. Brit. med. Bull. **5**, 142—148 (1947b).
— Neuro-hormonal mechanisms in lactation. J. Endocr. **6**, XVI—XXV (1949).
— Aspects of pituitary-mammary gland relationships. Recent Progr. Hormone Res. **7**, 107—131 (1952).
— The physiology of suckling and milking. In: Physiology and biochemistry of lactation. Edinburgh: Oliver & Boyd 1956.
—, and G.S. KNAGGS: Observations on oxytocin release in ruminants. J. Reprod. Fertil. **8**, 265—266 (1964).
— — Oxytocin levels in the blood of ruminants with special reference to the milking stimulus. In: Advances in oxytocin research, pp. 37—49. Ed. by J.H.M. PINKERTON. Oxford: Pergamon Press 1965a.
— — Levels of oxytocin in the jugular vein blood of goats during parturition. J. Endocr. **33**, 301—315 (1965b).
— — Milk-ejection activity (oxytocin) in the external jugular vein blood of the cow, goat and sow, in relation to the stimulus of milking or suckling. J. Endocr. **34**, 197—214 (1966).
FORD, H.D., and S. KANTOUNIS: Localization of neurosecretory secretions and pathways in male albino rabbit. J. comp. Neurol. **108**, 91—101 (1957).
FOSKER, A.P., and H.D. LAW: Oxytocin and 4-glycine oxytocin. J. chem. Soc. **907**, 4922—4929 (1965).
FRIEDMAN, E.A.: Direct measurement of milk-ejection pressure in unanaesthetized lactating humans. Amer. J. Obstet. Gynec. **80**, 119—123 (1960).
—, and M.R. SACHTLEBEN: Oxytocin in lactation: clinical applications. Amer. J. Obstet. Gynec. **82**, 846—855 (1961).
FUCHS, A.R., and G. WAGNER: Quantitative aspects of release of oxytocin by suckling in unanaesthetized rabbits. Acta endocr. (Kbh.) **44**, 581—592 (1963a).
— — The effect of ethyl alcohol on the release of oxytocin in rabbits. Acta endocr. (Kbh.) **44**, 593—605 (1963b).
— — Effect of alcohol on release of oxytocin. Nature (Lond.) **198**, 92—94 (1963c).
GAINES, W.L.: A contribution to the physiology of lactation. Amer. J. Physiol. **38**, 285—312 (1915).
—, and F.P. SANMANN: The quantity of milk present in the udder of the cow at milking time. Amer. J. Physiol. **80**, 691—701 (1927).
GAITAN, E., E. COBO, and M. MIZRACHI: Evidence for the differential secretion of oxytocin and vasopressin in man. J. clin. Invest. **43**, 2310—2322 (1964).
GALE, C.C., and B. LARSSON: Radiation induced "hypophysectomy" and hypothalamic lesions in lactating goats. Acta physiol. scand. **59**, 299—318 (1963).
—, S. TALEISNIK, H.M. FRIEDMAN, and S.M. MCCANN: Hormonal basis for impairments in milk synthesis and milk ejection following hypothalamic lesions. J. Endocr. **23**, 303—316 (1961).
GAVIN, W.: On the effects of administration of extracts of pituitary body and corpus luteum to milch cows. Quart. J. exp. Physiol. **6**, 13—16 (1913).
GERSCHENFELD, G., H.M. TRAMEZZANI, and E.D.P. DE ROBERTIS: Ultrastructure and function in neurohypophysis of the toad. Endocrinology **66**, 741—762 (1960).
GINSBURG, M., and L.M. BROWN: Effect of anaesthetics and haemorrhage on the release of neurohypophysial antidiuretic hormone. Brit. J. Pharmacol. **11**, 236—244 (1956).
GOFMAN, M.A.: Reflex regulation of milk ejection. Trans. Inst. Fiziol. (Moska). **4**, 22—33 (1955) (in russian).
GOMEZ, E.T.: The relation of the posterior hypophysis in the maintenance of lactation in hypophysectomized rats. J. Dairy Sci. **22**, 488 (1939).
— The effect of post hypophyseal extract on lactation in hypophysectomized post-gravid rats. J. Dairy Sci. **23**, 537—538 (1940).
GOWEN, J.W., and E.R. TOBEY: Udder size in relation to milk secretion. J. gen. Physiol. **10**, 949—960 (1927).
GREVING, R.: Zur Anatomie, Physiologie und Pathologie der vegetativen Zentren im Zwischenhirn. Z. ges. Anat. **24**, 348—413 (1923).
— Beitrag zur Innervation der Hypophyse. Klin. Wschr. **4**, 2181—2182 (1925).
— Beiträge zur Anatomie der Hypophyse und ihrer Funktion. I. Eine Faserverbindung zwischen Hypophyse und Zwischenhirnbasis (Tr.-Supraoptico-hypophysens). Dtsch. Z. Nervenheilk. **89**, 179—195 (1926).
— Das Zwischenhirn-Hypophysensystem. Seine Morphologie, Phylogenese und klinische Bedeutung. Klin. Wschr. **7**, 734—737 (1928).
GREWAL, R.S., F.C. LU, and M.G. ALLMARK: The release of posterior pituitary hormone in the rat by nicotine and lobeline. J. Pharmacol. exp. Ther. **135**, 84—88 (1962).

GROSVENOR, C. E.: Some effects of ergotamine on milk-ejection in lactating rat. Proc. Soc. exp. Biol. (N.Y.) **91**, 294—296 (1956a).

— Some effects of ergotamine tartrate upon lactation in the rat. Amer. J. Physiol. **186**, 211—215 (1956b).

— Lactation in rat mammary glands after spinal cord section. Endocrinology **74**, 548—553 (1964).

— Contraction of lactating rat mammary gland in response to direct mechanical stimulation. Amer. J. Physiol. **208**, 214—218 (1965a).

— Evidence that exteroceptive stimuli can release prolactin from pituitary gland of lactating rat. Endocrinology **76**, 340—342 (1965b).

— Effect of nursing and stress upon prolactin-inhibiting activity of the rat hypothalamus. Endocrinology **77**, 1037—1042 (1965c).

—, and C. W. TURNER: Ergotamine, oxytocin and milk let-down in lactating rat. Proc. Soc. exp. Biol. (N.Y.) **93**, 466—468 (1956).

— — A method for evaluation of milk "let-down" in lactating rat. Proc. Soc. exp. Biol. (N.Y.) **94**, 816—817 (1957a).

— — Estimation of amount of oxytocin released as result of nursing stimuli in lactating rat. Proc. Soc. exp. Biol. (N.Y.) **95**, 131—133 (1957b).

— — Evidence for adrenergic and cholinergic components in milk let-down reflex in lactating rat. Proc. Soc. exp. Biol. (N.Y.) **97**, 719—722 (1957c).

— — Milk let-down activity of synthetic oxytocin (syntocinon) and relaxin in lactating rats. Proc. Soc. exp. Biol. (N.Y.) **97**, 189—190 (1958a).

— — Effect of oxytocin and blocking agents upon pituitary lactogen discharge in lactating rats. Proc. Soc. exp. Biol. (N.Y.) **97**, 463—465 (1958b).

GUNTHER, M.: The posterior pituitary and labour. Brit. med. J. **1**, 567 (1948).

GUTTMANN, ST., and R. A. BOISSONNAS: Synthese de la Ser^4-oxytocine, de l'Ala^4-oxytocine, de la Ser^5-oxytocine et de l'Ala-oxytocine. Helv. chim. Acta **46**, 1626—1636 (1963).

HAEGER, K., and D. JACOBSOHN: A contribution to the study of milk ejection in women. Acta physiol. scand. **30**, Suppl. 111, 152—160 (1953).

HALDAR, J.: The problem of independent release of the neurohypophysial hormones. University of London Ph. D. Thesis 1966.

HAMMOND, J.: The physiology of milk and butter fat secretion. Vet. Rec. **16**, 519—527 (1936).

HARRIS, G. W.: The innervation and actions of the neurohypophysis; an investigation using the method of remote control stimulation. Phil. Trans. B. **232**, 385—441 (1947).

— The central nervous system, neurohypophysis and milk ejection. Proc. roy. Soc. B. **149**, 336—353 (1958).

—, and D. JACOBSOHN: Functional grafts of anterior pituitary. Proc. roy. Soc. B. **139**, 263—276 (1951).

—, and V. R. PICKLES: Reflex stimulation of neurohypophysis (posterior pituitary gland) and nature of posterior pituitary hormone(s). Nature (Lond.) **172**, 1049 (1953).

HAUN, C. K.: Induction of lactation in the rabbit with oxytocin. Anat. Rec. **133**, 286—287 (1959).

HAWKER, R. W.: Oxytocin and an unidentified oxytocic substance in extracts of blood. In: Oxytocin, pp. 425—436. Ed. by H. HELLER and R. CALDEYRO-BARCIA. Oxford: Pergamon Press 1961.

—, and P. A. ROBERTSON: Some properties of an oxytocic substance found in blood extracts. Endocrinology **63**, 242—249 (1958).

—, C. F. WALMSLEY, V. S. ROBERTS, and P. A. ROBERTSON: Oxytocin and oxytocic substance in blood extracts before and after hypothalamic stimulation in rats. Med. J. Aust. **2**, 524—525 (1959).

HAYS, R. L., and N. L. VANDEMARK: Effect of stimulation of the reproductive organs of cow on release of oxytocin-like substance. Endocrinology **52**, 634—637 (1953).

HEANEY, N. S.: A contribution to the study of pituitrin. Surg. Gynec. Obstet. **17**, 103—109 (1913).

HEBB, C. O., and J. L. LINZELL: Some conditions affecting the blood flow through the perfused mammary gland, with special reference to the action of adrenaline. Quart. J. exp. Physiol. **36**, 159—175 (1951).

HOLLAND, R. C., and B. A. CROSS: (unpublished). Quoted by B. A. CROSS. In: Oxytocin, pp. 24—47. Ed. by R. CALDEYRO-BARCIA and H. HELLER. London: Pergamon Press 1961.

— —, and C. H. SAWYER: Milk ejection in the rabbit in response to intracarotid injections of hypertonic saline. Fed. Proc. **17**, 73 (1958).

— — — Effects of intracarotid injections of hypertonic solutions on the neurohypophyseal milk-ejection mechanism. Amer. J. Physiol. **196**, 791—795 (1959a).

— — — EEG correlates of osmotic activation of the neurohypophyseal milk-ejection mechanism. Amer. J. Physiol. **196**, 796—802 (1959b).

HOLMES, R.C., and F.G.W. KNOWLES: Synaptic vesicles in the neurohypophysis. Nature (Lond.) **185**, 710—711 (1960).
HOPE, D.B., V.V.S. MURTI, and V. DU VIGNEAUD: A highly potent analogue of oxytocin, desamino-oxytocin. J. biol. Chem. **237**, 1563—1566 (1962).
HUANG, J.J.: A vagus-post-pituitary reflex. Chin. J. Physiol. **13**, 367—382 (1938).
HUGUENIN, R.C., and R.A. BOISSONNAS: (1963, unpublished). Quoted by B. BERDE and R.A. BOISSONNAS. In: The pituitary gland, pp. 624—661. Ed. by G.W. HARRIS and B.T. DONOVAN. London: Butterworths 1966.
HYNEK, B., J. BÍLEK, and M. LIS: Introduction of a permanent electrode into the pituitary gland of the cow. Influence of electrical stimulation on milk ejection. Nature (Lond.) **208**, 690—691 (1965).
INGELBRECHT, P.: Influence du système nerveux central sur la mamelle lactante chez le rat blanc. C.R. Soc. Biol. (Paris) **120**, 1369—1371 (1935).
ISBISTER, C.: A clinical study of the draught reflex in human lactation. Arch. Dis. Childh. **29**, 66—72 (1954).
ISHIKAWA, T., K. KOIZUMI, and C. MCBROOKS: Electrical activity recorded from the pituitary stalk of the cat. Amer. J. Physiol. **210**, 427—431 (1966).
JAQUENOUD, P.-A., and R.A. BOISSONNAS: Synthèse de la Phe^2-oxytocine. Helv. chim. Acta **42**, 788—793 (1959).
— — Synthèse de la Ileu^8-oxytocine et de la Val^8-oxytocine, deux analogues de l'oxytocine modifies dans la chaine laterale. Helv. chim. Acta. **44**, 113—122 (1961).
— — Synthèse de l'Asp $(NH_2)^4$-oxytocine, de la Glu $(NH_2)^4$-oxytocine et de l'Asp $(NH_2)^4$-Glu (NH_2) 5^2-oxytocine. Helv. chim. Acta. **45**, 1601—1607 (1962).
— — (1963, unpublished). Quoted by B. BERDE and R.A. BOISSONNAS. In: The pituitary gland, pp. 624—661. Ed. by G.W. HARRIS and B.T. DONOVAN. London: Butterworths 1966.
— — (1964, unpublished). Quoted by B. BERDE. In: The pituitary gland, pp. 624—661. Ed. by G.W. HARRIS and B.T. DONOVAN. London: Butterworths 1967.
JOŠT, K., J. RUDINGER, and F. ŠORM: Amino acids and peptides. XXXVIII. Structural analogues of oxytocin modified in position 2 of the peptide chain. Preparation and some chemical and biological properties. Coll. Czechoslov. Chem. Commun. **28**, 1706—1714 (1963a).
— — — Amino acids and peptides. XXXIX. Analogues of oxytocin exerting protracted biological effects. Coll. Czechoslov. Chem. Commun. **28**, 2021—2030 (1963b).
JUNG, H.: The effect of oxytocin on the mechanism of uterine excitation. In: Oxytocin, pp. 87—99. Ed. by R. CALDEYRO-BARCIA and H. HELLER. London: Pergamon Press 1961.
KALLIALA, H., and M.J. KARVONEN: Antidiuresis during suckling in lactating women. Ann. Med. exp. Fenn. **29**, 233—241 (1951).
— —, and V. LEPPÄNEN: Release of antidiuretic hormone during nursing in the dog. Ann. Med. exp. Fenn. **30**, 96—107 (1952).
KAMM, O., T.B. ALDRICH, I.W. GROTE, L.W. ROWE, and E.P. BUGBEE: The active principles of the posterior lobe of the pituitary gland. J. Amer. chem. Soc. **50**, 573—601 (1928).
KANDEL, E.R.: Electrical properties of hypothalamic neuroendocrine cells. J. gen. Physiol. **47**, 691—717 (1964).
KAY, H.D.: The science and practice of milking. Sci. Progr. **37**, 609—624 (1949).
— Milk liberation. Advanc. Sci. **12**, 83—88 (1955).
KIERNON, J.A.: Carboxylic esterases of the hypothalamus and neurohypophysis of the hedgehog. J. roy. micr. Soc. **83**, 297—306 (1964).
KNAGGS, G.S.: Blood oxytocin levels in the cow during milking and in the parturient goat. J. Endocr. **26**, XXIV-XXV (1963).
KOELLA, W.: Die Beeinflussung der Harnsekretion durch hypothalamische Reizung. Helv. physiol. pharm. Acta. **7**, 498—514 (1949).
KOELLE, G.B.: A proposed dual neurohumoral role of acetylcholine: its functions at the pre- and postsynaptic sites. Nature (Lond.) **190**, 208—211 (1961).
— A new general concept of the neurohumoral functions of acetylcholine and acetylcholinesterase. J. Pharm. Pharmacol. **14**, 65—90 (1962).
—, and C.N. GEESEY: Localization of acetylcholinesterase in the neurohypophysis and its functional implications. Proc. Soc. exp. Biol. (N.Y.) **106**, 625—628 (1961).
KOIZUMI, K., T. ISHIKAWA, and C. McC. BROOKS: Control of activity of neurones in the supraoptic nucleus. J. Neurophysiol. **27**, 878—892 (1964).
KONZETT, H., and B. BERDE: The biological activity of a new analogue of oxytocin in which the tyrosyl group is replaced by phenylalanyl. Brit. J. Pharmacol. **14**, 133—136 (1959).
KREJČÍ, I., I. POLÁČEK, B. KUPKOVÁ, and J. RUDINGER: Dose-response analysis of the action of some oxytocic analogues on the isolated uterus; the effect of ions. In: Oxytocin, vasopressin and their structural analogues. Ed. by J. RUDINGER. Proc. 2nd Int. Pharmacological Meeting, 117—123. Oxford: Pergamon Press 1964.

Kullander, S.: Studies on the hormonal control of the milk-ejection activity in lactating rabbits. Acta endocr. (Kbh.) **44**, 313—324 (1963).

Kuriyama, H., and A. Csapo: A study of the parturient uterus with the microelectrode technique. Endocrinology **68**, 1010—1025 (1961).

Labouche, C.: Action des extraits posthypophysaires à activité ocytocique sur la retention physiologique du lait chez la femelle bovine en milieu tropical. C.R. Soc. Biol. (Paris) 151, 1171—1176 (1957).

Langer, E., and S. Huhn: Der Submikroskopische Bau der Myoepithelzelle. Z. Zellforsch. Abt. Histochem. **47**, 507—516 (1958).

Laqueur, G.L.: Neurosecretory pathways between the hypothalamic paraventricular nucleus and the neurohypophysis. J. comp. Neurol. **101**, 543—554 (1954).

Laruelle, M.L.: Le système végétatif méso-diencéphalique partie anatomique. Rev. Neurol. **1**, 809—842 (1934).

Law, H.D., and V. du Vigneaud: Synthesis of 2-p-methoxyphenylalanine oxytocin (O-methyl-oxytocin) and some observations on its pharmacological behavior. J. Amer. chem. Soc. **82**, 4579—4581 (1960).

Lederis, K.: Vasopressin and oxytocin in the mammalian hypothalamus. Gen. comp. Endocr. **1**, 80—89 (1961).

— The distribution of vasopressin and oxytocin in hypothalamic nuclei. In: Neurosecretion, pp. 227—235. Ed. by H. Heller and R.B. Clark.Mem. Soc. Endocr. London: Pergamon Press 1962.

— Fine structure and hormone content of the hypothalamo-neurohypophysial system of the rainbow trout (*Salmo irideus*) exposed to sea water. Gen. comp. Endocr. **4**, 638—661 (1964).

— An electron-microscopical study of the human neurohypophysis. Z. Zellforsch. Abt. Histochem. **65**, 847—868 (1965).

—, and A. Livingston: Acetylcholine content in the rabbit neurohypophysis. J. Physiol. (Lond.) **185**, 37—38 (1966).

Levitskaya, E.S.: Study of the functioning of the ejection mechanism in the living mammary gland of a white mouse. Tr. Inst. Fiziol. (Mosk.) **4**, 58—62 (1955) (in russian).

Levy, B., and S. Tozzi: The adrenergic receptive mechanism of the rat uterus. J. Pharmacol. exp. Ther. **142**, 178—184 (1963).

Lewis, A.A.G., and T.M. Chalmers: A nicotine test for the investigation of diabetes insipidus. **10**, 137—144 (1951).

Linzell, J.L.: Vasomotor nerve fibres to the mammary glands of the cat and dog. Quart. J. exp. Physiol. **35**, 295—319 (1950).

— The silver staining of myoepithelial cells, particularly in the mammary gland and their relation to the ejection of milk. J. Anat. (Lond.) **86**, 49—57 (1952).

— The contractility of the alveoli of the mammary gland. J. Physiol. (Lond.) **123**, 32P (1954).

— Some observations on the contractile tissue of the mammary glands. J. Physiol. (Lond.) **130**, 257—267 (1955).

— Evidence against a parasympathetic innervation of the mammary glands. J. Physiol. (Lond.) **133**, 66—67P (1956).

— Physiology of the mammary glands. Physiol. Rev. **39**, 534—576 (1959).

— Transplantation of mammary glands. Nature (Lond.) **188**, 596—598 (1960).

— Recent advances in the physiology of the udder. Vet. Ann. **2**, 44—53 (1961).

— Some effects of denervating and transplanting mammary glands. Quart. J. exp. Physiol. **48**, 34—60 (1963).

Macaulay, M.H.I.: Factors involved in the ejection of milk from the mammary gland. Coll. int. Cent. nat. Rech. Sci. **32**, 145—155 (1950).

Mackenzie, K.: An experimental investigation of the mechanism of milk secretion, with special reference to the action of animal extracts. Quart. J. exp. Physiol. **4**, 305—330 (1911).

MacLean, P.D.: The limbic system with respect to self-preservation and the preservation of the species. J. nerv. ment. Dis. **127**, 1—11 (1958).

—, D.W. Ploog, and B.W. Robinson: Circulatory effects of limbic stimulation, with special reference to the male genital organ. Physiol. Rev. **40**, Suppl. 4, 105—112 (1960).

Marshall, J.M., and A.I. Csapo: Hormonal and ionic influences on the membrane activity of uterine smooth muscle cells. Endocrinology **68**, 1026—1035 (1961).

McCann, S.M., R. Mack, and C. Gale: The possible role of oxytocin in stimulating the release of prolactin. Endocrinology **64**, 870—888 (1959).

Meites, J.: Hormonal prolongation of lactation for 75 days after litter removal in parturient rats. Fed. Proc. **18**, 103 (1959).

—, and T.F. Hopkins: Mechanism of action of oxytocin in retarding mammary involution. Study in hypophysectomized rats. J. Endocr. **22**, 207—213 (1961).

—, and C.S. Nicoll: Hormonal prolongation of lactation for 75 days after litter withdrawal in postpartum rats. Endocrinology **65**, 572—579 (1959).

MEITES, J., C.S. NICOLL, and P.K. TALWALKER: Induction and maintenance of lactation in rats by electricalstimulation of uterine cervix. Proc. Soc. exp. Biol. (N.Y.) **102**, 127—131 (1959).
— — — Local action of oxytocin on mammary glands of postpartum rats after litter removal. Proc. Soc. exp. Biol. (N.Y.) **103**, 118—122 (1960).
— — —, and T.F. HOPKINS: Induction and maintenance of mammary growth and lactation by neurohormones, drugs, nonspecific stresses and hypothalamic tissue. Proc. 1st Int. Congr. Endocr., Copenhagen, Abstr. No. 573, 1137, 1960.
—, P.K. TALWALKER, and C.S. NICOLL: Failure of oxytocin to initiate mammary secretion in rabbits or rats. Proc. Soc. exp. Biol. (N.Y.) **105**, 467—469 (1960).
—, and C.W. TURNER: Studies concerning the mechanism controlling the initiation of lactation at parturition. Endocrinology **30**, 726—733 (1942).
MENA, F., and C. BEYER: Effect of high spinal section on established lactation in the rabbit. Amer. J. Physiol. **205**, 313—316 (1963).
MÉNDEZ-BAUER, C., H.M. CABOT, and R. CALDEYRO-BARCIA: A new test for the biological assay of oxytocin. Science **132**, 299—300 (1960).
MOON, R.C., and C.W. TURNER: Effect of reserpine on oxytocin and lactogen discharge in lactating rats. Proc. Soc. exp. Biol. (N.Y.) **101**, 332—335 (1959).
MOORE, R.D., and M.X. ZARROW: Contraction of the rabbit mammary strip in vitro in response to oxytocin. Acta endocr. (Kbh.) **48**, 186—198 (1965).
MORITA, H., T. ISHIBASHI, and S. YAMASHITA: Synaptic transmission in neurosecretory cells. Nature (Lond.) **191**, 183 (1961).
MUNSICK, R.A.: Effect of magnesium ion on the response of the rat uterus to neurohypophysial hormones and analogues. Endocrinology **66**, 451—457 (1960).
—, and C. JERONIMUS: Effects of diethylstilboestrol and magnesium on the rat oxytocic potencies of some neurohypophysial hormones and analogues. Endocrinology **76**, 90—96 (1965).
NESVADBA, H., J. HONZL, and J. RUDINGER: Amino acids and peptides. XXXVII. Some structural analogues of oxytocin modified in position 3 of the peptide chain: synthesis and some chemical and biological properties. Coll. Czechoslov. Chem. Commun. **28**, 1691—1705 (1963).
NEWTON, M., and N.R. NEWTON: The let-down reflex in human lactation. J. Pediat. **33**, 698—704 (1948).
— — Postpartum engorgement of the breast. Amer. J. Obstet. Gynec. **61**, 664—667 (1951).
— — Relation of the let-down reflex to the ability to breast feed. Pediatrics **5**, 726—733 (1950).
NIBBELINK, D.W.: Paraventricular nuclei, neurohypophysis and parturition. Amer. J. Physiol. **200**, 1229—1232 (1961).
NICKERSON, K., R.W. BONSNES, R.G. DOUGLAS, P. CONDLIFFE, and V. DU VIGNEAUD: Oxytocin and milk ejection. Amer. J. Obstet. Gynec. **67**, 1028—1034 (1954).
NICOLL, C.S., and J. MEITES: Prolongation of lactation in the rat by litter replacement. Proc. Soc. exp. Biol. (N.Y.) **101**, 81—82 (1959).
O'CONNOR, W.J., and E.V. VERNEY: Effect of increased activity of sympathetic system in inhibition of water-diuresis by functional stress. Quart. J. exp. Physiol. **33**, 77—90 (1945).
OLIVECRONA, H.: Relation of the paraventricular nucleus to the pituitary gland. Nature (Lond.) **173**, 1001 (1954).
— Paraventricular nucleus and pituitary gland. Acta physiol. scand. **40**, Suppl. 136, 1—178 (1957).
OTT, I., and J.C. SCOTT: The action of infundibulin upon the mammary secretion. Proc. Soc. exp. Biol. (N.Y.) **8**, 48 (1910).
PASETTO, N.: Sul meccanismo colinergico delle ipotalamo postipofisarie. Arch. Fisiol. **52**, 1—6 (1952).
PAVLOV, G.N.: Study of the reflex of milk-ejection in goats with the aid of localized cooling of the spinal cord. Tr. Inst. Fiziol. (Mosk.) **4**, 17—21 (1955) [in russian].
PEETERS, G.: Proprietes physiologiques et pharmacologiques du trayon. Arch. int. Pharmacodyn. **77**, 100—103 (1948).
—, J.H. BOUCKAERT, and W. OYAERT: The influence of unilateral lumbar sympathectomy on the udder of the sheep. Arch. int. Pharmacodyn. **89**, 197—203 (1952).
—, and R. COUSSENS: The influence of the milking act on the diuresis of the lactating cow. Arch. int. Pharmacodyn. **84**, 209—219 (1950).
— —, J.H. BOUCKAERT, and W. OYAERT: L'influence de la traite sur la diurèse de la vache gravide. Arch. int. Pharmacodyn. **80**, 355—358 (1949).
— —, and W. OYAERT: Physiology of the cistern of the bovine mammary gland. Arch. int. Pharmacodyn. **79**, 113—122 (1949).

Peeters, G., R. Coussens, and G. Sierens: Physiology of the nerves in the bovine mammary gland. Arch. int. Pharmacodyn. **79**, 75—82 (1949).
—, and M. Debackere: The effect on diuresis of vaginal distension, milking and suckling in the sheep. J. Physiol. (Paris) **55**, 481—493 (1963).
—, G. Genie, and R. Coussens: The autonomic innervation of the udder in sheep and cows. Arch. int. Pharmacodyn. **85**, 152—158 (1951).
—, and L. Massart: La perfusion de la glande mammaire isolee. Arch. int. Pharmacodyn. **74**, 83—89 (1947).
— — Artificial lactation and perfusion of the bovine mammary gland. Research (Lond.) **3**, 217—221 (1950).
— —, and R. Coussens: L'ejection du lait chez les bovides. Arch. int. Pharmacodyn. **75**, 85—89 (1947a).
— — — L'influence du calcium sur la glande mammaire isolee. Arch. int. Pharmacodyn. **74**, 151—154 (1947b).
— —, W. Oyaert, and R. Coussens: Plethysmography applied to the teats of the bovine mammary gland. Arch. int. Pharmacodyn. **75**, 243—255 (1948).
—, G. Sierens, and M. Silver: L'Expulsion du lait dans la glande mammaire bovine isolee. Ann. Endocr. (Paris) **12**, 255—257 (1951).
— — — Expulsion of milk in the isolated perfused udder of the cow. Arch. int. Pharmacodyn. **88**, 413—424 (1952).
—, H. Stormorken, and F. Vanschoubroek: The effect of different stimuli on milk ejection and diuresis in the lactating cow. J. Endocr. **20**, 163—172 (1960).
Petersen, W. E.: Effect of certain hormones and drugs on the perfused mammary gland. Proc. Soc. exp. Biol. (N.Y.) **50**, 298—300 (1942).
— Lactation. Physiol. Rev. **24**, 340—364 (1944).
—, and T.M. Ludwick: The humoral nature of the factor causing the let down of milk. Fed. Proc. **1**, 66—67 (1942).
—, L. G. Palmer, and C.H. Eckles: The synthesis and secretion of milk fat. Amer. J. Physiol. **90**, 573—599 (1929).
—, J.C. Shaw, and M.B. Visscher: Perfusion of the excised mammary gland as a method of studying milk secretion. J. Dairy Sci. **22**, 439—440 (1939).
— — — A technique for perfusing excised bovine mammary glands. J. Dairy Sci. **24**, 139—146 (1941).
Pickford, M.: The inhibitory effect of acetylcholine on water diuresis in the dog and its pituitary transmission. J. Physiol. (Lond.) **95**, 226—238 (1939).
— The action of acetylcholine on the supraoptic nucleus of the chloralosed dog. J. Physiol. (Lond.) **106**, 264—270 (1947).
— Milk ejection in the unanaesthetized dog. J. Physiol. (Lond.) **149**, 41—42 P (1959).
— Factors affecting milk release in the dog and the quantity of oxytocin liberated by suckling. J. Physiol. (Lond.) **152**, 515—526 (1960).
—, and J.A. Watt: A comparison of the effect of intravenous and intracarotid injections of acetylcholine in the dog. J. Physiol. (Lond.) **114**, 333—335 (1951).
Pickles, V.R.: Blood-flow estimations as indices of mammary activity. J. Obstet. Gynaec. Brit. Emp. **60**, 301—311 (1953).
Poláček, I., I. Krejčí, and J. Rudinger, Personal communication.
Popenoe, E.A., J.G. Pierce, V. du Vigneaud, and H.B. van Dyke: Oxytocic activity of purified vasopressin. Proc. Soc. exp. Biol. (N.Y.) **81**, 506—508 (1952).
Ratner, A.: Studies on the relation of prolactin-inhibiting activity of the hypothalamus to pituitary prolactin release in the rat. Diss. Abstr. **26**, 4771 (1966).
—, and J. Meites: Removal of prolactin inhibiting activity of rat hypothalamus by oestrogen, reserpine and suckling. Fed. Proc. **23**, 110 (1964a).
— — Depletion of prolacting-inhibiting activity of rat hypothalamus by estradiol or suckling stimulus. Endocrinology **75**, 377—382 (1964b).
Richardson, K.C.: Some structural features of the mammary tissues. Brit. med. Bull. **5**, 123—129 (1947).
— Contractile tissues in the mammary gland with special reference to myoepithelium in the goat. Proc. roy. Soc. B **136**, 30—45 (1949).
— The effector contractile tissues of the mammary gland. J. Endocr. **6**, XXV (1950a).
— Structural investigation of the contractile tissues in the mammary gland. Colloq. int. Cent. nat. Rech. Sci. **32**, 167—169 (1950b).
Rioch, D., G.B. Wislocki, and J.L. O'Leary: Précis of preoptic, hypothalamic and hypophysial terminology with atlas. Res. Publ. Ass. nerv. ment. Dis. **20**, 3—30 (1940).
de Robertis, E.: Ultrastructure and function in some neurosecretory systems. In: Neurosecretion, pp. 3—20. Ed. by H. Heller and R.B. Clark. Mem. Soc. Endocr. London: Academic Press 1962.

de Robertis, E.: Electron microscope and chemical study of binding sites of brain biogenic amines. Progr. Brain Res. **8**, 118—136 (1964a).
— Histophysiology of synapses and neurosecretion. London: Pergamon Press 1964b.
Robinson, M.: Failing lactation. Lancet **1**, 66—68 (1943).
Rudinger, J., and I. Krejčí: Dose-response relations for some synthetic analogues of oxytocin, and the mode of action of oxytocin on the isolated uterus. Experientia (Basel) **18**, 585 (1962).
Rydén, G., and I. Sjöholm: Assay of oxytocin by rat mammary gland in vitro. Brit. J. Pharmacol. **19**, 136—141 (1962).
Rydin, H., and E.B. Verney: Inhibition of water-diuresis by functional stress and by muscular exercise. Quart. J. exp. Physiol. **27**, 343—374 (1938).
Schäfer, E.A.: On the effect of pituitary and corpus luteum extracts on the mammary gland in the human subject. Quart. J. exp. Physiol. **6**, 17—19 (1913).
— Note on preceding paper by Simpson and Hill: The mode of action of pituitary extract on the mammary gland. Quart. J. exp. Physiol. **8**, 379—381 (1915).
—, and K. Mackenzie: The action of animal extracts on milk secretion. Proc. roy. Soc. B **84**, 16—22 (1912).
Selye, H., J.B. Collip, and D.C. Thomson: Nervous and humoral factors in lactation. Endocrinology **18**, 237—247 (1934).
Selye, H.L.: On the nervous control of lactation. Amer. J. Physiol. **107**, 535—538 (1934).
Shute, C.C.O., and P.R. Lewis: Cholinergic and monoaminergic pathways in the hypothalamus. Brit. med. Bull. **22**, 221—226 (1966).
Sica-Blanco, Y., C. Méndez-Bauer, N. Sala, H.M. Cabot, y R. Caldeyro-Barcia: Nuevo metodo para el estudio de la funcionalidad mamaria en la mujer. Arch. Ginec. Obstet. **17**, 63—72 (1959).
Silver, I.A.: Myoepithelial cells in the mammary and parotid glands. J. Physiol. (Lond.) **125**, 8 P (1954).
— Vascular changes in the mammary gland during engorgement with milk. J. Physiol. (Lond.) **133**, 65 P (1956).
Simpson, S., and R.L. Hill: The mode of action of pituitary extract on the mammary gland. Quart. J. exp. Physiol. **8**, 377—378 (1915).
Sjöholm, I., and G. Rydén: Improved method for quantitative estimation of oxytocin. Nature (Lond.) **193**, 77—78 (1962).
Smith, D.M., W.G. Whittlestone, and J. Allen: The design and use of a milking machine for sows. J. Dairy Res. **18**, 31—33 (1951).
Smith, M.W.: Some properties of rat mammary tissue. Nature (Lond.) **190**, 541—542 (1961).
Somlyo, A.V., C. Woo, and A.F. Somlyo: Effect of magnesium on posterior pituitary hormone action on vascular smooth muscle. Amer. J. Physiol. **210**, 705—714 (1966).
Stürmer, E., and B. Berde: A comparative pharmacological study of synthetic eledoisin and synthetic bradykinin. J. Pharmacol. exp. Ther. **140**, 349—355 (1963).
Sundsten, J.W., and C.H. Sawyer: Osmotic activation of neurohypophysial hormone release in rabbits with hypothalamic islands. Exp. Neurol. **4**, 548—561 (1961).
Supek, Z., and V. Eisen: The action of nervous depressants on the antidiuretic and chloruretic effect of nicotine. Arch. int. Pharmacodyn. **93**, 75—82 (1953).
Swanson, E.W., and C.W. Turner: Evidence for the presence of smooth muscle elements surrounding the alveoli of the mammary gland. J. Dairy Sci. **24**, 635—638 (1941).
Taleisnik, S., and R.P. Deis: Influence of cerebral cortex in inhibition of oxytocin release induced by stressful stimuli. Amer. J. Physiol. **207**, 1394—1398 (1964).
Talwalker, P.K., A. Ratner, and J. Meites: In vitro inhibition of pituitary prolactin synthesis and release by hypothalamic extract. Amer. J. Physiol. **205**, 213—218 (1963).
Taylor, N.B.G., and J.M. Walker: Antidiuretic substance in human urine after smoking. J. Physiol. (Lond.) **113**, 412—418 (1951).
Theobald, G.W.: The separate release of oxytocin and antidiuretic hormone. J. Physiol. (Lond.) **149**, 443—461 (1959).
Thorn, N.A.: Role of calcium in the release of vasopressin and oxytocin from posterior pituitary protein. Acta endocr. (Kbh.) **50**, 357—364 (1965).
Tindal, J.S., and A. Yokoyama: Assay of oxytocin by the milk-ejection response in the anaesthetized lactating guinea-pig. Endocrinology **71**, 196—202 (1962).
Tsakhaev, G.A.: Problem of reflex regulation of milk ejection. Tr. Inst. Fiziol. (Mosk.) **4**, 5—16 (1955) [in russian].
Turner, C.W., and W.D. Cooper: Assay of posterior pituitary factors which contract the lactating mammary gland. Endocrinology **29**, 320—323 (1941).
Turner, R.A., J.G. Pierce, and V. du Vigneaud: The purification and the amino acid content of vasopressin preparations. J. biol. Chem. **191**, 21—28 (1951).

TVERSKOI, G.B.: Sensitivity of the muscles of ducts, cistern and the teat sphincter of a cow's udder to nervous stimuli and pituitrin. Tr. Inst. Fiziol. (Mosk.) **4**, 51—57 (1955a) [in russian].

— The role of pressure fluctuations in the cavity system of the udder in the stimulation of milk secretion. Tr. Inst. Fiziol. (Mosk.) **4**, 68—74 (1955b) [in russian].

— Role of sensory innervation of udder in reflex regulation of milk secretion and butterfat synthesis. Zh. obshch. Biol. (Mosk.) **18**, 169—184 (1957) [in russian].

— Secretion of milk in goats after complete severance of the spinal cord. Dokl. Akad. Nank. SSSR. **123**, 1137—1139 (1958) [in russian].

VERNEY, E.B.: The antidiuretic hormone and the factors which determine its release. Proc. roy. Soc. B **135**, 25—106 (1947).

— Renal excretion of water and salt. Lancet **2**, 1237—1242, 1295—1298 (1957).

DU VIGNEAUD, V.: The hormones of the posterior pituitary gland with special reference to their milk-ejecting ability. Bull. N.Y. Acad. Med. **41**, 802—803 (1965).

—, G.S. DENNING, jr., S. DRABAREK, and W.Y. CHAN: The synthesis and pharmacological study of 4-decarboxamido-oxytocin (4-α-aminobutyric acid-oxytocin) and 5-decarboxamido-oxytocin (5-alanine-oxytocin). J. biol. Chem. **239**, 472—477 (1964).

—, P.S. FITT, M. BODANSZKY, and M. O'CONNELL: Synthesis and some pharmacological properties of a peptide derivative of oxytocin: glycyloxytocin. Proc. Soc. exp. Biol. (N.Y.) **104**, 653—656 (1960).

WALKER, J.M.: The effect of smoking on water diuresis in man. Quart. J. Med. **18**, 51—55 (1949).

— The release of vasopressin and oxytocin in response to drugs. In: The neurohypophysis, pp. 229—232. Ed. by H. HELLER. London: Butterworths 1957.

WALLER, H.K.: A reflex governing the outflow of milk from the breast. Lancet **1**, 69—72 (1943).

— Breast feeding and the early phase of lactation. Mth. Bull. Minist. Hlth Lab. Serv. **6**, 73—81 (1947a).

— Incidence, causes and prevention of failure of breast-feeding. Brit. med. Bull. **5**, 181—183 (1947b).

WHITTLESTONE, W.G.: The characteristics of the milk-ejection curve of normal dairy cows under standard milking conditions. N.Z. J. sci. Technol. **28—29**, 188—205 (1946—1948).

— Some recent experiments on the problem of milk-ejection. Proc. N.Z. Soc. Anim. Prod. 67—77 (1950a).

— Nature of the milk-ejection process. Nature (Lond.) **166**, 994 (1950b).

— Studies on milk-ejection in the dairy cow. N.Z. J. sci. Technol. **32**, 1—20 (1951).

— The milk-ejecting activity of extracts of the posterior pituitary gland. J. Endocr. 8, 89—95 (1952).

— Intramammary pressure changes in the lactating sow. J. Dairy Res. **21**, 19—30 (1954a).

— Intramammary pressure changes in the lactating sow. II. The effects of vasopressin and acetylcholine. J. Dairy Res. **21**, 183—187 (1954b).

— Intramammary pressure changes in the lactating sow. III. The effects of level of dose of oxytocin and the influence of rate of injection. J. Dairy Res. **21**, 188—193 (1954c).

— The effect of adrenaline on the milk-ejection response of the sow. J. Endocr. **10**, 167—172 (1954d).

—, E.G. BASSETT, and C.W. TURNER: Source of secretion of milk "let-down" hormone in domestic animals. Proc. Soc. exp. Biol. (N.Y.) **80**, 197—199 (1952).

—, and C.W. TURNER: Effect of acetylcholine on mammary gland of the lactating sow. Proc. Soc. exp. Biol. (N.Y.) **80**, 194—196 (1952).

WIEDERMAN, J., M. FREUND, and M.L. STONE: Oxytocin effect on myoepithelium of the breast throughout pregnancy. J. appl. Physiol. **19**, 310—314 (1964).

—, and M.L. STONE: Effect of oxytocin on myoepithelium of the breast. J. appl. Physiol. **17**, 539—542 (1962).

YOKOYAMA, A.: Milk-ejection responses following administration of "tap'" stimuli and posterior pituitary extracts. Endocr. jap. **3**, 32—37 (1956).

—, and K. OTA: The effect of hypothalamic lesions on litter growth in rats. Endocr. jap. **6**, 14—20 (1959a).

— — Effects of administration of oxytocin and prolactin on lactating activity of mammary glands in rats. Endocr. jap. **6**, 259—267 (1959b).

ZAKS, M.G.: Reflex regulation of the tonus of the walls of the udder cistern and of the intramammary pressure. Tr. Inst. Fiziol. (Mosk.) **4**, 34—50 (1955) [in russian].

ZHUZE, A.L., K. JOŠT, E. KASAFÍREK, and J. RUDINGER: Amino acids and peptides. XLV. Analogues of oxytocin with o-ethyltyrosine, p-methylphenylalanine, and p-ethylphenylalaline replacing tyrosine. Coll. Czechoslov. Chem. Commun. **29**, 2648—2662, (1964).

ZOTIKOVA, I.N.: Effect of the nervous system on secretion and ejection of milk in the white mouse. Tr. Inst. Fiziol. (Mosk.) **4**, 63—67 (1955) [in russian].

The Circulatory Actions of the Neurohypophysial Hormones and Similar Polypeptides

K. Saameli

I. Introduction

This chapter deals with the effects of neurohypophysial and some related peptides on the cardiovascular system in different mammalian species. No attempt is made to elucidate the reversed relationship, namely the action of cardiovascular changes on the production and/or the release of the hormones (for this subject see chapter by M. Ginsburg). According to the editor's suggestion this article is confined to the recent literature and does not include older papers, unless they are of more than merely historical interest. It is hoped, however, that most of the relevant papers published later than 1947 are reviewed.

In view of the distinct differences in circulatory action between vasopressin and oxytocin the two neurohypophysial principles are discussed in separate sections. On some occasions, however, the combined discussion is thought to be an advantage, and therefore overlapping between the two main sections is not always avoided. This holds true particularly for that part of the literature which gives results obtained with posterior pituitary extracts rather than with one of the two purified principles. The terms "vasopressin" and "oxytocin" will be used for the antidiuretic-pressor and the oxytocic principle of the mammalian neurohypophysis when general topics are discussed, or when a more specific designation for a drug mentioned in a given paper could not be found. Otherwise, if possible, the drugs will be referred to specifically (e.g. Pituitrin, Pitressin, lysine-vasopressin, arginine-vasopressin, Octapressin = phenylalanine-lysine-vasopressin, Pitocin, Syntocinon = synthetic oxytocin etc.).

II. Vasopressin

A. In Vitro Studies

1. The actions of vasopressin on the *isolated myocardium* have been studied in spontaneously beating atria and in electrically stimulated papillary muscles of the guinea-pig, as well as in isolated perfused hearts of guinea-pigs and rabbits. According to Heeg and Meng (1965) vasopressin (Vasopressin Hoechst), in doses of 0.5 and 1 IU, added to the perfusion fluid of the guinea-pig heart produced almost no change in rate (— 2%), but decreased contractile force by 6—20% and diminished coronary flow by 16—40%. The latter observation confirms an earlier report from Karp et al. (1960) who found a reduction of coronary flow by vasopressin in normal and in atherosclerotic hearts of rabbits. On the isolated cat heart (Langendorff), however, posterior pituitary extract in amounts from 0.02—0.1 IU very often causes dilatation of the coronary vessels (Kordik, 1951). Results obtained by different investigators on the isolated guinea-pig atrium are conflicting: using lysine-vasopressin, arginine-vasopressin or Octapressin in concentrations from 10—320 mU/ml on the electrically driven organ Nakano and Shackford (1965)

observed a clearly dose related reduction in contractile force, whereas Heeg and Meng (1965) described a positive inotropic effect (Vasopressin Hoechst 500 mU/ml) in the same species, not only on the spontaneously beating atrium (+ 24%) but also on the driven papillary muscle (+ 16%).

2. The effect of vasopressin on *arterial strips* depends upon the species and the anatomical site of the vessel: Pitressin in concentrations of 60 mU/ml constricts the aorta of the rat and the femoral artery of the dog and man, but does not contract the aorta of rabbit, dog or cat (Dodd and Daniel, 1960). Aortic strips from the rabbit have been found to be insensitive also to Octapressin in concentrations up to 500 mU/ml (Altura et al., 1965). Working with strips of bovine coronary arteries from different segments (right coronary, left coronary, and circumflex arteries) Altura (1966) did not observe any contraction after the addition of arginine-vasopressin or Octapressin to the bath although the concentrations used had been high (1000 and 500 mU/ml resp.). Only slight and inconsistent vasoconstriction was induced by lysine-vasopressin on helically cut arteries from human umbilical cords (Somlyo et al., 1965).

3. If vasopressin is applied to *isolated perfused organs* its vasoconstricting property can easily be demonstrated. The intraarterial infusion of Pitressin (e.g. 650 mU/kg/min) on the isolated dog hind limb had a pronounced vasoconstrictor effect (Diana and Masden, 1965). The same action was shown in the isolated spleen of the cat by Hertting and Suko (1966), in the isolated perfused rabbit ear by Berde et al. (1961) with single doses of 20—160 mU, and by Schmidt et al. (1962) with much smaller doses (1 or 2 mU) of lysine-vasopressin and Octapressin.

The fact that the constrictor action of vasopressin is more likely to appear when the drug is tested in a perfusion system rather than when given to an arterial strip, which for technical reasons can be obtained only from relatively large vessels, points to the conclusion that the main site of the constrictor action lies in the small peripheral vessels.

B. In Situ Studies

Cardiac output and systemic arterial blood pressure may be considered as the fundamental haemodynamic parameters: both are controlled by cardiac and peripheral factors. The cardiac regulating mechanism involves heart rate and contractility of the myocardium, the peripheral regulation is connected with changes in resistance and venous return.

Any alteration in cardiac output and/or systemic blood pressure caused by vasopressin originates from a change in one or more of the above-mentioned parameters (rate, contractility, peripheral resistance, venous return). Before describing the effects of vasopressin on cardiac output and blood pressure we therefore shall review its influence on each of the regulating factors.

1. Peripheral Resistance

Total peripheral resistance is the sum of the single resistances in many different vascular beds. As in most investigations the sensitivity to vasopressin was found to be different in various vascular beds, a separate discussion of the findings in some particular sections of the circulation is necessary.

a) In the *Femoral Vascular Bed* vasopressin causes a reduction in blood flow when given intraarterially. This was shown by Potter and Sutfin (1961) in the dog under barbiturate anaesthesia, using a canulating type electromagnetic flowmeter and simultaneous blood pressure recording distal to the flowmeter probe. 0.1—5 mU of vasopressin given as single injections decreased femoral flow by 7—64% proportional to the dose without affecting blood pressure, and increased femoral vascular resistance by 8—206%. Similar results have been obtained in cats under chloralose or barbiturate anaesthesia with lysine-vasopressin in doses of 5—90 mU (BARER, 1961; BISSET and LEWIS, 1962).

The effects of intravenous injections are more complicated. Single doses of 10 mU/kg and higher of lysine-vasopressin and Octapressin increased femoral flow in cats under urethane chloralose anaesthesia, and tended to biphasic reaction in dogs under barbiturate anaesthesia where the initial augmentation of femoral flow was often followed by a secondary diminution (BERDE et al., 1961). The same phenomenon was observed also in dogs by POTTER and SUTFIN (1961) with Pitressin: 5—100 mU given intravenously first increased the femoral flow by 14—63% and then reduced it by 9—34%. In another series (WAKIM et al., 1954) the initial augmentation of femoral flow in dogs after 0.1—1 IU/kg of Pitressin given intravenously was less pronounced and followed by a greater (> 50%) reduction. From blood pressure recordings and flow measurements in other vascular beds it may be concluded that the initial increase in flow is related to a changed distribution of cardiac output on one hand and possibly to reflex vasomotor activity on the other.

No biphasic reaction was seen in the dog when Octapressin was applied by constant intravenous infusion: 0.5—10 mU/kg/min led to a dose-related reduction of femoral flow from —32 to —50% (LONGO et al., 1965).

The femoral vascular bed may be subdivided into two major parts, the vascular bed of the skin and that of the musculature. As there is good evidence that the skin participates predominantly in the haemodynamic effects of vasopressin (and oxytocin) its responsiveness to vasopressin will be discussed separately.

b) *The Vascular Bed of the Skin.* In man profound skin pallor after the administration of vasopressin is a well known phenomenon. PICKFORD (1964) observed skin pallor which persisted for some hours following a 10 min intravenous infusion of 50 mU/min. Similar effects from either Pitressin or Octapressin in doses between 0.5 and 20 IU given as single intravenous injections or constant infusions over 30—40 min have been reported by RIBOT et al. (1961), RIBOT et al. (1963), SHANKS (1963) and TSAKIRIS and BÜHLMANN (1962). The fact that this action occurred also with relatively small doses which did not alter blood pressure or cardiac output, points to a particular affinity of vasopressin for skin vessels. This was clearly demonstrated in anaesthetized rats by BERDE (1965) using rubidium^{86} as a radioactive tracer following Sapirstein's method for the synchronous estimation of regional blood flow — or more precisely — for the estimation of the relative distribution of cardiac output on various organs including the skin. In these experiments the most prominent action of lysine-vasopressin as well as Octapressin consisted in a decreased blood flow in the skin; for Octapressin the dose-related reduction was from 15—65% with doses between 13 and 360 mU/kg. A reduction in skin blood flow of the rat without alteration of blood pressure and without flow changes in other organs was found by TAKACS and ALBERT (1963) after intraperitoneal doses from 10—1000 mU of lysine-vasopressin.

Finally it may be of interest that in man the local vasoconstrictor action of lysine-vasopressin and Octapressin, when injected intradermally on the volar aspect of the forearm, is accompanied by an increased rate of lymph flow in the superficial lymphatics. The mechanism of this action is unknown. Possible factors include dilation of the lymph channels, increase in peristaltic activity of the smooth muscle of the lymphatics and closure of lymphatico-venous communications (BURCH and DE PASQUALE, 1963, 1964).

c) *The Vascular Bed of the Splanchnic Area* is another region of the body for which it is claimed that the constrictor action of vasopressin is more or less selective (SHALDON et al., 1961; TSAKIRIS and BÜHLMANN, 1962). This statement derives essentially from the clinical observation in man that systemically applied vasopressin exerts a beneficial effect in the treatment of bleeding oesophageal varices by reducing portal pressure. A selective redistribution of blood away from the portal system would be responsible for this effect. At the present time it may be said that the evidence for such a selectivitiy is not convincing, either for the naturally occurring vasopressins, or for the phenylalanine-analogue Octapressin. The mechanism concerned in the fall in portal venous pressure and in splanchnic blood flow cannot be deduced reliably in the absence of simultaneous measurements of cardiac output. The above mentioned clinical concept is not supported by studies in man and dogs, in which cardiac output and/or blood flow to vascular beds other than the splanchnic area have been measured simultaneously with splanchnic blood flow. They indicate that the decrease of splanchnic blood flow and the consequent reduction of portal venous pressure produced by vasopressin reflect its generalized systemic and cardiac effects, rather than a selective or preferential action on the splanchnic arterioles (DRAPANAS et al., 1961; RUSHMER et al., 1961; SEGEL et al., 1963).

Regardless of this controversy one can say that under clinical and experimental conditions vasopressin constricts the splanchnic blood vessels. Details are given in Table 1 which is restricted to results obtained by direct measurement or observation. In addition to these data some information on changes in splanchnic blood flow due to vasopressin was gained by other authors less directly, mainly by the interpretation of changes in the oxygen content of hepatic venous blood or of alterations in portal venous pressure.

In patients with or without liver disease the splanchnic resistance, derived from systemical arterial pressure, intrasplenic pressure, wedged hepatic venous pressure and estimated hepatic blood flow, decreased by 87 $\pm$ 13 (SD) % during a 10 min intravenous infusion of 20 IU of Pitressin (SHALDON et al., 1961). TSAKIRIS and BÜHLMANN (1962) reported that 10 IU of Octapressin intravenously infused over a 10 min period decreased portal flow and portal pressure in patients with hepatic cirrhosis. These changes have been attributed to a reduction in splanchnic blood flow. The fact that the oxygen consumption in the splanchnic vascular bed did not change considerably led to the conclusion that the splanchnic organ functions were not impaired by the drug.

In another study done in man with hepatic cirrhosis an intravenous infusion of Octapressin (0.1—0.16 IU/min over a 32 min period) produced a 41% reduction of splanchnic blood flow which was calculated from changes in hepatic A-V oxygen difference assuming that there was no change in splanchnic oxygen uptake during the experiment. From the observation that the fall in simultaneously recorded cardiac output was of the same magnitude (—37%) as the reduction in splanchnic flow it was concluded that Octapressin had no greater constrictive effect upon the splanchnic blood vessels than elsewhere (SEGEL et al., 1963).

d) In discussing the effects of vasopressin on the vascular bed of the limbs, skin and splanchnic area (a, b, c) no emphasis was put on its *site and mode of action*. As practically all information on this problem, including changes in the *microcirculation* has been obtained in one of these three vascular beds, this topic will be reviewed before going on to other vascular beds.

A great deal of microcirculatory studies with vasopressin, and particularly with its phenylalanine analogue Octapressin, have been performed by direct microscopic visualization of the exteriorized mesoappendix in anaesthetized rats. In this preparation it was shown that the microvascular effects of vasopressin are different from those produced by other constrictor agents, such as catecholamines and

Table 1. *Effect of vasopressin on the splanchnic vascular bed*

Species	Condition	Drug	Dose	Form of application	Type of measurement	Effect	Ref.
Rat	dioestrous, anaesthetised (barbiturate)	vasopressin	0.05 to 0.5 mU	single i.v.-injection	direct microscopic observation of the vessels of the meso-appendix	constriction of mesenteric arterioles and capillaries	1
			0.25 mU/ml	topically on mesoappendix			
Cat	anaesthetised (chloralose)	lysine-vasopressin	50—1,000 mU	single i.v.-injection	canulating type electromagnetic flowmeter in the main mesenteric vein	decrease in mesenteric blood flow (e.g. approx. — 40% after 500 mU)	2
Cat	anaesthetised (urethane-chloralose)	lysine-vasopressin, Octapressin	20 mU/kg and lower	single i.v.-injection	Thermostromuhr (Rein) on superior mesenteric vein	decrease in mesenteric blood flow of the same magnitude as after epinephrine 1 μg/kg i.v., but of longer duration	3
Dog	anaesthetised (barbiturate)	Pitressin	16—340 mU/min	i.a.-infusion into perfused superior mesenteric artery	perfusion of the superior mesenteric artery at constant rate. Measurement of perfusion pressure and "small mesenteric artery pressure". Calculation of total mesenteric and "small mesenteric artery" resistance	increase in "total mesenteric resistance" (R_T) less than in "small mesenteric artery resistance" (R_{SV}): R_T + 62%, R_{SV} + 103% with 340 mU/min	4
Dog	anaesthetised (barbiturate)	Pitressin	0.5 IU/kg over 15 to 20 min (25—33 mU/kg/min)	i.v.-infusion	electromagnetic flowmeter probe around superior mesenteric artery	decrease in mesenteric blood flow by approx. 50%	5
Dog 20–30 kg	non-anaesthetised	Pitressin	1 IU	single i.v.-injection	chronically implanted ultrasonic type flowmeter probe on superior mesenteric or hepato-gastric artery	abrupt reduction in flow through the splanchnic vascular bed	6
Man	non-anaesthetised	Pitressin	3—8.6 IU (average 1 IU/min) or	i.v.-infusion	calorimetric estimation of blood flow in the sigma	decrease in sigma blood flow by 83%	7
			3 IU	i.m.-injection		by 51%	

References: 1: LLOYD (1959a); 2: BARER (1961); 3: BERDE et al. (1961); 4: TEXTER et al. (1964); 5: DRAPANAS et al. (1961); RUSHMER et al. (1961); 7: GROMOTKA and DEMLING (1962)

angiotensin (ALTURA et al., 1965; HERSHEY et al., 1965): topical application of 0.05 IU of Octapressin produced constriction of arterioles, precapillaries, metarterioles and venules with restriction of overall capillary blood flow. Smaller doses (0.02—0.03 IU) did not constrict arterioles, but resulted in some metarteriolar, precapillary and venular constriction which restricted postcapillary outflow; 0.01 IU affected only the venules, and doses below 0.01 IU were ineffective. These results indicate that the gradient of reactivity for Octapressin progresses from the venular toward the arteriolar side in contrast to the arteriolar to venular gradient for epinephrine and norepinephrine. The dose-graded constriction of the various vessel types induced by locally applied natural vasopressin (B.W. ZWEIFACH, 1961, cited by ALTURA et al., 1965) closely resembled the effects observed with Octapressin. In the same preparation single intravenous injections of Octapressin, in doses from 0.01—0.1 IU, produced a transient increase in capillary circulation and a definite narrowing of the arteriolar vessels while systemic blood pressure was not affected. Intravenous infusion of the synthetic peptide, at a rate of 0.03 μg/min (approximately 1.7 mU/min) over a 60 min period, constricted small arteries and arterioles less than did norepinephrine. It increased the speed of overall blood flow, did not dilate the venules, and did not produce stasis, leucocytic sticking, red cell agglutination or other unfavourable events in the microcirculation.

When given to rats in the state of experimental shock (haemorrhagic or intestinal ischemic shock) Octapressin created favourable microcirculatory blood flow and venous return by improving capillary inflow, decreasing sensitivity to epinephrine, and sustaining vasomotion and venular tone (ALTURA and HERSHEY, 1965; HERSHEY et al., 1965; MAZZIA et al., 1964). These results confirm earlier findings by ZWEIFACH (1950) who showed that vasopressin, in doses which did not increase systemic blood pressure, produced tonic narrowing of the terminal arterioles of the omentum and improved blood flow through the omental vessels in dogs under haemorrhagic shock. A constrictor action of vasopressin on arterioles was microscopically seen also by LANDESMAN and MENDELSOHN (1956) who studied the effects of topically applied neurohypophysial peptides on the uterine omentum of the rat.

The above mentioned results from microcirculatory studies in the rat, indicating that the constrictor action of vasopressin and Octapressin is more accentuated in the venous limb of peripheral circulation than on the arterial side, finds support from some microcirculatory studies done in other species. On the basis of experiments performed in a Mellander cat preparation (MELLANDER, 1960), in which alterations in peripheral flow reflect vascular changes in the arterial side of peripheral circulation and plethysmographically measured alterations of tissue volume indicate vascular changes in the venous side, CERLETTI et al. (1963) conclude that intraarterially injected Octapressin led to an accentuated and sustained constriction of venous vessels but had only a moderate constrictor activity on arterial vessels. This was in contrast to angiotensin which was a potent arterial vasoconstrictor with almost no action on the venous section of the vascular bed. In anaesthetized open-chest dogs the intravenous infusion of Pitressin (0.5—4 IU/min over a 5 min period) sometimes produced a transient increase of venous return (EMERSON, 1966) possibly caused by venous constriction. Further evidence for a predominant active venous constriction in the dog is given by DIANA and MASDEN (1965), who found that under the influence of lysine-vasopressin the venous outflow from a completely separated and artificially perfused hind limb exceeded the constant arterial inflow. In contrast to these results HADDY et al. (1961), using perfused dog forelimb preparations, observed decreases in small vein pressures during intra-arterial infusion of vasopressin and concluded that the arterioles were constricted relatively more than veins. TEXTER et al. (1964, 1965) measuring "large and small vessel pressures" in the perfused mesenteric bed of the dog, found that Pitressin and Octapressin, intraarterially infused at rates up to 0.36 IU/min, markedly increased small vessel resistance whereas venous resistance of the same vascular bed was not altered.

Very little is known about microcirculatory actions of vasopressin other than actions on vascular smooth muscle. When injected intradermally in a concentration of 0.25 IU/ml, lysine-vasopressin did not increase capillary permeability in guinea-pigs pretreated with a protein-bound dye (BISSET and LEWIS, 1962). In another study local tissue oxygen tension in the skin was measured when Octapressin was used as vasoconstrictor in local anaesthetic agents injected subcutaneously on the forearms of human subjects (KLINGENSTRÖM and WESTERMARK, 1964). In contrast to adrenaline and noradrenaline Octapressin did not lower tissue oxygen tension and did not produce local cyanosis as did the catecholamines. This might indicate that local vasoconstriction by Octapressin is achieved without increase in local oxygen consumption.

e) Despite considerable technical difficulties the effect of vasopressin on the *vascular bed of the liver* has been studied more extensively than the effects on most other vascular beds, not only in animals but also in man. The obvious reason for this lies in the wellknown clinical use of vasopressin in the treatment of bleeding oesophageal varices, a life-threatening condition usually caused by portal hypertension due to cirrhosis of the liver. In view of the fact that portal circulation is part of the hepatic circulation, results on these vascular beds will be given in the same table (Table 2).

As evident from these data the consistent finding is that vasopressin depresses portal and hepatic circulation in all species tested and does it under a variety of experimental conditions. It is generally accepted that reduction in splanchnic blood flow (resulting either from generalized systemic and cardiac effects or from a preferential constrictor action on the splanchnic arterioles, see p. 548) is the main causative factor for the reduction of portal vein pressure and flow. Studies in which splenic pulp pressure and splenic vein flow have been recorded in man (DAVIS jr. et al., 1957; SELDINGER and SUNDBLAD, 1963) suggest that in addition to the mesenteric vascular area the vascular bed of the spleen is also involved. When total hepatic venous return in the dog was measured simultaneously with portal flow, it was noted that the flow reducing effect of vasopressin was less pronounced and shorter in the total hepatic circulation than it was in the portal circulation. This was interpreted as being the result of an increasing flow of blood into the liver from the hepatic artery during the infusion of vasopressin (HEIMBURGER et al., 1960). However, studies in which hepatic artery flow of the dog was directly measured by means of an electromagnetic flowmeter and was compared with portal vein flow showed a significant reduction in arterial inflow to the liver caused by vasopressin. They are therefore at variance with the above-mentioned results despite the fact that hepatic arterial flow was not altered to the same extent as portal vein flow (DRAPANAS et al., 1961). Free hepatic venous pressure was found to be increased in man during and after constant intravenous infusion of Octapressin, and it was assumed that this phenomenon reflects a rise in right ventricular end-diastolic pressure and indicates relative heart failure (SEGEL et al., 1963).

f) Results on the action of vasopressin on the *renal vascular bed* are conflicting and so are the interpretations given by different investigators. It seems that the qualitative and quantitative response of the renal circulation to vasopressin depends strongly on dosage, species and type of anaesthesia.

Table 2. *Effect of vasopressin on the vascular bed of the liver*

Species	Condition	Drug	Dose	Form of application	Type of measurement	Effect on portal circulation	Effect on hepatic circulation	Ref.
Dog	anaesthetised (barbiturate)	Pituitrin	4 IU	single i.v.-injection	pressure measurement and sampling and reinfusion of portal vein blood;	decrease of portal pressure by approx. 26%, decrease of portal blood flow by 72%	decrease of hepatic blood flow by 34%	1
					sampling and reinfusion of total hepatic venous return	(the same as above)	(the same as above)	
			40 IU over 30 min (1.33 IU/min)	i.v.-infusion		decrease of portal pressure by approx. 50%, decrease of portal blood flow by approx. 60%	decrease of hepatic blood flow by approx. 60%	
Dog	anaesthetised (barbiturate)	Octapressin and lysine-vasopressin	2—20 mU/kg	single i.v.-injection	portal vein pressure after splenectomy	dose-related decrease of portal pressure up to "some cm H_2O"		2
Cat	anaesthetised (urethane-chloralose)	(as above)	10—1,000 mU/kg	(as above)	(as above)	(as above)		
Dog	anaesthetised (barbiturate)	Pitressin	10 IU over 15—20 min (e.g. 33 mU/kg/min)	i.v.-infusion	electromagnetic flow-meter on portal vein and hepatic artery	marked depression of portal vein flow (> 50%)	decrease of total hepatic blood flow (= portal vein flow and hepatic artery flow) by 49%	3
Man	normal	Pituitrin	2 IU	single i.v.-injection	hepatic vein catheter, bromsulphalein technique		decrease of hepatic blood flow	4
Man	cirrhosis	Pituitrin	20 IU over e.g. 24 min (approx. 1 IU/min)	i.v.-infusion or i.m.-injection	splenic pulp pressure and wedge hepatic vein pressure, hepatic blood flow by isotope technique	decrease of splenic pulp pressure and wedge hepatic vein pressure indicating pronounced reduction of portal vein pressure	decrease of total hepatic blood flow	5

Table 2 (Continuation)

Species	Condition	Drug	Dose	Form of application	Type of measurement	Effect on portal circulation	Effect on hepatic circulation	Ref.
Man	anaesthetised, shunt operation for oesophageal varices	Pituitrin	20 IU over 4—9 min (2.2—5 IU/min)	i.v.-infusion	pressure in portal or splenic vein	marked reduction of elevated portal pressure, e.g. from 300—150 mm H_2O		6
Man	cirrhosis	Pitressin		i.v.-infusion	wedge hepatic vein pressure	reduction of wedge hepatic vein pressure, indicating decrease of portal vein pressure		7
Man	normal	Octapressin	10—20 IU over 10 min (1—2 IU/min)*	i.v.-infusion	wedge hepatic vein pressure and bromsulphalein technique		decrease of hepatic blood flow by 25—62% (mean 46%)	8
	cirrhosis		10 IU over 10 min (1 IU/min)		(as above)	reduction of wedge hepatic vein pressure, indicating decrease of portal vein pressure by 2—14 mm Hg (mean 6 mm Hg)	decrease of hepatic blood flow by 24—51% (mean 37%)	
Man	normal and cirrhosis	Pitressin	20 IU over 10 min (2 IU/min)	i.v.-infusion	wedge hepatic vein and/or intrasplenic pressure, bromsulphalein technique	reduction of wedge hepatic vein pressure, indicating decrease of portal vein pressure by 39% (S.D. 7%)	decrease of hepatic blood flow by 40% (S.D. 6%), increase of calculated hepatic arteriolar resistance by 76% (S.D. 20%), no change in calculated postsinusoidal resistance	9
Man	normal and with portal hypertension during abdominal surgery	Pitressin	20 IU over 4—6 min (3.3—5 IU/min)	i.v.-infusion	omental vein pressure	reduction of omental (= portal) vein pressure by approx. 50% (—46% in patients with normal portal pressure, —60% in patients with portal hypertension)		10

* or 15—20 IU over 30—40 min (approx. 0.5 IU/min)

Table 2 (Continuation)

Species	Condition	Drug	Dose	Form of application	Type of measurement	Effect on portal circulation	Effect on hepatic circulation	Ref.
Man	cirrhosis	Octapressin	approx. 5 IU (0.1—0.16 IU/min over 32 min)	i.v.-infusion	wedge and free hepatic venous pressure	reduction of wedge hepatic vein pressure, indicating decrease of portal vein pressure by 6 mm Hg	increase of free hepatic venous pressure by 5 mm Hg	11
Man	normal, splenic vein thrombosis, cirrhosis	Octapressin	2.5—5 IU	single i.v.-injection	splenic pulp pressure and/or intrahepatic portal branch pressure, radiologic splenoportography	decrease of intrasplenic pressure, decrease of lienoportal and portal flow		12

References: 1: HEIMBURGER et al. (1960); 2: BERDE et al. (1961); 3: DRAPANAS et al. (1961); 4: BEARN et al. (1951); 5: DAVIS et al. (1957); 6: SCHWARTZ et al. (1959); 7: BABER et al. (1960), cited by DRAPANAS et al. (1961); 8: TSAKIRIS and BÜHLMANN (1962); 9: SHALDON et al. (1961); 10: EDMUNDS and WEST (1962); 11: SEGEL et al. (1963); 12: SELDINGER and SUNDBLAD (1963).

In non-anaesthetized dogs weighing from 20—30 kg the intravenous injection of 1 IU of Pitressin caused an abrupt reduction of renal blood flow as measured with an ultrasonic type flowmeter. This reduction was of the same magnitude as that produced in a splanchnic artery or in the lower part of the abdominal aorta (RUSHMER et al., 1961). Using smaller doses, e.g. 10 mU/kg i.v. of lysine-vasopressin or Octapressin in dogs under barbiturate anaesthesia BERDE et al. (1961) working with a "Thermo-Stromuhr", observed a slight increase of renal vein flow, whereas 100mU/kg led to a short decrease. In dogs anaesthetized with pentobarbital constant i.v. infusion of Octapressin, 0.5 to 10 mU/kg for 30—60 min, produced a reduction in renal circulation, renal blood flow being measured by means of an electromagnetic flowmeter. As blood flow through the renal artery fell to a lesser extent than the cardiac output, the conclusion was drawn that Octapressin increases the renal fraction of cardiac output (LONGO et al., 1964). A similar interpretation is given by BERDE et al. (1961) for the clearly observed augmentation of renal blood flow in cats under urethane-chloralose anaesthesia, following relatively small doses (10 mU/kg and more) of lysine-vasopressin or Octapressin; the increase in renal blood flow is not thought to be caused by vasodilatation in the renal vascular bed, but is attributed to a redistribution of blood flow due to vasoconstriction in other regions. Indeed with higher doses the renal blood flow increase was preceeded by a transient reduction which appeared to be the direct result of renal vasoconstriction. In contrast to the se investigators BARER (1961, 1963) assumes that the dose-related increase of renal blood flow, observed with a canulating type electromagnetic flowmeter in cats under chloralose anaesthesia, following intravenous injections of either lysine-vasopressin, arginine-vasopressin or Octapressin in doses from 5—1500 mU, reflects a direct dilating action of the peptides in the renal vessels. This statement is essentially based on the fact that the increase in renal blood flow occurred without change in arterial blood pressure. The validity of this argument might be questioned.

g) Only few investigations on the effects of vasopressin in the *uterine vascular bed* have been undertaken. Measuring blood flow by means of an optically recording rotameter in a uterine artery from anaesthetized pregnant or post partum dogs, AHLQUIST and WOODBURY (1947) found that a greater reduction of uterine blood flow occurred with vasopressin than with oxytocin. In view of the fact that the oxytocic activity of vasopressin is much smaller than that of oxytocin, it may be concluded that the decrease in uterine blood flow after vasopressin is not mediated only through mechanical constriction of the blood vessels due to uterine contraction but also, and probably to a much greater extent, through active vasoconstriction. These results have been confirmed by CARTER et al. (1966) in pregnant and non-pregnant rabbits under barbiturate anaesthesia. Continuous monitoring of uterine blood flow by diverting the outflow from a uterine vein through the dropping chamber of a photoelectric flowmeter, revealed a marked and sustained reduction of flow during and after short intravenous infusions (0.2 IU/min over 5 min) of lysine-vasopressin. Because of complete dissociation of the reduction in uterine vein flow from the general pressure response of the animals, carotid pressure increase being of much shorter duration than the change in uterine flow, it has been suggested that the vascular bed of the uterus is particularly sensitive to the constrictor action of vasopressin. It should be noticed, however, that the dosages used in this study are relatively high, so that any consideration of a possible pathophysiological relevance of the results is hardly justified.

h) Studies on the action of vasopressin in the *pulmonary circulation* are reviewed in Table 3. It is not surprising that the results obtained under different experimental and/or clinical conditions, in different species, with different peptides, and at different dose levels, show some variation. As an overall picture, however, it may be seen that vasopressin has only little influence on the circulation of the lung. No significant pulmonary changes have been observed by BARER (1961) in the cat after lysine-vasopressin, by MAXWELL (1965) in the dog with Octapressin, and by NELSON et al. (1955) and RIBOT et al. (1961) in man with Pitressin, although the doses used have been sufficient to affect general systemic circulation. When either one of the peptides increased pulmonary artery pressure and/or pulmonary wedge pressure, the latter being assumed to be indicative for pulmonary capillary or venous pressure, these changes were only slight and are assumed to be passive in nature. Coronary constriction with subsequent heart failure and a direct cardiodepressor action of vasopressin have been mentioned as causative factors. The pulmonary pressure rise would then be the consequence of the reduced pumping ability of the right ventricle, and of the increase in left ventricular end-diastolic and left atrial pressure. The concept of such a passive type reaction is supported by the common observation that pulmonary artery pressure and pulmonary wedge pressure rise simultaneously and to about the same extent, indicating that the arterio-venous gradient is not changed. In none of the studies is any convincing evidence given for active pulmonary vasoconstriction by vasopressin (CARLIER et al., 1960; RIBOT et al., 1963; SEGEL et al., 1963; TSAKIRIS and BÜHLMANN, 1963; WAKIM et al., 1954). It should be noted that the absence of pulmonary vasoconstriction in doses which are highly active in the peripheral circulation is so far a unique feature for vasopressin; other endogeneous pressure agents such as angiotensin, adrenaline and noradrenaline, do not show this discrepancy (NELSON et al.,

Table 3. *Action of vasopressin on pulmonary circulation*

Species	Condition	Drug	Dose	Form of application	Type of measurement	Effect	Ref.
Cat	anaesthetised (chloralose)	lysine-vasopressin	60—300 mU	single i.v.-injection or single injection into pulmonary artery	pulmonary artery pressure	no significant effect on the pulmonary arterial pressure	1
Dog	anaesthetised (morphin-chloralose)	Pituitrin	4 IU over 10 min (0.4 IU/min) or 4 IU	i.v.-infusion or single injection into pulmonary artery	pulmonary artery and pulmonary wedge pressure and cardiac output (FICK)	decrease in pulmonary artery pressure by 34% without considerable change of pulmonary wedge pressure (= capillary pressure), no change in pulmonary resistance	2
Dog	anaesthetised (barbiturate)	Pitressin	0.1—1 IU/kg	single i.v.-injection	pulmonary artery and pulmonary wedge pressure, retrograde catheter in left atrium	increase in pulmonary artery and wedge pressure (e.g. by 15 mm Hg after 0.5 IU/kg) simultaneously with pressure increase in the left atrium	3
Dog	anaesthetised (chloralose)	lysine-vasopressin, Pitressin	0.05—0.3 IU/kg or 0.075—0.4 IU/kg/min for 8—20 min	single i.v.-injection i.v.-infusion	pulmonary artery and pulmonary wedge pressure and cardiac output	variable changes in mean pulmonary artery pressure, increase in pulmonary wedge pressure due to cardiac depression	4
Dog	anaesthetised (morphine-urethane-barbiturate)	Octapressin	4 IU priming dose, followed by an infusion sufficient to maintain an increased systemic blood pressure	single i.v.-injection and i.v.-infusion	pulmonary artery pressure and cardiac output (FICK)	no significant change in pulmonary artery pressure, increase of pulmonary resistance by 57%	5
Dog	anaesthetised (chloralose)	Posterior Pituitary Extract	105 mU/kg over 7 min (15 mU/kg/min)	i.v.-infusion	pulmonary blood volume by dye dilution method	increase of pulmonary blood volume by 39%	6
Dog	anaesthetised (barbiturate) open chest	Pitressin	0.5—2 IU/min over 5 min (0.1—0.4 IU/min)	i.v.-infusion	pulmonary artery pressure at variable or constant cardiac inflow ("venous return preparation")	slight decrease of pulmonary artery pressure (approx. — 3 mm Hg) when cardiac inflow was variable, distinct increase of pulmonary artery pressure (approx. +15 mm Hg) when cardiac inflow was kept constant. Evidence for blood pooling in the cardio-pulmonary vasculature	7

Table 3 (Continuation)

Species	Condition	Drug	Dose	Form of application	Type of measurement	Effect	Ref.
Man	weak sedation or no premedication	Pitressin	20—30 IU	intramuscular injection	pulmonary artery and pulmonary wedge pressure	no change of pulmonary artery and pulmonary wedge pressure	8
Man	pulmonary tuberculosis, right heart catheterization	Pitressin	20 IU over 30 min (0.67 IU/min)	i.v.-infusion	pulmonary artery and pulmonary wedge pressure and cardiac output (Fick)	no significant change of pulmonary artery pressure, pulmonary wedge pressure, and pulmonary resistance except in patients with far-advanced pulmonary tuberculosis: increase of pulmonary artery pressure by approx. 5 mm Hg	9
Man	pulmonary tuberculosis, right heart catheterization	Octapressin	2—3 IU	i.v.-infusion or subcutaneous injection	pulmonary artery and pulmonary wedge pressure and cardiac output (Fick)	increase in pulmonary artery pressure, wedge pressure and total pulmonary resistance of greater magnitude in patients with faradvanced pulmonary tuberculosis than in patients with minimal to moderately advanced pulmonary tuberculosis	10
Man	cirrhosis of the liver, right heart catheterization	Octapressin	approx. 5 IU over 32 min (0.1—0.16 IU/min)	i.v.-infusion	pulmonary artery and pulmonary wedge pressure	slight significant increase of pulmonary artery pressure and pulmonary wedge pressure by approx. 5 mm Hg	11
Man	right heart catheterization	Octapressin	10 IU over 10 min (1 IU/min)	i.v.-infusion	pulmonary artery and pulmonary wedge pressure	increase in pulmonary artery and pulmonary wedge pressure by approx. 9 mm Hg, augmentation of pulmonary blood volume suspected	12

References: 1: Barer (1961); 2: Van der Straeten and Leusen (1954); 3: Wakim et al. (1954); 4: Carlier et al. (1960); 5: Maxwell (1965); Paulet et al. (1965); 7: Emerson (1966); 8: Nelson et al. (1955); 9: Ribot et al. (1961); 10: Ribot et al. (1963); 11: Segel et al. (1963); 12: Tsakiris and Bühlmann (1963).

1955). A marked decrease in pulmonary artery pressure with intravenous Pituitrin was noted in dogs by VAN DER STRAETEN and LEUSEN (1954); but again this alteration was thought to be related to a marked decrease in cardiac output rather than to a local action in the pulmonary vascular bed. The fact that injections of the drug directly into the pulmonary artery produced no greater effects on pulmonary circulation than did intravenous injections is strongly in favour of a passive mechanism.

In view of the great distensibility of pulmonary vessels the significance of pressure measurements may be questioned. Studies in which pulmonary blood volume in dogs was measured by a dye dilution method are therefore of particular interest. They show that during and after an intravenous infusion with posterior pituitary extract there is a remarkable increase in pulmonary blood volume (PAULET et al., 1965). Evidence for blood pooling in the cardio-pulmonary vasculature was also found by EMERSON (1966) using Pitressin in an open-chest dog preparation and by TSAKIRIS and BÜHLMANN (1963) testing Octapressin in man during right heart catheterization.

i) Studies, in which the *action of vasopressin on the coronary vascular bed* has been measured in a more or less direct way, have been performed in the dog and a few other species but not in man. Results are given in Table 4; they show a nearly uniform picture in that vasopressin decreased myocardial blood flow under a great variety of experimental conditions. Although relatively large doses up to 1000 mU/kg have been used in some instances, it may be said that effective doses given by single intravenous injection were below 100 mU/kg and in one study (BÜLBRING et al., 1949) doses of a few mU/kg still produced a slight reduction of coronary flow. This indicates that the sensitivity of the vascular bed of the heart to the constrictor action of vasopressin is relatively high. The significance of this feature will be stressed in more detail when the influences of vasopressin on contractility and electrical activity of the heart are discussed (see p. 561, 562). Indirect evidence for a coronary constrictor action of vasopressin is available also for man; it can be deduced from electrocardiographic studies as well as from clinical cases reported by SLOTNIK and TEIGLAND (1951), in which subcutaneous injection of 20 IU of Pitressin in elderly patients led to myocardial infarction. An increase in myocardial blood flow after intravenous injections of lysine-vasopressin or Octapressin was observed in rats using rubidium^{86} as radioactive tracer (BERDE, 1965); it should be noted, however, that the information gained by this experimental setup is restricted to relative changes in the distribution of cardiac output, and it may be concluded that the relative increase of myocardial blood flow after vasopressin reflects a passive mechanism rather than an active vasodilatation in the coronary vascular bed.

k) *Vasopressin as "Vasodilator"*. Based on the information given in the foregoing section of this chapter one finds that the most prominent action of vasopressin on peripheral circulation is to constrict blood vessels. Some exceptions to this rule have already been mentioned: absence of active vasoconstriction in the lung (e.g. CARLIER et al., 1960; RIBOT et al., 1963; TSAKIRIS and BÜHLMANN, 1963), evidence for active or passive vasodilation in the liver (HEIMBURGER et al., 1960) and in the kidney (BARER, 1961, 1963; BERDE, 1961). In addition to this there are a few other reports pointing to a paradoxic action of vasopressin: AHLQUIST and WOODBURY (1945) and WOODBURY and AHLQUIST (1946) noted cutaneous flushing after intravenous administration of Pitressin in man. Measuring oxygen and carbon dioxide content in the femoral venous blood from dogs, they found after intravenous injection of 0.1 or 0.5 IU/kg of Pitressin a transient "arterial shift" (increase in O_2, decrease in CO_2) usually attributed to vasodilation. As no "arterial shift" was observed in the femoral venous blood when the skin had been completely

Table 4. *Action of vasopressin on the coronary vascular bed*

Species	Condition	Drug	Dose	Form of application	Type of measurement	Effect	Ref.
Rat	anaesthetised (urethane)	lysine-vasopressin, Octapressin	120 mU/kg	single i.v.-injection	regional distribution of cardiac output (tracer method)	increase in myocardial blood flow by approx. 40%	1
Cat	anaesthetised (barbiturate), open chest	vasopressin	1 IU/kg	single i.v.-injection	heat clearance probe in the left ventricular myocardium	reduction of myocardial blood flow	2
Dog	anaesthetised and non-anaesthetised, open chest	Pitressin	0.5—2 IU	single i.v.-injection	Thermostromuhr	decrease in coronary blood flow by 64—82%	3
Dog	anaesthetised (morphine-barbiturate, morphine-chloralose), open chest	Pitressin	0.1—2 IU	single injection into left coronary artery	canulating type flowmeter on perfused coronary artery	reduction of coronary blood flow, e.g. by 70% after 1 IU	4
Dog	anaesthetised (chloralose)	Pituitrin	10—50 mU	single i.v.-injection	Morawitz canula in coronary sinus	slight decrease in coronary blood flow	5
Dog	anaesthetised (barbiturate), open chest	posterior pituitary extract	10 and 20 IU	single injection into perfused coronary artery	perfusion of the anterior descending branch of the left coronary artery, continuous flow recording	decrease in coronary blood flow by 15 and 30% respectively	6
			150 mU and higher	single i.v.-injection	(the same as above)	decrease in coronary blood flow (150 mU being a threshold dose)	
Dog	anaesthetised (barbiturate), open chest	Pitressin	15 IU over 15 min (e.g. 25 IU/kg/min)	i.v.-infusion	electromagnetic flowmeter on circumflex branch of left coronary artery	drastic fall in coronary blood flow e.g. by 70%	7
Dog	anaesthetised (barbiturate), open chest	lysine-vasopressin, Octapressin	2—250 mU	single injection into circumflex branch of left coronary artery or	bubble flowmeter on circumflex branch of left coronary artery	reduction of coronary blood flow	8
			0.12 IU/kg	single i.v.-injection	(the same as above)	(the same as above)	

Table 4 (Continuation)

Species	Condition	Drug	Dose	Form of application	Type of measurement	Effect	Ref.
Dog	anaesthetised (barbiturate), open chest	vasopressin	0.2 IU/kg	single i.v.-injection	electromagnetic flowmeter on circumflex branch of left coronary artery	decrease of coronary blood flow by 49%, increase in coronary resistance by 131%	9
Dog	anaesthetised (morphine-urethane-barbiturate)	Octapressin	4 IU priming dose, followed by infusion sufficient to maintain an increased systemic blood pressure	single i.v.-injection and i.v.-infusion	coronary sinus catheterization, nitrous oxide saturation method	decrease in coronary blood flow from 89 ± 16 to 68 ± 10 ml/100 g/min (= —24%), increase in coronary vascular resistance by 39%	10

References: 1: BERDE (1965); 2: BETZ et al. (1965); 3: ESSEX et al. (1940); 4: GREEN et al. (1942); 5: BÜLBRING et al. (1949); 6: SCHOFIELD and WALKER (1953); 7: DRAPANAS et al. (1961); 8: SCHMIDT et al. (1962); 9: NASH (1965); 10: MAXWELL (1965).

removed from the leg, it was concluded that vasodilation occurred mainly in the skin; a passive dilatation originating from elevation of arterial pressure and an actively dilating mechanism have been suggested. These findings are supported by results from forearm plethysmography in man which showed that the intravenous infusion of Pitressin (167 mU/min over 25 min) caused an increase in forearm blood flow (BARCROFT and COBBOLD, 1956).

Under very special conditions a depressor effect of vasopressin can be observed not only for a single vascular bed but also for the total circulation of an intact animal. This was shown by HONORÉ and LLOYD (1961a, b) who found an initial vasodepressor response to vasopressin in castrated male rats between the sixth and tenth day but at no other time after the operation.

Whenever a paradoxic action of vasopressin, e.g. increase in blood flow through a given body area, is seen, a passive type reaction should be considered (displacement of parts of the circulating blood volume from some body regions to other areas which are less sensitive to the constrictor action of vasopressin). For those reports in which this possibility has been excluded or in which an additional active vasodilator action has been claimed (AHLQUIST and WOODBURY, 1945; BARER, 1961, 1963; WOODBURY and AHLQUIST, 1946) one should bear in mind that vasodilatation is a characteristic action of vasopressin in birds (COON, 1939). It is not unlikely that the predominant action seen in a non-mammalian species may occur under special experimental conditions also in mammals.

2. *Venous Return*

Although venous return, which is the flow of blood into the heart from the peripheral circulation, plays an important rôle in regulating cardiac contractility and cardiac output, its experimental assessment under the influence of vasopressin has rarely been done. In a study on anaesthetized dogs, in which venous return was measured directly by sampling and re-infusing the outflow from the superior and inferior venae cavae, intravenous Pitressin at infusion rates from 0.5—2 IU/min nearly always caused a decrease from a mean initial value of 70 to a mean value of 42 ml/min/kg (EMERSON, 1966). The fall began shortly after the onset of the infusion and reached a maximum by the end of the 5 min infusion period. In some instances, however, a slight and transient increase of venous return was observed immediately after the onset of the infusion. It was suggested that this change could be due to venous constriction. In view of the fact that under steady state conditions, such as during intravenous infusions of a vasoactive agent, venous return must be equal to cardiac output, it is not surprising that the occasional observation of an increased venous return is limited to the very early phase of the infusion, i.e. to a phase in which steady state conditions are not yet reached. Only at this time of transient haemodynamic changes is a divergent behaviour of venous return and cardiac output conceivable.

3. Actions on the Heart

a) Effects on the *contractility of the heart* can easily be evaluated *in vitro*, working with isolated hearts, atria or papillary muscles. Results obtained in such preparations with vasopressin have already been mentioned (see p. 545). The problem is much more complex if *in situ* actions are to be discussed. This of course, is due to the rather complex nature of cardiac regulating factors on one hand and to the almost inevitable lack of well defined and constant experimental conditions on the other. Most statements regarding vasopressin induced changes in cardiac contractility *in situ* are derived from combined interpretations of changes in cardiac output, systemic blood pressure, central venous or atrial pressure and end-diastolic ventricular pressure. Even when myocardial contractile force is directly measured by means of a strain gauge arch sutured to the surface of one of the ventricles, or when the rate of pressure increase in the left ventricle (dp/dt) is used as parameter for inotropic actions, the results obtained may be influenced by extracardiac factors.

VAN DER STRAETEN and LEUSEN (1954) noted a reduction of cardiac output by 42%, as calculated by the Fick principle in dogs under morphine-chloralose anaesthesia during 10 min infusions of Pitressin at a rate of 0.4 IU/min. As simultaneously occurring changes in systemic arterial blood pressure have been variable, and did not always show an increase, the reduction of cardiac output cannot be attributed solely to increased peripheral resistance, and therefore a direct cardiodepressor action of vasopressin may be suggested.

A similar conclusion was drawn by CARLIER et al. (1960) from the observation that single intravenous injections of 0.05—0.3 IU/kg of synthetic lysine-vasopressin or Pitressin, as well as constant intravenous infusions at rates from 0.075 to 0.4 IU/kg/min, produced marked peripheral vasoconstriction in dogs under chloralose anaesthesia without increasing arterial blood pressure.

Evidence for a possible cardiotoxic effect from relatively high doses of Lysine-vasopressin and Octapressin (0.1—1 IU/kg intravenously) was seen by BERDE et al. (1961) in dogs anaesthetized with barbiturate, on the basis of a transient pressure increase in the right atrium. In open-chest dogs under halothane anaesthesia arginine-vasopressin, lysine-vasopressin, Octapressin, and other analogues (ornithine^8-vasopressin, phenylalanine^2-ornithine^8-oxytocin) sometimes decreased contractile force of the left ventricle as measured by the strain-gauge method, slowed ventricular systolic pressure rise and increased end-diastolic pressure in the left ventricle at relatively high dose levels, e.g. 60—180 mU/kg single intravenous injections or 5 min intravenous infusions at rates from 8—50 mU/kg/min (SAAMELI, 1966, unpublished).

Indications of inhibition of myocardial contractility by vasopressin have also been found in man. Octapressin has been given as intravenous infusions at rates from 0.1—0.16 IU/min over about half an hour to patients with cirrhosis of the liver and portal hypertension. This caused a reduction of cardiac output by 36% as measured by the Fick method, and slowing of heart rate by an average of 16 beats per minute. Pretreatment with atropine prevented the fall in heart rate but had no considerable influence on the decrease in cardiac output. This was taken as evidence that the fall in cardiac output is not reflexly determined but due to a direct depressant action of vasopressin upon the myocardium, acting either directly on the muscle or indirectly through coronary vasoconstriction (SEGEL et al., 1963).

Other investigators, however, using even higher doses of either vasopressin (TSAKIRIS and BÜHLMANN, 1962, 1963) or Pitressin (WAGNER and BRAUNWALD, 1956) observed no change in cardiac output in man. Their results therefore do not suggest any negative inotropic activity of vasopressin.

To make the picture still more puzzling, a very recent report on cardiovascular effects of Octapressin in the rat under urethane anaesthesia should be mentioned: single intravenous injections of 2—16 mU produced a dose-related increase in blood pressure without affecting cardiac output, the latter being measured by the thermo-dilution method. This was interpreted as a possible stimulating effect of Octapressin on myocardial contractility (DE JONG and MC LEOD, 1967).

Despite the fact that some of the results obtained in man, dog and rat are at variance, the overall impression is that vasopressin, at least under certain conditions, can exert a depressant action on the myocardium. Further support for this statement will be given when effects on systemic blood pressure are discussed.

b) Vasopressin usually decreases *heart rate* (see Table 5). This action occurs in rat, rabbit, cat, dog, and man and possibly in many other species which so far have not been studied. Only in two reports has an occasional slight increase in cardiac rate, during short intravenous infusions of Pitressin (GROMOTKA and DEMLING, 1962) or after local infiltration of Octapressin (KULLANDER and WIDE, 1966), been mentioned in man. As the bradycardic effect usually coincides with the pressor effect of vasopressin, it may be assumed that baroreceptor mechanisms are involved (e.g. MAXWELL, 1965; PERRONI et al., 1965; TSAKIRIS and BÜHLMANN, 1963). In man the bradycardic effect of an Octapressin intravenous infusion was reduced by pretreatment with atropine (SEGEL et al., 1963). In rats, however, atropine did not prevent bradycardia following single i.v. injections of the same peptide (DE JONG and MC LEOD, 1967). This latter observation indicates that apart from increasing vagal activity vasopressin, under certain conditions, may also exert a direct slowing effect on the heart.

c) The influence of vasopressin on the *electrocardiogram* has been studied mainly in rabbit, dog, and man.

In non-anaesthetized rabbits large intravenous doses of Pitressin (2—4 IU/kg) caused biphasic changes of the electrocardiogram as recorded from a bipolar chest lead (BLACK, 1960). The first phase immediately followed the injection of vasopressin, lasted for 20—30 sec, and was characterized by elevated T-waves and S-T-segments and shortened Q-T intervals. These alterations have been interpreted as the result of a brief period of accelerated repolarisation involving the whole apical myocardial mass. The second phase succeeded phase 1, lasted for several minutes and was characterized by depressed S-T-segment, depressed or inverted T-wave and relatively normal or prolonged Q-T intervals. Injury in the subendo-

Table 5. *Effect of vasopressin on heart rate*

Species	Type of anaesthesia, other conditions in brackets	Drug	Dose	Form of application	Effect on heart rate	Ref.
Rat	barbiturate	Pitressin	0.07—0.8 IU/kg/min over 6—13 min	i.v.-infusion	variable changes	1
Rat	urethane	Octapressin	18 mU	single i.v.-injection	decrease by 17 ± 6 beats/min	2
Rabbit	urethane-barbiturate	Pitressin	0.014—0.33 IU/kg/min over 11—60 min	i.v.-infusion	marked and sustained reduction, e.g. by 60 beats/min during 0.09 IU/kg/min	1
Rabbit	none	Pitressin	2 or 4 IU/kg	single i.v.-injection	decrease from 300—100 beats/min approx. (combined with a shock-like state during maximal effect)	3
Cat	urethane-barbiturate	Pitressin	0.1 IU/kg/min	i.v.-infusion	transient decrease during the first few minutes and back to normal for the remaining part of the infusion	1
Cat	urethane-chloralose	lysine-vasopressin, Octapressin	0.1—1 IU/kg	single i.v.-injection	slight reduction after 0.1 IU/kg, more prominent after 1 IU/kg	4
Dog	barbiturate	Pitressin	0.1—1 IU/kg	single i.v.-injection	poorly dose-related reduction by 7—68 (mean 30) beats/min	5
Dog	morphine-chloralose	Pitressin	4 IU or	single i.v.-injection	mean reduction by 36 beats/min	6
			4 IU over 10 min (0.4 IU/min)	i.v.-infusion	mean reduction by 36 beats/min	
Dog	chloralose	lysine-vasopressin, Pitressin	0.05—0.3 IU/kg or	single i.v.-injection	reduction; e.g. by approx. 30 beats/min after 0.1 IU/kg injection or during 0.1 IU/kg/min infusion	7
			0.075—0.4 IU/kg/min over 7—12 min	i.v.-infusion	(the same as above)	
Dog	barbiturate	Pitressin	e.g. 0.5 IU/kg over 15 min (0.033 IU/kg/min)	i.v.-infusion	reduction from 175—75 beats/min	8
Dog	barbiturate	lysine-vasopressin, Octapressin	20—100 mU/kg	single i.v.-injection	slight reduction after 20 mU/kg, more prominent after 100 mU/kg	4
Dog	barbiturate	Octapressin	0.5—10 mU/kg/min over 30—60 min	i.v.-infusion	dose-related reduction by 17—50%	9

Table 5 (Continuation)

Species	Type of anaesthesia, other conditions in brackets	Drug	Dose	Form of application	Effect on heart rate	Ref.
Dog	morphine-urethane	Octapressin	4 IU priming dose, followed by infusion sufficient to maintain increased blood pressure	single i.v.-injection and i.v.-infusion	reduction from 87 ± 15 to 67 ± 17 beats/min	10
Dog	barbiturate	Pitressin	2.5—10 IU over 5 min (0.5—2 IU/min)	i.v.-infusion	reduction by approx. 10—15 beats/min	11
Man	none (heart catheterization)	Pitressin	20—30 IU	intramuscular injection	no change in 5/8 patients, reduction by approx. 20 beats/min in 3 patients	12
Man	none	Pitressin	approx. 6 IU over 3—9 min (approx. 1 IU/min)	i.v.-infusion	variable effect: decrease by 8—20 beats/min, increase by 8 beats/min, or no change	13
Man	none	lysine-vasopressin	0.5 IU	single i.v.-injection	reduction by 6—34 (mean 18) beats/min	14
Man	none (heart catheterization, pulmonary tuberculosis)	Octapressin	3 IU over 40 min (75 mU/min)	i.v.-infusion	reduction	15
Man	none (heart catheterization, cirrhosis of the liver)	Octapressin	approx. 5 IU over 32 min (0.1—0.16 IU/min)	i.v.-infusion	mean reduction from 104—88 beats/min	16
Man	none	Octapressin	0.5—3 IU	single i.v.-injection	dose-related reduction by 15—28 beats/min (3 IU i.v. act supramaximally)	17
			10 IU over 10 min (1 IU/min)	i.v.-infusion	reduction	
Man	none	Octapressin	3—80 mU/min	i.v.-infusion	dose-related reduction by 8—24 beats/min	9
Man	none	Octapressin	0.4 IU slowly	i.v.-injection	reduction	18
Man	general anaesthesia (vaginal operation)	Octapressin	1.5 IU	infiltration of uterine cervix	reduction in 15/18 patients by 5—20 beats/min and more; occasionally slight increase	19

References: 1: FRIEDMAN and PAULS (1952); 2: DE JONG and MC LEOD (1967); 3: BLACK (1960); 4: BERDE et al. (1961); 5: WAKIM et al. (1954); 6: VAN DER STRAETEN and LEUSEN (1954); 7: CARLIER et al. (1960); 8: DRAPANAS et al. (1961); 9: LONGO et al. (1964); 10: MAXWELL (1965); 11: EMERSON (1966); 12: NELSON et al. (1955); 13: GROMOTKA and DEMLING (1962); 14: LIPTON et al. (1962); 15: RIBOT et al. (1963); 16: SEGEL et al. (1963); 17: TSAKIRIS and BÜHLMANN (1963); 18: PERRONI et al. (1965); 19: KULLANDER and WIDE (1966).

cardial layers of the left ventricle which are known to be particularly susceptible to anoxaemia is thought to be the basis for phase 2. Changes in the S-T segment and in the T-wave after intravenous vasopressin (1 IU/kg) in the rabbit have also been reported by MELVILLE and VARMA (1961).

In non-anaesthetized dogs Pitressin, injected intravenously in doses from 0.1—1 ml, caused a prolonged period of cardiac slowing during which the following electrocardiographic alterations have been observed: shifting pacemaker, prolongation of the auriculo-ventricular conduction time, sino-auricular block, partial auriculo-ventricular block, extrasystoles, high T-waves, high branching T-waves and bigeminal pulse (GRUBER and KOUNTZ, 1930). Not all of these changes are attributable to coronary vasoconstriction; reflex vagal stimulation may play an important rôle. On the other hand, since pretreatment with atropine or dissection of both vagi did not prevent the cardiac changes completely, a direct action of vasopressin upon the heart muscle is assumed.

Bradycardia associated with ventricular extrasystoles, first or second degree heart block, and T-wave changes were frequently noted when Pitressin was infused intravenously at relatively high rates, e.g. 33 mU/kg/min into dogs under barbiturate anaesthesia (DRAPANAS et al., 1961).

Similar changes in the electrocardiogram of anaesthetized dogs occurred after single intravenous injections of 50 or 500 mU/kg of lysine-vasopressin, the smaller dose being less effective.

When Octapressin was applied by constant intravenous infusion at rates from 0.5—10 mU/kg/min to dogs under barbiturate anaesthesia the animals showed bradycardia, but this was without evident ECG alterations (LONGO et al., 1964). It should be noticed, however, that the doses used in this study have been considerably lower than those used by other investigators, and this may be responsible for the lack of electrocardiographic changes rather than a fundamental difference in action between naturally occurring vasopressin and its phenylalanine^2-analogue.

Reports on electrocardiographic observations following the administration of vasopressin in man show either no or only slight influences. This may be explained by the fact that in most instances, for obvious reasons, only relatively small single doses or low infusion rates have been used. Results are summarized in Table 6.

d) As was already mentioned in the foregoing section, vasopressin may exert an *action on cardiac rhythm*. Since great emphasis is often put on this topic particularly in papers dealing with the clinical use of vasopressin, the problem will be briefly discussed.

As early as 1898 VON CYON (cited by GRUBER and KOUNTZ, 1930) reported that pulsus bigeminus was common after the injection of pituitary extract in experimental animals. This has been confirmed afterwards by many investigators using purified or synthetic material.

In non-anaesthetized dogs intravenous injections of Pitressin (0.1—1 ml) sometimes produced, among other profound changes in the electrocardiogram, extrasystoles and bigeminal pulse (GRUBER and KOUNTZ, 1930). Similar observations have been made in dogs under barbiturate anaesthesia after single intravenous injections of 0.1—1 IU/kg of Pitressin (WAKIM et al., 1954), lysine-vasopressin or Octapressin (BERDE et al., 1961), as well as during constant intravenous infusions of Pitressin at rates in the range of 30 mU/kg/min (DRAPANAS et al., 1961). Occasionally occurring brief arrhythmia after i.v. injections of 0.05—0.3 IU/kg of lysine-vasopressin or Pitressin was noted in dogs also when chloralose anaesthesia was employed (CARLIER et al., 1960). No arrhythmia was seen in cats during halothane or cyclopropane anaesthesia with i.v. injections of 1—2 IU/kg of Octapressin (KATZ, 1965).

Table 6. *Influence of vasopressin on human electrocardiogram*

Condition	Drug	Dose	Form of application	Effect on ECG	References
Right heart catheterization, pulmonary tuberculosis	Pitressin	20 IU over 30 min (0.67 IU/min)	i.v.-infusion	no electrocardiographic changes during or after vasopressin	RIBOT et al. (1961)
normal or with cirrhosis of the liver	Octapressin	10—20 IU over 10—40 min	i.v.-infusion	no electrocardiographic evidence for myocardial hypoxia	TSAKIRIS and BÜHLMANN(1962)
normal	lysine-vasopressin	0.5 IU	single i.v.-injection	bradycardia and sinus arrhythmia without changes in the S-T segment or in the T-wave	LIPTON et al. (1962)
right heart catheterisation, mitral stenosis or normal	Octapressin	10 IU over 10 min (1 IU/min)	i.v.-infusion	bradycardia, occasionally atrio-ventricular or sinu-auricular block, no evidence for myocardial hypoxia	TEXTER et al. (1964)
halothane anaesthesia (1%) for minor surgery	Octapressin	0.5—6.5 IU repeatedly up to a total of 10 IU	single i.v.-injections	no electrocardiographic changes to suggest myocardial ischemia, occasional arrhythmia probably not due to Octapressin	SHANKS (1963)
episiotomy in local anaesthesia	Octapressin	10 IU	local infiltration of the perineum	no pathologic ECG alterations due to Octapressin	ORENGO (1965)
vaginal surgery (conisation of uterine cervix) under general anaesthesia	Octapressin	1.5 IU	local infiltration of the uterine cervix	no change in S-T segment, T-wave flattening in 2/18 patients, extrasystoles in 2/18 patients, occasional conduction disturbances	KULLANDER and WIDE (1966)

In man the tendency to arrhythmia after vasopressin seems to be less pronounced than in animals. The rapid i.v. injection of 0.5 IU of lysine-vasopressin in non-anaesthetized individuals produced only sinus-arrhythmia associated with bradycardia but no extrasystoles (LIPTON et al., 1962). During halothane anaesthesia the incidence of rhythm disturbances was not significantly increased after repeated intravenous injections of Octapressin in doses from 0.5—6.5 IU (SHANKS, 1963). In another clinical study in which Octapressin in doses from 3—5 IU was tested during different types of general anaesthesia, including cyclopropane and halothane, no arrhythmia was observed (KATZ, 1965). However, when Octapressin (1.5 IU) was used as a local haemostatic agent during cone biopsy of the uterine cervix under general anaesthesia, 2 out of 18 patients showed supraventricular or ventricular extrasystoles (KULLANDER and WIDE, 1966); it is not clear whether this was caused by the drug or was due to other circumstances. Despite the predominantly negative findings in human studies, in which relatively small doses have been employed, it can be taken for granted that vasopressin under certain conditions may lead to arrhythmia. The mode of action is not clear. Several different factors such as sudden rise of intraventricular pressure, myocardial hypoxia and delayed sinu-atrial and/or atrio-ventricular conduction seem to be involved. Delayed atrio-ventricular conduction was clearly demonstrated in electrocardiographic studies (see p. 565). It may be considered to be the result of a quinidine-like action, and under this aspect it is of interest to note that according to BRODEUR and BEAULNES (1964) lysine-vasopressin in doses of 50 or 500 mU/kg intravenously prevented ventricular fibrillation usually occurring in dogs under chloroform anaesthesia after large doses of adrenaline.

4. Systemic Arterial Blood Pressure, Cardiac Output and Total Peripheral Resistance

Having discussed the actions of vasopressin on single vascular beds and on the heart we shall now review the resulting effects on blood pressure and cardiac output; results on total peripheral resistance, which is defined as the ratio between arterial mean pressure and cardiac output, will also be included. Findings concerning one or more of these three parameters in different species (rat, rabbit, cat, dog, monkey, man) are tabulated in Table 7.

Bearing in mind that the most prominent action of vasopressin on peripheral circulation is to constrict blood vessels, and that bradycardia and depression of myocardial contractility is another common observation, it is not surprising that whenever sufficiently high doses of vasopressin have been used, increase in systemic blood pressure often associated with a decrease in cardiac output has been observed in most instances.

From studies in which relatively low doses of vasopressin were given by single i.v. injection, it can be deduced that at least in some species amounts as little as a few milliunits per kilogram may be sufficient to produce a slight pressure rise (BERDE et al., 1961; BISSET and LEWIS, 1962; DE JONG and MC LEOD, 1967; GUHL, 1961; HONORÉ, 1961 a and b; LIPTON et al., 1962; LLOYD, 1959b; PERRONI et al., 1965; POTTER and SUTFIN, 1961; TSAKIRIS and BÜHLMANN, 1963). If 10 mU/kg of synthetic lysine-vasopressin (with a pressor activity of approximately 270 IU/mg) are taken as a threshold dose and are compared with 0.1 μg/kg of noradrenaline, which also may be considered to be a threshold dose, it can be calculated that the pressor activity of vasopressin is 2.7 times higher on a weight basis, and 16 times higher on a molecular basis than that of noradrenaline. The result of such a calculation may be without any significance with regard to a possible physiological rôle; it simply underlines the remarkable high potency

Table 7. *Action of vasopressin on blood pressure, cardiac output and totat peripheral resistance*

Species	Condition	Drug	Dose	Form of application	Type of measurement	Effect on blood pressure	Effect on cardiac output (CO) and/or stroke volume (SV)	Effect on total peripheral resistance	Ref.
Rat	lightly anaesthetised (barbiturate)	Pitressin	0.07—0.8 IU/kg/min over 6—13 min	i.v.-infusion	aortic pressure	increase by 55—90 mm Hg systolic and 40—67 mm Hg diastolic			1
Rat	anaesthetised (urethane), eventually atropine/ dibenamine pretreatment	vasopressin	4 mU	single i.v.-injection	carotid artery pressure	"satisfactory pressure response", e.g. increase by approx. 20 mm Hg			2
Rat	anaesthetised (barbiturate), dioestrus	Pitressin or arginine-vasopressin	0.4 mU	single i.v.-injection	carotid artery pressure	increase by approx. 10 mm Hg			3
Rat	anaesthetised (barbiturate), dioestrus	Pitressin or arginine-vasopressin	0.6—1.0 mU	single i.v.-injection	carotid artery pressure	increase by 10 mm Hg			4
Rat	anaesthetised (barbiturate) male	vasopressin	1 mU/200 g	single i.v.-injection	carotid artery pressure	increase by 10 mm Hg			5
Rat	anaesthetised (urethane), dibenamin pretreatment	lysine-vasopressin, Octapressin	2—8 mU/ 420 g	single i.v.-injection	carotid artery pressure	dose-related increase by approx. 10—30 mm Hg			6
Rat	anaesthetised (?)	lysine-vasopressin, Octapressin	50 mU/min	i.v.-infusion	aortic pressure	sharp initial increase followed by continuous decrease during the remainder of the infusion			7
Rat	anaesthetised (barbiturate)	lysine-vasopressin	0.5—1,000 mU/100 g	single i.v.-injection	carotid artery pressure	increase by 6—62 mm Hg. Effects from doses 5 mU/ 100 g and higher are close to maximal effects			8

Table 7 (Continuation)

Species	Condition	Drug	Dose	Form of application	Type of measurement	Effect on blood pressure	Effect on cardiac output (CO) and/or stroke volume (SV)	Effect on total peripheral resistance	Ref.
Rat	anaesthetised (ethyl alcohol), water loaded	lysine-vasopressin	0.1—8 mU	single i.v.-injection	carotid artery pressure	dose-related increase by approx. 5—45 mm Hg			9
Rat	anaesthetised (barbiturate), exteriorized mesoappendix	Octapressin	0.01—0.1 IU	single i.v.-injection		no effect			10
Rat	anaesthetised (urethane)	Octapressin	2—18 mU	single i.v.-injection	femoral artery pressure, thermodilution	dose-related increase by approx. 10—30 mm Hg	no significant change of CO	considerable increase	11
Rabbit	lightly anaesthetised (urethane-barbiturate)	Pitressin	0.02—0.12 IU/kg	single i.v.-injection	femoral artery pressure	sharp rise followed by temporary fall, then secondary rise to a peak level (+35 to +55 mm Hg) followed by rapid fall back to normal			1
	(as above)	(as above)	0.014—0.33 IU/kg/min over 11—60 min	i.v.-infusion	(as above)	similar to i.v.-injections; maximal increase within the first few minutes then continuous fall close to normal during the remainder of the infusion			
Rabbit	anaesthetised (barbiturate)	Pitressin	1 IU/kg	single i.v.-injection	femoral artery pressure	prompt rise (e.g. +20 mm Hg) followed by a temporary sharp fall and a secondary rise			12
Cat	lightly anaesthetised (urethane-barbiturate)	Pitressin	0.1 IU/kg/min over 60 min	i.v.-infusion	femoral artery pressure	sharp increase (+30 mm Hg approx.) in the beginning, slight tendency to normal during the remainder of the infusion			1

Table 7 (Continuation)

Species	Condition	Drug	Dose	Form of application	Type of measurement	Effect on blood pressure	Effect on cardiac output (CO) and/or stroke volume (SV)	Effect on total peripheral resistance	Ref.
Cat	anaesthetised (chloralose), open chest	lysine-vasopressin	24—1,000 mU	single i.v.-injection	arterial blood pressure, pulmonary artery flow (canulating type electromagnetic flowmeter)	no increase with doses below 120 mU, dose-related increase with doses from 120—300 mU up to 30 mm Hg, no further increase with higher doses	no constant change in CO		13
Cat	anaesthetised (urethane-(chloralose)	lysine-vasopressin, Octapressin	10—1,000 mU/kg	single i.v.-injection	carotid artery pressure	sharp increase often followed by a rapid fall and secondary increase up to 60 mm Hg			6
Cat	anaesthetised (halothane or cyclopropane)	Octapressin	1—2 IU/kg	single i.v.-injection	femoral artery pressure	increase (systolic and diastolic) by 15—25%			14
Dog	non-anaesthetised	Pitressin	0.1—1 ml	single i.v.-injection	arterial blood pressure	e.g. with 0.3 ml slight primary increase, followed by a temporary rapid fall below control (—100 mm/Hg) and a secondary increase above control (+50 mm Hg)			15
Dog	anaesthetised (morphine-chloralose)	Pituitrin	0.4 IU/min over 10 min	i.v.-infusion	femoral artery pressure, Fick method	variable effects	decrease in CO by 42%	increase by 64%	16
Dog	anaesthetised (barbiturate)	Pitressin	0.1—1 IU/kg	single i.v.-injection	femoral artery pressure, Fick method	slight initial increase followed by decrease below control	reduction in CO by 34—71%		17
Dog	anaesthetised (barbiturate)	Pituitrin	4 IU	single i.v.-injection	femoral artery pressure	increase by 45 mm Hg			18
	(as above)	(as above)	1.33 IU/min over 30 min	i.v.-infusion	(as above)	increase by 12 mm Hg			

Table 7 (Continuation)

Species	Condition	Drug	Dose	Form of application	Type of measurement	Effect on blood pressure	Effect on cardiac output (CO) and/or stroke volume (SV)	Effect on total peripheral resistance	Ref.
Dog	anaesthetised (chloralose)	lysine-vasopressin, Pitressin	0.05—0.3 IU/kg	single i.v.-injection	left ventricular pressure, Fick method	initial increase followed by decrease in systolic pressure, increase in diastolic pressure with 0.1 IU/kg and higher			19
	(as above)	(as above)	0.075—0.4 IU/kg/min	i.v.-infusion	(as above)	initial decrease in systolic pressure followed by increase back to normal or higher, increase in diastolic pressure	reduction in CO by 45—60%		
Dog	anaesthetised (barbiturate)	lysine-vasopressin, Octapressin	5—100 mU/kg	single i.v.-injection	carotid artery pressure	sharp initial increase followed by rapid decrease and secondary increase up to 40 mm Hg			6
Dog	anaesthetised (barbiturate), open chest	Pitressin	33 mU/kg/min over 15 min	i.v.-infusion	carotid artery pressure, electromagnetic flowmeter on ascending aorta	increase by approx. 40 mm Hg within the first 5 min followed by some decrease (not below control) during the remainder of the infusion	reduction in CO by approx. 40%		20
Dog	anaesthetised (barbiturate)	Pitressin	5—100 mU	single i.v.-injection	femoral artery pressure	slight but significant increase by 3—12%			21
Dog	anaesthetised (barbiturate), open chest	lysine-vasopressin, Octapressin	e.g. 0.12 IU/kg	single i.v.-injection	femoral artery pressure	initial increase followed by decrease below control			7
	(as above)	(as above)	5—20 mU	single injection into coronary artery	(as above)	dose-related decrease			
Dog	anaesthetised (barbiturate), open chest, "venous return preparation"	Pitressin	0.5—2 IU/min over 5 min	i.v.-infusion	femoral artery pressure	moderate increase (+20 mm Hg approx.) when cardiac inflow was variable, marked increase (+80 mm Hg approx.) when cardiac inflow was kept constant		increase by approx. 100%	22

Table 7 (Continuation)

Species	Condition	Drug	Dose	Form of application	Type of measurement	Effect on blood pressure	Effect on cardiac output (CO) and/or stroke volume (SV)	Effect on total peripheral resistance	Ref.
Dog	anaesthetised (barbiturate), open chest	Octapressin	0.5—10 mU/kg/min over 30—60 min	i.v.-infusion	aortic pressure, electromagnetic flowmeter on ascending aorta	dose-related increase by 22—37%	dose-related decrease in CO by 40—71%		23
Dog	anaesthetised (morphine-urethane-barbiturate)	Octapressin	4 IU priming dose followed by constant infusion sufficient to maintain blood pressure	single i.v.-injection and i.v.-infusion	femoral artery pressure, Fick method	increase from 114 ±23 to 124 ±14 mm Hg (+ 9%)	decrease in CO from 2.7 ±0.4 to 1.1 ±0.6 litre/min (—50%), decrease in SV from 26 ±5 to 19 ±5 ml (—27%)	increase from 4140 ± 1210 to 8557 ±5280 dyn sec cm^{-5} (+ 107%)	24
Dog	anaesthetised (chloralose)	vasopressin	15 mU/kg/min over 7 min	i.v.-infusion	carotid artery pressure, dye dilution	increase by 10%	decrease in CO by 12.5—60%, mean 38%	increase by 30—134%, mean 85%	25
Monkey	anaesthetised (barbiturate)	vasopressin	0.5 IU	single i.v.-injection	carotid artery pressure	increase by 24—44 mm Hg			26
Man	slightly premedicated (barbiturate, morphine), right heart catheterization	Pitressin	20—30 IU	intramuscular injection	brachial cuff	increase (by 8—57 mm Hg) in only one-half the cases			27
Man	normal	Pitressin	57—260 mU/min over 120 min	i.v.-infusion	femoral artery pressure	no significant effect			28
	(as above)	(as above)	0.5—1 IU	single i.v.-injection	(as above)	mean increase by 15 mm Hg systolic and 18 mm Hg diastolic			

Table 7 (Continuation)

Species	Condition	Drug	Dose	Form of application	Type of measurement	Effect on blood pressure	Effect on cardiac output (CO) and/or stroke volume (SV)	Effect on total peripheral resistance	Ref.
Man	cirrhosis of the liver	Pituitrin	20 IU	slow i.v.-infusion		little change	no significant change in CO		29
Man	post partum	Pitressin	1 IU	single i.v.-injection	femoral artery pressure	increase by approx. 30 mm Hg			30
	(as above)	Pituitrin	(as above)	(as above)	(as above)	increase preceded by short decrease			
Man	anaesthetised, during abdominal surgery for portal hypertension	Pituitrin, Pitressin	20 IU over 4—9 min	i.v.-infusion	brachial cuff	significant increase in only 1 out of 9 patients			31
Man	cirrhosis of the liver	Pituitrin	60 IU over 32 min	i.v.-infusion	brachial cuff	decrease from 110—80 mm Hg toward the end of infusion			18
Man	normal and with cirrhosis of the liver	Pitressin	20 IU over 10 min	i.v.-infusion	brachial cuff	increase by 19 ±8%			32
Man	pulmonary tuberculosis, right heart catheterisation	Pitressin	20 IU over 30 min	i.v.-infusion	brachial artery pressure, Fick method	no significant change, tendency toward reduction	no significant change		33
Man	normal	lysine-vasopressin, Octapressin	0.2—5 IU or 0.02—0.1 IU/min over 15—20 min	single i.v.-injection i.v.-infusion	brachial cuff or brachial artery pressure	dose-related increase up to 35 mm Hg, 0.2 IU of Octapressin and 1 IU of lysine-vasopressin being a threshold dose			34
Man	normal	Pitressin	approx. 1 IU over 3—9 min	i.v.-infusion	brachial cuff	increase by 8—47 mm Hg systolic and 14—45 mm Hg diastolic			35
Man	anaesthetised for abdominal surgery	Pitressin	20 IU over 4—6 min	i.v.-infusion	systemic arterial blood pressure	slight increase (+ 20 mm Hg approx.) in all patients			36

Table 7 (Continuation)

Species	Condition	Drug	Dose	Form of application	Type of measurement	Effect on blood pressure	Effect on cardiac output (CO) and/or stroke volume (SV)	Effect on total peripheral resistance	Ref.
Man	normal	lysine-vasopressin	0.5 IU	single i.v.-injection	brachial cuff	increase by 5—30 (mean 18) mm Hg systolic and 10—30 (mean 22) mm Hg diastolic			37
Man	anaesthetised (halothane 1%) for minor surgery	Octapressin	0.5—6.5 IU	repeated i.v.-injections	brachial cuff	slight increase (e.g. + 10 mm Hg), rarely decrease			38
Man	normal	Octapressin	0.5—3 IU	single i.v.-injection	femoral artery pressure, Fick method	dose-related increase by 15 to 75 mm Hg systolic and by 10—35 mm Hg diastolic			39
	(as above)	(as above)	1 IU/min over 10 min	i.v.-infusion	(as above)	increase by 37 mm Hg systolic and by 25 mm Hg diastolic	no signifi cant change in CO	increase by approx. 35%	
Man	pulmonary tuberculosis, right heart catheterization	Octapressin	3 IU over 40 min	i.v.-infusion	brachial artery pressure, Fick method	increase	decrease		40
Man	cirrhosis of the liver	Octapressin	0.1—0.16 IU/min over 32 min	i.v.-infusion	brachial artery pressure	sustained increase during infusion by 26 mm Hg systolic, and by 21 mm Hg diastolic	decrease in by 36%, significant decrease in SV		41
Man	normal	Octapressin	0.4 IU	slow (1 min) single i.v.-injection	brachial cuff oscillometry	sharp increase systolic and diastolic	evidence for increase in SV		42
Man	local haemostasis for obstetrical or gynecological operations	Octapressin	up to 10 IU	local tissue infiltrations	brachial cuff	increase by 10—30 mm Hg			43

Table 7 (Continuation)

Species	Condition	Drug	Dose	Form of application	Form of measurement	Effect on blood pressure	Effect on cardiac output (CO) and/or stroke volume (SV)	Effect on total peripheral resistance	Ref.
Man	anaesthetised (halothane, cyclopropane and other)	Octapressin	3—5 IU	single i.v.-injection	brachial cuff	increase by 15—40%			14
Man	general anaesthesia, local haemostasis for cone biopsy of uterine cervix	Octapressin	1.5 IU	local tissue infiltration	brachial cuff	increase rarely more than 30 mm Hg, in 9 out of 18 patients increase in diastolic pressure without or with only minal increase of systolic pressure			44

References; 1: Friedman and Pauls (1952); 2: van Dyke et al. (1955); 3: Lloyd (1959a); 4: Lloyd (1959b); 5: Honoré and Lloyd (1961a); 6: Berde et al. (1961); 7: Schmidt et al. (1962); 8: Lipton et al. (1962); 9: Bisset and Lewis (1962); 10: Altura et al. (1965); 11: De Jong and Mc Leod (1967); 12: Melville and Varma (1961); 13: Barer (1961); 14: Katz (1965); 15: Gruber and Kountz (1930); 16: Van der Straeten and Leusen (1954); 17: Wakim et al. (1954); 18: Heimburger et al. (1960); 19: Carlier et al. (1960); 20: Drapanas et al. (1961); 21: Potter and Sutfin (1961); 22: Emerson (1966); 23: Longo et al. (1964); 24: Maxwell (1965); 25: Paulet et al. (1965); 26: Chaudhury and Tarak (1965); 27: Nelson et al. (1955); 28: Wagner and Braunwald (1956); 29: Davis et al. (1957); 30: Caldeyro-Barcia and Poseiro (1958); 31: Schwartz et al. (1959); 32: Shaldon et al. (1961); 33: Ribot et al. (1961); 34: Guhl (1961); 35: Gromotka and Demling (1962); 36: Edmunds and West (1962); 37: Lipton et al. (1962); 38: Shanks (1963); 39: Tsakiris and Bühlmann (1963); 40: Ribot et al. (1963); 41: Segel et al. (1963); 42: Perroni et al. (1965); 43: Orengo (1965); 44: Kullander and Wide (1966).

of vasopressin. This fact is often neglected in circulatory studies, and it suggests the possibility that the huge amount of vasopressin used in some of the experimental and clinical work is not always free from deleterious effects. Indeed, in some species it is a common observation that the initial pressure increase occurring after an i.v. injection of vasopressin is often followed by a short and transient pressure fall toward or below control levels. This type of reaction was seen by FRIEDMAN and PAULS (1952) and MELVILLE and VARMA (1961) in the rabbit, by BERDE et al. (1961) in the cat, and by BERDE et al. (1961), GRUBER and KOUNTZ (1930), SCHMIDT et al. (1962) in the dog. The nature of the transient pressure fall is not quite clear. In a study in dogs in which femoral blood pressure was recorded simultaneously with coronary blood flow (using a bubble flowmeter on the circumflex branch of the left coronary artery), SCHMIDT et al. (1962) were able to demonstrate that the transient decrease in arterial blood pressure following the sharp initial increase was accompanied by a marked reduction in coronary blood flow. This suggests that weakening of myocardial force, caused by coronary constriction and consequent myocardial hypoxia, is involved, but it does not exclude the possibility of an additional direct depressant effect on the heart muscle itself. Further evidence for cardiac depression resulting in blood pressure fall is available from experiments in which vasopressin, when applied in high doses by constant intravenous infusion to the rat (SCHMIDT et al., 1962), rabbit and cat (FRIEDMAN and PAULS, 1952), or to the dog (DRAPANAS et al., 1961), produced hypertension only during the initial phase of the infusion period. The decrease in blood pressure observed during the remaining course of the infusion, toward or even below control values, could again be attributed to coronary constriction and/or direct negative inotropic action. However, developing refractoriness to the drug should also be considered as a possible explanation. That vasopressin at high dose levels may decrease blood pressure also in man was reported by ANREP and STACEY (1927) and more recently by HEIMBURGER et al. (1960) who observed a rather drastic drop in systolic arterial blood pressure in a patient with hepatic cirrhosis toward the end of a 32 min intravenous infusion of 60 IU (!) of Pituitrin.

For all of the studies which are included in Table 7, whether they describe an increase or a reduction in blood pressure, the site of action of vasopressin is usually assumed to be either the vascular tree or the heart. That the central nervous system, at least theoretically, should be regarded as a possible additional site of action is suggested by experiments in lightly anaesthetized cats. Injection of Pituitrin (1—3.5 IU) or Octapressin (0.5 IU) into the left lateral ventricle of the brain caused a fall in carotid artery pressure by 10—30 mm Hg, whereas higher doses of both drugs increased blood pressure up to 50 mm Hg (NASHOLD jr. et al., 1962). According to these authors the intraventricular injection of small amounts of the drugs may cause a local metabolic or vascular change in the hypothalamus with fall in the blood pressure, while large amounts of drug may result in the release of pressor agents into the circulation.

As pointed out before the most frequently observed response to intravenous or intramuscular vasopressin is an increase in systemic blood pressure caused by vasoconstriction in the major parts of the total vascular bed. Its immediate consequence for the heart is an increased load which could not be overcome unless the heart were able to increase its pumping power either by increasing force or rate. Since neither of these two possible compensatory mechanisms are likely to occur, the common action of vasopressin on cardiac output is expected to be a decrease. This is confirmed by most investigations in which cardiac output was measured or estimated using one of the wellknown methods (Fick principle, dilution method, electromagnetic flowmeter).

In some studies in dogs (e.g. MAXWELL, 1965; VAN DER STRAETEN and LEUSEN, 1954; WAKIM et al., 1954) the observed reduction in cardiac output after vasopressin was greater than would have been expected from relatively small changes in blood pressure. This indicates that increased cardiac load is not the only factor responsible for the usual decrease in cardiac output, cardiac depression may also participate. Not all of the results presented in Table 7 agree with this concept. In rats in which cardiac output was measured by thermo-dilution (DE JONG and MC LEOD, 1967), as well as in human studies in which the Fick method was applied (TSAKIRIS and BÜHLMANN, 1963), Octapressin did not decrease cardiac output despite the occurrence of a marked pressor effect. Similar results have been obtained with lysine-vasopressin in the cat, when cardiac output was measured in the pulmonary artery by means of an electromagnetic flowmeter (BARER, 1961). These findings suggest that under certain conditions an additional stimulating effect of vasopressin on myocardial contractility may play a rôle in maintaining a constant cardiac output with the heart pumping against an increased peripheral resistance.

5. Clinical Use of Vasopressin in Man

The constrictor activity of vasopressin is clinically used under several different conditions. They will be briefly mentioned, but since this chapter deals with pharmacological actions of vasopressin rather than with its clinical aspects, the discussion will not go into details and the review will be restricted to a small part of the literature.

Haemostasis and prolongation of local anaesthesia in surgery are probably the most frequently and most successfully used clinical applications for vasopressin. The drug is added in suitable amounts either to a dilute solution of a commonly employed local anaesthetic or to physiological saline and is applied by local infiltration to the tissue area in which surgery will be performed. Good results have been reported for arginine-vasopressin in uterine surgery by DILLON et al. (1958) and more recently for Octapressin by HOCHULI (1962), FERRARI and VANDONE (1964), ORENGO (1965), KULLANDER and WIDE (1966), and MUNSICK (1966) in obstetrics and/or gynecology, by MUNCHOW and KURZE (1966) in cranial surgery and by FISHER et al. (1965) in dental surgery. The advantage of vasopressin over other vasoconstrictors such as adrenaline and noradrenaline apparently lies in the lack of unfavourable cardiovascular effects especially when general anaesthetics (e.g. halothane) are simultaneously employed. The relatively lower antidiuretic potency of Octapressin in comparison with the natural occurring vasopressins (see chapter by BERDE and BOISSONNAS) points to a particular usefulness of this drug.

Another field for the clinical use of vasopressin lies in the treatment of bleeding oesophageal varices. The mode of action has already been discussed (see p. 548). However, the usefulness of this procedure is not generally accepted, since rather large amounts of the drug (e.g. 20 IU) are necessary to produce a therapeutic effect, and such doses may cause unfavourable cardiovascular reactions (e.g. SEGEL et al., 1963). Satisfactory results have been described by SCHWARTZ et al. (1959) and SHALDON and SHERLOCK (1960) for the use of Pituitrin and Pitressin and by TSAKIRIS et al. (1964) for Octapressin. The value of such treatment was doubted by KATZ et al. (1965).

A rare, but nevertheless highly interesting therapeutical application of vasopressin in man has been mentioned by WAGNER and BRAUNWALD (1956). They found Pitressin at extraordinary low dose levels to be therapeutically effective in patients with orthostatic hypotension due to primary autonomic insufficiency, which is an uncommon diffuse autonomic nervous system disease.

Untoward effects of vasopressin in man, as reported by several authors, are mainly connected with coronary vasoconstriction (e. g. LIPTON et al., 1962; SLOTNIK and TEIGLAND, 1951) or with contraction of intestinal smooth muscle (e. g. LONGO et al., 1964; SHALDON et al., 1961; TSAKIRIS and BÜHLMANN, 1963). It should be noted, however, that according to the majority of reports even large doses of vasopressin have been well tolerated. For instance 60 IU of Pituitrin, given as an intravenous infusion over a 32 min period in a 55 years old man with hepatic cirrhosis and marked depression of liver function, may be considered an extremely high dose. Though toward the end of the infusion it produced a fall in systemic blood pressure which could be counteracted by Aramine, it caused no other apparent side effects (HEIMBURGER et al., 1960).

C. Are there Qualitative and/or Quantitative Differences Between Various Vasopressins?

A frequent source of misunderstanding may be eliminated by reference to data given in the chapter by BERDE and BOISSONNAS, Table 5. There it is shown that the pressor potencies (rat blood pressure) of various vasopressins, if expressed in IU per mg, show considerable differences, the values being approximately 400 IU/mg for arginine-vasopressin, 270 $\pm$ 20 IU/mg for lysine-vasopressin and 55 $\pm$ 7 IU/mg for Octapressin. However, if quantitative comparisons between different vasopressin drugs are discussed in this chapter, this will always be done on a relative potency (= unit per unit) basis.

Qualitative and/or quantitative similarity in the cardiovascular action of different vasopressin drugs has been reported by many investigators: VAN DYKE et al. (1956) found lysine-vasopressin and arginine-vasopressin to be equally potent as an intravenous pressor agent in the dog and rat. No differences between Pitressin, and synthetic lysine-vasopressin have beeen seen by CARLIER et al. (1960) with regard to the haemodynamic responses in the dog. Actions of Pitressin and synthetic arginine-vasopressin were practically indistinguishable when the drugs were applied to a perfused isolated hind limb preparation of the dog (DIANA and MASDEN, 1965). Comparing the effects of Octapressin with those of lysine-vasopressin on a variety of cardiovascular parameters (heart rate, pressure in the carotid artery, the portal vein and right atrium, blood flow in the femoral artery, lienal, superior mesenteric and renal veins) in dogs and cats, BERDE et al. (1961) and BERDE and BOISSONNAS (1966) were unable to demonstrate any significant differences. The same drugs proved to be similar in action in rats on the basis of practically identical dose-pressure response curves (BERDE et al., 1961) and also on the basis of results obtained with the Sapirstein method, which indicated a very similar regional distribution of cardiac output (BERDE, 1965). According to SCHMIDT et al. (1962) Octapressin and lysine-vasopressin when given to the dog produce not only a comparable increase of systemic blood pressure, they also produce a similar reduction in coronary blood flow. No quantitative differences between Octapressin and lysine-vasopressin have been found by BARER (1963) with regard to increased renal circulation.

Reports on dissimilarities in circulatory actions of different vasopressin drugs are also available. They concern quantitative differences more than qualitative aspects: when Pitressin and arginine-vasopressin have been locally applied to the uterine omentum of the rat, the microscopically observed constrictor action of arginine-vasopressin on arterioles was found to be about 10 times stronger than that of Pitressin (LANDESMAN and MENDELSOHN, 1956). Pituitrin was more effective than Pitressin in decreasing portal pressure in patients with hepatic cirrhosis (HEIMBURGER et al., 1960). In a quantitative comparison between Octapressin and lysine-vasopressin on the isolated perfused rabbit ear, the vasoconstrictor potency of the analogue was 2.5 times lower than that of the natural vasopressin (BERDE et al., 1961). In man, however, Octapressin was found to be about five times more effective than lysine-vasopressin; this statement being based on i.v. threshold doses required to produce a slight increase in blood pressure (GUHL, 1961). NAKANO and SHACKFORD (1965) report that in isolated guinea-pig atria the negative inotropic action produced by lysine-vasopressin is less pronounced than that of arginine-vasopressin or Octapressin, the latter two being about equal. Evidence for qualitative differences between Octapressin and Pitressin was seen by TEXTER et al. (1965) on a dog preparation in which the mesenteric vascular bed was artificially perfused and blood pressure was measured simultaneously in small and larger arteries and veins. Octapressin constricted both the larger and the small vessels, whereas Pitressin constricted only small vessels.

From the foregoing it can be seen that opinions on whether different vasopressins have similar or different cardiovascular actions are far from being uniform. However, it may be recognized that dissimilarity is somewhat less frequently reported and that the quantitative differences, as indicated by several authors, are not very pronounced. Furthermore it should be said that only a small part of the given information is based on pharmacologically evaluated dose-response curves. With these restrictions in mind one tends to the conclusion that at the present time, at least for practical purposes, the circulatory actions of different vasopressins can be considered to be similar. It is almost certain, however, that further and more sophisticated work, especially in the field of microcirculation, will reveal important differences.

III. Oxytocin

A. In Vitro Studies

1. In order to study the action of Oxytocin on the *isolated myocardium* of different species fairly large amounts had to be added to the perfusion bath. Concentrations up to 40 mU/ml of Syntocinon had no influence on the amplitude of electrically stimulated guinea-pig atria or on dog papillary muscle; concentrations from 80—320 mU/ml, however, decreased contractility in proportion to the concentration, both in experiments with guinea-pig atria and dog papillary muscles. In no instance with either preparation was an increase in contractility observed (NAKANO and FISHER, 1963). This is in contrast with effects seen on the driven cat papillary muscle by COVINO (1963), who reported a 30% increase in the amplitude of contraction with concentrations of 15 and 30 mU/ml. According to this author, Syntocinon had no influence on rate and contractility of the spontaneously beating cat atrium in doses up to 60 mU/ml; at 90 mU/ml there was still no change in amplitude, but a significant fall in atrial rate occurred. When Pitocin was tested on perfused isolated hearts from rabbits and cats it decreased the amplitude of cardiac contractions at concentrations of 0.01 or 0.1 IU/ml in the perfusate; in the rabbit heart there was some evidence for coronary dilatation (WOODBURY and ABREU, 1944).

As will be discussed later (see page 589) oxytocin owns antiarrhythmic properties *in situ*. This interesting action was also investigated in the isolated myocardium.

In isolated rabbit atria oxytocin (Syntocinon) did not prevent or arrest arrhythmia induced by electrical stimulation, administration of acetylcholine and lowering of the potassium concentration. However, when administered in concentrations from 0.1—0.3 IU/ml either during the arrhythmia or before its induction, this substance reduced the frequency of arrhythmic action potentials and shortened the duration of arrhythmia (PANISSET and BEAULNES, 1961). More convincing evidence for antiarrhythmic actions of oxytocin is given by the same authors on the basis of experiments performed on isolated perfused rabbit hearts (Langendorff preparation) in which fibrillation was induced by electrical stimulation. When Syntocinon (2 IU) was administered during ventricular fibrillation, 70% of the hearts ceased to fibrillate within a few minutes, and when the drug was contained in the perfusate in a concentration of 50 mU/ml the resistance of the preparation to electrical stimuli was markedly increased, so that in about half of the experiments fibrillation could not be induced. The above mentioned increase in amplitude of contraction, observed by COVINO (1963) in the electrically driven cat papillary muscle preparation during exposure to oxytocin (15 and 30 mU/ml), occurred without significant change in stimulus threshold and in conduction velocity, but was accompanied by a marked prolongation of refractory period. The latter effect has also been reported to be seen in the isolated rabbit atrium by BRODEUR (1962). In isolated perfused cat hearts Syntocinon (e. g. 2 IU) was able to restore atrioventricular conduction after A-V block had been induced either by temporary anoxia or by the administration of noradrenaline (KLASSEN et al., 1963).

Considering all these observations one has to point out that the doses required to produce antiarrhythmic and antifibrillatory effects have been remarkably high.

2. Little information is available on the *action of oxytocin on isolated blood vessels*. The contractility of isolated human uterine artery sections or spiral strips as obtained from Cesarean hysterectomy, was not influenced by oxytocin in bath concentrations known to have a marked oxytocic effect on myometrial tissues from pregnant animals (CUTCHIN et al., 1964). However, when tested on helically cut strips from human umbilical arteries and veins, Pitocin and Syntocinon are highly effective vasoconstrictors. It should be remembered that in the same preparation interestingly enough the action of vasopressin was less pronounced and rather inconsistent (SOMLYO et al., 1965).

B. In Situ Studies

Discussing cardiovascular effects of oxytocin *in situ* we shall follow the same approach as with vasopressin. This means that once more the combined discussion of actions on systemic blood pressure and cardiac output, the two fundamental haemodynamic parameters, will be preceded by a review of the underlying peripheral and cardiac effects.

1. The Action of Oxytocin on Different Vascular Beds

a) The normal effect of oxytocin on the *vascular bed of the extremities* (*skin and musculature*) is dilatation. This was shown in the cat, dog, monkey and man, in all of which oxytocin at sufficiently high dose levels produced an increase in blood flow through the femoral or brachial circulation without increasing systemic arterial blood pressure. No change in femoral flow was observed in the pregnant sheep (ASSALI et al., 1961). Details are presented in Table 8.

In man single intrabrachial-artery injections of 25—50 mU of oxytocin caused an increase in blood flow through the hand and forearm with no change in systemic

Table 8. *Action of oxytocin on the femoral and brachial vascular bed*

Species	Condition	Drug	Dose	Form of application	Type of measurement	Effect	Ref.
Cat	anaesthetised (barbiturate)	Syntocinon	1.4 IU	single i.a.-injection into femoral artery	femoral vein flow (photoelectric drop recorder)	marked increase in femoral vein flow, accompanied by slight reduction in systemic arterial blood pressure	1
Dog	anaesthetised (barbiturate)	Syntocinon	250—500 mU or 50 mU	single i.v.-injection single i.a.-injection into femoral artery	femoral vein flow (Pavlov-Stromuhr) (as above)	increase in femoral vein flow, e.g. by approx. 25% after 250 mU i.v. (as above)	2
Dog	anaesthetised (barbiturate), open-chest, female dogs in oestrus or pregnant	Syntocinon	5 mU/kg	single i.a.-injection into brachial or femoral artery	brachial and femoral arterial blood flow (rotameter), or perfusion pressure at constant pump perfusion	increase in brachial flow by $55 \pm 13\%$, decrease in brachial vascular resistance by $33 \pm 5\%$; increase in femoral flow by $42 \pm 13\%$, decrease in femoral vascular resistance by $24 \pm 1\%$	3
Dog	anaesthetised (barbiturate)	Syntocinon	e.g. 750 mU	single i.v.-injection	femoral vein flow (Pavlov-Stromuhr)	increase	4
Sheep	spinal anaesthesia, pregnant at different periods of gestation or in labour	Syntocinon or Pitocin	100—800 mU/kg or 3—60 mU/kg/min	single i.v.-injection i.v.-infusion	femoral artery flow (electromagnetic flowmeter)	no significant change	5
Monkey	anaesthetised (barbiturate)	Syntocinon	e.g. 200 mU	single i.v.-injection	femoral vein flow (Pavlov-Stromuhr)	increase	4
Man	normal	Pitocin or Syntocinon	200—800 mU	single i.v.-injection	hand and forearm blood flow (venous occlusion plethysmography)	dose-related increase by 15—150% in hand flow and by 0—60% in forearm flow	6
	(as above)	(as above)	10—100 mU	single i.a.-injection into brachial artery	(as above)	increase in hand flow up to 100%, decrease in vascular resistance up to 50%	
	(as above)	(as above)	150, 500 or 1000 mU/min over 6—10 min	i.v.-infusion	(as above)	no change in hand and forearm blood flow with 150 mU/min, moderate increase (up to 55%) with the higher doses	

Table 8 (Continuation)

Species	Condition	Drug	Dose	Form of application	Type of measurement	Effect	Ref.
Man	normal	Syntocinon, valine^3-oxytocin	300—500 mU	single i.v.-injections	hand and forearm blood flow (venous occlusion plethysmography)	increase in hand and forearm blood flow, valyl^3-oxytocin being about 1.5—2 times more effective than Syntocinon	7
	(as above)	(as above)	or 20—50 mU	single i.a.-injection into brachial artery	(as above)	(as above)	
	(as above)	(as above)	or 1000 mU/min	i.v.-infusion	(as above)	(as above)	
Man	normal, men and women	Syntocinon	50—75 mU	single i.a.-injection into brachial artery	hand and forearm blood flow (venous occlusion plethysmography)	increase in hand and forearm blood flow	8
	(as above)	(as above)	or 25 or 50 mU/min over 3—10 min after 25 or 50 mU priming dose	i.a.-infusion into brachial artery following i.a.-injection	(as above)	(as above)	
Man	normal	Syntocinon	500 mU	single i.v.-injection	hand blood flow (venous occlusion plethysmography)	increase in hand blood flow	9
	(as above)	(as above)	or 50 mU	single i.a.-injection into brachial artery	(as above)	(as above)	
	(as above)	(as above)	or 25 mU/min	i.v.-infusion	(as above)	(as above)	

References: 1: BISSET and LEWIS (1962); 2: LLOYD and PICKFORD (1962); 3: NAKANO and FISHER (1963); 4: HAIGH et al. (1965); 5: ASSALI et al. (1961); 6: KITCHIN, LLOYD, and PICKFORD (1959); 7: KITCHIN, KONZETT, and PICKFORD (1959); 8: HAIGH et al. (1963); 9: DEIS et al. (1963).

pressure. In order to produce a comparable effect by the intravenous route of administration considerably higher doses (200—800 mU) had to be given. In this case the increase in peripheral flow was accompanied by a drop in systolic and diastolic blood pressure corresponding in time with the peripheral vasodilatation (KITCHIN et al., 1959). In contrast to man no pressure fall was observed in the dog after single i. v. doses which definitely increased blood flow through the hind leg (LLOYD and PICKFORD, 1962). This was interpreted as being either the consequence of a very rapid adjustment of cardiac output or the result of vasoconstriction occurring in some other region (PICKFORD, 1966).

It is a clinically well-known fact that in man large amounts of oxytocin may cause flushing of the skin especially that of the face, neck and hands. This points to an accentuated susceptibility of skin vessels to the dilator action of oxytocin. Experimental evidence for such an affinity is given by KITCHIN et al. (1959) who demonstrated that after single i. v. injections of oxytocin the relative increase of blood flow in the hand is greater than in the forearm. Since the skin participates in the vascular bed of the hand to a much greater extent than it does in the forearm, the above mentioned conclusion seems to be valid at least for man. In dogs, however, it was shown that the increase in hind limb flow occurring after intravenous injections of oxytocin was not changed when the foot was excluded from the circulation, suggesting that the action of oxytocin is not confined to the skin vessels alone (LLOYD and PICKFORD, 1962); blood vessels of the musculature may be equally or even more involved.

The general statement that oxytocin has a vasodilator action in the extremities cannot be made without some restrictions: in dogs pretreated with an oestrogen, or given i.v. oestrogen during the course of an acute experiment, oxytocin decreased hind limb flow in doses which under normal conditions showed a dilator effect. A similar modification was seen after sympathetic interference either by unilateral lumbar sympathectomy or by administration of sympathetic blocking agents such as dihydroergotamine, bretylium tosylate and hexamethonium (LLOYD and PICKFORD, 1962). Measuring hand blood flow by venous occlusion plethysmography, HAIGH et al. (1963) were able to demonstrate a vasoconstrictor action of intraarterially applied oxytocin also in men and women, some 45 min after intraarterial injection or infusion of oestriol (1 mg). Similar results, also in man and using the same method, have been obtained by DEIS et al. (1963) when total nerve block was induced by infiltration of lignocain around the brachial nerves, or when bretylium tosylate (15—50 mg) had previously been infused into the brachial artery. In dog and monkey the usual dilator response to oxytocin, seen in the innervated hind limb, was converted to a constrictor response by pretreatment with reserpine (16.5 mg) or promazine (4 mg/kg) (HAIGH et al., 1965).

It should be noted that practically all information on the relationship between the action of oxytocin on the femoral and brachial vascular bed and hormonal or nervous conditions comes from the same group of investigators. A different experimental set-up was employed in dogs by others (NAKANO and FISHER, 1963) and arterial inflow to the limb was either directly measured by means of a rotameter or was kept constant by means of a pump. Here intraarterially applied oxytocin caused vasodilatation in oestrous female and pregnant dogs, as well as it did in males.

b) There is relatively little information on the action of oxytocin in *vascular beds other than that of the limbs.*

Mesenteric vessels of the rat are dilated by intravenous (10—30 mU), or locally (50 mU/ml) applied oxytocin in males and dioestrous females. In contrast to this there is a constrictor response to the same doses when the animals have been pretreated with stilboestrol and/or progesterone, or when they are in natural oestrous (LLOYD, 1959a). In male and oestrous female dogs anaesthetized with pentobarbital, intraarterial injections of 5 mU/kg of Syntocinon increased blood flow through the superior mesenteric artery by 28 ± 7%, and decreased vascular resistance by 22 ± 3%. As this occurred without any alterations in heart rate, mean arterial blood pressure, left atrial pressure, and myocardial contractility, the change was attributed to a direct vasodilator action of oxytocin in the mesenteric vascular bed (NAKANO and FISHER, 1963).

Portal blood flow, when evaluated in anaesthetized dogs by sampling and reinfusing the blood passing through the portal vein, was not influenced by the intravenous administration of Pitocin (4 IU) (HEIMBURGER et al., 1960).

Very little is known about the action of oxytocin on *renal vessels*. BYROM and PRATT (1959) report that in spayed rats large amounts of oxytocin (e. g. 7 IU i. v.) caused blanching of the kidney surface; however, the same was produced with relatively small doses (20—30 mU) if the rats had been treated with ovarian hormones, and very large doses (i. e. from 4—20 or more units per 100 g body weight subcutaneously) led to massive renal cortical necrosis. In pregnant sheep under spinal anaesthesia at different periods of gestation, including parturition, single i.v. injections (from 60—800 mU/kg) or continuous infusion (from 3—60 mU per kg) of oxytocin did not produce significant changes of renal artery flow as measured by means of an electromagnetic flowmeter (ASSALI et al., 1961).

In the same experiments *blood flow through a main uterine artery* was also measured. Whereas in animals not in labour the above mentioned dosages had no influence, they caused a clearly dose-related reduction in uterine blood flow when given to animals in labour. Under these conditions oxytocin also enhanced uterine contractions and it was assumed that the contracting muscle surrounding the uterine arterioles caused an increase in vascular resistance, and thus a decrease in uterine blood flow. Similar results have been reported in the same paper for parturient dogs under barbiturate anaesthesia. They do not fully agree with earlier findings published by AHLQUIST and WOODBURY (1947) who measured uterine artery flow in pregnant and post partum dogs by means of an optically recording rotameter. In these studies oxytocin produced active uterine vasodilatation in pregnant dogs and vasoconstriction in post partum animals.

The action of oxytocin on the *vascular bed of the lung* has been investigated in man during right heart catheterization by RIBOT et al. (1964). Single i.v. injections of 1 IU of Syntocinon did not change pulmonary artery pressure. When higher doses have been given by constant intravenous infusion (10—15 IU over a 30 min period) a slight but statistically significant increase in pulmonary artery pressure by an average of 1.6 mm Hg was observed. This occurred without significant change in pulmonary wedge pressure and pulmonary vascular resistance.

On the basis of other experimental data obtained in the same studies, such as recordings of ECG and cardiac output, the authors conclude that oxytocin had no constrictor action on *coronary vessels*. This agrees with findings in the anaesthetized open chest dog in which intracoronary injections of 5 mU/kg of Syntocinon even increased coronary blood flow by 78 ± 14%, and decreased coronary vascular resistance by 41 ± 6% without essentially altering heart rate, mean arterial blood pressure, left atrial pressure, and myocardial contractility (NAKANO and FISHER, 1963). However, when oxytocin or De-Amino^1-oxytocin (a powerful synthetic oxytocin analogue) were studied for influences on regional blood flow in rats using Sapirstein's method, no characteristic change in the myocardial fraction of cardiac output was observed with intravenous doses up to 360 mU/kg (BERDE, 1965). This indicates that under the given conditions in rats the response of the coronary vascular bed to oxytocin is qualitatively and quantitatively similar to the overall response of the entire circulation.

2. *Actions on the Heart*

a) *Influence on Cardiac Contractility.* In some of the older work oxytocin (Pitocin) has been said to decrease blood pressure, in various species including man, by decreasing myocardial contractile force and cardiac output rather than by dilating peripheral vessels. Since there was no evidence for coronary artery constriction it was assumed that interference with oxidative processes of the heart was responsible for the weakening of myocardial contractions (Woodbury and Abreu, 1944; Woodbury et al., 1944). More recent studies do not agree with the above mentioned conclusions. When cardiovascular effects of extremely large doses of oxytocin (e. g. 30 min constant i. v. infusion of Syntocinon at a rate of 16 IU/min) have been evaluated in women with a dead foetus in utero or in the early postpartum period the transient initial fall in systemic arterial blood pressure was accompanied by an increase in cardiac output (Cournand's method) and a slight reduction of central venous pressure, indicating that even large doses of oxytocin failed to depress the cardiac muscle (Bieniarz, 1961). According to Andersen et al. (1965) the intravenous injection of 10 IU of Syntocinon to patients undergoing Cesarean section or Cesarean hysterectomy caused an increase in cardiac output and stroke volume (dye-dilution) by 24 and 15% resp. whilst decreasing mean arterial pressure by 19 mm Hg. The positive-inotropic effect seen with oxytocin in isolated papillary muscle (Covino, 1963) and its strong stimulating effect on uterine smooth muscle suggested that the observed increase in cardiac output in man might not be entirely due to peripheral vasodilation but to a certain extent also to a stimulating effect on the myocardium. A careful and sophisticated study performed in open-chest dogs by Nakano and Fisher (1963) confirmed neither a considerable negative-inotropic nor a direct positive-inotropic effect; changes in myocardial contractile force, as measured with a Walton-Brodie strain gauge arch sutured to the left ventricle, and changes in cardiac output, as measured by means of a Shipley-Wilson rotameter, have been attributed to peripheral vasodilatation and to reflexly increased sympathetic activity. Doses of Syntocinon used in these experiments were from 0.05—1.6 IU/kg given by intravenous injections. In anaesthetized cats there was either no change in myocardial contractile force (Walton-Brodie strain gauge arch) or a slight passive increase after large intravenous doses from 1—20 IU/kg of Syntocinon (Katz, 1964).

b) Effects of oxytocin on *cardiac rate* are presented in Table 9. Most of these studies are confined to the action in man, i.e. a species in which oxytocin in high i.v. doses usually produces a rapid and short blood pressure fall. Since the increase in rate and the decrease in pressure follow a similar time course, it has often been said that tachycardia is likely to be reflex in nature, being the consequence of either an increase in sympathetic activity or of a decrease in vagal tone (Brotanek and Kazda, 1965; Caldeyro-Barcia and Poseiro, 1958; Klassen et al., 1963; Mayes and Shearman, 1956). In contrast to this it was observed that tachycardia occurred whether or not there was a drop in blood pressure, and therefore it was concluded that the increase in rate was not due to a baroreceptor-reflex mechanism (Katz, 1964). Since oxytocin failed to produce cardiac acceleration in the presence of general anaesthesia (an observation which has been confirmed by Brotanek and Kazda (1965) but which does not agree with reports from Lipton et al. (1962), Katz (1963, 1964) and Andersen et al. (1965)) it was thought that

Table 9. *Effect of oxytocin on heart rate*

Species	Type of anaesthesia, other conditions in brackets	Drug	Dose	Form of application	Effect on heart rate	References
Rabbit	morphine	Pitocin	e.g. 10—15 IU/kg	single i.v.-injection	slowing, sometimes accompanied by pulsus alternans	Woodbury and Abreu (1944)
Cat	halopropane or cyclopropane	Syntocinon	20 IU/kg	single i.v.-injection	decrease by 15—30 beats/min	Katz (1965)
	(as above)	synthetic oxytocin without chlorbutanol	(as above)	(as above)	no change	
Dog	barbiturate (open chest)	Syntocinon	0.05—1.6 IU/kg	single i.v.-injection	slight increase, e.g. by 7 ± 4 beats/min with 0.5 IU/kg in male dogs	Nakano and Fisher (1963)
Man	none	Pitocin	e.g. 3 IU	single i.v.-injection	increase	Woodbury et al. (1944)
	ether or cyclopropane	(as above)	(as above)	(as above)	no change	
Man	none	Syntocinon	2—5 IU	single i.v.-injection	marked tachycardia	Mayes and Shearman (1956)
Man	none	Syntocinon	2 IU	single i.v.-injection	increase (e.g. by approx. 25 beats/min)	Caldeyro-Barcia and Poseiro (1958)
Man	none	Syntocinon, Pitocin	0.2—0.8 IU or 0.5—1 IU/min over 6—10 min	single i.v.-injection i.v.-infusion	tachycardia	Kitchin, Lloyd, and Pickford (1959)
Man	none	Syntocinon, valine³-oxytocin	0.3—0.5 IU or	single i.v.-injection	increase, valyl³-oxytocin being more effective	Kitchin, Konzett, and Pickford (1959)
	(as above)	(as above)	1 IU/min over 5 min	i.v.-infusion	(as above)	
Man	none (6 hours to 7 days post partum)	Syntocinon	10 IU	single i.v.-injection	mean increase by 30—35 beats/min	Bergquist and Kaiser (1959)

Table 9 (Continuation)

Species	Type of anaesthesia, other conditions in brackets	Drug	Dose	Form of application	Effect on heart rate	References
Man	none (?) (with dead foetus in utero or post partum)	Syntocinon	8—16 IU/min for up to 30 min	i.v.-infusion	increase from 95—125 to 115—165 beats/min during the initial fall of blood pressure, sometimes followed by a decrease to 85—136 beats/min when blood pressure was elevated	BIENIARZ (1961)
Man	none	Syntocinon, Pitocin	10 IU	single i.v.-injection	mean increase by 34 (24—43) beats/min	LIPTON et al. (1962)
	general or spinal anaesthesia for different surgical procedures	(as above)	(as above)	(as above)	mean increase by 12 (0—60) beats/min	
		(as above)	30 mU/min over 30 min and longer	i.v.-infusion	no change	
Man	none	Syntocinon	10 IU	slow (1 min) i.v.-injection	increase by 33 (24—46) beats/min	KLASSEN et al. (1963)
Man	halothane or methoxyfluorane (ventricular arrhythmia)	Syntocinon	10—20 IU	single i.v.-injection	increase by 10—20 beats/min in 3 out of 10 patients	KATZ (1963)
Man	general anaesthesia various volatile anaesthetics)	Syntocinon	10—20 IU	single i.v.-injection	increase by 10—20 beats/min	KATZ (1964)
Man	none	synthetic oxytocin	3 IU	single i.v.-injection	increase (by 60 beats/min at the most)	BROTANEK and KAZDA (1965)
	pentothal sodium	(as above)	(as above)	(as above)	practically no increase	
Man	general anaesthesia or spinal or epidural analgesia for cesarean section or hysterectomy	Syntocinon	10 IU	single i.v.-injection	mean increase by 14 beats/min	ANDERSEN et al. (1965)
Man	none (right heart catheterization in patients with pulmonary disease)	Syntocinon	1 IU	single i.v.-injection	increase from 88—96 beats/min	RIBOT et al. (1964)
		(as above)	0.33—0.5 IU/min over 30 min	i.v.-infusion	slight increase	

tachycardia usually seen in nonanaesthetized human individuals could be psychic in origin (WOODBURY et al., 1944).

In the anaesthetized dog a slight increase in cardiac rate after intravenous injections of oxytocin was also seen and has been related to simultaneously occurring hypotension (NAKANO and FISHER, 1963). However, given in high doses (up to 15 IU/kg) to morphinized rabbits, Pitocin led to a marked slowing of the heart, sometimes accompanied by pulsus alternans (WOODBURY and ABREU, 1944). This has been interpreted as a direct effect of the drug upon the heart itself. Using 20 IU per kg of Syntocinon as single i.v. injections in anaesthetized cats, KATZ (1964) observed a decrease in rate also in this species. When pure synthetic oxytocin was given instead of commercial Syntocinon, which contains chlorbutanol as a preservative, there was no change in cardiac rate. This, of course, leads to the conclusion that chlorbutanol, which is contained in Pitocin too, could have been involved in the above mentioned bradycardic effect in rabbits.

c) *The influence of oxytocin on the electrocardiogram* has been studied mostly in man and only occasionally in other species. The results reported by different investigators are not quite consistent.

Essentially no ECG changes have been observed in man by CARTER and SHAW (1960) with low rate i.v. infusions of Pitocin in women sub partu and after delivery, by RIBOT et al. (1964) with 30 min i.v. infusions of Syntocinon up to 0.5 IU/min in patients during heart catheterization, and by KATZ (1964) with single i.v. injections of 10—20 IU of Syntocinon in anaesthetized patients. When extremely large doses of Syntocinon (8—16 IU/min) have been given by constant intravenous infusion to women with intrauterine foetal demise or postpartum, no effects on ECG other than those resulting from changes in heart rate have been seen by BIENIARZ (1961). According to FELDMAN et al. (1958) there were no electrocardiographic abnormalities after i.v injections of 1 IU/kg of Syntocinon in dogs under cyclopropane anaesthesia; and in pregnant sheep no significant ECG changes were found during continuous i.v. infusions of Pitocin or Syntocinon at rates up to 60 mU/kg/min (ASSALI et al., 1961).

However, there are also studies in which oxytocin did produce alterations of the electrocardiogram. If this was the case flattening and sometimes inversion of the T-wave was the most frequent change. It has been observed in man under various conditions (e.g. anaesthetized and non-anaesthetized, male, female, pregnant and non-pregnant) following single intravenous injections of Pitocin or Syntocinon in doses from 3—10 IU (ANDERSEN et al., 1965; BERGQUIST and KAISER, 1959; BROTANEK and KAZDA, 1965; ICHIYANAGI and MORRIS, 1959; LIPTON et al., 1962; MAYES and SHEARMAN, 1956; WOODBURY et al., 1944). In addition to T-wave alterations occasional depression of the S-T segment was noted when 10 IU of oxytocin were injected intravenously in women postpartum (BERGQUIST and KAISER, 1959) or in normal young adults of both sex (LIPTON et al., 1962).

Different explanations have been given for the observed electrocardiographic changes: T-wave flattening was thought to be due to direct interference of oxytocin with oxidative processes in the myocardium itself, rather than to a reduction in coronary blood flow secondary to hypotension (WOODBURY et al., 1944). According to BERGQUIST and KAISER (1959) and BROTANEK and KAZDA (1965), however, poor coronary filling resulting from hypotension and/or tachycardia would mainly be responsible. From the observation that in healthy young people exercise produced a much more marked tachycardia than i.v. oxytocin, but resulted in less flattening of the T-wave and did not change the S-T segment, LIPTON et al. (1962) concluded that tachycardia was not the only factor responsible. Since adrenaline may cause similar T-wave alterations it was suggested that release of catecholamines as the usual response to sudden hypotension might also be involved.

Be this as it may, all of the electrocardiographic changes observed with oxytocin have been of short duration and are not likely to be of great functional significance. Indeed there is a report on a study performed in anaesthetized atherosclerotic and normal rabbits which shows that Syntocinon in single i.v. doses from 1—5 IU/kg was able to prevent or antagonize S-T changes experimentally induced by hypoxia, ergometrine or vasopressin (MELVILLE and VARMA, 1961).

d) *Actions of Oxytocin on Cardiac Rhythm.* Posterior pituitary preparations used as oxytocic agents at parturition have been reported to cause deleterious cardiovascular effects some of which have resulted in death (e.g. BELINKOFF, 1944). Since many of these accidents occurred when anaesthetics were being used it was thought that the adverse effects might have been due to arrhythmia resulting from incompatibility between the oxytocic and the anaesthetic drug. Cyclopropane has been especially suspected. In order to determine whether such incompatibility exists PARSLOE et al. (1960) studied the effects of various pituitary fractions combined with several anaesthetic agents, including cyclopropane in dogs. Their results do not support the above-mentioned concept. Indeed general anaesthesia decreased the incidence of deleterious cardiac effects caused by Pituitrin (1 IU/kg i.v.), and Pitocin (1 IU/kg i.v.) did not produce any disturbances of cardiac rhythm. In women sub partu anaesthetized with cyclopropane, intramuscularly injected Pitocin did not cause electrocardiographic irregularities while Pituitrin under the same conditions was possibly responsible for some of the cases in which arrhythmia of ventricular or supraventricular origin was observed (MORRIS et al., 1952). In another study Syntocinon or Pitocin have been given to postpartum women under cyclopropane anaesthesia in single i.v. doses of 10 IU. This did not increase the incidence of rhythm disturbances usually seen with cyclopropane alone (ICHIYANAGI and MORRIS, 1959).

On the basis of these reports and since Syntocinon and Pitocin are widely used in today's clinical obstetrics apparently without untoward effects on cardiac rhythm, it may be said that oxytocin at least in its synthetic or highly purified form does not produce arrhythmia.

As already mentioned for the in vitro actions (see p. 580) there is good evidence that oxytocin may even exert antiarrhythmic and antifibrillatory effects. In rabbits in which cardiac arrhythmia or ventricular fibrillation was induced by injections of picrotoxin into the lateral cerebral ventricle, Syntocinon in relatively large doses (2 IU/kg i.v.) was able to restore normal rhythm (MELVILLE and VARMA, 1961). Even larger doses (20 IU/kg) were required to abolish experimental arrhythmia induced in cats by a combination of halopropane or cyclopropane with noradrenaline or hypercapnia (KATZ, 1964; KATZ et al., 1963). Also in dogs under cyclopropane and trichlorethylene anaesthesia, intravenous injections of 1 IU/kg of Syntocinon afforded some protection against adrenaline induced arrhythmia (FELDMAN et al., 1958). In the same species 3—5 IU/kg i.v. have been able to reverse arrhythmia caused by a combination of halopropane and carbon dioxide (KATZ, 1964; KATZ et al., 1963), and repeated i.v. doses of 2 IU/kg have been effective against rhythm disturbances induced by digoxin (BRODEUR and BEAULNES, 1963). High rate intravenous infusions of Syntocinon (1 IU/kg/min) reduced the incidence of ventricular fibrillation in hypothermic dogs from 83—25% (COVINO, 1963). In man, according to KATZ (1963), Syntocinon has been successfully used as an antiarrhythmic agent during halothane or methoxyfluorane anaesthesia. In 8 out of 10 patients showing premature ventricular contractions, bigeminus or multifocal ventricular extrasystoles, the rapid intravenous infusion of 10 or 20 IU of Syntocinon restored normal sinus rhythm.

Neither the site nor mechanism of antiarrhythmic action of oxytocin is known. Several different factors may be involved, one of them being the ability of oxytocin to promote atrioventricular conduction. This was shown by KLASSEN et al. (1963) under various experimental and clinical circumstances such as A-V block induced by anoxia or noradrenaline administration in the isolated heart of the cat, A-V block induced by digitalis in the intact cat and certain forms of clinical heart block or atrial fibrillation due to digitalis therapy in man. According to MELVILLE and VARMA (1961) the antiarrhythmic and antifibrillatory effects of oxytocin could be related to a metabolic action, enabling the heart to utilize oxygen more effectively. PANISSET and BEAULNES (1961) suggested a quinidine-like action of oxytocin. COVINO (1963), however, observed that oxytocin, unlike quinidine, increased refractory period in the papillary muscle preparation of the cat without affecting exitability or conduction velocity.

3. *Actions of Oxytocin on Blood Pressure, Cardiac Output, Stroke Volume, and Total Peripheral Resistance*

Alterations in blood pressure, cardiac output, stroke volume and total peripheral resistance after oxytocin are secondary to the above-mentioned cardiac and peripheral actions of the drug. Results obtained under many different conditions in different species are presented in Table 10. There is so much variation not only quantitatively but also qualitatively, that generalisations can hardly be made. Oxytocin-induced changes in systemic blood pressure as reported for the rat, rabbit, cat, and dog included increases as well as decreases. In man the most frequently reported effect on blood pressure is transient hypotension, sometimes followed by slight secondary hypertension. There is no question that considerable species differences do exist. However, they can explain only a part of the marked discrepancies in results. Differences in the dosage of oxytocin and differences in the type of anaesthesia (if any was used) as well as differences in sex and hormonal conditions should also be considered as important factors determining the direction and the magnitude of the evoked response.

If oxytocin produces a fall in blood pressure, it is now generally accepted that this effect is caused by a widespread peripheral vasodilatation, which visibly involves the skin in man, and was shown to include the vessels of the muscles in various species. Earlier findings (WOODBURY and ABREU, 1944; WOODBURY et al., 1944) which suggested that the hypotensive action of oxytocin was related to myocardial depression of unknown mechanism have not been confirmed (e.g. BIENIARZ, 1961). It should be noticed in this respect that results on the action of oxytocin on cardiac output indicate either no significant change or an increase but never a significant reduction, the only exception being reported by NAKANO and FISHER (1963) who attributed the slight secondary reduction of cardiac output which occurred in dogs after an initial increase to peripheral pooling of blood. If cardiac depression were involved in the mechanism of the hypotensive action of oxytocin one would expect primary reduction in cardiac output to be the usual response. Further evidence for the absence of a cardiodepressant action may be seen in the fact that the increase in cardiac output occurring during the hypotensive phase was due not only to concomittant tachycardia alone, but also to an increase in stroke volume (ANDERSEN et al., 1965; BIENIARZ, 1961). The increase in heart rate after i.v. oxytocin can be explained on the basis of reflex sympathetic stimulation secondary to the hypotension. This mechanism may also be responsible for the frequently observed phenomenon in man of a secondary rise in blood

Table 10. *Action of oxytocin on blood pressure, cardiac output and total peripheral resistance*

Species	Condition	Drug	Dose	Form of application	Type of measurement	Effect on blood pressure	Effect on cardiac output (CO) and/or stroke volume (SV)	Effect on total peripheral resistance	Ref.
Rat	anaesthetised (urethane), pretreated with dibenamine	oxytocin	300 mU	single i.v.-injection	carotid artery pressure	increase by approx. 20 mm Hg, sometimes preceded by a slight fall	—	—	1
Rat	anaesthetised (barbiturate)	oxytocin	10—30 mU	single i.v.-injection	carotid artery pressure	no change	—	—	2
	♂ and dioestrous ♀	(as above)	(as above)	(as above)	(as above)	(as above)	—	—	
	♂ pretreated with ovarian hormones, and oestrous ♀	(as above)	(as above)	(as above)	(as above)	increase	—	—	
Rat	anaesthetised (barbiturate), dioestrous	Syntocinon	5—100 mU/200 g	single i.v.-injection	carotid artery press.	no change, or very slight decrease	—	—	3
Rat	anaesthetised (barbiturate), after decerebration or pithing or ganglionic blockade or peripheral sympathetic blockade	Syntocinon	50 mU	single i.v.-injection	carotid artery pressure	increase	—	—	4
Rat	anaesthetised (barbiturate)	Syntocinon	20—500 mU/100 g	single i.v.-injection	carotid artery press.	dose-related increase by 8—32 mm Hg	—	—	5
Rat	anaesthetised (barbiturate), ♂ and pregnant ♀	Syntocinon	0.05—3.2 IU/kg	single i.v.-injection	femoral artery pressure	dose-related increase up to +20 mm Hg	—	—	6
Guinea-pig	anaesthetised (barbiturate)	Syntocinon	0.05—3.2 IU/kg	single i.v.-injection	carotid artery press.	dose-related increase up to +15 mm Hg	—	—	6
Rabbit	morphinized	Pitocin	e.g. 10 IU/kg	single i.v.-injection	femoral artery press.	average decrease from 130/95 to 50/43 mm Hg	—	—	7
Rabbit	anaesthetised (barbiturate)	Syntocinon	5 IU/kg	single i.v.-injection	femoral artery press.	increase	—	—	8

Table 10 (Continuation)

Species	Condition	Drug	Dose	Form of application	Type of measurement	Effect on blood pressure	Effect on cardiac output (CO) and/or stroke volume (SV)	Effect on total peripheral resistance	Ref.
Rabbit	anaesthetised (barbiturate)	Syntocinon	0.05—3.2 IU/kg	single i.v.-injection	femoral artery press.	dose-related increase up to +15 mm Hg	—	—	6
Cat	anaesthetised (barbiturate)	Pitocin	15—20 IU/kg	single i.v.-injection	—	decrease from 120/75 to 80/50 mm Hg	—	—	7
Cat	anaesthetised (halo-prane or cyclopropane)	Syntocinon	1—20 IU/kg	single i.v.-injection	femoral artery press.	variable changes (in crease or decrease)	—	—	9
Dog	anaesthetised (barbi-turate), normal	Pitocin	10 IU/kg	single i.v.-injection	—	increase	—	—	7
	pregnant or pretreated with oestrogen	(as above)	(as above)	(as above)	—	decrease	—	—	
Dog	anaesthetised (cyclopropane)	Syntocinon	1 IU/kg	single i.v.-injection	femoral artery press.	mainly decrease by 10—40 mm Hg	—	—	10
	(trichlorethylene)	(as above)	(as above)	(as above)	(as above)	increase by 10—35 mm Hg	—	—	
	(barbiturate)	(as above)	(as above)	(as above)	(as above)	mainly slight increase	—	—	
Dog	anaesthetised (barbi-turate), pregnant	Syntocinon Pitocin	up to 0.8 IU/kg or up to 60 mU/kg/min	single i.v.-injection i.v.-infusion	carotid artery pres-sure, dye dilution	no significant change	no signifi-cant change in CO	—	11
Dog	anaesthetised (barbiturate)	Syntocinon	1 IU	single i.v.-injection	carotid artery press.	slight decrease	—	—	12
Dog	anaesthetised (barbiturate)	Syntocinon	0.05—1.6 IU/kg	single i.v.-injection	carotid artery pres-sure, rota-meter	dose-related decrease of mean pressure up to —45 mm Hg	biphasic re-action in CO: after 0.5 IU/kg increase by 12±2%, followed by 8±2% decrease	after 0.5 IU/kg de-crease by 24±4%	13

Table 10 (Continuation)

Species	Condition	Drug	Dose	Form of application	Type of measurement	Effect on blood pressure	Effect on cardiac output (CO) and/or stroke volume (SV)	Effect on total peripheral resistance	Ref.
Dog	anaesthetised (barbiturate)	Syntocinon	2 IU/kg	single i.v.-injection	carotid artery press.	mainly increase	—	—	14
Dog	anaesthetised (barbiturate), hypothermia	Syntocinon	1 IU/kg/min	i.v.-infusion	—	initial increase by 10 to 20 mm Hg, followed by decrease to control values for the remainder of the infusion	—	—	15
Sheep	spinal analgesia, pregnant	Syntocinon, Pitocin	up to 0.8 IU/kg or up to 60 mU/kg/min	single i.v.-injection i.v.-infusion	carotid artery pressure, dye dilution	no significant change	no significant change in CO	no significant change	11
Monkey	anaesthetised (barbiturate)	oxytocin	1 IU	single i.v.-injection	carotid artery press.	decrease by 20—70 mm Hg	—	—	16
Man	anaesthetised (ether, cyclopropane), or non anaesthetised, ♂ and ♀, pregnant or non-pregnant	Pitocin	1—10 IU	single i.v.-injection	brachial artery pressure	dose-related decrease; e.g. —30 to —50 mm Hg after 3 IU, 10 IU being supramaximal	—	—	17
Man	non-anaesthetised, normal	oxytocin	20—40 IU over 120 min (= 167 to 334 mU/min)	i.v.-infusion	brachial or femoral artery press.	no significant change	—	—	18
	orthostatic hypotension	(as above)	1 IU	single i.v.-injection	(as above)	marked initial decrease followed by slight hypertension			
Man	non-anaesthetised, ♂ and ♀	Syntocinon, Pitocin	2—5 IU	single i.v.-injection	brachial cuff	decrease	—	—	19
Man	non-anaesthetised, ♀ post partum	Syntocinon	0.2—2 IU	single i.v.-injection	femoral artery press.	dose-related decrease; e.g. —3 mm Hg after 2 IU	—	—	20

Table 10 (Continuation)

Species	Condition	Drug	Dose	Form of application	Type of measurement	Effect on blood pressure	Effect on cardiac output (CO) and/or stroke volume (SV)	Effect on total peripheral resistance	Ref.
Man	non-anaesthetised, ♀ post partum	Syntocinon, Orasthin	3 IU	slow (1 min) i.v.-injection	brachial cuff	increase by 10—25 mm Hg	—	—	21
Man	non-anaesthetised, ♀ post partum and puerperium	Syntocinon	10 IU	single i.v.-injection	brachial cuff	initial decrease followed by slight hypertension	—	—	22
Man	non-anaesthetised, ♀ pregnant at term, induction of labour	Syntocinon	low rate i.v.-infusion		brachial cuff	increase in 17% of all patients	—	—	23
Man	non-anaesthetised, normal	Syntocinon, valine³-oxytocin	0.3—0.5 IU or 1 IU/min	single i.v.-injection i.v.-infusion	brachial artery pressure	decrease, valyl³-oxytocin being somewhat more effective	—	—	24
Man	non-anaesthetised, normal ♂ and ♀	Syntocinon Pitocin	20—800 mU	single i.v.-injection	brachial artery pressure, Fick method	decrease with doses of 300 mU and higher; e.g. up to —40% (average —21%) with 500 mU	increase in CO by 0—42% (average +21%) with 500 mU	decrease by 19—46% (average —32%) with 500 mU	25
Man	non-anaesthetised, ♂ and ♀ (non-pregnant)	Syntocinon	1—8 IU/min	i.v.-infusion	femoral artery pressure	decrease during the first 30 min of infusion, back to control values during the remainder of the infusion	—	—	26
	♀ pregnant	(as above)	(as above)	(as above)	(as above)	initial decrease, followed by increase above control values during the remainder of the infusion	—	—	
Man	non-anaesthetised or light anaesthesia (N_2O, ether), sub partum and post partum	Syntocinon	5 IU or 10 IU	single i.v.-injection i.m.-injection	brachial cuff	no change in 62% of the patients, decrease by 17/10 mm Hg in 24%, and increase up to +30 mm Hg in 14%	—	—	27

Table 10 (Continuation)

Species	Condition	Drug	Dose	Form of application	Type of measurement	Effect on blood pressure	Effect on cardiac output (CO) and/or stroke volume (SV)	Effect on total peripheral resistance	Ref.
Man	non-anaesthetised, ♀ pregnant (foetal demise), post partum, and during menstruation	Syntocinon	8—16 IU/min	i.v.-infusion	femoral artery pressure, Cournand's method for cardiac output (mixed venous blood O_2-saturation)	initial decrease by 20—43 mm Hg systolic and 11—26 mm Hg diastolic, followed by sustained increase by 15—47 mm Hg systolic and 8—28 mm Hg diastolic	increase in CO during the hypotensive and early hypertensive phase, then tendency toward control values. Increase in SV	decrease by 50% during the first 4 min and back to control values during the remainder of an 8 IU/min infusion	28
Man	non-anaesthetised, therapeutic abortion at midtrimester pregnancy	Syntocinon	up to 3.4 IU/min	i.v.-infusion	brachial cuff	increase by 15 mm Hg	—	—	29
Man	non-anaesthetised	Syntocinon	—	single i.v.-injection	brachial cuff	decrease by 20—40 (mean 26) mm Hg systolic and 10—40 (mean 21) mm Hg diastolic	—	—	5
	anaesthetised (e.g. cyclopropane)	(as above)	10 IU	(as above)	(as above)	marked initial decrease (average —44 mm Hg systolic and —22 mm Hg diastolic) followed by slight increase above control values	—	—	
	anaesthetised (e.g. cyclopropane)	Syntocinon	30 mU/min	i.v.-infusion	brachial cuff	no decrease; slight increase in 50% of the patients	—	—	

Table 10 (Continuation)

Species	Condition	Drug	Dose	Form of application	Type of measurement	Effect on blood pressure	Effect on cardiac output (CO) and/or stroke volume (SV)	Effect on total peripheral resistance	Ref.
Man	♂ and ♀, pregnant and non-pregnant	oxytocin	3 IU	single i.v.-injection	brachial cuff	decrease	increase in CO	decrease	30
Man	non-anaesthetised	Syntocinon	10 IU	slow (1 min) i.v.-injection	brachial cuff	decrease by 18—40 (mean 22) mm Hg systolic and 29—50 (mean 39) mm Hg diastolic	—	—	31
Man	anaesthetised (halothane or methoxyfluorane)	Syntocinon	10—20 IU	single i.v.-injection	brachial cuff	decrease in mean pressure by 15—20 mm Hg in 5 from 10 patients	—	—	32
Man	caudal or spinal analgesia, ♀ post partum	Syntocinon, Pitocin	10 IU	single i.v.- or i.m.-injection	brachial cuff	no significant differences during the first 60 min after injection when compared with control group	—	—	33
Man	anaesthetised (halothane, cyclopropane and others)	Syntocinon	10—20 IU	single i.v.-injection	brachial cuff	initial decrease, followed by a slight increase by 5 to 15 mm Hg above control values	—	—	9
Man	non-anaesthetised, right heart catherization	Syntocinon	1 IU	single i.v.-injection	brachial artery pressure, Fick method	decrease by 13 mm Hg	—	—	34
		Syntocinon	0.33—0.5 IU/min	i.v.-infusion		no significant change	increase in CO by 18%, no significant change in SV	no significant change	

Table 10 (Continuation)

Species	Condition	Drug	Dose	Form of application	Type of measurement	Effect on blood pressure	Effect on cardiac output (CO) and/or stroke volume (SV)	Fffect on total peripheral resistance	Ref.
Man	non-anaesthetised, ♂	oxytocin	3 IU	single i.v.-injection	brachial cuff	decrease diastolic by: 25—45 (mean 31) mm Hg	—	—	35
	♀ non-pregnant	(as above)	(as above)	(as above)	(as above)	20—90 (mean 52) mm Hg	—	—	
	1st trimester pregnancy					15—30 (mean 24) mm Hg	—	—	
	3rd trimester pregnancy					5—30 (mean 16) mm Hg	—	—	
	post partum					5—25 (mean 10) mm Hg in 50% of the patients followed by increase up to +30 mm Hg systolic and +15 mm Hg diastolic	—	—	
	anaesthetised	(as above)	(as above)	(as above)	(as above)	no secondary increase	—	—	
Man	anaesthetised (e.g. cyclopropane) or spinal or epidural analgesia, cesarian section and hysterectomy	Syntocinon	10 IU	single i.v.-injection	radial artery pressure, dye dilution	decrease by 41 mm Hg systolic and 28 mm Hg diastolic; no secondary increase	increase in CO by approx. 25%, increase in SV by approx. 12%	decrease by approx. 35%	36

References: 1: Van Dyke et al. (1955); 2: Lloyd (1959a); 3: Lloyd (1959b); 4: Lloyd and Pickford (1961); 5: Lipton et al. (1962); 6: Nakano (1964); 7: Woodbury and Abreu (1944); 8: Melville and Varma (1961); 9: Katz (1964); 10: Feldman et al. (1958); 11: Assali et al. (1961); 12: Lloyd and Pickford (1962); 13: Nakano and Fisher (1963); 14: Brodeur and Beaulnes (1963); 15: Covino (1963); 16: Chaudhury and Tarak (1965); 17: Woodbury et al. (1944); 18: Wagner and Braunwald (1956); 19: Mayes and Shearman (1956); 20: Caldeyro-Barcia and Poseiro (1958); 21: Siener (1958); 22: Bergquist and Kaiser (1959); 23: Engstrom (1959); 24: Kitchin, Konzett, and Pickford (1959); 25: Kitchin, Lloyd, and Pickford (1959); 26: Caldeyro-Barcia (1960); 27: Mc Gee (1960); 28: Bieniarz (1961); 29: Burnhill et al. (1962); 30: Brotánek et al. (1963); 31: Klassen et al. (1963); 32: Katz (1963); 33: Poppy (1963); 34: Ribot et al. (1964); 35: Brotanek and Kazda (1965); 36: Andersen et al. (1965).

pressure slightly above control values following the marked initial decrease (BERGQUIST and KAISER, 1959; BIENIARZ, 1961; BROTANEK and KAZDA, 1965; KATZ, 1964; LIPTON et al., 1962; WAGNER and BRAUNWALD, 1956). It is not clear whether this "over-shoot"-reaction is favoured or depressed by general anaesthesia. According to BROTANEK and KAZDA (1965) secondary hypertension was seen after the intravenous injection of 3 IU of oxytocin in 50% of non-anaesthetized patients but was always absent in anaesthetized individuals. Conversely LIPTON et al. (1962) have observed that an over-shooting secondary reaction to 10 IU i.v. of Syntocinon occurred only in anaesthetized patients.

In species other than man the hypotensive action of oxytocin is less consistent and there is a rather large number of reports indicating either no significant change or a primary increase in blood pressure. The fact that in some studies in dogs oxytocin fails to lower the blood pressure although it causes a distinct peripheral vasodilatation, shown by an increased blood flow through the hind leg, could be explained on the basis of a very rapid cardiac adjustment (PICKFORD, 1966). However, this hypothesis cannot be applied in the interpretation of the frequently observed primary hypertensive action of oxytocin, and one might assume that a vasoconstrictor action, possibly related to the intrinsic slight pressure activity of oxytocin (see chapter by BERDE and BOISSONNAS, Table 2), could be involved. From the extensive work of PICKFORD and her collaborators (DEIS et al., 1963); HAIGH et al., 1963, 1965; HONORÉ and LLOYD, 1961a and b; LLOYD, 1959a and b; LLOYD and PICKFORD, 1961a, 1962) it is well known that the vascular responses to neurohypophysial hormones are influenced by ovarian hormones and sympathetic denervation or blockade (for review see PICKFORD, 1966). With regard to oxytocin it is suggested that its inherent vasoconstrictor action is unmasked by sympathetic blockade or by the action of ovarian hormones. In rat, dog and man sympathetic denervation converted the dilator action of oxytocin to a constrictor action, and in the same species oestrogen appeared to act in the same direction as sympathetic interference. According to BROTANEK and KAZDA (1965) the depressor effect of oxytocin (3 IU intravenously) is decreased during pregnancy, and some authors report a slight hypertensive effect in women in the course of therapeutic abortion (BURNHILL et al., 1962), induction of labour (ENGSTROM, 1959) and postpartum (SIENER, 1958). It is tempting to suggest that in these studies the action of oxytocin was influenced by the large amounts of placental hormones. However, it should also be considered that oxytocin may cause uterine contractions which expel blood from that organ into the general circulation, thus leading to a rise in pressure (HENDRICKS, 1958).

Although there is no doubt that the main site of action for the circulatory effects of oxytocin lies in the peripheral blood vessels, it is at least theoretically of interest that its direct application to the left lateral ventricle of the brain in cats was not without influence on systemic blood pressure. Doses from 0.2—0.4 IU of Syntocinon decreased blood pressure by approximately 10 mm Hg, higher doses (0.5—1.5 IU) led to an increase by 10—30 mm Hg (NASHOLD jr. et al., 1962).

IV. General Aspects

A. Cardiovascular Interactions Between Neurohypophysial Peptides and Other Drugs

The relationship between neurohypophysial peptides and other drugs is complex. While vasopressin and oxytocin may interfere with the cardiovascular effects of various substances, their own circulatory actions may be altered by the presence of either exogenous or endogenous substances.

1. Autonomic Nervous System

In non-anaesthetized man the intravenous infusion of Octapressin at a rate of 0.1—0.6 IU/min produced cardiac slowing which was less pronounced when *atropine* had been given before. It was concluded that bradycardia was partially due to a vagal reflex mechanism (SEGEL et al., 1963). However, the typical direct vascular actions of neurohypophysial peptides are usually not influenced by atropine. This drug did not interfere with femoral blood flow changes caused by synthetic oxytocin or lysine-vasopressin in the cat (BISSET and LEWIS, 1962), nor did it prevent the rapid and transient fall in blood pressure seen after intravenous injections of 3 IU of Pitocin in man (WOODBURY et al., 1944). Controversial results have been reported by DE JONG and MC LEOD (1967) who observed that in anaesthetized rats the pressor response to Octapressin was increased by atropine while bradycardia was not affected.

The pressor action of *adrenaline* or *noradrenaline* was shown to be potentiated by vasopressin or oxytocin in the rat, cat and dog (BARTELSTONE and NASMYTH, 1965; LOCKETT, 1957; STAVRAKY and OLIVER, 1952). Doses as low as 20 μU/kg/min of arginine-vasopressin or 1 mU/kg of Pitocin, i.e. doses which were far below threshold for a direct circulatory effect, have been sufficient for this potentiation. Since enhancement of the reactivity to pressor amines by neurohypophysial peptides was demonstrated not only in intact animals but also in isolated organs (aortic strip, atrium, papillary muscle) it may be concluded that this action is a direct one and is not related to central nervous influences. In contrast vasodilator effects of β-adrenergic stimulation are not potentiated but inhibited by the neurohypophysial peptides. In anaesthetized cats 20 IU/kg of synthetic oxytocin produced partial or total inhibition and sometimes reversal of the blood pressure lowering effect of *isoproterenol* (KATZ, 1964). Reversal of the isoproterenol induced pressure fall into a pressure increase was also observed in dogs during constant i.v. infusion of Pitressin at a rate of 8 mU/kg/min, or after single i.v. injections of the same drug in doses from 0.5—1 IU/kg (NASH et al., 1961). In order to explain this phenomenon it was suggested that vasopressin blocked peripheral vasodilating receptors without antagonising the cardiac stimulating action of isoproterenol.

When the interactions between neurohypophysial peptides and catecholamines have been studied in the field of microcirculation distinct differences in the action of various peptides have been established. During microscopical observation of the small vessels in the mesoappendix of anaesthetized rats (ZWEIFACH test) it was seen that synthetic oxytocin (0.05—0.5 IU/100 g i.v. injection) diminished the microvascular effects of locally applied adrenaline, while lysine-vasopressin in doses from 0.0005—1.0 IU/100 g increased the reactivity to adrenaline (LIPTON et al., 1962). Results obtained in the same preparation with Octapressin are particularly interesting. Octapressin, although it may potentiate the action of locally applied adrenaline in normal rats (ALTURA et al., 1965; HERSHEY et al., 1965), was shown to decrease the abnormally high reactivity to adrenaline in rats under the condition of intestinal ischemic shock (ALTURA et al., 1966).

CHENOWETH et al. (1958) noticed in anaesthetized dogs subjected to a short asphyxial stimulus that the administration of some pressor amines (e.g. noradrenaline) greatly sensitized the vascular system to the pressor effect of a substance arising in the head; there were reasons for believing that the active material was vasopressin, since there was a similarly increased sensitivity to this hormone. This example shows not only that neurohypophysial peptides influence the action of sympathomimetic amines, but also that their own circulatory action may be altered by these substances.

Considering the above mentioned interactions between neurohypophysial peptides and sympathomimetic amines it is not surprising that *chemical interference with the sympathetic system* at the receptor-, neuron- or ganglionsite may markedly alter the circulatory actions of vasopressin and oxytocin.

According to LLOYD and PICKFORD (1962) and DE JONG and McLEOD (1967) the pressor response of rats to Octapressin or Pitressin is enhanced when the animals have been pretreated with propranolol, chlorpromazine, phenoxybenzamine, dibenamine, dihydroergotamine, bretylium, and TEA. In dogs an increased pressor response to vasopressin was observed after the administration of dibenamine, tolazoline, hydergine, chlorpromazine, and reserpine (FRIEDEN and KELLER, 1954; NASH, 1965; SUPEK et al., 1960, 1962; WEIDMANN and CERLETTI, 1961). In patients with orthostatic hypotension caused by primary autonomic insufficiency the doses of vasopressin required to produce an increase in blood pressure are much lower than in normal individuals, and when a state similar to orthostatic hypotension was induced in normal subject by ganglionic blockade with TEA, the sensitivity to vasopressin was greatly increased (WAGNER and BRAUNWALD, 1956).

Alterations of the circulatory effects of oxytocin caused by chemical sympathetic blockade have also been reported. Its usual vasodilator action in rats was converted to a vasoconstrictor action under the influence of dibenamine, dihydroergotamine, bretylium, and TEA (LLOYD and PICKFORD, 1961a). In another study performed in rats in which Syntocinon had a pressor effect, this action was potentiated in reserpinised animals. It was suggested that there was greater response of the vessels simply because the vascular smooth muscles were more relaxed by reserpine (NAKANO and FISHER, 1963). In the dog, monkey and man, oxytocin applied intraarterially into a brachial or femoral artery causes an increase in blood flow through the extremity. Under the influence of dihydroergotamine, chlorpromazine, bretylium, reserpine or hexamethonium, oxytocin acts as a vasoconstrictor and thus decreases blood flow (DEIS et al., 1963; HAIGH et al., 1965; LLOYD and PICKFORD, 1962).

2. Hormonal State

Similar alterations in the cardiovascular effects of neurohypophysial peptides as were caused by sympathetic interference have been reported to occur under the influence of ovarian hormones. In rats the sensitivity to the pressor action of vasopressin increases during pregnancy, and doses of oxytocin which in the non-pregnant dioestrous state are either without effect on blood pressure or cause a slight fall, are able to increase the pressure during the second half of pregnancy (LLOYD, 1959b). The same type of reaction may be observed when rats are in natural oestrous or have been treated by oestrogens (LLOYD and PICKFORD, 1961a). In the dog and monkey oestrogens are able to depress or reverse the vasodilating action of oxytocin. This was shown in studies in which limb blood flow was measured (HAIGH et al., 1965; LLOYD and PICKFORD, 1961a; LLOYD and PICKFORD, 1962).

The existence of a distinct relationship between the cardiovascular actions of oxytocin and the hormonal state has also been demonstrated in man. The results are in agreement with animal studies. In non-anaesthetized men and women the intraarterial injection or infusion of relatively small amounts of Syntocinon (e.g. 50 mU single injection or 50 mU/min infusion) caused an increase in hand blood flow on the side of injection, as measured by venous occlusion plethysmography; some 45 min after intraarterial oestriol (1 mg) oxytocin caused a reduction in blood flow on the side of injection, and flow through the other, control, hand was not affected (HAIGH et al., 1963). In pregnant women the vascular sensitivity to oxytocin decreases in the course of pregnancy. This was shown by BROTANEK and KAZDA (1965) on the basis of threshold doses required for producing a fall in blood pressure; in men and non-pregnant women this threshold was of 25—100 mU i.v., it increased during pregnancy and reached a maximum of 150—900 mU in the post partum period. When extremely large amounts of oxytocin have been given by constant intravenous infusion (1000—8000 mU/min) the pattern of blood pressure changes has been different in pregnant and non-pregnant individuals. In man and non-pregnant woman there was hypotension during the first 30 min of the infusion followed by normalisation during the remaining part of the infusion; in pregnant women the hypotensive phase was considerably shorter and was followed by a pressure increase above control values which lasted until the end of the infusion (CALDEYRO-BARCIA, 1960).

3. *Miscellaneous*

The sensitivity to the pressor action of vasopressin was found to be reduced in male and female rats treated with *DOCA* when the peptide was given at a time before hypertension had developed; *cortisone* reduced the sensitivity to vasopressin of oestrous females but increased that of males and dioestrous females (HONORÉ, 1962a and b). In pithed rats *prostaglandin* was able to inhibit the pressor increase after vasopressin; since this antagonism existed also for the pressor action of angiotensin and catecholamines it was said to be a nonspecific mechanism (HOLMES et al., 1963). In cats and dogs it was shown that the vasomotor action of *histamine* and lysine-vasopressin neutralize each other (BAISSET et al., 1965). However, in rats this substance as well as two other endogenous vasodilators, namely *acetylcholine*, and *serotonin*, did not influence the blood pressure response to neurohypophysial peptides (LLOYD and PICKFORD, 1961a). According to BISSET and LEWIS (1962) neither the vasodilator action of oxytocin nor the vasoconstrictor action of vasopressin have been altered in cats by mepyramine, a potent *antihistamine*. Vasopressin reduced the pressor response to single injections of *angiotensin* in dogs; since it did not alter the pressor response to noradrenaline it was suggested that vasopressin and angiotensin may compete for a common receptor (LOUIS and DOYLE, 1966). Under this aspect it may be of interest that vasopressin and angiotensin (but not oxytocin) share another remarkable property: both peptides inhibit the release of *renin* induced in dogs by lowering renal perfusion pressure. As in some experiments with vasopressin inhibition of renin release occurred without changes in systemic blood pressure, the inhibitory action could not be related to haemodynamic alterations (BUNAC et al., 1967).

In sections B and C of this chapter it has repeatedly been mentioned that *anaesthesia* may modify the cardiovascular actions of neurohypophysial peptides. For details it can be referred to Tables 1—10. A characteristic example of circulatory interactions between oxytocin and general anaesthesia in man is given by LIPTON et al. (1962), who found that the rapid intravenous injection of 10 IU of Syntocinon produces greater hypotension but less tachycardia in patients under cyclopropane anaesthesia than it does in the non-anaesthetized subject. It is most likely that in this case as in many others, the interaction between the neurohypophysial peptide and the anaesthetic agent is not a direct one but is related to alterations in circulatory reflex mechanisms.

B. Duration of the Circulatory Actions

Most cardiovascular actions of the neurohypophysial peptides which are discussed in this chapter are of relatively short duration. At least two different factors may be responsible: First, biological half-life of the neurohypophysial hormones is likely to be short (rapid destruction or elimination from the body); second, in the intact organism fast adaptation to an altered circulatory situation by means of central nervous reflex mechanisms is a commonly observed phenomenon.

The most prominent example for a short circulatory action of neurohypophysial peptides is given by oxytocin in regard to its vasodilator effect. The duration of action never exceeded a few minutes, whether it was evaluated by blood flow measurement in dog (LLOYD and PICKFORD, 1962) and man (KITCHIN et al., 1959), or was judged on the basis of a reduced systemic arterial blood pressure in the cat (WOODBURY and ABREU, 1944) and in man (e.g. ANDERSEN et al., 1965; BERGQUIST and KAISER, 1959; BROTANEK and KAZDA, 1965; KATZ, 1964; KLASSEN et al., 1963; LIPTON et al., 1962; MAYES and SHEARMAN, 1956; RIBOT et al., 1964). In a study in which femoral arterial blood pressure was directly measured in a post partum woman, the pressure drop started 14 sec after the rapid intravenous injection of 2 IU of Syntocinon, reached its maximum at the 24th second, and the pressure returned to its original level 80 sec after the injection (CALDEYRO-BARCIA and POSEIRO, 1958). The fact that vasodilatation starts almost immediately after the injection, and according to all reports is fully established within less than 1 min, may suggest that the vascular action of oxytocin is a direct one, and not likely to be related to the release of other dilator substances. From results reported by BROTANEK and KAZDA (1965) it is evident that the duration of the hypotensive action of oxytocin depends not only on the dose but also, and possibly to a greater extent, on the individual sensitivity to the dilator action. In men and non-pregnant women in which the threshold dose of oxytocin required for producing a fall in blood pressure was low (25—100 mU i.v.), the hypotension caused by intravenous injection of 3 IU lasted from 102—152 (mean 129) sec and from 74—289 (mean 148) sec respectively; however, in women post partum in which the threshold dose was higher (150—900 mU i.v.), the hypotensive effect of 3 IU of oxytocin was considerably shorter, lasting from 8—35 (mean 25) sec.

Cardiovascular actions of oxytocin other than vasodilatation, have also been reported to be of short duration. This holds for tachycardia, which follows essentially the same time pattern as hypotension and therefore may be regarded as a secondary phenomenon (e.g. CALDEYRO-BARCIA et al., 1957; KATZ, 1963, 1964; KLASSEN et al., 1963; RIBOT et al., 1964), and it can also be applied to changes sometimes observed in the electrocardiogram (ICHIYANAGI and MORRIS, 1959; LIPTON et al., 1962; MAYES and SHEARMAN, 1956). It should be noticed, however, that in some animal studies in which the antiarrhythmic action of oxytocin was investigated this effect lasted considerably longer, e.g. up to 90 min (BRODEUR and BEAULNES, 1963; FELDMAN et al., 1958; MELVILLE and VARMA, 1961).

Another interesting point was brought up by NAKANO and FISHER (1963) who found cardiovascular refractoriness of the dog to repeated doses of oxytocin to be of relatively long duration (e.g. 45 min), although the directly measured circulatory changes after the effective initial dose were short. They suggest that oxytocin may be retained in the cardiovascular tissues of the dog for a considerably longer period than is usually assumed on the basis of half-life measurements in man (see chapter by M. GINSBURG.

If vasopressin or Octapressin is given by single i.v. injection the onset of its vasoconstrictor action is equally rapid as the onset of the vasodilator effect after i.v. oxytocin. When 0.5—3 IU of Octapressin had been given intravenously to patients the blood pressure started to rise within 15—20 sec (TSAKIRIS and BÜHLMANN, 1963), and in anaesthetized dogs which were given a rapid i.v. injection of either lysine-vasopressin, arginine-vasopressin, Octapressin or ornithine[8]-vasopressin in doses from 20—180 mU/kg, the time from the injection to the onset of pressure increase was less than 20 sec (SAAMELI, 1966, unpublished). Another similarity between vasopressin and oxytocin with regard to the time course of their circulatory actions, may be seen in the fact that with both hormones the maximal blood pressure change following single i.v. injections is usually reached within a minute or less (e.g. POTTER and SUTFIN, 1961; SAAMELI, 1966, unpublished). However, when the duration of the vasomotor action of vasopressin is compared with that of oxytocin considerable differences will be noted. Although vasopressin cannot be called a long-acting drug, its main circulatory actions last markedly longer than those of oxytocin. Before going into details it should be pointed out that in the case of vasopressin the duration of hypertension is not a valuable indicator for the duration of the vasoconstrictor action. Since vasoconstriction also occurs in the coronary vascular bed this may lead to myocardial hypoxia, with consequent reduction of myocardial contractility which may be responsible for an early return of the elevated blood pressure to, or even below, control values. A possible direct cardiodepressor effect, independent from coronary constriction, should also be taken into account. Furthermore it should be remembered that different vascular beds may have a different affinity for vasopressin, and that vasopressin may alter the redistribution of cardiac output without affecting total peripheral resistance.

On the basis of these considerations it is not surprising that the values as given in the literature for the duration of the circulatory actions of vasopressin show great variations. As a rule one can say that in dog and man the hypertensive phase following intravenous or intramuscular doses of vasopressin or Octapressin lasts about 10—30 min (e.g. BERDE et al., 1961; BRODEUR and BEAULNES, 1964; NELSON et al., 1955; PERRONI et al., 1965; SEGEL et al., 1963; SHANKS, 1963; TSAKIRIS and BÜHLMANN, 1963). However, a hypertensive effect of less than 10 min is reported by WAGNER and BRAUNWALD (1956) and GROMOTKA and DEMLING (1962) in man after intravenous injections of 0.5—1 IU and after rapid intravenous infusions of 3—9 IU of vasopressin, and in a study in dogs in which vasopressin was intravenously infused up to a total dose of 0.5 IU/kg, the elevation of blood pressure lasted longer than 45 min (DRAPANAS et al., 1961).

Compared with the relatively short hypertensive effect of vasopressin, its action on peripheral blood flow lasts somewhat longer. This is indicated by studies in which either cardiac output or blood flow through a particular vascular bed have been measured. The depression of cardiac output caused in man by a 32 min intravenous infusion of Octapressin up to a total dose of 5 IU lasted more than 1 hour (SEGEL et al., 1963), and values given by several authors for the duration of reduced blood flow in the femoral-, splanchnic- or coronary vascular bed were usually of more than 30 min (e.g. BÜLBRING et al., 1949; DRAPANAS et al., 1961; ESSEX et al., 1940; GROMOTKA and DEMLING, 1962; RUSHMER et al., 1961). In a study performed in dogs the intravenous injection of 0.1—1 IU/kg of Pitressin led to a marked decrease in femoral blood flow lasting for about 2 hours (WAKIM et al., 1954). Indirect evidence for a relatively long lasting vasoconstriction in a particular vascular bed can be gained from the observation that in man skin pallor occurring during a 10 min intravenous infusion of vasopressin, at a rate of 50 mU/min, lasted for several hours after the infusion had been stopped (PICKFORD, 1966).

C. Tachyphylaxis

Many reports on the cardiovascular actions of vasopressin and oxytocin indicate that repeated doses of the two hormones produce smaller circulatory effects than the initial dose. This was shown in the case of oxytocin with regard to its vasodilator and hypotensive action in the rabbit (WOODBURY and ABREU, 1944), dog (NAKANO and FISHER, 1963) and man (BIENIARZ, 1961; KATZ, 1964; WOODBURY et al., 1944). Since decreasing responsiveness to repeated doses of oxytocin was observed in man with intraarterial, as well as with intravenous injections, it has been suggested that the phenomenon is due to a change in the responsiveness of the blood vessels to the direct effect of the hormone (KITCHIN et al., 1959). There is no question that the degree of tachyphylaxis depends on many factors such as species, type of anaesthesia, dosage, time interval, and number of repeated applications. This may account for considerable differences in results and may also be responsible for the fact that in some studies in man there was no tachyphylaxis to oxytocin (e.g. ANDERSEN et al., 1965; RIBOT et al., 1964).

Tachyphylaxis to the vasoconstrictor action of vasopressin or Octapressin has been found in the rat (SCHMIDT et al., 1962), rabbit (FRIEDMAN and PAULS, 1952; KARP et al., 1960; MELVILLE and VARMA, 1961; SCHMIDT et al., 1962), cat (BISSET and LEWIS, 1962), dog (CARLIER et al., 1960; DIANA and MASDEN, 1965; NASH, 1965; SCHMIDT et al., 1962) and man (e.g. SHANKS, 1963). A characteristic example is reported by NASH (1965): In dogs under barbiturate anaesthesia the average initial blood pressure response to an intravenous injection of 0.2 IU/kg of vasopressin was an increase of 50 mm Hg. When the same dose was repeated every 30 min there was a progressive decrease in pressure response and by the fourth dose the increase in blood pressure averaged only 6 mm Hg. In animals pretreated with reserpine the development of tachyphylaxis was markedly inhibited. It has been suggested that autonomic innervation is not likely to play an essential rôle in vasopressin tachyphylaxis since this is not influenced by ganglionic blockade with chlorisondamine. The antitachyphylactic effect of reserpine was thought to be the result of a quicker recovery of the systemic circulation, due to a reduced binding of vasopressin in the peripheral vascular tissue.

In other studies, particularly those in dog and man, tachyphylaxis to the circulatory effects of vasopressin, Octapressin and other analogues was absent or not pronounced (BERDE et al., 1961; HEIMBURGER et al., 1960; TSAKIRIS and BÜHLMANN, 1962, 1963; SAAMELI, 1966, unpublished). In view of the therapeutic use of Octapressin in the treatment of bleeding oesophageal varices it should be noted that repeated short i.v. infusions of 10 IU of this drug, given in man at 30 min intervals, produced approximately equal quantitative effects on hepatic blood flow (TSAKIRIS and BÜHLMANN, 1962).

D. Mechanism of Action

The mode of the circulatory actions of neurohypophysial peptides at the cellular- and subcellular level is virtually unknown. Although a distinct relationship between their vascular effects and sympathetic activity has been demonstrated, it is generally accepted that adrenergic α- and β-receptors are not involved (e.g. PICKFORD, 1964). Studies performed on the perfused isolated cat spleen did not give evidence for release of noradrenaline by vasopressin (HERTTING and SUKO, 1966), and in anaesthetized rats which responded to i.v. oxytocin with a pressure increase, this action was still present or even accentuated after pretreatment with reserpine, indicating that hypertension was not due to release of catecholamines (NAKANO, 1964). As was mentioned before, vasopressin may potentiate the pressure response to catecholamines in intact animals as well as in isolated arterial strips. According to BARTELSTONE and NASMYTH (1965) this action may be related to a change in the availability of cyclic adenosine 3', 5'-monophosphate.

Some insight into the mechanism by which vasopressin constricts blood vessels was gained by studies of electrolytes. It has been suggested that vasopressin affects the intra- and extra-cellular distribution of ions. When sodium and potassium concentrations in the inulin space of dogs and rats have been measured before, during and after the administration of vasopressin (and noradrenaline) a close relationship was found between the pressor action and the distribution of these ions. As blood pressure rose sodium disappeared from the inulin space and potassium entered it, and when pressure fell the reverse occurred. It was assumed that the ions moved in and out of the vascular smooth muscle cells (FRIEDMAN et al., 1957a and b). Acute elevation of plasma sodium concentration in the rat reduced the pressure response to injected vasopressin, both in normal rats and those given a sympathetic blocking agent (FRIEDMAN et al., 1959), and in oestrous rats in which oxytocin caused blood pressure increase, this effect was inhibited when the sodium concentration in the plasma had been raised by approximately 10% with an intravenous infusion of sodium phosphate (LLOYD, 1964).

These observations suggest that one stage in the vasoconstrictor action of neurohypophysial peptides is linked with a shift in the intra- and extra-cellular balance of ions, and that this shift itself is dependent on the electrolyte environment.

E. Possible Physiological and Pathophysiological Significance of the Neurohypophysial Peptides in the Circulatory System

At the present time it is still an open question whether the circulatory effects of vasopressin and oxytocin, which can be observed in animals and in man under certain conditions are of biological significance.

The doses of both hormones usually required to produce detectable changes in the cardiovascular system are high when compared with those known to be effective in other biological systems (antidiuresis, uterine stimulation, milk-ejection). This may be taken as strong evidence against an important physiological rôle of the two peptides in the field of circulation.

However, there are observations which suggest that at least one of the hormones, namely vasopressin, in some way might be involved in vascular phenomena.

In patients with orthostatic hypotension due to primary autonomic insufficiency, blood pressure was raised by relatively small doses of Pitressin, such as 10 mU i.v. injections, or 1 mU/min i.v. infusions (WAGNER and BRAUNWALD, 1956). Using a standardized haemorrhage procedure FRIEDEN and KELLER (1954) showed that dogs with diabetes insipidus were more susceptible to haemorrhage than normal animals. When Pitressin was administered in subpressor doses (50—200 mU) this susceptibility to haemorrhage was reversed to, or toward, normal. Since Pitressin did not increase the intact dog's resistance to haemorrhage it has been claimed that the neurohypophysial pressor principle serves a physiologic rôle in maintaining blood pressure during haemorrhage. When hepatic blood flow was measured in man, during and after fainting, the observed changes have been similar to those seen after the administration of Pitressin (BEARN et al., 1951). Since fainting is also known to be associated with the occurrence of an antidiuretic substance in the urine, it is tempting to speculate that the haemodynamic changes in the hepatic circulation are caused by the release of vasopressin. A possible rôle of vasopressin in the aetiology of hypertension should also be considered. It is a common observation that in man with hypertensive disease the increase in systemic arterial blood pressure occurs without increase in pulmonary pressure. NELSON et al. (1955) demonstrated that among various pressor agents, including angiotensin, adrenaline and noradrenaline, vasopressin was the only one capable of raising the systemic pressure without increasing pulmonary pressure. Another interesting point in this respect was brought up by PHELAN et al. (1962) who have been able to establish a colony of rats with a high incidence of spontaneous hypertension by selective breeding. When vasopressin was given to animals with manifested hypertension the pressor response was smaller than in normal control animals. However, when vasopressin was injected into rats of the same colony, with a blood pressure within the upper range of control rat blood pressures (inherited latent hypertension ?), the pressor response was enhanced. The same phenomenon was shown with adrenaline but was not present with angiotensin and noradrenaline. As mentioned before (see p. 599) vasopressin may potentiate the pressor action of catecholamines under various experimental conditions. With regard to its possible physiological or pathophysiological significance in the circulatory system, it is an interesting fact that this potentiation occurred in the dog, rat and cat at dose levels which had no direct action on circulation, and which may be assumed to be in the physiological range of secretory rates. For example it was found that an intravenous infusion of vasopressin at a rate of only 20 μU/kg/min was capable of inducing a definite potentiation of the noradrenaline pressor response in a 12 kg dog, after a total amount of only 3.8 mU had been infused during 16 min. It has been suggested that endogenously liberated vasopressin may play a rôle in the responsiveness of vascular smooth muscle to endogenously liberated catecholamines in dog, rat and cat (BARTELSTONE and NASMYTH, 1965).

On the basis of the above-mentioned observations the assumption seems to be justified that endogenous vasopressin, under certain conditions, does play a rôle in the cardiovascular system. It is not clear whether this assumption should be restricted to pathological conditions or may also be applicable to the normal circulation. No convincing evidence indicating that oxytocin is of physiological importance to the vascular system is available.

References

AHLQUIST, R.P., and R.A. WOODBURY: The cutaneous vasodilating action of pitressin. Fed. Proc. **4**, No. 1 (1945).

— — Influence of drugs and uterine activity upon uterine blood flow. Fed. Proc. **6**, 305 (1947).

ALTURA, B.M.: Differential actions of polypeptides and other drugs on coronary inflow vessels. Amer. Heart J. **72**, 709 (1966).

—, and S.G. HERSHEY: Effects of vasoactive drug therapy on microvascular injury in shock. Pharmacologist **7**, 144 (1965).

— —, and V.D.B. MAZZIA: Microcirculatory approach to vasopressor therapy in intestinal ischemic (SMA) shock. Amer. J. Surg. **111**, 186 (1966).

— —, and B.W. ZWEIFACH: Effects of a synthetic analogue of vasopressin on vascular smooth muscle. Proc. Soc. exp. Biol. (N.Y.) **119**, 258 (1965).

ANDERSEN, T.W., C.B. DE PADUA, and V. STENGER: Cardiovascular effects of rapid intravenous injection of synthetic oxytocin during elective section. Clin. Pharmacol. Ther. **6**, 345 (1965).

ANREP, G.U., and R.S. STACEY: Comparative effects of various drugs upon coronary circulation. J. Physiol. (Lond.) **64**, 187 (1927).

ASSALI, N.S., L. HORM, and H. PARKER: Regional blood flow and vascular resistance in response to oxytocin in the pregnant sheep and dog. J. appl. Physiol. **16**, 1087 (1961).

BABER, J.J., M. CHAFIZADEH, E.J. HALLIGAN, and C.M. LEEVY: Hemodynamic effects of posterior pituitrin in cirrhosis. Surg. Forum **11**, 354 (1960); Clin. Congr. Chicago, 1960.

BAISSET, A., M. CARTON, J. COTONAT, et P. MONTASTRUC: Recherche d'un antagonisme entre l'histamine et la fibre lisse vasculaire et bronchique. Thérapie **20**, 41 (1965).

BARCROFT, H., and A.F. COBBOLD: On the action of intravenous pitressin on forearm blood flow and blood lactate in man. J. Physiol. (Lond.) **132**, 10 P (1956).

BARER, G.R.: A comparison of the circulatory effects of angiotensin, vasopressin and adrenaline in the anaesthetised cat. J. Physiol. (Lond.) **156**, 49 (1961).

— The action of vasopressin, a vasopressin analogue (PLV_2), oxytocin, angiotensin, bradykinin and theophylline ethylene diamine on renal blood flow in the anaesthetised cat. J. Physiol. (Lond.) **169**, 62 (1963).

BARTELSTONE, H.J., and P.A. NASMYTH: Vasopressin potentiation of catecholamine action in dog, rat, cat, and rat aortic strip. Amer. J. Physiol. **208**, 754 (1965).

BEARN, A.G., B. BILLING, O.G. EDHOLM, and S. SHERLOCK: Hepatic blood flow and carbohydrate changes in man during fainting. J. Physiol. (Lond.) **115**, 442 (1951).

BELINKOFF, ST.: Cyclopropane-pituitrin incompatibility. Amer. J. Obstet. Gynec. **48**, 109 (1944).

BERDE, B.: Some observations on the circulatory effects of oxytocin, vasopressin and similar polypeptides. In: Advances in oxytocin, p. 11. Oxford: Pergamon Press 1965.

—, and R.A. BOISSONNAS: Synthetic analogues and homologues of the posterior pituitary hormones. In: The pituitary gland, p. 624. Ed. by G.W. HARRIS and B.T. DONOVAN. London: Butterworths & Co. Ltd. 1966.

—, H. WEIDMANN u. A. CERLETTI: Über Phenylalanin²-Lysin-Vasopressin. Helv. physiol. pharmacol. Acta **19**, 285 (1961).

BERGQUIST, J.R., and I.H. KAISER: Cardiovascular effects of intravenous Syntocinon. Obstet. gynec. Surv. **13**, 360 (1959).

BETZ, E., W. NIESEL, F.W. SCHMAHL u. K. SCHMIDT: Lokale Durchblutung und capilläre Sauerstoffsättigung des Myokards unter Hypoxie und Hyperkapnie sowie nach Einwirkung von Adrenalin, Noradrenalin und Vasopressin. Pflügers Arch. ges. Physiol. **285**, 55 (1965).

BIENIARZ J.: In: Oxytocin p. 80. Ed. by R. CALDEYRO-BARCIA and H. HELLER. Oxford: Pergamon Press 1961.

BISSET G.W. and G.P. LEWIS: A spectrum of pharmacological activity in some biologically active peptides. Brit. J. Pharmacol. **19**, 168 (1962).

BLACK, J.W.: Electrocardiographic changes produced in rabbits by vasopressin (pitressin) and their alteration by prolonged treatment with a commercial heart extract. J. Pharm. Pharmacol. **12**, 87 (1960).

BRODEUR, J.: Etude des propriétés antiarythmiques de quelques polypeptides hormonaux (Thèse, 1962).

— Effets de la lysyl⁸-vasopressine synthétique sur les arythmies adrénalino-chloroformiques chez le chien anesthésié. Rev. canad. Biol. **23**, 37 (1964).

—, et A. BEAULNES: Effets de l'ocytocin sur les arythmies digitaliques chez le chien. Rev. canad. Biol. **22**, 275 (1963).

BROTÁNEK, V., and S. KAZDA: Differences in the vasodepressor reaction to oxytocin in men and nonpregnant and pregnant women. Amer. J. Obstet. Gynec. **93**, 547 (1965).

— —, and Č. JUNGMANNOVA: Differences in the vascular reaction to oxytocin in man and their causes. Biochem. Pharmacol. **12**, Suppl., 256 (1963).

BÜLBRING, E., J.H. BURN, and J.M. WALKER: Reduction in coronary flow by pituitary (posterior lobe) extract in relation to the action of nicotine and to smoking. Quart. J. Med. **18**, 73 (1949).

BUNAC, R.D., I.H. PAGE, and J.W. MC CUBBIN: Inhibition of renin release by vasopressin and angiotensin. Cardiovasc. Res. **1**, 67 (1967).

BURCH, G.E., and N.P. DE PASQUALE: Response of the superficial lymphatics of man to phenylalanine²-lysine⁸-vasopressin (PLV_2). Circulation **28**, 697 (1963).

— — Response of the superficial lymphatics of the arm of intact man to synthetic vasopressin. Proc. Soc. exp. Biol. (N.Y.) **117**, 141 (1964).

BURNHILL, M.S., J.A. GAINES, and A.F. GUTTMACHER: Concentrated oxytocin solution for therapeutic interruption of midtrimester pregnancy. Obstet. gynec. surv. **20**, 94 (1962).

BYROM, F.M., and O.E. PRATT: Oxytocin and renal cortical necrosis. Lancet **1959 I**, 753.

CALDEYRO-BARCIA, R.: Oxytocin in pregnancy and labour. Acta endocr. (Kbh.) **34**, 41, Suppl. 50 (1960).

—, H. ALVAREZ, J.J. POSEIRO, C.H. HENDRICKS, Y. SICA-BLANCO, S.V. POSE, L.A. CIBILS, M.A. CARBALLO, V. GONZALEZ-PANIZZA, C. FIELITZ, C. MENDEZ-BAUER, y E.A. DE TELIAS: La induccion del parto con ocitocina sintética (Syntocinon). 2º Congreso Uruguayo de Ginecotocologia, October 1957.

—, and J.J. POSEIRO: Fetal and maternal dangers due to misuse of oxytocin. Extrait du Deuxième Congrès International de Gynécologie et d'Obstétrique de Montréal, en 1958, Tome II, page 450.

CARLIER, J., G. LEJEUNE-LEDANT, et G. BARAC: Effets hémodynamiques comparés d'une vasopressine synthétique et de la pitressine chez le chien. Arch. int. Pharmacodyn. **125**, 287 (1960).
CARTER, A.M., P.J. LEWIS, and L.P. BENGTSSON: Effects of vasopressin on uterine blood flow in the rabbit. Acta pharmacol. (Kbh.) **24**, 435 (1966).
CARTER, E.R., and G.P. SHAW: Cardiovascular effects of common intravenous oxytocics. Obstet. gynec. Surv. **16**, 47 (1960).
CERLETTI, A., H. WEBER u. H. WEIDMANN: Zur Wirkung von Phenylalanin²-Lysine-Vasopressin (Octapressin) auf den arteriellen und venösen Anteil eines peripheren Gefäßgebietes. Helv. physiol. pharmacol. Acta **21**, 394 (1963).
CHAUDHURY, R.R., and T.K. TARAK: Action of the neurohypophysial hormones on the vascular system of the male monkey and the rooster. J. Pharm. Pharmacol. **17**, 316 (1965).
CHENOWETH, M.B., G.L. ELLMAN, R.C. REYNOLDS, and P.J. SHEA: A secondary response to pressor stimuli caused by sensitization to an endogenous pituitary hormone. Circulat. Res. **6**, 334 (1958).
COON, J.M.: A new method for the assay of posterior pituitary extracts. Arch. int. Pharmacodyn. **62**, 79 (1939).
COVINO, B.G.: Cardiac effects of synthetic oxytocin (Syntocinon). Amer. Heart J. **66**, 627 (1963).
CUTCHIN jr., J.H., H.S. MC GAUGHEY jr., W.A. SCOGGIN, G.M. HARBERT jr., and N.W. THORNTON jr.: Contractility of the isolated human uterine artery. Amer. J. Obstet. Gynec. **90**, 143 (1964).
DAVIS jr., W.D., R. GORLIN, S. REICHMAN, and J.P. STORAASLI: Effect of pituitrin in reducing portal pressure in the human being. New Engl. J. Med. **256**, 108 (1957).
DEIS, R.P., A.H. KITCHIN, and M. PICKFORD: The effect of oxytocin on hand blood flow in man following total and sympathetic nerve block. J. Physiol. (Lond.) **166**, 489 (1963).
DIANA, J.N., and R.R. MASDEN: Effect of vasopressin infusion and sciatic nerve stimulation in isolated dog hindlimb. J. Physiol. (Lond.) **209**, 390 (1965).
DILLON, T.F., B.E. MARBURY, R.W. BONSNES, R.G. DOUGLAS, and V. DU VIGNEAUD: Vasopressin as a hemostatic in gynecologic surgery. Obstet. and Gynec. **11**, 363 (1958).
DODD, W.A., and E.E. DANIEL: Vascular muscle reactivity. Circulat. Res. **8**, 446 (1960).
DRAPANAS, T., C.P. CROWE, W.K.T. SHIM, and W.G. SCHENK jr.: The effect of pitressin on cardiac output and coronary, hepatic, and intestinal blood flow. Surg. Gynec. Obstet. **113**, 484 (1961).
DYKE, H.B. VAN, K. ADAMSONS jr., and S.L. ENGEL: Aspects of the biochemistry and physiology of the neurohypophysial hormones. Recent Progr. Hormone Res. **9**, 1 (1955).
—, S.L. ENGEL, and K. ADAMSONS jr.: Comparison of pharmacological effects of lysine and arginine vasopressins. Proc. Soc. exp. Biol. (N.Y.) **91**, 484 (1956).
EDMUNDS, R., and J.P. WEST: A study of the effect of vasopressin on portal and systemic blood pressure. Surg. Gynec. Obstet. **114**, 458 (1962).
EMERSON jr., T.E.: Effects of angiotensin, epinephrine, nor-epinephrine, and vasopressin on venous return. Amer. J. Physiol. **210**, 933 (1966).
ENGSTROM, L.: Induction of labour around full term, especially by means of synthetic oxytocin intravenous drip. Acta obstet. gynec. scand. **38**, Suppl. **3** (1959).
ESSEX, H.E., R.G.E. WEGRIA, J.F. HERRICK, and F.C. MANN: The effect of certain drugs on the coronary blood flow of the trained dog. Amer. Heart J. **19**, 554 (1940).
FELDMAN, S.A., D.M. FORGAARD, and L.E. MORRIS: Compatibility of a synthetic oxytocin (Syntocinon) with anesthesia in dogs. Anesthesiology **19**, 878 (1958).
FERRARI, G., and A. VANDONE: Octapressin als lokaler Vasoconstrictor in Geburtshilfe und Gynaekologie. Minerva ginec. **16**, 629 (1964) (in Italian).
FISHER, S.J., J. GEHRIG, and H. GREEN: Non-catechol amine vasopressor (PLV_2) for use as adjunct to local anesthesia. J. Amer. dent. Ass. **70**, 1189 (1965).
FRIEDEN, J., and A.D. KELLER: Decreased resistance to hemorrhage in neurohypophysectomized dogs. Circulat. Res. **2**, 214 (1954).
FRIEDMAN, S.M., R.M. BUTT, and C.L. FRIEDMAN: Cation shifts and blood pressure regulation in the dog. Amer. J. Physiol. **190**, 507 (1957b).
—, C.L. FRIEDMAN, and M. NAKASHIMA: Cationic shifts and blood pressure regulation. Circulat. Res. **5**, 261 (1957a).
—, J.D. JAMIESON, and C.L. FRIEDMAN: Sodium gradient, smooth muscle tone, and blood pressure regulation. Circulat. Res. **7**, 44 (1959).
—, and H. PAULS: The effect of pitressin infusion on blood pressure of the rabbit, cat and rat. Amer. Heart J. **44**, 131 (1952).
GREEN, H.D., R. WEGIRA, and N.H. BOYER: Effects of epinephrine and pitressin on the coronary artery inflow in anesthetized dogs. J. Pharm. Pharmacol. **76**, 378 (1942).

Gromotka, R., u. L. Demling: Der Einfluß von Vasopressin auf die Darmdurchblutung des Menschen. Klin. Wschr. **40**, 456 (1962).

Gruber, C.M., and W.B. Kountz: The electrocardiogram of non-anesthetized dogs as modified by the intravenous injection of pitressin, atropine sulphate and vagus section. J. Pharmacol. exp. Ther. **40**, 253 (1930).

Guhl, U.: Die antidiuretische und pressorische Wirksamkeit von Arginin⁸-Vasopressin, Lysin⁸-Vasopressin und Phenylalanin²-lysin⁸-Vasopressin beim Menschen. Schweiz. med. Wschr. **91**, 798 (1961).

Haddy, F.J., J.I. Molnar, and R.W. Campbell: Effects of denervation and vasoactive agents on vascular pressures and weight of dog forelimb. Amer. J. Physiol. **201**, 631 (1961).

Haigh, A.L., A.H. Kitchin, and M. Pickford: The effect of oxytocin on hand blood flow in man following the administration of an oestrogen and isoprenaline. J. Physiol. (Lond.) **169**, 161 (1963).

—, S. Lloyd, and M. Pickford: A relationship between adrenaline and the mode of action of oxytocin and oestrogen on vascular smooth muscle. J. Physiol. (Lond.) **178**, 563 (1965).

Heeg, E., u. K. Meng: Die Wirkung des Bradykinins, Angiotensins und Vasopressins auf Vorhof, Papillarmuskel und isoliert durchströmte Herzpräparate des Meerschweinchens. Arch. exp. Path. Pharmakol. **250**, 35 (1965).

Heimburger, I., S. Teramoto, and H.B. Shumacker jr.: Effect of surgical pituitrin upon portal and hepatic circulation. Surgery **48**, 706 (1960).

Hendricks, C.H.: The hemodynamic of a uterine contraction. Amer. J. Obstet. Gynec. **76**, 969 (1958).

Hershey, S.G., V.D.B. Mazzia, B.M. Altura, and L. Gyure: Effects of vasopressors on the microcirculation and on survival in hemorrhagic shock. Anesthesiology **26**, 179 (1965).

Hertting, G., and J. Suko: Influence of angiotensin, vasopressin or changes in flow rate on vasoconstriction, changes in volume and [^{3}H]-noradrenaline release following postganglionic sympathetic nerve stimulation in the isolated cat spleen. Brit. J. Pharmacol. **26**, 686 (1966).

Hochuli, E.: Klinische Erfahrungen mit der lokalen Anwendung von Octapressin in der Gynäkologie und in der Geburtshilfe. Schweiz. med. Wschr. **92**, 654 (1962).

Holmes, S.W., E.W. Horton, and I.H.M. Main: The effect of prostaglandin E, on responses of smooth muscle to catechol amines, angiotensin and vasopressin. Brit. J. Pharmacol. **21**, 538 (1963).

Honoré, L.H.: The effects of single doses of deoxycorticosterone acetate (DOCA) and cortisone on the vascular response of female rats to posterior pituitary hormones. Quart. J. exp. Physiol. **47**, 334 (1962a).

— The vascular responses of male rats to post-pituitary hormones after treatment with deoxycorticosterone acetate (DOCA) and cortisone. Quart. J. exp. Physiol. **47**, 345 (1962b).

—, and S.M. Lloyd: Posterior lobe hormones on the vascular response of the male rat after castration. J. Physiol. (Lond.) **155**, 61 P (1961a).

— — The effects of castration on the vascular responses of male rats to posterior pituitary hormones. J. Physiol. (Lond.) **159**, 183 (1961b).

Ichiyanagi, K., and L.E. Morris: Effect of cyclopropane and various oxytocics on cardiac rhythm in the parturient woman. Anesthesiology **20**, 669 (1959).

de Jong, W., and St. M. McLeod: Effect of autonomic blocking agents on the cardiovascular effects of Octapressin in the rat. Europ. J. Pharmacol. **1**, 93 (1967).

Karp, D., S.H. Rinzler, and J. Travell: Effects of ergometrine (ergonovine) on the isolated atherosclerotic heart of the cholesterol-fed rabbit. Brit. J. Pharmacol. **15**, 333 (1960).

Katz, D., D.J. Paulo, W.S. Rosenthal, and H. Weisbert: Selective therapy in bleeding esophageal varices. Gastroenterology **48**, 826 (1965).

Katz, L.N., and E. Lindner: The reaction of the coronary vessels to drugs and other substances. J. Amer. med. Ass. **113**, 2116 (1939).

Katz, R.L.: Antiarrhythmic action of synthetic oxytocin in anesthetized man. Experientia (Basel) **19**, 160 (1963).

— Antiarrhythmic and cardiovascular effects of synthetic oxytocin. Anesthesiology **25**, 653 (1964).

— Epinephrine and PLV_2: cardiac rhythm and local vasoconstrictor effects. Anesthesiology **26**, 619 (1965).

—, R.P. Bircher, E.M. Papper, and S.C. Wang: Effects of synthetic oxytocin on cardiac arrhythmias. Scientific Exhibit, Amer. med. Ass., Atlantic City (N.J.), June 16—20, 1963.

Kitchin, A.H., H. Konzett, and M. Pickford: Comparison of effects of valyl³-oxytocin and Syntocinon in the cardiovascular system of man. Brit. J. Pharmacol. **14**, 567 (1959).

—, S.M. Lloyd, and M. Pickford: Some actions of oxytocin on the cardiovascular system in man. Clin. Sci. **18**, 399 (1959).

Klassen, G.A., J.W. Rubin, and M. Mc Gregor: The effect of synthetic oxytocin on impaired atrioventricular conduction. Amer. J. Cardiol. **12**, 523 (1963).

KLINGENSTRÖM, P., and L. WESTERMARK: Local tissue-oxygen tension after adrenaline, noradrenaline and Octapressin in local anaesthesia. Acta anaesth. scand. **8**, 261 (1964).
KORDIK, P.: Responses of coronary vessels to pituitary (posterior lobe) extract and to adrenaline. Brit. J. Pharmacol. **6**, 75 (1951).
KULLANDER, S., and E. WIDE: A synthetic vasopressin (Octapressin Sandoz) for haemostasis during cone biopsy of the cervix. Acta obstet. gynec. scand. **45**, 102 (1966).
LANDESMAN, R., and B. MENDELSOHN: The uterine omentum of the rat and its response to vasoconstrictor drugs. Amer. J. Obstet. Gynec. **72**, 84 (1956).
LIPTON, B., S.G. HERSHEY, and S. BAEZ: Compatibility of oxytocics with anesthetic agents. J. Amer. med. Ass. **179**, 410 (1962).
LLOYD, S.: The vascular responses of the rat during the reproductive cycle. J. Physiol. (Lond.) **148**, 625 (1959a).
— Changes in the vascular responses of the rat during pregnancy. J. Physiol. (Lond.) **149**, 586 (1959b).
—, and M. PICKFORD: The action of posterior pituitary hormones and oestrogens on the vascular system of the rat. J. Physiol. (Lond.) **155**, 161 (1961a).
— — Renal response to oxytocin and vasopressin in the presence of stilboestrol. J. Physiol. (Lond.) **158**, 40 P (1961b).
— — The effect of oestrogens and sympathetic denervation on the response to oxytocin of the blood vessels in the hind limb of the dog. J. Physiol. (Lond.) **163**, 362 (1962).
LLOYD, S.M.: Mode of action of oxytocin on blood vessels. In: Oxytocin, vasopressin and their structural analogues, p. 37. Ed. by J. RUDINGER. Oxford: Pergamon Press 1964.
LOCKETT, M.F.: An action of oxytocin on the cardiovascular system. J. Physiol. (Lond.) **136**, 26 P (1957).
LONGO, L.D., J.A. MORRIS, R.W. SMITH, R. BECK, and N.S. ASSALI: Hemodynamic and renal effects of Octapressin. Proc. Soc. exp. Biol. (N.Y.) **115**, 766 (1964).
LOUIS, W.J., and A.E. DOYLE: The relationship between the vascular responses to the peptides Angiotensin and Pitressin. Clin. Sci. **31**, 255 (1966).
MAXWELL, G.M.: The cardiovascular effects of Octapressin. Arch. int. Pharmacodyn. **158**, 17 (1965).
MAYES, B.T., and R.P. SHEARMAN: Experience with synthetic oxytocin. The effects on the cardiovascular system and its use for the induction of labour and control of the third stage. J. Obstet. Gynaec. Brit. Emp. **63**, 812 (1956).
MAZZIA, V.D.B., J.M.MC KENNA, and L. GYURE: Influence of a synthetic analogue of vasopressin on the microcirculation and on survival in shock. Fed. Proc. **23**, 539 (1964).
McGEE, J.E.: Effect of Syntocinon on blood pressure in the second and third stages of labor. Obstet. gynec. Surv. **16**, 44 (1960).
MELLANDER, S.: Comparative studies on the adrenergic neurohormonal control of resistance and capacitance blood vessels in the cat. Acta physiol. scand. **50**, Suppl. 176, 1 (1960).
MELVILLE, K.I., and D.R. VARMA: Synthetic oxytocin as an antagonist of experimental cardiac anoxic changes in rabbits. Brit. J. Pharmacol. **17**, 218 (1961).
MORRIS, L.E., M.J. THORNTON, and J.W. HARRIS: Comparison of the effect of pituitrin, pitocin, and ergonovine on cardiac rhythm during cyclopropane anesthesia for parturition. Amer. J. Obstet. Gynec. **63**, 171 (1952).
MUNCHOW, O.B., and T. KURZE: Hemostatic effectiveness of infiltration with felypressin prior to skin incisions. J. Amer. med. Ass. **196**, 625 (1966).
MUNSICK, R.A.: Local hemostasis in gynecologic surgery. Rocky Mtn med. J. **63**, 33 (1966).
NAKANO, J.: Cardiovascular effect of oxytocin in rodents and a marsupial. Proc. Soc. exp. Biol. (N.Y.) **115**, 707 (1964).
—, and R.D. FISHER: Studies on the cardiovascular effects of synthetic oxytocin. J. Pharmacol. exp. Ther. **142**, 206 (1963).
—, and J.S. SHACKFORD: Effect of synthetic vasopressins on the myocardial contractile force in the isolated guinea-pig atria. Experientia (Basel) **21**, 474 (1965).
NASH, C.B.: Alteration of vasopressin tachyphylaxis by reserpine pretreatment. Arch. int. Pharmacodyn. **155**, 90 (1965).
—, L.D. BOYAJY, and E.S. MANLEY: Vasopressin antagonism of adrenergic vasodilation. Arch. int. Pharmacodyn. **133**, 433 (1961).
NASHOLD jr., B.S., E. MANNARINO, and M. WUNDERLICH: Pressor-depressor blood pressure responses in the cat after intraventricular injection of drugs. Nature (Lond.) **193**, 1297 (1962).
NELSON, R.A., L.G. MAY, A. BENNETT, M. KOBAYASHI, and R. GREGORY: Comparison of the effects of pressor and depressor agents and influences on pulmonary and systemic pressures of normotensive and hypertensive subjects. Amer. Heart J. **50**, 172 (1955).
ORENGO, F.: Anwendung eines synthetischen Vasopressinanalogon als Haemostatikum in der geburtshilflichen und gynäkologischen Chirurgie. Gynaecologia (Basel) **160**, 221 (1965).

PANISSET, J.C., and A. BEAULNES: The effect of oxytocin on experimental cardiac arrhythmia. Rev. canad. Biol. **20**, 47 (1961).
PARSLOE, C.P., L.E. MORRIS, and O.S. ORTH: The relationship of various anesthetic agents to the action of pituitrin, pitressin and pitocin. Anesthesiology **11**, 76 (1950).
PAULET, G., J.P. BERNARD, et R. LE BARS: Action de la vasopressine sur la masse sanguine pulmonaire chez le chien. C.R. Soc. Biol. (Paris) **159**, 2485 (1965).
PERRONI, G., F. BERNAVA, F.S. BRIGUGLIO, e A. BERTOLAMI: Studio di alcuni effetti dell'Octapressina sul sistema cardiovascolare nell'uomo. Minerva med. sicil. **10**, 3 (1965).
PHELAN, E.L., I. ERYETISHIR, M. DAH, and F.H. SMIRK: Observations on the responses of rats with spontaneous hypertension and control rats to pressor drugs and to hexamethonium. Circulat. Res. **10**, 817 (1962).
PICKFORD, M.: Effects of neurohypophysial hormones on the vascular system. In: Oxytocin, vasopressin and their structural analogues, p. 31. Ed. by J. RUDINGER. Oxford: Pergamon Press 1964.
— Neurohypophysis and vascular reactions. In: The pituitary gland, vol. III, p. 399. Ed. by G.W. HARRIS and B.T. DONOVAN. London: Butterworths 1966.
POPPY, J.H.: Pressor and emetic effects of oxytocics in the fourth stage of labor. Obstet. gynec. Surv. **22**, 185 (1963).
POTTER, H.D., and D.C. SUTFIN: Effects of vasopressin on femoral arterial blood flow and pressure in the anesthetized dog. Proc. Soc. exp. Biol. (N.Y.) **106**, 511 (1961).
RIBOT, S., S. ABRAMOWITZ, H. GREEN, M.J. SMALL, and I. SCHWARTZ: Cardiovascular effects of oxytocin and comparison with related polypeptides. Amer. J. med. Sci. **248**, 61 (1964).
— —, W.S. KELHOFFER, H. GREEN, M.J. SMALL, and I. SCHWARTZ: Cardiovascular effects of phenylalanyl-2-lysyl-8-vasopressin (PLV-2). Amer. J. med. Sci. **246**, 479 (1963).
—, H. GREEN, M.J. SMALL, and S. ABRAMOWITZ: Cardiovascular effects of vasopressin. Amer. J. med. Sci. **242**, 612 (1961).
RUSHMER, R.F., D.L. FRANKLIN, R.L. VAN CITTERS, and O.A. SMITH: Changes in peripheral blood flow distribution in healthy dogs. Circulat. Res. **9**, 675 (1961).
SCHMIDT, L., W. BERNAUER u. H. MENZEL: Die Wirkung von Phenylalanin-2-Lysin-8-Vasopressin and Lysin-8-Vasopressin auf Coronardurchblutung und Blutdruck des Hundes und den Rattenuterus. Arzneimittel-Forsch. **12**, 1019 (1962).
SCHOFIELD, B.M., and J.M. WALKER: Perfusion of the coronary arteries of the dog. J. Physiol. (Lond.) **122**, 489 (1953).
SCHWARTZ, S.I., H.W. BALES, G.L. EMERSON, and E.B. MAHONEY: The use of intravenous pituitrin in treatment of bleeding esophageal varices. Surgery **45**, 72 (1959).
SEGEL, N., T.J. BAYLEY, A. PATON, P.W. DYKES, and J.M. BISHOP: The effects of synthetic vasopressin and angiotensin on the circulation in cirrhosis of the liver. Clin. Sci. **25**, 43 (1963).
SELDINGER, S.I., and R. SUNDBLAD: Splenic regulation of portal flow in man. Scand. J. clin. Lab. Invest. **15**, 380 (1963).
SHALDON, ST., W. DOLLE, L. GUEVARA, F.L. IBER, and S. SHERLOCK: Effect of pitressin on the splanchnic circulation in man. Circulation **24**, 797 (1961).
—, and S. SHERLOCK: The use of vasopressin ("Pitressin") in the control of bleeding from oesophageal varices. Lancet **1960 II**, 222.
SHANKS, C.A.: Intravenous Octapressin during halothane anaesthesia. A pilot study. Brit. J. Anaesth. **35**, 640 (1963).
SIENER, H.: Vergleichende Untersuchungen über die uteruswirksamen und blutdrucksteigernden Eigenschaften von Syntocinon (Sandoz), Orasthin (Hoechst) und Oxystin (A.W.D.). Zbl. Gynäk. **80**, 903 (1958).
SLOTNIK, I.L., and J.D. TEIGLAND: Cardiac accidents following vasopressin injection (Pitressin). J. Amer. med. Ass. **146**, 1127 (1951).
SOMLYO, A.V., C.Y. WOO, and A.P. SOMLYO: Responses of nerve-free vessels to vasoactive amines and polypeptides. Amer. J. Physiol. **208**, 748 (1965).
STAVRAKY, G.W., and R.J. OLIVER: Influence of the posterior pituitary on the pressor action of epinephrine. Fed. Proc. **11**, 392 (1952).
VAN DER STRAETEN, M., et I. LEUSEN: Influence de la pituitrine sur la circulation pulmonaire. Arch. int. Pharmacodyn. **96**, 487 (1954).
SUPEK, Z., B. UROIĆ u. V. GJURIŠ: Über den Mechanismus der verstärkenden Wirkung des Chlorpromazins auf die Blutdruckerhöhung durch Vasopressin. Arch. exp. Path. Pharmakol. **238**, 139 (1960).
— — —, and N. MARIJAN: The effect of adrenergic blocking agents and of chlorpromazine on blood pressure increase by vasopressin and angiotensin. J. Pharm. Pharmacol. **14**, 284 (1962).
TAKÁCS, L., and K. ALBERT: The effect of vasopressin on the circulation of the rat organs, with special consideration of the skin. Experientia (Basel) **19**, 365 (1963).

TEXTER, E.C., C.C. CHOU, and H.C. LAURETA: Local effects of Octapressin and vasopressin on segmental resistance of the mesenteric and portal circulations. Gastroenterology **48**, 497 (1965).

TEXTER jr., E.C., C.C. CHOU, ST. L. MERRILL, H.C. LAURETA, and E.D. FRÖHLICH: Direct effects of vasoactive agents on segmental resistance of the mesenteric and portal circulation. J. Lab. clin. Med. **64**, 624 (1964).

TSAKIRIS, A., u. A. BÜHLMANN: Experimentelle Untersuchungen beim Menschen über die Wirkung von Vasopressin auf die Leberdurchblutung und den portalen Druck. Schweiz. med. Wschr. **92**, 147 (1962).

— — Kreislaufwirkungen eines neuen synthetischen Vasopressins. Experimentelle Untersuchungen mit (2-Phenylalanin-8-Lysin) Vasopressin. Dtsch. med. Wschr. **88**, 46 (1963).

—, U.P. HAEMMERLE, and A. BÜHLMANN: Reduction of portal venous pressure in cirrhotic patients with bleeding from oesophageal varices, by administration of a vasopressin derivative, phenylalanine^2-lysine^8-vasopressin. Amer. J. Med. **36**, 825 (1964).

WAGNER, H.N., and E. BRAUNWALD: The pressor effect of the antidiuretic principle of the posterior pituitary in orthostatic hypotension. J. clin. Invest. **35**, 1412 (1956).

WAKIM, K.G., C. DENTON, and H.E. ESSEX: Certain cardiovascular effects of vasopressin (Pitressin). Amer. Heart J. **47**, 77 (1954).

WEIDMANN, H., u. A. CERLETTI: Verstärkung des Blutdruckeffektes von Vasopressin durch Reserpin. Helv. physiol. pharmacol. Acta **19**, C 119 (1961).

WOODBURY, R.A., and B.E. ABREU: Influence of oxytocin (Pitocin) upon the heart and blood pressure of the chicken, rabbit, cat, dog and turtle. Amer. J. Physiol. **142**, 114 (1944).

—, and R.P. AHLQUIST: The cutaneous vasodilating action of Pitressin. J. Pharmacol. exp. Ther. **86**, 14 (1946).

—, W.F. HAMILTON, P.P. VOLPITTO, B.E. ARBREU, and H.T. HARPER: Cardiac and blood pressure effects of Pitocin (oxytocin) in man. J. Pharmacol. exp. Ther. **81**, 95 (1944).

ZWEIFACH, B.W.: Peripheral circulatory changes as criteria for hemorrhagic shock therapy. Circulation **1**, 433 (1950).

Metabolic Effects of the Neurohypophyseal Hormones and Related Polypeptides

I.A. Mirsky

With 6 Figures

I. Introduction

There are no known disorders of carbohydrate, fat or protein metabolism in clinical or experimental conditions associated with derangements in neurohypophyseal function. Yet, a very impressive array of reports can be marshalled to demonstrate that the administration of neurohypophyseal extracts may influence a variety of metabolic regulations (Schaumann, 1937; van Dyke, 1936, 1939; Harris, 1948; Stehle, 1950; Shull and Mayer, 1956).

In the almost 60 years since Borchardt (1908) first reported that the injection of an extract of the posterior (infundibular) hypophysis produced hyperglycemia and glycosuria in rabbits, numerous studies led to the consensus that the neurohypophyseal hormones exert a significant effect on the regulation of carbohydrate and fat metabolism. While most investigators found that crude or partially purified posterior pituitary extracts induced a persistent hyperglycemia in many species, including man (Cushing, 1910; Geiling and Eddy, 1928; Draper and Hill, 1929; Bacq and Dworkin, 1930; Houssay and Benedetto, 1933; Schroeder, 1933; Thaddea, 1933), and inhibited the hypoglycemic action of insulin (Burn, 1923; Blotner and Fitz, 1927; Gurd, 1934; Stenstrom, 1913; Thaddea, 1933; La Barre, 1930), some have shown that hypoglycemia, and an inhibition of the hyperglycemic action of epinephrine (van Dyke, 1936, 1939; Stenstrom, 1913; Silver and Mislowitzer, 1931), may ensue from the administration of such extracts. Likewise, while some have shown that posterior pituitary extracts produce a decrease in the concentration of neutral fat or fatty acids in the blood (Raab, 1930; Blix and Ohlin, 1927; Long et al., 1932) and a deposition of fat in the liver (Coope and Chamberlain, 1925), others have reported negative results (van Dyke, 1936, 1939).

Critical evaluation of the older literature reveals many inconsistencies and contradictions about the action of the neurohypophyseal extracts as well as little agreement as to whether the active factor is the vasopressor or oxytocic agent. These discrepancies may be attributed to a variety of factors such as the species of animal employed, the relative purity and quantity of the extract injected, the route of administration, the time of observation, the presence or absence of anesthesia, etc. The availability of pure natural and synthetic vasopressin and oxytocin in recent years promised clarification of some of the effects of the neurohypophyseal hormones and related polypeptides on carbohydrate and fat metabolism. To date, however, very few studies with pure or synthetic hormones have appeared which would permit definite conclusions about their metabolic effects.

II. Metabolic Rate

A reduction in body temperature (OKUNO et al., 1965) and oxygen consumption (TSUKADA et al., 1965) is produced in both normal and alloxan-diabetic rats by the intraperitoneal injection of synthetic lysine vasopressin in a single dose of from 20—100 mU/100 g. No changes ensue from the administration of either smaller doses of vasopressin or larger doses of synthetic oxytocin. The reduction in oxytocin consumption is associated with an increase in respiratory quotient (RQ) which is interpreted to denote a decrease in the oxidation of fat. Further, lysine-vasopressin inhibits the calorigenic action of norepinephrine (TSUKADA et al., 1965). Since the latter may be related to an increase in the rate of mobilization (STEINBERG et al., 1964) and utilization (HANNON and LARSON, 1962) of free fatty acids, it has been suggested that the effect of lysine-vasopressin on the oxygen consumption of the rat is due to a reduction in the oxidation of fat by peripheral tissues. Although a relatively high concentration of Lys-vasopressin (0.5 IU/ml) *in vitro* decreases oxygen consumption of rat brown adipose tissue, liver slices and diaphragm (ITOH et al., 1966), there is no evidence that a reduction in fat oxidation is responsible.

III. Carbohydrate Metabolism

In accord with earlier studies on the action of vasopressin-rich extracts of the posterior pituitary (pitressin), the intravenous or subcutaneous injection of a single dose of Arg- or Lys-vasopressin induces a prompt, relatively transient hyperglycemic response in the unanesthetized and anesthetized male and female dog (BERGEN et al., 1960; MIRSKY, 1962; HEIDENREICH et al., 1962, 1963; MIRSKY, 1963a; BAISSET et al., 1965; BALASSE et al., 1966), cat (HEIDEN-

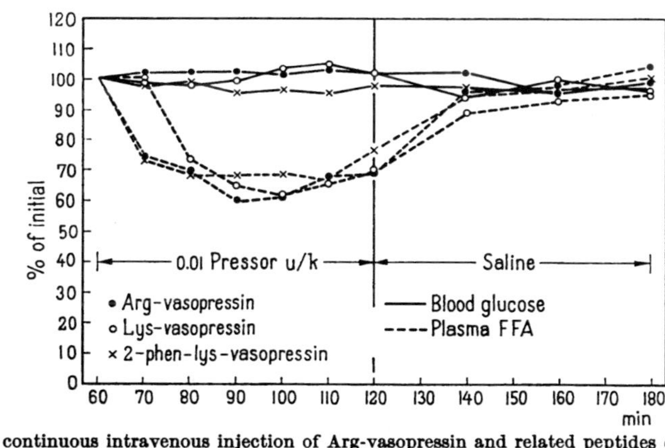

Fig. 1. Effect of continuous intravenous injection of Arg-vasopressin and related peptides on the blood glucose and plasma FFA of nondiabetic dogs. Data presented as per cent of the mean of values obtained during continuous injection of saline in the first 60 min. Each curve represents the average of data from three dogs (MIRSKY, 1963a)

REICH et al., 1962, 1963), rabbit (CASH and KAPLAN, 1964), rat (HEIDENREICH et al., 1962, 1963), guinea-pig (HEIDENREICH et al., 1962), and frog (HEIDENREICH et al., 1962). The magnitude of the hyperglycemic response is directly related to the dosage injected (HEIDENREICH et al., 1962) and the rate at which the hormone enters the circulation (MIRSKY, 1963a). Thus, a significant hyperglycemia ensues in the dog after the rapid intravenous injection of from 0.01—1.0 IU Arg- or Lys-vasopressin per kilogram body weight but no significant change in the blood glucose concentration occurs when the same quantity of hormone is administered as a continuous intravenous injection during a period of 1 h (Fig. 1) (MIRSKY, 1962; HEIDENREICH et al., 1962, 1963; MIRSKY, 1963a, b). Likewise, although the rapid injection of a single dose of pitressin in man induces a hyperglycemic response (SCHAUMANN, 1937; VAN DYKE, 1939; HARRIS, 1948; STEHLE, 1950; SHULL and MAYER, 1956), no significant change in the blood glucose concentration is noted during the continuous intravenous injection of pitressin in a dose of 0.01 IU/kg/h (GOLDMAN, 1964).

Species differ markedly in their responsiveness. Whereas the dog exhibits a significant rise in blood glucose after the rapid intravenous injection of even less than 0.1 IU vasopressin per kilogram, the rabbit shows a similar response only when about 1 IU/kg body weight is injected.

There is a paucity of data on the relative hyperglycemic actions of the various analogues of vasopressin. Such data as are available suggest that pharmacologically equivalent doses of Arg- and Lys-vasopressin are equally potent in their hyperglycemic action in the dog (MIRSKY, 1963a) and rabbit (CASH and KAPLAN, 1964).

Essentially the same hyperglycemic response occurs in the dog after the rapid intravenous injection of pharmacologically equivalent doses of Arg-vasopressin, Lys-vasopressin and Phe[2]-Lys[8]-vasopressin (Fig. 1) (MIRSKY, 1963a). Mole for mole, however, the latter is not as effective as Arg- or Lys-vasopressin. Likewise,

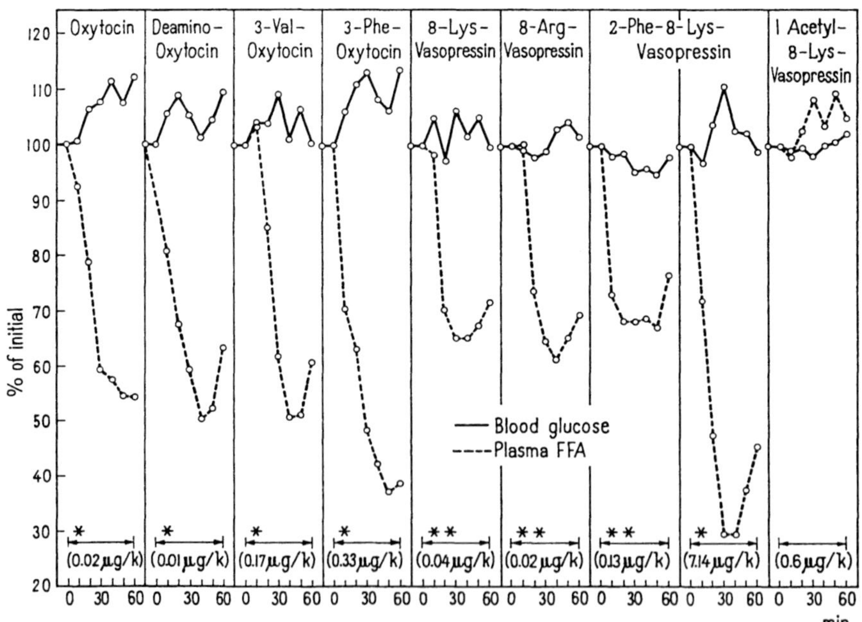

Fig. 2. Effect of oxytocin and related peptides on blood glucose and plasma FFA of dogs. Each set of curves represents the data obtained in from five to ten dogs expressed as in Fig. 1 (* designates the intravenous injection of 0.01 vasodepressor unit/kg/h; ** designates the injection of 0.01 pressor unit/kg/h) (MIRSKY, 1965)

whereas the hyperglycemic response of rabbits to the rapid injection of Deamino[1]-Lys[8]-vasopressin differs little from that induced by Lys-vasopressin, the response to Acetyl-Lys[8]-vasopressin is reduced (CASH and KAPLAN, 1964). However, as with Arg- and Lys-vasopressin, no significant change in the blood glucose concentration of the dog is produced when Phe[2]-Lys[8]-vasopressin or l-Acetyl-Lys[8]-vasopressin is infused in pharmacologically equivalent doses during the course of 1 h (Fig. 2) (MIRSKY, 1965).

Synthetic oxytocin, like vasopressin, may induce a prompt but transient increase in the blood glucose concentration when given intravenously or subcutaneously to the dog (MIRSKY, 1962; HEIDENREICH et al., 1962, 1963; MIRSKY, 1963a; BAISSET et al., 1965; BALASSE and RASIO, 1965b), cat (HEIDENREICH et al., 1962, 1963), rabbit (CHAUDHURY and NAYYAR, 1962), chicken (KOOK et al., 1964), and frog (HEIDENREICH et al., 1962). As with vasopressin, the responsiveness to oxytocin varies with the species (HEIDENREICH et al., 1962), the quantity administered (HEIDENREICH et al., 1962; BALASSE et al., 1966; MIRSKY, 1965) and the rate at which the hormone is introduced into the circulation (MIRSKY, 1963a, b). Thus, the rapid intravenous administration of oxytocin in a dose of from 0.01—1.0 IU/kg induces a significant hyperglycemic response while the same dose administered during the course of 1 h may induce no significant change ($\pm$ 10%) in the blood glucose concentration.

Synthetic analogues of oxytocin (Deamino^1-oxytocin, Val^3-oxytocin, and Phe^3-oxytocin) infused intravenously in pharmacologically equivalent doses of 0.01 vasodepressor units per kilogram per hour exert essentially the same negligible effect on the blood glucose concentration (Fig. 2) (MIRSKY, 1965).

Since most investigators find that both vasopressin and oxytocin can induce a hyperglycemic response when given in adequate dosage to responsive animals, it is of interest to note that the administration of Arg^8-oxytocin (vasotocin) also results in an increase in the blood glucose concentration of cyclostome fishes (BENTLEY and FOLLETT, 1965) and toads (BENTLEY, 1965).

In contrast to the observations of others, are the reports by one group of investigators that the rapid intravenous administration of from 0.01—0.4 IU oxytocin per kilogram body weight induces a relatively insignificant transient increase in blood glucose concentration which is followed by a highly significant hypoglycemia in dogs and man (BURT and LEAKE, 1962; BURT et al., 1963; BURT et al., 1964a, b; BURT, 1964). Of some interest also is the report that the injection of 20—40 IU oxytocin directly into the liver via a catheter in the portal vein induces no change in concentration of glucose in the hepatic vein blood (BERGEN et al., 1960). It is quite difficult to reconcile these observations with the data depicted in Fig. 3 which are derived from a more recent replication of the studies discussed above.

The mechanism whereby vasopressin and oxytocin may exert a hyperglycemic effect is still obscure. Most of the available data support the conclusions derived from the many earlier studies with pitressin and pitocin (VAN DYKE, 1936, 1939; HARRIS, 1948; STEHLE, 1950), viz., that vasopressin and oxytocin stimulate hepatic glycogenolysis. Thus, concomitant with their hyperglycemic effect in the dog, synthetic vasopressin and oxytocin induce a decrease in liver glycogen (HEIDENREICH et al., 1963). Such findings are difficult to reconcile with the demonstration that whereas the intraportal injection of Lys-vasopressin induces an immediate release of glucose into the hepatic vein, the injection of a massive dose of oxytocin produces no change (BERGEN et al., 1960). Yet, studies with perfused livers of rats reveal that both agents stimulate the output of glucose by the liver into the perfusate (VAISLER et al., 1965). In accord is the demonstration that relatively minute concentrations of Lys-vasopressin (HEIDENREICH et al., 1963; HOROWITZ et al., 1966) and oxytocin (HEIDENREICH et al., 1963) stimulate glycogen breakdown in liver slices *in vitro*. In contrast with the action of epinephrine, neither vasopressin nor oxytocin stimulates the breakdown of glycogen of the rat diaphragm *in vitro* (HEIDENREICH et al., 1963; MIRSKY and PERISUTTI, 1962).

The role of the adrenal and hypophyseal glands in the hyperglycemic response to vasopressin and oxytocin remains unsettled. Thus, one group found that adrenalectomy did not affect the hyperglycemic response of cats and rats to exogenous vasopressin and oxytocin (HEIDENREICH et al., 1963). Others, however, showed that adrenalectomy or hypophysectomy induced a hypoglycemic instead of a hyperglycemic response of the dog to vasopressin (BAISSET et al., 1963, 1965). The hyperglycemic response to oxytocin, however, was not altered by such ablations. Yet, the rapid hyperglycemic response of anesthetized female rabbits to the injection of oxytocin (1 IU) is inhibited by adrenalectomy or treatment with dehydroergotamine (CHAUDHURY and NAYYAR, 1962). Even more confusing is the observation that the hypoglycemic response of the adrenalectomized or hypophysectomized dog to vasopressin is inhibited by the concomitant administration of actinomycin (BAISSET et al., 1967).

IV. Fat Metabolism

The rapid intravenous injection of pure natural or synthetic vasopressin and of oxytocin in a single dose of from 0.01—1.0 IU/kg body weight results in a rapid decrease in the concentration of the free fatty acids (FFA) of the plasma of unanesthetized and anesthetized, male and female dogs (MIRSKY, 1962, 1963a; HEIDENREICH et al., 1963; BALASSE et al., 1966; BALASSE and RASIO, 1965a, b) and anesthetized rats (ITOH et al., 1966). The same response occurs in alloxan-diabetic (MIRSKY, 1963a) and depancreatized (BAISSET et al., 1965) dogs. Likewise, the rapid injection of a variety of analogues of oxytocin and vasopressin results in a reduction in the concentration of the FFA of the plasma (MIRSKY, 1963a). In contrast to these observations are the reports by one group of investigators that whereas the rapid injection of oxytocin in a dosage of from 0.01—0.4 IU/kg body weight induces a progressive decrease in the plasma FFA of male dogs, young men and postmenopausal women, the administration of the same dosage to male dogs, young women and puerperal women results in a rapid, progressive increase in plasma FFA concentration (BURT and LEAKE, 1962; BURT, 1964; BURT et al., 1963, 1964a, b). As noted above, the data obtained from a recent replication of previous studies reveal no sex-differences in the response of dogs to oxytocin (Fig. 3).

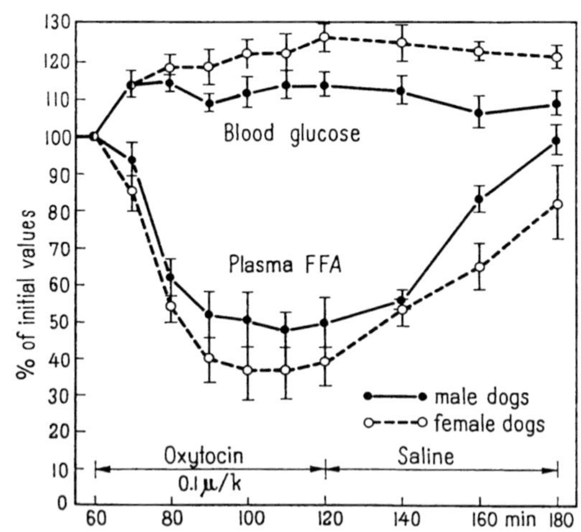

Fig. 3. Effect of oxytocin on blood glucose and plasma FFA of male and female dogs. The data from six dogs of each sex expressed as in Fig. 1

Since vasopressin and oxytocin are rapidly inactivated *in vivo* (Chapter by M. GINSBURG in this volume), it is probable that the response to the rapid injection of these hormones represents the effect of only a small fraction of the quantity administered. In accord is the demonstration that whereas the rapid intravenous injection of 0.1 IU oxytocin per kilogram body weight produces a small but significant decrease in the plasma FFA concentration, a greater decrease occurs when even 0.01 IU/kg is injected into normal or alloxan-diabetic dogs during the course of 1 h (Fig. 1, 2 and 3) (MIRSKY, 1963a). Thus, with the slow infusion, a significant decrease of plasma FFA occurs within 30 min by which time only 0.005 IU/kg had been introduced into the circulation. Such data suggest that endogenous neurohypophyseal hormones may play a role in the physiologic mechanisms responsible for the regulation of the plasma FFA.

The data depicted in Fig. 2 reveal that the slow intravenous infusion of pharmacologically equivalent doses (0.01 pressor units per kilogram body weight) of Arg-vasopressin, Lys-vasopressin Phe^2-Lys^8-vasopressin results in essentially the same significant decrease in the plasma FFA (Mirsky, 1963a) while Acetyl-Lys^8-vasopressin produces no change (Mirsky, 1965). Essentially similar reductions in the plasma FFA ensue from the slow infusion of equivalent doses (0.01 vasodepressor units per kilogram) of oxytocin, Deamino-oxytocin and Val^3-oxytocin while a significantly greater response is produced by Phe^3-oxytocin. Mole for mole, however, the potencies of the various compounds differ markedly. Thus, in decreasing order, the potencies of the various compounds in reducing the plasma FFA are deamino-oxytocin, oxytocin, Arg-vasopressin, Lys-vasopressin, Phe^2-Lys^8-vasopressin, Val^3-oxytocin, Phe^2-oxytocin, and Acetyl-Lys^8-vasopressin.

Definitive studies on species differences in the plasma FFA response to vasopressin and oxytocin are not available. The only available data, other than those discussed above, reveal that rabbits given a massive subcutaneous dose of vasopressin (40 IU) exhibit an increase in plasma FFA in 2 h; a similar injection of 30 IU oxytocin results in a decrease in the same interval (Di Girolama et al., 1961).

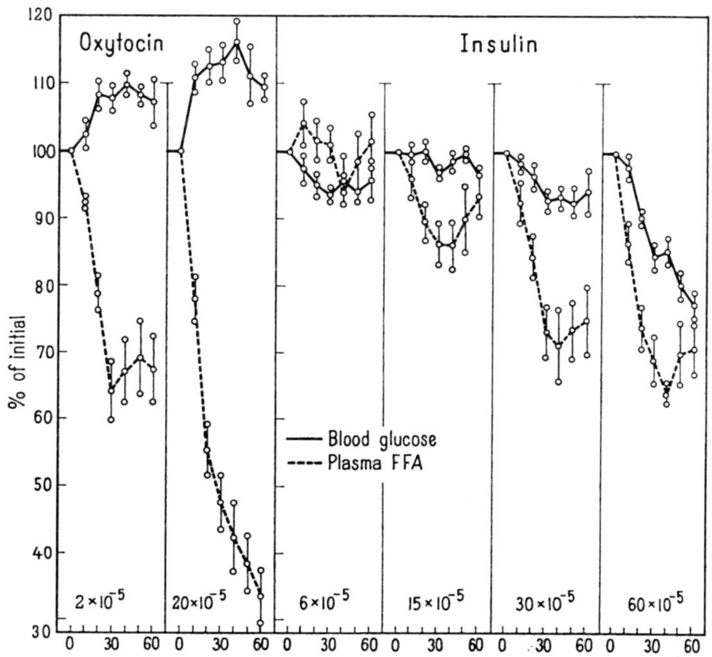

Fig. 4. Comparison of the effects of oxytocin and insulin on the blood glucose and plasma FFA of dogs. Data from five to eight dogs expressed as in Fig. 1 (Mirsky, 1965)

Vasopressin and oxytocin mimic insulin in their effects on the concentration of plasma FFA of the dog (Fig. 4). A dose of insulin which does not produce an appreciable change in blood glucose can induce a prompt decrease in the FFA concentration of the plasma of both nondiabetic and alloxan-diabetic dogs. Thus, the intravenous injection of insulin at a rate of 15×10^{-5} μmoles/kg/h produces a significant decrease in the plasma FFA without affecting the blood glucose concentration (MIRSKY, 1963b). The injection of oxytocin or Lys-vasopressin at a rate of 2×10^{-5} μmoles/kg/h induces a statistically highly significant decrease in plasma FFA without a statistically significant change in the blood glucose concentration. Accordingly, mole for mole, oxytocin and vasopressin appear to be at least 15 times more effective than insulin in their action on plasma FFA.

The degradation of insulin by liver extracts (MIRSKY and PERISUTTI, 1957) and kidney slices (CAMU and CONARD, 1966) is inhibited by oxytocin and vasopressin. Accordingly, their action on the plasma FFA may be due to an increase in the availability of endogenous insulin consequent to an inhibition of its rate of degeneration *in vivo*. This possibility receives some support in the observation that an increase in the insulin-like activity (ILA) of the plasma occurs within 10 min after the onset of the infusion of 1 IU oxytocin/kg/h and is back to the initial level by the 20th min (BALASSE and RASIO, 1965a, b). Such a transient increase in plasma ILA is not noted during the continuous injection of vasopressin (BALASSE et al., 1966). Moreover, the plasma FFA response to oxytocin, vasopressin and related peptides exhibited by the alloxan-diabetic dog suggests that an increased availability of endogenous insulin is not essential for the reduction of plasma FFA of the normal dog.

The mechanism whereby the neurohypophyseal hormones induce a decrease in the concentration of the plasma FFA has not been established. Such a decrease can be due to a reduction in the release of FFA from adipose tissues, to an increase in their removal from the circulation, or to both. That the former is more likely is suggested by the evidence that the decrease in the concentration of the FFA of the plasma produced by the administration of glucose or insulin to animal or man is due to a decrease in the release of FFA from the depots (GORDON and CHERKES, 1956; BIERMAN et al., 1957; ESTES et al., 1959) such as occurs *in vitro* in the presence of insulin (GORDON and CHERKES, 1958; CAHILL et al., 1959; RENOLD and CAHILL, 1965). Likewise, as is discussed below, the effects of oxytocin and related peptides on the concentration of plasma FFA is in accord with their insulin-likeaction on adipose tissue *in vitro*.

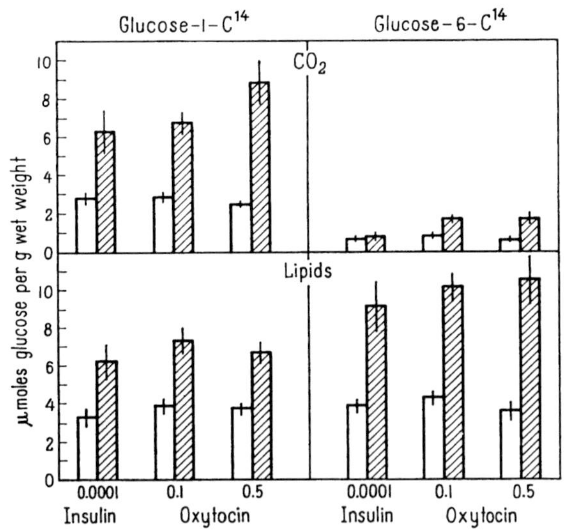

Fig. 5. Effect of oxytocin on the utilization of glucose-1-C^{14} and glucose-6-C^{14} by rat epididymal adipose tissue. The adipose tissue was incubated with glucose-1-C^{14} or glucose-6-C^{14} without and with oxytocin (unit per ml) or glucagon-free insulin (unit per ml). The data are expressed as the mean ± SE μmole glucose oxidized to $C^{14}O_2$ or incorporated into the total lipids (MIRSKY, 1965)

Like insulin, oxytocin acts on rat epididymal adipose tissue *in vitro* to increase glucose uptake, glucose oxidation, lipogenesis from glucose and acetate, and protein synthesis (MIRSKY and PERISUTTI, 1961, 1962; PITTMAN et al., 1961; KRAHL, 1964; GOODMAN, 1965; MIGLIOVINI and LINDER, 1966). Fat cells isolated from rat epididymal adipose tissue respond in a similar manner on incubation with oxytocin (RODBELL, 1964). The data depicted in Fig. 5 reveal that like insulin, oxytocin stimulates the production of $C^{14}O_2$ from glucose 1-C^{14} to a much greater degree than from glucose-6-C^{14}. Like insulin, oxytocin enhances the incorporation of labeled carbon into triglycerides from both glucose-1-C^{14} and glucose-6-C^{14}. Furthermore, like insulin, oxytocin stimulates the incorporation of acetate-1-C^{14} into fatty acids and of histidine-C^{14} into a protein fraction of rat epididymal adipose tissue (Krahl, 1964). The action of oxytocin on this tissue, however, differs from that of insulin in that mole for mole, the latter is nearly 300 times more active than oxytocin.

Comparison of the action of oxytocin on rat adipose tissue *in vitro* with that of related disulfide peptides reveal significant differences (Fig. 6). Whereas pharmacologically equivalent concentrations of oxytocin and related analogues stimulate the oxidation of glucose to CO_2 to the same degree, Arg-vasopressin, Lys-vasopressin and 1-Acetyl-Lys-vasopressin are relatively ineffective. When sufficiently

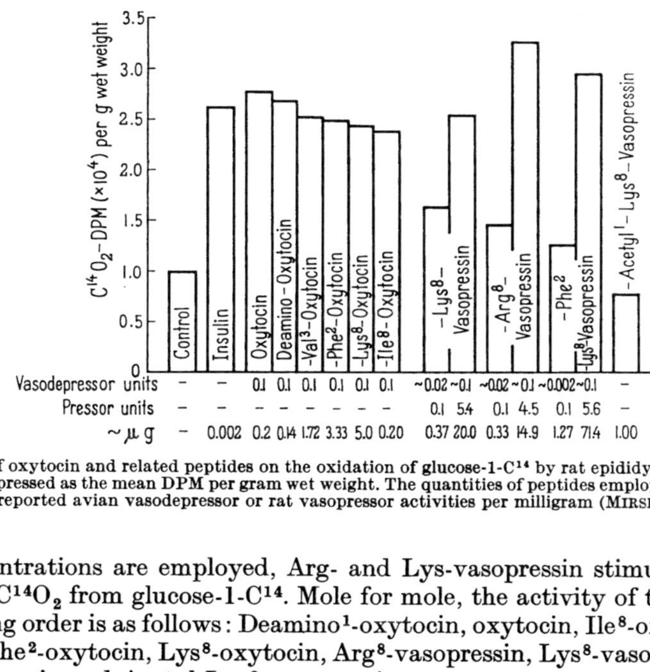

Fig. 6. Effect of oxytocin and related peptides on the oxidation of glucose-1-C^{14} by rat epididymal adipose tissue. The data are expressed as the mean DPM per gram wet weight. The quantities of peptides employed were computed from reported avian vasodepressor or rat vasopressor activities per milligram (Mirsky, 1965)

large concentrations are employed, Arg- and Lys-vasopressin stimulate the production of $C^{14}O_2$ from glucose-1-C^{14}. Mole for mole, the activity of these peptides in decreasing order is as follows: Deamino^1-oxytocin, oxytocin, Ile^8-oxytocin, Val^3-oxytocin, Phe^2-oxytocin, Lys^8-oxytocin, Arg^8-vasopressin, Lys^8-vasopressin, Phe^2-Lys^8-vasopressin and Acetyl-Lys^8-vasopressin.

The data derived from both *in vivo* and *in vitro* studies suggest a positive correlation between the oxytocic and insulin-like activities of the disulfide peptides insofar as their action on fat metabolism is concerned. Thus, the absence of the free amino group in position I results in a marked enhancement of both oxytocic and insulin-like activity; the substitution for isoleucine in position 3 results in some loss of both activities, and the acetylation of the amino group of the half-cystine residue in position 1 results in a complete loss of both activities.

The insulin-like action of oxytocin and vasopressin *in vitro* is not restricted to rat epididymal adipose tissue. Like insulin, oxytocin and vasopressin can stimulate the uptake of glucose and the rate of its oxidation to CO_2 by slices of mammary gland from lactating rats, rabbits and mice (Goodfriend and Topper, 1961; Cohen et al., 1962). Since the mammary gland in late lactation is practically devoid of adipose tissue (Goodfriend and Topper, 1961), the effects of oxytocin and vasopressin are attributed to stimulation of the secretory tissue. Unlike insulin, however, oxytocin and vasopressin do not stimulate the incorporation of leucine-1-C^{14} into total protein of mammary gland slices (COHEN et al., 1962). Yet, the action of these neurohypophyseal peptides on glucose oxidation by adipose tissue *in vitro* is inhibited by puromycin (COHEN et al., 1962).

In addition to their actions on rat adipose tissue and mammary gland slices *in vitro*, oxytocin and vasopressin stimulate the production of $C^{14}O_2$ from C^{14} labeled glucose, pyruvate, lactate and palmitate by toad bladder strips (GOODFRIEND and KIRKPATRICK, 1963). The selectivity of the action of these hormones is indicated by their inability to stimulate the oxidation of acetate and succinate by toad bladder slices.

In contrast with its action on other tissues *in vitro*, vasopressin inhibits the production of CO_2 and lipogenesis from acetate-1-C^{14} and pyruvate-2-C^{14} by slices and homogenates of rat liver, rabbit kidney and rabbit liver (HOROWITZ et al., 1966).

It must be emphasized that the *in vitro* insulin-like effect of either Arg- or Lys-vasopressin on rat adipose tissue occurs only with relatively massive concentrations of the hormone. In more "physiological" concentrations, natural or synthetic Arg- and Lys-vasopressin do not affect either the utilization of glucose (MIRSKY and PERISUTTI, 1962) or the release of FFA from triglycerides by rat adipose tissue (ITOH et al., 1966). Yet, similar concentrations of Arg-vasopressin, but not Lys-vasopressin, have been reported to increase the release of FFA *in vitro* from rabbit and guinea-pig adipose tissues (RUDMAN et al., 1963). Pitressin, consisting of a mixture of Arg- and Lys-vasopressin plus oxytocin and other contaminants, has been reported by some to have no effect on the release of FFA by rat adipose tissues *in vitro* (RUDMAN et al., 1963; WHITE and ENGEL, 1958), while others have reported a lipolytic action (VAUGHAN, 1964). A similar mixture of vasopressins has been reported to exert no lipolytic action on adipose tissue from the hamster, pig and dog (RUDMAN et al., 1963).

It is apparent from the preceding that the information available at the present time suggests that purified natural or synthetic vasopressins and oxytocin do not exert an adipokinetic action on adipose tissue from any species other than rabbit and guinea-pig. Many more *in vivo* and *in vitro* studies on the action of synthetic hormones in a variety of species are essential before their role in the regulation of fat metabolism is established.

Any discussion of the adipokinetic action of neurohypophyseal hormones must consider the role of agents other than vasopressin and oxytocin. Thus, the intravenous injection of a dialyzable material ("lipid mobilizing factor") extracted from the posterior pituitary of pigs has been reported to produce a lipemia within 1 h in mice, guinea-pigs, rabbits and dogs (SEIFTER and BAEDER, 1957). The nature of this factor and its action on adipose tissue *in vitro* is unknown.

Another potent adipokinetic factor, "Peptide II", has recently been extracted from porcine posterior pituitary lobes (FRIESEN and ASTWOOD, 1967). This peptide appears to be identical with "Fraction H", isolated from anterior pituitary glands (RUDMAN et al., 1962). It has been proposed that both factors may be identical to the so-called van Dyke protein or "neurophysin" (Chapter by M. GINSBURG in this volume) which has a highly specific binding capacity for both vasopressin and oxytocin. Both "Peptide II" and "Fraction H" are adipokinetic only in the rabbit and exhibit a high lipolytic activity *in vitro* only with rabbit adipose tissue (RUDMAN et al., 1962). This hitherto unsuspected function of neurophysin opens intriguing possibilities about the role of neurosecretory material in the hypothalamus.

Summary

Discrepancies between the data obtained by various investigators and discrepancies between *in vivo* and *in vitro* effects of the various agents preclude any definitive conclusions about the metabolic action of the neurohypophyseal hormones. The only consensus that can be gained from a review of studies with natural or synthetic vasopressins and oxytocin is that both hormones and related disulfide peptides can induce hyperglycemia when administered in adequate dosage to responsive species. Both hormones, as well as neurophysin, may play a role in the regulation of the FFA concentration of the plasma of some species. The mechanisms whereby these various actions are attained and the factors that determine the responsiveness to some and not to other species remain unknown. Consequently, little can be stated at the present time concerning the physiological significance, if any, of the metabolic actions of the neurohypophyseal hormones. Nevertheless, it is quite possible that in addition to their known vascular, muscular, mammary secretory, and other actions, the neurohypophyseal hormones play a central or peripheral role in the regulation of carbohydrate and fat metabolism.

References

BACQ, Z. M., and S. DWORKIN: The heart rate after sympathectomy and vagotomy and the blood sugar as affected by posterior hypophyseal extracts (Pitressin and Pitocin). Amer. J. Physiol. **95**, 605 (1930).

BAISSET, A., L. DANG TRAN, et P. MONTASTRUC: Action hypoglycémiante de la vasopressine chez le chien surrénalectomisé ou hypophysectomisé. C.R. Soc. Biol. (Paris) **157**, 877 (1963).

— — — Effets comparés de la vasopressine et de l'ocytocine sur la glycémie du chien normal ou privé de divers systèmes endocriniens. C.R. Soc. Biol. (Paris) **159**, 477 (1965).

— — — Influence de l'actinomycine D sur l'action hypoglycémiante de la vasopressine chez le chien surrénalectomisé ou hypophysectomisé. C.R. Soc. Biol. (Paris) **160**, 1084 (1967).

BALASSE, E., et E. RASIO: Action insulino-libératrice de l'ocytocine chez le chien. Arch. Int. Physiol. Biochim. **73**, 27 (1965a).

— — Mécanisme d'action de l'ocytocine sur la concentration plasmatique des acides gras libres (A.G.L.) chez le chien. Arch. int. Pharmacodyn. **157**, 356 (1965b).

— —, et V. CONARD: Action insulino-mimétique de la vasopressine chez le chien. Arch. int. Pharmacodyn. **161**, 392 (1966).

LA BARRE, J.: A propos des variations glycémiques consécutives à l'administration d'extrait hypophysaire postérieur. Arch. int. Pharmacodyn. **38**, 409 (1930).

BENTLEY, P. J.: Hyperglycemic effect of vasotocin in toads. Nature (Lond.) **206**, 1053 (1965).

—, and B. K. FOLLETT: The effects of hormones on the carbohydrate metabolism of the Lamprey Lampetra Fluviatilis. J. Endocr. **31**, 127 (1965).

BERGEN, S. S., R. SULLIVAN, J. G. HILTON, S. W. WILLIS jr., and T. B. VAN ITALLIE: Glycogenolytic effect of vasopressin in the canine liver. Amer. J. Physiol. **199**, 136 (1960).

BIERMAN, E. L., I. L. SCHWARTZ, and V. P. DOLE: Action of insulin on release of fatty acids from tissue stores. Amer. J. Physiol. **191**, 359 (1957).

BLIX, G., u. C. A. OHLIN: Pituitrin und Blutlipoide. Skand. Arch. Physiol. **51**, 167 (1927).

BLOTNER, H., and R. FITZ: The effect of insulin, pituitrin and adrenalin on the blood-sugar level. J. clin. Invest. **5**, 51 (1927).

BORCHARDT, L.: Experimentelles über den Diabetes bei der Akromegalie. Dtsch. med. Wschr. **34**, 946 (1908).

BURN, J. H.: The modification of the action of insulin by pituitary extract and other substances. J. Physiol. (Lond.) **57**, 318 (1923).

BURT, R. L.: Influence of sex and gonadal function on metabolic effects of oxytocin. Obstet. and Gynec. **24**, 559 (1964).

—, and N. H. LEAKE: Metabolic activity of oxytocin. Preliminary observations. Obstet. and Gynec. **20**, 442 (1962).

— —, and W. N. DANNENBURG: Effect of synthetic oxytocin on plasma nonesterified fatty acids, triglycerides and blood glucose. Obstet. and Gynec. **21**, 708 (1963).

— — — Comparative metabolic effects of certain oxytocic preparations and related compounds on blood glucose and plasma NEFA. Obstet. and Gynec. **23**, 574 (1964a).

— — — Sex differences in metabolic effects of oxytocin. Nature (Lond.) **201**, 829 (1964b).

CAHILL jr., G.F., B. JEANRENAUD, B. LE BOEUF, and A.E. RENOLD: Effects of insulin on adipose tissue. Ann. N.Y. Acad. Sci. **82**, 403 (1959).
CAMU, F., et V. CONARD: Effet de l'ocytocine sur l'inactivation de l'insuline par le rein de rat normal *in vitro*. Arch. int. Pharmacodyn. **162**, 247 (1966).
CASH, W.D., and M.H. KAPLAN: Comparison of 8-lysine-vasopressin, 1-deamino-8-lysine-vasopressin and 1-acetyl-8-lysine-vasopressin on the blood glucose level in rabbits. Endocrinology **74**, 803 (1964).
CHAUDHURY, R.R., and P.P. NAYYAR: The hyperglycemic action of synthetic oxytocin. Toxicol. appl. Pharmacol. **4**, 174 (1962).
COHEN, J., A.R. BRENNEMAN, and Y.J. TOPPER: The stimulation by oxytocin and acetylcholine of glucose oxidation by lactating — rat mammary — gland slices: Inhibition of the hormone effects by puromycin. Biochim. biophys. Acta (Amst.) **63**, 554 (1962).
COOPE, R., and E.N. CHAMBERLAIN: The effects of pituitrin on the fatty acid of the liver. J. Physiol. (Lond.) **60**, 67 (1925).
CUSHING, H.: The pituitary body and its disorders. Philadelphia: Lippincott 1910.
DRAPER, W.B., and R.M. HILL: Pituitary extract and the CO_2 combining power of the blood plasma. Proc. Soc. exp. Biol. (N.Y.) **27**, 33 (1929).
VAN DYKE, H.B.: The physiology and pharmacology of the pituitary body. Vols 1 and 2. Chicago: University of Chicago Press 1936 and 1939.
ESTES jr., E.H., M.D. BOGDONOFF, S.J. FRIEDBERG, W.R. HARLAN, and D.L. TROUT: The effect of insulin on nonesterified fatty acid release from the human leg. J. clin. Invest. **38**, 2131 (1959).
FRIESEN, H.G., and E.B. ASTWOOD: Changes in neurohypophyseal proteins induced by dehydration and ingestion of saline. Endocrinology **80**, 278 (1967).
GEILING, E.M.K., and C.A. EDDY: The hyperglycemic effect of vasopressin, oxytocin and pituitrin. Proc. Soc. exp. Biol. (N.Y.) **26**, 146 (1928).
DI GIROLAMA, M., D. RUDMAN, M. REID, and F. SEIDMAN: Effect of pituitary hormones upon serum fatty acid concentration of the rabbit. Endocrinology **68**, 457 (1961).
GOLDMAN, J.K.: Effect of pitressin infusion on plasma free fatty acid levels in man. Proc. Soc. exp. Biol. (N.Y.) **117**, 164 (1964).
GOODFRIEND, T., and J. KIRKPATRICK: Effect of neurohypophyseal hormones on oxidative metabolism of the toad bladder *in vitro*. Endocrinology **72**, 742 (1963).
—, and Y.J. TOPPER: Effects of oxytocin, vasopressin and acetylcholine on glucose metabolism in mammary tissue *in vitro*. J. biol. Chem. **236**, 1241 (1961).
GOODMAN, H.M.: Effects of insulin on water uptake by adipose tissue during incubation *in vitro*. Endocrinology **76**, 531 (1965).
GORDON jr., R.S., and A. CHERKES: Unesterified fatty acid in human blood plasma. J. clin. Invest. **35**, 206 (1956).
— — Production of unesterified fatty acids from isolated rat adipose tissue incubated *in vitro*. Proc. Soc. exp. Biol. (N.Y.) **97**, 150 (1958).
GURD, M.R.: The effect of oxytocin and vasopressin on the action of insulin. Quart. J. Pharm. **7**, 661 (1934).
HANNON, J.P., and A.M. LARSON: Fatty acid metabolism during norepinephrine induced thermogenesis in the cold-acclimatized rat. Amer. J. Physiol. **203**, 1055 (1962).
HARRIS, G.W.: Neural control of the pituitary gland. Physiol. Rev. **28**, 139 (1948).
HEIDENREICH, O., Y. KOOK, L. BAUMEISTER u. P. KELLER: Untersuchungen über die Wirkungsweise der Hypophysenhinterlappenhormone auf den Kohlenhydrat- und Fettstoffwechsel. Naunyn-Schmiedebergs Arch. exp. Path. Pharmak. **245**, 321 (1963).
— — u. E. REUS: Quantitative Untersuchungen über die blutzuckersteigernde Wirkung von synthetischem Oxytocin und Vasopressin sowie über das Auftreten dieses Hormoneffektes unter physiologischen Bedingungen. Naunyn-Schmiedebergs Arch. exp. Path. Pharmak. **243**, 136 (1962).
HOROWITZ, I., J.C. BECK, and D. RUBINSTEIN: The effect of vasopressin on lipogenesis *in vitro*. J. biol. Chem. **241**, 1031 (1966).
HOUSSAY, B.A., et E. DI BENEDETTO: Action hyperglycémiante de l'extrait réptropituitaire. C.R. Soc. Biol. (Paris) **114**, 793 (1933).
ITOH, S., M. TSUKADA, A. OKUNO, and T. YOSHINARI: Effects of vasopressin on the plasma concentration of free fatty acids and *in vitro* oxygen consumption of tissues of the rat. Jap. J. Physiol. **16**, 23 (1966).
KOOK, Y., K.B. CHO, and K.O. YUN: Metabolic effects of oxytocin in the chicken. Nature (Lond.) **204**, 385 (1964).
KRAHL, M.E.: Specificity of insulin or oxytocin stimulation of protein synthesis in adipose tissue. Amer. J. Physiol. **207**, 1169 (1964).
LONG, C.N.H., E. HILL, and F. BISCHOFF: The posterior pituitary hormone in metabolism. III. The effect of pitressin and pituitrin upon the lipoid distribution. Amer. J. Physiol. **102**, 402 (1932).

Migliovini, R. H., and C. Linder: Oxytocin and lipogenesis by adipose tissue *in vitro*. Biochim. biophys. Acta (Amst.) **125**, 392 (1966).
Mirsky, I. A.: Effect of oxytocin on plasma free fatty acids on non-diabetic and diabetic dogs. Proc. Soc. exp. Biol. (N.Y.) **110**, 42 (1962).
— Effect of oxytocin, vasopressin, and related peptides on plasma FFA of non-diabetic and diabetic dogs. Amer. J. Physiol. **204**, 842 (1963a).
— Relative effects of insulin, oxytocin and vasopressin on the free fatty acid concentration of the plasma of non-diabetic and diabetic dogs. Endocrinology **73**, 613 (1963b).
— Effect of biologically active peptides on adipose tissue. Handbook of physiology — Adipose tissue. American Physiological Society, Washington, D.C., 1965, p. 407.
—, and G. Perisutti: Insulinase-inhibitory activity of protein hydrolysates. Proc. Soc. exp. Biol. (N.Y.) **94**, 589 (1957).
— — The insulin-like action of oxytocin on adipose tissue. Biochim. biophys. Acta (Amst.) **50**, 603 (1961).
— — The action of oxytocin and related peptides on epididymal adipose tissue of the rat. Endocrinology **71**, 158 (1962).
Okuno, A., M. Yamamoto, and S. Itoh: Lowering of the body temperature induced by vasopressin. Jap. J. Physiol. **15**, 378 (1965).
Pittman, J. A., B. R. Boshell, B. H. Williams, D. Hamner, and P. Hill: Insulin-like activity of vasopressin and oxytocin. Biochem. biophys. Res. Commun. **6**, 29 (1961).
Raab, W.: The role of the pituitary posterior hormone in fat metabolism. Endocrinology **14**, 385 (1930).
Renold, A. E., and G. F. Cahill jr.: Metabolism of isolated adipose tissue: A summary. Handbook of physiology — Adipose tissue. American Physiological Society, Washington, D.C., 1965, p. 483.
Rodbell, M.: Metabolism of isolated fat cells. I. Effects of hormones on glucose metabolism and lipolysis. J. biol. Chem. **239**, 375 (1964).
Rudman, D., S. J. Brown, and M. F. Malkin: Adipokinetic actions of adrenocorticotropin, thyroid-stimulating hormone, vasopressin, α- and β-melanocyte-stimulating hormones, fraction H, epinephrine and norepinephrine in the rabbit, guinea-pig, hamster, rat, pig and dog. Endocrinology **72**, 527 (1963).
—, R. L. Hirsch, F. F. Kendall, F. Seidman, and S. J. Brown: An adipokinetic component of the pituitary gland: purification, physical, chemical and biological. Recent Progr. Hormone Res. **18**, 89 (1962).
Schaumann, O.: Heffter's Handbuch der experimentellen Pharmakologie. Berlin 1937.
Schroeder, H.: Über die blutzuckersteigernde und insulinantagonistische Wirkung des Tonephins bzw. Pitressins und Orasthins. Klin. Wschr. **12**, 1766 (1933).
Seifter, J., and D. H. Baeder: Lipid mobilizer (LM) from posterior pituitary of hogs in rat adipose tissue. Proc. Soc. exp. Biol. (N.Y.) **95**, 318 (1957).
Shull, K. H., and J. Mayer: Experimental hyperglycemic states not primarily due to a lack of insulin. Vitam. u. Horm. **14**, 187 (1956).
Silver, S., u. E. Mislowitzer: Studien über die Adrenalinhyperglykämie. II. Mitt. Die Beeinflussung der Adrenalinhyperglykämie durch die getrennten Hypophysenhinterlappensubstanzen. Z. ges. exp. Med. **78**, 741 (1931).
Stehle, R. L.: The physiological actions of the hormones of the posterior lobe of the pituitary gland. Vitam. u. Horm. **8**, 215 (1950).
Steinberg, D., P. J. Nestel, E. R. Buskirk, and R. H. Thompson: Calorigenic effect of norepinephrine correlated with plasma free fatty acid turnover and oxidation. J. clin. Invest. **43**, 167 (1964).
Stenstrom, T.: Das Pituitrin und die Adrenalinhyperglykämie. Biochem. Z. **58**, 472 (1913).
Thaddea, S.: Über Beziehungen der isolierten Hypophysenhinterlappenhormone zum Kohlehydratstoffwechsel beim Menschen. Z. klin. Med. **125**, 175 (1933).
—, u. A. Waly: Zur Frage der Wirkungsweise und des Angriffspunktes der isolierten Hypophysenhinterlappenhormone auf den Kohlehydratstoffwechsel. Arch. Exptl. Pathol. Pharmakol. **172**, 535 (1933).
Tsukada, M., A. Okuno, and S. Itoh: Influence of vasopressin on the metabolic rate in rats. Jap. J. Physiol. **15**, 388 (1965).
Vaisler, L., E. Costiner, and C. Gheorghin: Actiunea hyperglicemianta a oxitocinei in sistemul de fiscat perfuzat *in vitro*. Stud. Cercet. Endocr. **16**, 557 (1965).
Vaughan, M.: Effects of pitressin on lipolysis and on phosphorylase activity in rat adipose tissue. Amer. J. Physiol. **207**, 1166 (1964).
White, J. E., and F. L. Engel: Lypolytic action of corticotropin on rat adipose tissue *in vitro*. J. clin. Invest. **37**, 1556 (1958).

The Influence of Neurohypophysial Polypeptides on Adenohypophysial Function

W. DOEPFNER

I. Introduction

The possibility that neural control of the adenohypophysis might be humorally transmitted to the pars distalis was suggested relatively early. On the basis of his own very elegant investigations and a critical appraisal of all the known facts and literature references, HARRIS (1948) in a brilliant review expressed his conviction that: "The pars distalis of the pituitary may, in general terms, be described as a gland under nervous control, but lacking a nerve supply."

This view was a logical one, since but few nerve fibres can be detected in the pars distalis — too few to support a postulated nervous control mechanism (RASMUSSEN, 1938). By contrast the posterior lobe of the hypophysis is quite richly supplied with nerve fibres which have their origin in the supraoptic nucleus and paraventricular nucleus in the hypothalamus. This fibre tract can be traced along the infundibular stem as far as the infundibular process and is generally called the supraoptico-hypophysial tract. A second fibre tract, taking its origin in the hypothalamus also, terminates in the median eminence where the nerve endings are in intimate contact with capillary vessels. For a time the fibres of this tubero-hypophysial tract were assumed to have a vasomotor function, regulating adenohypophysial secretion by such a mechanism. This difference between the two lobes of the pituitary is also explained by their embryological development. The posterior lobe originates from a diverticulum of the third ventricle, the infundibular recess, whereas the anterior lobe develops from an evagination of the oral epithelium, the so-called Rathke's pouch. Later this tissue forms the tuberal portion and distal portion of anterior lobe of the hypophysis.

In addition to the composite structure of the gland and the histology of its parts the hypophysis has a very unusual vascular system. POPA and FIELDING (1930, 1933) first described the vascular system of the human hypophysis, showing it to be a portal system. Their investigations were confirmed by many authors, and further findings were reported by WISLOCKI (1937, 1938) and by GREEN and HARRIS (1947). This portal system receives its blood supply from the internal carotid artery and ramifies into a first capillary bed which extends as far as the median eminence. The blood from this primary plexus collects in the portal trunk and is again distributed in a second capillary bed (sinusoids) in the pars distalis, the glandular part of the adenohypophysis. Moreover, the adenohypophysis and the neurohypophysis are directly connected by short vessels, and blood vessels pass back into the region of hypothalamus. The discovery of this portal system was a sine qua non for the hypothesis of humoral control of anterior pituitary function. Subsequent developments were decisively influenced by the elegant researches of B. and E. SCHARRER (1940, 1954a, b; E. SCHARRER, 1966) and of BARGMANN (1949, 1954) who showed how, using a suitable staining technique, the material stored in the posterior lobe of the hypophysis could be traced in its passage along nerve fibres from its place of origin in certain hypothalamic nuclei (BARGMANN and SCHARRER, 1951). The transported matter which is now generally called neurosecretory material is probably identical with the protein described by VAN DYKE et al. (1942), and later given the name neurophysin by ACHER (1963). This substance is a high molecular weight protein to which vasopressin and oxytocin are attached. On the basis of their investigations BARGMANN and SCHARRER assumed that vasopressin and oxytocin were produced in the hypothalamic nuclei and transported along the nerve fibres to the posterior lobe of the hypophysis, where they were merely stored. Support for such a view was forthcoming in the findings of HILD and ZETLER (1951, 1952, 1953a, b), who investigated the occurrence and distribution of the postpituitary hormones in the posterior lobe of the pituitary and in the hypothalamic nuclear areas using a bioassay procedure.

Once these prerequisite conditions, anatomical and functional, had been satisfied, a humoral hypothesis could be put forward to explain the mechanism by which the secretion of the anterior pituitary hormones was regulated. It is quite conceivable that neurosecretory material from a hypothalamic nuclear area could reach the capillary bed in the region of median eminence along the nerve fibres and find its way via the portal circulation to the pars distalis, i.e. to the hormone-producing cells of the adenohypophysis. Subsequently interest was focussed on the analysis of this neurosecretory mechanism and on the transmitter substances possibly involved.

Extracts of posterior lobe and of tissue from the region of the median eminence as well as hypothalamic extracts exhibited a stimulant effect on the secretion of most anterior lobe hormones when administered parenterally to many different species. The ensuing investigations and much work directed towards isolating these hypothalamic releasing factors and elucidating their chemical structure — work which is still in progress — suggests that they are peptides of low molecular weight which differ but little in their chemical and physical properties from vasopressin and oxytocin. For this reason their preparation in a pure state, i.e. their separation from these latter hormones, is fraught with considerable difficulties. Although in most cases the secretion of the anterior pituitary hormones is regulated by stimulating factors, it now seems certain that the secretion of one of these hormones, namely prolactin, is controlled by a hypothalamic pituitary-inhibiting factor. Moreover, it is possible that these factors also influence the synthesis of the anterior pituitary hormones. The "releasing factors" have been dealt with in numerous reviews, and, in particular, their importance within the ensemble of regulatory and feedback mechanisms controlling the individual anterior pituitary hormones has been analysed. The reader is referred to the reviews listed in the references (EVERETT, 1964; FRASCHINI et al., 1966; GLICK et al., 1965; GUILLEMIN, 1964; HARRIS and DONOVAN, 1966; MCKENZIE, 1966; KNOBIL and HOTCHKISS, 1964; LLOYD and WEISZ, 1966; MARTINI, 1966; MARTINI and GANONG, 1966; MCSHAN and HARTLEY, 1965; MEITES and NICOLL, 1966; NALBANDOV, 1963; SAFFRAN, 1966; SMITH, 1965; SZENTAGOTHAI et al., 1962; VERNIKOS-DANELLIS, 1965). The present discussion will thus be confined to the effect on the individual anterior pituitary hormones of the post-pituitary hormones occurring in mammals, and of such analogues as have so far been investigated.

II. Adrenocorticotrophic Hormone (ACTH)

ACTH is the most thoroughly investigated anterior lobe hormone. Its importance for the control of adrenocortical function was recognized fairly early, as was the fact that noxious stimuli, which SELYE (1936) referred to collectively as stress, would induce hypersecretion. Moreover it was the only anterior lobe hormone which allowed of relatively accurate standardisation. The methods most frequently employed are adrenal ascorbic acid depletion (SAYERS et al., 1948) or estimation of steroids in blood or urine. It is understandable, therefore, that the effect of neurohypophysial hormones on ACTH secretion should have been the subject of the first, and, subsequently, the most numerous investigations.

These studies may be divided into three groups, which will serve as a convenient framework for presentation of the findings and observations. Let it be stated from the outset that these results are in some cases contradictory: (a) On the one hand attempts were made to analyse the functional significance of *endogenous vasopressin or oxytocin* in the hypothalamus or in the neurohypophysis in relation to ACTH secretion. (b) On the other, the effects of *exogenous hormone* were studied, i.e. the effects of postpituitary extracts or synthetic vasopressin and oxytocin, administered in various ways and under different experimental conditions. (c) Similar experiments were carried out using *analogues* of these hormones.

A. Endogenous Neurohypophysial Hormones

1. Stress (Noxious Stimuli)

As mentioned earlier SELYE (1936) showed in the mid-thirties that a number of noxious treatments of a highly diverse nature led to hypertrophy of the adrenals and to involution of the thymus. The most frequently applied stimuli are: surgery, loud noises, bacterial toxins, restraint, insulin, ether, histamine, acetylcholine and adrenaline (MUNSON and BRIGGS, 1955). The three last-named substances were believed for a while to be transmitter substances (LONG, 1952), since they occur in a fairly high concentration in the hypothalamus and lead to release of ACTH in a matter of minutes when administered systemically (GRAY and MUNSON, 1951). It was shown that these substances, unlike emotional or neurotropic stimuli, exerted an effect on a hypophysis transplanted in, say, the anterior chamber of the eye and thus remote from any hypothalamic nervous or blood supply (FORTIER, 1951). This being the case a dual control mechanism was postulated. However, it was later shown that histamine, acetylcholine or adrenaline could not be the true hypothalamic transmitter substances sought after (GUILLEMIN, 1955).

Practically all the noxious stimuli mentioned and any sufficiently powerful emotional stimulus lead to the release of ACTH as well as of antidiuretic hormone (MIRSKY et al., 1954). However, this occurs only in animals with an intact hypothalamo-hypophysial axis. Suffice it to mention here but a few of the numerous investigations which set out to demonstrate a correlation between these two hormones, i.e. to show that ACTH secretion was dependent upon the antidiuretic function of the hypothalamo-neurohypophysial axis.

In dehydrated rats, whose posterior lobe has been completely depleted of neurosecretory material, the effect of a pure neurogenic stimulus, such as a strange environment or loud noise, on plasma corticosterone levels is markedly diminished (DE WIED, 1961b). In posterior lobectomised rats with a markedly depressed antidiuretic response adrenal activation, measured by the increase of plasma corticosterone levels in response to a strange environment, noise or pain (mild electric shocks) is significantly less than that of normal controls (DE WIED, 1961b; SMELIK et al., 1962).

After hypophysectomy, stalk section, hypothalamic lesions or transplantation of the pituitary to the anterior chamber of the eye or to beneath the kidney capsule (all of these procedures disconnecting the pars distalis from its humoral supply), most of the stimuli mentioned are without effect.

Two exceptions to this generalisation have, however, been described. In man, insulin-induced hypoglycaemia appears to release ACTH, as evidenced by an increase in plasma corticosteroids, even though vasopressin is not released (McDONALD et al., 1957). In water-loaded dogs NICHOLS and GUILLEMIN (1959) observed the expected antidiuresis on infusion of hypertonic saline, but the blood cortisone level did not rise in most of the animals.

2. *Influences (Interactions) of Steroids*

SAYERS and SAYERS (1945) discovered that the response of the pituitary anterior lobe to certain stressful stimuli could be blocked to a greater or less extent by previous administration of adrenocortical extract or pure cortical steroids. These findings suggested that the ACTH secretion was regulated by a feedback-mechanism, which depends upon the plasma corticosteroid level (YATES et al., 1961). Presumably the non-protein-bound steroids have to be held mainly responsible (KAWAI and YATES, 1966; DAUGHADAY, 1959; YATES and URQUHART, 1962). Corticosteroids which are preferentially accumulated in posterior pituitary tissue (COURRIER and ZIZINE, 1956; SCHAPIRO and KATZ, 1959) diminish the antidiuretic as well as the adrenal response of rats to a mild electric shock stimulus (McCANN et al., 1958). Moreover in rats undergoing dehydration less pituitary vasopressin depletion is observed in animals pretreated with methylprednisolone (MOSES, 1963). Furthermore, CAVALLERO et al. (1954) were able to demonstrate that the pituitary content of antidiuretic hormone was reduced by adrenalectomy and could be restored to varying degrees by replacement treatment with corticosteroids. These observations, showing an interrelation between ACTH secretion and the antidiuretic hormone or neurosecretory material, could have an important bearing upon a possible role played by vasopressin as a transmitter.

Histological observations said to demonstrate alterations in the amount of neurosecretory material in relation to the circulating blood level of corticosteroids have also been reported (MALANDRA and CORBETTA, 1953; ROTHBALLER, 1953), but have been called into question by others (DE GROOT, 1957; RENNELS and RUSSEL, 1957; DE GROOT and HARTFIELD, 1961).

RINNE (1960) in a very thorough histological study, compared changes in the neurosecretory material around the portal vessels and in the hypothalamus and the infundibular process, under normal conditions as well as under acute or chronic stress. He concluded that as far as the secretion of posterior pituitary hormones is concerned, the hypothalamo-neurohypophysial system is not necessarily important in the regulation of ACTH release.

Quantitative data, based on the biological estimation of the oxytocin and vasopressin content of the pituitary posterior lobe of rats were reported by BARNAFI and CROXATTO (1966). The pituitaries of female rats contained significantly more of both hormones but no change was observed after adrenalectomy. However, vasopressin and oxytocin were depleted by 40% and 37% respectively in males after adrenalectomy compared with sham operated controls.

3. *Physiological Changes*

Young rats respond normally to exogenous ACTH and contain physiologically active ACTH in their pituitaries (RINFRET and HANE, 1955). But it has been reported by several investigators that their response to stressful stimuli is underdeveloped (JAILER, 1950; LEVINE et al., 1957; LEVINE and LEWIS, 1959; SCHAPIRO et al., 1961; SCHAPIRO, 1965). Similar observations have been made in mice, dogs and rabbits (MILKOVIC and MILKOVIC, 1959; THOMPSON and BLOUNT, 1954). Since the posterior pituitary mechanism is known to be immature at birth (HELLER and

LEDERIS, 1959) a degree of parallelism in the development of the two functions would be meaningful.

However, it has been shown that handling or mild stimulation during infancy hastens the appearance of the stress-response (LEVINE et al., 1957; LEVINE and LEWIS, 1959). Unfortunately in most of these experiments an indirect criterion, ascorbic acid depletion, was taken as an index of ACTH release, and different noxious stimuli were applied. Moreover, it was shown recently that even two day old rats display a significant increase in plasma corticosterone in response to electric shock or heat (ZARROW et al., 1966). In general it seems that the immaturity of the hypothalamo-adenohypophysial system is only a matter of degree. Its function, which can be trained, depends upon the intensity and type of stressful stimulus used.

In this connection, two hitherto little correlated phenomena are the very marked diurnal rhythms of the anterior and posterior pituitary hormones. The pituitary-adrenal rhythm is one of the best known and most thoroughly analysed. It is common to all mammals studied, its pattern varying with the habits of the species, but it is relatively immune to environmental changes (HALBERG et al., 1961). In the rat and in the mouse it is characterised by a peak peripheral corticosterone level at about 4 p.m. (GUILLEMIN et al., 1959b; HALBERG et al., 1958, 1959). In man, peak adrenal activity, reflected by 17-hydroxy-corticosteroid levels in blood and urine occurs in the early morning, while the individual is usually still asleep (PERKOFF et al., 1959). The diurnal rhythm of diuresis in man has been studied under various conditions, it shows a maximum in the early afternoon and a minimum in the early morning (MILLS, 1951; LEWIS and LOBBAN, 1958; ASCHOFF, 1963). In the rat urine excretion is maximal during the day and minimal during the night (KÖNIG and MEYER, 1967). Whereas the time pattern of diuresis is similar in man and in the rat, the steroid maxima occur at different times. However, more systematic investigations are needed, if further conclusions are to be drawn.

4. Pathological Changes

Diabetes insipidus due to impaired or abolished release of antidiuretic hormone can be induced experimentally by extirpating the pituitary posterior lobe or by interrupting the supraoptical tract. If the antidiuretic hormone were involved in the regulation of ACTH secretion an inverse relationship would be expected to exist between the severity of the diabetes insipidus and the release of ACTH. The findings reported in the extensive literature are conflicting. A correlation has been observed by some authors (MCCANN and BROBECK, 1954; MCCANN et al., 1958; GOLDMAN et al., 1962), but has not been seen by others (DAILY and GANONG, 1958; NICHOLS et al., 1959; MCCANN and HABERLAND, 1960). Rats with little or no diabetes insipidus can have impaired ACTH secretion and conversely rats with an extremely high water turnover, are reported to have normal ACTH secretion (MCCANN and HABERLAND, 1960; KENNEDY et al., 1963). Also hypertrophy of the adrenals after hypothalamic lesions or posterior lobectomy has been reported (NOWELL, 1959; SMELIK, 1960; DE WIED, 1961b; DEAR and GUILLEMIN, 1960). The main reason for these discrepancies may be the difficulty in interrupting the supraoptical tract or in inflicting appropriate lesions capable of preventing any neurosecretory material from reaching the pars distalis of the adenohypophysis. The development of diabetes insipidus in rats after lesions in the pituitary stalk and the influence of these lesions on the pituitary-adrenal function have been studied in detail (KOVACS et al., 1962; LASZLO and DE WIED, 1966a, b). Bearing in mind the complicated anatomical situation and the various ways by which neurosecretory material can reach the pars distalis, it is hardly surprising that only slightly different experimental approaches may lead to completely different functional disturbances (MARTINI, 1966).

The discovery of rats with hereditary diabetes insipidus by VALTIN and SCHROEDER (1964) may facilitate the examination of this problem. Analysis of the hypothalamo-hypophysial regions of these rats (Brattleboro strain) revealed a complete absence of stored vasopressin, not only in the pituitary gland but almost certainly in the hypothalamus as well (VALTIN et al., 1965). MCCANN et al. (1966) showed that two different types of stress, i.e. etherisation and restraint, raised the plasma corticosterone levels of these animals, but to a significantly smaller degree than in normal animals. On the other hand, the corticotrophin-releasing activity in the median eminence and the pituitary ACTH concentration were not significantly different in these diabetes insipidus and normal rats. This would suggest that, although vasopressin is not the corticotrophin-releasing factor, it may play a minor role in adrenocortical response to stress.

B. Exogenous Neurohypophysial Hormones

NAGAREDA and GAUNT (1951) and ESER and SIPAHIOGLU (1951) were the first to demonstrate that injection of postpituitary extracts in rats led to ascorbic acid depletion of the adrenals and to a reduction in eosinophil count. Since this effect was not observed in hypophysectomised animals, ESER and SIPAHIOGLU assumed that the primary mechanism must consist in stimulation of the adrenocorticotrophic function of the anterior lobe of the pituitary. The two postpituitary extracts employed by ESER and SIPAHIOGLU possessed different antidiuretic activities, and the authors concluded from this that the factor responsible for stimulation must be identical with the antidiuretic-vasopressor principle. These findings were subsequently confirmed by BERTELLI and MARTINI (1952) and by a number of other investigators. Stimulation of ACTH secretion by natural or synthetic vasopressin has been demonstrated in other species, such as the intact dog (KWAAN and BARTELSTONE, 1959) and the intact guinea-pig (SOBEL et al., 1955; SIDEMAN and SOBEL, 1960).

Stress, even the mere handling of the animals leads to stimulation of ACTH secretion. Thus investigation of a substance or extract is complicated by interference with endogenously released corticotrophin-releasing factor. MCCANN and BROBECK (1954) and MCCANN and FRUIT (1957) were the first to use chronic lesions to the median eminence. This rendered the animal unresponsive to environmental stimuli, but Pitressin would still induce adrenal ascorbic acid depletion.

Various operative procedures, such as hypophysectomy and transplantation of the pituitary remote from the hypothalamic nerve and blood supply, posterior lobectomy, pituitary stalk section and hypothalamic lesions have been used to eliminate interference with endogenous releasing factor and to characterise the effect of the natural or synthetic pituitary posterior hormone in question. Unfortunately the pituitary is damaged by most of these procedures (ADAMS et al., 1964; DAVID et al., 1965a). For the pharmacological elimination or suppression of stress responses the drugs which have been most widely used are corticosteroids (BARRETT, 1961; MCCANN, 1957; MCCANN et al., 1958; CARRARO et al., 1961; CASENTINI et al., 1959; CHAUVET and ACHER, 1959; DE WIED and MIRSKY, 1959; DE WIED, 1964; FRASCHINI et al., 1964; KENDALL, 1961; LEEMAN et al., 1962; MARTINI et al., 1962; RERUP, 1964; RUMSFELD and PORTER, 1962), pentobarbital/morphine (BRIGGS and MUNSON, 1955; MCCANN, 1957; DE WIED et al., 1958; DOEPFNER et al., 1963; MUNSON and BRIGGS, 1955; MUNSON, 1962, 1963; GUILLEMIN et al., 1959a), chlorpromazine (SEVY et al., 1957) and α-ethyltryptamine (GANONG et al., 1965).

Methods which avoid all uncontrolled stimuli in loco are organ culture of the anterior pituitary (GUILLEMIN and ROSENBERG, 1955) or short-term incubation of anterior pituitary tissue in Ringer solution (SAFFRAN et al., 1955). However, these *in vitro* methods must be viewed with caution, because of the possibility of non-specific effects (GUILLEMIN and SCHALLY, 1959; GUILLEMIN et al., 1957).

In all these methods natural or synthetic arginine- and lysine-vasopressin have been found to possess considerable ACTH-releasing activity. By contrast, natural or synthetic oxytocin showed only very weak activity if any, whether administered to steroid- or pentobarbital/morphine-blocked animals (CARRARO et al., 1961; CASENTINI et al., 1959; DOEPFNER et al., 1963; FRASCHINI et al., 1964; RINNE et al., 1959), to hypophysectomised animals with the pituitary transplanted into the anterior chamber of the eye (CASENTINI et al., 1959), or to animals with hypothalamic lesions (DE WIED, 1961a). A similar lack of activity was also found in the *in vitro* assay (SAFFRAN, 1962). In man also intravenous infusion of Pitocin or highly purified oxytocin did not increase plasma concentration or urinary excretion of 17-hydroxycorticosteroids (MCDONALD and WEISE, 1956a).

The accumulated evidence, indicating that vasopressin might have a direct and possibly physiological corticotrophin-releasing action has been called into question by some controversial findings and arguments. ROYCE and SAYERS (1958) have shown that Pitressin depletes adrenal ascorbic acid and potentiates the action of ACTH in hypophysectomised rats. However, rather high doses had to be used and CASENTINI et al. (1959) could not reproduce this effect. Furthermore, even very large doses of vasopressin fail to increase corticosterone secretion in the hypophysectomised rat (HEARN et al., 1961; SMEETS and DE WIED, 1962). — Vasopressin also causes increased secretion of 17-hydroxycorticosteroids in the hypophysectomised dog (HUME and NELSON, 1957). This direct effect on the adrenals has been further substantiated by direct injection of arginine- and lysine-vasopressin *in vivo* into the blood supply perfusing the adrenals (HILTON, 1960; HILTON et al., 1959, 1960; ANDERSEN and EGDAHL, 1964). Oxytocin was inactive in this test. Since this direct effect of vasopressin on the adrenals occurs only in a limited number of species, some results obtained in recent years may be called into question, but this does not disprove the concept as a whole.

A further argument against the hypothesis that vasopressin might be involved in the physiological regulation of ACTH secretion is that although the doses which elicit ACTH secretion are small, they are still larger than those required to produce maximal antidiuresis. For example, NICHOLS and GUILLEMIN (1959) estimated that the minimal intravenous dose of lysine-vasopressin that would produce ACTH release was more than 3000 times the amount necessary to produce maximal antidiuresis in the dog. These figures may be misleading, for if vasopressin were liberated into the portal vessels in the median eminence, minute amounts would result in a high concentration in the portal blood reaching the adenohypophysis. GOLDMAN and LINDNER (1962) measured rat neural lobe blood flow and calculated that the concentration of vasopressin in the effluent from the neural lobe of the rat subjected to stress increased 300-fold over the resting level to a concentration of the order of about 2 units per ml of neural lobe blood. They also calculated that to achieve concentration levels of this magnitude by peripheral i.v. injection it would be necessary to administer rather heroic doses: in a normal rat, 80 mU for the basal state and 28 units for extreme stress. The first dose is well within the range provoking ACTH secretion, the second is lethal.

Experimentally also it has been shown that very low doses of vasopressin can be effective. KWAAN and BARTELSTONE (1959) obtained enhanced adrenal 17-hydroxycorticosteroid secretion in conscious dogs after the injection of only 2 mU highly purified arginine-vasopressin into the third ventricle. And as shown by GRINDELAND et al. (1962) vasopressin in amounts as low as 0.001 mU, a dose which does not produce antidiuresis, causes ACTH release when injected directly into the arterial supply of an ACTH-secreting pituitary tumor transplanted to the hind leg of hypophysectomised rats. An even more convincing answer to criticism of the large doses of vasopressin needed by the parenteral route was obtained by GAVAZZI et al. (1964) who injected synthetic lysine-vasopressin directly into the carotid artery of dexamethasone-blocked rats. The threshold dose was 2.5 mU per 100 g body weight, which is about 10 times less than the dose required by i.v. injection.

To evaluate the site of action of vasopressin HEDGE et al. (1966) injected synthetic lysine-vasopressin or porcine pituitary extract into the median eminence or into the pituitary gland of dexamethasone-blocked rats. The doses were below the minimal dose capable of eliciting an increase in adrenal secretion of corticosterone after i.v. injection. Vasopressin provoked marked release of ACTH when it was placed in the median eminence of the hypothalamus, as did the pituitary extract. When the two substances were tested by intra-adenohypophysial injection, the vasopressin caused much less ACTH release and the extract caused more ACTH release than observed after intra-hypothalamic injections. Morphine abolished the ACTH release after vasopressin injections at either site, as well as after the injection of the extract into the median eminence. However, morphine failed to abolish, or even diminish appreciably, the ACTH release observed after injection of the extract into the anterior pituitary. From these results it was concluded that the extract contained activity resembling that of a corticotrophin-releasing factor, but that vasopressin did not have such activity at the doses used. The vasopressin apparently acted directly on the hypothalamus to cause release of endogenous corticotrophin-releasing factor.

C. Synthetic Neurohypophysial Hormones and Analogues

The two mammalian vasopressins, the one with arginine the other with lysine, in position 8, have almost identical corticotrophin-releasing activity *in vitro* (SAFFRAN, 1962) as *in vivo* in pentobarbital/morphine-blocked rats (DOEPFNER et al., 1963) and in dexamethasone-blocked rats (FRASCHINI et al., 1964).

One analogue of vasopressin and one analogue of oxytocin each with substituents in position 8 have been compared with the corresponding natural hormone *in vitro* by SAFFRAN (1962). Replacement of lysine or arginine in position 8 of vasopressin by histidine reduced the activity of vasopressin tremendously. By contrast, the very low activity of oxytocin was enhanced 100 times on substituting arginine for leucine in position 8. The *in vitro* activity of Arg^8-oxytocin obtained by this modification, equals that of Arg^8-vasopressin. This is of some interest since Arg^8-oxytocin contains the side chain of Arg^8-vasopressin and the peptide ring of oxytocin, and occurs physiologically in some non-mammalian vertebrates (vasotocin). The reverse combination, i.e. a peptide which contains the peptide ring of vasopressin and the side chain of oxytocin (Phe^3-oxytocin = oxypressin), also has ACTH-releasing activity as measured by the adrenal ascorbic acid depletion method (DE WIED et al., 1961). But surprisingly enough, neither vasotocin nor oxypressin produced any significant increase in adrenal corticosteroid secretion when injected into the third ventricle in dogs (KWAAN and BARTELSTONE, 1959).

The differences in potency between vasopressin and oxytocin and some of their analogues have been elucidated by CARRARO et al. (1961) and by MARTINI et al. (1962) in dexamethasone-blocked rats, using corticosterone secretion as the criterion of activity. They showed, that Lys^8-vasopressin and its Phe^2-analogue have very high and almost equal activity, whereas oxytocin as well as its Val³- and Ile⁸-analogues are very weak ACTH releasers.

Physiological corticotrophin-releasing factor would appear to be distinct from oxytocin and vasopressin, but it resembles them closely in its physico-chemical properties (SAFFRAN et al., 1955, 1958). On analysing the amino acid composition of partially purified corticotrophin-releasing factor, SCHALLY et al. (1958) found that it had most of amino acids in common with lysine-vasopressin but contained, in addition, amounts of serine and histidine.

In this connection a detailed study by DOEPFNER et al. (1963) of synthetic neurohypophysial hormones and a number of analogues including some whose molecule has been enlarged by attaching a histidine/serine side chain to the N-terminal end is of interest. The dosage in this study was based on pressor units since comparison of the corticotrophin-releasing and pressor activities affords a measure of the specificity of such peptides. The amount of each peptide eliciting a 100% increase in plasma corticosterone (ED 100%) was arbitrarily defined as 1 CR unit (U). For convenience of comparison the values obtained (U/mg peptide) have been recalculated and are given in the table.

Corticotrophin-releasing activity and specificity of synthetic neurohypophysial hormones and some related peptides

	Rat	Pentobarbital/morphine-blocked rats*		Dexamethasone-blocked rats**	
	Pressor IU/mg	CR Activity/mg	Ratio $\frac{CR}{pressor}$ Specificity Index	CR Activity/mg	Ratio $\frac{CR}{pressor}$ Specificity Index
Arg⁸-vasopressin	300	300	1	300	1
Lys⁸-vasopressin	270	235	0.87	264	0.98
Phe²-Arg⁸-vasopressin	102	71.5	0.70		
Phe²-Lys⁸-vasopressin	55	31.3	0.57	42.6	0.78
De-Amino¹-Lys⁸-vasopressin	126			118.5	0.94
Ile³-Lys⁸-vasopressin	125			106.5	0.85
Val⁷-Lys⁸-vasopressin	0.66	2.22	0.34		
Ac-Ser-Tyr-Ser-Lys⁸-vasopress.	0.06	0.24	0.4		
(His-Ser-Cys)¹-Arg⁸-vasopressin	11	10.6	0.97		
(His-Ser-Cys)¹-Lys⁸-vasopress.	11	22.5	2.04	13.2	
(Ser-His-Cys)¹-Lys⁸-vasopress.	2	3.9	1.95		
Oxytocin	5	5.7	1.14		
(His-Ser-Cys)¹-oxytocin	0.27	0.49	1.81		

* DOEPFNER et al. (1963)
** FRASCHINI et al. (1964)

The activity of Arg⁸-vasopressin, the most potent peptide, was assigned the arbitrary value 300, and the potencies of the other peptides were related to this value. With this procedure the ratio CR/pressor activity for Arg⁸-vasopressin becomes 1. Ratios higher than 1 indicate that the peptide in question is more specific than Arg⁸-vasopressin and accordingly ratios less than 1 indicate a lower specificity. Although the three mammalian neurohypophysial hormones show considerable differences in absolute CR activity, their CR specificities are remarkably uniform. Thus, the CR activities of Arg⁸-vasopressin, Lys⁸-vasopressin and oxytocin are in the ratio 53:41:1, whereas their indices of specificity are 1.0, 0.87 and 1.14.

All the synthetic analogues mentioned in this study exhibit biological activities lower than those of the natural parent hormones from which they are derived.

However, the CR specificity of some of the analogues is higher than that of the natural hormones. In two instances (His-Ser-Cys)^1-Lys^8-vasopressin and (His-Ser-Cys)^1-oxytocin enlarging the molecule by attaching a histidine/serine side chain to the N-terminal end enhanced the CR specificity. However, the same modification applied to Arg^8-vasopressin [(His-Ser-Cys)^1-Arg^8-vasopressin] did not affect CR specificity. An N-terminal side chain comprising the same amino acid residues in reverse sequence and attached to Lys^8-vasopressin [(Ser-His-Cys)^1-Lys^8-vasopressin] brought about the same increase of specificity as the His-Ser side chain, but a greater loss of absolute CR activity. Removal of the phenolic OH group in position 2 (Phe^2-Lys^8-vasopressin and Phe^2-Arg^8-vasopressin) decreased both CR activity and specificity. (Acetyl-Ser-Tyr-Ser-Cys)^1-Lys^8-vasopressin and Val^7-Lys^8-vasopressin are very weak and have the lowest CR specificity of all the peptides investigated.

Since then four of these peptides (and, in addition, De-Amino^1-Lys^8-vasopressin and Ile^3-Lys^8-vasopressin) have been characterised by FRASCHINI et al. (1964) in dexamethasone-blocked rats, their values have been recalculated for convenience of comparison to fit in this scheme and are also presented in the table. The figures agree well, showing that the two methods of blockade used give comparable results. De-Amino^1-Lys^8-vasopressin and Ile^3-Lys^8-vasopressin have about half the absolute CR activity of Lys^8-vasopressin, but practically the same specificity.

Lys^8-vasopressin and (His-Ser-Cys)^1-Lys^8-vasopressin were also tested in dexamethasone-blocked mice (RERUP, 1964) as well as in normal and dexamethasone-blocked human subjects (CLAYTON et al., 1963, 1965). In mice the absolute potency as well as the specificity of (His-Ser-Cys)^1-Lys^8-vasopressin was found to be less than that of Lys^8-vasopressin, and in man identical effects were obtained after administration of equipressor doses of both peptides. These differences in the results obtained by the various methods in different species may stem from the experimental error of the procedures used. However, they may also be due to species differences, since the dosages in all species used were based on pressor units measured in rats.

None of the peptides reported may be structurally related to the physiological corticotrophin-releasing factor. But the figures given in the table show, that it is possible by structural modification to separate pressor and CR activity to a certain extent.

D. Clinical Application

It has been shown that natural or synthetic vasopressin as well as a non-pressor fraction from commercial extracts of posterior pituitary also stimulate corticotrophin release in man (CLAYTON et al., 1957; McDONALD et al., 1956; McDONALD and WEISE, 1956b, c). Since this is the only way of stimulating the anterior pituitary without having to stimulate a higher level directly, it has been adopted for clinical use. This CRF or vasopressin test permits evaluation of anterior pituitary responsiveness in respect to corticotrophic function and localises defects in the hypothalamo-hypophysial-adrenal axis. Several authors have made use of this test, giving Lys^8-vasopressin, Phe^2-Lys^8-vasopressin or Pitressin i.m. or by i.v. infusion and estimating plasma or urinary corticosteroid levels (GWINUP, 1965a, b; LANDON et al., 1965; BERNARD-WEIL et al., 1967; VAN DER WAL, 1965; STROTT et al., 1967).

III. Thyroid-stimulating Hormone (TSH)

Many attempts have been made to relate neurosecretory phenomena with functional alteration in the pituitary-thyroid system. In 1940 UOTILA expressed the view that external stimuli, such as cold, reaching the adenohypophysis through a hypothalamic-hypophysial connection, were capable of modifying basal TSH secretion ordinarily regulated by a humoral mechanism. During the last 25 years much work has been devoted to analysis of the nervous and humoral regulation of TSH secretion. This has been discussed in some excellent, for the most part recent reviews, the reader is referred to (D'ANGELO, 1963; BROWN-GRANT, 1966; HARRIS, 1964; MCKENZIE, 1966; PURVES, 1964; REICHLIN, 1964, 1966a).

Several investigators have succeeded in obtaining TSH-releasing material in a more or less purified state by extraction of hypothalamic or neurohypophysial tissue (GUILLEMIN, 1964; SCHALLY et al., 1966). But characterisation of this TRF, as well as elucidation of the role played by the neurohypophysial hormones themselves has been complicated by several factors: There appear to be rather pronounced species differences, unspecific or direct effects on the thyroid, interference by other hormones. Moreover, methods have been used whose specificity has not been proved.

The most frequently employed parameters are the increase of protein bound iodide (PBI) in blood, increase of plasma TSH concentration, elevation of the thyroid uptake or release of I^{131}, and changes in blood radioactivity in animals treated with I^{131} and thyroxine (ADAMS and PURVES, 1955; MCKENZIE, 1958). A further improvement of these methods has been suggested by REDDING et al. (1966a and b) who inject codeine in addition to thyroxine to obtain a better blockade of basal TSH secretion. The *in vitro* incubation of isolated pituitaries, by analogy with the method introduced and used for the measurement of CRF, has also been adopted for the analysis of TRF effects. The criterion of TSH stimulation used is TSH released in the medium, or acid phosphatase activity, this enzyme being involved in TSH biosynthesis.

A. Endogenous Neurohypophysial Hormones

Electrical stimulation of the hypothalamus in the region of the supraoptico-hypophysial tract in unanaesthetised rabbits is known to be effective in releasing neurohypophysial hormones and also results in increased thyroid activity (HARRIS and WOODS, 1958). Similar results were obtained in other species. It has also been shown that hypothalamic lesions which block TSH release, almost invariably result in atrophy of the paraventricular nucleus which is associated with the release of posterior pituitary hormones (GREER and ERWIN, 1954). A cold environment, a well-known form of stress, stimulates TSH release, whereas exposure to a hot environment inhibits it (SMITH and HOIJER, 1962). However, there is now much evidence suggesting that stresses of various kinds, whether emotional or physical, inhibit TSH secretion. This contrasts with the stimulating effect of stress due to noxious treatments on ACTH secretion which has been correlated in most instances with increased vasopressin secretion. This reciprocal relationship between TSH and ACTH secretion under the conditions of stress (HARRIS, 1955, 1956) does not favour the view that vasopressin plays an important role as a physiological TSH-releasing factor.

In rats deprived of water, a state which is known to be associated with hypersecretion of vasopressin, thyroid function is depressed, but the change observed may be atributable to an accompanying decline in food intake (REICHLIN, 1957).

If vasopressin were involved in TSH release an inverse relationship might be expected between severity of diabetes insipidus and thyroid activity. In rats with experimental diabetes insipidus produced by hypothalamic lesions, thyroid function was low, but Pitressin administered in amounts sufficient to restore water balance did not restore thyroid function (REICHLIN, 1966a; CROSSON et al., 1960). This may be interpreted as indicating that neurohypophysial deficiency and TSH deficiency are independent sequelae of the hypothalamic lesions. Even more convincing evidence that vasopressin is not involved in thyroid regulation has been obtained by GALTON et al. (1966): In rats with hereditary diabetes insipidus, thyroid function measured by various methods is normal.

A circadian rhythm of the TSH content of the pituitary of normal rats has also been reported. A peak occurs at 8 a.m. and the TSH content then declines until noon (BAKKE and LAWRENCE, 1965). This situation is the reverse of that seen with ACTH, but further work is necessary to elucidate whether or not a correlation exists.

B. Exogenous Neurohypophysial Hormones

The first evidence that the neurohypophysial hormones exerted a TSH-releasing effect was obtained by FRAJA and MARTINI (1953) who reported increased TSH blood levels after suboccipital administration of oxytocin and vasopressin in dogs. Oxytocin was more effective than vasopressin. Stimulating effects of Pitressin in the rabbit were also described relatively early (BOTTARI, 1957), but could not be confirmed later using improved methods (GARCIA et al., 1964). Using a more sensitive method based on the acute release of I^{131}-labelled compounds from the thyroid gland as determined by measurements of blood radioactivity, GARCIA et al. (1964) were able to demonstrate that neither natural nor synthetic Arg^8-vasopressin and Lys^8-vasopressin nor synthetic oxytocin provoke TSH release. However vasopressin exerted a direct action on the thyroid gland almost identical to that of TSH itself (GARCIA et al., 1964). An analogous observation had been made earlier in the dog (LIPSCOMB et al., 1961).

An interesting finding is the sensitising effect of oestrogen on male rats which renders them responsive to subsequent administration of vasopressin, so that the latter elicits thyroid stimulation (HARRIS et al., 1964). This and the inhibitory effect of cortisone on TSH secretion for example (INGBAR and FREINKEL, 1956) demonstrate the interrelationship between TSH release and steroid hormones which are regulated by other adenohypophysial hormones. Using the *in vitro* method both oxytocin and vasopressin were found by GUILLEMIN et al. (1963) to be without significant effect. In another *in vitro* procedure using slices of the bovine anterior pituitary gland, up to ten-fold increase of TSH release occurred in the presence of low concentrations (10^{-11}—10^{-9} M) of each of the neurohypophysial hormones (LA BELLA, 1964). Concentrations greater than 10^{-9} M were less effective, ineffective or even inhibitory. Vasopressin stimulated at lower concentrations than did oxytocin. In addition, direct effects on the thyroid *in vitro* have been reported. PETROVIC and HAY (1961) and PETROVIC and PORTE (1963) were able to show that the activity of thyroid tissue is enhanced if incubated together with hypothalamic or neurohypophysial tissue. This finding as well as the strong dose dependence reported by LA BELLA (1964) indicate how difficult it can be to draw firm conclusions from *in vitro* experiments.

In mice vasopressin either had no or only a very small and irregular thyroid-stimulating effect as measured by the MCKENZIE assay (BOWERS et al., 1964; WERNER et al., 1964; YAMAZAKI, 1963). Similarly only small and variable effects were observed with oxytocin (BOWERS et al., 1964; WERNER et al., 1964). Neither Pitressin nor synthetic oxytocin influenced the thyroid I^{131} release rate in normal rats, adrenalectomised rats or rats with hypothalamic lesions (CROSSON et al., 1960).

In man no effect was reported after two hours infusion with a large dose of Pitressin or oxytocin (MOSES et al., 1961). Nevertheless, a small, but significant effect was seen with a vasopressin depot preparation (MERTZ, 1959), and long-term treatment with Pitressin-tannate was reported to stimulate thyroid function (ROSNER et al., 1962).

C. Synthetic Neurohypophysial Hormones and Analogues

Data in the literature on this subject are rather scant, and there are no comparable values from different laboratories.

WERNER et al. (1964) compared Arg^8-vasopressin, Lys^8-vasopressin, Phe^2-Lys^8-vasopressin and oxytocin, using a slightly modified McKENZIE assay in mice. Oxytocin proved to be inactive, whereas the three vasopressins gave positive results. However, the response was of the more prolonged type, resembling that elicited by LATS.

The conversion ratio of free iodide^{131} to hormonal iodide^{131} after i.p. injection of Lys^8-vasopressin, Phe^2-Lys^8-vasopressin and (His-Ser-Cys)^1-Lys^8-vasopressin as well as oxytocin and Ile^8-oxytocin were reported by CROIZET et al. (1963) to be accelerated in male rats, the activities of the vasopressins increasing in that order. The His-Ser-Cys^1-analogue was the most potent. Oxytocin and Ile^8-oxytocin were equipotent, and both were more potent than Lys^8-vasopressin.

The effect of synthetic oxytocin and four analogues [Val^3-oxytocin, Nva^3-oxytocin, Phe^3-oxytocin, (Leu-Gly-Gly-Cys)^1-oxytocin] on the acid phosphatase activity of isolated rat pituitaries, incubated *in vitro*, was measured by SCHREIBER and his group (SCHREIBER et al., 1964a, b, 1965). When the pituitaries were obtained from normal rats, none of the peptides showed an effect, but using pituitaries from hypothyroid rats which have a greatly increased acid phosphatase activity, Val^3-oxytocin exerted a significant inhibitory effect. Following up this line of investigation the authors were able to demonstrate that Val^3-oxytocin also inhibited acid phosphatase activation provoked by purified bovine hypothalamic extracts which were assumed to contain natural TRF. This inhibition of TSH release has been further substantiated by direct measurement of the TSH concentration in the medium.

IV. Growth Hormone (GH)

Research on growth hormone itself, the amino acid sequence of which was evaluated quite recently by LI et al. (1966) as well as work on the factors and influences responsible for its control gained impetus only slowly over the years for various reasons: growth hormone has a high species specificity, its action is not directed towards a single gland, whose activity could be used as criterion in a biological assay, instead, it affects various metabolic processes, and these metabolic effects are mimicked, modified or antagonised by a number of other hormones.

Evidence of hypothalamic control of GH secretion has been forthcoming from experiments in which growth retardation was demonstrated as a sequel to hypothalamic lesions (HINTON and STEVENSON, 1962; REICHLIN, 1959, 1960a, b, 1961; BACH et al., 1964). However, the general conclusion that can be drawn from these studies is that impairment of growth is obtained only after large defects in the hypothalamus. Hypothalamic extracts containing GH-releasing activity have been prepared by a number of investigators (DEUBEN and MEITES, 1964; FRANZ et al., 1962; PECILE et al., 1965; MUELLER and PECILE, 1966). The estimation of GH should, for preference, be based on measurements of its effect on tibia cartilage width in normal animals. The *in vitro* procedure in which the amount of GH released into the medium is estimated, as well as experiments on animals with hypothalamic lesions were used to evaluate GH-releasing effects, since no feedback controllers of GH secretion were known which would be able to reduce or block unspecific stresses. The pituitary depletion method, a new and more sensitive method, is based on measurement of pituitary GH and its depletion in normal male recipient rats after a single intracarotid injection of the extract or hormone in question (Pecile et al., 1965; Meites and Fiel, 1965). The sensitivity and precision of GH measurements in plasma has greatly increased with the development of new immunological and radioimmunological methods (Potts et al., 1967; Glick et al., 1965). Influences on and control of growth hormone secretion as well as bioassay methods are the subject of a number of recent reviews (Reichlin, 1966b; Pecile and Müller, 1966; Fraschini et al., 1966; Knobil and Hotchkiss, 1964).

A. Endogenous Neurohypophysial Hormones

It has been reported that environmental stimuli or stressful treatments known to release vasopressin increase the number of acidophil cells in the adenohypophysis (Knigge, 1958) and the intensity of their granulation (Shanklin, 1956). Moreover, such stimuli have been found to raise the growth hormone concentration of the plasma and of the pituitary in various species including man (Glick et al., 1965; Roth et al., 1963b; Meyer and Knobil, 1967; Greenwood and Landon, 1966). Hypoglycaemia provoked by insulin has been found to be a very potent stimulus of growth hormone release in man (Roth et al., 1963a, b; Cornblath et al., 1965), monkeys (Abrams et al., 1966) as well as in rats (Müller et al., 1967; Krulich and McCann, 1966), an effect which can be reduced or abolished by pituitary stalk section (Roth et al., 1963b) or hypothalamic lesions (Abrams et al., 1966).

Elevation of plasma growth hormone concentration in man, as measured by radioimmunoassay (Roth et al., 1963a, b; Marks and Howorth, 1965), and decrease of pituitary growth hormone content as well as of the amount of GH-releasing material present in the hypothalamus, in rats (Friedman and Reichlin, 1965; Meites and Fiel, 1965) can also be brought about by starvation. Strangely enough, blood GH levels after fasting are much higher in females than in males (Unger, 1965). Fasting and food intake may be assumed to be one of the factors regulating diurnal growth hormone secretion.

It has been shown that growth failure in rats with hypothalamic lesions is roughly proportional to the degree of polyuria (Reichlin, 1960a, b). But this observation is not very conclusive since, as already mentioned lesions which impair the growth rate are of necessity relatively extensive and may influence other hypothalamic functions as well. More convincing evidence in favour of the view that vasopressin is a growth hormone releasing factor has been obtained with hereditary diabetes insipidus rats of the Brattleboro strain. The body weight and length of these diabetes insipidus rats which show complete absence of vasopressin, but only moderate reduction of oxytocin content in the hypothalamo-hypophysial region, were consistently less than for normal rats of the same age (Valtin and Schroeder, 1964; McCann et al., 1966). This could be interpreted as indicating that vasopressin plays a physiological role in growth hormone secretion. But since the weights of the adrenal and pituitary glands were lower in these rats than in healthy control rats it is difficult to rule out the possibility that other hormonal disturbances may have influenced growth.

B. Exogenous Neurohypophysial Hormones

In 1958 Del Vecchio et al., using tibial cartilage width as criterion, demonstrated that Pitressin given daily i.p. for 10 days exerted a growth hormone stimulating effect. Pitocin was ineffective, and Pitressin was also devoid of activity in hypophysectomised rats. These findings could not be confirmed by Reichlin and Brown (1961) following the same procedure. However, it was argued that they used rats whose cartilage width was already large (MARTINI, 1966). Later BERNARDIS and SKELTON (1964) using normal rats as well as rats with hypothalamic lesions, and HJALMARSON and AHRÉN (1965) using normal rats and rats whose pituitary had been transplanted to the kidney, did not observe stimulation by Pitressin. By the more sensitive pituitary GH-depletion method MÜLLER et al. (1967) obtained a rather small effect, but had to administer relatively large doses of lysine-vasopressin. Moreover, replacement therapy with Pitressin failed to restore normal growth in rats with hereditary vasopressin deficiency (McCANN et al., 1966) or with hypothalamic lesions (REICHLIN, 1960b). It has also been observed that daily treatment of normal and hypophysectomised rats with Pitressin tannate resulted in equal body weight gain in both types of rats over a period of 63 days (WEXLER, 1963). In the light of these findings it might be assumed that little if any GH-stimulating effect can be ascribed to vasopressin, at all events in the rat.

Nevertheless, more recent findings have shown that a single i.v. injection of Pitressin or Lys^8-vasopressin provokes an instant several-fold increase in plasma growth hormone concentration as measured by radioimmunoassay in monkeys (MEYER and KNOBIL, 1966). In human subjects, curiously enough only in women, a pronounced rise in plasma growth hormone concentration lasting for almost 2 h was observed using the same method (GREENWOOD and LANDON, 1966).

These findings well illustrate the need to bear in mind species differences as well as the possibility of sex differences, since sex differences have also been observed after starvation, as already mentioned (UNGER, 1965). Furthermore, as far as the sequence of events is concerned it has to be remembered that vasopressin induces hypoglycaemia (BAÏSSET et al., 1963) as well as a decrease of free fatty acids in plasma (MIRSKY, 1963) and these changes might, in turn, exert secondary effects.

V. Gonadotrophic Hormones

The two gonadotrophic hormones — luteinizing hormone (LH) and follicle-stimulating hormone (FSH) — first described as Prolan A and Prolan B by ZONDEK and ASCHHEIM (1927, 1928) and ZONDEK (1930), both act on the gonads. Their combined and separate actions on the ovaries and feedback control exerted by the ovarian steroid hormones in response to LH and FSH are well known. The influence of emotional stimuli or physical stress on this highly sensitive and well-balanced hormone system was borne out by the experience of physicians and physiologists alike. Excellent reviews on the regulation and control of gonadotrophin secretion have been published during the last few years. (EVERETT, 1964; LLOYD and WEISZ, 1966; HARRIS and CAMPBELL, 1966; DONOVAN, 1966; SAWYER et al., 1966).

Until recently no specific methods were available for estimating LH and FSH separately. However, many observations were made and indirect evidence was obtained which demonstrated or failed to demonstrate that the neurohypophysial hormones oxytocin or vasopressin stimulated the adenohypophysis to release LH and/or FSH. They will be mentioned briefly before discussing the data obtained for LH and FSH by the more or less specific bioassay methods which were developed later.

An increase in gonadotrophin excretion in the urine was observed by MARTINI et al. (1959) after i.v. injection of neurohypophysial hormones in rabbits. In the same species KAWAKAMI and SAWYER (1959) observed EEG changes of a closely similar pattern after the injection of pituitary gonadotrophin, LH, prolactin, Pitressin and Pitocin. Pitressin was less active than Pitocin. In rats whose normal cycle had been suppressed by steroid treatment SUCHOWSKY (1962) was able to reverse this effect by daily administration of synthetic oxytocin. Ovulation as a criterion of stimulation by gonadotrophic hormones, more especially LH secretion, has been used by several authors. In rabbits BRINKLEY and NALBANDOV (1963) blocked ovulation by i.v. or s.c. injection of oxytocin 4—19 min before copulation. Injections closer to or after copulation did not interfere with ovulation and did not affect normal development of the corpora lutea in those animals which did ovulate. Two papers are concerned with a very elegant technique which afforded negative results. NIKITOVITCH-WINER (1962) infused synthetic Arg^8-vasopressin directly into the pituitary of pentobarbital-blocked pre-oestrous rats, and no ovulation occurred. Using the same technique, i.e. intrapituitary infusion, but employing rabbits CAMPBELL et al. (1964) failed to induce ovulation with synthetic Lys^8-vasopressin, oxytocin or Lys-vasotocin. Similarly, in androgenised rats neither Pitressin nor Pitocin administered i.v. were able to provoke ovulation (JOHNSON, 1963). As measured by an indirect criterion of LH-release, namely the *in vitro* synthesis of progesterone by porcine (DUNCAN et al., 1961) and bovine (MARES and CASIDA, 1963) luteal tissue, oxytocin did not exert a stimulant effect. The *in vivo* secretion of progesterone by the ovary was not significantly stimulated by intrapituitary or intrahypothalamic injection of Lys^8-vasopressin or oxytocin in pregnant or pseudopregnant rabbits (ENDRÖCZI and HILLIARD, 1965). Oxytocin given by i.v. drip infusion or in the form of buccal tablets for several days to four women with amenorrhoea of long standing led to increased urinary gonadotrophin excretion, as measured by an immunological method, in two cases (WENNER, 1965).

Indirect, but positive evidence for a functional role of the neurohypophysial hormones in gonadotrophin secretion was obtained by BARNAFI and CROXATTO (1966). Orchidectomy lowered the vasopressor activity of the posterior lobe of the hypophysis in male rats, but had no effect on oxytocic activity. Ovariectomy decreased oxytocic activity, but produced no significant changes in vasopressor activity in female rats.

A. Luteinizing Hormone (LH)

The most frequently used method of estimating LH is the ovarian ascorbic acid depletion test, introduced by PARLOW (1958, 1961). It is also widely used to assay LH-releasing activity. However, its specificity has been questioned, since vasopressin was found to deplete ovarian ascorbic acid, presumably by a direct action on the ovary (McCANN and TALEISNIK, 1960). Moreover, it was shown by SAKIZ and GUILLEMIN (1963) that Arg^8-vasopressin potentiates the ovarian ascorbic acid depletion activity of a purified LH-releasing hypothalamic fraction. For evaluation of LH-releasing activity it is preferable to use rats with hypothalamic lesions or rats whose endogenous LH-secretion has been blocked by pretreatment with high doses of oestrogen (McCANN, 1962) or oestrogen and progesterone (RAMIREZ and McCANN, 1963.

The presence of LH-releasing activity in hypothalamic extracts has been demonstrated by numerous investigators, and such extracts have yielded highly purified material, which was characterised as a peptide with a molecular weight of about 1200—1400 (McCANN and DHARIWAL, 1966). As soon as the ovarian ascorbic acid depletion (OAAD) method became available, there was an upsurge of interest in possible LH-releasing effects of neurohypophysial hormones. PARLOW (1958) in the first report on his new method mentioned that oxytocin was devoid of effect, whereas Pitressin caused depletion. The inactivity of oxytocin was confirmed in normal (McCANN et al., 1960; McCANN and TALEISNIK, 1960) as well as in steroid blocked animals (RAMIREZ and McCANN, 1963). When it was shown that the depleting effect of Pitressin was not diminished by hypophysectomy (McCANN et al., 1960), this problem was investigated in greater detail by McCANN and TALEISNIK

(1960). To ascertain whether vasopressin acts directly on the ovary, Pitressin was administered by retrograde injection into the ovarial vein. The dose-response curve for ascorbic acid depletion so obtained was indistinguishable from that obtained after systemic injection, but the sensitivity was increased about tenfold. From these findings it was assumed that vasopressin acts directly on the ovary. These authors also found that vasopressin was slightly more active in adult rats than in immature rats and that synthetic Lys^8-vasopressin was about twice as potent as Arg^8-vasopressin. According to SCHALLY and BOWERS (1964), Arg^8-vasopressin was the more potent: Twice as active as Lys^8-vasopressin.

To evaluate the influence of endogenously released neurohypophysial hormones on the ovary MCCANN and TALEISNIK (1960) used stressful stimuli such as haemorrhage and nicotine, known to release vasopressin. No ascorbic acid depletion was observed. These findings as well as the observation of SCHALLY and BOWERS (1964), who showed that Lys^8-vasopressin had no LH-releasing effect when added to isolated pituitaries *in vitro*, would appear to indicate that vasopressin should not be regarded as a potent LH-releasing hormone.

B. Follicle-stimulating Hormone (FSH)

The classical procedure for the bioassay of FSH is the Steelman-Pohley method which is based on augmentation of ovarian weight in rats (STEELMAN and POHLEY, 1953). More recently a method has been devised by IGARASHI and MCCANN (1964a) based on augmentation of mouse uterine weight. This method is more sensitive but less specific.

For estimation of FSH-releasing activity *in vivo* use is made of rats whose endogenous FSH secretion has been blocked by hypothalamic lesions or by pretreatment with large doses of oestrogen and progesterone (IGARASHI and MCCANN, 1964a). An even more sensitive method is the pituitary depletion method (DAVID et al., 1965b) in which male rats are given an intracarotid injection of the extract or substance in question. The *in vitro* culture of rat pituitaries can also be used (MITTLER and MEITES, 1964).

The FSH-releasing activity of hypothalamic extracts was first demonstrated quite recently by IGARASHI and MCCANN (1964b). Their findings have been confirmed by other methods and for hypothalamic tissue from various species. In these studies neurohypophysial hormones were administered in parallel with hypothalamic extracts, in an attempt to establish or disprove identity with the unknown active substance. In steroid blocked rats up to 500 mU synthetic oxytocin or Arg^8-vasopressin failed to stimulate FSH release as revealed by measurement of plasma FSH levels (IGARASHI et al., 1964). Lys^8-vasopressin was also found to be devoid of FSH-releasing activity either *in vivo* or *in vitro* (KUROSHIMA et al., 1965). Even after intracarotid injection of as much as 100 mU Lys^8-vasopressin per rat, KUROSHIMA et al. (1966) did not observe depletion of pituitary FSH content as measured by the STEELMAN and POHLEY assay, though bovine and porcine hypothalamic extracts were effective. However, as already mentioned, investigations on FSH release have just been started and further work is needed.

VI. Prolactin

The mammary gland is assumed to be the principal target organ of prolactin in mammals. Mammary growth and lactation constitute an integral part of the reproduction process and prolactin is one of the factors involved. However, in one way or another, all the pituitary hormones or the hormones of their respective peripheral endocrine glands can or do influence mammary function. The hormonal aspects of mammary physiology (Folley, 1956; Lyons et al., 1958; Cowie and Folley, 1961) and the factors and influences regulating the secretion of prolactin (Meites et al., 1963; Meites and Nicoll, 1966; Everett, 1966) have recently been reviewed.

The suckling stimulus during lactation provokes reflex discharge of oxytocin from the neurohypophysis into the circulation. The oxytocin causes the myoepithelial elements surrounding the alveoli and finer ducts to contract and milk-ejection ensues (Petersen, 1944; Cross and Harris, 1951/1952). However, prolactin and ACTH are released at the same time. Prolactin is assumed to initiate and maintain lactation and evoke milk secretion. Since these effects are interlinked, this makes for difficulties, when an attempt is made to use them as criteria for one specific hormone. Initiation and maintenance of lactation are frequently used to demonstrate prolactin activity, but the pigeon crop sac method or one of its modifications is the classical quantitative method for the bioassay of prolactin (Riddle et al., 1933; Bates et al., 1963).

Secretion of hormones by the mammary gland itself has not been demonstrated, hence there is no feedback mechanism of the classical type between the anterior pituitary and the breast which could be made use of for suppression or blockade of external stimuli to prolactin secretion. It will be seen below that the regulation of prolactin secretion is unique, since it is the only anterior pituitary hormone which appears to be chronically inhibited by the hypothalamus in mammals. In view of this, the isolated pituitary anterior lobe (or parts of it), cultured or incubated *in vitro*, affords a very convenient and useful approach in the study of direct effects on prolactin synthesis and release (Meites et al., 1961). Generally speaking, lactation will continue as long as the suckling stimulus is applied (Bruce, 1958; Nicoll and Meites, 1959). It may thus be assumed that oxytocin as well as prolactin play a part in preventing the mammary gland from involution. The role of these two hormones and their interdependence in this activity has been studied intensively during the last few years.

It has been shown that the injection of natural or synthetic oxytocin can postpone involution of the mammary gland in normal rats or rats with hypothalamic lesions, an effect comparable with that achieved by injection of prolactin (Benson and Folley, 1956, 1957; McCann et al., 1959; Yokoyama and Ota, 1959). Pitressin was less effective, and in rats with hypothalamic lesions no correlations were observed between severity of diabetes insipidus and litter weight gain (McCann et al., 1959). It was logical to assume that oxytocin stimulated the pituitary anterior gland causing the release of prolactin. However, this postulated direct stimulatory effect of oxytocin on prolactin secretion by the anterior pituitary was called into question by Meites and Hopkins (1961a, b) who observed that oxytocin retarded mammary involution but by a direct action on the mammary gland. Furthermore, it was demonstrated that oxytocin did not initiate lactation in oestrogen-primed or pseudopregnant rabbits, whereas prolactin did. Besides, in rats pretreated with oestrogen, neither oxytocin nor vasopressin inhibited mammary gland involution or induced milk-secretion (Meites et al., 1960b; Meites, 1961, 1962). These findings were in harmony with observations by Grosvenor and Turner (1958) who obtained pituitary prolactin discharge in lactating rats after nursing but not after the i.v. injection of physiological doses of oxytocin. Only a slight effect was observed after injection of rather high doses. On the basis of histological studies in postpartum rats which were treated with oxytocin and prolactin according to various dosage schedules after removal of their litters, Meites et al. (1960a) concluded that the milk-ejecting effect of oxytocin would adequately account for oxytocin's capacity to maintain milk-secretion. This opinion found further support in the investigations of Ota et al. (1965). Their measurements of the nucleic acid and phosphoprotein content and their histological studies of the mammary gland after three days treatment of lactating rats deprived of their litters with oxytocin suggested that the hormone exerted a direct action on the mammary gland.

In studies using cultured anterior pituitary tissue able to synthesise prolactin actively *in vitro* (Meites et al., 1961), addition of vasopressin or oxytocin to the culture medium did not stimulate the synthesis or release of prolactin (Nicoll and Meites, 1962). These results were not confirmed by Gala and Reece (1963, 1965), who found enhanced prolactin release *in vitro* in response to oxytocin. Incidental to these studies which set out to answer the question of whether or not oxytocin does in fact bring about the release of prolactin from the adenohypophysis and could be considered to be a releasing factor, evidence accumulated that in mammals prolactin secretion was controlled not by a hypothalamic stimulating factor, but, just the reverse, by a prolactin-inhibiting factor (PIF). Everett (1954) had already observed continuous secretory function of the corpora lutea in rats after transplantation of the pituitary and suggested that prolactin secretion may even be promoted by isolation of the pituitary. Increased prolactin secretion was also observed in mice after pituitary transplantation, but did not occur when the hypothalamus was transplanted together with the pituitary (Montemurro and Gardner, 1961). Further, it was shown in *in vitro* studies that the addition of hypothalamic tissue to cultured anterior pituitary tissue significantly reduced the amount of prolactin synthesised and released into the medium (Pasteels, 1961; Talwalker et al., 1963; Gala and Reece, 1964).

The inhibitory activity of hypothalamic tissue on prolactin release *in vitro* was confirmed by *in vivo* experiments conducted by Grosvenor et al. (1965). These authors showed that acid extracts of bovine stalk-median eminence administered i.p. 1—2 min before nursing and ether anaesthesia inhibited the fall in prolactin concentration which follows the combined stimuli of nursing and stress.

Ratner and Meites (1964) observed that hypothalamic tissue obtained from rats after suckling no longer inhibited prolactin release when incubated together with pituitaries, whereas normal hypothalamic tissue did. They concluded that depletion of prolactin-inhibiting activity had occurred in the hypothalamus due to inhibition of PIF synthesis by the suckling stimulus. Nevertheless, Gala and Reece (1964) also using an *in vitro* system found that neither aqueous extracts of hypothalamus nor hypothalamic fragments obtained from lactating rats showed lessened prolactin-inhibiting activity: their activity was roughly the same as for non-lactating female rats. Grosvenor (1965) in similar experiments, this time *in vivo* obtained results which suggested that the acute stimuli of nursing and stress bring about the discharge of prolactin in the rat by suppressing the release of PIF from the hypothalamus. Thus we are left with cogent evidence that the stimulus of suckling and stress causes discharge of prolactin by inhibiting the release and perhaps also the synthesis of PIF. Whether the neurohypophysial hormones which are released simultaneously during suckling or stress or some other factor are involved in this mechanism will have to be elucidated by further experimentation.

References

Abrams, R. L., M. L. Parker, S. Blanco, S. Reichlin, and W. H. Daughaday: Hypothalamic regulation of growth hormone secretion. Endocrinology **78**, 605 (1966).

Acher, R.: The comparative chemistry of neurohypophysial hormones. Symp. zool. Soc. (Lond.) No. 9, 83 (1963).

ADAMS, D.D., and H.D. PURVES: A new method of assay for thyrotrophic hormone. Endocrinology **57**, 17 (1955).

ADAMS, J.H., P.M. DANIEL, and M.M.L. PRICHARD: Distribution of hypophysial portal blood in the anterior lobe of the pituitary gland. Endocrinology **75**, 120 (1964).

ANDERSEN, R.N., and R.H. EGDAHL: Effect of vasopressin on pituitary-adrenal secretion in the dog. Endocrinology **74**, 538 (1964).

ASCHOFF, J.: Gesetzmäßigkeiten der biologischen Tagesperiodik. Dtsch. med. Wschr. **88**, 1930 (1963).

BACH, L.M.N., C.P. O'BRIEN, and G.P. COOPER: Some observations concerning the hypothalamic regulation of growth and of food intake. In: Progress in Brain Research, Vol. 5: Lectures on the Diencephalon, p. 114. Ed. by W. BARGMANN and J.P. SCHADÉ. Amsterdam: Elsevier 1964.

BAÏSSET, A., LAC DANG TRAN, et P. MONTASTRUC: Mise en évidence chez le chien d'un effet hypoglycémiant de la vasopressine après ablation de l'hypophyse ou des surrénales. C.R. Acad. Sci. (Paris) **257**, 766 (1963).

BAKKE, J., and N. LAWRENCE: Circadian periodicity in thyroid stimulating hormone titer in the rat hypophysis and serum. Metabolism **14**, 841 (1965).

BARGMANN, W.: Über die neurosekretorische Verknüpfung von Hypothalamus und Neurohypophyse. Z. Zellforsch. **34**, 610 (1949).

— Das Zwischenhirn-Hypophysensystem. Berlin-Göttingen-Heidelberg: Springer 1954.

—, and E. SCHARRER: The site of origin of the hormones of the posterior pituitary. Amer. Scientist **39**, 255 (1951).

BARNAFI, L., and H. CROXATTO: Vasopressor and oxytocic activities in the posterior lobe of the pituitary gland of male and female rats following adrenalectomy and gonadectomy. Acta endocr. (Kbh.) **52**, 3 (1966).

BARRETT, M.: The effect of cortisone and hydrocortisone on the plasma levels of corticotrophin in the rat, after an acute stress. J. Pharm. Pharmacol. **13**, 20 (1961).

BATES, R.W., M.M. GARRISON, and J. CORNFIELD: An improved bioassay for prolactin using adult pigeons. Endocrinology **73**, 217 (1963).

BENSON, G.K., and S.J. FOLLEY: Oxytocin as stimulator for the release of prolactin from the anterior pituitary. Nature (Lond.) **177**, 700 (1956).

— — The effect of oxytocin on mammary gland involution in the rat. J. Endocrinology **16**, 189 (1957).

BERNARDIS, L.L., and F.R. SKELTON: Contribution to the problem of growth hormone-releasing effect of antidiuretic hormone. Growth **28**, 263 (1964).

BERNARD-WEIL, E., J. DECOURT, G. DREYFUS, M. DAVID, J. SEBAOUN, and Y. ADAM: Evaluation of hypothalamo-pituitary-adrenal function by the vasopressin (or C.R.F.) test. Proc. 2nd Int. Congr. on Hormonal Steroids 23/28th May, 1966, Milan (Ed. by L. MARTINI, F. FRASCHINI, and M. MOTTA). Int. Congr. Ser. No. 132, p. 1149. Excerpta crim. (Amst.) 1967.

BERTELLI, A., and L. MARTINI: Caduta dell'acido ascorbico surrenalico in animali trattati con ormoni postipofisari — Nota 3ª. Atti Soc. lombarda Sci. med.-biol. **7**, 430 (1952).

BOTTARI, P.M.: The concentration of thyrotropic hormone in the blood of the rabbit under different experimental conditions. Ciba Found. Colloq. Endocrinol. **11**, 52 (1957).

BOWERS, C.Y., R.W. REDDING, and A.V. SCHALLY: Effects of α- and β-melanocyte stimulating hormones and other peptides on the thyroid in mice. Endocrinology **74**, 559 (1964).

BRIGGS, F.N., and P.L. MUNSON: Studies on the mechanism of stimulation of ACTH secretion with the aid of morphine as a blocking agent. Endocrinology **57**, 205 (1955).

BRINKLEY, H.J., and A.V. NALBANDOV: Effect of oxytocin on ovulation in rabbits and rats. Endocrinology **73**, 515 (1963).

BROWN-GRANT, K.: The control of TSH Secretion. In: The pituitary gland, Vol. 2, p. 235. Ed. by G.W. HARRIS and B.T. DONOVAN. London: Butterworths 1966.

BRUCE, H.M.: Suckling stimulus and lactation. Proc. roy. Soc. B **149**, 421 (1958).

CAMPBELL, H.J., G. FEUER, and G.W. HARRIS: The effect of intrapituitary infusion of median eminence and other brain extracts on anterior pituitary gonadotrophic secretion. J. Physiol. (Lond.) **170**, 474 (1964).

CARRARO, A., F. CLEMENTI, F. FRASCHINI, L. MARTINI, and E. MULLER: Neurohumoral control of the anterior pituitary gland. Proc. Sci. Soc. Bosnia and Herzegovina **1**, 123 (1961).

CASENTINI, S., A. DE POLI, S. HUKOVIC, and L. MARTINI: Studies on the control of corticotrophin release. Endocrinology **64**, 483 (1959).

CAVALLERO, C., E. DOVA, and L. ROSSI: Antidiuretic activity in the neurohypophysis of rats after adrenalectomy and replacement therapy. J. Endocr. **10**, 228 (1954).

CHAUVET, J., and R. ACHER: Influence de la vasopressine sur la sécrétion de la corticotropine (ACTH). Ann. Endocr. (Paris) **20**, 111 (1959).

Clayton, G.W., W.R. Bell, and R. Guillemin: Stimulation of ACTH-release in humans by non-pressor fraction from commercial extract of posterior pituitary. Proc. Soc. exp. Biol. (N.Y.) **96**, 777 (1957).
—, L. Librik, R.L. Gardner, and R. Guillemin: Studies on the circadian rhythm of pituitary adrenocorticotrophin release in man. J. clin. Endocr. **23**, 975 (1963).
— —, A. Horan, and L. Sussman: Effect of corticosteroid administration on vasopressin-induced adrenocorticotropin release in man. J. clin. Endocr. **25**, 1156 (1965).
Cornblath, M., M.L. Parker, S.H. Reisner, A.E. Forbes, and W.H. Daughaday: Secretion and metabolism of growth hormone in premature and full-term infants. J. clin. Endocr. **25**, 209 (1965).
Courrier, R., et L. Zizine: Sur la distribution de la cortisone marquée chez le lapin. C.R. Acad. Sci. (Paris) **242**, 315 (1956).
Cowie, A.T., and S.J. Folley: The mammary gland and lactation. In: Sex and Internal Secretions. 3rd ed., Vol. 1, p. 590. Ed. by W.C. Young. Baltimore/Maryland: Williams and Wilkins 1961.
Croizet, M., P. Blanquet, C. Vrignaud, A. Brandrick, et G. Meyniel: A propos de l'action thyréostimulante de quelques hormones synthétiques posthypophysaires. C.R. Soc. Biol. (Paris) **157**, 1264 (1963).
Cross, B.A., and G.W. Harris: The role of the neurohypophysis in the milk-ejection reflex. J. Endocr. **8**, 148 (1951/52).
Crosson, J., J. Falch, and S. Reichlin: Failure to demonstrate TSH-releasing activity of Pitressin and oxytocin. Endocrinology **66**, 777 (1960).
Daily, W.J.R., and W.F. Ganong: The effect of ventral hypothalamic lesions on sodium and potassium metabolism in the dog. Endocrinology **62**, 442 (1958).
D'Angelo, S.A.: Central nervous regulation of the secretion and release of thyroid stimulating hormone. In: Advances in Neuroendocrinology, p. 158. Ed. by A.V. Nalbandov. Urbana, Illinois: Univ. of Illinois Press 1963.
Daughaday, W.H.: Steroid protein interactions. Physiol. Rev. **39**, 885 (1959).
Dávid, M.A., L. Csernay, F.A. László, and K. Kovács: Hypophysial blood flow in rats after destruction of the pituitary stalk. Endocrinology **77**, 183 (1965a).
—, F. Fraschini, and L. Martini: An in vivo method for evaluating the hypothalamic follicle stimulating hormone releasing factor. Experientia (Basel) **21**, 483 (1965b).
Dear, W.E., and R. Guillemin: Adrenal sensitivity to ACTH as a function of time after hypothalamic lesion and after hypophysectomy. Proc. Soc. exp. Biol. (N.Y.) **103**, 356 (1960).
Deuben, R.R., and J. Meites: Stimulation of pituitary growth hormone release by a hypothalamic extract *in vitro*. Endocrinology **74**, 408 (1964).
Doepfner, W., E. Stürmer, and B. Berde: On the corticotrophin-releasing activity of synthetic neurohypophysial hormones and some related peptides. Endocrinology **72**, 897 (1963).
Donovan, B.T.: The regulation of the secretion of follicle-stimulating hormone. In: The pituitary gland, Vol. 2, p. 49. Ed. by G.W. Harris and B.T. Donovan. London: Butterworths 1966.
Duncan, G.W., A.M. Bowerman, L.L. Anderson, W.R. Hearn, and R.M. Melampy: Factors influencing *in vitro* synthesis of progesterone. Endocrinology **68**, 199 (1961).
Dyke, H.B. van, B.F. Chow, R.O. Greep, and A. Rothen: The isolation of a protein from the pars neuralis of the ox pituitary with constant oxytocic, pressor and diuresis-inhibiting activities. J. Pharmacol. exp. Ther. **74**, 190 (1942).
Endröczi, E., and J. Hilliard: Luteinizing hormone releasing activity in different parts of rabbit and dog brain. Endocrinology **77**, 667 (1965).
Eser, S., et U. Sipahioglu: Action des extraits posthypophysaires sur le système hypophyse antérieure corticosurrénale. La Sem. Hôp. **27**, 3570 (1951).
Everett, J.W.: Luteotrophic function of autografts of the rat hypophysis. Endocrinology **54**, 685 (1954).
— Central neural control of reproductive functions of the adenohypophysis. Physiol. Rev. **44**, 373 (1964).
— The control of the secretion of prolactin. In: The pituitary gland, Vol. 2, p. 166. Ed. by G.W. Harris and B.T. Donovan. London: Butterworths 1966.
Folley, S.J.: The physiology and biochemistry of lactation. Springfield, Illionois: Thomas 1956.
Fortier, C.: Dual control of adrenocorticotrophin release. Endocrinology **49**, 782 (1951).
Fraja, A., e L. Martini: Alcune osservazioni sul passaggio in circolo dell'ormone tireotropo. Arch. int. pharmacodyn. **93**, 167 (1953).
Franz, J., C.H. Haselbach, and O. Libert: Studies of the effect of hypothalamic extracts on somatotrophic pituitary function. Acta endocr. **41**, 336 (1962).

Fraschini, F., G. Mangili, L. Martini, and M. Motta: Neurohypophysial principles and anterior pituitary function. Proc. 2nd Int. Pharmacol. Meeting, Prague 1963, Vol. 10. In: Oxytocin, vasopressin and their structural analogues, p. 75. Ed. by J. Rudinger. Pergamon Press 1964.
—, M. Motta, and L. Martini: Methods for the evaluation of hypothalamic hypophysiotropic principles. In: Methods in Drug Evaluation, p. 424. Ed. by P. Mantegazza and F. Piccinini. Amsterdam: North-Holland Publ. Co. 1966.
Friedman, R.C., and S. Reichlin: Growth hormone content of the pituitary gland of starved rats. Endocrinology **76**, 787 (1965).
Gala, R.R., and R.P. Reece: Effect of neurohumors on lactogen (LTH) production by the anterior pituitary *in vitro*. Fed. Proc. **22**, 506 (1963).
— — Influence of hypothalamic fragments and extracts on lactogen production *in vitro*. Proc. Soc. exp. Biol. (N.Y.) **117**, 833 (1964).
— — Influence of neurohurmors on anterior pituitary lactogen production *in vitro*. Proc. Soc. exp. Biol. (N.Y.) **120**, 220 (1965).
Galicich, J.H., F. Halberg, L.A. French, and F. Ungar: Effect of cerebral ablation on a circadian pituitary adrenocorticotropic rhythm in C mice. Endocrinology **76**, 895 (1965).
Galton, V.A., H. Valtin, and D.G. Johnson: Thyroid function in the absence of vasopressin. Endocrinology **78**, 1224 (1966).
Ganong, W.F., B.L. Wise, R. Shackleford, A.T. Boryczaka, and B. Zipf: Site at which α-ethyltryptamine act to inhibit the secretion of ACTH. Endocrinology **76**, 526 (1965).
Garcia, J., G.W. Harris, and W.J. Schindler: Vasopressin and thyroid function in the rabbit. J. Physiol. (Lond.) **170**, 487 (1964).
Gavazzi, G., G. Mangili, L. Martini, and M. Motta: Role of vasopressin in ACTH release. In: Major problems in neuroendocrinology, p. 196. Ed. by E. Bajusz and G. Jasmin. Basel/New York: S. Karger 1964.
Glick, S.M., J. Roth, R.S. Yalow, and S.A. Berson: The regulation of growth hormone secretion. Recent Progr. Hormone Res. **21**, 241 (1965).
Goldman, H., M. Alpert, S. Levine, and A. Wetzel: Production of persistent diabetes insipidus and panhypopituitarism in rats. Endocrinology **71**, 36 (1962).
—, and L. Lindner: Antidiuretic hormone concentration in blood perfusing the adenohypophysis. Experientia (Basel) **18**, 279 (1962).
Gray, W.D., and P.L. Munson: The rapidity of the adrenocorticotropic response of the pituitary to the intravenous administration of histamine. Endocrinology **48**, 471 (1951).
Green, J.D., and G.W. Harris: The neurovascular link between the neurohypophysis and adenohypophysis. J. Endocr. **5**, 136 (1947).
Greenwood, F.C., and J. Landon: Growth hormone secretion in response to stress in man. Nature (Lond.) **210**, 540 (1966).
Greer, M.A., and H. Erwin: The location of the hypothalamic area controlling the secretion of thyrotropin by the pituitary. J. clin. Invest. **33**, 938 (1954).
Grindeland, R.E., F.E. Wherry, and E. Anderson: Vasopressin and ACTH release. Proc. Soc. exp. Biol. (N.Y.) **110**, 377 (1962).
Groot, J. de: Neurosecretion in experimental conditions. Anat. Rec. **127**, 201 (1957).
—, and J.E. Hartfield: Quantitative changes in rat pituitary neurosecretory material in altered adrenocortical function. Acta neuroveg. (Wien) **22**, 177 (1961).
Grosvenor, C.E.: Effect of nursing and stress upon prolactin-inhibiting activity of the rat hypothalamus. Endocrinology **77**, 1037 (1965).
—, S.M. McCann, and R. Nallar: Inhibition of nursing-induced and stress-induced fall in pituitary prolactin concentration in lactating rats by injection of acid extracts of bovine hypothalamus. Endocrinology **76**, 883 (1965).
—, and C.W. Turner: Effects of oxytocin and blocking agents upon pituitary lactogen discharge in lactating rats. Proc. Soc. exp. Biol. (N.Y.) **97**, 463 (1958).
Guillemin, R.: A re-evaluation of acetylcholine, adrenaline, nor-adrenaline and histamine as possible mediators of the pituitary adrenocorticotrophic activation by stress. Endocrinology **56**, 248 (1955).
— Hypothalamic factors releasing pituitary hormones. Recent Progr. Hormone Res. **20**, 89 (1964).
—, W.E. Dear, B. Nichols jr., and H.S. Lipscomb: ACTH releasing activity *in vivo* of a CRF preparation and lysine vasopressin. Proc. Soc. exp. Biol. (N.Y.) **101**, 107 (1959a).
— —, and R.A. Liebelt: Nychthermal variations in plasma free corticosteroid levels of the rat. Proc. Soc. exp. Biol. (N.Y.) **101, 394** (1959b).
—, W.R. Hearn, W.R. Cheek, and D.E. Housholder: Control of corticotrophin release: Further studies with *in vitro* methods. Endocrinology **60**, 488 (1957).
—, and B. Rosenberg: Humoral hypothalamic control of anterior pituitary: a study with combined tissue cultures. Endocrinology **57**, 599 (1955).

GUILLEMIN. R., and A.V. SCHALLY: Re-evaluation of a technique of pituitary incubation *in vitro* as an assay for corticotropin releasing factor. Endocrinology **65**, 555 (1959).

—, E. YAMAZAKI, D.A. GARD, M. JUTISZ, and E. SAKIZ: *In vitro* secretion of thyrotropin (TSH): stimulation by a hypothalamic peptide (TRF). Endocrinology **73**, 564 (1963).

GWINUP, G.: Test for pituitary function using vasopressin. Lancet **II**, 572 (1965a).

— Studies on the mechanism of vasopressin-induced steroid secretion in man. Metabolism **14**, 1282 (1965b).

HALBERG, F., P.G. ALBRECHT, and J.J. BITTNER: Corticosterone rhythm of mouse adrenal in relation to serum corticosterone and sampling. Amer. J. Physiol. **197**, 1083 (1959).

—, C.P. BARNUM, R.H. SILBER, and J.J. BITTNER: 24-hour-rhythms at several levels of integration in mice on different lighting regimens. Proc. Soc. exp. Biol. (N.Y.) **97**, 897 (1958).

—, R. FRANK, J. HARNER, H. MATTHEWS, H. AAKER, H. GRAVEM, and J. MELBY: The adrenal cycle in men on different schedules of motor and mental activity. Experientia (Basel) **17**, 282 (1961).

HARRIS, G.W.: Neural control of the pituitary gland. Physiol. Rev. **28**, 139 (1948).

— The reciprocal relationship between the thyroid and adrenocortical responses to stress. Ciba Found. Colloq. Endocrinol. **8**, 531 (1955).

— Hypothalamic regulation of anterior pituitary secretion. Schweiz. med. Wschr. **86**, 1252 (1956).

— A summary of some recent research on brain-thyroid relationships. In: Brain-thyroid relationships, p. 3. Ed. by M.P. CAMERON, M.A. and M. O'Connor, B.A. London: J. and A. Churchill, Ltd. 1964.

—, and H.J. CAMPBELL: The regulation of the secretion of luteinizing hormone and ovulation. In: The pituitary gland, Vol. 2, p. 99. Ed. by G.W. HARRIS and B.T. DONOVAN. London: Butterworths 1966.

—, and B.T. DONOVAN: The pituitary gland, Vol. 2. London: Butterworths 1966.

—, S. LEVINE, and W.J. SCHINDLER: Vasopressin and thyroid function in the rat: The effect of oestrogens. J. Physiol. (Lond.) **170**, 516 (1964).

—, and J.W. WOODS: The effect of electrical stimulation of the hypothalamus or pituitary gland on thyroid activity. J. Physiol. (Lond.) **143**, 246 (1958).

HEARN, W.R., E.J. WEBER, P.W. RANDOLPH, and N.E. BARKS: Corticotropin releasing activity of synthetic lysine vasopressin. Proc. Soc. exp. Biol. (N.Y.) **107**, 515 (1961).

HEDGE, G.A., M.B. YATES, R. MARCUS, and F.E. YATES: Site of action of vasopressin in causing corticotropin release. Endocrinology **79**, 328 (1966).

HELLER, H., and K. LEDERIS: Maturation of the hypothalamo-neurohypophysial system. J. Physiol. (Lond.) **147**, 299 (1959).

HILD, W., u. G. ZETLER: Über das Vorkommen der Hypophysenhinterlappenhormone im Zwischenhirn. Arch. exp. Path. Pharmakol. **213**, 139 (1951).

— — Neurosekretion und Hormonvorkommen im Zwischenhirn des Menschen. Klin. Wschr **30**, 433 (1952).

— — Experimenteller Beweis für die Entstehung der sog. Hypophysenhinterlappenwirkstoffe im Hypothalamus. Pflügers Arch. ges. Physiol. **257**, 169 (1953a).

— — Über die Funktion des Neurosekrets im Zwischenhirn-Neurohypophysensystem als Trägersubstanz für Vasopressin, Adiuretin und Oxytocin. Z. ges. exp. Med. **120**, 236 (1953b).

HILTON, J.G.: Adrenocorticotropic action of antidiuretic hormone. Circulation **21**, 1038 (1960).

—, L.F. SCIAN, C.D. WESTERMANN, and O.R. KRUESI: Direct stimulation of adrenocortical secretion by synthetic vasopressin. Proc. Soc. exp. Biol. (N.Y.) **100**, 523 (1959).

— — —, J. NAKANO, and O.R. KRUESI: Vasopressin stimulation of the isolated adrenal glands: Nature and mechanism of hydrocortisone secretion. Endocrinology **67**, 298 (1960).

HINTON, G.G., and J.A.F. STEVENSON: The effect of hypothalamic lesions on growth. Canad. J. Biochem. **40**, 1239 (1962).

HJALMARSON, A., and K. AHRÉN: Studies on growth hormone secretion in rats with the hypophysis autotransplanted to the kidney capsule. Acta endocr. (Kbh.) **49**, 17 (1965).

HUME, D.M., and D. NELSON: Abstr. 39th Endocrine Soc. Meeting, 98 (1957), quoted by SMEETS and DE WIED, 1962.

IGARASHI, M., and S.M. MCCANN: A new sensitive bio-assay for follicle-stimulating hormone (FSH). Endocrinology **74**, 440 (1964a).

— — A hypothalamic follicle stimulating hormone-releasing factor. Endocrinology **74**, 446 (1964b).

—, R. NALLAR, and S.M. MCCANN: Further studies on the follicle-stimulating hormone-releasing action of hypothalamic extracts. Endocrinology **75**, 901 (1964).

INGBAR, S.H., and N. FREINKEL: ACTH, cortisone and the metabolism of iodine. Metabolism **5**, 652 (1956).

JAILER, J.W.: The maturation of the pituitary-adrenal axis in the newborn rat. Endocrinology **46**, 420 (1950).

JOHNSON, D.C.: Hypophysial LH release in androgenized female rats after administration of sheep brain extracts. Endocrinology **72**, 832 (1963).
KAWAI, A., and F.E. YATES: Interference with feedback inhibition of adrenocorticotropin release by protein binding of corticosterone. Endocrinology **79**, 1040 (1966).
KAWAKAMI, M., and C.H. SAWYER: Induction of behavioral and electroencephalographic changes in the rabbit by hormone administration or brain stimulation. Endocrinology **65**, 631 (1959).
KENDALL, J.W.: Quantitative and temporal studies on effect of dexamethasone on corticosterone secretion in the rat. Proc. Soc. exp. Biol. (N.Y.) **107**, 926 (1961).
KENNEDY, G.C., H. LIPSCOMB, and P. HAGUE: Plasma corticosterone in rats with experimental diabetes insipidus. J. Endocr. **27**, 345 (1963).
KNIGGE, K.M.: Cytology and growth hormone content of rat's pituitary gland following thyroidectomy and stress. Anat. Rec. **130**, 543 (1958).
KNOBIL, E., and J. HOTCHKISS: Growth hormone. Ann. Rev. Physiol. **26**, 47 (1964).
KÖNIG, A., u. A. MEYER: Tagesperiodische Schwankungen der Urinausscheidung und des Adiuretingehaltes im Hypophysenhinterlappen männlicher Wistar-Ratten. Acta Endocr. **54**, 275 (1967).
KOVÁCS, K., M.A. DÁVID, and F.A. LÁSZLÓ: Adrenocortical function in rats after lesion of the pituitary stalk. J. endocr. (Kbh.) **25**, 9 (1962).
KRULICH, L., and S.M. MCCANN: Effect of alterations in blood sugar on pituitary growth hormone content in the rat. Endocrinology **78**, 759 (1966).
KUROSHIMA, A., A. ARIMURA, T. SAITO, Y. ISHIDA, C.Y. BOWERS, and A.V. SCHALLY: Depletion of pituitary follicle-stimulating hormone by beef and pig hypothalamic extracts. Endocrinology **78**, 1105 (1966).
—, Y. ISHIDA, C.Y. BOWERS, and A.V. SCHALLY: Stimulation of release of follicle-stimulating hormone by hypothalamic extracts *in vitro* and *in vivo*. Endocrinology **76**, 614 (1965).
KWAAN, H.C., and H.J. BARTELSTONE: Corticotropin release following injections of minute doses of arginine vasopressin into the third ventricle of the dog. Endocrinology **65**, 982 (1959).
LABELLA, F.S.: Release of thyrotropin *in vivo* and *in vitro* by synthetic neurohypophysial hormones. Canad. J. Physiol. Pharmacol. **42**, 75 (1964).
LANDON, J., V.H.T. JAMES, and D.J. STOKER: Plasma-cortisol response to lysine-vasopressin. Comparison with other tests of human pituitary-adrenocortical function. Lancet, 1156 (1965).
LÁSZLÓ, F.A., and D. DE WIED: Pituitary-adrenal system in rats bearing lesions in the pituitary stalk. Endocrinology **79**, 547 (1966a).
— — Antidiuretic hormone content of the hypothalamo-neurohypophysial system and urinary excretion of antidiuretic hormone in rats during the development of diabetes insipidus after lesions in the pituitary stalk. J. Endocr. **36**, 125 (1966b).
LEEMANN, S.E., D.W. GLENISTER, and F.E. YATES: Characterization of a calf hypothalamic extract with adrenocorticotropin-releasing properties. Evidence for a central nervous system site for corticosteroid inhibition of adrenocorticotropin release. Endocrinology **70**, 249 (1962).
LEVINE, S., M. ALPERT, and G.W. LEWIS: Infantile experience and the maturation of the pituitary-adrenal axis. Science **126**, 1347 (1957).
—, and G.W. LEWIS: Critical period for effects of infantile experience on maturation of stress response. Science **129**, 42 (1959).
LEWIS, P.R., and M.C. LOBBAN: The effect of exercise on diurnal excretory rhythms in man. J. Physiol. (Lond.) **143**, 8P (1958).
LI, C.H., W.K. LIU, and J.S. DIXON: Human pituitary growth hormone. XII. The amino acid sequence of the hormone. J. Amer. chem. Soc. **88**, 2050 (1966).
LIPSCOMB, H., D. HATHAWAY, and D. GARD: Direct effect of vasopressin on thyroid. Clin. Res. **9**, 20 (1961).
LLOYD, C.W., and J. WEISZ: Some aspects of reproductive physiology. Ann. Rev. Physiol. **28**, 267 (1966).
LONG, C.N.H.: Regulation of ACTH secretion. Recent Progr. Hormone Res. **7**, 75 (1952).
LYONS, W.R., C.H. LI, and R.E. JOHNSON: The hormonal control of mammary growth and lactation. Recent Progr. Hormone Res. **14**, 219 (1958).
MALANDRA, B., e S. CORBETTA: La sostanza Gomori-positiva della neuroipofisi del ratto dopo surrenectomia e trattamento con corticoidi surrenali e sale. Z. Zellforsch. **39**, 318 (1953).
MARES, S.E., and L.E. CASIDA: Effect of exogenous oxytocin on the progestogen content of the bovine corpus luteum. Endocrinology **72**, 78 (1963).
MARKS, V., and N. HOWORTH: Plasma growth-hormone levels in chronic starvation in man. Nature (Lond.) **208**, 686 (1965).

MARTINI, L.: Neurohypophysis and anterior pituitary activity. In: The pituitary gland, Vol. 3, p. 535. Ed. by G.W. HARRIS and B.T. DONOVAN. London: Butterworths 1966.
—, and W.F. GANONG: Neuroendocrinology, Vol. 1. New York and London: Academic Press 1966.
—, L. MIRA, A. PECILE, and S. SAITO: Neurohypophysial hormones and release of gonadotrophins. J. Endocr. **18**, 245 (1959).
—, A. PECILE, G. GIULIANI, F. FRASCHINI, and A. CARRARO: Neurohumoral control of the anterior pituitary gland. 8. Symposium der Deutschen Gesellschaft für Endokrinologie, München, 1.—3. 3. 1961 über „Gewebs- und Neurohormone, Physiologie des Melanophorenhormons", p. 117, 1962.
MCCANN, S.M.: The ACTH-releasing activity of extracts of the posterior lobe of the pituitary *in vivo*. Endocrinology **60**, 664 (1957).
— A hypothalamic luteinizing-hormone-releasing factor. Amer. J. Physiol. **202**, 395 (1962).
—, J. ANTUNES-RODRIGUES, R. NALLAR, and H. VALTIN: Pituitary-adrenal function in the absence of vasopressin. Endocrinology **79**, 1058 (1966).
—, and J.R. BROBECK: Evidence for a role of the supraoptico-hypophysial system in regulation of adrenocorticotrophin secretion. Proc. Soc. exp. Biol. (N.Y.) **87**, 318 (1954).
—, and A.P.S. DHARIWAL: Hypothalamic releasing factors and the neurovascular link between the brain and the anterior pituitary. Neuroendocrinology, Vol. 1. 261 (1966).
—, and A. FRUIT: Effect of synthetic vasopressin on release of adrenocorticotrophin in rats with hypothalamic lesions. Proc. Soc. exp. Biol. (N.Y.) **96**, 566 (1957).
— —, and B.D. FULFORD: Studies on the loci of action of cortical hormones in inhibiting the release of adrenocorticotrophin. Endocrinology **63**, 29 (1958).
—, and P. HABERLAND: Further studies on the regulation of pituitary ACTH in rats with hypothalamic lesions. Endocrinology **66**, 217 (1960).
—, R. MACK, and C. GALE: The possible role of oxytocin in stimulating the release of prolactin. Endocrinology **64**, 870 (1959).
—, and S. TALEISNIK: Effect of luteinizing hormone and vasopressin on ovarian ascorbic acid. Amer. J. Physiol. **199**, 847 (1960).
— —, and H.M. FRIEDMAN: LH-releasing activity in hypothalamic extracts. Proc. Soc. exp. Biol. (N.Y.) **104**, 432 (1960).
MCDONALD, R.K., H.N. WAGNER, and V.K. WEISE: Relationship between endogenous antidiuretic hormone activity and ACTH release in man. Proc. Soc. exp. Biol. (N.Y.) **96**, 652 (1957).
—, and V.K. WEISE: Effect of oxytocin on adrenocortical activity in man. Proc. Soc. exp. Biol. (N.Y.) **92**, 109 (1956a).
— — Effect of Pitressin on adrenocortical activity in man. Proc. Soc. exp. Biol. (N.Y.) **92**, 107 (1956b).
— — Effect of arginine-vasopressin and lysine-vasopressin on plasma 17-hydroxycorticosteroid levels in man. Proc. Soc. exp. Biol. (N.Y.) **92**, 481 (1956c).
— —, and R.W. PATRICK: Effect of synthetic lysine-vasopressin on plasma hydrocortisone levels in man. Proc. Soc. exp. Biol. (N.Y.) **93**, 348 (1956).
MCKENZIE, J.M.: The bioassay of thyrotropin in serum. Endocrinology **63**, 372 (1958).
— The thyroid-activating hormones and hypothalamic control. Res. Publ. Ass. nerv. ment. Dis. **43**, 47 (1966).
MCSHAN, W.H., and M.W. HARTLEY: Production, storage and release of anterior pituitary hormones. Ergebn. Physiol. **56**, 264 (1965).
MEITES, J.: Pharmacological control of prolactin secretion and lactation. Biochem. Pharmacol. **8**, 27 (1961).
— Pharmacological control of prolactin secretion and lactation. Proc. 1st Int. Pharmacol. Meeting August 22—25, 1961, Vol. 1, p. 151. Ed. by R. GUILLEMIN and P. LINDGREN. Oxford: Pergamon Press 1962.
—, and N.J. FIEL: Effect of starvation on hypothalamic content of somatotropin releasing factor and pituitary growth hormone content. Endocrinology **77**, 455 (1965).
—, and T.F. HOPKINS: Retardation of mammary involution in hypophysectomized, postpartum rats by oxytocin. Fed. Proc. **20**, 186 (1961a).
— — Mechanism of action of oxytocin in retarding mammary involution. Study in hypophysectomized rats. J. Endocr. **22**, 207 (1961b).
—, R.H. KAHN, and C.S. NICOLL: Prolactin production by rat pituitary *in vitro*. Proc. Soc. exp. Biol. (N.Y.) **108**, 440 (1961).
—, and C.S. NICOLL: Adenohypophysis: Prolactin. Ann. Rev. Physiol. **28**, 57 (1966).
— —, and P.K. TALWALKER: Local action of oxytocin on mammary glands of postpartum rats after litter removal. Proc. Soc. exp. Biol. (N.Y.) **103**, 118 (1960a).
— — — The central nervous system and the secretion and release of prolactin. In: Advances in Neuroendocrinology, p. 238. Ed. by A.V. NALBANDOV. Urbana, Illinois: Univ. of Illinois Press 1963.

MEITES, J., P.K. TALWALKER, and C.S. NICOLL: Failure of oxytocin to initiate mammar seycretion in rabbits or rats. Proc. Soc. exp. Biol. (N.Y.) **105**, 467 (1960b).
MERTZ, D.P.: Über den Einfluß von Pitressin und Oxytocin auf die Schilddrüsenfunktion. Z. klin. Med. **156**, 138 (1959).
MEYER, V., and E. KNOBIL: Stimulation of growth hormone secretion by vasopressin in the rhesus monkey. Endocrinology **79**, 1016 (1966).
— — Growth hormone secretion in the unanesthetized rhesus monkey in response to noxious stimuli. Endocrinology **80**, 163 (1967).
MILKOVIC, K., and S. MILKOVIC: Reactiveness of the postnatal period in some laboratory mammals. Endokrinologie **37**, 301 (1959).
MILLS, J.N.: Diurnal rhythm in urine flow. J. Physiol. (Lond.) **113**, 528 (1951).
MIRSKY, I.A.: Effect of oxytocin, vasopressin, and related peptides on plasma free fatty acids. Amer. J. Physiol. **204**, 842 (1963).
—, M. STEIN, and G. PAULISCH: The secretion of an antidiuretic substance into the circulation of adrenalectomized and hypophysectomized rats exposed to noxious stimuli. Endocrinology **55**, 28 (1954).
MITTLER, J.C., and J. MEITES: *In vitro* stimulation of pituitary follicle-stimulating-hormone release by hypothalamic extract. Proc. Soc. exp. Biol. (N.Y.) **117**, 309 (1964).
MONTEMURRO, D.G., and W.U. GARDNER: The effect of subcutaneous transplants of hypothalamus and pituitary gland on the estrous cycle of the mouse. Fed. Proc. **20**, 188 (1961).
MOSES, A.M.: Adrenal-neurohypophysial relationships in the dehydrated rat. Endocrinology **73**, 230 (1963).
—, F. LOBOVSKY, R.B. CHODOS, and C.W. LLOYD: Failure of vasopressin or oxytocin to stimulate thyroid function in the normal male. J. clin. Endocr. **21**, 1543 (1961).
MÜLLER, E.E., and A. PECILE: Growth hormone-releasing activity in the hypothalamus of primates. Endocrinology **79**, 448 (1966).
—, T. SAITO, A. ARIMURA, and A.V. SCHALLY: Hypoglycemia, stress and growth hormone release. Blockade of growth hormone release by drugs acting on the central nervous system. Endocrinology **80**, 109 (1967).
MUNSON, P.L.: Pharmacological control of the secretion of ACTH. Proc. 1st Int. Pharmacological Meeting, Stockholm 1961, Vol. 1, p. 11. Oxford: Pergamon Press 1962.
— Pharmacology of neuroendocrine blocking agents. In: Advances in Neuroendocrinology, p. 427. Ed. by A.V. NALBANDOV. Urbana: University of Illinois Press 1963.
—, and F.N. BRIGGS: The mechanism of stimulation of ACTHs ecretion. Recent Progr. Hormone Res. **11**, 83 (1955).
NAGAREDA, C.S., and R. GAUNT: Functional relationship between the adrenal cortex and posterior pituitary. Endocrinology **48**, 560 (1951).
NALBANDOV, A.V.: Advances in Neuroendocrinology. Urbana: University of Illinois Press 1963.
NICHOLS, B.L., W. DEAR, S.W. ROBINSON, and R. GUILLEMIN: Diabetes insipidus and inhibition of stress induced ACTH-release after hypothalamic lesions. Fed. Proc. **18**, 113 (1959).
—, and R. GUILLEMIN: Endogenous and exogenous vasopressin on ACTH release. Endocrinology **64**, 914 (1959).
NICOLL, C.S., and J. MEITES: Prolongation of lactation in the rat by litter replacement. Proc. Soc. exp. Biol. (N.Y.) **101**, 81 (1959).
— — Failure of neurohypophysial hormones to influence prolactin secretion *in vitro*. Endocrinology **70**, 927 (1962).
NIKITOVITCH-WINER, M.B.: Induction of ovulation in rats by direct intrapituitary infusion of median eminence extracts. Endocrinology **70**, 350 (1962).
NOWELL, N.W.: Studies in the activitation and inhibition of adrenocorticotrophin secretion. Endocrinology **64**, 191 (1959).
ÔTA, K., Y. SHINDE, and A. YOKOYAMA: Relationship between oxytocin and prolacting secretion in maintenance of lactation in rats. Endocrinology **76**, 1 (1965).
PARLOW, A.F.: A rapid bioassay method for LH and factors stimulating LH secretion. Fed. Proc. **17**, 402 (1958).
— Bio-assay of pituitary luteinizing hormone by depletion of ovarian ascorbic acid. In: Human pituitary gonadotropins, p. 300. Ed. by A. ALBERT. Springfield/Ill.: Ch. C. Thomas 1961.
PASTÉELS, J.L.: Premiers résultats de culture combinée *in vitro* d'hypophyse et d'hypothalamus, dans le but d'en apprécier la sécrétion de prolactine. C.R. Acad. Sci. (Paris) **253**, 3074 (1961).
PECILE, A., and E.E. MUELLER: Control of growth hormone secretion. Neuroendocrinology, Vol. 1. 537 (1966).
— —, G. FALCONI, and L. MARTINI: Growth hormone-releasing activity of hypothalamic extracts at different ages. Endocrinology **77**, 241 (1965).

PERKOFF, G.T., K. EIK-NES, C.A. NUGENT, H.L. FRED, R.A. NIMER, L. RUSH, L.T. SAMUELS, and F.H. TYLER: Studies of the diurnal variation of plasma 17-hydroxycorticosteroids in man. J. clin. Endocr. **19**, 432 (1959).

PETERSEN, W.E.: Lactation. Physiol. Rev. **24**, 340 (1944).

PETROVIC, A., et D. HAY: Action directe de fragments d'hypothalamus de cobaye sur la thyroide de l'embryon de Poulet de 14 jours en culture organotypique. C.R. Acad. Sci. (Paris) **253**, 1867 (1961).

—, et A. PORTE: Nouvelles données sur l'activité thyréostimulante en culture organotypique de fragments d'hypothalamus de cobaye adulte normal. C.R. Soc. Biol. (Paris) **157**, 1051 (1963).

POPA, G.T., and U. FIELDING: A portal circulation from the pituitary to the hypothalamic region. J. Anat. (Lond.) **65**, 88 (1930).

— — Hypophysis portal vessels and their colloid accompaniment. J. Anat. (Lond.) **67**, 227 (1933).

POTTS jr., J.T., L.M. SHERWOOD, J.L.H. O'RIORDAN, and G.D. AURBACH: Radioimmunoassay of polypeptide hormones. In: Advances in internal medicine, Vol. 3, p. 183. Ed. by W. DOCK and I. SNAPPER. Year Book Medical Publishers, 1967.

PURVES, H.D.: Control of thyroid function. In: The thyroid gland, Vol. 2, p. 1. Ed. by R. PITT-RIVERS and W.R. TROTTER. London and Washington, D.C.: Butterworths 1964.

RAMIREZ, V.D., and S.M. MCCANN: A highly sensitive test for LH-releasing activity. The ovariectomized, estrogen progesterone-blocked rat. Endocrinology **73**, 193 (1963).

RASMUSSEN, A.T.: Innervation of the hypophysis. Endocrinology **23**, 263 (1938).

RATNER, A., and J. MEITES: Depletion of prolactin-inhibiting activity of rat hypothalamus by estradiol or suckling stimulus. Endocrinology **75**, 377 (1964).

REDDING, T.W., C.Y. BOWERS, and A.V. SCHALLY: The effects of morphine and other narcotics on thyroid function in mice. Acta endocr. (Kbh.) **51**, 391 (1966a).

— — — An *in vivo* assay for thyrotropin releasing factor. Endocrinology **79**, 229 (1966b).

REICHLIN, S.: The effect of dehydration, starvation, and Pitressin injections on thyroid activity in the rat. Endocrinology **60**, 470 (1957).

— Mechanism of growth failure in rats with lesion of the hypothalamus. J. Lab. clin. Med. **54**, 937 (1959).

— Thyroid function, body temperature regulation and growth in rats with hypothalamic lesions. Endocrinology **66**, 340 (1960a).

— Growth and the hypothalamus. Endocrinology **67**, 760 (1960b).

— Growth hormone content of pituitaries from rats with hypothalamic lesions. Endocrinology **69**, 225 (1961).

— Function of the hypothalamus in regulation of pituitary-thyroid activity. In: Brain-thyroid relationships, p. 17. Ed. by M.P. CAMERON, M.A., and M. O'CONNOR, B.A. London: J. and A. Churchill, Ltd. 1964.

— Control of thyrotropic hormone secretion. Neuroendocrinology, Vol. 1, 445 (1966a).

— Regulation of somatotrophic hormone secretion. In: The pituitary gland, Vol. 2, p. 270. Ed. by. G.W. HARRIS and B.T. DONOVAN. London: Butterworths 1966b.

—, and J.G. BROWN: Failure to confirm the report that Pitressin has a growth stimulating effect. Endocrinology **69**, 394 (1961).

RENNELS, E.G., and G.V. RUSSEL: Effect of electroshock on the neurohypophysis of the rat. Tex. Rep. Biol. Med. **15**, 411 (1957).

RERUP, C.: The determination of corticotrophin-releasing activity in steroid-blocked mice. Acta endocr. (Kbh.) **46**, 71 (1964).

RIDDLE, O., R.W. BATES, and S.W. DYKSHORN: The preparation, identification, and assay of prolactin — a hormone of the anterior pituitary. Amer. J. Physiol. **105**, 191 (1933).

RINFRET, A.P., and S. HANE: The adrenal ascorbic acid-depleting capacity of extracts of the infant rat pituitary gland. Endocrinology **56**, 341 (1955).

RINNE, U.K.: Neurosecretory material around the hypophysial portal vessels in the median eminence of the rat. Acta endocr. (Kbh.) **35**, Suppl. 57, 5 (1960).

—, E. KIVALO, and K. LAHTINEN: Studies on the corticotrophin releasing activity of synthetic oxytocin. Acta endocr. (Kbh.) **32**, 589 (1959).

ROSNER, J.M., A.B. HOUSSAY, and J.H. ROTMISTROVSKY: Diabetes insipidus and pituitary myxedema. Effect of Pitressin on thyroid function. J. clin. Endocr. **22**, 449 (1962).

ROTH, J., S.M. GLICK, R.S. YALOW, and S.A. BERSON: Hypoglycemia. A potent stimulus to secretion of growth hormone. Science **140**, 987 (1963a).

— — — — Secretion of human growth hormone. Physiologic and experimental modification. Metabolism **12**, 577 (1963b).

ROTHBALLER, A.B.: Changes in the rat neurohypophysis induced by painful stimuli with particular reference to neurosecretory material. Anat. Rec. **115**, 21 (1953).

ROYCE, P.C., and G. SAYERS: Extrapituitary interaction between Pitressin and ACTH. Proc. Soc. exp. Biol. (N.Y.) **98**, 70 (1958).
RUMSFELD, H.W., and J.C. PORTER: ACTH-releasing activity of bovine posterior pituitaries. Endocrinology **70**, 62 (1962).
SAFFRAN, M.: Mechanisms of adrenocortical control. Brit. med. Bull. **18**, 122 (1962).
— Hypothalamic regulation of ACTH secretion. Res. Publ. Ass. nerv. ment. Dis. **43**, 36 (1966).
—, A.V. SCHALLY, and B.G. BENFEY: Stimulation of the release of corticotropin from the adenohypophysis by a neurohypophysial factor. Endocrinology **57**, 439 (1955).
— —, M. SEGAL, and B. ZIMMERMANN: Characterization of the corticotrophin releasing factor in the neurohypophysis. 2. Int. Symposium über Neurosekretion, Lund 1957. Ed. by W. BARGMANN et al., p. 55. Berlin-Göttingen-Heidelberg: Springer 1958.
SAKIZ, E., et R. GUILLEMIN: Potentiation de l'activité biologique du facteur hypothalamique LRF d'origine bovine ou ovine par l'arginine-vasopressin de synthèse. C.R. Acad. Sic. (Paris) **259**, 237 (1963).
SAWYER, C.H., M. KAWAKAMI, and S. KANEMATSU: Neuroendocrine aspects of reproduction. Res. Publ. Ass. nerv. ment. Dis. **43**, 59 (1966).
SAYERS, G., and M.A. SAYERS: Regulatory effect of adrenocortical extract on elaboration of pituitary ACTH. Proc. Soc. exp. Biol. (N.Y.) **60**, 162 (1945).
— —, and L.A. WOODBURY: The assay of adrenocorticotrophic hormone by the adrenal ascorbic acid depletion method. Endocrinology **42**, 379 (1948).
SCHALLY, A.V., and C.Y. BOWERS: *In vitro* and *in vivo* stimulation of the release of luteinizing hormone. Endocrinology **75**, 312 (1964).
— —, and T.W. REDDING: Purification of thyrotropic hormone-releasing factor from bovine hypothalamus. Endocrinology **78**, 726 (1966).
—, M. SAFFRAN, and B. ZIMMERMANN: A corticotrophin-releasing factor. Partial purification and amino acid composition. Biochem. J. **70**, 97 (1958).
SCHAPIRO, S.: Adrenal cortical hormones and resistance to histamine stress in the infant rat. Acta endocr. (Kbh.) **48**, 249 (1965).
—, E. GELLER, and S. EIDUSON: Neonatal adrenal cortical response to stress and vasopressin. Proc. Soc. exp. Biol. (N.Y.) **109**, 937 (1961).
—, and J. KATZ: Preferential concentration of C^{14} in posterior pituitary following hydrocortisone C^{14} injection. Proc. Soc. exp. Biol. (N.Y.) **102**, 609 (1959).
SCHARRER, E.: Principles of neuroendocrine integration. Res. Publ. Ass. nerv. ment. Dis. **43**, 1 (1966).
—, and B. SCHARRER: Secretory cells within the hypothalamus. Res. Publ. Ass. nerv. ment. Dis. **20**, 170 (1940).
— — Hormones produced by neurosecretory cells. Recent Progr. Hormone Res. **10**, 183, (1954a).
— — Neurosekretion. In: Handbuch der mikroskopischen Anatomie des Menschen. Hrsg. von W. VON MÖLLENDORF u. W. BARGMANN. Berlin-Göttingen-Heidelberg: Springer 1954b.
SCHREIBER, V., V. KMENTOVÁ, and A. ECKERTOVÁ: Inhibition of *in vitro* release of thyreotrophin by an analogue of oxytocin, 3-valine-oxytocin. Experientia (Basel) **20**, 673 (1964b).
— —, M. RYBÁK, and A. ECKERTOVÁ: Anti-thyrotrophin releasing factor (TRF) activity of synthetic 3-valine-oxytocin. Physiol. bohemoslov. **14**, 53 (1965).
—, Z. LOJDA, et V. KMENTOVÁ: Activité anti-TRF de la valine^3-ocytocine. Effet inhibiteur sur les phosphatases acides adénohypophysaires du rat. Étude bio- et histochimique. C.R. Acad. Sic. (Paris) **259**, 1222 (1964a).
SELYE, H.: Syndrome produced by diverse nocuous agents. Nature (Lond.) **138**, 32 (1936).
SEVY, R.W., E.A. OHLER, and A. WINER: Effect of chloropromazine on stress induced adrenal ascorbic acid depletion. Endocrinology **61**, 450 (1957).
SHANKLIN, W.M.: The human hypophysis in cases of burns. Acta Endocr. **21**, 1 (1956).
SIDEMAN, M., and H. SOBEL: ACTH releasing factor active in the guinea pig. Proc. Soc. exp. Biol. (N.Y.) **103**, 274 (1960).
SMEETS, E.H.J., and D. DE WIED: Effect of intra-arterial infusion of lysine vasopressin or U.S.P. ACTH on the corticosterone content of the adrenal venous effluent of hypophysectomized rats. Acta physiol. pharmacol. neerl. **11**, 295 (1962).
SMELIK, P.G.: Mechanism of hypophysial response to psychic stress. Acta endocr. (Kbh.) **33**, 437 (1960).
—, J.H. GAARENSTROOM, W. KONIJNENDIJK, and D. DE WIED: Evaluation of the role of the posterior lobe of the hypophysis in the reflex secretion of corticotrophin. Acta physiol. pharmacol. neerl. **11**, 20 (1962).
SMITH, G.P.: Neural control of the pituitary-adrenocortical system. In: Physiological control and regulations, p. 117. Ed. by WS. YAMAMOTO and J.R. BROBECK. Philadelphia: W.B. Saunders 1965.

SMITH, P.E., and D.J. HOIJER: Metabolism and cellular function in cold acclimation. Physiol. Rev. **42**, 60 (1962).
SOBEL, H., R.S. LEVY, J. MARMORSTON, S. SCHAPIRO, and S. ROSENFELD: Increased excretion of urinary corticosteroids by guinea pigs following administration of Pitressin. Proc. Soc. exp. Biol. (N.Y.) **89**, 10 (1955).
STEELMAN, S.L., and F.M. POHLEY: Assay of the follicle stimulating hormone based on the augmentation with human chorionic gonadotropin. Endocrinology **53**, 604 (1953).
STROTT, C.A., K. NAKAGAWA, H. NANKIN, and C.A. NUGENT: A phenylalanine-lysine-vasopressin test of ACTH release. J. clin. Endocr. **27**, 448 (1967).
SUCHOWSKY, G.K.: Einfluß von Hypophysenwirkstoffen auf den Sexualcyclus der Ratte. In: Gewebs- und Neurohormone — Physiologie des Melanophorenhormons, S. 411. Hrsg. von H. NOWAKOWSKI. Berlin-Göttingen-Heidelberg: Springer 1962.
SZENTÁGOTHAI, J., B. FLERKÓ, B. MESS, and B. HALÁSZ: Hypothalamic control of the anterior pituitary. Budapest: Akademiai Kiado, Publ. House of the Hungarian Acad. of Sci. 1962.
TALWALKER, P.K., A. RATNER, and J. MEITES: *In vitro* inhibition of pituitary prolactin synthesis and release by hypothalamic extract. Amer. J. Physiol. **205**, 213 (1963).
THOMPSON, J.C., and R.F. BLOUNT: The age of beginning reactivity of the pituitary-adrenocortical system to stress in the mouse. Endocrinology **54**, 620 (1954).
UNGER, R.H., A.M. EISENTRAUT, L.L. MADISON, and M.D. SIPERSTEIN: Fasting levels of growth hormone in men and women. Nature (Lond.) **205**, 804 (1965).
UOTILA, U.U.: Hypothalamic control of anterior pituitary function. Res. Publ. Ass. Res. nerv. ment. Dis. **20**, 580 (1940).
VALTIN, H., W.H. SAWYER, and H.W. SOKOL: Neurohypophysial principles in rats homozygous and heterozygous for hypothalamic diabetes insipidus. Endocrinology **77**, 701 (1965).
—, and H.A. SCHROEDER: Familial hypothalamic diabetes insipidus in rats (Brattleboro strain). Amer. J. Physiol. **206**, 425 (1964).
DEL VECCHIO, A., E. GENOVESE, and L. MARTINI: Hypothalamus and somatotrophic hormone release. Proc. Soc. exp. Biol. (N.Y.) **98**, 641 (1958).
VERNIKOS-DANELLIS, J.: The regulation of the synthesis and release of ACTH. In: Vitamins and hormones, Vol. 23, p. 97. New York: Academic Press 1965.
VAN DER WAL, B., T. WIEGMAN, J.F. JANSSEN, A. DELVER, and D. DE WIED: Evaluation of pituitary-adrenal function in children. Acta endocr. (Kbh.) **48**, 81 (1965).
WENNER, R.: Test zur Stimulation der gonadotropen Funktion des Hypophysenvorderlappens mit Oxytocin. Arch. Gynäk. **202**, 191 (1965).
WERNER, S.C., J. TIERNEY, and T. TALLBERG: Thyrotropic and "long-acting thyroid stimulator" effects from certain polypeptides. J. clin. Endocr. **24**, 339 (1964).
WEXLER, B.C.: Histologic alterations in the adrenal cortex of intact and hypophysectomized rats following ACTH, pitressin and adrenal steroids. Endocrinology **72**, 149 (1963).
WIED, D. DE: An assay of corticotrophin-releasing principles in hypothalamic lesioned rats. Acta endocr. (Kbh.) **37**, 288 (1961a).
— The significance of the antidiuretic hormone in the release mechanism of corticotropin. Endocrinology **68**, 956 (1961b).
— The site of the blocking action of dexamethasone on stress-induced pituitary ACTH release. J. Endocr. **29**, 29 (1964).
—, P.R. BOUMAN, and P.G. SMELIK: The effect of a lipide extract from the posterior hypothalamus and of pitressin on the release of ACTH from the pituitary gland. Endocrinology **62**, 605 (1958).
—, and I.A. MIRSKY: The action of delta-1-hydrocortisone on the antidiuretic and adrenocorticotropic responses to noxious stimuli. Endocrinology **64**, 955 (1959).
—, P. SIDERIUS, and I. A. MIRSKY: The antidiuretic- and ACTH-releasing effect of various octapeptides. Arch. int. Pharmacodyn. **83**, 50 (1961).
WISLOCKI, G.B.: The vascular supply of the hypophysis cerebri of the cat. Anat. Rec. **69**, 361 (1937).
— The vascular supply of the hypophysis cerebri of the rhesus monkey and man. Res. Publ. Ass. nerv. ment. Dis. **17**, 48 (1938).
YAMAZAKI, E., E. SAKIZ, and R. GUILLEMIN: An *in vivo* bioassay for TSH-releasing factor (TRF). Experientia (Basel) **19**, 480 (1963).
YATES, F.E., S.E. LEEMAN, D.W. GLENISTER, and M.F. DALLMAN: Interaction between plasma corticosterone concentration and adrenocorticotropin-releasing stimuli in the rat. Evidence for the reset of an endocrine feedback control. Endocrinology **69**, 67 (1961).
—, and J. URQUHART: Control of plasma concentrations of adrenocortical hormones. Physiol. Rev. **42**, 359 (1962).
YOKOYAMA, A., and K. OTA: Effects of administration of oxytocin and prolactin on lactating activity of mammary glands in rats. Endocr. jap. **6**, 259 (1959).

ZARROW, M. X., G. C. HALTMEYER, V. H. DENENBERG, and J. THATCHER: Response of the infantile rat to stress. Endocrinology **79**, 631 (1966).

ZONDEK, B.: Über die Hormone des Hypophysenvorderlappens. I. Wachstumshormon, Follikelreifungshormon (Prolan A), Luteinisierungshormon (Prolan B), Stoffwechselhormon. Klin. Wschr. **9**, 245 (1930).

—, u. S. ASCHHEIM: Hypophysenvorderlappen und Ovarium. Beziehungen der endokrinen Drüsen zur Ovarialfunktion. Arch. Gynäk. **130**, 1 (1927).

— — Das Hormon des Hypophysenvorderlappens. Darstellung, chemische Eigenschaften, biologische Wirkungen. Klin. Wschr. **7**, 831 (1928).

Actions and Functions of the Neurohypophysial Hormones and Related Peptides in Lower Vertebrates

FRANÇOIS MOREL and SERGE JARD

With 3 Figures

Introduction

This chapter deals with the physiological role and effects of neurohypophysial hormones in lower vertebrates, and also with the mechanism of the hormonal action at the cellular level, as revealed by *in vitro* studies on amphibian target organs. It falls into two separate parts: the first concerns comparative endocrinology and physiology of homeostasis in lower vertebrates; the second has to do with general physiology at the cellular level and molecular endocrinology. As will appear to the reader, our understanding of the regulatory role exerted by neurohypophysial hormones is very much less advanced in lower vertebrates than in mammals. On the other hand, the epithelial cells of amphibians have been widely used as convenient and simple structures in order to analyse the mechanism of action of the hormone at the cellular level on a biochemical, biophysical and molecular basis; in this respect the functioning of these cells is used as a model for the homologous mammalian target organs (especially the kidney tubule).

In order to understand fully the regulatory role played by a hormone in a given function, several steps of the feed-back mechanism have to be established or demonstrated, i.e. 1. the nature of the physiological stimulus, 2. the change in the hormonal concentration within the systemic blood resulting from the stimulus, and 3. the regulatory response of the target organ to the hormone; moreover 4. the removal of the endocrine gland must supress the response of the effector to the stimulus, and 5. intravenous injection of exogeneous hormone must mimic the effect of the specific input stimulus on the target organ.

Each of these steps has been clearly established in the case of the role of ADH in mammals, for example. Unfortunately, there is no such a well understood example in lower vertebrates, and our knowledge in these groups is quite incomplete, at best. Most of the published results concern experiments in which neurohypophysial hormones or neurohypophysial extracts have been injected into animals and the resulting changes in given functions have been observed. In such experiments, it is often very difficult to decide if the observed effects correspond to physiological actions of the hormone or are purely pharmacological ones. The criterion of the dose range of hormone to be injected in order to elicit an effect has been widely used to distinguish between physiological and pharmacological actions. This criterion is far from absolute, since, in most cases, even the order of magnitude of the physiological concentrations in blood is unknown; of course, if tremendous amounts of hormone have to be injected, this is an indication that the effects cannot be physiological. Finally, it has appeared to us that, when possible, the safest way to establish the possible roles or actions of neurohypophysial hormones in lower vertebrates was to compare the data obtained under various conditions and from different methods (endocrinology, morphology, ecology and so on) and then, to demonstrate that there is a physiological convergence in these respective results.

Another difficulty results from the fact that, in most of the experiments — with the exception of those published in very recent years —, either crude extracts of neurohypophysis (that is a mixture of unknown hormones) or pure mammalian hormones have been used. All these experiments have to be carefully discussed, since we know to day that the hormonal peptides present in the neurohypophysis of lower vertebrates are different from those of the mammals. Although outside the topic of the present chapter, this point is so closely related to physiology, that it will be briefly recalled now.

That lower vertebrates could have different neurohypophysial hormones than those of mammals was first suggested by HELLER (1941), who presented pharmacological evidence for the occurence of a "water balance principle." More recently, it has been reported (MAETZ et al., 1959a, b; MOREL and MAETZ, 1959) that the neurohypophysis of most groups of vertebrates, with the exception of the mammals and presumably of the Elasmobranchii, contains a "natriferic principle" (i.e. a principle very powerful in stimulating the active transport of sodium by the frog skin *in vitro*). At the same time, KATSOYANNIS and DU VIGNEAUD (1958) synthesized a peptide called vasotocin (Arg^8-oxytocin), the chemical structure of which is intermediate between those of oxytocin and vasopressin; it appeared that this artificial peptide has remarkable pharmacological properties and, more precisely, very high water balance and toad bladder activities (SAWYER et al., 1959), so that it was suggested that vasotocin is a naturally occuring hormone (SAWYER et al., 1959). By isolating from frog neurohypophysis (ACHER et al., 1960a) and from fowl neurohypophysis (CHAUVET et al., 1960) a peptide with amino-acid composition and sequence identical to those of vasotocin, ACHER has given conclusive evidence that vasotocin is a hormone in lower vertebrates; since that time, this hormone has also been found in several species of Teleosts (ACHER et al., 1961; HELLER and PICKERING, 1961; RASMUSSEN and CRAIG, 1961). On the other hand, it has been concluded from pharmacological evidence that the oxytocic principle of Teleosts cannot be oxytocin itself (HELLER et al., 1961); the structure of this second new hormone, isotocin (Ser^4-$Ileu^8$-oxytocin), has been chemically established by ACHER et al. (1962) from hypophysis of several kinds of Teleost fishes; more recently, ACHER has demonstrated that the oxytocic fraction present in the frog neurohypophysis is $Ileu^8$-oxytocin, a third new hormone that has been called mesotocin (ACHER et al., 1964b). Quite recently, a fourth new hormone, glumitocin (Ser^4-$Glu(NH_2)^8$-oxytocin) has been reported to exist in several species of Elasmobranchii (ACHER et al., 1965b, CHAUVET et al., 1965); conversely, the mammalian hormones seem to be absent from lower vertebrates, with the exception of the birds, in which oxytocin has been chemically identified in the fowl neurohypophysis (ACHER et al., 1960b). In summary, the distribution of the neurohypophysial hormones known at the present time among the main groups of vertebrates is as follows: Elasmobranchii: glumitocin; Teleosts: isotocin and vasotocin; Amphibians: mesotocin and vasotocin; Reptiles: vasotocin (presumably); Birds: oxytocin and vasotocin; Mammals: oxytocin and vasopressin. It must be pointed out that these hormones have been characterized in very few species only in each group, and that other hormones as yet unidentified probably exist (see, for example, MOREL et al., 1961a).

The first part of this chapter has been divided on the basis of physiology rather than zoology, so that the main functions in which neurohypophysial hormones could be involved are successively discussed; nevertheless, each function has been further subdivided by following the main zoological groups. Moreover, on several occasions, reference has been made in a few words to comparative physiology and to ecology, in order to discuss the role of neurohypophysial hormones on as wide a biological basis as possible. Quantitative indications concerning the amount of hormone used have been given very often; when possible, the hormonal concentrations are expressed as molar concentrations, and the injected doses are expressed as weight of peptide per unit of body weight. When crude extract (and not pure peptides) have been used, the doses have been indicated as usual, by reference to the oxytocic or vasopressic activities injected.

First Part

Comparative Physiology

I. Control of Adenohypophysial Activity by Neurohypophysial Hormones

There is much evidence indicating that adenohypophysial activity is controlled by chemical mediators of hypothalamic origin in all groups of vertebrates, with the possible exception of Cyclostomata and Elasmobranchii for which no experimental data are available. In mammals, it has been demonstrated that hormones of the *pars nervosa*, when injected intravenously, can act as "releasing factors" (STUTINSKY et al., 1952; SOBEL et al., 1955; MARTINI and DE POLI, 1956; MC CANN, 1957; MC CANN and FRUIT, 1957; SMELIK and DE WIED, 1958; BENSON and FOLLEY, 1956, 1958). Therefore, it has been suggested that neurohypophysial hormones could exert a double function, i.e. a central control of adenohypophysial activity and a peripheral action on specific target organs (FULFORD and MC CANN, 1955; MC CANN, 1957; MC CANN and BROBECK, 1954; MC CANN and FRUIT, 1957).

Before discussing the situation in lower vertebrates, it is important to define what is meant by "neurohypophysial hormones" so that the problem to be analysed in this section may be clearly delimited. An anatomical definition, that is, reference to the *pars nervosa*, is no longer sufficient, since these hormones are synthetized in hypothalamic nuclei and are only stored in the neurohypophysial tissue. A chemical definition is useless as well, since new active peptides have been isolated from the neurohypophysis of lower vertebrates during recent years (see above) and since it is probable that further hormones remain to be discovered. By analogy with what is known in mammals, neurohypophysial hormones could be defined as those active peptides which are formed in the hypothalamus, which reach the neurohypophysial tissue through a neurosecretory pathway, which are stored in that tissue, and which after release into the blood exert a specific action on one or several peripheral target organs. On this definition, our discussion is limited to the possibility that some active peptides (vasopressin, oxytocin or vasotocin for example) have a further physiological effect on the function and activity of the *pars distalis*.

In mammals, despite the fact that injected vasopressin may show a powerful CRF like activity (STUTINSKY et al., 1952; MARTINI and DE POLI, 1956; MC CANN, 1957; MC CANN and FRUIT, 1957; SMELIK and DE WIED, 1958), it appears very probable that C.R.F. itself is a peptide(s) of related, but different structure (SCHALLY and SAFFRAN, 1956; GUILLEMIN, 1957; GUILLEMIN et al., 1957; SCHALLY et al., 1958; SAFFRAN et al., 1958). The hypothalamic releasing factors controlling the *pars distalis* are probably formed in different hypothalamic nuclei than the supraoptic and paraventricular nuclei; they do not accumulate in the *pars nervosa* but exert their action from the median eminence through the portal vessels of the pituitary stalk; finally, they have no known peripheral actions.

Unfortunately, it may be much more difficult to make such distinctions in the case of lower vertebrates, especially for the most primitive groups. In all vertebrates, the neurohypophysis develops from an evagination of the diencephalic floor and from the floor itself in an area located between the evagination and the optic chiasma (GREEN, 1951), but the size and the development of that structure vary greatly from one group to the other. In the Cyclostamata, the neurohypophysis is very poorly developed and appears to be only a thickening of the ventricular floor. In the Elasmobranchii and Teleostei, the neurohypophysial tissue derives from both the diverticulum and the floor of the diencephalon (WINGSTRAND, 1951, 1959); it is well developed and is closely associated with the adenohypophysial tissue; nevertheless, there are not yet two well distinct parts, the median eminence and the *pars nervosa*. In the Dipnoi, as well as in the tetrapods, the neurohypophysis is anatomically and morphologically differentiated into these two parts. The median eminence is always chacterized by its close vascular connections with the *pars distalis* (WINGSTRAND, 1956). In the Urodela, the median eminence is relatively simple, whereas in Anura the portal system is fully developed, as in the other groups of superior vertebrates (GREEN, 1951; WINGSTRAND, 1951). It must be stressed that vascular connections exist between neurohypophysial tissue and the *pars distalis* in all classes of vertebrates, even when there is no well-characterized portal system. In the tetrapods, the blood flowing to the *pars distalis* comes mostly from the median eminence, whereas in Teleostei (GREEN, 1951) and Elasmobranchii (MELLINGER et al., 1962; MELLINGER, 1960, 1965; MEURLING, 1960) it comes from the whole neurohypophysial tissue of the gland.

There are only a few experimental observations which suggest that the same active peptide could both act as a hormone on a peripheral target organ and play a separate physiological role by directly controlling the activity of some adenohypophysial function. Furthermore, the observation that, when injected in large amounts, exogenous neurohypophysial hormone may act as a specific releasing factor, as in some of the experiments to be reported here, is obviously unsufficient to demonstrate that these hormones have this physiological role.

A. Fishes

It has been suggested from morphological observations that, in this group, the main physiological role of neurohypophysial hormones is to control the activity of the *pars distalis* (JØRGENSEN and LARSEN, 1963; SAWYER et al., 1960; SAWYER, 1961a, b, 1964a); but, as far as we know, there is no physiological evidence supporting such a view. Spawning behaviour in *Fundulus*, for example (as it will be discussed later), can be induced by injecting hypophysial extracts from fish (PICKFORD, 1952; WILHELMI et al., 1955; SAWYER and PICKFORD, 1963) as well as very large doses (20—60 IU/kg) of oxytocin and vasopressin (WILHELMI et al., 1955). The observed effect, however, does not seem to result from a gonadotrophin releasing action of the hormone, since it is produced in the immature animal as well as after both hypophysectomy and gonadectomy (PICKFORD, unpublished observations quoted by WILHELMI et al., 1955). In many species of fishes it has been reported that gonadotrophin is released under stimulation by light (HOOVER and HUBBARD, 1937; BULLOUGH, 1940; HARRINGTON, 1950; BAGGERMAN, 1957; EGAMI, 1959a) and that ACTH is released as a response to several kind of stress (CHAVIN, 1956; BALL, 1960; LELOUP-HATEY, 1958); but the nature of the chemical mediators involved in these responses as well as their mechanism of action are completely unknown. Thus, the observation by RASQUIN and STOLL (1957) that injection of pitressin (1 IU) to the Characin results in a hypertrophy of the adrenal tissue has not been confirmed by CHAVIN (1959) in *Carassius*.

B. Amphibians

Many data indicate that most functions of the *pars distalis* are under the control of the hypothalamus. Such a control has been suggested for gonadotrophin release (VIVIEN and SCHOTT, 1957; MAZZI and PEYROT, 1960; JØRGENSEN and LARSEN, 1963), prolactin release (ETKIN and LEHRER, 1960; MASUR, 1962), thyreostimulin release (JØRGENSEN and LARSEN, 1963) and corticotrophin release (JACOBSOHN and JØRGENSEN, 1956; JØRGENSEN and NIELSEN, 1958; JØRGENSEN et al., 1960; JØRGENSEN and LARSEN, 1960a), but a clear effect of injected neurohypophysial hormone has been observed only on ACTH release. Thus, in toads in which there is an adrenal insufficiency resulting from either the destruction of the median eminence (JØRGENSEN et al., 1960), or from hypophysial transplantation (JACOBSOHN and JØRGENSEN, 1956), the injection of lysine-vasopressin restores moulting (JØRGENSEN and NIELSEN, 1958; JØRGENSEN and LARSEN, 1960a) in the same way as ACTH does (JØRGENSEN and LARSEN, 1960b); when lysine-vasopressin is injected in hypophysectomized toads, the moulting effect is no longer present, whereas ACTH is still effective (JØRGENSEN and LARSEN, 1960b—1963); these observations unequivocally indicate that vasopressin exerts its action via the release of ACTH. Oxytocin (JØRGENSEN and LARSEN, 1960a), arginine-vasopressin (AVP) and arginine-vasotocin (AVT) (JØRGENSEN and LARSEN, 1963), when injected in the same conditions, all produce the same moulting effect as lysin-vasopressin (LVP). The amounts of hormone required to produce moulting in 50% of the toads are respectively 5 (AVP), 20 (LVP), 200 (AVT) and 1000 mμg (oxytocin). It must be noted that AVT, which is presumably the natural hormone in this species, is about forty times less active than AVP on this test; on the other hand, the amount of AVT required is about 400 times higher than that required to produce an antidiuretic effect in the same species (JØRGENSEN and LARSEN, 1963); but, in this particular case, the necessity of injecting relatively large amounts of the hormone is not an argument against a possible role of AVT on ACTH release, since the local concentration of AVT into the blood of the pituitary vessels could be relatively high even when physiological amounts are released from the *pars nervosa*. Nevertheless it remains quite possible that, in the case of the amphibians as in mammals (see above), the CRF activitiy of vasopressin only results from the fact that its structure is chemically closely related to that of the physiological hypothalamic CRF.

C. Reptiles

As far as we know, there is no data available concerning this group.

D. Birds

The existence of a hypothalamic control of hypophysial function has been clearly established in the case of gonadotrophic hormones (BENOIT and ASSENMACHER, 1953, 1955; ASSENMACHER, 1958), prolactin (RIDDLE, 1963; ASSENMACHER and TIXIER VIDAL, 1964; LEHRMAN, 1964; NICOLL, 1965; KRAGT and MEITES, 1965; MEITES and NICOLL, 1965), thyreotropic hormone (SHIRLEY and NALBANDOV, 1956a; ASSENMACHER, 1958) and corticotrophic hormone (ASSENMACHER, 1958). But there is no direct experimental evidence suggesting that neurohypophysial hormones could act as the releasing factor of any these adenohypophysial hormones.

According to CHAUDHURY and CHAUDHURY (1962), systemic or intramuscular injection of oxytocin in the pigeon results in an increase in the weight of the crop gland similar to that produced by prolactin injection (RIDDLE and BATES, 1939), an observation which was interpreted as suggesting that oxytocin could act via the release of prolactin; nevertheless, these results were not confirmed (HOHN, 1963; MIZUNO and MEITES, 1963); more precisely, it seems that the morphological changes induced in the crop gland by the injection of oxytocin and by the injection of prolactin are not similar; MIZUNO and MEITES (1963) conclude that the effect of oxytocin is not a specific one.

It is well known in the birds that an increase in daylight-length induces an enlargement of the gonad due to an increase in the release of gonadostimulin (BENOIT and ASSENMACHER, 1953, 1955; ASSENMACHER, 1958; OKSCHE et al., 1959). It has been observed by ISHII et al. (1962) on the passerine bird *Zosterops palbebrosa japonica* that, in that experimental situation, there is also an increase in the hormonal content of the median eminence, as judged by the activities of extracts on rat uterus and toad bladder. Moreover the ratio of these two biological activities suggests that the hormone present is arginine-vasotocin; therefore, ISHII and coworkers conclude that vasotocin could be involved in the regulation of the release of gonadotrophin in this bird species. However, the evidence supporting such an interpretation remains somewhat indirect.

II. Action of Neurohypophysial Hormones on Reproductive Functions in Lower Vertebrates

It is likely that neurohypophysial peptides are involved to some extent in the reproductory functions of all classes of vertebrates; in the most evolved lower vertebrates, the observed effect results from a peripheral action equivalent to the uterotonic and galactobolic action of oxytocin in mammals; however, in some fishes, it is possible that the hormone exerts its effect via the central nervous system.

A. Fishes

Many histophysiological data suggest that neurohypophysial hormones are involved in reproductive functions. A decrease of neurosecretory material in the neurohypophysial tissue during the period of reproduction has been described in several species: *Fundulus heteroclitus* (SOKOL, 1961), sturgeon (POLENOV and BARANNIKOVA, 1958; BARANNIKOVA and POLENOV, 1960), *Oryzias latipes* (EGAMI and ISHII, 1961). These morphological observations have been confirmed by bioassay of the hormonal content of the gland (SAWYER and PICKFORD, 1963). According to these last authors, isotocin (Ser^4-$Ileu^8$-oxytocin) would be the physiological "oxytocic" principle in this group; it disappears more or less completely from the hypophysis in female *Fundulus* during the reproductive period, whereas it remains at a high level during the other periods in the female and throughout the year in the male. On the other hand, injections of crude or partially purified extracts of *Pollachius* hypophysis induce typical spawning behaviour in *Fundulus*. There is a close correlation between the activity of the different fractions assayed on that test and their content in oxytocic and vasopressic activities (WILHELMI et al., 1955). Extracts of *Perca* hypophysis also show the same kind of biological activity (SWIFT and PICKFORD, 1965). Arginine-vasopressin and oxytocin (natural and synthetic), when injected in very large doses (20—60 IU/kg), produce similar effect, as mentioned before. These results have been confirmed in other species than *Fundulus: Oryzias latipes* (EGAMI, 1959b; EGAMI and ISHII, 1962; EGAMI and NAMBU,

1961) and *Rhodeus ocellatus* (Shirai, quoted from Egami and Ishii, 1962). In a viviparus species, *Gambusia*, frog or mammalian neurohypophysial extracts, injected into the pregnant female, induce the delivery of the youngs (Ishii, 1961). In all these experiments, the amount of injected hormone was very large, so that the observed effect could be a pharmacological one. In any case, the mechanism of action involved is still unknown. We have already mentioned that it cannot be a gonadotrophin releasing action, since the hormone produces the same effect in the hypophysectomized fish (Pickford, quoted by Wilhelmi et al., 1955). Some specific action on a peripheral target organ seems to be equally out of question, since, in fishes, the wall of the oviduct contains mostly connective tissue and elastic fibers with very few, if any, smooth muscle fibers; oviposition in this group mainly results from the contractions of the striated muscular wall of the abdomen, and depends of the central nervous system (see, for example, Aronson, 1957). This kind of remark applies to the induction of spawning behaviour by the injection of hormones as well, since a highly coordinated muscular activity is also involved in this action. Thus, according to Wilhelmi et al. (1955), it appears that, if neurohypophysial hormones do play a role in reproductive function, they may well act directly on the central nervous system itself. The mechanism of such an action remains completely unknown.

B. Amphibians

There are only a few experimental data available. According to Bentley and Heller (unpublished observations in Heller, 1965a), arginine-vasotocin induces parturition of the viviparus Salamander *(Salamandra maculosa)*. If the oviduct of a pregnant female is maintained *in vitro*, the addition of the hormone to the medium enhances the contractions.*

C. Birds

It has been repeatedly claimed that neurohypophysectomy (Shirley and Nalbandov, 1956b) or the destruction of the supraoptic area (Yasuda, 1957; Ralph, 1960) does not necessarely supress a normal rythm of laying in the hen. Nevertheless, cyclical changes in the hormonal content of the neurohypophysis in direct relation to the laying period, as well as the induction of oviposition by injections of exogeneous neurohypophysial hormones, strongly suggest the role of the neurohypophysis in oviposition in the birds. Thus, the hormonal content of the gland, when tested both on toad bladder and rat uterus, decreases at the time of laying in the hen (Tanaka and Nakajo, 1960; see also Legait, 1959); moreover, this drop of activity is more pronounced on the toad bladder test than on the rat uterus test (Tanaka and Nakajo, 1962), indicating that the hormone released is vasotocin and not oxytocin, since vasotocin has a much higher toad bladder to rat uterus ratio of activities than oxytocin. Recently, Sturkie and Yu-Chong (1966) have shown that the hormonal concentration in systemic blood of the hen increases up to 50 times at the time of oviposition. Stimulation of the preoptic area of the brain of hen causes a premature oviposition associated with the release of vasotocin (Opel, 1964, 1966). Injections of neurohypophysial extracts in the dove (Riddle, 1921) or the hen (Burrows and Byerly, 1942), result in the early laying of the eggs present in the oviduct. Arginine-vasotocin, injected intravenously

* Added in proof: Even very low concnntrations induce *in vitro* concentrations of the oviducts in several species of urodeles as well as anurans, arginine-vasoticin being more active than mesotocin, oxytocin or arginine-vasopressin (Heller H., E. Ferreri and D. H. G. Leathers: the effect of neurohypophysial hormones on the amphibian oviduct. J. Endocr. *37*, XXXIX, 1967).

to a hen in a dose of 30 mU (vasopressic activity), induced oviposition in about 90 sec (MUNSICK et al., 1960); such a dose is about 7% of the neurohypophysial content; it is 10—50 times higher than the dose sufficient to produce a definite antidiuretic action in the same species (SKADHAUGE, 1964). When added *in vitro* to the uterine portion of the oviduct of laying hens, neurohypophysial hormones induce contractions (MUNSICK et al., 1959—1960; MUNSICK, 1965); among the peptides tested, AVT has the highest "hen oxytocic activity"; it is 2.6, 22 and 34 times more active than AVP, oxytocin and LVP respectively.

All these results clearly demonstrate that AVT is physiologically involved in the control of oviposition in birds by stimulating uterine contractions; the possible role of oxytocin in this group remains to be solved. As will be mentioned later, AVT is most probably the physiological antidiuretic hormone in birds, and by the way also plays a role in the control of the water balance in this group. The question thus arises as to how a single hormone can act independently on two different functions in the same animal. An explanation could be that antidiuresis is a more or less permanent state requiring a sustained secretion of small amounts of AVT, the range of which is much to low to induce oviposition; on the other hand, oviposition is a transient process resulting from a phasic release of a relatively larger amount of AVT; due to the short biological half-life of the circulating hormone (SUSKA-BRZEZINSKA and EWY, 1965), the associated antidiuretic effect will be of short duration, without any significant effect on the water balance of the body.

D. Reptiles

MUNSICK et al. (1960) indicate that AVT induces contractions of the isolated oviduct of the turtle *(Chrysemis picta)*, and suggest that in the reptiles this hormone could play a role in reproduction similar to that just described in birds.

III. Action of Neurohypophysial Hormones on the Vascular System of Lower Vertebrates

The change in blood pressure resulting from the injection of neurohypophysial extract was the first peripheral action of these hormones to have been recognized both in mammals (OLIVER and SCHÄFER, 1895) and in birds. The vasodepressor effect of crude neurohypophysial extract in both the duck and the hen has been described by PATON and WATSON (1912) and HOGBEN and SCHLAPP (1924). It has been shown by GADDUM (1928) that the effect is actually produced by oxytocin. More recently, this vasodepressor action of oxytocin has been observed in several other species of birds: the pigeon (WARING et al., 1956), the emu, the penguin and the cormorant (WOOLEY, 1959), as well as in reptiles: the alligator, a species of turtle, *Chelonia oblonga*, and a species of lizard, *Tachysaurus rugosus* (WOOLEY, 1959). Depending on the experimental condition and the injected doses, vasopressin may show either vasopressor or vasodepressor effects (STRAHAN and WARING, 1954; WARING et al., 1956; WOOLEY, 1959). Vasotocin, like oxytocin, is vasodepressor in birds, but it is about 3 times less potent per unit of weight than oxytocin (KATSOYANNIS and DU VIGNEAUD, 1958; MUNSICK et al., 1960).

The vasodepressor action of oxytocin in the hen is quite reproducible and its intensity is a function of the injected amount, so that it is widely used as a bioassay for oxytocin and related peptides (avian vasodepressor test). The pharmacological data of importance which have been obtained with this test, as well as the bioassay technique itself, are discussed in another section of this book.

Within the amphibians, the vascular responses observed seem to bee rather variable and inconstant: a vasopressor action of both pitressin and pitocin (dose range from 1—10 IU/kg) has been described in *Bufo marinus* by WOOLEY (1959); a vasopressor effect has also been recorded when arginine-vasotocin was injected in *Rana macrodon* (VAN DYKE and YEOH, 1965). On the other hand, a diphasic response to pituitrin, pitocin and pitressin (SAWYER and SAWYER, 1952) and to oxytocin (1 IU/kg) (URANGA and SAWYER, 1960) has been observed in *Rana castesbiana*; a diphasic response to pitressin, pitocin and arginine-vasotocin has also been reported in *Bufo arenarum* (LICO, 1963). All these effects on blood pressure are obtained with amounts of hormone which are much larger (about 100 times) than those required to produce physiological responses such as the antidiuretic action. Thus, they are probably pharmacological effects resulting from a more or less generalized action on the smooth muscle of the arteriolar media (WOOLEY and WARING, 1959). Nevertheless, as will be discussed later, it remains quite possible that the vasomotor muscles of some specific target organs or areas in the body have a particularly high sensitivity to neurohypophysial hormones. Thus, they could mediate physiological responses to these hormones by changing the local haemodynamic conditions and (or) blood flow rate, without involving any changes at the systemic level.

There is no data available concerning fishes at the present time. Systemic vascular effects in response to neurohypophysial peptides can be expected in this group, at least with large doses, since after hormonal administration changes in glomerular filtration rate, probably of vascular origin, have been reported (see below).

IV. Action of Neurohypophysial Hormones on Osmoregulation in Lower Vertebrates

There is much evidence, from physiological, ecological and histological studies, which clearly demonstrates that neurohypophysial hormones are physiologically involved in osmoregulation in all — or at least nearly all — groups of vertebrates. As far as we know, the mechanisms of the hormonal action at the cellular level are quite similar, an observation which contrasts with the variability of the target organs concerned in osmoregulation. These mechanisms of action, which will be discussed in detail in a later section, always result in an increase in water permeability and (or) a stimulation of active transport of sodium across the layer of epithelial cells separating the body fluids from the external medium. Since the osmoregulatory pattern appears to be highly variable from one group to another depending on the phylogenetic degree of evolution and the ecological mode of life, it seems suitable to analyse the role of neurohypophysial hormones in osmoregulation within the different zoological groups in succession: fishes, amphibians, reptiles and birds.

A. Fishes

The osmoregulatory pattern in fishes has been clearly elucidated by the well-known pioneering work of H. W. SMITH and A. KROGH. With the exception of the sea water Elasmobranchii (the body fluids of which are kept almost isosmotic with sea water by the accumulation of urea), all fishes are able to maintain the osmotic pressure of their body fluids at a value different from that of the surrounding medium. As a result of this osmotic pressure gradient, fresh water fishes are exposed to overhydration and sea water fishes to dehydration, resulting from a passive osmotic flow of water through the body surface, and especially through the gills. In all cases, osmoregulation is achieved by mechanisms of active transport of salt against concentration gradients, that is, by energy consuming processes separating salt from water. In the fresh water fishes of all classes — Agnathii, Chondrycthii, Actinopterygii and Choanichthii, — most of this work is performed by the kidneys, which excrete a large volume (up to 300 ml/kg B.W./day) of a very dilute urine (see SMITH, 1932; KROGH, 1939; FONTAINE and KOCH, 1950; WIKGREN, 1953; FONTAINE, 1956; MORRIS, 1956, 1958; BENTLEY and FOLLET, 1963b). In addition, there is an active uptake of salt from the external medium by the gills (KROGH, 1937a), which balances the salt losses due to the excretion of solutes by the kidney and to the passive diffusion into the external medium through the outer surface. In the sea water fishes, the osmoregulatory pattern is quite different. The kidney is unable to excrete a hypertonic urine. Marine Teleostei drink large amounts of sea water (up to 25% of their body weight per day according to SMITH, 1930—1932); both salt and water are absorbed through the intestinal wall. Finally, the excess of salt is extruded into the external medium through the gills by a process of active transport. According to MORRIS (1958, 1960), the osmoregulatory mechanisms in Agnathii seem to be quite similar (see also BENTLEY, 1962c).

It must be stressed at this point that, as far as the control of osmoregulation is concerned, stenohaline species and euryhaline species are in completely different situations. In stenohaline species, osmoregulatory active transports can proceed at a relatively constant speed, since the chemical composition of the external medium is constant. On the other hand, in euryhaline species, the intensity and even the direction and the site of the active transports involved must be able to change greatly in response to changes in the salinity of the external medium.

Thus, for example, when euryhaline fishes adapted to fresh water are transferred into sea water (or partially diluted sea water), drastic physiological changes are observed: the animals start drinking water, urine flow and glomerular filtration rate are reduced 5—10 times (HOLMES and MAC BEAN, 1963; SHARRATT et al., 1964; FLEMING and STANLEY, 1965; LAHLOU, 1966), and the osmotic pressure of the excreted urine increases to a value near that of the plasma (FLEMING and STANLEY, 1965); moreover, the direction of the net flux of sodium transport through the gills is reversed from inwards to outwards. Simultaneously the polarity (as defined from histological criteria) of the so-called chloride cells of the gills of *Fundulus* is reversed (COPELAND, 1950). By using radioactive sodium as a tracer in several species of euryhaline fishes such as *Gasterosteus* (MULLINS, 1950), *Platichthys* (MOTAIS, 1961a, b—1967), *Blemnius* (HOUSE, 1963), it has been repeatedly observed that the turnover rate of the exchangable sodium pool increases from very low values of about 1% per hour in fresh water to values as high as 20%, and even 50—60% per hour in *Blemnius*, when the fishes are adapted to sea water. A large part of this enormous outflux of sodium is thought to result from a sodium exchange diffusion process occuring in the epithelial cells of the gills (MAETZ, 1964; MOTAIS, 1967; MOTAIS et al., 1966). Moreover, in the flounder, MOTAIS (1961a, b) has clearly shown that an almost instantaneous reduction in the outflux of sodium occurs when fishes adapted to sea water are transferred to fresh water; this is followed by a further, progressive, reduction corresponding to the adaptation of the fish to fresh water. When they are transferred from fresh to sea water, the reverse change is rather progressive; moreover, the longer the adaptation period to fresh water, the slower is the rate of change in the sodium outflux when the fishes are returned to sea water.

The possible role of neurohypophysial hormones in the regulation of volume or osmotic pressure of body fluids may now be considered. *A priori*, it appears that a hormonal action increasing the osmotic permeability coefficient to water of the epithelial cells in contact with the external medium (as observed in other groups such as amphibians) would be of no help at all in either sea water or fresh water fishes, since such an effect would in fact enhance the passive net flow of water in a direction opposite to that required for osmoregulation. An action of the hormone stimulating the active transport of sodium (at the level of the gill and (or) of the kidney) would constitute an efficient mechanism of osmoregulation. It must be stressed, nevertheless, that the mechanism of active ion transport that is working in the gill of the fresh water fishes seems to be rather different from those known in other epithelial structures of vertebrates; it has thus been demonstrated in *Carassius* that the uptakes of Cl^- and Na^+ ions are independent and respectively result from both a $Cl^- \rightleftarrows HCO_3^-$ anionic and a $Na^+ \rightleftarrows NH_4^+$ cationic exchange mechanisms (KROGH, 1939; GARCIA ROMEU and MAETZ, 1964; MAETZ and GARCIA ROMEU, 1964).

There are two main kinds of evidence which suggest that neurohypophysial hormones may be involved in osmoregulation in the fishes: firstly, the observation of peripheral effects in response to exogeneous hormone, and, secondly, the description of morphological and functional changes in the neurohypophysis which result from osmotic stimulation.

It has long been established that administration of neurohypophysial extracts (from fishes or mammals) does not have any significant effect on the water balance in fresh water Teleostei (BOYD and DINGWALL, 1939; FONTAINE and RAFFY, 1950; CALLAMAND et al., 1951), marine Teleostei (FONTAINE and RAFFY, 1950), the lungfish (HELLER, 1956), or the lamprey (BENTLEY, 1962c). These negative results have been recently confirmed for large doses of arginine-vasotocin (HELLER and BENTLEY, 1965). It has also been established that neurohypophysial extracts from Elasmobranchii administered to Elasmobranchii have no effect on water balance (HELLER and BENTLEY, 1965). Despite the relatively poor sensitivity and specificity of the water balance test which has been used in all these experiments (the effect measured was a change in body weight), it seems clearly established that neurohypophysial hormones do not produce any large increase of the osmotic permeability of the gill to water.

As far as the kidney is concerned, the data seem to be rather variable, depending upon conditions, species, hormones and dose range: no change in urine flow rate in the catfish after injection of 0.2—2 IU/kg of vasopressin (BURGESS et al., 1933); diuretic effect of injected vasopressin in the goldfish (SEXTON, 1955); antidiuretic effect of vasopressin in the trout (HOLMES, 1959; CHESTER JONES et al., 1959). According to MAETZ (1963) and to MAETZ et al. (1964), both urine flow rate and inulin clearance in the goldfish increase when vasotocin or oxytocin is injected intraperitoneally without any disturbance to the animal. There is no simultaneous change in the osmotic pressure or salt concentration of the excreted urine, so that the relative free water clearance (C_{H_2O}/C_{In}) remains unchanged. This observation suggests that the injected hormone has no tubular action, but only increases GFR. Glomerular recruitment could be the mechanism by which GFR controls the urine flow rate in fishes (FORSTER, 1953). LAHLOU (1966) has recently given arguments supporting such a point of view. In similar conditions, isotocin (Ser^4-$Ileu^8$-oxytocin) produced a slight antidiuretic effect and a significant decrease in sodium excretion (MAETZ et al., 1964). In the lungfish, arginine-vasotocin has been reported to be both diuretic and natriuretic, whereas oxytocin and isotocin lacked any clearcut action (SAWYER, 1966). The relatively small doses of vasotocin required to obtain a diuretic response, as well as the time course of this response, suggest a direct action of the hormone on the kidney, which could be of physiological importance. There is no information available concerning a possible action of neurohypophysial hormones on the kidney of marine Teleostei.

As far as the salt balance through the gill is concerned, it is well known that stress, for example handling or injections, may considerably disturb the sodium exchanges in fishes (see for instance KROGH, 1939; MEYER, 1948—1951; MAETZ, 1956—1963), so that one has to be especially careful when looking for a possible hormonal action on the fluxes of ions through the gill. MAETZ and JULIEN (1961) first reported that, when measured 12 h after the injection to goldfishes of: *Carassius* neurohypophysial extract (45—90 mU oxytocic activity), oxytocin (150—1000 mU) or saline, the influx of sodium was greater in the fishes injected with hormone than in the controls. The outflux of sodium was unchanged, so that the overall action observed was a gain of sodium by the fish. In similar experiments, lysine-vasopressin appeared to be much less active. Such a protracted effect of neurohypophysial hormones on sodium balance has also been observed in *Fundulus kansae* (MEIER and FLEMING, 1962). The possibility that these effects could result from an indirect action of the injected hormone via the *pars distalis* of the hypophysis has been suggested, but later experiments have shown that the effect can be elicited during the first hour after the intraperitoneal injection of vasotocin or isotocin (MAETZ, 1963; MAETZ et al., 1964), an observation compatible with a direct action of the hormone on the gill epithelium. Further experiments on hypophysectomized fishes or, even better, on isolated gills *in vitro*, seem required to demonstrate unequivocally whether neurohypophysial hormones act directly on these epithelial cells. Qualitative differences have been reported between the effects of the two hormones occurring naturally in the fishes on sodium fluxes through the gills. In *Carassius*, arginine-vasotocin enhances both the influx and the outflux of sodium, whereas isotocin increases the influx only and leaves the outflux unchanged (MAETZ et al., 1964). Both hormones are active in a dose range (i.e.: 2—4 μg/kg B.W.) which seems to be at the upper limit compatible with a direct physiological effect.

Since the observation by KEYS and BATEMAN (1932) that vasopressin has no effect on the salt balance of the eel, interesting experiments have been reported in a euryhaline Teleost, the flounder *(Platichthys flesus)*: oxytocin (300 mU/100 g) stimulates the sodium influx in flounders adapted to fresh water and increases the turnover rate of the sodium pool in flounders adapted to sea water (MOTAIS and MAETZ, 1964). Moreover, oxytocin, but not vasopressin, accelerates the rate of adaptation to sea water when flounders are transferred from fresh water into sea water (MOTAIS, 1967).

In the lamprey (BENTLEY and FOLLET, 1962—1963a), arginine-vasotocin or isotocin increases the negative net flux of sodium. Oxytocin and vasotocin have been reported to produce similar effects in the lungfish (HELLER and BENTLEY, 1965). Finally, a possible action of glumitocin [a physiological hormone in the Elasmobranchii (ACHER et al., 1965b)] on the osmoregulatory target organs in this group requires to be investigated.

In summary, the experiments in which neurohypophysial hormones (or related peptides) have been injected in fresh water fishes suggest two different peripheral actions of the hormone, i.e. an increase in GFR (vascular effect on the kidney) and a stimulation of the active uptake of sodium by the gill. Whether these two effects correspond to physiological actions of the endogenous hormone is far from established and remains to be discussed. As pointed out by MAETZ (1963) and BOURGUET et al. (1964), both effects would result in an increase in the salt concentration of body fluids (increased output of free water by the kidney and increased net uptake of salt by the gill). The hormone would thus enhance the effectiveness of the active osmoregulatory mechanisms of the fresh water fishes. BOURGUET et al. (1964) report that an experimental decrease in the salt concentration of the body fluids (by injection of hypotonic saline or isosmotic mannitol solution) in the goldfish induces both a diuretic response and an increase in the sodium influx through the gills. Injections of hyperosmotic sodium chloride solutions induce reverse responses. MAETZ (1963) has suggested that dilution (or expansion) of body fluids in fresh water fishes could act as a stimulus for the release of neurohypophysial hormones; but there is unfortunately no evidence suggesting that these responses result from an increase in the concentration of the circulating hormone. Moreover, such a mechanism seems to be in opposition with a number of histophysiological studies which indicate, on the contrary, that Gomori positive material disappears from the neurohypophysial tissue in response to environmental changes which lead to an increased concentration of body fluids (ARVY and GABE, 1954; TUURALA, 1957; ARVY et al., 1954; FRIDBERG and OLSON, 1959; SCHIEBLER and BREHM, 1958; KOBAYASHI et al., 1959; STUTINSKY, 1952—1953; ENAMI, 1954; ARVY et al., 1955, 1956, 1959). Since parallel variations in the content of Gomori stainable material and in the amount of biological activity measured by classical bioassays have been observed in a few instances (CARLSON and HOLMES, 1962; LEDERIS, 1963), these experiments suggest an increased release of neurohypophysial hormones as a response to the osmotic stimulation. Unfortunately, the exact nature of the stimulus as well as its specificity remain an open question in many cases. Many different kinds of stress may induce similar changes in the preoptic nuclei (RASQUIN and STOLL, 1955); moreover, strong osmotic stimuli of reversed direction (transfer from fresh water to diluted sea water and vice versa) produce changes in the histological aspect of the neurohypophysial tissue which cannot be distinguished each other (FRIDBERG and OLSSON, 1959).

Even the experiments of hypophysectomy in euryhaline Teleostei have given somewhat different results from species to species. The hypophysectomized eel is able to support repeated and rapid transfers from fresh to sea water (FONTAINE et al., 1949; CALLAMAND et al., 1951), whereas the hypophysectomized *Fundulus heteroclitus* (PICKFORD, 1953; BURDEN, 1956; PICKFORD and ATZ, 1957; PICKFORD et al., 1965), *Poecilia latipinna* and *Poecilia formosa* (BALL, 1962; BALL et al., 1965), *Xiphophorus maculatus* and *Xiphophorus helleri* (SCHREIBMAN and KALLMAN, 1963), all fail to survive after a rapid transfer from sea to fresh water. Administration of large doses of neurohypophysial extracts (BURDEN, 1956) or pure arginine-vasotocin and isotocin (PICKFORD et al., 1965; SAWYER, 1965), does not allow the hypophysectomized fish to survive in fresh water. On the other hand, transplantation of the hypophysis (BALL and KALLMAN, 1962; BALL et al., 1965) as well as injections of prolactin (BURDEN, 1956; PICKFORD and PHILLIPS, 1959; BALL and OLIVEREAU, 1964; PICKFORD et al., 1965) can reverse the effects of hypophysectomy. While these observations strongly suggest that prolactin or some related adenohypophysial hormone could be involved in the mechanism of adaptation of euryhaline fishes to fresh water, there is no available evidence indicating the nature of the action of prolactin on the organs involved in osmoregulation (see for example MEITES and NICOLL, 1965).

In conclusion, many data indicate that injected neurohypophysial hormones may act on both kidney and gill functions, but it is not yet unequivocally demonstrated either that this action is a direct one or that it corresponds to a physiological role of the hormone in osmoregulation. Part of our ignorance probably results from the fact that osmoregulatory mechanisms are quite different in this purely aquatic group of vertebrates than in the other groups. Moreover, with the exception of the euryhaline species (which are of most interest in this respect) it does not seem necessary, *a priori*, that "phasic" hormones with a short biological half-life are required for the control of the osmoregulatory processes, which may work at a more or less constant rate, since the external medium remains remarkably constant.

B. Amphibians

The physiological role of neurohypophysial hormones in osmoregulation among vertebrates appears clearly in amphibians, and especially in those species that frequent terrestrial habitats. Considerable attention has been given to this transitional group, so that to day the osmoregulatory mechanisms, the actions of neurohypophysial hormones on the target organs, and (to a lesser extent) the feed-back mechanisms of release are relatively well established.

As far as osmoregulatory mechanisms are concerned, there are three different ecological situations to be discussed: a) the animal in water; b) the animal during a period of life in a terrestrial habitat; and c) the animal returning from a terrestrial habitat to water.

a) During long periods of life in water, the amphibians are in a situation similar to that of the fresh water fishes; there is a tendency for continuous overhydration to occur, as a result of the gradient of osmotic pressure that exists across the skin. This passive water gain is balanced by the excretion of large volumes of dilute urine. Salt losses (by excretion in the urine and by diffusion through the skin) are balanced by an uptake of external NaCl by the skin. Such an uptake of sodium ions may occur from a very dilute external medium, that is, it works against a high chemical gradient and must therefore results from active transport (KROGH, 1937b, 1939; JØRGENSEN et al., 1946).

b) During periods of life in a terrestrial habitat, the amphibians loose water by evaporation through the skin (ADOLPH, 1932); when there is no water available, this results in a progressive increase in the osmotic pressure and sodium concentration of body fluids (SHOEMAKER, 1964). The extent of dehydration that the animal can tolerate varies from one species to another and constitutes one of the factors determining adaptation to a terrestrial habitat in amphibians (see CHEW, 1961; HELLER, 1965b; BENTLEY, 1966b). Generally there appears to be a close correlation between the ability to tolerate dehydration and the adaptation to terrestrial life in both the anurans (THORSON and SVIHLA, 1943; THORSON, 1955) and the urodeles (LITTLEFORD et al., 1947; COHEN, 1952). Nevertheless, for a few species this correlation does not hold (see, for example, BENTLEY et al., 1958), an observation which indicates that regulatory factors are also of importance in adaptation. Thus, during dehydration, the urinary output of water is greatly decreased (ADOLPH, 1927; POHLE, 1920; SCHMIDT-NIELSEN and FORSTER, 1954; JØRGENSEN et al., 1956; SAWYER, 1956, 1957a; SHOEMAKER, 1965). Moreover, the tendency for the osmolarity of the body fluids to increase is partly balanced by the reabsorption of water from the dilute bladder urine, which may be stored in very large amounts, especially in some anuran species (STEEN, 1929; EWER, 1952a; SAWYER and SCHISGALL, 1956; URANGA and QUINTANA, 1958). The physiological importance of this mechanism, first suggested by DARWIN (1839) (quoted by HELLER, 1965b), is demonstrated by the old observation of OVERTON (1904) that animals *(Hyla arborea)* with a full bladder tolerate a period of dehydration much better than those whose bladder had been emptied when starting the experiment. Likewise, in *Bufo cognatus* (RUIBAL, 1962) or *Bufo marinus* (SHOEMAKER, 1964), the increase in plasma osmolarity resulting from dehydration is much delayed in the animal with a full bladder as compared to the control with an emptied bladder. In addition, the ability of the animals to absorb water through the skin very efficiently, even when the area of skin in contact with water is very small (ADOLPH, 1927, 1933), is a factor of importance in the natural conditions of life which helps some amphibian species to live for long periods in relatively dry habitats.

c) When put into fresh water, anurans like *Bufo carens* (EWER, 1952a) or *Rana pipiens* (LEVINSKY and SAWYER, 1953) increase more rapidly in weight if they have been previously dehydrated than if they are normally hydrated, indicating that the permeability of the skin to water increases as a result of dehydration.

The action of neurohypophysial hormones in osmoregulation in amphibians was discovered by BRUNN (1921), who showed that normally hydrated anurans injected with neurohypophysial extracts gain weight when placed in water (water balance effect). Since that time, it has been clearly and repeatedly shown that this overall effect results from the action of the hormone on the water permeability at three levels: the kidney, the bladder* and the skin. More recently, it has been demonstrated that the hormone not only enhances the permeability to water, but also stimulates the active uptake of sodium that takes place through the skin (JØRGENSEN et al., 1946; FUHRMAN and USSING, 1951; MOREL et al., 1958) and the bladder (LEAF, 1960; BOURGUET and MAETZ, 1961), as well as the active reabsorption of sodium by the tubules of the kidney (JARD and MOREL, 1963); these observations suggest that neurohypophysial hormones could be involved in the regulation of both the water (1) and the sodium (2) metabolisms. These two aspects will now be discussed separately.

1. Regulation of the Water Metabolism

Action on the Water Balance. The water balance effect of neurohypophysial hormones, as judged by the gain in body weight, has been observed in many amphibian species; Table 1 summarizes these results and indicates the corresponding references. The data are difficult to compare, since the results depend on the experimental conditions and on the nature of the peptide injected. Nevertheless, it is obvious that there are species differences in sensitivity, and that there appears to be a rough correlation between the intensity of the water balance effect and the usual ecological conditions of the species (STEGGERDA, 1937; EWER, 1952a; BENTLEY and HELLER, 1964; HELLER and BENTLEY, 1965): the response to the hormone is almost zero in the strictly aquatic species, like *Xenopus laevis;* on the other hand, the weight change may be tremendous (up to 50% of the body weight) in the most terrestrial species. However, water balance effects of similar magnitude may result from different sites of hormonal action. Thus, it has been recently demonstrated by BENTLEY and HELLER (1964) that the water balance effect observed in *Triturus* chiefly results from an antidiuretic action, without any change in the osmotic permeability to water either of the skin or of the bladder (which is poorly developed in this species), whereas, in the salamander, the water balance effect seems to result from an increased reabsorption of water by the bladder (BENTLEY and HELLER, 1965). HELLER (1965b) suggests that the term "water balance effect" should be used only for the anurans, in which actions on the three sites (kidney, bladder and skin) seem to be simultaneously present in most cases. The table also indicates the relative activities of the different peptides used in this bioassay. In every instance, arginine-vasotocin, when tested, was the most active compound. We know that it is a naturally occuring hormone in the frog (ACHER et al., 1960a) and other species of amphibians (ACHER et al., 1964a). The amounts required to observe an effect vary from species to species, the order of magnitude being about 10^{-11} M/kg in *Ambystoma* and about 10^{-9} M/kg in *Triturus* (BENTLEY and HELLER, 1964). This dose range is high, but the very low sensitivity of the test used must be pointed out; it is obvious, for example, that an antidiuretic effect is much easier to observe

* It is obvious that an increased reabsorption of water from the bladder can contribute to the observed water balance effect only if the bladder is carefully emptied, both at the beginning and at the end of the water balance test, before weighing the animals.

Table 1. *Maximal water uptake by amphibians injected with neurohypophysial hormones*

Species	Maximal Water Retention g/100 g initial BW	Hormone	References
Anurans:			
Xenopus laevis	0	Pitressin, Pitocin	EWER (1952a)
	0	arginine-vasotocin (164 mμM/kg)	HELLER and BENTLEY (1965)
Neobatrachus	10	Pitressin	BENTLEY et al. (1958)
Leptodactylus	16	Pitressin, Pitocin	BIASSOTI (1923),
	—	Pitressin, Pitocin	EWER (1952a)
Discoglossus pictus	19	arginine-vasotocin (328 mμM/kg)	HELLER and BENTLEY (1965)
Pelobates cultripes	13	arginine-vasotocin (328 mμM/kg)	HELLER and BENTLEY (1965)
Rana clamitans	14	Pitocin > Pitressin	EWER (1952a)
Rana pipiens	14—19	Pitocin > Pitressin	EWER (1952a),
	18	Pituitrin	STEGGERDA (1937)
Rana esculenta	12—24	Pitocin > Pitressin	EWER (1952a)
		AVT > AVP > Oxy > LVP	HELLER and BENTLEY
	20.4	arginine-vasotocin (36 mμM/kg)	(1965)
Rana temporaria	28	Pitocin > Pitressin	EWER (1952a)
Bufo bufo		AVT > AVP > Oxy > LVP	HELLER and BENTLEY
	18.3	arginine-vasotocin (70 mμM/kg)	(1965)
	40	Pitressin > Pitocin	EWER (1952a), JØRGENSEN (1950)
Bufo carens	22	Pitressin > Pitocin	EWER (1952a)
Bufo regularis	22	Pitressin > Pitocin	EWER (1952a),
	45	Pituitrin	STEGGERDA (1937)
Bufo americanus	45	Pitressin > Pitocin	EWER (1952a)
Hyla hyla	53	arginine-vasotocin (410 mμM/kg)	HELLER and BENTLEY (1965)
Urodeles:			
Necturus	4	Pituitrin	STEGGERDA (1937)
	1.7	arginine-vasotocin (24 mμM/kg)	BENTLEY and HELLER (1964)
Ambystoma	6—8	arginine-vasotocin	ALVARADO and JOHNSON (1965)
	—	vasopressin	DOW and ZUCKERMAN (1939)
	—	Pituitrin	BELEHRADEK and HUXLEY (1927)
	7	—	JØRGENSEN et al. (1946)
	6	—	SCHREIBER and SCHREIBER (1950)
	7	arginine-vasotocin (36 mμM/kg)	BENTLEY and HELLER (1964)
Triturus alpestris	8	arginine-vasotocin (7 mμM/kg)	BENTLEY and HELLER (1964)
Triturus cristatus	10	arginine-vasotocin (7 mμM/kg)	BENTLEY and HELLER (1964)
Salamandra maculosa	0	arginine-vasotocin (180 mμM/kg)	BENTLEY and HELLER (1965)

by recording the urine flow rate than the total body weight! It has been observed that arginine-vasopressin is more active than oxytocin in several species of *Bufo*, whereas the reverse is true for several species of *Rana;* this kind of observation remains of limited physiological importance, since most probably neither oxytocin nor vasopressin are natural hormones for amphibians. The pharmacological differences reported could indicate that there are species variations in the steric configuration of the receptor molecule to which the active peptides bind in the target organs.

Action on the Permeability of the Skin to Water. The first experimental demonstration of the action of neurohypophysial hormones on the permeability of the skin itself was that the water balance effect is still present after removal of the kidneys (BRUNN, 1921), ligation of the ureters (BIASOTTI, 1923) or ligation of the cloaca (HOUSSAY and POTICK, 1929a–b; STEGGERDA, 1931; REY, 1935), whereas it disappears after removal of the skin (STEGGERDA, 1931; NOVELLI, 1936). It has later been shown (FUHRMAN and USSING, 1951; SAWYER, 1951b; KOEFOED-JOHNSEN and USSING, 1953) that the action can be elicited *in vitro* on isolated pieces of skin. Several techniques for quantitative recording of the net flux of water through the skin have been described (KOEFOED-JOHNSEN and USSING, 1953; MOREL et al., 1958; BOURGUET and MAETZ, 1961; BOURGUET and JARD, 1964). Table 2 indicates the values of the net flux of water measured *in vitro* through the skin of about 10 different amphibian species before and after addition of neurohypophysial hormone. All data are expressed as μl of water per hour per square centimeter of skin area, and for an osmotic pressure difference of 220 mOsm/l. It is quite clear that neurohypophysial hormones increase the permeability of the skin to water in the terrestrial anuran species (*Bufo* and *Rana*), but is ineffective in the purely aquatic anuran species *Xenopus* (MAETZ, 1963), as well as in all the urodele species tested (BENTLEY and HELLER, 1964, 1965). In *Rana esculenta*, it has been observed (BOURGUET and MAETZ, 1961) that arginine-vasotocin is much more active on that test than lysine-vasotocin or oxytocin, the active concentration for AVT lying between 10^{-10} and 10^{-9} M.

Action on the Permeability of the Bladder to Water. This effect was first demonstrated *in vivo* by EWER (1952b) and confirmed by SAWYER and SCHISGALL (1956). BENTLEY (1958) showed that the effect of the hormone can be elicited *in vitro* and is easily and precisely measured by the change in weight of closed bladders, filled with hyposmotic solutions and immerged in a Ringer solution. In the absence of neurohypophysial hormone, the net flux of water reabsorption is very low: .5—5 μl/min for the whole bladder of *Bufo bufo* and *Rana esculenta* (MAETZ, 1963), .5—1 μl/min for *Bufo marinus* (RASMUSSEN et al., 1963). For an osmotic gradient of 160 mOsm/l, HAYS and LEAF (1962a) give for the bladder of *Bufo marinus* a net flux of .07 $\mu l\ min^{-1}\ cm^{-2}$, a figure which is at the lower end of the range of values measured on the skin (Table 2). Addition of hormone to the medium bathing the serosal side of the bladder results in a tremendous increase in the net flux of water, much higher than for the skin. Thus, maximal fluxes as high as 150 μl/min in *Bufo bufo* (MAETZ, 1963), 50 μl/min in *Rana esculenta* (BOURGUET and MAETZ, 1961; MAETZ, 1963), 70 μl/min in *Bufo marinus* (RASMUSSEN et al., 1963) have been reported; when expressed per unit of bladder area, the corresponding figures are 1.5 $\mu l\ min^{-1}\ cm^{-2}$ in *Rana catesbiana* (SAWYER, 1960a) and 3.5 $\mu l\ min^{-1}\ cm^{-2}$ (160 mOsm/l osmotic gradient) in *Bufo marinus* (HAYS and LEAF, 1962a). This correspond to an about fifty fold increase as compared to the control values without hormone. As far as physiology is concerned, the amount of water which can be reabsorbed by this process depends upon the anatomical development of the bladder, which is highly variable from species to species (see BENTLEY, 1966a): in anurans, the full bladder may represent up to 25—30% of the body weight in *Bufo bufo* and 10% in *Rana esculenta*, whereas it is very small in *Xenopus laevis;* there is a similar correlation in urodeles; the more terrestrial species have a larger bladder (20% of body weight in *Ambystoma*, 12—34% in *Salamandra maculosa*) than the purely

Table 2. *Osmotic permeability to water of isolated skin of amphibians and action of neurohypophysial hormones*

Species	Fn H_2O ($\mu l \cdot h^{-1} \cdot cm^{-2}$) Gradient: 200 mOsm/l control	after hormone		Hormone	Ref.
Bufo bufo	9.2	20.9		Whale neurohypophysial extract	1
	21.4	45.7		Oxy 10^{-8} M, Pollachius Extract (200 μU/ml)	2
Rana esculenta.	9.3	17		Oxy 10^{-8} M, Pollachius Extract (80 μU/ml)	2
Rana pipiens	4.7	19		Pituitrin (500 mU/ml)	3
Xenopus	5	5	NS	Oxy 5×10^{-7} M, LVP 10^{-7} M, Pollachius Extract (15 mU/ml)	2
Triturus alpestris	7	8	NS	AVT: 2.9×10^{-8} M	4
Triturus cristatus. . . .	7	7	NS	AVT: 4.6×10^{-8} M	4
Ambystoma before metamorphosis	4	7	NS	AVT: 8.2×10^{-8} M	4
Ambystoma after metamorphosis	2	5	NS	AVT: 4.6×10^{-8} M	4
Necturus	3	4	NS	AVT: 1.12×10^{-7} M	4
Salamandra maculosa . .	7.3	10.9	NS	AVT: 4×10^{-8} M	5

References. 1: Koefed-Johnsen and Ussing (1953); 2: Maetz (1963); 3: Sawyer (1951b); 4: Bentley and Heller (1964); 5: Bentley and Heller (1965).

Abbreviations: Fn = net flux; Oxy = oxytocin; LVP = lysine-vasopressin; AVT = arginine-vasotocin; NS = non significant

aquatic ones (2% of body weight in *Triturus*, 5% in *Necturus;* Bentley and Heller, 1964). There are also species differences in the response of the bladder to neurohypophysial hormones which appear to show a correlation with the ecological conditions: thus, when tested on the bladder of *Triturus*, *Ambystoma* and *Necturus*, AVT had no effect (Bentley and Heller, 1964), whereas it increased fivefold the permeability to water of the bladder of *Salamandra* (Bentley and Heller, 1965) and that of the most terrestrial anuran species by up to fifty-fold. On the other hand, arginine-vasotocin is by far the most powerful hormone on the amphibian bladder; in *Rana esculenta*, for example, it is 30—35 times more active than oxytocin (Jard et al., 1960) and about 25 times more active than oxytocin in *Bufo marinus* (Rasmussen et al., 1963). Moreover, the minimal concentration of arginine-vasotocin which has to be reached in the bathing medium in order to observe an effect is remarkably low, since it is of the order of 10^{-12} M for the most sensitive bladders of *Rana esculenta* (see, for example, Bourguet and Maetz, 1961). The other naturally occuring hormone of the frog, mesotocin (Acher et al., 1964b), which is probably present in the other amphibians species (Acher et al., 1965a; Follet and Heller, 1964b), is about 12 times less active than arginine-vasotocin on the bladder.

Actions on Water Excretion by the Kidney. The first observations reported (Oehme, 1919; Brunn, 1921; Biasotti, 1923; Steggerda, 1931) were negative, as well as the experiments of Burgess, Harvey and Marshall (1933) on *Rana catesbiana:*

Table 3. *Distribution of antidiuretic action of neurohypophysial hormones in amphibians*

Species	Hormone	Antidiuretic action	Nature of the effect	Ref.
Bufo arenarum	Mammalian neurohypophysial extract	+	Tubular action	1
	Mammalian neurohypophysial extract	+	Constriction of afferent glomerular vessels	2
	Mammalian neurohypophysial extract	+	—	3
Bufo carens	vasopressin, oxytocin	+	—	4
Bufo regularis	vasopressin, oxytocin	+	—	5
Bufo marinus	Pituitrin, Pitressin	+	Tubular action	6
		+	Glomerular effect	7
	oxytocin	—	Glomerular diuretic effect	8
Bufo bufo	AVT, AVP, LVP, Oxyt.	+	—	9
Rana pipiens	Pitocin, Pituitrin	+	Glomerular effect	10
	Pituitrin	+ —	Increase with larges doses or decrease with small doses of the number of active glomeruli	11
	Pituitrin	+	Inhibition of water diuresis	12
	Pituitrin	+	Decrease in the rate of dehydration	13
	Hypophysial extracts	+	Inhibition of salt diuresis	14
Rana catesbiana	AVT, oxytocin	+ —	Glomerular and tubular antidiuresis Glomerular diuretic effect	15
	Pitocin, Pituitrin	+	Glomerular effect	16
	Pituitrin-Pitressin	0	—	17
	Frog neurohypophysial extract	+	Tubular action	18
Rana temporaria	Mammalian neurohypophysial extract	0	—	19
	oxytocin, vasopressin	+	—	20
		+	—	21
Rana esculenta	Pituitrin-Pitressin	+	Tubular action	22
	arginine-vasotocin	+	Glomerular and tubular antidiuresis	23
Xenopus		0	—	24
Ambystoma	arginine-vasotocin	+	Glomerular effect	25
	arginine-vasotocin	0	—	26
Triturus alpestris	arginine-vasotocin	+	—	26
Triturus cristatus	arginine-vasotocin	+	—	26
Necturus	arginine-vasotocin	0	—	26
Salamandra maculosa	arginine-vasotocin	0	—	27

References: 1: Pasqualini (1938a, b); 2: Adolph (1936); 3: Novelli (1936); 4: Ewer (1952a); 5: Ewer (1951); 6: Sawyer (1957a, b); 7: Sawyer and Sawyer (1952); 8: Uranga (1961); 9: Jørgensen and Larsen (1963); 10: Sawyer (1951a); 11: Richards and Schmidt (1924); 12: Boyd and Whyte (1939); 13: Boyd and Whyte (1938); 14: Oldham (1936); 15: Uranga and Sawyer (1960); 16: Sawyer and Sawyer (1952); 17: Burgess et al. (1933); 18: Sawyer (1956); 19: Oehme (1919), Brunn (1921), Biasotti (1923), Steggerda (1931); 20: Jørgensen (1950); 21: Rey (1935); 22: Jancso (1955a, b); 23: Jard and Morel (1961 and 1963), Jard (1966); 24: Ewer (1952a); 25: Alvarado and Johnson (1965); 26: Bentley and Heller (1964); 27: Bentley and Heller (1965).

these last authors did not observe any antidiuretic effect after injections of large doses of either pituitrin or pitressin to hydrated or dehydrated animals. Later publications, the references of which are given on Table 3, indicate a more or less pronounced antidiuretic response according to the nature and doses of the hormone injected, to the species tested, and to the experimental conditions. The observed antidiuresis resulted sometimes from an increased tubular water reabsorption, sometimes from a decreased glomerular filtration rate, and sometimes from a combination of these two mechanisms. These results deserve further comments:

1. The renal effects of the hormone can be observed only *in vivo* in the whole animal, that is in conditions in which many parameters and factors may change kidney function qualitatively or quantitatively; it is well known, for example, that GFR may vary over a large range in amphibians in response to an increase in the volume of the extracellular fluid (RICHARDS and SCHMIDT, 1924), to an injection of adrenalin (BIETER, 1930; FORSTER, 1943), to the stimulation of splanchnic nerves (RICHARDS et al., 1927; WHITE, 1929), as well as to many other kinds of stress and stimuli; thus, it may well be that many of the effects observed after injection of very large doses of neurohypophysial peptides (especially with mammalian hormones which are unphysiological in amphibians) are pharmacological ones, indirectly mediated via vascular actions for example.

2. The experiments in which the final urine only has been collected and analysed remain difficult to interpret, since it is impossible to distinguish between the renal and the bladder actions of the hormone.

3. All the reported experiments have been performed on animals with the neurohypophysis present; if neurohypophysial hormones do exert a physiological action on the kidney, it is to be expected that the observed effects of injected hormone will be completely different, depending on whether there is a release of endogeneous hormone during the experiment or not, that is, depending on whether the animals are well hydrated or dehydrated.

In experiments performed on well hydrated animals, and in which urine samples were collected from ureteral catheters, the administration of fresh amphibian neurohypophysial extract (in doses equivalent to one hundreth of a gland) to *Rana catesbiana* and to *Bufo marinus* (SAWYER, 1957a,b) or the injection of arginine-vasotocin (in doses of 10^{-11} M/kg B.W.) to *Rana catesbiana* (URANGA and SAWYER, 1960) and to *Rana esculenta* (JARD et al., 1960; JARD and MOREL, 1963), all produced a well pronounced antidiuretic effect. This effect results both from a decrease in GFR — the relative magnitude of which is highly variable from experiment to experiment — and from an increase in tubular free water reabsorption (as indicated by an increased urinary osmolarity and a decreased relative free water clearance (SAWYER, 1957a,b; URANGA and SAWYER, 1960; JARD and MOREL, 1963). The osmotic pressure of the urine may be equal to that of the plasma, as in *Bufo marinus* (SAWYER, 1957a), or it may remain hyposmotic, as in *Rana esculenta* (JARD and MOREL, 1963); it is never hyperosmotic to the plasma. The decrease in GFR produced by arginine-vasotocin in anurans most probably results from a diminution in the number of active glomeruli. This has been noted at the surface of the kidney by direct microscopic observation after injection of low doses of pituitrin (RICHARDS and SCHMIDT, 1924) or pitocin (SAWYER, 1951a) to *Rana pipiens;* this has also been recently demonstrated by JARD (1966) for arginine-vasotocin in *Rana esculenta* by using a functional technique proposed by FORSTER (1942), that is, by measuring the maximal transport capacity of glucose: both GFR and Tm_G decrease similarly during AVT perfusion, indicating that a fraction of the nephrons is functionally excluded. Several other arguments, on the other hand, demonstrate that the observed tubular effects of the hormone are not secondary to its glomerular action, but result from a direct action on the permeability of the tubule. Thus, a) the tubular effect is present even in the animals in which the glomerular action is lacking (SAWYER, 1957a,b; JARD et al., 1960); b) there is no correlation between the magnitudes of the two actions (JARD, 1966), and c) in *Rana esculenta*, oxytocin inhibits the tubular effects of vasotocin but does not modify its glomerular effect (MOREL and JARD, 1963a). The site of the tubular action is probably located at the level of the distal tubule in amphibians as in mammals (WIRZ 1956, 1957). The tubular fluid is hyposmotic to the plasma along this segment (WALKER et al., 1937), so that an increase in the osmotic permeability of the tubular cells to water — a mechanism of hormonal action similar to that described on the epithelial cells of the skin and the bladder, as will be discussed later — would account for the observed antidiuretic effect (SAWYER, 1957b; JARD and MOREL, 1963; see also WHITTEMBURY et al., 1960). But, in great contrast with the mammals, the osmotic pressure of the urine delivered to the ureter is not in equilibrium with the surrounding fluid. This suggests either that the segment of the distal tubule, the permeability of which is enhanced by the hormone, is a very short one (so that tubular fluid does not reach osmotic equilibrium when flowing along), or that there is an even more distal segment which further dilutes the urine (by actively reabsorbing solutes through walls impermeable to water, JARD, 1966).

An antidiuretic action of vasotocin has also been reported in several species of urodeles by BENTLEY and HELLER (1964); the mechanism of this action has not been studied; nevertheless, according to the authors, it could be a purely glomerular one.

There are almost no data available concerning the possible action of mesotocin on the amphibian kidney. In *Rana esculenta* (JARD and MOREL, 1963; JARD, 1966), injections of mesotocin in minute amounts (equal to those in which arginine-vasotocin is active) do not change urine flow rate, GFR, or urinary composition. When injected in large amounts, mesotocin is diuretic, natriuretic and kaliuretic, all these effects probably being secondary to a large increase in GFR, as revealed by inuline clearance measurements.

2. Regulation of the Sodium Metabolism

As already mentioned, the neurohypophysial hormone stimulates the active transport of sodium by epithelial cells (natriferic action) in the same target organs in which it enhances the permeability to water, namely, the skin, the bladder and the kidney tubule.

The net flux of sodium through the skin, as measured *in vitro* by the short-circuit current technique (USSING and ZERAHN, 1951), has been observed to increase in response to neurohypophysial hormones in many anuran species: *Rana temporaria* (USSING and ZERAHN, 1951), *Rana esculenta* (MOREL and MAETZ, 1958; MAETZ, 1959; MOREL et al., 1958, 1961b), *Bufo bufo* (MAETZ et al., 1959b), *Xenopus laevis* (MAETZ, 1963), as well as in some species of urodele, like *Triturus*, but not in others, like *Necturus* or *Ambystoma*, in which both the spontaneous potential difference and the short-circuit current are very low (BENTLEY and HELLER, 1964).

The action of neurohypophysial hormone on sodium transport by the bladder has been clearly observed in anuran species like *Bufo marinus* (LEAF et al., 1958; BENTLEY, 1960; LEAF, 1960) and *Rana esculenta* (BOURGUET and MAETZ, 1961), whereas it was not present in the three urodele species studied by BENTLEY and HELLER (1964): *Ambystoma*, *Necturus* and *Triturus*.

When measured in the ureteral urine, the sodium excretion (in *Rana esculenta*) is markedly reduced in response to low doses of arginine-vasotocin. This effect is closely associated with the tubular antidiuretic effect and has the same time course; it does not result from the concomitant change in GFR, since, during the hormonal action, the relative sodium clearance (C_{Na}/C_{In}) decreases whereas the relative osmotic clearance (C_{Osm}/C_{In}) and the relative potassium clearance (C_K/C_{In}) remain unchanged (JARD and MOREL, 1963).

Arginine-vasotocin is the most potent natriferic peptide tested on each of these three structures, skin, bladder and kidney tubule. In *Rana esculenta*, for example, arginine-vasotocin is about 15 and 2.5 times more active than oxytocin on the bladder (BOURGUET and MAETZ, 1961) and on the skin (JARD et al., 1960) respectively. On the skin, mesotocin has a very high natriferic activity, in between those of oxytocin and vasotocin (MOREL and BASTIDE, 1964; MOREL et al., 1965). In all these structures, the amounts of arginine-vasotocin required to produce a natriferic response are comparable to those required to elicit an effect on the osmotic water flow; the correlation between the two effects is striking but not absolute as it will be discussed further in a later section. An example of dissociation of the two effects, which could be of physiological importance, has been reported by BENTLEY and HELLER (1962, 1964): the skin of aquatic urodeles responds to arginine-vasotocin *in vitro* by a stimulation of the Na transport without increase in water permeability.

With the exception of the kidney tubule of the frog, the natriferic action of neurohypophysial hormones seems to be more difficult to observe *in vivo* than *in vitro*; this probably results from technical limitations. Nevertheless, arginine-vasotocin, oxytocin, vasopressin or neurohypophysial extract have been reported to increase *in vivo* the net flux of sodium absorption through the skin in *Triturus* (BENTLEY and HELLER, 1964), *Ambystoma* (JØRGENSEN et al., 1946; ALVARADO and JOHNSON, 1965) and *Bufo regularis* (MAETZ, 1963). When the sodium balance of the whole body was measured, administration of the hormone sometimes resulted in no effect, as in *Xenopus*, *Rana esculenta* (HELLER and BENTLEY, 1965) or *Necturus* (BENTLEY and HELLER, 1964), and sometimes in a reduction of the negativity of the Na balance, as in *Triturus* according to BENTLEY and HELLER (1964). The excretion of a salt load, on the contrary, has been reported to be improved by neurohypophysial hormones in *Rana pipiens* (BOYD and WHYTE, 1939; SAWYER and SAWYER, 1952).

Thus, the experiments in which the hormone is injected *in vivo* or added *in vitro* indicate that arginine-vasotocin is involved in the control of the salt and water balance by acting at three levels: the skin, the bladder and the kidney (on both glomerular filtration rate and tubular function). Other kinds of experiments give support to such an interpretation. There is much evidence that the release of neurohypophysial hormones is increased during dehydration: dehydration results in a reduction in the amount of Gomori positive material present within the neurohypophysial tissue (HILD, 1951; TRAMEZZANI and URANGA, 1954; RIDLEY, 1964a) and in a reduction in the number of neurosecretory granules which can be observed by electron microscopy (GERSCHENFELD et al., 1960). The hormonal content of the gland, as judged by the rat uterus, the rat antidiuretic and the water balance activities, is decreased during dehydration (LEVINSKY and SAWYER, 1953; TRAMEZZANI and URANGA, 1954; JØRGENSEN et al., 1956) as well as by keeping frogs in isotonic saline for weeks (MAETZ et al., 1959b). Such a diminution most probably results from an increased hormonal release into the general circulation, since blood plasma removed from dehydrated toads elicits an antidiuretic effect and a water balance effect, when injected into control hydrated toads (SHOEMAKER, 1964). On the other hand, the injection of hyperosmotic solutions of sodium chloride or sucrose mimics the effects of the water deprivation, as judged by the reduction of neurosecretory granules in the gland (GERSCHENFELD et al., 1960) and by the change in water permeability of the target organs (SHOEMAKER, 1965). These last observations suggest (but do not prove) that changes in plasma osmolarity could control the release of neurohypophysial hormones into the general circulation in amphibians as in mammals (VERNEY, 1947). Unfortunately, the general picture just described concerning the possible role of neurohypophysial hormone in the osmoregulation of amphibians is not clearly supported by the experiments on hypophysectomized animals. Removal of the hypophysis in amphibians does not produce an experimental condition which could be compared to the diabetes insipidus resulting from neurohypophysectomy in mammals and birds. In fact, the published results show many discrepancies. It must be stressed that most of these results have been observed in animals in which the whole hypophysis had been removed. It is well known in mammals that the removal of the *pars distalis* can obscure the peripheral effects resulting from the absence of neurohypophysial hormones. This phenomenon could occur in amphibians as well, since the effects of injected neurohypophysial hormone are markedly reduced in adenohypophysectomized animals (STEGGERDA and JONES, 1935; CHEN et al., 1943; LEVINSKY and SAWYER, 1952). An increased diuresis has only been reported in a few instances, in *Bufo marinus* (HOUSSAY et al., 1925) and in *Bufo arenarum* (DEL CHIARAVIGLIO, 1961a, b). On the contrary, the urine flow rate was reported to decrease in the frog according to POHLE (1920) or to remain unchanged in *Rana temporaria* and *Rana viridis* according to REY (1937). Similar discrepancies concerning the changes in the water permeability of the skin in response to hypophysectomy have been published. LEVINSKY and SAWYER (1953) have observed that, when dehydrated hypophysectomized *Rana pipiens* are placed in water, they do not increase in weight as fast as dehydrated control frogs. On the contrary, in the experiments of JØRGENSEN et al. (1956) on *Bufo bufo* in which the pituitary stalk only was destroyed (with subsequent degenerescence of the neurohypophysis), the animals did not show any difference in the permeability of the skin to water, or in the response to dehydration when compared to the controls. Removal of the gland did not result in any change of the chloride net flux through the skin (JØRGENSEN and ROSENKILDE, 1957), as well as in any modification of the urinary sodium excretion (RIDLEY, 1964b). In order to account for these negative results, it could be suggested that some neurohypophysial hormone was directly released from functional tissue remaining in the hypothalamus.

Many other questions remain unsolved or difficult to understand. Thus, if the role of arginine-vasotocin in the regulation of the water balance of terrestrial anuran species seems clearly established, its physiological role in the regulation of the sodium balance is not so easy to figure out; it is quite clear that other hormones are involved in the sodium regulation too, especially aldosterone. It is well established that, by adrenalectomizing frogs (MYERS et al., 1956—1961; BISHOP et al., 1961) or by keeping them for weeks in saline (MAETZ et al., 1958), one markedly reduces the active transport of sodium through the skin; injections of aldosterone restore the transport to normal values (MAETZ et al., 1958; CRABBE, 1961a). Aldosterone acts directly on the epithelial cells, since the effect may be elicited in the bladder (CRABBE, 1961b; PORTER and EDELMAN, 1964; SHARP and LEAF, 1964), or in the skin (CRABBE and DE WEER, 1964) by adding the hormone *in vitro*; the mechanism of this action of aldosterone has been much analysed recently (see for example EDELMAN et al., 1963; SHARP and LEAF, 1966).

Among the other unsolved questions, the physiological functions of mesotocin, as well as the role of arginine-vasotocin in osmoregulation of urodeles, deserve mention.

Osmoregulation in marine amphibians has been partly analysed during the last years (Gordon et al., 1961; Gordon, 1962; Schmidt-Nielsen and Lee, 1962), but there is no data yet available concerning the physiological role of neurohypophysial hormones in these species.

C. Reptiles

There are only few data concerning the role of neurohypophysial hormones on osmoregulation in reptiles. Osmoregulation, in this group, seems to depend mostly from kidneys without participation neither of the skin nor of the bladder; the permeability of the skin to water and solutes is very low as compared to that of amphibians (Bogert and Cowles, 1947; Bentley, 1959a; Templeton, 1960; Chew and Dammann, 1961; Bentley and Schmidt-Nielsen, 1965, 1966). The kidney of reptiles is characterized by the presence of few and relatively small glomeruli (Marshall and Smith, 1930). As it is well known, the excretion of uric acid in large amounts (Needham, 1931) allows the terrestrial species to excrete their metabolic nitrogen in a low volume of iso- or even hyposmotic urine (Smith, 1932). GFR, urinary flow rate and urinary osmotic pressure appear to be a function of the degree of hydration of the animals. Overhydration, for example, results in a large polyuria for many species of the main classes of reptiles: Crocodilians (Burgess et al., 1933; Sawyer and Sawyer, 1952), Apodes (Le Brie and Sutherland, 1962), Lacertilians (Bentley, 1959a), Chelonians (Dantzler and Schmidt-Nielsen, 1966). Dehydration, on the reverse, markedly reduces the urine flow rate, by sometimes mostly decreasing GFR, as in alligators (Shannon, 1942), horned toads and Galapagos lizards (Roberts and Schmidt-Nielsen, 1966), and sometimes both decreasing GFR and enhancing tubular free water reabsorption, as in the turtle *Pseudemys scripta* (Dantzler and Schmidt-Nielsen, 1966), in which there is a concomitant increase in urinary osmotic pressure. According to Dantzler and Schmidt-Nielsen (1966), the observed changes in GFR seem to reflect changes in the number of functioning glomeruli.

Injections of neurohypophysial hormone to reptiles produce renal effects the nature and the intensity of which appear to vary with the species under study. In the alligator, relatively low doses of vasopressin (0.01—1 IU/kg B.W.) induce a large antidiuretic response or sometimes even an anuria; the response entierly results from a decrease in GFR (Burgess et al., 1933; Sawyer and Sawyer, 1952). The antidiuretic action of pitressin, pitocin or pituitrin has been confirmed in several instances, for example in *Tachysaurus* (Bentley, 1959a), in several species of *Natrix* (Le Brie and Sutherland, 1962), in a turtle, *Pseudemys scripta* (Dantzler and Schmidt-Nielsen, 1966). Within this last species, the antidiuretic action produced by low doses of hormone results from an increase in tubular water reabsorption without change in GFR, whereas the action produced by large doses seems mostly to result from a decrease in GFR. The renal actions of vasotocin, which is most probably a natural hormone in reptiles (see Sawyer et al., 1961a), have not been so far investigated. There is, at the present time, no evidence suggesting an action of neurohypophysial hormones on extrarenal osmoregulatory mechanisms in the reptiles. The active transport of sodium which occurs through the turtle bladder (Bentley, 1962a; Bricker et al., 1962; Brodsky et al., 1963) and the intestinal wall (Baillien and Schoffeniels, 1961a, b) is not affected by neurohypophysial hormones (Bentley, 1962a); nor is the water permeability of the bladder (Brodsky and Schilb, 1960; Bentley, 1962a).

To summarize, it seems probable that the antidiuretic action of neurohypophysial hormones in reptiles could be a physiological one, since it closely mimics the effects produced by dehydration. But further experiments are needed in order to ascertain the respective roles of the golmeruli and of the tubules in the response, as well as to establish which is the hormone involved, and how its rate of secretion into the general circulation is controlled.

D. Birds

Birds and mammals appear to be roughly similar when the main aspects of the osmoregulatory mechanisms and the role of neurohypophysial hormones in osmoregulation are compared. In both of them, the kidney is not only the principal organ involved in osmoregulation, but it contains loops of Henle and it is able to elaborate an urine of an osmotic pressure higher than that of the plasma (CADE, 1964; BARTHOLOMEW and CADE, 1963); nevertheless, these anatomical and functional characters are much more developed in mammals than in birds. The most striking difference between the two groups remains that birds are uricotelic (SHANNON, 1938) and mammals ureotelic.

The experimental data concerning osmoregulation and neurohypophysial hormones in birds are not very numerous, but they appear to be univocal and complementary, so that relatively precise conclusions can be drawn.

The experimental destruction of the neurohypophysial tissue in birds — obtained in pigeon by ablation of the ventral thalamus (ROGERS, 1924), or in the hen by lesions of the hypothalamus (MC FARLAND, 1959), by electrocoagulation of the supraoptic area (RALPH, 1960) and by neurohypophysectomy (SHIRLEY and NALBANDOV, 1956b) — always resulted in large polyuria and polydypsia. Experimental water overloading in birds induces a diuretic response with an associated decrease of the osmotic pressure of the urine (up to values as low as 50—60 mOsm/l, according to DICKER and HASLAM, 1966). These responses are quite similar to the diabetes insipidus and to the water diuresis observed in mammals under the same experimental conditions.

Dehydration of birds results in a state of antidiuresis; the osmotic pressure of the urine increases, so that the urine over plasma ratio of osmotic pressure may reach values of the order of 2 in the hen (DICKER and HASLAM, 1966) and in the pigeon (SCOTHORNE, 1959), and even values as high as 4.5 in a desert species of granine passerine (POULSON and BARTHOLOMEW, 1962). There is a simultaneous reduction in the content of the gland both in neurosecretory material (LEGAIT, 1959; OKSCHE et al., 1959; BERN et al., 1966) and in biological activity (ISHII et al., 1962).

Injection of neurohypophysial hormone in hydrated animals produces a typical antidiuretic response (GIBBS, 1929; BURGESS et al., 1933; KORR, 1939; HESTER et al., 1940; HOLMES and ADAMS, 1963). Both SAWYER et al. (1959) and SKADHAUGE (1964) have demonstrated in the water-loaded hen that arginine-vasotocin is a much more powerful antidiuretic peptide than vasopressin and oxytocin. A significant response can be elicited with intravenously injected amounts of arginine-vasotocin as low as 7—58 mμg per hen (SKADHAUGE, 1964). On the contrary, oxytocin injected in large doses produces a diphasic response, including a week and irregular antidiuretic effect of (probably) glomerular origin (SAWYER et al., 1959). These observations suggest that the hormone physiologically involved in the control of water excretion by the kidney in birds is vasotocin and not oxytocin. The mechanism of the vasotocin antidiuretic action entirely results from an increase in the free water reabsorption along the tubules. The excreted urine becomes hyperosmotic to plasma, without any significant change neither in plasma flow rate through the kidney (as judged by PAH clearance) nor in the glomerular filtration rate (as judged by inulin clearance), (SKADHAUGE, 1964). When vasotocin is perfused directly into the portal vein of one of the two kidneys, the resulting antidiuretic effect is significantly more pronounced in the perfused side than in the control side, an observation which demonstrates the direct effect of vasotocin on the permeability of the tubule to water (SKADHAUGE, 1964).

It thus seems probable that the glomerular effects which have been reported in birds after relatively large amounts of either pitressin (BURGESS et al., 1933) or oxytocin (SAWYER et al., 1960), are purely pharmacological ones.

The mechanisms by which hyperosmotic urine is formed within the kidney of some species of birds are probably quite similar to those which are now well known to operate within the mammalian kidney (WIRZ et al., 1951; WIRZ, 1956). If the first anatomical descriptions of the avian nephron (D'ERRICO, 1907; HUBER, 1917; see also SPERBER, 1960) reported only very poorly developed loops of henle, more recent data show that the loops are relatively well developed in these desert species which are able to form an urine of high concentration. Moreover, the interrelationships between loops of Henle and collecting ducts, as well as the disposition of the blood supply, seem to suggest that these structures could function as a countercurrent concentration multiplier system (POULSON, 1965; see also VOGEL, 1964; VOGEL and STOECKERT, 1965).

There is actually no indication available in birds indicating an extrarenal action of neurohypophysial hormone, except a transient secretory effect on the salt gland of the duck produced by the injection of oxytocin or vasopressin, according to HOLMES and ADAMS (1963). Since the salt gland is involved in the regulation of the salt balance in birds (SCHMIDT-NIELSEN et al., 1958; SCHMIDT-NIELSEN, 1960), further studies on its possible control by neurohypophysial hormone would be of high interest. The same is true for the water reabsorption that occurs in the cloaca (HESTER et al., 1940).

Second Part

Cellular Mechanisms of Action

As it has been discussed in the previous section, neurohypophysial hormones are able to elicit their specific effects on amphibian epithelial cells even when added *in vitro* to the bathing fluid. It is well known that both the amphibian skin and the amphibian bladder appear to be relatively simple structures, in which active sodium transport as well as water permeability can be quantitatively measured as a function of time. That is the reason why these two structures have been so widely used as very suitable and simple systems for further analysis of the permeability and transport properties of the epithelial cells. Several general reviews have recently been published concerning the physiology and biophysics of these cells (USSING, 1960; LEAF, 1965; BENTLEY, 1966a). In this section, we shall briefly recall these general considerations which must be kept in mind in order to understand the nature and the mechanism of the hormonal action. Since it has been found that the cellular aspects of the hormonal action are similar in the bladder and in the skin, these two structures will be discussed together. Three different points will successively be presented:

I. The final effect of the hormonal action, i.e. the nature of the change in water permeability (A) and of the stimulation of the active transport of sodium (B), as well as their relationships (C).

II. The possible metabolic steps leading from the first molecular interaction between hormone and target cell, up to the final observed effect.

III. The discussion of the interaction between the hormone and its molecular receptor.

I. Final Effects

A. Nature of the Change in Water Permeability

The net fluxes of water occuring through the skin and bladder are always entierly passive in nature; this net flux results both *in vivo* (HEVESY et al., 1935; NOVELLI, 1936; STEWART, 1949; SAWYER, 1951b; BENTLEY, 1957) and *in vitro* (USSING, 1952; SAWYER, 1960a; HAYS and LEAF, 1962a) from a difference in osmotic pressure between the fluids bathing the two sides of the structure. In the presence of neurohypophysial hormone as well as in the absence of hormone, the actual value of the net flux is proportional to the difference between the water activities in the two solutions (SAWYER, 1960a; HAYS and LEAF, 1962a). If the direction of the osmotic pressure difference is reversed, by using a hyperosmotic solution as the outside (mucosal) bathing solution, the direction of the net flux of water is also reversed (NOVELLI, 1936; SAWYER, 1960a; BENTLEY, 1961, 1965a). But there is some degree of rectification, i.e., for the same difference in osmotic pressure the value of the net flux is lower in the outward direction than in the inward direction, so that the proportionality constant linking the net flux to the osmotic driving force is greater when the flux is inwards directed (BENTLEY, 1961 and 1965a). The rectification of flow persists when sodium transport is abolished by using sodium-free Ringer solutions. It could result from the presence of two non-homogeneous barriers in series (BENTLEY, 1966a). Such a rectification can be demonstrated with artificial membranes (PATLAK et al., 1963). In the absence of osmotic gradient, one observes a small inwards directed net flow of water, which is associated with the active net transport of salt; this residual net flux of water is supressed when the active sodium transport is stopped, a situation which can be achieved by using isosmotic mannitol or choline Ringer solutions as mucosal bathing medium (MAETZ, 1960). When neurohypophysial hormone is added to the serosal medium (the hormone is inactive on both skin and bladder when added to the mucosal medium; FUHRMAN and USSING, 1951; LEAF et al., 1958), the net flux of water increases. The maximum increase which can be observed depends upon species and structures, as it has already been mentioned: it amounts to 2—3 times the control net flux for the skin of *Rana temporaria* (KOEFOED-JOHNSEN and USSING, 1953) and up to 50 times for the bladder of *Bufo marinus* (HAYS and LEAF, 1962a; LEAF and HAYS, 1962).

When unidirectional fluxes of water are measured with labelled water in the absence of any osmotic pressure difference across the preparation, both fluxes are equal (HEVESY et al., 1935; KOEFOED-JOHNSEN and USSING, 1953; HAYS and LEAF, 1962a). Addition of the hormone increases the absolute value of the unidiurectional fluxes, but to a much lesser extent (about 10% on the frog skin and 100% on the toad bladder) than the net flux; in other words, the hormone produces in the membrane a much larger increase in the osmotic permeability coefficient to water than in the diffusion permeability coefficient to water. In any case — in the absence of the hormone and even more so in its presence — net diffusion of water, alone, cannot account for the observed osmotic flux of water (USSING, 1952); a large drag effect of water molecules on water molecules in the direction of the net flux must exist, in order to account for the measured values. Such a drag effect indicates that water crosses the cellular membrane which acts as the limiting factor by flowing along water filled channels, rather than by diffusing through a continuous lipoid membrane (USSING, 1952; KOEFOED-JOHNSEN and USSING, 1953). By making the assumption that these channels are cyclindrical pores, and further assuming that the flow along these pores is laminar and obeys Poiseuille's law, it is possible to calculate the pore diameter necessary to account for both the diffusional and osmotic water permeabilities. The observation that the hormone increases the osmotic permeability much more than the diffusional one, would suggest that the radius of the "pores" but not their number would be increased as a result of the hormonal action. Such calculation indicates that the "mean pore radius", would increase from 8—12 Å within the frog skin (KOEFOED-JOHNSEN and USSING, 1953) and from 8—40 Å within the toad bladder (HAYS and LEAF, 1962a). The validity of such calculations has been frequently questioned (see for example HAYS and LEAF, 1962a; DAINTY and HOUSE, 1966); in any case it is evident that such values of "pore" diameters should only be regarded as an expression of the functional permeability of the membrane to water and not as a possible description of its actual structure. That the drag effect is an important factor which contributes to the osmotic flow of water through epithelial cells has been clearly demonstrated by ANDERSEN and USSING (1957): the two unidirectional fluxes through the skin of small water soluble molecules, such as acetamide or thiourea, are identical in the absence of chemical gradient and of net flux of water; when there is an osmotic pressure difference across the skin, the unidirectional flux of these indicators in the direction of the osmotic flow of water surpasses the unidirectional flux in the reverse direction; this drag effect is enhanced by the addition of neurohypophysial hormone. An increased diffusion permeability to urea, acetamide and other small polar molecules has also been reported on the toad bladder under the action of vasopressin (MAFFLY et al., 1960; LEAF and HAYS, 1962). Several kinds of experimental evidence suggest that the structure limiting the water fluxes through the skin and the bladder (which is necessarily also the site of the final action of the neurohypophysial hormone on the permeability to water) is the membrane located at the mucosal border of the epithelial cells. Thus, when the osmotic behaviour of skin epithelial cells is observed under a light microscope, it appears that these cells, in the absence of hormone, are near osmotic equilibrium with the serosal bathing medium and not with the mucosal one; when hormone is added, there is an increase in cellular volume if the mucosal bathing medium is of low osmotic pressure, indicating an increase in the osmotic permeability to water of the mucosal border (MC ROBBIE and USSING, 1961). Such a cellular swelling, as a result of the hormonal action, has also been reported for frog and toad bladders incubated with an hypotonic solution on the mucosal side (NATOCHIN et al., 1965). On the other hand, when isolated toad bladders are incubated with tritiated water added in one of the two bathing media, the specific activity of the cellular water reaches a steady state value very much closer to that of the serosal medium than to that of the other. In the presence of hormone, this steady state value is significantly shifted towards the specific activity within the mucosal medium (LEAF and HAYS, 1962). This observation indicates that the mucosal membrane acts as the limiting factor for diffusion of water, and that its permeability to water is increased by the hormone. When bladders incubated with a hypotonic mucosal medium are fixed and examined by electron microscopy (PAK POY and BENTLEY, 1960; PEACHEY and RASMUSSEN, 1961; CARASSO et al., 1962; JARD et al., 1966b), it is obvious that the epithelial cells are enlarged in those preparations which have been treated by neurohyplphysial hormones. Such a cellular swelling as a result of the hormonal action is depicted in the Fig. 1, which shows the structure of the bladder of *Rana esculenta* under differ-

---

Fig. 1. *Electron micrographs of the epithelial layer of the Frog (Rana esculenta) urinary bladder.* The structure of two hemibladders incubated with Ringer inside and half-Ringer outside are compared: one hemibladder was stimulated by a maximal dose of oxytocin (net flux of water: 1 μl min^{-1} cm^{-2} at the time the fixative was added), the second was used as a control (net flux of water 0,1 μl min^{-1} cm^{-2}). One can observe cellular swelling and enlargment of intercellular spaces in the stimulated hemibladder (lower graph) as compared to the resting hemibladder (upper graph)
× 8000. From CARASSO et al. (1966)

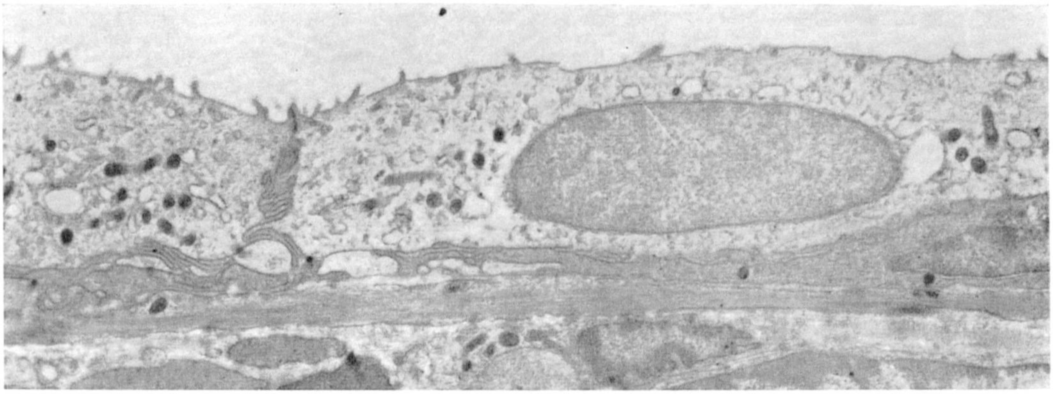

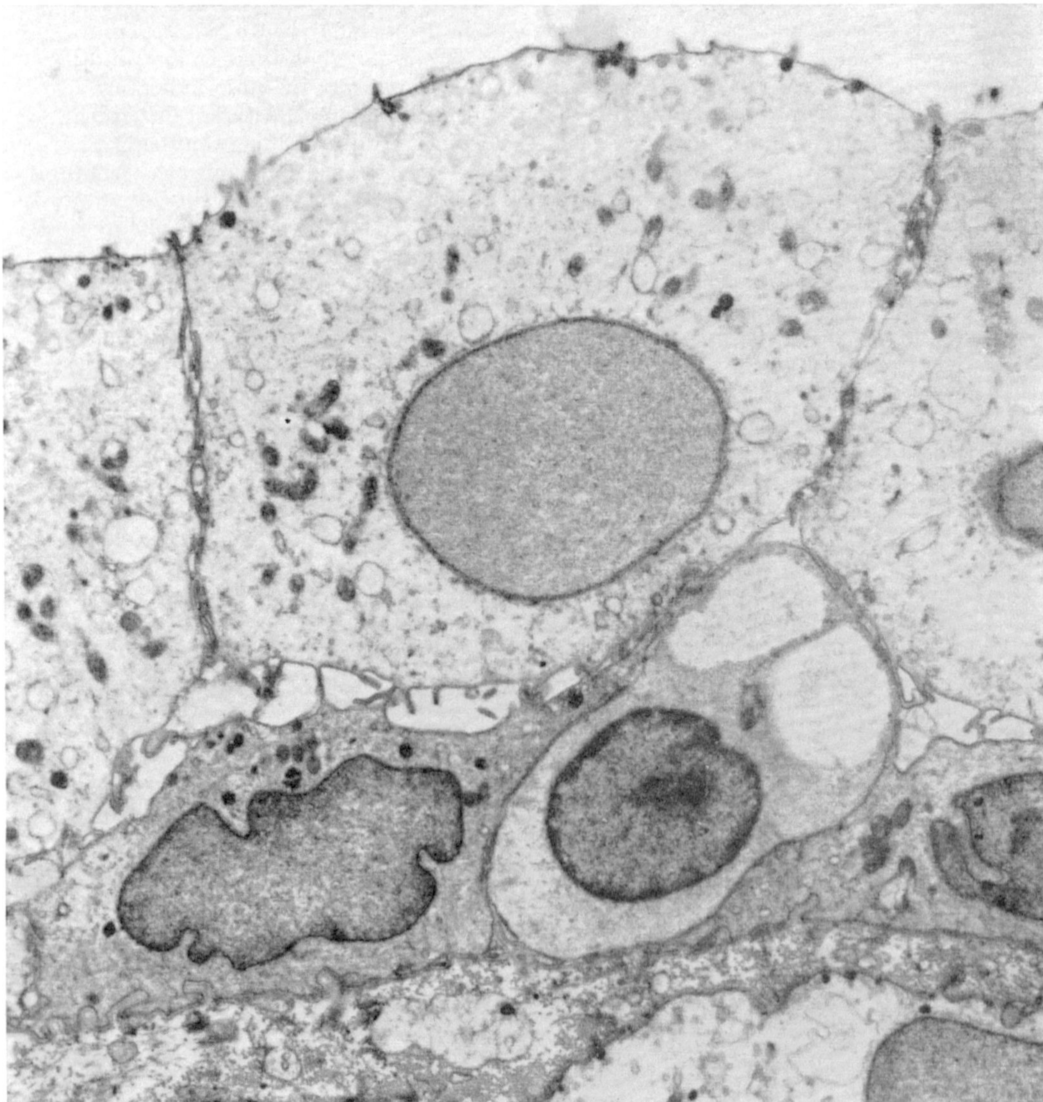

ent experimental conditions at the time the fixative was added. When fixed in the presence of an osmotic pressure difference across the cells, the hemibladder treated with oxytocin (through which a large osmotic flow of water was measured just

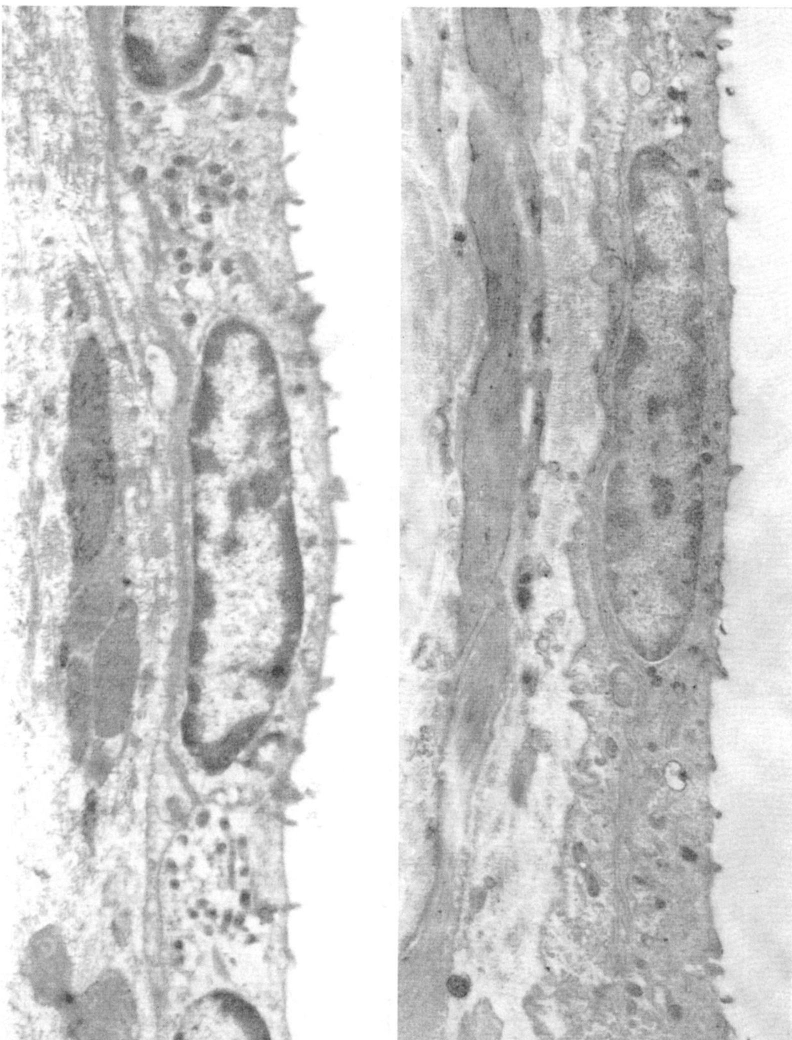

Fig. 2. *Electron micrographs of two hemibladders of Rana esculenta fixed in the absence of an osmotic flow of water (Ringer on both sides).* One hemibladder (lower graph) was stimulated by oxytocin, the second (upper graph) was used as a control. In both cases the net flux of water remains very low (measured value at the time the fixative was added: 0.06 μl min^{-1} cm^{-2}. In these experimental conditions oxytocin does not produce cellular swelling or enlargment of intercellular spaces.
$\times$ 8000. From CARASSO et al. (1966)

prior to fixation) shows enlarged cells with dilated intercellular spaces, as compared to the untreated control hemibladder. There are no visible differences between the two hemibladders, either with respect to the plasma membrane, or to tight-junctions. As shown on Fig. 2, when hemibladders are fixed during incubation with Ringer solution on both sides, the effects of oxytocin on the dimensions of the cells and intercellular spaces are absent (CARASSO et al., 1966; FAVARD et al.,

1966). Thus these effects appear to be indirect ones, and probably result from changes in both the cellular osmolarity and the net flux of water induced by the hormone. There is no indication of any pores in the mucosal plasma membrane, despite the curious observation that the increase in osmotic permeability produced by the hormone is maintained to some extent even after the preparation has been fixed (PEACHEY and RASMUSSEN, 1961; JARD et al., 1966b).

B. Nature of the Stimulation of the Active Transport of Sodium

The mechanisms by which the sodium ions are actively transported by the epithelial cells of the amphibian skin and bladder have been discussed on many occasions (USSING, 1960; LEAF, 1965; BENTLEY, 1966a). The main points will be briefly summarized. In the absence of electrochemical gradient for any ion across the cells (short-circuited condition), the net flux of sodium — equal to the difference between the two unidirectional fluxes as measured (simultaneously) with two isotopes of Na^+ — has been shown to be identical to the electrical current (short-circuit current) passing through the skin (USSING and ZERAHN, 1951) or the bladder (LEAF et al., 1958). Thus, sodium ions are the only ones to be actively transported (from mucosal to serosal side), whereas chloride ions, for example, diffuse down their electrochemical gradient (KOEFOED-JOHNSEN et al., 1952b). Moreover, both the net flux and the short-circuit current are equally increased by addition of neurohypophysial hormone (USSING and ZERAHN, 1951; MOREL and MAETZ, 1958; LEAF and DEMPSEY, 1960). The spontaneous electrical polarity of the skin, which can be observed even when the preparation is bathed by the same solution on the two sides, results from the difference in ionic permeabilities of the apical and basal borders of the cells for sodium and potassium ions. Thus, when measured in appropriate conditions, it has been shown that the outer border behaves more or less like a sodium reversible electrode, whereas the inner border behaves like a potassium reversible electrode (USSING and KOEFOED-JOHNSEN, 1956; KOEFOED-JOHNSEN and USSING, 1958); this indicates that the outer membrane is much more permeable to the diffusion of sodium than of potassium ions, and that this situation is reversed in the inner membrane. Such differences in the permeability of the two cellular faces for potassium ions have been confirmed by other methods (MC ROBBIE and USSING, 1961; USSING et al., 1965). According to this view, a neutral cationic pump located in the inner border and exchanging one sodium ion (actively extruded) for one potassium ion (entering the cell) would be responsible for the low Na and high K concentrations within the cell and, therefore, for the diffusion potentials measured at the two cellular borders (KOEFOED-JOHNSEN and USSING, 1958). As shown recently (BRICKER et al., 1963; BRICKER and KLAHR, 1963; ESSIG and LEAF, 1963; FRAZIER and LEAF, 1963), it is also possible that the sodium pump located in the inner border is an electrogenic one, and that potassium ions are entering the cells passively down the electrical field created by the active extrusion of the sodium ions. Moreover, it could be that the active pumping system is not only located within the inner border but also within the intercellular membrane of the epithelial cells (see for example USSING, 1965), as suggested by the histochemical evidence for ATPase activity along the intercellular spaces (FARQUHAR and PALADE, 1964—1966). This general description of the permiselectivity of the two membranes for alcali metal ions was confirmed by electrophysiological methods. Using Ling Gerard type of microelectrodes, several authors (ENGBAEK and HOSHIKO, 1957; HOSHIKO, 1961; WHITTEMBURY and HERRERA, 1964) have observed two positive electrical jumps located within the skin at the level of the *stratum germinativum*. More recently, this simple description of the epithelium of the skin has been somewhat complicated by assuming that several layers of epithelial cells and not only the *stratum germinativum* are actually involved in the process of active transport of sodium (USSING, 1965); this refinment accounts for the observation that frequently more than two electrical jumps are observed through the skin (USSING and WINDHAGER, 1964a, b), but does not greatly change the general picture just described. In any case, there is a single layer of epithelial cells in the bladder, and, according to FRAZIER (1962) and FRAZIER and LEAF (1963), only two positive electrical jumps corresponding to the mucosal and serosal borders of these cells.

It is generally accepted that the sodium concentration within the cells is kept low or even very low, so that the net flux directed from the cells to the serosal medium has to be an active one, since it occurs both against a chemical and an electrical gradient. According to most authors, it is assumed, on the contrary, that the net flux of sodium through the mucosal border is a passive one, that is, occurs down the electrochemical gradient (KOEFOED-JOHNSEN and USSING, 1958; LEAF, 1960). This assumption seems to be justified by the observation, already mentioned, that the mucosal border behaves like a sodium reversible electrode. Nevertheless, in order to be absolutely sure of this point, it would be necessary to know the exact chemical activity of Na ions within the cells, what is not possible at the present time. Indirect measurements of the cellular sodium pool of the bladder as a function of the sodium concentration in the mucosal bathing solution suggest that the cellular concentration is always lower than that in the mucosal medium when the net flux is inwards directed (FRAZIER, DEMPSEY and LEAF, 1962). On the other hand, it has been shown (FRAZIER and LEAF, 1964) that the kinetics of the unidirectional flux Fin (from mucosal to serosal border), as well as the size of the cellular pool of exchangeable sodium, when measured as functions of the outside concentration, show evidence of saturation. This would indicate that the entry of sodium ions into the cells through their mucosal border is not a simple diffusional process, but involves some interaction with specific sites of limited number within the membrane (carrier mediated process). Similar mechanisms would account for the entry of sodium ions into the frog skin (CEREIJIDO et al., 1964). It must be stressed that there is to day no unequivocal evidence demonstrating that the movements of Na^+ ions through the mucosal border are purely passive.

As mentioned previously, addition of neurohypophysial hormones to the serosal bathing medium results in an increase of the short-circuit current through both the skin (USSING and ZERAHN, 1951; FUHRMAN and USSING, 1951) and the bladder (LEAF et al., 1958; BOURGUET and MAETZ, 1961), the magnitude of which is entirely accounted for by the stimulation of the active transport of sodium (USSING, 1955; MOREL and MAETZ 1958; LEAF and DEMPSEY, 1960). The mechanism of this response is not yet clearly understood. According to the majority of the authors, the hormone would enhance the permeability to the passive movement of sodium ions at the mucosal border, this factor being rate limiting for the net flux of sodium (see for instance USSING, 1952; LEAF, 1960; CRABBE and DE WEER, 1965). An increase in the Na cellular content will result, so that, at the serosal border, more sodium will be available to the active transporting mechanism. On such a view, a single site of action, and possibly even a single mechanism of action of the hormone on the permeability of the mucosal barrier could account for both the increase in water permeability and in active sodium transport (LEAF, 1960; FRAZIER et al., 1961). Such a mechanism of action on the net flux of sodium was supported by the experiments of USSING and ZERAHN (1951), indicating that the addition of hormone does not change the calculated electromotive force of the transporting system (E_{Na}), whereas the resistance exerted by the skin to Na^+ diffusion was lowered, and by the observations of FRAZIER et al. (1962) indicating that the sodium pool of the bladder which can be exchanged through the mucosal border is effectively increased as a result of the hormonal action. However, the assumed proportionality between the so called sodium pool measured in the bladder and the sodium concentration within the cells remains open to discussion, since an unknown fraction of this sodium could be located in the intercellular and/or interstitial spaces. On the other hand, it has been repeatedly observed, both on the skin (see for example Morel and Maetz, 1958) and the bladder (see Leaf, 1961), that neurohypophysial hormone stimulates the influx of sodium ions, without any significant change in the outflux, suggesting an action on the driving force of the transporting system rather than on the resistance to Na diffusion. Finally, the best evidence favouring an action of the hormone on the permeability to sodium at the mucosal barrier, — i.e., the increase in the mucosal outflux of radiosodium without change in the serosal outflux as a response to the addition of hormone during the washout period of bladders loaded with radiosodium (Frazier and Hammer, 1963) — has not been confirmed (Leaf, 1965). On the other hand, it has been observed on frog skin (Bourguet and Maetz, 1961; Morel and Bastide, 1965) and toad bladder (Civan et al., 1966) that, when the mucosal sodium concentration is kept at very low levels, both the short-circuit current and the net flux of sodium are outwards directed; if hormone is now added to the preparation, the direction of the net flux may reverse. This would indicate either that the electrochemical gradient for Na ions at the mucosal border is reversed by the hormone (suggesting a stimulating action on an active step of transport) (Morel and Bastide, 1965) or that there are two types of channels for Na diffusion through the mucosal border, that is: a) intercellular channels with an outwards directed passive net flux (along the chemical gradient in the conditions of these experiments) and b) an inwards downhill net penetration into the cells through the cell membrane itself. If the active transport process located at the serosal border is equivalent to an electromotive force of 180 mV, i.e. is capable of creating a electrochemical gradient of 180 mV across the mucosal border, then even the change in direction observed could result from a hormonal action on the passive mucosal permeability to sodium ions (Civan et al., 1966; Morel and Bastide, 1967).

C. Interrelations Between the Hormonal Effects on Water Permeability and on Sodium Transport

Several kinds of experimental evidence indicate that a single change in the structure (or the properties) of the mucosal border as a result of the hormonal action cannot alone account for both the increase in osmotic permeability and the increase in sodium transport.

It has been reported (Lichtenstein and Leaf, 1965) that the addition of amphotericin to the mucosal medium bathing the toad bladder results in an increase in permeability of the mucosal border to sodium and urea, without change in the osmotic flow of water, an observation which indicates that the factors limiting the permeability to sodium and to water are different. On the other hand, Petersen and Edelman (1964) and Bentley (1959b—1960) have shown on the toad bladder that, when the calcium concentration in the bathing medium is high, the effect of vasopressin on water flow and urea permeability is inhibited, whereas the effect of the hormone on the sodium transport remains unchanged. Furthermore, calcium inhibits the increase in water permeability produced by vasopressin but not that produced by theophylline or 3'-5'-cyclic AMP (Petersen and Edelman, 1964). These observations suggest that the calcium effect is located a) to an early step in the mechanism of action of the hormone on water permeability, and

b) that this step is different from those involved in the mechanism of its action on sodium transport. Moreover, as already mentioned in a previous section, in some amphibian species, the addition of the hormone to skin preparations may result in only one of the two effects (BENTLEY and HELLER, 1964, see also MOREL, 1964). All these experiments clearly indicate that the two final effects of the hormone may be dissociated. An other kind of evidence suggests that the dissociation is not only between the final effects or between one intermediate step, but also between the corresponding hormonal receptors: thus, when the relative potencies of both oxytocin and Arginine-vasotocin are compared by measuring the two effects on the frog bladder *(Rana esculenta)*, it appears (BOURGUET and MAETZ, 1961) that the

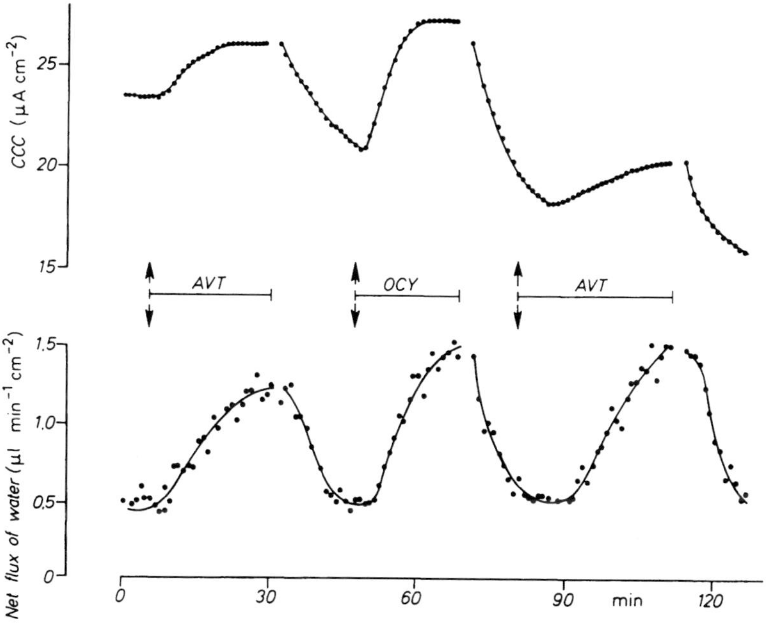

Fig. 3. *Relative potencies of oxytocin (ocy) and Arginine-vasotocin (AVT) on active sodium transport and water permeability of the frog bladder (Rana esculenta L.).* The short circuited current (ccc) and the net flux of water are registred simultaneously on the same preparation. Ringer is used as inside medium and 20 fold diluted Ringer as outside medium (in these experimental conditions short-circuited current represents a good estimation of the active transport of sodium). One can observe that the doses of oxytocin (625 μU/ml) and vasotocin (3.2 μU/ml: oxytocic units) used in this experiment produce an increase of the same magnitude in the net flux of water while oxytocin produces a much larger effect on short-circuited current than arginine-vasotocin does. From BOURGUET and MOREL (1967)

activity of arginine-vasotocin (relative to that of oxytocin) is higher when measured on water flow than when measured on sodium transport (see Table 4). A similar dissociation has been observed when the two effects are recorded simultaneously on the same preparation, as shown by Fig. 3 (BOURGUET and MOREL, 1967). The most likely explanation for the observed difference in the arginine-vasotocin relative activities is to assume that the two effects result from the interaction of the hormone with two different kinds of receptors, the relative affinities of which for both oxytocin and arginine-vasotocin are different.

II. Intermediate Steps

The sequence of events which occur within the epithelial cells between the first step of the hormonal action, — that is, the binding of the hormone with its specific molecular receptor — and the final observed effect — i.e., the increase in permeability to water or the stimulation of the sodium transport — is far from completely solved.

One theory of the mechanism of action of the antidiuretic hormone involves the secretion of hyaluronidase by the epithelial target cells. The enzyme is supposed to increase the permeability to water by depolymeryzing mucopolysaccharids within the intercellular spaces and the basal membrane (GINETZINSKY, 1958). This theory has been discussed in detail by BERLYNE (1960) in the case of the mammalian kidney (see also DICKER and EGGLETON, 1961; GINETZINSKY and BERLYNE, 1961; HELLER, 1963b). In the case of the amphibian bladder, neither LEAF (1960) nor BENTLEY (1962b) were able to observe any effect after addition of hyaluronidase to the bathing medium. Nevertheless, NATOCHIN (1963) reports that inhibitors of hyaluronidase activity, such as $FeCl_3$, heparin and $CuSO_4$, also inhibit the action of the hormone on the water permeability of the frog bladder *(Rana temporaria)*. At the present time, this theory is rejected by most authors (see ORLOFF and HANDLER, 1964a), at least for the case of amphibian epithelial cells.

Another theory was suggested a few years ago by SCHWARTZ et al. (1960), FONG et al. (1959—1960) and RASMUSSEN et al. (1960). According to this theory the hormone molecule could bind to proteins of the cell membrane by a sulfhydryl-disulfide exchange mechanism. This hormonal fixation would be directly responsible for the observed permeability change by a sequence of SH S–S exchange reactions within the proteins of the membrane. Recently, such a hypothetical mechanism has been rejected by these authors, as will be discussed later, since analogues of the hormone lacking the disulfide bridge (RUDINGER and JOST, 1964) are not completely devoid of biological activity (SCHWARTZ et al., 1964). Moreover, there is no evidence available at the present time which indicates that the hormone binds to these molecular structures, the modifications of which are responsible for the final hormonal effect.

On the contrary, indirect arguments suggest that intermediate steps are probably involved. It has been repeatedly observed that changes in the actual value of the physicochemical parameters of the system may greatly modify the hormonal response. The analysis of such effects may help in elucidating the metabolic aspects of the hormonal action. They will be briefly discussed now.

A. Influence of the pH

It has been observed, *in vitro* (BENTLEY, 1958; RASMUSSEN et al., 1963; GULYASSY and EDELMAN, 1965), that acidification of the Ringer bathing the serosal border of the toad bladder results in a strong inhibition of the increase in osmotic permeability to water produced by the hormone. At pH 6.4, the inhibition is almost complete (BENTLEY, 1959b). There is an optimum pH value of about 8. When the pH stays between 7 and 8, there is some reduction in the responses to non-maximal doses of hormone, but the maximal effect remains unchanged (RASMUSSEN et al., 1963; GULYASSY and EDELMAN, 1965). Lowering the pH equally reduces the responses to oxytocin and deamino-oxytocin (RASMUSSEN et al., 1963), to oxytocin, arginine-vasopressin and deamino-oxytocin (GULYASSY and EDELMAN, 1965). Since these peptides have different charged groups (*a* amino group of cystein, pK = 5.3, hydroxyl group of tyrosin, pK = 11; guanidin group of arginine, pK = 12.5), it can be concluded that ionic groups of the receptor proteins (or of proteins involved in some other rate limiting step), and not ionic groups of the hormone itself, are responsible for the observed pH inhibition. Acidification of the medium bathing the serosal border of the frog skin produces a large inhibition of the natriferic response to oxytocin (BASTIDE, unpublished observations), similar to that just described for the bladder.

B. Influence of Temperature

When the osmotic response of the bladder to the hormone is recorded *in vitro* at different temperatures, one observes that the magnitude of the response is only weakly temperature dependent, whereas the time course of the response is markedly temperature dependent (Rasmussen et al., 1960; Bourguet, 1966). Using, as an index of the kinetics of the hormonal action, the time required for the response to reach half of its maximum value, it has been shown by Bourguet (1966) that the Q_{10} of the reaction has a value as high as 2.3 for temperature variations between 15 and 25° C. Such a value strongly indicates that the factor limiting the time course of the hormonal response is not a physical one, such as the diffusion of the hormone through the preparation, but a step involving some chemical interaction or reaction of high activation energy. On the other hand, the magnitude of the response is only slightly affected by the temperature, an observation which confirms the fact that the osmotic flow of water through the epithelial cells results from low energy physical interactions only (Hays and Leaf, 1962b; Leaf, 1962).

C. Oxygen Consumption

If intermediate chemical steps are involved in the hormonal action, it would be of importance to determine the metabolic energy expenditure corresponding to these reactions. Such an experimental determination is difficult, since the hormone enhances the rate of active sodium transport, which, in normal conditions, corresponds to the larger part of the oxygen consumption of the cells for both the skin (Zerahn, 1956; Leaf and Renshaw, 1957) and the bladder (Leaf et al., 1959; Leaf, 1960; Leaf and Dempsey, 1960). When the hormonal action is studied by the change in osmotic flow of water under experimental conditions in which the active transport of sodium has been stopped (either by suppressing the sodium ions in the mucosal bathing medium, or by adding metabolic inhibitors to the serosal bathing medium), contradictory results have been reported. According to Rasmussen et al. (1960), there is no increase in oxygen consumption after addition of vasopressin when the bladder of *Bufo marinus* is incubated in Ringer choline medium; moreover, the suppression of O_2 or the addition of inhibitors of glycolysis do not change the response of the bladder to the hormone. On the contrary, according to Bentley (1958) and Orloff and Handler (1964b), addition of DNP, iodoacetamide, or other metabolic inhibitors inhibits the response to the hormone. The discrepancy could result from the concentrations used and from the duration of the experiments. Nevertheless, it remains difficult from these experiments to decide if the hormonal action requires the presence of oxygen or energy-rich chemical intermediates, since the negative results of the last authors could result from irreversible non-specific damage to the cell produced by an anoxia of long duration. On the other hand, according to Goodfriend and Kirkpatrick (1963), neurohypophysial hormones increase the rate of glucose, pyruvate, lactate and palmitate utilization, even in conditions in which active sodium transport is reduced to very low values.

Another metabolic effect of vasotocin in toads has recently been observed by Bentley (1965b): minute amounts of arginine-vasotocin (0.4—40×10^{-9} M/kg), injected to toads, result in a 60—70% increase of the concentration of glucose in the blood.

D. Role of 3'-5' Cyclic AMP

It has been reported (Hilton et al., 1959) that the perfusion of vasopressin into the adrenal artery is able to mimic the effects of the perfusion of ACTH, which are most probably mediated through the cellular production of 3'-5' cyclic AMP

(HAYNES and BERTHET, 1957). From that and similar observations, ORLOFF and HANDLER (1961—1962) have suggested that neurohypophysial hormones could produce their specific actions on epithelial cells via an increased release of cyclic AMP within these cells; there is actually much evidence supporting such a mechanism of action, which can be summarized as follows:

a) 3'-5' cyclic AMP, when added to the medium bathing the serosal border of the toad bladder, induces, as vasopressin does, both an increase in osmotic water permeability and a stimulation of the active transport of sodium (ORLOFF and HANDLER, 1961—1962); the required concentrations are very high (10^{-2} to 10^{-3} M), but such a weak activity could result both from the well known low permeability of most cellular membranes to nucleotides, and from the existence of an efficient enzymatic mechanism for cyclic-AMP breakdown within the cells (BUTCHER and SUTHERLAND, 1959). It has been established, for example, that the cyclic AMP concentrations required, in order to stimulate phosphorylase activity in liver from mammals, are much higher when tissue slices are used than when tissue homogenates are used (see, for example, SUTHERLAND and RALL, 1960).

b) Theophylline, which, like other compounds of the methylxanthine group, is a powerful inhibitor of the phosphodiesterases (BUTCHER and SUTHERLAND, 1959), mimics the effect of neurohypophysial hormones when added to the serosal bathing medium in concentrations ranging from 10^{-2} to 10^{-3} M (ORLOFF and HANDLER, 1961—1962). According to the authors, this effect would indicate an increased cellular concentration of cyclic AMP resulting from an inhibition of its rate of destruction by a theophylline sensitive phosphodiesterase, without change in its rate of endogenous production. Moreover, there is an additivity in the effects of theophylline and of low doses of either vasopressin or 3'-5' cyclic AMP (ORLOFF and HANDLER, 1962).

c) It has been observed by BOURGUET (1968) on the frog bladder that, when low concentrations of theophylline and oxytocin, or of theophylline and 3'-5' cyclic AMP are used together, an almost maximal increase in the net flux of water might be achieved, whereas, when used alone in the same concentrations, these compounds elicit only very low responses. This potentiating effect of theophylline on both the hormonal and the 3'-5' cyclic AMP actions suggests that the hormone acts via an increased production of cyclic AMP by the epithelial cells.

d) Both vasopressin and 3'-5' cyclic AMP have been reported to increase the phosphorylase activity, the rate of glycogen hydrolysis, and the oxygen consumption of the toad bladder (HANDLER and ORLOFF, 1963). In experimental conditions in which the active transport of sodium had been stopped by removing the external sodium, the stimulation of the phosphorylase activity by the hormone is still present, as is the increase in permeability to water, whereas the changes in glycogen hydrolysis and in oxygen consumption disappear (HANDLER and ORLOFF, 1963). This last result, however, has not been confirmed by SCHOESSLER (1964); according to SCHOESSLER, vasopressin enhances the phosphorylase activity of the toad bladder only when sodium is present; on the other hand, she was unable to stimulate this enzyme activity with cyclic AMP. Another discrepancy has been observed by HANDLER, PETERSEN and ORLOFF (quoted by ORLOFF and HANDLER, 1964a): the phosphofructokinase activity of the toad bladder is unaffected by the addition of vasopressin, whereas the addition of exogenous 3'-5' cyclic AMP (even in low concentration unable to increase the permeability to water) results in a powerful stimulation.

e) Finally, it has been demonstrated (and this is the most important evidence favouring the theory) that both vasopressin and theophylline increase the cellular content of the bladder in 3'-5' cyclic AMP; this effect of the hormone is potentiated by theophylline and is still present when a sodium free solution is used as bathing medium (Handler et al., 1965).

All these experimental results strongly suggest that 3'-5' cyclic AMP is involved in the mechanism of action of vasopressin on the amphibian bladder. There is also experimental evidence indicating that cyclic AMP could be involved in the mechanism of the ADH action on the mammalian kidney (Brown et al., 1963; Grantham and Burg, 1966) and in the natriferic action of oxytocin on the frog skin (Bastide and Jard, 1968). It has to be pointed out that catecholamines, which are known to enhance 3'-5' cyclic AMP production within hepatic cells and avian red blood cells (Sutherland and Rall, 1957), induce effects on the frog skin similar to those of oxytocin, namely a stimulation of the active transport of sodium and an increase in osmotic permeability to water (Bastide and Jard, 1968).

It thus appears that 3'-5' cyclic AMP could act as an intracellular mediator of the action of various hormones (catecholamines: Sutherland and Rall, 1957; corticotrophin: Haynes and Berthet, 1957; glucagon: Rall and Sutherland, 1958; neurohypophysial hormones: see above) on many different target organs. Moreover, 3'-5' cyclic AMP has been reported to control the activity of several enzyme systems: phosphorylase (Rall and Sutherland, 1958), phosphofructokinase (see Mansour, 1963), lipase (Rizack, 1964). In these circumstances the problem of the specificity of the hormonal action must be briefly discussed in two respects. Firstly, it is necessary to assume that there is, in each target organ, a specific adenylcyclase, the activity of which is selectively stimulated by the corresponding hormone. Such a specificity has been observed in several systems; thus, glucagon activates the production of cyclic AMP by liver fractions, but does not do so on muscle fractions (Rall and Sutherland, 1958); ACTH activates adenylcyclase from adrenal cortex, whereas catecholamines, insulin and glucagon are inactive on the same substrate (Haynes, 1958); serotonin, but not catecholamines, stimulates the cyclic AMP accumulation in microsome suspensions of *Fasciola hepatica* (Mansour et al., 1960). It must be pointed out that there are no data available at the present time demonstrating a similar direct stimulating action of neurohypophysial hormones on the adenylcyclase activity of roughly purified subcellular fractions. Secondly, it appears necessary to explain how the same 3'-5' cyclic AMP may induce very specific and different effects in the different target organs, and, more precisely, how it could be responsible within the amphibian epithelial cells for both the increase in permeability to water and the stimulation of the sodium transport, if, as already discussed, these two effects are functionally dissociated and involve two different molecular receptors of the hormone ? Such a dissociation could be explained either a) if there is not a uniform pool of cyclic AMP within the cells, but several pools in relation to different cyclases and to each of the physiological functions of cyclic AMP; or, b) if different types of epithelial cells were responsible for the two observed hormonal effects, a possibility which has been recently discussed for other purposes (Leaf, 1965) and which is compatible with the various types of cells observed in the electron microscopy of the amphibian bladder (Keller, 1960; Carasso et al., 1962; Choi, 1963).

On the other hand, the mechanisms by which 3'-5'- cyclic AMP could — directly or indirectly — change the permeability to water, and increase the active transport of sodium are completely unknown. If the metabolic actions of the catecholamines and glucagon can be accounted for by a stimulating action of cyclic AMP on the phosphorylase and phosphofructokinase activities, such a mechanism does not seem to be sufficient in the case of neurohypophysial hormones. Finally, it remains quite possible that the neurohypophysial hormone has different cellular sites of action, and that the observed change in cyclic AMP production reflects only part of the mechanism, that is, the direct (or secondary) adaptation of the cell metabolism to the increased energy expenditure which is the ordinary counterpart of the hormonal action.

III. Interactions Between the Hormonal Peptides and their Molecular Receptors

Whatever the metabolic and final steps of the hormonal action at the cellular level could be, the first step involved, which will be briefly discussed now from experimental evidence obtained in amphibians, obviously consists of some interaction between the active peptide and a molecular receptor. The specificity of the biological "information" carried in the blood by a hormone finally results from the specificity of this interaction and is related to the configuration or the structure of the hormonal molecule. Moreover, in normal conditions, the intensity of the final effect elicited by the hormone appears to be a function of the hormonal concentration; this indicates that, in the physiological range of hormonal concentrations, it is the interaction between the hormone and its molecular receptor which limits the rate of the whole sequence of events up to the final observed effect.

Three different kinds of experimental approach have been used on amphibian structures, as on mammalian structures, in order to analyse further this molecular interaction: a) the presence (and the nature) of the binding mechanism has been studied by using radioactive hormone, b) the kinetics of the reaction has been indirectly approached by careful observation of the dose-response curves, and c) the stereospecificity of the reaction has been established by studying structure-activity relationships.

A. Nature of the Binding Mechanism

As shown by Schwartz et al. (1960), when toad bladders are exposed to tritiated vasopressin, a significant amount of radioactivity binds to a protein fraction. The radioactivity is not removed by several treatments, such as electrodialysis or hypertonic urea, suggesting that the binding does not correspond to simple adsorption or electrovalent bonds, but could result from covalent bonds. Moreover, by reducing the disulfide bridges by cysteine, part of the radioactivity is released, an observation which would indicate, according to Schwartz et al. (1960), that binding of the hormone to its molecular receptor could involve the formation of mixed disulfide bridges between the active peptide and the receptor protein. A similar mechanism has been suggested by Fong et al. (1960) for binding of vasopressin to the mammalian kidney. Such a mechanism would account for the observations of Ames and van Dyke (1951) and Audrain and Clauser (1960) that reduction of the disulfide bond of vasopressin and oxytocin results in a complete loss of biological activity. Since, on the other hand, the chemical agents which block the free SH groups of the proteins inhibit the action of the hormone on the water permeability of the toad bladder (Rasmussen et al., 1960; Bentley, 1964; Handler and Orloff, 1964), it was assumed by Rasmussen and Schwartz, as already mentioned, that binding of the hormone could be directly responsible of the observed permeability change. In order to account both for the specificity in the biological activities of the different neurohypophysial peptides, and for the reversibility of the binding (suggested by the reversibility of the action), the authors assume, firstly, that the binding mechanism involves two successive steps, i.e. a stereospecific binding by low energy bonds, followed by the covalent sulfhydryl-disulfide exchange reaction, and, secondly, the presence of an enzymatic splitting of the hormone-receptor complex. This possible mechanism of binding has been recently questioned (SCHWARTZ et al., 1964) by the observation that analogues of oxytocin lacking the disulfide bridge (that is, in the molecule of which one or both of the sulphur atoms have been substituted by methylene radicals) still have some biological activity (SCHWARTZ et al., 1964). Similarly, seleno-oxytocin has a rat uterus activity about as high as oxytocin itself (RODERICH and DU VIGNEAUD, 1966). It would thus appear that the formation of covalent disulfide bridges between the hormone and the receptor protein is not a prerequisite for hormonal action.

B. Dose-Response Relationships on Amphibian Skin, Bladder and Kidney

To a first approximation, the quantitative relation between the concentration (or administred amount) of hormone, and the magnitude of the observed effect, can be described as a Langmuir isotherm of absorption. This has been reported for the effect of vasopressin on the osmotic flow of water through the toad bladder *in vitro* (EDELMAN and PETERSEN, 1962; EDELMAN et al., 1964; RASMUSSEN et al., 1963) and for the tubular effects (water and sodium reabsorption) of vasotocin on the frog kidney *in vivo* (JARD, 1966). Such a relation is compatible with the hypothesis of a one to one reversible binding of the hormone to its molecular receptor. However, more precise *in vitro* kinetic analysis of the skin natriferic and bladder water responses to oxytocin in *Rana esculenta* show a significant deviation from the hyperbolic relation, especially in the range of low hormonal concentrations (JARD et al., 1966a). The experimental curves are S-shaped, an observation which could be accounted for by interactions between hormone-binding sites of the receptor molecule. Similar kinetics are known to occur in regulatory enzymes in which allosteric transitions take place (see MONOD et al., 1965). It must be pointed out, however, that the use of the Michaelis-Menten equation or of other enzyme kinetic equations in order to describe hormonal dose-effect curves is limited by the fact that several hypotheses have to be introduced; for example, it has to be assumed 1. that the hormonal concentration at the site of the binding is equal (or proportional) to that introduced in the bathing fluid, and 2. that the magnitude of the observed final effect is proportional to the concentration of the hormone-receptor complex; this second assumption is, most likely, an arbitrary oversimplification, which obviously limits the interpretation of the dose-response kinetics curves. On the other hand, the production of inhibitors of the hormone within the structure (KARLIN, 1963) or its destruction by intracellular peptidases (CAMPBELL et al., 1965) may modify the concentration of the active hormone introduced in the bathing fluid.

C. Structure-activity Relationships

Table 4 shows the biological activities of neurohypophysial hormones and related peptides as measured on the best known target organs in lower vertebrates. The avian depressor activities have not been reported in the table, since they are discussed in an other chapter of this book. The most numerous data refer to the natriferic test (increase in the sodium transport by the frog skin) and to the amphibian bladder test (increase in water permeability of the isolated bladder of the toad or of the frog). Examination of the table suggests a few general comments:

1. There is a high structural specificity in the hormonal action, since chemically closely related peptides may show very different biological activities;

2. As pointed out in the case of mammalian bioassays (see for instance BOISSONNAS, 1965), the activity of the hormonal peptide does not seem to result from the presence of chemically reactive groups within the molecule, since the analogues

Table 4. *Relationships between the chemical structure and the biological activities of the posterior pituitary hormones and their synthetic analogues in lower vertebrates*

	Fowl oviduct	Fowl antidiuresis	Frog natriferic	bladder permeability to water		Frog antidiuresis
				Frog	Toad	
Posterior Pituitary hormones occuring in nature						
Arg^8-Oxy (arginine-vasotocin)	640 [11]	880 [11]	1100 [5] 1140 [8, 9] 1150 [1] 4400 [13]	10000 [13, 14, 15] 14000 [5] 16000 [1] 34000 [20]	100 [12]	100 [4, 5, 6] 100 [13] b
Ileu^8-Oxy (Mesotocin)	—	—	507 [8, 9]	—	8 [12]	0 [4, 6]
Ser^4-Ileu^8-Oxy (Isotocin)	—	—	5.3 [8, 9]	—	1.6 [12]	0 [4]
Ser^4-Glu$(NH_2)^8$-Oxy (Glumitocin)	—	—	—	—	—	—
Oxytocin	29 [11] 34 [19] 47 [10] a	—	450 [8, 9, 1] 360 [13]	450 [1, 5] 500 [20] 420 [3] 360 [13, 14, 15]	4 [12]	0 [4, 5, 6] 1.9 [13] b
Phe^3-Arg^8-Oxy (arginine-vasopressin)	240 [11] 320 [19]	300 [11]	32.6 [8, 9] 30 [5] 70 [13]	26 [3] 70 [13] 80 [5] 90 [20]	1.3 [12]	0 [5]
Phe^3-Lys^8-Oxy (lysine-vasopressin)	15 [11]	—	5.4 [8, 9] 8 [5]	5 [14] 7.5 [3] 12.5 [5]	0.4 [12]	0 [4, 5, 6]
Substitution in position 1						
Deamino-Oxy	14.9 [10] a	—	190 [8, 9]	—	0.45 [12]	0 [4, 6]
Me-Cys^1-Oxy	—	—	9.1 [8, 9]	—	0.033 [12]	—
D Cys^1-Oxy	—	—	23.7 [8, 9]	—	0.016 [12]	—
Homo Cys^1-Oxy	—	—	—	—	0.015 [12]	—
Substitutions in positions 1 and 2						
Deamino^1-Phe^2-Oxy	—	—	—	—	0.02 [18]	—
Substitutions in positions 1, 3 and 8						
1 N-acetyl Phe^3-Arg^8-Oxy	—	—	—	—	0.002 [18]	—
1 Deamino-Phe^3-Lys^8-Oxy	—	—	—	—	0.036 [12]	—
1 N-acetyl Phe^3-Lys^8-Oxy	—	—	—	—	0.003 [17]	—

Table 4 (Continuation)

	Fowl oviduct	Fowl antidiuresis	Frog natriferic	bladder permeability to water		Frog antidiuresis
				Frog	Toad	
Substitution in position 2						
Phe^{2}-Oxy	—	—	36.0 [8, 9]	20 [14], 18 [13]	0.098 [12]	—
Tyr(Me)^{2}-Oxy	—	—	8.6 [8, 9]	—	0.085 [12]	—
Leu^{2}-Oxy	—	—	8.2 [8, 9]	—	0.0007 [12]	—
Substitutions in positions 2, 3 and 8						
Phe^{2,3}-Lys^{8}-Oxy	—	—	1.9 [8, 9]	—	—	0 [4, 6]
(ITyr)^{2}-Phe^{3}-Arg^{8}-Oxy	—	—	—	—	0.013 [2,18]	—
Ser^{2}-Phe^{3}-Lys^{8}-Oxy	—	—	—	—	0 [12]	—
Substitution in position 3						
aIle^{3}-Oxy	—	—	8.9 [8, 9]	—	0.34 [12]	—
Leu^{3}-Oxy	—	—	17.1 [8, 9]	—	0.16 [12] 0.224 [18]	0 [4]
			61.6 [8, 9]			
Nle^{3}-Oxy	—	—	1.45 [8, 9]	—	0.013 [12]	—
Val^{3}-Oxy	—	—	49 [8, 9]	—	0.12 [18]	0 [4, 6]
N Val^{3}-Oxy	—	—	2.8 [8, 9]	—	0.048 [12]	—
Phe^{3}-Oxy	0.9 [11]	—	1.8 [8, 9]	20 [13]	0.012 [12]	0 [4, 6]
Substitutions in position 3 and 8						
Phe^{3}-Hist^{8}-Oxy	0.2 [11]	—	—	12 [11, 14]	—	—
Phe^{3}-Cit^{8}-Oxy	—	—	—	4 [20]	0.16 [12]	—
Substitutions in positions 3, 7 and 8						
Phe^{3}-Val^{7}-Lys^{8}-Oxy	—	—	0.135 [8, 9]	—	—	—
Substitution in position 4						
Asp(NH$_2$)^{4}-Oxy	—	—	18 [8, 9]		4.0 [12]	—
Ala^{4}-Oxy	—	—	13 [8, 9]	—	—	—
Substitution in position 5						
Glu(NH$_2$)^{5}-Oxy	—	—	2.6 [8, 9]	—	—	0 [4]
Substitution in position 8						
Lys^{8}-Oxy	75 [15]	—	940 [8, 9]	380 [13, 14]	25 [12]	100 [4, 6, 7]
			1015 [5] c	975 [5] c		100 [5] c
			935 [1] c	1015 [1] c		
Val^{8}-Oxy	—	—	610 [8, 9]	—	—	—
Cit^{8}-Oxy	—	—	—	800 [20]	6.6 [12]	—
Substitution in position 9						
Sar^{9}-Oxy	—	—	—	—	2.5 [12]	—

Table 4 (Continuation)

	Fowl oviduct	Fowl antidiuresis	Frog natriferic	bladder permeability to water: Frog	bladder permeability to water: Toad	Frog antidiuresis
Modification of the disulfide bridge						
1—6 Djenkolic Phe^3-Lys^8-Oxy	—	—	—	—	0.001 [16]	—
LengLengthening of the peptidic chain						
Sar-Cys^1-Oxy	—	—	2.7 [8, 9]	—	0.004 [12]	—
Leu-Gly-Gly-Cys^1-Oxy	—	—	2.1 [8, 9]	—	0.0031 [12]	—
Gly-Cys^1-Oxy	—	—	—	—	0.004 [12]	—
Phe^3-Val^7-Val^7-Lys^8-Oxy	—	—	1.25 [8, 9]	—	—	—
Shortening of the peptidic chain						
de- Pro^7-Oxy	—	—	18.3 [8, 9]	—	—	0 [4]
de Leu^8-Oxy	—	—	660 [8, 9]	—	—	0 [4]
de Gly^9-Oxy	—	—	1100 [8, 9]	—	—	—
de(Pro^7-Leu^8-Gly^9)-Oxy	—	—	—	—	0.02 [12]	—

1 Bourguet and Maetz (1961)
2 Fong et al. (1960)
3 Heller (1963a)
4 Jard (1966)
5 Jard et al. (1960)
6 Jard and Morel (1963)
7 Morel and Jard (1963a)
8 Morel and Bastide (1964)
9 Morel et al. (1965)
10 Munsick (1965)
11 Munsick et al. (1960)
12 Rasmussen et al. (1963)
13 Sawyer (1960b)
14 Sawyer (1961b)
15 Sawyer et al. (1961b)
16 Schwartz et al. (1964)
17 Schwartz and Rasmussen (1964)
18 Schwartz and Livingston (1964)
19 van Dyke (1959)
20 van Dyke et al. (1963)

Biological activities are expressed as units per mg except for toad bladder and frog antidiuretic activities which are expressed as per cent of the activity of arginine-vasotocin.

One fowl oviduct or fowl antidiuretic unit is the activity countained in 0.5 mg of U.S.P., International Standard of ox posterior Pituitary powder.

By definition, one frog natriferic or one frog bladder unit is the activity on these tests of one unit of synthetic oxytocin; since several values for the actual potency of pure oxytocin have been used by the different authors, it results a proportional variation in the biological activities of the analogues tested. In each case, the numbers in brackets may help to found the corresponding reference activity used for oxytocin.

a = values calculated from author's data assuming for absolute rat oxytocic activities of oxytocin and deamino-oxytocin, 486 IU/mg and 684 IU/mg respectively (Chan and du Vigneaud, 1962).

b = values recalculated as per cent of arginine-vasotocin activity.

c = values recalculated by using for Lys^8-oxytocin a rat uterus activity of 78 IU/mg (Boissonnas et al., 1961) and not 20 IU/mg (Boissonnas and Huguenin, 1960).

lacking one or another of these groups still show high biological activities. The activity seems, more likely, to result from the shape and the steric configuration of the whole molecule. Moreover, generally speaking, the artificial analogues in which the peptidic chain — or one of the side chain — has been increased in size (as compared to the natural hormone) have a much lower biological activity than those analogues in which the size of the molecule has been decreased at the same site.

3. There must be some chemical or steric differencies from target organ to target organ within the receptor molecules, since the relative activities of most peptides vary in large limits according to the bioassay under study. This point is especially striking in the case of the three test organs of the frog, the skin, the bladder and the kidney tubule. These three test organs belong to the same species, they are involved in the same osmoregulatory function, and they all respond to vasotocin by eliciting the same two effects, namely an increase in the osmotic to permeability water and a stimulation of the active transport of sodium. However, there are obvious differences in the structure-activity relationships between these three receptors. Let us consider, for example, the series of analogues tested, in which an amino-acid substitution has been introduced in position 8 of the peptidic chain of the oxytocin molecule. It is apparent that, in the natriferic test, all these analogues have the same high activity as oxytocin. As judged by the bladder test, the presence of a basic amino-acid (lysine or arginine) in position 8 increases the biological activity up to 20 times as compared to the other analogues. Finally, on the kidney tubule, the presence of the basic amino-acid in position 8 is a prerequisite for the hormonal action: Arg^8- and Lys^8-oxytocin (i.e. the vasotocins) are the only active peptides. Thus, the "receptor" molecules must be different within these three target organs. As already mentioned, similar dissociations have even been observed between the water and sodium responses of the same structure (BOURGUET and MAETZ, 1961; BOURGUET and MOREL, 1967), suggesting separate cellular receptors and pathways for the two responses.

4. When the structure-activity relationships obtained on the frog skin natriferic test (MOREL and BASTIDE, 1964) and on the mammalian bioassays (see for instance BOISSONNAS et al., 1961; SCHWARTZ and LIVINGSTON, 1964, see also chapter by Berde and Boissonnas in this volume) are compared, two general differences may be observed. Firstly, the peptides with an amino-acid substitution in the fourth position preserve most of their oxytocic activity whereas their natriferic activity is very low. Secondly, the peptides with an amino-acid substitution in position 8 (or a shortened side chain), always show a highly decreased rat uterus activity, whereas their natriferic activity is equal or even higher than that of oxytocin.

5. In the case of the frog natriferic and toad bladder tests, the differences in activity observed from one peptide to the other seem to result from differences in their binding affinities for the molecular receptor, since, with large concentrations, maximal effects of the same magnitude are elicited (RASMUSSEN et al., 1963; MOREL et al., 1965). Moreover, it has not been possible to observe any inhibition of the effect of the most active peptides by large amounts of analogues of low activity, either on the bladder (RASMUSSEN et al., 1963) or on the skin (MOREL et al., 1965).

6. The kidney tubule of the frog, on the contrary, shows extremely specific structural requirements: among all the peptides tested, only vasotocin (both lysine and arginine) elicited the increase in free water and in sodium reabsorptions. But, when injected before vasotocin, large amounts of oxytocin (which is inactive on this test) completely inhibit the vasotocin action, whereas large amounts of vasopressin (which is also inactive on this test) do not change the magnitude

of the response to vasotocin (Jard and Morel, 1961; Morel and Jard, 1963a, b). Oxytocin also inhibits vasotocin induced antidiuresis and cutaneous water uptake in *Bufo bufo* (Jørgensen and Larsen, 1962). The inhibition of the vasotocin action by oxytocin in the frog is reversible and results from competition for binding, since maximal effects of the same magnitude can be elicited with very large amounts of vasotocin in the presence of oxytocin and with vasotocin alone (Jard, 1966). From kinetic analysis of the inhibition, it may be concluded that both the active hormone (vasotocin) and the inhibitor (oxytocin) have similar affinities for the binding site (Jard, 1963, 1966). Among the inactive peptides tested, some (like oxytocin) are inhibitors of the vasotocin actions, and the others (like vasopressin) are not (Morel and Jard, 1963). The first group of peptides (which show a high affinity for the tubular receptor) includes analogues with a structure of the cyclic part of their molecules identical (or closely related) to that of vasotocin but with a substitution of the basic amino acid of the side chain in the eighth position. The second group of peptides (which are devoid of affinity for the tubular receptor) includes analogues with a structure of the cyclic part of their molecules different from that of vasotocin (for example, by substitution of isoleucine by phenylalanine in the third position), regardless the structure of the side chain, i.e. even in the presence of a basic amino acid in the eighth position. The structural requirements for binding to the receptor molecule are not very different for the frog kidney tubule and the frog skin (Morel et al., 1965). But, although binding of the peptide to its molecular receptor is a necessary condition for biological activity, it is not a sufficient condition in the case of the tubule. For the receptor-hormone complex to be active, the presence of arginine or lysine in the eighth position of the hormonal molecule appears necessary.

Readers who are interested in the mechanisms of the molecular interactions between neurohypophysial hormones and their target organs will find more general and extensive discussions of this important problem in other chapters of this book.

Conclusion

The physiological part of this review deals with a very large field — fishes alone, for example, constitute quite a world when compared to the small group of mammals! It is not surprising that our understanding of the role of neurohypophysial hormones in lower vertebrates is yet really poor at the present time, as is our knowledge of the physiology of these animals in general. There is no doubt that the situation will change rapidly in the near future, since the natural hormones involved in lower vertebrates are now either known or being actively investigated, and since the experimental methods of comparative endocrinology are constantly improving. A few points only seem to be firmly established today, for example, the role of vasotocin in the control of water excretion and oviposition in birds, or the role of vasotocin in the osmoregulation of terrestrial anurans; however, even in these groups, obscure points (such as the functions of oxytocin in birds or the functions of mesotocin in amphibians, if any!) remain to be solved. For aquatic species, and especially for all groups of fishes, the solution of the question is made even more difficult by the fact that what is known from mammals cannot be used by analogy, even for the construction of working hypotheses, since the ecological conditions and the osmoregulatory problems have nothing in common between the two classes. This is probably the reason why, in the aquatic groups, no regulatory mechanism involving neurohypophysial hormones has ever been clearly established, even though some of the effects observed in response to injected hormones may possibly represent physiological actions.

There is a field, however, in which lower vertebrates have been and remain of great help for understanding what happens in mammals. This field concerns the mechanism of action of neurohypophysial hormones at the cellular level.

The sequence of events which occurs, from the first interaction between the hormone and its molecular receptor to the final observed effects, is, yet, far from completely solved; nevertheless, many steps have been clarified, and rapid progress is being made towards the understanding of others.

It is apparent that, as far as the problems related to neurohypophysial hormones are concerned — as, indeed, for many other physiological problems — our knowledge about the world of lower vertebrates is quite insufficient. Almost everything still remains to be done; the questions are numerous, the clearcut responses only very few. But it is also apparent that the world of lower vertebrates may help greatly in the solution of basic problems of cellular physiology and molecular endocrinology, by furnishing highly suitable biological structures. This is one of the reasons why comparative physiology needs to be vigorously developed.

References

Acher, R., R. Beaupain, J. Chauvet, M.T. Chauvet, and D. Crepy: The neurohypophysial hormones of the amphibians. Comparison of the hormones of *Rana esculenta* and *Xenopus laevis*. Gen. comp. Endocr. **4**, 596—602 (1964a).

—, J. Chauvet, M.T. Chauvet, et D. Crepy: Les hormones neurohypophysaires des poissons. Isolement d'une vasotocine du tacaud (*Gadus Luscus* L.). Biochim. biophys. Acta (Amst.) **51**, 419—420 (1961).

— — — — Isolement d'une nouvelle hormone neurohypophysaire, l'isotocine préśente chez les poissons osseux. Biochim. biophys. Acta (Amst.) **58**, 624—625 (1962).

— — — — Phylogenie des peptides neurohypophysaires. Isolement de la mésotocine (Ileu 8-ocytocine) de la grenouille; intermédiaire entre la Ser 4-Ileu 8- ocytocine des poissons osseux et l'ocytocine des mammifères. Biochim. biophys. Acta (Amst.) **90**, 613—615 (1964b).

— — — — Les hormones neurohypophysaires des vertébrés. Variations des structures au cours de l'évolution. Ann. Endocr. (Paris) **26** (suppl.), 662—669 (1965a).

— — — — Phylogénie des peptides neurohypophysaires. Isolement d'une nouvelle hormone; la glumitocine (Ser 4 Gln 8-ocytocine) présente chez un poisson cartilagineux, la raie *(Raia clavata)*. Biochim. biophys. Acta (Amst.) **107**, 393—396 (1965b).

— —, et M.T. Lenci: Isolement de l'ocytocine du Poulet. Biochim. biophys. Acta (Amst.) **38**, 344—345 (1960b).

— — —, F. Morel, et J. Maetz: Présence d'une vasotocine dans la neurohypophyse de la grenouille (*Rana esculenta* L.). Biochim. biophys. Acta (Amst.) **42**, 379—380 (1960a).

Adolph, E.F.: The excretion of water by the kidneys of frogs. Amer. J. Physiol. **81**, 315— 324 (1927).

— The vapor tension relations of frogs. Biol. Bull. **62**, 112—125 (1932).

— Exchanges of water in the frog. Biol. Rev. **8**, 224—240 (1933).

— Control of urine formation in the frog by the renal circulation. Amer. J. Physiol. **117**, 366—379 (1936).

Alvarado, R.H., and S.R. Johnson: The effects of arginine-vasotocin and oxytocin on sodium and water balance in *Ambystoma*. Comp. Biochem. Physiol. **16**, 531—546 (1965).

Ames, R.G., and H.B. van Dyke: Thioglycollate inactivation of posterior pituitary antidiuretic principle as determined in the rat. Proc. Soc. exp. Biol. (N.Y.) **76**, 576—578 (1951).

Andersen, B., and H.H. Ussing: Solvent drag on non electrolytes during osmotic flow through isolated toad skin and its response to antidiuretie hormone. Acta physiol. scand. **39**, 228 to 239 (1957).

Aronson, L.R.: Reproductive and parental behavior. In: The physiology of fishes, Vol. II, pp. 271—304. Ed. by M.E. Brown. New York: Academic Press 1957.

Arvy, L., M. Fontaine, et M. Gabe: Action des solutions salines hypertoniques sur le système hypopholamo-hypophysaire chez *Phoximus laevis* Agass. et chez *Anguilla anguilla* (L.). C.R. Soc. Biol. (Paris) **148**, 1759—1761 (1954).

— — — Action des solutions salines hypertoniques sur la neurosecretion chez l'anguille hypophysectomisée. C.R. Soc. Biol. (Paris) **149**, 225—227 (1955).

— — — Modifications de la voie neurosecretrice hypothalamo-hypophysaire de *Salmo solar* L. au cours du cycle évolutif. C.R. Ass. Anat. **89**, 224—233 (1956).

ARVY, L., M. FONTAINE, et M. GABE: La voie neurosecretrice hypothalamo-hypophysaire des Teleosteens. J. Physiol. (Paris) **51**, 1031—1085 (1959).

—, et M. GABE: Modifications du système hypothalamo-hypophysaire chez *Callionymus lyra* et *Ammodytes lanceolatus* au cours des variations de l'equilibre osmotique. C. R. Ass. Anat. **41**, 843—849 (1954).

ASSENMACHER, I.: Recherches sur le contrôle hypothalamique de la fonction gonadotrope préhypophysaire chez le canard. Arch. Anat. micr. Morph. exp. **47**, 448—572 (1958).

—, et A. TIXIER VIDAL: Repercussion de la section des veines portes hypophysaires sur la prehypophyse du canard pekin male entier ou castré. Arch. Anat. micr. Morph. exp. **53**, 83 à 108 (1964).

AUDRAIN, L., et H. CLAUSER: Mécanisme de l'inactivation de l'ocytocine par le tissu uterin. Biochim. biophys. Acta (Amst.) **38**, 494—501 (1960).

BAILLIEN, M., et E. SCHOFFENIELS: Origine des potentiels bioelectriques de l'épithélium intestinal isolé de la tortue grecque. Biochim. biophys. Acta (Amst.) **53**, 537—548 (1961a).

— — Origin of the potential difference in the intestinal epithelium of the turtle. Nature (Lond.) **190**, 1107—1108 (1961b).

BAGGERMAN, B.: An experimental study of the timing of breeding and migration in the 3-spined stickleback. Arch. Neerl. Zool. **7**, 105—317 (1957).

BALL, J. N.: Reproduction in female bony fishes. Symp. Zool. Soc. (Lond.) **1**, 105—135 (1960).

— Brood production after hypophysectomy in the viviparus teleost *Mollienesia latipinna*. Le Sueur. Nature (Lond.) **194**, 787—787 (1962).

—, and K. D. KALLMAN: Functional pituitary transplants in the all female gynogenetic teleost, *Mollienesia formosa* (Girard). Amer. Zool. **2**, 389 (1962).

—, et M. OLIVEREAU: Role de la prolactine dans la survie en eau douce de *Poecilia latipinna* hypophysectonisé et arguments en faveur de sa synthèse par les cellules erythrosinophiles D de l'hypophyse des Teleostéens. C. R. Acad. Sci. (Paris) **259**, 1443—1446 (1964).

— —, A. M. SLICHER, and K. D. KALLMAN: Functional capacity of ectopic pituitary transplants in a teleost fish, *Poecilia formosa*, with a comparative discussion on the transplanted pituitary. Phil. Trans. Roy. Soc. London, Ser. B: **249**, 66—99 (1965).

BARANNIKOVA, I. A., and A. L. POLENOV: An ecological and histophysiological analysis of the preoptico-hypophyseal neurosecretory system in the sturgeon. Dokl. Akad. Nauk SSR, Otl. Biokh. **133**, 719—721 (1960).

BARTHOLOMEW, G. A., and T. J. CADE: The water economy of land birds. The Auk. **80**, 504—539 (1963).

BASTIDE, F., et S. JARD: Actions de la noradrenaline et de l'ocytocine sur le transport actif de sodium et la permeabilité à l'eau de la peau de la grenouille: role de l'adenosine 3'-5' monophosphate cyclique. Biochim. biophys. Acta. (Amst.) **150**, 113—123 (1968).

BĚLEHRÁDEK, T., and J. S. HUXLEY: The effects of pituitrin and narcosis on water regulation in larval and metamorphosed *Ambystoma*. J. exp. Biol. **5**, 89—96 (1927).

BENOIT, J., et I. ASSENMACHER: Action des facteurs externes et plus particulièrement du facteur lumineux sur l'activité sexuelle des Oiseaux. Extrait de la IIème Reunion d'Endocrinologie de Langue Franç. Paris: Mason et Cie, 33—80 (1953).

— — Le contrôle hypothalamique et hypophysaire de l'activité préhypophysaire gonadotrope. J. Physiol. (Paris) **47**, 427—567 (1955).

BENSON, G. K., and S. J. FOLLEY: Oxytocin as stimulator for the release of prolactin from the anterior pituitary. Nature (Lond.) **177**, 700—701 (1956).

— — The effect of oxytocin on mammary gland involution in the rat. J. Endocr. **16**, 189—201 (1958).

BENTLEY, P. J.: The effects of vasopressin on water uptake of the toad *Bufo marinus* while bathed in different hypotonic solutions. J. Endocr. **16**, 126—134 (1957).

— The effects of neurohypophysial extracts on water transfer across the wall of the isolated urinary bladder of the toad *Bufo marinus*. J. Endocr. **17**, 201—209 (1958).

— Studies on the water and electrolyte metabolism of the lizard *Trachysaurus rugosus* (Gray). J. Physiol. (Lond.) **145**, 37—47 (1959a).

— The effects of ionic changes on water transfer across the isolated urinary bladder of the toad *Bufo marinus*. J. Endocr. **18**, 327—333 (1959b).

— The effects of vasopressin on the short-circuit current across the wall of the isolated bladder of the toad *Bufo marinus*. J. Endocr. **21**, 161—170 (1960).

— Directional differences in the permeability to water of the isolated urinary bladder of the toad *(Bufo marinus)*. J. Endocr. **22**, 95—100 (1961).

— Studies on the permeability of the large intestine and urinary bladder of the tortoise *(Testudo Graeca)* with special reference to the effects of neurohypophysial and adrenocortical hormones. Gen. comp. Endocr. **2**, 323—328 (1962a).

— Hyaluronidase, corticosteroids and the action of neurohypophysial hormone on the urinary bladder of the frog. J. Endocr. **24**, 407—414 (1962b).

BENTLEY, P. J.: Permeability of the skin of the cyclostome *Lampetra fluviatilis* to water and electrolytes. Comp. Biochem. Physiol. **6**, 95—98 (1962c).
— The effect of N-ethylmaleimide and glutathione on the isolated rat uterus and frog bladder with special reference to the action of oxytocin. J. Endocr. **30**, 103—113 (1964).
— Rectification of water flow across the bladder of the toad; effect of vasopressin. Life Sci. **4**, 133—140 (1965a).
— Hyperglycaemic effect of vasotocin in toads. Nature (Lond.) **206**, 1053—1054 (1965b).
— The physiology of the urinary bladder of amphibia. Biol. Rev. **41**, 275—316 (1966a).
— Adaptations of amphibia to arid environments. Science **152**, 619—623 (1966b).
—, and B. K. FOLLETT: The action of neurohypophysial and adrenocortical hormones on sodium balance in the cyclostome *Lampetra fluviatilis*. Gen. comp. Endocr. **2**, 329—335 (1962).
— — Control of water and electrolyte metabolism in the cyclostome *Lampetra fluviatilis*. Gen. comp. Endocr. **3**, 685 (1963a).
— — Kidney function in a primitive vertebrate, the cyclostome *Lampetra fluviatilis*. J. Physiol. (Lond.) **169**, 902—918 (1963b).
—, and H. HELLER: The sites of actions of neurohypophysial hormones in urodeles. Gen. comp. Endocr. **2**, 601 (1962).
— — The action of neurohypophysial hormones on the water and sodium metabolism of urodele amphibians. J. Physiol. (Lond.) **171**, 434—453 (1964).
— — The water retaining action of vasotocin on the fire salamander *(Salamandra maculosa)*: the role of the urinary bladder. J. Physiol. (Lond.) **181**, 124—129 (1965).
—, A. K. LEE, and A. R. MAIN: Comparison of dehydration and hydration of two genera of frogs *(Heleioporus* and *Neobatrachus)* that live in areas of varying aridity. J. exp. Biol. **35**, 677 to 684 (1958).
—, and K. SCHMIDT-NIELSEN: Permeability to water and sodium of the crocodilian *Caiman selerops*. J. cell. comp. Physiol. **66**, 303—310 (1965).
— — Cutaneous water loss in reptiles. Science **151**, 1547—1549 (1966).
BERLYNE, G. M.: Urinary hyaluronidase, a method of assay and investigation of its relationship to the urine concentrating mechanism. Clin. Sci. **19**, 12—25 (1960).
BERN, H. A., R. S. NISHIOKA, L. R. MEWALDT, and D. S. FARNER: Photoperiodic and osmotic influences on the ultrastructure of the hypothalamic neurosecretory system of the white-crowned sparrow *Zonotrichia leucophrys gambelii*. Z. Zellforsch. **69**, 198—227 (1966).
BIASOTTI, A.: Influence de l'extrait d'hypophyse sur l'imbibition des tissus. C.R. Soc. Biol. (Paris) **88**, 361—362 (1923).
BIETER, R. N.: The effects of the splanchics upon glomerular blood flow in the frog's kidney. Amer. J. Physiol. **91**, 436—460 (1930).
BISHOP, W. R., M. M. MUMBACH, and B. T. SCHEER: Interrenal control of active sodium transport across frog skin. Amer. J. Physiol. **200**, 451—453 (1961).
BOGERT, C. M., and R. B. COWLES: Moisture loss in relation to habitat selection in some Floridian reptiles. Amer. Museum Novitates **40**, No 1358, 1—34 (1947).
BOISSONNAS, R. A.: Les bases chimiques de l'interprétation du mécanisme d'action des hormones peptidiques. Ann. Endocr. (Paris) **26**, 635—642 (1965).
—, ST. GUTTMANN, B. BERDE, and H. KONZETT: Relationships between the chemical structures and the biological properties of the posterior pituitary hormones and their synthetic analogues. Experientia (Basel) **17**, 377—391 (1961).
—, et R. L. HUGUENIN: Synthèse de la Lys^8-ocytocine (lysine-vasotocine) et nouvelle synthèse de la lysine-vasopressine. Helv. chim. Acta **43**, 182—190 (1960).
BOURGUET, J.: Influence de la temperature sur la cinétique de l'augmentation de permeabilité à l'eau de la vessie de grenouille sous l'action de l'ocytocine. J. Physiol. (Paris) **58**, 476—477 (1966).
— Cinétique de la perméabilisation de la vessie de grenouille par l'ocytocine. Rôle du 3'-5' adenosine monophosphate cyclique. Biochim. biophys. Acta. (Amst.) **150**, 104—112 (1968).
—, et S. JARD: Un dispositif automatique d'enregistrement du flux net d'eau à travers la peau et la vessie des amphibiens. Biochim. biophys. Acta (Amst.) **88**, 442—444 (1964).
—, B. LAHLOUH, et J. MAETZ: Modifications expérimentales de l'équilibre hydrominéral et osmorégulation chez *Carassius auratus*. Gen. comp. Endocr. **4**, 563—576 (1964).
—, et J. MAETZ: Arguments en faveur de l'indépendance des mécanismes d'action de divers peptides neurohypophysaires sur le flux osmotique d'eau et sur le transport actif de sodium au sein d'un même recepteur, études sur la vessie et la peau de *Rana esculenta* L. Biochim. biophys. Acta (Amst.) **52**, 552—565 (1961).
—, et F. MOREL: Indépendance des variations de permeabilité à l'eau et au sodium produites par les hormones neurohypophysaires sur la vessie de grenouille. (Biochim. biophys. Acta (Amst.) **135**, 693—700 (1967).

Boyd, E.M., and M. Dingwall: The effect of pituitary (posterior lobe) extract on the body water of fish and reptiles. J. Physiol. (Lond.) **95**, 501—507 (1939).

—, and S.W. Whyte: The effect of extract of the posterior hypophysis on loss of water by frogs in a dry environment. Amer. J. Physiol. **124**, 759—766 (1938).

— — The effect of posterior hypophysial extract on retention of water and salt injected into frogs. Amer. J. Physiol. **125**, 415—422 (1939).

Bricker, N.S., and T. Biber: Active "downhill" sodium transport across the isolated frog skin. J. clin. Invest. **41**, 1348 (1962).

— —, and H.H. Ussing: Exposure of the isolated frog skin to high potassium concentrations at the internal surface. I. Bioelectric phenomena and sodium transport. J. clin. Invest. **42**, 88—99 (1963).

—, and S. Klahr: On the electrogenic nature of active sodium transport across the isolated frog skin. J. clin. Invest. **42**, 920 (1963).

— —, H.V. Murdauch, E.D. Robin, and P.S. Soteres: Persistence of transcellular sodium transport by an epithelial cell membrane in the absence of oxidative phosphorylation. J. Lab. clin. Med. **60**, 861—862 (1962).

Brodsky, W.A., and T.P. Schilb: Electrical and osmotic characteristics of the isolated turtle bladder. J. clin. Invest. **39**, 974—975 (1960).

— —, and A.K. Spafford: Anion transport in the isolated turtle bladder. Fed. Proc. **22**, 322 (1963).

Brown, E., D.L. Clarke, V. Roux, and G.H. Sherman: The stimulation of adenosine 3'-5' monophosphate production by antidiuretic factors. J. biol. Chem. **238**, PC 852 (1963).

Brunn, F.: Beitrag zur Kenntnis der Wirkung von Hypophysenextrakten auf den Wasserhaushalt des Frosches. Z. ges. exp. Med. **25**, 170—175 (1921).

Bullough, W.S.: The effect of the reduction of light in spring on the breeding season of the minnow (*Phoximus laevis* Linn.). Proc. Zool. Soc. (Lond.) **110**, 149—157 (1940).

Burden, C.E.: The failure of hypophysectomized *Fundulus heteroclitus* to survive in freshwater. Biol. Bull. **110**, 8—28 (1956).

Burgess, W.W., A.M. Harvey, and E.K. Marshall: The site of the antidiuretic action of pituitary extract. J. Pharmacol. exp. Ther. **49**, 237—248 (1933).

Burrows, W.H., and T.C. Byerly: Premature expulsion of eggs by hens following injection of whole posterior pituitary preparations. Poultry Sci. **21**, 416—420 (1942).

Butcher, R.W., jr., and E.W. Sutherland: Enzymatic inactivation of adenosine 3'-5' phosphate by preparations from heart. Pharmacologist **1**, 63—71 (1959).

Cade, T.J.: Water and salt balance in granivorous birds. In: Thirst, pp. 237—256. New York: Pergamon Press 1964.

Callamand, O., M. Fontaine, M. Olivereau, et A. Raffy: Hypophyse et osmoregulation chez les poissons. Bull. Inst. Oceanog. **984**, 1—7 (1951).

Campbell, B.J., B. Thysen, and F.S. Chu: Peptidase catalysed hydrolysis of antidiuretic hormone in toad bladder. Life Sci. **4**, 2129—2140 (1965).

Carasso, N., P. Favard, J. Bourguet, et S. Jard: Rôle du flux net d'eau dans les modifications ultrastructurales de la vessie de Grenouille stimulée par l'ocytocine. J. Microscopie **5**, 519—522 (1966).

— —, et J. Valerien: Variations des ultrastructures dans les cellules épitheliales de la vessie du Crapaud après stimulation par l'hormone neurohypophysaire. J. Microscopie **1**, 143—158 (1962).

Carlson, I.H., and W.N. Holmes: Changes in the hormone content of the hypothalamo-hypophysial system of the rainbow trout *(Salmo gaidneri)*. J. Endocr. **24**, 23—32 (1962).

Cereijido, M., F.C. Herrera, W.J. Flanigan, and P.F. Curran: The influence of Na concentration on Na transport across frog skin. J. gen. Physiol. **47**, 879—894 (1964).

Chan, W.Y., and V. du Vigneaud: Comparison of the pharmacologic properties of oxytocin and its highly potent analogue, desamino oxytocin. Endocrinology **71**, 977—982 (1962).

Chaudhury, R.R., and M.R. Chaudhury: Action of synthetic oxytocin on the crop gland of the pigeon. Nature (Lond.) **13**, 179—180 (1962).

Chauvet, J., M. T. Chauvet, D. Beaupain, et R. Acher: Les hormones neurohypophysaires des raies: comparaison des hormones du pocheteau blanc *(Raia batis)* et de la raie bouclée *(Raia clavata)*. Nature (Lond.) **208**, 4234—4236 (1965).

—, M. T. Lenci, et R. Acher: Présence de deux vasopressines dans la neurohypophyse du Poulet. Biochim. biophys. Acta (Amst.) **38**, 571—573 (1960).

Chavin, W.: Pituitary-adrenal control of melanization in xanthic goldfish *(Carassius auratus* L.). J. exp. Zool. **133**, 1—46 (1956).

— Pituitary hormones in melanogenesis. In: Pigment cell biology. Ed. by M. Gordon. New York: Academic Press 1959.

CHEN, G., F.K. OLDHAM, and E.M.K. GEILING: Effect of posterior pituitary extract on water uptake in frogs after hypophysectomy and infundibular lesions. Proc. Soc. exp. Biol. (N.Y.) **52**, 108—111 (1943).

CHESTER JONES, I., J.G. PHILLIPS, and W.N. HOLMES: Comparative physiology of the adrenal cortex. In: Comparative endocrinology. pp. 582—612. Ed. by A. GORBMAN. New York: J. Wiley 1959.

CHEW, R.M.: Water metabolism of desert inhabiting vertebrates. Biol. Rev. **36**, 1—31 (1961).

—, and A.E. DAMMANN: Evaporation water loss of small vertebrates, as measured with an infrared analyser. Science **133**, 384—385 (1961).

DEL CHIARAVIGLIO, E.: Elimination et retention hydrique chez *Bufo Arenarum* Hensel hypophysectomisé. C.R. Soc. Biol. (Paris) **155**, 150 (1961a).

— Action de l'hypophysectomie sur l'absorption cutanée d'eau et la volémie du crapaud. C.R. Soc. Biol. (Paris) **155**, 405—406 (1961b).

CHOI, J.K.: The fine structure of the urinary bladder of the toad, *Bufo marinus*. J. Cell. Biol. **16**, 53—72 (1963).

CIVAN, M.M., O. KEDEM, and A. LEAF: Effect of vasopressin on toad bladder under conditions of zero net sodium transport. Amer. J. Physiol. **211**, 569—575 (1966).

COHEN, N.W.: Comparative rates of dehydration and hydration in some California salamanders. Ecology **33**, 462—479 (1952).

COPELAND, D.E.: Adaptive behaviour of the chloride cell in the gill of *Fundulus heteroclitus*. J. Morph. **87**, 369—379 (1950).

CRABBE, J.: Stimulation of active sodium transport across the isolated toad bladder after injection of aldosterone to the animal. Endocrinology **69**, 673—682 (1961a).

— Stimulation of active sodium transport by the isolated toad bladder with aldosterone *in vitro*. J. clin. Invest. **40**, 2103—2110 (1961b).

—, and P. DE WEER: Action of aldosterone on the bladder and skin of the toad. Nature (Lond.) **202**, 298—299 (1964).

— — Action of aldosterone and vasopressin on the active transport of sodium by the isolated toad bladder. J. Physiol. (Lond.) **180**, 560—567 (1965).

DAINTY, J., and C.R. HOUSE: An examination of the evidence for membrane pores in frog skin. J. Physiol. (Lond.) **185**, 172—184 (1966).

DANTZLER, W.H., and B. SCHMIDT-NIELSEN: Excretion in fresh water turtle *(Pseudemys scripta)* and desert tortoise *(Gopherus agassizii)*. Amer. J. Physiol. **210**, 198—210 (1966).

DARWIN, C.: The voyage of the beagle. New York: Bantam 1958 (1st edit. 1839).

DICKER, S.E., and M.G. EGGLETON: Renal excretion of hyaluronidase and calcium in man during the antidiuretic action of vasopressins and some analogues. J. Physiol. (Lond.) **157**, 351—362 (1961).

—, and J. HASLAM: Water diuresis in the domestic fowl. J. Physiol. (Lond.) **183**, 225—235 (1966).

DOW, D., and S. ZUCKERMAN: The effect of vasopressin, sex hormones and adrenal cortical hormone on body water in axolotls. J. Endocr. **1**, 387—398 (1939).

VAN DYKE, H.B.: The nature of the vasopressins and their secretion. Proc. XXIth Int. Congr. Physiol., pp. 61—70, Buenos Aires 1959.

—, W.H. SAWYER, and N.I.A. OVERWEG: Pharmacological activities of the 8-citrulline analogues of oxytocin and vasopressin. Endocrinology **73**, 637—639 (1963).

—, and T.S. YEOH: Effects of Arginine vasotocin and other pharmacologically active substances on the cardiovascular system of the frog *(Rana macrodon)*. Endocrinology **77**, 716—724 (1965).

EDELMAN, I.S., R. BOGOROCH, and G.A. PORTER: On the mechanism of action of aldosterone on sodium transport. The role of protein synthesis. Proc. nat. Acad. Sci. (Wash.) **50**, 1169 to 1177 (1963).

—, and M.J. PETERSEN: A kinetic analysis of the antidiuretic action of vasopressin. J. clin. Invest. **41**, 1356 (1962).

— —, and P.F. GULYASSY: Kinetic analysis of the antidiuretic action of vasopressin and adenosine-3'-5' monophosphate. J. clin. Invest. **43**, 2185—2194 (1964).

EGAMI, N.: Effect of removal of eyes on oviposition of the fish *Oryzias latipes*. Zool. Mag. (Tokyo) **68**, 379—385 (1959a).

— Preliminary note on the induction of the spawning reflex and oviposition in *Oryzias latipes* by the administration of neurohypophysial substances. Annot. Zool. Jap. **32**, 13—17 (1959b).

—, and S. ISHII: Hypophyseal factors controlling ovarian activities in several fresh water fishes. Abstr. Symp. Papers 10th Pacific Sci. Congr. Honolulu, Hawaï, pp. 156—157 (1961).

— — Hypophyseal control of reproductive functions in teleost fishes. Gen. comp. Endocr. Suppl. **1**, 248—253 (1962).

—, and H. NAMBU: Factors initiating mating behavior and oviposition in the fish. *Oryzias latipes*. J. Fac. Sci. Univ. Tokyo **9**, 263—278 (1961).

Enami, M.: Studies on neurosecretion. Praeoptico-subcommissural neurosecretory system in the eeal *(Anguilla japonica)*. Endocr. jap. **1**, 133—145 (1954).
Engbaek, L., and T. Hoshiko: Electrical potential gradients through the frog skin. Acta physiol. scand. **39**, 348—355 (1957).
D'Errico, G.: Über die physiko-chemischen Verhältnisse und die Harnsekretion bei Hühnern. Beitr. Chem. Physiol. Path. **9**, 453—469 (1907).
Essig, A., and A. Leaf: The role of potassium in active transport of sodium by the toad bladder. J. gen. Physiol. **46**, 505—515 (1963).
Etkin, W., and R. Lehrer: Excess growth in tadpoles after transplantation of the adenohypophysis. Endocrinology **67**, 457—466 (1960).
Ewer, R.F.: The effect of pitressin and pitocin on water balance in *Bufo regularis*. Reuss. J. exp. Biol. **28**, 374—384 (1951).
— The effects of posterior pituitary extracts of water balance in *Bufo carens* and *Xenopus laevis*, together with some general considerations of anuran water economy. J. exp. Biol. **29**, 429—439 (1952a).
— The effect of pituitrin on fluid distribution in *Bufo regularis*. Reuss. J. exp. Biol. **29**, 173 to 177 (1952b).
Farquhar, M.G., and G.E. Palade: Functional organization of amphibian skin. Proc. nat. Acad. Sci. (Wash.) **51**, 569—577 (1964).
— — Adenosine triphosphatase localization in amphibian epidermis. J. Cell. Biol. **30**, 359—379 (1966).
Favard, P., N. Carasso, J. Bourguet, et S. Jard: Origine des modifications ultrastructurales observées sur la vessie de grenouille au cours de sa permeabilisation à l'eau par les peptides neurohypophysaires. J. Physiol. (Paris) **58**, 519 (1966).
Fleming, W.R., and J.G. Stanley: Effects of rapid changes in salinity on the renal function of a euryhaline teleost. Amer. J. Physiol. **209**, 1025—1030 (1965).
Follett, B.K., and H. Heller: The neurohypophysial hormones of bony fishes and cyclostomes. J. Physiol. (Lond.) **172**, 74—91 (1964a).
— — The neurohypophysial hormones of lungfishes and amphibians. J. Physiol. (Lond.) **172**, 92—106 (1964b).
Fong, C.T.O., I.L. Schwartz, E.A. Popenoe, L. Silver, and M.A. Schoessler: On the molecular binding of lysine-vasopressin at its renal receptor site. J. Amer. chem. Soc. **81**, 2592 to 2593 (1959).
—, L. Silver, D.R. Christman, and I.L. Schwartz: On the mechanism of action of the antidiuretic hormone vasopressin. Proc. nat. Acad. Sci. (Wash.) **46**, 1273—1277 (1960).
Fontaine, M.: The hormonal control of water and salt electrolyte metabolism in fishes. Mem. Soc. Endocr. **5**, 69—82 (1956).
—, O. Callamand, et M. Olivereau: Hypophyse et euryhalinité chez l'Anguille. C.R. Acad. Sci. (Paris) **228**, 513—514 (1949).
—, et H. Koch: Les variations d'euryhalinité et d'osmoregulation chez les Poissons. Leur rapport possible avec les migrations. J. Physiol. (Paris) **42**, 287—318 (1950).
—, et A. Raffy: Le facteur hypophysaire de retention d'eau chez les Teleosteens. C.R. Soc. Biol. (Paris) **144**, 6—7 (1950).
Forster, R.P.: The nature of the glucose reabsorptive process in the frog renal tubule. Evidence for intermittency of glomerular function in the intact animal. J. cell. comp. Physiol. **20**, 55—68 (1942).
— The effect of ephinephrine upon frog renal hemodynamics in the intact animal. Amer. J. Physiol. **140**, 221—225 (1943).
— A comparative study of renal function in marine teleosts. J. cell. comp. Physiol. **42**, 487—509 (1953).
Frazier, H.S.: The electrical potential profile of the isolated toad bladder. J. gen. Physiol. **45**, 515—528 (1962).
—, E.F. Dempsey, and A. Leaf: The initial step in active sodium transport by the toad bladder. J. clin. Invest. **40**, 1039 (1961).
— — — Movement of sodium across the mucosal surface of the isolated toad bladder and its modification by vasopressin. J. gen. Physiol. **45**, 529—543 (1962).
—, and E.I. Hammer: Efflux of sodium from isolated toad bladder. Amer. J. Physiol. **205**, 718—722 (1963).
—, and A. Leaf: The electrical characteristics of active sodium transport in the toad bladder. J. gen. Physiol. **46**, 491—503 (1963).
— — Cellular mechanisms in the control of body fluids. Medicine **43**, 281—289 (1964).
Fridberg, G., and R. Olsson: The preoptical hypophysial system, *nucleus tuberis lateralis* and the subcommissural organ of *gasterosteus aculeatus* after changes in osmotic stimuli. Z. Zellforsch. **49**, 531—540 (1959).

Fulford, B.D., and S.M. McCann: Suppression of adrenal compensatory hypertrophy by hypothalamic lesions. Proc. Soc. exp. Biol. (N.Y.) **90**, 78—80 (1955).
Fuhrman, F.A., and H.H. Ussing: A characteristic response of the isolated frog skin potential to neurohypophysial principles and its relations to the transport of sodium and water. J. cell. comp. Physiol. **38**, 109—130 (1951).
Gaddum, J.H.: Some properties of the separated active principles of the pituitary (posterior lobe). J. Physiol. (Lond.) **65**, 434—440 (1928).
Garcia Romeu, F., and J. Maetz: The mechanism of sodium and chloride uptake by the gills of a fresh water fish *Carassius auratus*. I. Evidence for an independant uptake of sodium and chloride ions. J. gen. Physiol. **47**, 1195—1208 (1964).
Gerschenfeld, H.M., J.H. Tramezzani, and E. de Robertis: Ultrastructure and function in neurohypophysis of the toad. Endocrinology **66**, 741—762 (1960).
Gibbs, O.S.: The function of the fowl's ureter. Amer. J. Physiol. **87**, 545—601 (1929).
Ginetzinsky, A.G.: Role of hyaluronidase in the reabsorption of water in renal tubules. The mechanism of action of the antidiuretic hormone. Nature (Lond.) **182**, 1218—1219 (1958).
—, and G.M. Berlyne: Relationships between urinary hyaluronidase and diuresis. Nature (Lond.) **189**, 235—237 (1961).
Goodfriend, T., and J. Kirkpatrick: Effects of neurohypophysial hormones on oxidative metabolism of the toad bladder *in vitro*. Endocrinology **72**, 742—748 (1963).
Gordon, M.S.: Osmotic regulation in the green toad *(Bufo viridis)*. J. exp. Biol. **39**, 261—270 (1962).
—, K. Schmidt-Nielsen, and H.M. Kelly: Osmotic regulation in the crab-eating frog *(Rana cancrivora)*. J. exp. Biol. **38**, 659—678 (1961).
Grantham, J.J., and M.B. Burg: Effect of vasopressin and cyclic AMP on permeability of isolated collecting tubules. Amer. J. Physiol. **211**, 255—259 (1966).
Green, J.D.: The comparative anatomy of the hypophysis with special reference to its blood supply and innervation. Amer. J. Anat. **88**, 225—311 (1951).
Guillemin, R.: Über die hypothalamische Kontrolle der ACTH-Sekretion betrachtet an den Ergebnissen von *in-vitro*-Versuchen. Endocrinology **34**, 193—201 (1957).
—, W.R. Hearn, W.R. Check, and D.E. Housholder: Control of corticotrophin release. Further studies with *in vitro* methods. Endocrinology **60**, 488—506 (1957).
Gulyassy, P.F., and I.S. Edelman: Hydrogen-ion dependence of the antidiuretic action of vasopressin, oxytocin and deamino oxytocin. Biochim. biophys. Acta (Amst.) **102**, 185—197 (1965).
Handler, J.S., R.W. Butcher, E.W. Sutherland, and J. Orloff: The effect of vasopressin and of theophyllin on the concentration of adenosine 3'-5'-phosphate in the urinary bladder of the toad. J. biol. Chem. **240**, 4524—4526 (1965).
—, and J. Orloff: Activation of phosphorylase in toad bladder and mammalian kidney by antidiuretic hormone. Amer. J. Physiol. **205**, 298—302 (1963).
— — Cysteine effect on toad bladder response to vasopressin, cyclic A.M.P. and theophylline. Amer. J. Physiol. **206**, 505—509 (1964).
Harrington, R.W.: Preseasonal breeding by the bridled shiner *Notropis bifrenatus*, induced under light-temperature control. Copeia No. 304 (1950).
Haynes, R.C., jr.: The activation of adrenal phosphorylase by the adrenocorticotropic hormone. J. biol. Chem. **233**, 1220—1222 (1958).
—, and L. Berthet: Studies on the mechanism of action of the adrenocorticotropic hormone. J. biol. Chem. **225**, 115—124 (1957).
Hays, R.M., and A. Leaf: Studies on the movement of water through the isolated toad bladder and its modifications by vasopressin. J. gen. Physiol. **45**, 905—920 (1962a).
— — The state of water in the isolated toad bladder in the presence and absence of vasopressin. J. gen. Physiol. **45**, 933—948 (1962b).
Heller, H.: Differentiation of an (amphibian) water balance principle from the antidiuretic principle of the posterior pituitary gland. J. Physiol. (Lond.) **100**, 125—141 (1941).
— The comparative physiology of the neurohypophysis. Experientia (Basel) **6**, 368—376 (1950).
— The hormonal control of water and salt electrolyte metabolism with special reference to higher vertebrates. Mem. Soc. Endocrinol. **5**, 25—43 (1956).
— Neurohypophyseal hormones. In: Comparative endocrinology, Vol.I, pp. 26—72. Ed. by Euler and Heller. New York: Academic Press 1963a.
— Hypophysenhinterlappenhormone. Naunyn-Schmiedebergs Arch. exp. Path. Pharmak., Bd. **245**, Heft 11, S. 142—153 (1963b).
— Chairman's introduction. In: Advances in oxytocin. Oxford: Pergamon Press 1965a.
— Osmoregulation in amphibia. Arch. Anat. micr. Morph. exp. **54**, 471—490 (1965b).
—, and P.J. Bentley: Phylogenetic distribution of the effects of neurohypophysial hormones on water and sodium metabolism. Gen. comp. Endocr. **5**, 96—108 (1965).

HELLER, H., and T.B. PICKERING: Neurohypophysial hormones of non-mammalian vertebrates. J. Physiol. (Lond.) **155**, 98—114 (1961).

— —, J. MAETZ, and F. MOREL: Pharmacological characterization of the oxytocic peptides in the pituitary of a marine teleost fish *(Pollachius virens)*. Nature (Lond.) **191**, 670—671 (1961).

HESTER, H.R., H.E. ESSEX, and F.C. MANN: Secretion of urine in the chicken *(Gallus domesticus)*. Amer. J. Physiol. **128**, 592—602 (1940).

HEVESY, G.V., E. HOFER, and A. KROGH: The permeability of the skin of frogs to water as determined par D_2O and H_2O. Skand. Arch. Physiol. **72**, 199—214 (1935).

HILD, W.: Experimentelle morphologische Untersuchungen über das Verhalten der „neurosekretorischen Bahn“ nach Hypophysenstieldurchtrennung, Eingriffen in den Wasserhaushalt und Belastung der Osmoregulation. Virchows Arch. path. Anat. **319**, 526—546 (1951).

HILTON, J.G., L.F. SCIAN, C.D. WESTERMANN, and O.R. KRUESI: Effect of synthetic lysine-vasopressin on adrenocortical secretion. Science **129**, 971 (1959).

HOGBEN, L.T., and W. SCHLAPP: The vasomotor activity of pituitary extracts throughout the vertebrate series. Quart. J. exp. Physiol. **14**, 229—258 (1924).

HOHN, E.O.: Failure of oxytocin to produce a prolactin-like response in the pigeon's crop sac. J. Endocr. **26**, 177—178 (1963).

HOLMES, W.N.: Studies on the hormonal control of sodium metabolism in the rainbow trout *(Salmo gairdnerii)*. Acta endocr. (Kbh.) **31**, 587—602 (1959).

—, and B.M. ADAMS: Effects of adrenocortical and neurohypophysial hormones on the renal excretory pattern in the water-loaded duck *(Anas platyrhynchus)*. Endocrinology **73**, 5—10 (1963).

—, and R.L. MC BEAN: Studies on the glomerular filtration rate of rainbow trout. J. exp. Biol. **40**, 335—341 (1963).

HOOVER, E.E., and H.E. HUBBARD: Modification of the sexual cycle in trout by control of light. Copeia **1937**, 206.

HOSHIKO, T.: Electrogenesis in frog skin. Biophysics of physiological and pharmacological actions. Amer. Ass. Advanc. Sci. (Wash.), pp. 31—47 (1961).

HOUSE, C.R.: Osmotic regulation in the brackfish water teleost *(Blennius pholis)*. J. exp. Biol. **40**, 87—104 (1963).

HOUSSAY, B.A., L. GIUSTI, and G.P. GONALONS: Rev. Soc. argent. Biol. **1**, 237 (1925). Cited from B.A. HOUSSAY and D. POTICK: El antagonismo Hipofisis insuline in los sapos. Rev. Soc. argent. Biol. **5**, 66—76 (1929a).

—, et D. POTICK: Antagonisme entre l'hypophyse et l'insuline chez le Crapaud. C.R. Soc. Biol. (Paris) **101**, 940—942 (1929b).

— — El antagonismo hypofisis insuline in los sapos. Rev. Soc. argent. Biol. **5**, 66—76 (1929a).

HOWES, N.H.: The response of the water regulating mechanism of developmental stages of the commun toad *Bufo bufo* (L.) to treatment with extracts of the posterior lobe of the pituitary body. J. exp. Biol. **17**, 128—138 (1940).

HUBER, G.C.: On the morphology of the renal tubules of vertebrates. Anat. Rec. **13**, 305—339 (1917).

ISHII, S.: Artificial induction of parturition in the top minnow *Gambusia* sp. (Abstract in Japanese). Zool. Mag. (Tokyo) **70**, 3—4 (1961).

—, T. HIRANO, and H. KOBOYASHI: Neurohypophyseal hormones in the Avian median Eminence and *pars nervosa*. Gen. comp. Endocr. **2**, 433—440 (1962).

JACOBSOHN, D., and C.B. JØRGENSEN: Survival and function of auto and homografts of adenohypophysial tissue in the toad. Acta physiol. scand. **36**, 1—12 (1956).

JANCSÓ, N.: Storage of proteins and vinylpolymers in histiocytes and in the renal epithelium. Acta med. Acad. Sci. hung. **7**, 173—210 (1955a).

— Speicherung und Stoffanreicherung im Retikuloendothel und in der Niere. Budapest: Academiai Kiado 1955b.

JARD, S.: Inhibition par l'ocytocine des actions tubulaires de la vasotocine chez la grenouille. Arguments en faveur de sa nature compétitive. Excerpta Med. Int. Congr. Ser. **78**, 602—604 (1963).

— Etude des effects de la vasotocine sur l'excretion de l'eau et des electrolytes par le rein de la grenouille (*Rana esculenta* L.). Analyse à l'aide d'analogues artificiels de l'hormone naturelle des caractères structuraux requis pour son activité biologique. J. Physiol. (Paris) **58**, Suppl. 16, 123 p. (1966).

—, F. BASTIDE, et F. MOREL: Etude quantitative de la relation dose effet pour l'ocytocine sur deux de ses recepteurs. (Abstract no. **312**, Second Int. Biophys. Congress, Vienna, 5—9 Sept. 1966a.

—, J. BOURGUET, N. CARASSO, et P. FAVARD: Action de divers fixateurs sur la permeabilité et l'ultrastructure de la vessie de grenouille. J. Microscopie **5**, 31—50 (1966b).

JARD, S., J. MAETZ, et F. MOREL: Action de quelques analogues de l'ocytocine sur différents recepteurs intervenant dans l'osmorégulation de *Rana esculenta*. C.R. Acad. Sci. (Paris) **251**, 788—790 (1960).
—, et F. MOREL: Inhibition competitive de l'action antidiurétique de la lysine-vasotocine par l'ocytocine chez *Rana esculenta*. C. R. Acad. Sci. (Paris) **252**, 339—341 (1961).
— — Actions of vasotocin and some of its analogues on salt and water excretion by the frog. Amer. J. Physiol. **204**, 222—226 (1963).
JØRGENSEN, C.B.: The amphibian water economy with special regard to the effect of neurohypophysial extracts. Acta physiol. scand. **22**, Suppl. 78 (1950).
—, and L.O. LARSEN: Effect of neurohypophyseal principles on adenophyseal activity in toads. Proc. Soc. exp. Biol. (N.Y.) **103**, 685—688 (1960a).
— — Hormonal control of moulting in amphibians. Nature (Lond.) **185**, 244—245 (1960b).
— — Inhibition by oxytocin of vasotocin induced activities in toads. Proc. Soc. exp. Biol. (N.Y.) **110**, 293—294 (1962).
— — Neuro-adenohypophysial relationships. Symp. Zool. Soc. (Lond.) **9**, 59—82 (1963).
— —, P. ROSENKILDE, and K.G. WINGSTRAND: Effect of extirpation of median eminence on function of *pars distalis* of the hypophysis in the toad *Bufo bufo* (L.). Comp. Biochem. Physiol. **1**, 38—43 (1960).
—, H. LEVI, and H.H. USSING: On the influence of neurohypophysial principles on sodium metabolism in the axolotl *Ambystoma mexicanum*. Acta. physiol. scand. **12**, 350—371 (1946).
—, and L. NIELSEN: Effect of synthetic lysine-vasopressin on adenohypophysial activity in toads. Proc. Soc. exp. Biol. (N.Y.) **98**, 393—395 (1958).
—, and P. ROSENKILDE: Chloride balance in hypophysectomized frogs. Endocrinology **50**, 219—224 (1957).
—, K.G. WINGSTRAND, and P. ROSENKILDE: Neurohypophysis and water metabolism in the toad *Bufo bufo* (L.). Endocrinology **59**, 601—610 (1956).
KARLIN, A.: The *in vitro* release by the toad bladder of an inhibitor of oxytocin. Biochem. biophys. Res. Commun. **11**, 44—49 (1963).
KATSOYANNIS, P.G., and V. DU VIGNEAUD: Arginin-vasotocin a synthetic analogue of the posterior pituitary hormones containing the ring of oxytocin and the side chain of vasopressin. J. biol. Chem. **233**, 1352—1354 (1958).
KELLER, A.R.: An electron microscopic study of the bladder of the tropical toad *(Bufo marinus)*. Thesis. Dep. Biochem. Sci., Harvard Coll., Cambridge, Mass. (1960).
KEYS, A., and J.B. BATEMAN: Branchial responses to adrenalin and to pitressin in the eel. Biol. Bull. **63**, 327—336 (1932).
KOBAYASHI, H., A. GORBMAN, and S. ISHII: Hypothalamic neurosecretory apparatus of a young Goby *(Lepidogobius lepidus)*. Anat. Rec. **134**, 595 (1959).
KOEFOED-JOHNSEN, V., H. LEVI, and H.H. USSING: The mode of passage of chloride ions through the isolated frog skin. Acta physiol. scand. **25**, 150—163 (1952b).
—, and H.H. USSING: The contributions of diffusion and flow to the passage of D_2O through living membranes. Effect of neurohypophyseal hormone on isolated anuran skin. Acta physiol. scand. **28**, 60—76 (1953).
— — The nature of the frog skin potential. Acta physiol. scand. **42**, 298—308 (1958).
— —, and K. ZEHRAN: The origin of the short circuit current in the adrenaline stimulated frog skin. Acta physiol. scand. **27**, 38—48 (1952a).
KORR, I.M.: The osmotic function of the chicken kidney. J. cell. comp. Physiol. **13**, 175—194 (1939).
KRAGT, C.L., and J. MEITES: Stimulation of pigeon pituitary prolactin release by pigeon hypothalamic extract *in vitro*. Endocrinology **76**, 1169—1176 (1965).
KROGH, A.: Osmotic regulation in freshwater fishes by active absorption of chloride ions. Z. vergl. Physiol. **24**, 656—666 (1937a).
— Osmotic regulation in the frog *(Rana esculenta)* by active absorption of chloride ions. Skand. Arch. Physiol. **76**, 60—69 (1937b).
— Osmotic regulation in aquatic animals. Cambridge Univ. Press (1939).
LAHLOU, B.: Mise en évidence d'un recrutement glomerulaire dans le rein des teleosteens d'après la mesure du Tm glucose. C.R. Acad. Sci. (Paris) **262**, 1356—1358 (1966).
LEAF, A.: Some actions of neurohypophysial hormones on a living membrane. J. gen. Physiol. **43**, 175—189 (1960).
— Some observations on transport across the toad bladder *in vitro*. In: Symposium on membrane transport and metabolism, p. 247. Ed. by A. KLEINZELLER and A. KOTYK. Prague: Czech. Acad. Sciences 1961.
— Action of neurohypophyseal hormones on the toad bladder. Gen. comp. Endocr. **2**, 148—160 (1962).

LEAF, A.: Transepithelial transport and its hormonal control in toad bladder. Ergebn. Physiol. **56**, 216—264 (1965).
—, J. ANDERSON, and L.B. PAGE: Active sodium transport by the isolated toad bladder. J. gen. Physiol. **41**, 657—668 (1958).
—, and E. DEMPSEY: Some effects of mammalian neurohypophyseal hormones on metabolism and active transport of sodium by the isolated toad bladder. J. biol. Chem. **235**, 2160—2163 (1960).
—, and R.M. HAYS: Permeability of the isolated toad bladder to solutes and its modification by vasopressin. J. gen. Physiol. **45**, 921—932 (1962).
—, L.B. PAGE, and J. ANDERSON: Respiration and active sodium transport of isolated toad bladder. J. biol. Chem. **234**, 1625—1629 (1959).
—, and A. RENSHAW: Ion transport and respiration of isolated frog skin. Biochem. J. **65**, 82—90 (1957).
LE BRIE, S.J., and I.D.W. SUTHERLAND: Renal function in water snakes. Amer. J. Physiol. **203**, 995—1000 (1962).
LEDERIS, K.: Effects of salinity on hormone content and on ultrastructure of trout neurohypophysis. J. Endocr. **26**, 21—22 (1963).
LEGAIT, H.: Contribution à l'étude morphologique et expérimentale du système hypothalamo-neurohypophysaire de la Poule Rhode-Island. Thèse d'agrégation de l'enseignement superieur Louvain. Nancy: S.I.T. 1959.
LEHRMAN, D.S.: The reproductive behaviour of ring doves. Sci. Amer. **211**, No. 5, 48—54 (1964).
LELOUP-HATEY, J.: Influence de l'agitation motrice sur la teneur du plasma en 17-hydroxycorticosteroïdes du plasma d'un Teleosteen: la carpe (*Cyprinus carpio* L.). C.R. Acad. Sci. (Paris) **246**, 1088—1091 (1958).
LEVINSKY, N.G., and W.H. SAWYER: Influence of the adenohypophysis on frog water balance response. Endocrinology **51**, 110—116 (1952).
— — Significance of the neurohypophysis in regulation of fluid balance in the frog. Proc. Soc. exp. Biol. (N.Y.) **82**, 272—274 (1953).
LICHTENSTEIN, N.S., and A. LEAF: Effect of Amphotericin B on the permeability of the toad bladder. J. clin. Invest. **44**, 1328—1342 (1965).
LICO, M.C.: The role of the hypophysis in the regulation of arterial pressure in the toad. Acta physiol. lat.-amer. **12**, 375—380 (1963).
LITTLEFORD, R.A., W.F. KELLER, and N.E. PHILLIPS: Studies on the vital limits of water loss in the plethodont salamanders. Ecology **28**, 440—447 (1947).
MCCANN, S.M.: The ACTH-releasing activity of the posterior lobe of the pituitary. Endocrinology **60**, 664—676 (1957).
—, and J.R. BROBECK: Evidence for a role of the supraopticohypophyseal system in regulation of adrenocorticotrophin secretion. Proc. Soc. exp. Biol. (N.Y.) **87**, 318—324 (1954).
—, and A. FRUIT: Effect of synthetic vasopressin on release of adrenocorticotrophin in rats with hypothalamic lesions. Proc. Soc. exp. Biol. (N.Y.) **96**, 566—567 (1957).
MCFARLAND, L.Z.: Effects of an electric lesion in the avian hypothalamo-hypophysial tract. Anat. Rec. **133**, 411 (1959).
MCROBBIE, E.A.C., and H.H. USSING: Osmotic behaviour of the epithelial cells of frog skin. Acta physiol. scand. **53**, 348—366 (1961).
MAETZ, J.: Les échanges de sodium chez le poisson *Carassius auratus* L.; Action d'un inhibiteur de l'anhydrase carbonique. J. Physiol. (Paris) **48**, 1085—1099 (1956).
— Le controle endocrinien du transport actif de sodium à travers la peau de grenouille. In: La méthode des indicateurs nucleaires dans l'étude des transports actifs d'ions (1er colloque de Biologie de Saclay), p. 185—196. Paris: Pergamon Press 1959.
— Corrélation entre les actions des hormones neurohypophysaires sur le transport actif de sodium et le flux osmotique d'eau à travers la peau de divers amphibiens. Acta endocr. (Kbh.) **35**, Suppl. **51**, 133 (1960).
— Physiological aspects of neurohypophysial function in fishes with some reference to the amphibia. Symp. Zool. Soc. (Lond.) **9**, 107—140 (1963).
— Recherches sur la permeabilité aux electrolytes de la branchie des poissons et sa régulation endocrinienne. Bulletin d'Informations scientifiques et techniques du Commissariat à l'Energie atomique, No. 86 (1964).
—, J. BOURGUET, B. LAHLOUH, et J. HOURDRY: Peptides neurohypophysaires et osmoregulation chez *Carassius auratus*. Gen. comp. Endocr. **4**, 508—522 (1964).
—, and F. GARCIA ROMEU: The mechanism of sodium and chloride uptake by the gills of a fresh water fish *Carassius auratus*. II. Evidence of $NH\ 4^+/NA^+$ and HCO_3^-/CL^- exchanges. J. gen. Physiol. **47**, 1209—1228 (1964).
—, S. JARD, et F. MOREL: Action de l'aldosterone sur le transport actif de sodium de la peau de grenouille. C.R. Acad. Sci. (Paris) **247**, 516—518 (1958).

Maetz, J., and M. Julien: Action of neurohypophyseal hormones on the sodium fluxes of a fresh water teleost. Nature (Lond.) **189**, 152—153 (1961).
—, F. Morel, and B. Lahlouh: Natriferin. A new hormonal principle in the neurohypophysis of certain vertebrates. Nature (Lond.) **184**, 1236—1237 (1959a).
— —, et B. Race: Mise en évidence dans la neurohypophyse de *Rana esculenta* L., d'un facteur hormonal nouveau stimulant le transport actif de sodium. Biochim. biophys. Acta (Amst.) **36**, 317—326 (1959b).
Maffly, R.H., R.M. Hays, E. Lamdin, and A. Leaf: The effect of neurohypophyseal hormones on the permeability of the toad bladder to urea. J. clin. Invest. **39**, 630—641 (1960).
Mansour, T.E.: Studies on heart phosphofructokinase: purification inhibition and activation. J. biol. Chem. **238**, 2285—2292 (1963).
—, E.W. Sutherland, T.W. Rall, and E. Bueding: The effect of 5-hydroxytrypotamine (serotonin) on the formation of adenosine 3'-5'-phosphate by tissue particles from the liver fluke, *Fasciola hepatica*. J. biol. Chem. **235**, 466—470 (1960).
Marshall, E.K., jr., and H.W. Smith: The glomerular development of vertebrate kidney in relation to habitat. Biol. Bull. **59**, 135—153 (1930).
Martini, L., and A. de Poli: Neurohumoral control of the release of adrenocorticotrophic hormone. J. Endocr. **13**, 229—234 (1956).
Masur, S.K.: Autotransplantation of the pituitary in the red eft. Amer. Zool. **2**, 528 (1962).
Mazzi, V., e A. Peyrot: Effetti differenziali di lesioni ipotalamiche croniche sulla tyroide e sul testicolo di *Triturus cristatus carnifex*. Laur. trattati con tiouria. Arch. Ital. Anat. Embriol. **65**, 295—300 (1960).
Meier, A.H., and W.R. Fleming: The effects of pitocin and pitressin on water and sodium movements in the euryhaline killifish *Fundulus kansae*. Comp. Biochem. Physiol. **6**, 215 to 231 (1962).
Meites, J., and C.S. Nicoll: Adenohypophysis: prolactin. Ann. Rev. Physiol. **27**, 57—88 (1965).
Mellinger, J.: Esquisse structurale de l'appareil hypophysaire d'un selacien, *Scyliorhinus caniculus* (L.) pour servir de base à une étude expérimentale des correlations neuroendocriniennes. C.R. Acad. Sci. (Paris) **251**, 2422—2424 (1960).
— Observation *in vivo* de la circulation hypophysaire chez la Raie *(Raja undulata)* et la Torpille *(Torpedo marmorata)*. C.R. Acad. Sci. (Paris) **261**, 5671—5674 (1965).
—, E. Follenius, et A. Porte: Presence de terminaisons neurosecretoires sur les capillaires primaires du systeme Porte hypophysaire de la Roussette *(Scyliorhinus caniculus)*. Etude au microscope électronique. C.R. Acad. Sci. (Paris) **254**, 1158—1159 (1962).
Meurling, P.: Presence of a pituitary portal system in Elasmobranchs. Nature (Lond.) **187**, 336—337 (1960).
Meyer, D.K.: Physiological adjustments in chloride balance of the goldfish. Science **108**, 305—308 (1948).
— Sodium flux through the gills of goldfish. Amer. J. Physiol. **165**, 580—587 (1951).
Mizuno, H., and J. Meites: Failure of oxytocin to stimulate the pigeon (Crop gland). Nature (Lond.) **198**, 1209—1210 (1963).
Monod, J., J. Wyman, and J.P. Changeux: On the nature of allosteric transitions. A plausible model. J. molec. Biol. **12**, 88—118 (1965).
Morel, F.: Action of neurohypophyseal hormones on the active transport of sodium. In: Water and electrolyte metabolism. Part II. Ed. by De Graeff and Leijnse. Amsterdam: Elsevier Publ. Co. 1964.
—, and F. Bastide: Relationship between the structure of several analogues of oxytocin and their "natriferic" activity *in vitro*. In: Oxytocin, vasopressin and their structural analogues, pp. 47—55. Ed. by J. Rudinger. New York: Pergamon Press 1964.
— — Action de l'ocytocine sur la composante active du transport de sodium par la peau de grenouille. Biochim. biophys. Acta (Amst.) **94**, 609—611 (1965).
— — Relationships between the natriferic action of oxytocin and active transport of sodium through the frog's skin. Protoplasma **63**, 58—61 (1967).
—, and S. Jard: Inhibition of frog *(Rana esculenta)* antidiuretic action of vasotocin by some analogues. Amer. J. Physiol. **204**, 227—232 (1963a).
— — Experiments concerning the first steps of the mechanism of action of neurohypophysial hormones on the kidney. Mem. Soc. Endocrinol. **13**, 67—74 (1963b).
— —, et F. Bastide: Correlations entre la structure des peptides neurohypophysaires et leur activité biologique sur la peau et le rein de grenouille. Ann. Endocr. (Paris) **26**, 643—654 (1965).
—, et J. Maetz: Emploi de méthodes biophysiques pour l'étude du mécanisme d'action de certaines hormones. Colloque de biophysique. Journées médicales de Bordeaux. Sté. Edit. de l'enseignement superieur (1958).

MOREL, F., et J. MAETZ: Quelques ascpects du contrôle hormonal du transport de sodium à travers la peau de grenouille. J. Physiol. (Paris) **51**, 536—537 (1959).

— —, R. ACHER, J. CHAUVET, and M.T. LENCI: A "natriferic" principle other than arginine-vasotocin in the frog neurohypophysis. Nature (Lond.) **190**, 4778—4780 (1961a).

— —, et C. LUCARAIN: Action de deux peptides neurohypophysaires sur le transport actif de sodium et le flux net d'eau à travers la peau de divers batraciens anoures. Biochim. biophys. Acta (Amst.) **28**, 619—626 (1958).

—, M. ODIER, et C. LUCARAIN: Un dispositif de mesures multiples et simultanées du transport actif de sodium à travers plusieurs régions d'une même peau de grenouille. J. Physiol. (Paris) **53**, 757—762 (1961b).

MORRIS, R.: The osmoregulatory ability of the lampern (*Lampetra fluviatilis* L.) in sea water during the course of its spawning migration. J. exp. Biol. **33**, 235—248 (1956).

— The mechanism of marine osmoregulation in the lampern (*Lampetra fluviatilis* L.) and the cause of its breakdown during the spawning migration. J. exp. Biol. **35**, 649—658 (1958).

— General problems of osmoregulation with special reference to cyclostomes. Symp. Zool. Soc. (Lond.) **1**, 1—13 (1960).

MOTAIS, R.: Les échanges de sodium chez un teleosteen euryhalin *Platichthys flesus flesus* L.: cinétique de ces échanges lors des passages d'eau de mer en eau douce et d'eau douce en eau de mer. C.R. Acad. Sci. (Paris) **253**, 724—726 (1961a).

— Cinetique des échanges de sodium chez un teleosteen euryhalin (*Platichthys flesus* L.) au cours de passages successifs eau de mer-eau douce-eau de mer en fonction du temps de séjour en deau douce. C.R. Acad. Sci. (Paris) **253**, 2609—2611 (1961b).

— Les mécanismes d'échanges ioniques branchiaux chez les Teleosteens. Ann. Inst. Oceanog. (Paris) **45**, 1—83 (1967).

—, F. GARCIA ROMEU, et J. MAETZ: Mécanisme de l'euryhalinité. Etude comparée du flet (euryhalin) et du serran (stenohalin) au cours du transfert en eau douce. C.R. Acad. Sci. (Paris) **261**, 801—804 (1965).

— — — Exchange diffusion effect and euryhalinity in Teleosts. J. gen. Physiol. **50**, 391—422 (1966).

—, et J. MAETZ: Action des hormones neurohypophysaires sur les échanges de sodium (Mesurés à l'aide du radio-sodium Na^{24}) chez un teleosteen euryhalin: *Platichthys flesus* L.. Gen. comp. Endocr. **4**, 210—224 (1964).

— — Arginine-vasotocine et évolution de la perméabilité branchiale au sodium au cours du passage d'eau douce en eau de mer chez le Flet J. Physiol. (Paris) **59**, 271 (1967).

MUNSICK, R.A.: Hen oxytocic activities of oxytocin and l.-deamino-oxytocin. Endocrinology **76**, 161—162 (1965).

—, W.H. SAWYER, and H.B. VAN DYKE: Hormonal characteristics of avian neurohypophysis. Fed. Proc. **18**, 110 (1959).

— — — Avian neurohypophysial hormones, pharmacological properties and tentative identification. Endocrinology **66**, 860—871 (1960).

MULLINS, L.J.: Osmotic regulation in fish as studied with radioisotopes. Acta physiol. scand. **21**, 303—314 (1950).

MYERS, R.M., W.R. BISHOP, and B.T. SCHEER: Anterior pituitary control of active sodium transport across frog skin. Amer. J. Physiol. **200**, 444—450 (1961).

—, W.R. FLEMING, and B.T. SCHEER: Pituitary adrenal control of sodium flux across frog skin. Endocrinology **58**, 674—676 (1956).

NATOCHIN, J.W.: Mechanism of pituitrin action increasing permeability of the urinary bladder in *Rana temporaria*. Sechenov physiol. J. U.S.S.R. **49**, 525—531 (1963).

—, K. JANAECK, and R. RYBOVA: The swelling of frog bladder cells produced by oxytocin. J. Endocr. **33**, 171—177 (1965).

NEEDHAM, J.: Nitrogenous waste products. In: Chemical embryology **2**, Sect. 9, 1055—1145 (1931).

NICOLL, C.S.: Neural regulation of adenohypophysial prolactin secretion in Tetrapods: indications from *in vitro* studies. J. Exp. Zool. **158**, 203—210 (1965).

NOVELLI, A.: Lobulo posterior de hipofisis e imbibicion de los batracios. II. Mecanismo de su accion. Rev. Soc. argent. Biol. **12**, 163—164 (1936).

OEHME: Z. ges. exp. Med. **9**, 251 (1919). In: W.W. BURGESS, A.M. HARVEY, and E.K. MARSHALL: The site of the antidiuretic action of pituitary extract. J. Pharmacol. exp. Ther. **49**, 237—248 (1933).

OKSCHE, A., D.F. LAWS, F.I. KAMEMOTO, and D.S. FARNER: The hypothalamo-hypophysial neurosecretory system of the white crowned sparrow *(Zonotrichia leucophrys Cambelii)*. Z. Zellforsch. **51**, 1—42 (1959).

OLDHAM, F.K.: The action of the preparations from the posterior lobe of the pituitary gland upon the imbibition of water by frogs. Amer. J. Physiol. **115**, 275—280 (1936).

Oliver, G., and E. A. Schäfer: On the physiological action of extracts of pituitary body and certain other glandular organs. J. Physiol. (Lond.) **18**, 277—279 (1895).

Opel, H.: Premature oviposition following operative interference with the brain of the chicken. Endocrinology **74**, 193—200 (1964).

— Release of oviposition-inducing factor from the median eminence pituitary stalk region in neural lobectomized hens. Anat. Rec. **154**, 396 (1966).

Orloff, J., and J.S. Handler: Vasopressin-like effects of adenosine 3'-5'-phosphate (cyclic 3'-5' AMP) and theophylline in the toad bladder. Biochem. biophys. Res. Commun. **5**, 63—66 (1961).

— — The similarity of effects of vasopressin, adenosine 3'-5' phosphate (cyclic AMP) and theophylline on the toad bladder. J. clin. Invest. **41**, 702—709 (1962).

— — The cellular mode of action of antidiuretic hormone. Amer. J. Med. **36**, 686—697 (1964a).

— — The role of adenosine 3'-5' monophosphate (cyclic AMP) in the action of neurohypophysial hormones. In: Oxytocin, vasopressin and their structural analogues, pp. 133—139. Ed. by J. Rudinger. Prague. (1964b).

Overton, E.: Neununddreißig Thesen über die Wasserökonomie der Amphibien und die osmotischen Eigenschaften der Amphibienhaut. Verh. phys.-med. Ges. Würzb. **36**, 277—296 (1904).

Pak Poy, R.F.K., and P.J. Bentley: Fine structure of the epithelial cells of the toad urinary bladder. Exp. Cell Res. **20**, 235—237 (1960).

Pasqualini, R.Q.: Papel de la hipofisis en la regulation de la diuresis. Buenos Aires: El Aleneo (1938a).

— Estudios sobre el metabolismo hidrico en el Bufo arenarum. Hensel. V. Accion de los extractos hipofisarios. Rev. Soc. argent. Biol. **14**, 260—274 (1938b).

Patlak, C.S., D.A. Goldstein, and J.F. Hoffman: The flow of solute and solvent across a two membrane system. J. theor. Biol. **5**, 426—442 (1963).

Paton, D.N., and A. Watson: The actions of pituitrin, adrenalin and barium on the circulation of the bird. J. Physiol. (Lond.) **44**, 413—424 (1912).

Peachey, L.D., and H. Rasmussen: Structure of the toad's urinary bladder as related to its physiology. J. biophys. biochem. Cytol. **10**, 529—553 (1961).

Petersen, M., and I.S. Edelman: Calcium inhibition of the action of vasopressin on the urinary bladder of the toad. J. clin. Invest. **43**, 583—594 (1964).

Pickford, G.E.: Induction of a spawning reflex in hypophysectomized killifish. Nature (Lond.) **170**, 807—808 (1952).

— The hypophysectomized male killifish. Bull. Bingham. Oceanogr. Coll. **14**, 5—14 (1953).

—, and J.W. Atz: The physiology of the pituitary gland of fishes. New York: Zoological Society 1957.

—, and J.G. Phillips: Prolactin, a factor in promoting survival of hypophysectomized killifish in fresh water. Science **130**, 454—455 (1959).

—, E.E. Robertson, and W.H. Sawyer: Hypophysectomy replacement therapy, and the tolerance of the euryhaline killifish *Fundulus heteroclitus*, to hypotonic media. Gen. comp. Endocr. **5**, 160—180 (1965).

Pohle, E.: Arch. ges. Physiol. **182**, 215 (1920); cited from C.B. Jørgensen, K.G. Wingstrand, and P. Rosenkilde: Neurohypophysis and water metabolism in the toad (*Bufo bufo* L.). Endocrinology **59**, 601—610 (1956).

Polenov, A.L., and J.A. Barannikova: The preoptico neurohypophysial neurosecretory system in sturgeon. Dokl. Akad. Nauk SSR, Otd. Biokh. **123**, 1117—1120 (1958).

Porter, G.A., and I. Edelman: The action of aldosterone and related corticosteroids on sodium transport across the toad bladder. J. clin. Invest. **43**, 611—620 (1964).

Poulson, T.L.: Countercurrent multipliers in avian kidneys. Science **148**, 389—391 (1965).

—, and G.A. Bartholomew: Salt balance in the savannah sparrow. Physiol. Zool. **35**, 109 to 113 (1962).

Rall, T.W., and E.W. Sutherland: Formation of a cyclic adenine ribonucleotide by tissue particles. J. biol. Chem. **232**, 1065—1076 (1958).

Ralph, C.L.: Polydipsia in the hen following lesions in the supraoptic hypothalamus. Amer. J. Physiol. **198**, 528—530 (1960).

Rasmussen, H., and L. Craig: The isolation of arginine-vasotocin from fish pituitary glands. Endocrinology **68**, 1051—1055 (1961).

—, I.L. Schwartz, R. Young, and J. Marc-Aurele: Structural requirements for the action of neurohypophyseal hormones upon the isolated amphibian urinary bladder. J. gen. Physiol. **46**, 1171—1189 (1963).

— —, M.A. Schoessler, and G. Hochster: Studies on the mechanism of action of vasopressin. Proc. nat. Acad. Sci. (Wash.) **46**, 1278—1287 (1960).

Rasquin, P., and L.M. Stoll: Effects of pitressin and water injections on secretions of brain and hypophysis in a telest. J. comp. Neurol. **107**, 273—294 (1955).

REY, P.: La region tubero-hypophysaire et les echanges d'eau chez la grenouille. C.R. Soc. Biol. (Paris) **118**, 1132—1134 (1935).

— Recherches experimentales sur l'economie de l'eau chez les batraciens. Ann. Physiol. **13**, 1081—1144 (1937).

RICHARDS, A.N., J.B. BARNWELL, and R.C. BRADLEY: The effect of small amounts of adrenalin upon the glomerular blood vessels of the frog's kidney perfused at a constant rate. Amer. J. Physiol. **79**, 410—432 (1927).

—, and C.F. SCHMIDT: A description of the glomerular circulation in the frog's kidney and observations concerning the action of adrenalin and other substances upon it. Amer. J. Physiol. **71**, 178—208 (1924).

RIDDLE, O.: A simple method of obtaining premature eggs from birds. Science **54**, 664—666 (1921).

— Prolactin in vertebrate function and organization. J. nat. Cancer Inst. **31**, 1039—1110 (1963).

—, and R.W. BATES: Sex and internal secretions. Ed. by E. ALLEN. Baltimore: Williams & Wilkins Co. 1939.

RIDLEY, A.: Secretion in the brain of *Rana Catesbeiana* and its modification by osmotic stress and hypophysectomy. Gen. comp. Endocr. **4**, 486—492 (1964a).

— Effects of osmotic stress and hypophysectomy on ion distribution in bullfrogs. Gen. comp. Endocr. **4**, 481—486 (1964b).

RIZACK, M.A.: Activation of epinephrine sensitive lipolytric activity from adipose tissue by adenosine 3'-5'-phosphate. J. biol. Chem. **239**, 392—395 (1964).

ROBERTS, J.S., and B. SCHMIDT-NIELSEN: Renal ultrastructure and excretion of salt and water by three terrestrial lizards. Amer. J. Physiol. **211**, 476—486 (1966).

RODERICH, W., and V. DU VIGNEAUD: 1-Deamino-1, 6-L-selenocystine-oxytocin, a highly potent isolog of 1-Deamino-oxytocin. J. Amer. Chem. Soc. **88**, 1331 (1966).

ROGERS, F.T.: Studies on the brain stem. VIII. Diuresis and anhydremia following destruction of the thalamus. Amer. J. Physiol. **68**, 499—516 (1924).

RUDINGER, J., and K. JOST: A biologically active analogue of oxytocin not containing a disulfide group. Experientia (Basel) **20**, 570—571 (1964).

RUIBAL, R.: The adaptative value of bladder water in the toad *Bufo cognatus*. Physiol. Zool. **35**, 218—223 (1962).

SAFFRAN, M., A.V. SCHALLY, M. SEGAL, and B. ZIMMERMAN: Characterization of the corticotrophin releasing factor of the neurohypophysis. 2. Int. Symp. Neurosekretion, pp. 55—59. Berlin-Göttingen-Heidelberg: Springer 1958.

SAWYER, W.H.: Effect of posterior pituitary extracts on urine formation and glomerular circulation in the frog. Amer. J. Physiol. **164**, 457—466 (1951a).

— Effect of posterior pituitary extract on permeability of frog skin to water. Amer. J. Physiol. **164**, 44—48 (1951b).

— The hormonal control of water and salt metabolism with special reference to the amphibia. Mem. Soc. Endocr. **5**, 44—49 (1956).

— Increased renal absorption of osmotically free water by the toad *(Bufo marinus)* in response to neurohypophysial hormones. Amer. J. Physiol. **189**, 564—568 (1957a).

— The antidiuretic action of neurohypophysial hormones in amphibia. Colston papers, Vol. VIII. Proceedings of the Eighth Symposium of the Colston Research Society, Vol. VIII, pp. 171—179. London: Butterworths 1957b.

— Increased water permeability of the bullfrog *(Rana catesbiana)* bladder *in vitro* in response to synthetic oxytocin and Arginine vasotocin and to neurohypophysial extracts from nonmammalian vertebrates. Endocrinology **66**, 112—120 (1960a).

— Evidence for the identity of Natriferin, the frog water balance principle and Arginine vasotocin. Nature (Lond.) **187**, 1030—1031 (1960b).

— Comparative physiology and pharmacology of the neurohypophysis. Recent Progr. Hormone Res. **17**, 437—465 (1961a).

— Neurohypophysial hormones. Pharmacol. Rev. **13**, 225—277 (1961b).

— Vertebrate neurohypophysial principles. Endocrinology **75**, 981—990 (1964a).

— Phyletic distribution of neurohypophysial peptides. From "Protides of the biological fluids", pp. 135—142. Ed. by H. PEETERS. Amsterdam: Elsevier 1964b.

— Evolution of neurohypophysial principles. Arch. Anat. micr. Morph. exp. **54**, 295—312 (1965).

— Diuretic and natriuretic responses of lungfish *(Protopterus aethiopicus)* to Arginine-vasotocin. Amer. J. Physiol. **210**, 191—197 (1966).

—, R.A. MUNSICK, and H.B. VAN DYKE: Pharmacological evidence for the presence of Arginine-vasotocin and oxytocin in neurohypophysial extracts from cold blooded vertebrates. Nature (Lond.) 1464—1465 (1959).

— — — Antidiuretic hormones. Circulation. **21**, 1027—1037 (1960).

Sawyer, W. H., R. A. Munsick, and H. B. van Dyke: Evidence for the presence of Arginine-vasotocin (8-arginine-oxytocin) and oxytocin in neurohypophysial extracts from amphibians and reptiles. Gen. comp. Endocr. **1**, 30—36 (1961a).
— — — Pharmacological Characteristics of the active principles in neurohypophysial extracts from several species of fishes. Endocrinology **68**, 215—225 (1961b).
—, and G. E. Pickford: Neurohypophyseal principles of *Fundulus heteroclutus:* Characteristics and seasonal changes. Gen. comp. Endocr. **3**, 439—445 (1963).
—, and M. K. Sawyer: Adaptative responses to neurohypophyseal fractions in vertebrates. Physiol. Zool. **25**, 84—98 (1952).
—, and R. M. Schisgall: Increased permeability of the frog bladder to water in response to dehydration and neurohypophysial extracts. Amer. J. Physiol. **187**, 312—314 (1956).
Schally, A. V., and M. Saffran: Effect of histamine, hog vasopressin and corticotrophin releasing factor (CRF) on ACTH release *in vitro*. Proc. Soc. exp. Biol. (N.Y.) **92**, 636—667 (1956).
— —, and B. Zimmermann: A corticotrophin releasing factor. Partial purification and amino-acid composition. Biochem. J. **70**, 97—103 (1958).
Schiebler, T. H., u. V. H. Brehm: Über jahreszyklische und altersbedingte Veränderungen in den neurosekretorischen Systemen von Teleostiern. Naturwissenschaften **45**, 450—451 (1958).
Schmidt-Nielsen, B., and P. Lee: Kidney function in the crab-eating frog *(Rana cancrivora)*. J. exp. Biol. **39**, 167—177 (1962).
Schmidt-Nielsen, K.: The salt secreting gland of marine birds. Circulation **21**, 955—967 (1960).
—, and R. P. Forster: The effect of dehydration and low temperature on renal function in the bullfrog. J. cell. comp. Physiol. **44**, 233—246 (1954).
—, C. B. Jørgensen, and H. Osaki: Extrarenal salt excretion in birds. Amer. J. Physiol. **193**, 101—107 (1958).
Schoessler, M. A.: Metabolic effects of neurohypophysial hormones and adrenosine 3'-5' monophosphate. In: Oxytocin, vasopressin and their structural analogues, pp. 177—183. Ed. by J. Rudinger. Prague 1964.
Schreiber, B. V., et O. Schreiber: Réaction de Brunn chez les Axolotls. C.R. Soc. Biol. (Paris) **145**, 619—620 (1950).
Schreibman, M. P., and K. D. Kallman: Effects of hypophysectomy on *Xiphophorus*. Amer. Zool. **3**, 556 (1963).
Schwartz, I. L., and L. M. Livingston: Cellular and molecular aspects of the antidiuretic action of vasopressins and related peptides. Vitam. u. Horm. **22**, 261—359 (1964).
—, and H. Rasmussen: Unpublished data. In: Cellular and molecular aspects of the antidiuretic action of vasopressins and related peptides. Ed. by I. L. Schwartz and L. M. Livingston. Vitam. u. Horm. **22**, 261—359 (1964).
— —, and J. Rudinger: Activity of neurohypophysial hormone analogues lacking a disulfide bridge. Proc. nat. Acad. Sci. (Wash.) **52**, 1044—1045 (1964).
— —, M. A. Schoessler, L. Silver, and C. T. O. Fong: Relation of chemical attachment to physiological action of vasopressin. Proc. nat. Acad. Sci. (Wash.) **46**, 1288—1298 (1960).
Scothorne, R. J.: On the response of the duck and the pigeon to intravenous hypertonic saline solutions. Quart. J. exp. Physiol. **44**, 200—207 (1959).
Sexton, A. W.: Factors influencing the uptake of sodium against a concentration gradient in the goldfish gill. Thesis. Univ. Missouri (1955).
Shannon, J. A.: The excretion of uric acid by the chicken. J. cell. comp. Physiol. **11**, 135—148 (1938).
— The control of the renal excretion of water. II. The effect of variations in the state of hydration on water excretion in dogs with diabetes insipidus. J. exp. Med. **76**, 371—386 (1942).
Sharp, G. W. G., and A. Leaf: Biological action of aldosterone *in vitro*. Nature (Lond.) **202**, 1185—1188 (1964).
— — Mechanism of action of aldosterone. Physiol. Rev. **46**, 593—633 (1966).
Sharratt, B. M., I. Chester Jones, and D. Bellamy: Adaptation of the silver eel *(Anguilla anguilla)* to sea water and to artificial media together with observations on the role of the gut. Comp. Biochem. Physiol. **11**, 19—30 (1964).
Shirley, H. V., and A. V. Nalbandov: Effects of transecting hypophyseal stalks in laying hens. Endocrinology **58**, 694—700 (1956a).
— — Effects of neurohypophysectomy in domestic chickens. Endocrinology **58**, 477—483 (1956b).
Shoemaker, V. H.: The effects of dehydration on electrolyte concentrations in a toad, *Bufo marinus*. Comp. Biochem. Physiol. **13**, 261—271 (1964).
— The stimulus for the water balance response to dehydration in toads. Comp. Biochem. Physiol. **15**, 81—87 (1965).
Skadhauge, E.: Effects of unilateral infusion of arginine vasotocin into the portal circulation of the avian kidney. Acta endocr. (Kbh.) **47**, 321—330 (1964).

SMELIK, P.G., and D. DE WIED: Corticotrophin releasing action of adrenaline, serotonin and pitressin. Experientia (Basel) **14**, 17—18 (1958).
SMITH, H.W.: The absorption and excretion of water and salts by marine teleosts. Amer. J. Physiol. **93**, 480—505 (1930).
— Water regulation and its evolution in fishes. Quart. Rev. Biol. **7**, 1—26 (1932).
SOBEL, H., R.S. LEVY, J. MARMORSTON, S. SCHAPIRO, and S. ROSENFELD: Increased excretion of urinary corticoids by guinea pigs following administration of pitressin. Proc. Soc. exp. Biol. (N.Y.) **89**, 10—13 (1955).
SOKOL, H.W.: Cytological changes in the teleost pituitary gland associated with the reproductive cycle. J. Morph. **109**, 219—236 (1961).
SPERBER, I.: Excretion. In: Biology and comparative physiology of birds, pp. 469—492. Ed. by A.J. MARSHALL. New York and London: Academic Press 1960.
STEEN, W.B.: On the permeability of the frog's bladder to water. Anat. Rec. **43**, 215—220 (1929).
STEGGERDA, F.R.: The relation of Pitressin to water interchange in frogs. Amer. J. Physiol. **98**, 255—261 (1931).
— Comparative study of water metabolism in amphibians injected with pituitrin. Proc. Soc. exp. Biol. (N.Y.) **36**, 103—106 (1937).
—, and M.E. JONES: Studies on water metabolism in normal and hypophysectomized frogs. Amer. J. Physiol. **112**, 397—400 (1935).
STEWART, W.C.: Effect of mammalian (posterior lobe) pituitary extract on water balance of frogs when placed in different osmotic environments. Amer. J. Physiol. **157**, 412—417 (1949).
STRAHAN, R., and H. WARING: The effect of pituitary posterior lobe extracts on the blood pressure of the fowl. Aust. J. exp. Biol. med. Sci. **32**, 192—205 (1954).
STURKIE, P.D., and YU-CHONG LIN: Release of vasotocin and oviposition in the hen. J. Endocr. **35**, 325—326 (1966).
STUTINSKY, F.: Modalités de la neurosecretion dans le noyau préoptique de l'anguille. Bull. Soc. Zool. France **77**, 276—284 (1952).
— La neurosécrétion chez l'Anguille normale et hypophysectomisée. Z. Zellforsch. **173**, 1096 à 2008 (1953).
—, J. SCHNEIDER, et P. DENOYELLE: Dosage de l'ACTH sur le rat normal et influence de la présence des principes posthypophysaires. Ann. Endocr. (Paris) **13**, 641—650 (1952).
SUSKA-BRZEZINSKA, E., and Z. EWY: Oxytocinase in hen serum. Bull. Acad. polon. Sci. Biol. **13**, 17—21 (1965).
SUTHERLAND, E.W., and T.W. RALL: Fractionation and characterisation of a cyclic adenine ribonucleotide formed by tissue particles. J. biol. Chem. **232**, 1077—1091 (1957).
— — The relation of adenosine 3'-5' phosphate and phosphorylase to the actions of catecholamines and other hormones. Pharmacol. Rev. **12**, 265—299 (1960).
SWIFT, D.R., and G.E. PICKFORD: Seasonal variations in the hormone content of the pituitary gland of the perch (*Perca fluviatilis* L.). Gen. comp. Endocr. **5**, 354—365 (1965).
TANAKA, K., and S. NAKAJO: Oxytocin in the neurohypophysis of the laying hen. Nature (Lond.) **187**, 245 (1960).
— — Participation of neurohypophysial hormone in oviposition in the hen. Endocrinology **70**, 453—458 (1962).
TEMPLETON, J.A.: Respiration and water loss at the higher temperatures in the desert iguana *Dipsosaurus dorsalis*. Physiol. Zool. **33**, 136—145 (1960).
THORSON, T., and A. SVIHLA: Correlation of the habitats of amphibians with their ability to survive the loss of water. Ecology **24**, 374—381 (1943).
THORSON, T.B.: The relationship of water economy to terrestrialism in amphibians. Ecology **36**, 100—116 (1955).
TRAMEZZANI, J.H., y J.V. URANGA: Variaciones de la substancia Gomori positiva y activitad antidiuretica en la neurohypofisis de sapos hidratos y deshidratos. Rev. Soc. argent. Biol. **30**, 148—151 (1954).
TUURALA, O.: Über den Einfluß der osmotischen Belastung auf die Neurosekretion der Klein fische *Gasterosteus aculeatus* L. und *Phoxinus laevis*. Agass. aus dem Brackwasser des Finnischen Meerbusens. Ann. Acad. Sci. Fenn. Biol. **36**, 1—9 (1957).
USSING, H.H.: Some aspects of the application of tracers in permeability studies. Advanc. Enzymol. **13**, 21—65 (1952).
— The relation between active ion transport and bioelectric phenomena. Rio de Janeiro: Instituto de Biofisica 1955.
— The alkali metal ions in biology. I. The alkali metal ions in isolated systems and tissues, pp. 49—129. Berlin-Göttingen-Heidelberg: Springer 1960.
— Transport of electrolytes and water across epithelia. Harvey Lect. series **59** (1965).
—, T.U. BIBER, and N.S. BRICKER: Exposure of the isolated frog skin to high potassium concentrations at the internal surface. II. Changes in epithelial cell volume, resistance, and response to antidiuretic hormone. J. gen. Physiol. **48**, 425—434 (1965).

USSING, H.H., and V. KOEFOED-JOHNSEN: Nature of the frog skin potential. Abstr. Comm. 20th Int Physiol. Congr., p. 511. Brussels 1956.
—, and E.E. WINDHAGER: Active sodium transport at the cellular level. In: Water and electrolyte metabolism, part II. Ed. by J. DE GRAEFF and B. LEIJNSE. Amsterdam: Elsevier Publ. Co. 1964a.
— — Nature of shunt path and active sodium transport path through frog skin epithelium. Acta physiol. scand. **61**, 484—504 (1964b).
—, and K. ZERAHN: Active transport of sodium as the source of electric current in the short circuited isolated frog skin. Acta physiol. scand. **23**, 110—127 (1951).
URANGA, J.: Absorcion de Agua por la piel del sapo. Rev. Soc. argent. Biol. **34**, 233—238 (1958).
— Action de l'ocytocine et de la température sur le filtrat glomérulaire du crapaud. C.R. Soc. Biol. (Paris) **155**, 173—174 (1961).
—, y G. QINTANA: Absorcion de aqua en la vejiga del sapo. Rev. Soc. argent. Biol. **34**, 75—81 (1958).
—, and W.H. SAWYER: Renal responses of the bullfrog to oxytocin, Arginine vasotocin and frog neurohypophysial extract. Amer. J. Physiol. **198**, 1887—1890 (1960).
VERNEY, E.B.: The antidiuretic hormone and the factors which determine its release. Proc. roy. Soc. (Lond.) **135**, 25—106 (1947).
VIVIEN, J.H., et J. SCHOTT: Activité gonadotrope des autogreffes antéhypophysaires chez *Rana temporaria* L. C.R. Acad. Sci. (Paris) **244**, 1263—1265 (1957).
VOGEL, G.: Weitere Daten zur Physiologie der Harnbereitung beim Truthuhn *(Meleagris pavo)*, Konzentrierungsvermögen und Mechanismus. Pflügers Arch. ges. Physiol. **279**, R. 29 (1964).
—, u. I. STOECKERT: Vergleichende stop-flow-Untersuchungen an Nieren mit geringem und ausgeprägtem Konzentrierungsvermögen und wenig und gut ausgebildetem System Henlescher Schleifen-Versuche am Truthuhn (*Meleagris pavo* L.) und an der weißen Ratte *(Rattus rattus)*. Pflügers Arch. ges. Physiol. **283**, 160—170 (1965).
WALKER, A.M., C.L. HUDSON, T.J. FINDLEY, and A.N. RICHARDS: The total molecular concentration and the chloride concentration of fluid from different segments of the renal tubule of amphibia. The site of chloride reabsorption. Amer. J. Physiol. **118**, 121—129 (1937).
WARING, H., L. MORRIS, and G. STEPHENS: The effect of pituitary posterior lobe extracts on the blood pressure of the pigeon. Aust. J. exp. Biol. med. Sci. **34**, 235—238 (1956).
WHITE, H.L.: Observations on the nature of glomerular activity. Amer. J. Physiol. **90**, 689 to 704 (1929).
WHITTEMBURY, G.: Action of antidiuretic hormone on the equivalent pore radius at both surfaces of the epithelium of the isolated frog skin. J. gen. Physiol. **46**, 117—130 (1962).
—, and F.C. HERRERA: Electrical potential profile on the toad skin epithelium. J. gen. Physiol. **47**, 795—808 (1964).
—, N. SUGINO, and A.K. SOLOMON: Effect of antidiuretic hormone and calcium on the equivalent pore radius of kidney slices from Necturus. Nature (Lond.) **20**, 700—701 (1960).
WIKGREN, J.B.: Osmotic regulation on some aquatic animals with special reference to the influence of temperature. Acta Zool. fennica **71**, 1—102 (1953).
WILHELMI, A.E., G.E. PICKFORD, and W.H. SAWYER: Initiation of the spawning reflex response in *Fundulus* by the administration of fish and mammalian neurohypophysial preparations and synthetic oxytocin. Endocrinology **57**, 243—252 (1955).
WINGSTRAND, K.G.: The structure and development of the avian pituitary from a comparative and functional viewpoint. Lund: G.W.K. Gleerup 1951.
— The structure of the pituitary in the African lungfish, *Protopterus annecteus* (Owen). Vidensk. Medd. dansk naturhist. Foren **118**, 193—210 (1956).
— Attempts at a comparison between the neurohypophysial region in fishes and tetrapods with particular regard to amphibians. In: Comparative endocrinology, p. 393. Ed. by A. GORBMAN. New York: J. Wiley 1959.
WIRZ, H.: Der osmotische Druck in den corticalen Tubuli der Rattenniere. Helv. physiol. pharmacol. Acta **14**, 353—362 (1956).
— The location of antidiuretic action in the mammalian kidney. In: The neurohypophysis, pp. 157—159. Ed. by H. HELLER. London: Butterworths 1957.
—, B. HARGITAY u. W. KUHN: Lokalisation des Konzentrierungsprozesses in der Niere durch direkte Kryoskopie. Helv. physiol. pharmacol. Acta **9**, 196—207 (1951).
WOOLEY, P.: The effect of posterior lobe pituitary extracts on blood pressure in several vertebrate classes. J. exp. Biol. **36**, 453—458 (1959).
—, and H. WARING: Responses of the perfused fowl leg to posterior lobe pituitary extracts. Aust. J. exp. Biol. med. Sci. **36**, 447—456 (1959).
YASUDA, M.: The functional relationship between the diencephalon and the reproductive organs in the fowl. Jap. J. Zootech. Sci. **28**, 69—75 (1957).
ZERAHN, K.: Oxygen consumption and active sodium transport in the isolated and short circuited frog skin. Acta physiol. scand. **36**, 300—318 (1956).

Phylogenetic Aspects of the Neurohypophysial Hormones

WILBUR H. SAWYER

I. Introduction

A. General

The classic studies of DU VIGNEAUD and his collaborators led to the elucidation of the molecular structures of oxytocin, arginine-vasopressin and lysine-vasopressin in the early 1950's (summarized by DU VIGNEAUD, 1956a). Synthesis of peptides with biological properties identical with those of the natural hormones

Table 1. *Neurohypophysial principles found among the vertebrates*[1]

Vasopressor principles:

1. Cys · Tyr · Phe · Glu (NH_2) · Asp (NH_2) · Cys · Pro · Arg · Gly (NH_2)
   1 2 3 4 5 6 7 8 9
   arginine-vasopressin
2. Cys —— Phe —— Cys —— Lys ——
   lysine-vasopressin
3. Cys —— Ileu —— Cys —— Arg ——
   arginine-vasotocin

Oxytocin-like principles:

4. Cys —— Ileu —— Cys —— Leu ——
   oxytocin
5. Cys —— Ileu · Ser —— Cys —— Ileu ——
   4-serine, 8-isoleucine-oxytocin ("isotocin")
6. Cys —— Ileu —— Cys —— Ileu ——
   8-isoleucine-oxytocin ("mesotocin")
7. Cys —— Ileu · Ser —— Cys —— Glu (NH_2) ——
   4-serine, 8-glutamine-oxytocin ("glumitocin")
8. elasmobranch principle I
9. elasmobranch principle II

[1] The complete amino acid sequence of arginine-vasopressin is shown. Only those amino acids by which the other known principles differ are shown. These are in the 3, 4 and 8 positions

provided conclusive proof of their structures. This chemical identification of active peptides from cattle and swine provided the essential background for exploration of active neurohypophysial principles found among other vertebrates. The search has been rewarding. At least nine natural principles have now been tentatively characterized (Table 1). The structures of seven are known, and much information has accumulated concerning their phyletic distribution. Some recent reviews dealing with this subject are SAWYER (1961a, 1964, 1965a, b); HELLER (1963a, b); ACHER (1963), ACHER et al. (1965a); VLIEGENTHART and VERSTEEG (1965).

B. Early History

A vasopressor substance in the mammalian pituitary was first reported by OLIVER and SCHÄFER in 1895. Oxytocic, milk-ejecting, avian vasodepressor, and antidiuretic properties of pituitary extracts were described in the next two decades. HERRING (1908, 1913) examined pituitary extracts from a variety of nonmammalian vertebrates. Most of these contained at least some of the pharmacological properties of mammalian extracts. More detailed characterization of natural neurohypophysial principles in nonmammalian vertebrates only became possible after many years of experience had provided more information on the properties of the active principles in the mammalian pituitary.

HELLER (1941) was the first to demonstrate clearly that there were significant differences in the biological properties of pituitary extracts from different species. He found that extracts from birds, reptiles, amphibians and teleost fishes were much more active in causing increased water uptake by frogs than were mammalian extracts containing equivalent amounts of oxytocic and antidiuretic activities. Thus the "frog water balance" activity could not be due to oxytocin or vasopressin. HELLER suggested that there was a distinct "water balance principle" present in most vertebrates other than mammals. SAWYER (1957a, b) later reported that frog and toad pituitaries contained much more antidiuretic activity, when tested in frogs and toads, and much more activity in causing water reabsorption from the frog bladder (SAWYER and SCHISGALL, 1956) than they would if they contained only oxytocin and vasopressin. This was consistent with the presence of a peptide or peptides with activities differing from those of the mammalian principles. MAETZ et al. (1959) also found that pituitary extracts from amphibians and teleost fishes contained a principle ("natriferin") with high relative potency in causing increased sodium transport by frog skin. When arginine-vasotocin had been proposed as a possible natural principle in pituitaries from nonmammalian vertebrates (SAWYER et al., 1959) it was found to have properties quite similar to those of the natural "water balance principle" of frog pituitary extracts (SAWYER, 1960a, b; URANGA and SAWYER, 1960). The resemblance of the biological properties of nonmammalian pituitary extracts, as first reported by HELLER in 1941, to the properties of an analogue of oxytocin synthesized by KATSOYANNIS and DU VIGNEAUD in 1958 therefore provided the first major clue to the identity of an active nonmammalian neurohypophysial peptide.

II. Methods

A. Pharmacological Methods

Only detailed chemical analysis confirmed by synthesis can establish the molecular structure of a neurohypophysial peptide beyond doubt (DU VIGNEAUD, 1956a). Pharmacological methods are essential, however, in the investigation of naturally occurring principles. Biological activities are used for the initial localization of peptides and as guides to their chemical isolation. Once a structure has been proposed it must be proved by establishing pharmacological identity of synthetic and natural peptides.

Pharmacological methods are also extremely valuable in comparative studies. They have been repeatedly used to indicate where unknown active principles exist. Biological assays are infinitely more sensitive than currently practical methods for amino acid analysis, and can be applied to crude or partially purified extracts. Such methods are thus less demanding of both time and material. This makes them particularly useful in comparative studies involving a variety of species, and in investigations on small, rare or exotic species from which it would be impractical to isolate enough material for definitive chemical studies.

Although pharmacological methods are sensitive and convenient they may also be misleading. They can discriminate between peptides with widely differing biological properties, such as oxytocin and vasopressin, or the frog water balance principle and the mammalian hormones. Arginine-vasotocin was the first non-mammalian principle identified because it has a highly characteristic pharmacological activity "profile" (MUNSICK et al., 1960). Unfortunately the differences between the biological properties of oxytocin and many of its neutral analogues are less obvious. Progress toward identification of natural principles resembling oxytocin has, therefore, been slow.

One of the more widely used pharmacological methods for characterizing neutral oxytocin-like principles has been determination of the effects of magnesium ion on the responses of the isolated rat uterus (MUNSICK, 1960). Sensitivity of rat uteri to most oxytocin analogues is enhanced when 0.5 mM Mg^{++} is present in the bathing solution. Sensitivity to oxytocin changes less. Thus the activity of an analogue in the presence of Mg^{++} (RU_{Mg}) determined by assays against an oxytocincontaining standard appears greater than its activity in the absence of Mg^{++} (RU). RU_{Mg}/RU ratios have been used in characterizing many nonmammalian principles (MUNSICK et al., 1960; HELLER et al., 1961; HELLER and ROY, 1965a, b; CHAUVET et al., 1965; SAWYER, 1965a, d; MUNSICK. 1966).

The meaning of an RU_{Mg}/RU ratio is clear if it differs significantly from 1.0. This indicates that the oxytocic activity of a preparation cannot be due to oxytocin alone (HELLER et al., 1961). The varying degrees of variation of ratios from 1.0 are more difficult to interpret. Nevertheless the magnitude of such ratios has provided important information contributing to the identification of previously unrecognized natural principles (HELLER et al., 1961; FOLLETT and HELLER, 1964b; HELLER and ROY 1965a).

The endocrine status of the rats from which uteri are taken for use in assays may influence the RU_{Mg}/RU ratio of some analogues. MUNSICK and JERONIMUS (1965) found that the RU_{Mg}/RU ratio for arginine-vasotocin increases from 1.23 ± 0.04 when estimated on uteri from metestrous rats to 1.98 ± 0.06 when uteri came from rats injected with 10 μg of diethylstilbestrol 14—16 hours earlier. These authors properly point out that this "should serve as a warning to those employing this ratio for pharmacological identification of unknown peptides." They also suggest that the ratio "may also depend upon the strain of rat, the ionic milieu other than magnesium, and other variables which are not as yet known."

The validity of MUNSICK and JERONIMUS (1965) warning has been further documented by recent experiences in the author's laboratory. We have long used RU_{Mg}/RU ratios as a rapid means for distinguishing between oxytocin and mesotocin (isoleucine^8-oxytocin). We originally found that this ratio for mesotocin was relatively consistent and varied between 1.2 and 1.3. FOLLETT and HELLER (1964b) and MUNSICK (1966) also report this ratio as 1.3. Recently, however, we have obtained ratios averaging 1.02 ± 0.03. These were based on assays performed on uteri from rats pretreated with diethylstilbestrol. Ratios determined from assays on uteri from rats of the same group but in natural estrus averaged 1.23 ± 0.05. Diethylstilbestrol treatment appears to have abolished the difference between the effect of magnesium ion on responses to oxytocin and mesotocin. However, both

FOLLETT and HELLER (1964b) and MUNSICK (1966) used rats pretreated with diethylstilbestrol and obtained ratios significantly different from 1.0. This implies strain differences in rats that influence their responses to diethylstilbestrol and underline the risks involved in reliance on this particular pharmacological test.

As predicted by MUNSICK and JERONIMUS (1965) factors other than state of estrus can certainly influence RU_{Mg}/RU ratios. We have found this ratio for arginine-vasotocin to be as low as 1.6 ± 0.07 and as high as 3.2 ± 0.2 on different occasions. These variations do not depend only on the stage of estrus since they occurred among rats pretreated with diethylstilbestrol as well as in rats in natural estrus.

The exact magnitude of the RU_{Mg}/RU ratio is not, therefore, a consistent characteristic of uterine responses to specific neurohypophysial peptides. Fortunately, however, the ratios do tend to remain relatively stable over short periods of time when uteri are obtained from a homogeneous population of rats. Comparisons of activity ratios of natural principles to those of synthetic analogues are thus only reliable when the ratios have been determined repeatedly and as nearly simultaneously as possible, preferably on the same uteri.

Activity ratios other than RU_{Mg}/RU may also appear capricious at times. Fowl vasodepressor activity of the same solution of synthetic mesotocin, for example, has been found to vary rather widely when estimated from assays on different chickens. This again emphasizes that comparing activity ratios of unknowns to known peptides may be misleading unless these are based on assays performed on the same fowl or fowls.

B. Chromatographic and Chemical Methods for Separating Active Principles

Chromatographic methods have been useful for separating natural principles prior to pharmacological and chemical studies. Preliminary purification by molecular sieving on Sephadex G-25 columns can be very helpful in comparative studies (RASMUSSEN and GRAIG, 1961; SAWYER and VAN DYKE, 1963b). Basic peptides, such as the vasopressins and arginine-vasotocin, have characteristic mobilities on some paper and thin-layer chromatographic systems that make their separation from other active principles in natural extracts relatively easy (HELLER and LEDERIS, 1958; PICKERING and HELLER, 1959; FERGUSON, 1965). Column chromatography on ion exchange substrates is also convenient for separating basic principles from neurohypophysial extracts. Amberlite IRC-50 (XE-64) (TAYLOR, 1954), carboxymethylcellulose (CMC) (WARD and GUILLEMIN, 1957) and CM-Sephadex (PERKS and SAWYER, 1965) have been successfully used for this purpose. Ion exchange columns cannot, however, resolve mixtures of neutral principles resembling oxytocin which are only weakly adsorbed. Countercurrent distribution can effectively separate such neutral peptides but is impractical when starting material is limited in quantity. Column partition chromatography on Sephadex has recently been shown to separate closely related synthetic neutral analogues of oxytocin (YAMASHIRO, 1964; YAMASHIRO et al., 1966). This technique is useful for the separation and characterization, on a small scale, of naturally occurring principles resembling oxytocin (SAWYER, unpublished).

ACHER, LIGHT, and DU VIGNEAUD (1958) isolated the van Dyke protein as a first step in the purification of oxytocin and vasopressin. The van Dyke protein (VAN DYKE et al., 1941) can be precipitated from acid extracts of mammalian neurohypophyses with 10% NaCl. The precipitate can be washed, and then dissolved by dialyzing away the NaCl. The van Dyke protein can then be dissociated with trichloracetic acid which precipitates the protein moiety, "neurophysin," leaving the peptides in solution (ACHER et al., 1956). This method has been used successfully to provide preparations of mammalian oxytocin and vasopressin free from much of the nonspecific peptide present in the original extract (ACHER, LIGHT, and DU VIGNEAUD, 1958). This method is applicable to small quantities, and thus useful in comparative studies.

There are problems, however, in applying protein precipitation to the isolation of active neurohypophysial principles from nonmammalian vertebrates since their peptide-protein complexes do not appear to precipitate as readily. HELLER and PICKERING (1961) found that the NaCl concentration had to be raised to 25% before there was adequate precipitation of protein-peptide complex from pollack pituitary extract. SAWYER and VAN DYKE (1963b) abandoned NaCl precipitation as a useful step toward purification of pollack pituitary principles since the supernatant after trichloracetic acid treatment contained a high concentration of nonspecific peptide. ACHER et al. (1961) obtained precipitation of the active neurohypophysial peptides of several fishes at lower NaCl concentrations by adding mammalian neurophysin to the acid extract. This procedure entails an element of danger, however, in that it may introduce traces of the mammalian peptides which could interfere with subsequent analysis (MUNSICK, 1964, 1966).

III. Phyletic Distribution of Active Principles

A. Introduction

A logically constructed discussion of the distribution of neurohypophysial principles among the vertebrates should start with the most primitive species and attempt to follow phylogenetic lines toward the most specialized. This cannot be done effectively at this time. Most of the solid information available on the identities of active principles comes from highly evolved forms, mammals, birds, amphibians, and the teleost fishes. Knowledge of principles in less advanced vertebrates is meager, and identifications are largely tentative. It is therefore planned to outline the subject in more or less the manner in which it has been investigated, starting with mammals and then progressing to other vertebrate groups. After the available information on phyletic distribution has been presented it can then be related to vertebrate evolution in a more appropriately oriented fashion.

B. The Mammalian Principles

1. Vasopressins

Oxytocin isolated from both beef and hog pituitaries by DU VIGNEAUD and his co-workers appeared to be exactly the same. When they undertook to isolate and characterize vasopressin, however, they found that there was a clear difference between peptides from these species (see DU VIGNEAUD, 1956b). Partial hydrolysis indicated that bovine vasopressin contained arginine in the eighth position while porcine vasopressin contained lysine in this position (Table 1).

When highly purified samples of arginine and lysine-vasopressins were made available, VAN DYKE et al. (1956) demonstrated a clear pharmacological difference. Lysine-vasopressin had about $^1/_6$ of the antidiuretic activity, when assayed in dogs, of an equal vasopressor dose of arginine-vasopressin. This difference was exploited as a means of distinguishing the probable identity of vasopressins in crude pituitary extracts from several species of mammals. This general procedure, the measurement of activity ratios, has since become a primary tool for the investigation of naturally occurring vasopressins. It has the great advantage of requiring little material and, in many instances, of being informative when applied to crude pituitary extracts.

Other characteristics can distinguish between the two known mammalian vasopressins. They have slightly different mobilities on some paper (HELLER and LEDERIS, 1958) or thin-layer (FERGUSON, 1965) chromatographic systems. They differ in relative biological activities other than dog antidiuresis. Determination of other activity ratios can be used for their tentative identification. Arginine-vasopressin has much more activity on the isolated hen oviduct than does an amount of lysine-vasopressin with equal vasopressor activity (MUNSICK et al., 1960). The

Table 2. *Mammalian neurohypophysial principles*

Species investigated	Systems used for separation[1]	Evidence for identity of[2]: Arg VP	Lys VP	Oxy	Ref.
Prototheria: O. Monotremata:					
Spiny anteater (*Tachyglossus aculeatus*)	none	HO/VP	—	RU/VP	1
Theria: O. Marsupalia:					
Virginia opossum (*Didelphis virginiana*)	none	HO/VP	—	RU/VP	1
Australian opossum (*Trichosurus vulpecula*)	PC, CMC, AG	NF/VP	—	R_F	2
Wallaby (*Setonyx brachyuris*)	PC, TLC	NF/VP	—	R_F	2
Kangaroo (*Macropus rufus*)	PC, TLC	NF/VP	—	R_F	2
Eutheria:					
O. Insectivora:					
Hedgehog (*Erinaceus europaeus*)	TLC	NF/VP	—	R_F	2
O. Chiroptera:					
Fruit bat (*Eidolon helvum*)	TLC	NF/VP	—	R_F	2
O. Edentata:					
Armadillo (*Priodontes gigas*)	TLC	R_F	—	R_F	2
Armadillo (*Dasypus novemcintus*)	TLC	R_F	—	R_F	2
O. Primates:					
Monkey (*Macaca mulatta*)	none	DAD/VP	—	ME/VP	3
Monkey (species ?)	CMC, CCD	*Analysis*	—	R_F	4
Man	none	DAD/VP	—	ME/VP	3
Man	IRC, PE, PC	*Analysis*	—	*Analysis*	5
O. Cetacea:					
Finback whale (*Balaenoptera physalus*)	IRC, PE	*Analysis*	—	*Analysis*	6
Balaenoptera physalus	IRC, PC	*Analysis*	—	*Analysis*	7
O. Carnivora:					
Domestic dog	none	DAD/VP	—	ME/VP	3
Domestic cat	none	DAD/VP	—	ME/VP	3
Badger (*Meles meles*)	TLC	NF/VP	—	R_F	2
O. Rodentia:					
White rat	none	DAD/VP	—	ME/VP	3
Kangaroo rat (*Dipodomys merriami*)	none	DAD/VP	—	ME/VP	9
Gerbil (*Meriones unguiculatus*)	none	DAD/VP	—	ME/VP	9
Guinea pig	none	DAD/VP	—	ME/VP	9
O. Lagomorpha:					
Domestic rabbit	none	DAD/VP	—	ME/VP	9
O. Hyracoidea:					
Hyrax (*Procavia capensis*)	TLC	NF/VP	—	R_F	2
O. Proboscidae:					
Indian elephant (*Elephas elephas*)	TLC	R_F	—	R_F	2
African elephant (*Loxodontia afric.*)	TLC	NF/VP	—	R_F	2

Continuation Table 2

Species investigated	Systems used for separation[1]	Evidence for identity of[2]: Arg VP	Lys VP	Oxy	Ref.
O. Perissodactyla:					
Domestic horse	IRC, PE	*Analysis*	—	*Analysis*	10
Zebra *(Equus burchelli)*	PC, FLC	NF/VP	—	R_F	2
Tapir *(Tapirus terrestris)*	TLC	NF/VP	—	R_F	2
Rhinoceros *(Diceros bicornis)*	TLC	NF/VP	—	R_F	2
O. Artiodactyla:					
S. O. Suina:					
F. Suidae:					
Domestic pig *(Sus)*	CCD	—	*Analysis*	*Analysis*	11
Wild boar *(Sus scrofa)*	(1) PC, AG	DAD/VP	DAD/VP	R_F	2
	(4) PC, AG	—	NF/VP	R_F	2
Warthog *(Phacochoerus aethiop.)*	(1) PC	NF/VP	NF/VP	R_F	2
	(4) PC, CMC, AG	—	NF/VP	R_F	2
Bushpig *(Potamochoerus porcus)*	(1) TLC	—	NF/VP	R_F	2
Giant forest hog	(1) TLC	NF/VP	NF/VP	R_F	2
(Hylochoerus meinertzhageni)	(1) TLC	—	NF/VP	R_F	2
F. Dicotylidae:					
Collared peccary	none	DAD/VP	—	RU/VP	12
(Tayassu angulatus)	PC	R_F	NF/VP	R_F	2
White lipped peccary	(1) PC	DAD/VP	DAD/VP	R_F	2
(Tayassu pecari)	(1) TLC, CMC	NF/VP	—	R_F	2
F. Hippopotomidae:					
Hippopotamus	PC	—	DAD/VP	R_F	13
(Hippopotamus amphibius)	PC	—	NF/VP	R_F	2
S. O. Tylopoda:					
Camel	none	DAD/VP	—	ME/VP	8
Llama *(Lama glama)*	PC	NF/VP	—	R_F	2
S. O. Ruminantia:					
Domestic cattle	CCD	*Analysis*	—	*Analysis*	11
Domestic sheep	IRC, PE	*Analysis*	—	*Analysis*	14
African buffalo *(Syncerus caffer)*	TLC	NF/VP	—	R_F	2
Kongoni *(Alcephalus cokei)*	PC, TLC	NF/VP	—	R_F	2
Topi *(Damaliscus korrigum)*	PC	NF/VP	—	R_F	2
Bushbuck *(Tragelaphus scriptus)*	TLC	NF/VP	—	R_F	2
Kob *(Kobus kob)*	TLC	NF/VP	—	R_F	2

References: 1. Sawyer et al. (1960); 2. Ferguson and Heller (1965); 3. van Dyke et al. (1956); 4. Ward et al. (1962); 5. Light and du Vigneaud (1958); 6. Chauvet, Chauvet, and Acher (1963); 7. Vliegenthart (1964); 8. Adamsons et al. (1956); 9. van Dyke, Engel, and Adamsons (unpublished data); 10. Acher, Chauvet, and Lenci (1958a); 11. See du Vigneaud (1956a, b); 12. Sawyer (1961); 13. Heller and Lederis (1960); 14. Acher, Chauvet, and Lenci (1959).

[1] Primary methods used to separate active principles. Abbreviations used are: AG = agar gel electrophoresis; CCD = countercurrent distribution; CMC = column chromatography on CMC or CM-Sephadex; IRC = column chromatography on IRC-50 or equivalent resin; PC = paper chromatography; PE = paper electrophoresis; TLC = thin layer chromatography.

[2] Most important pharmacological or chemical information on which to base identification of the active peptides. Abbreviations used are:
Analysis = amino acid analysis with or without partial degradation studies.
R_F = activity with appropriate chromatographic mobility.
Activity ratios shown include these assays: ADH = rat antidiuresis; DAD = dog antidiuresis; FB = frog bladder in vitro; FD = fowl vasodepressor; GM = guinea pig milk-ejection; HO = hen oviduct in vitro; ME = rabbit milk-ejection; NF = natriferic, frog skin or toad bladder in vitro; RU = rat uterus in vitro, no Mg^{++} in bath; RU_{Mg} = rat uterus in vitro, 0.5 mM Mg^{++} in bath; VP = rat vasopressor; WB = frog water balance.

hen oviduct/vasopressor ratio can thus be exploited as a method for identifying vasopressins (SAWYER et al., 1960). Arginine-vasopressin also has higher relative natriferic activity when assayed on the toad bladder in vitro. Determination of toad bladder natriferic/vasopressor ratios has been effectively applied by FERGUSON and HELLER (1965) in their extensive survey of the vasopressins found among mammals.

A large number of mammalian species has been examined with respect to the vasopressin content of their pituitaries (Table 2). There is conclusive chemical evidence that arginine-vasopressin is the predominant vasopressor principle in man, monkey, whale, horse, sheep and cow. Chromatographic or pharmacological evidence, or both, indicates that arginine vasopressin is present in all mammals with the possible exception of some members of the family Suidae and the hippopotamus (FERGUSON and HELLER, 1965).

The members of the suborder Suina, which includes pigs, peccaries, and the hippopotamus, appear unusual in that some members, at least, of each species investigated, secrete lysine-vasopressin. FERGUSON and HELLER (1965) have carefully investigated individual pituitaries from several suiform species. They find that many posses both vasopressins (Table 2). Only the domestic hog, the bushpig and the hippopotamus appear to lack arginine vasopressin. There is individual variation among members of the other species. Some may possess only lysine-vasopressin, only arginine-vasopressin, or a mixture of both. Of five warthogs studied, for example, one appeared to have both vasopressins, the other four seemed to have lysine-vasopressin alone. Five wild boars showed the same pattern of vasopressin distribution. One pituitary from the white lipped peccary contained only arginine-vasopressin, while another contained both vasopressins. This type of distribution strongly suggests that the presence of arginine and lysine-vasopressins in a single species is genetically determined, and that the gene for neither vasopressin is dominant. This is an extremely interesting example of genetic determination of peptide structure and should be further investigated by studies on a larger sampling of individual pituitaries from one of these species.

2. *Oxytocin*

Oxytocin was first identified in beef and hog neurohypophysial preparations (DU VIGNEAUD, 1956a) and has since been chemically identified in man, whale, horse and sheep. It is generally assumed that it is present in all other mammals (SAWYER, 1965b). This assumption, however, is based on weak evidence. The presence of milk-ejection (VAN DYKE et al., 1956) or rat uterus (SAWYER et al., 1960) activity in excess of that possibly due to vasopressin (a high oxytocic to vasopressor activity ratio) merely indicates that there is a principle with oxytocic and milk-ejecting activity present in addition to vasopressin, nothing more. The presence of rat uterus activity with chromatographic mobility similar to that of oxytocin adds little towards identification (FERGUSON and HELLER, 1965). There are a great number of synthetic and natural peptides related to oxytocin that have similar mobilities on many chromatographic systems. The methods applied in most studies of mammalian pituitary extracts would probably fail to distinguish between oxytocin and mesotocin (isoleucine^{8}-oxytocin) or isotocin (serine^{4}-isoleucine^{8}-oxytocin). Since both of these analogues are known to occur as natural principles among other vertebrates it is dangerous to assume that an oxytocic principle, with chromatographic properties similar to those of oxytocin, is oxytocin. Chromatographic and pharmacological tests that can discriminate among neutral oxytocin analogues should be applied to some of these species in which the identity of the oxytocin-like peptide remains questionable.

C. Avian Principles

1. Vasopressor Principles

Studies on chicken pituitaries provided the first clear evidence for the identity of an active neurohypophysial principle differing from those found in mammals. MUNSICK et al. (1960) observed that chicken pituitary extracts were very active in causing contraction of the hen oviduct in vitro and in vivo. The hen oviduct/rat vasopressor activity ratio was much higher than that for either mammalian vasopressin. Arginine-vasopressin was the most active previously known natural principle when assayed on the hen oviduct. Oxytocin was about one tenth as active and lysine-vasopressin was even weaker. Oxypressin (phenylalanine^3-oxytocin) had undetectable activity. These observations suggested that both the isoleucine^3 of oxytocin and the arginine^8 of arginine vasopressin contributed to the hen oviduct activity of these peptides.

MUNSICK et al. (1960) were very fortunate in receiving a timely gift of synthetic arginine-vasotocin (arginine^8-oxytocin) from KATSOYANNIS and DU VIGNEAUD. This analogue had the ring structure of oxytocin and the side-chain of arginine-vasopressin (Table 1). It had been shown to have strong rat vasopressor and fowl vasodepressor activities, properties in common with both oxytocin and arginine-vasopressin (KATSOYANNIS and DU VIGNEAUD, 1958). When arginine-vasotocin was tested by the fowl oviduct assay it was about six times as active as an equal vasopressor dose of arginine-vasopressin. In fact, its hen oviduct/rat vasopressor activity ratio was exactly that found for chicken pituitary extracts (SAWYER et al., 1959; MUNSICK et al., 1960). Other assays were devised and applied to test further this pharmacological resemblance. Relative activities on turtle oviduct *in vitro*, chicken antidiuretic, isolated frog bladder, frog water-balance and dog and rat antidiuretic assays were essentially identical for both chicken extract and arginine-vasotocin.

The pharmacological profiles of chicken extract and arginine-vasotocin did not match perfectly, however. Chicken extract contained relatively greater rat uterus, fowl vasodepressor and rabbit milk-ejection activities than did arginine-vasotocin. This suggested that a principle resembling oxytocin was also present. MUNSICK et al. (1960) separated two active principles by paper chromatography of crude chicken neurohypophysial extracts. One contained the vasopressor activity and had an R_F similar to that of synthetic arginine-vasotocin. The other resembled oxytocin. PICKERING and HELLER (1959) had similarly separated a vasopressor-antidiuretic principle with high water-balance activity and an oxytocin-like principle from chicken pituitary extracts. It therefore seemed highly probable that the chicken neurohypophysis contained arginine-vasotocin and either oxytocin or a closely similar peptide (MUNSICK et al., 1960; HELLER and PICKERING, 1961). HELLER (1941) had found water-balance activity in pituitaries from many non-mammalian vertebrates. This suggested that if arginine-vasotocin was the frog water-balance principle it might be widely distributed. Pituitary extracts from representative vertebrate species were subjected to pharmacological analyses similar to that applied to chicken extracts. Activities characteristic of arginine vasotocin were found in species from all major nonmammalian groups except the elasmobranchs (SAWYER et al., 1959; SAWYER, 1961a; HELLER and PICKERING, 1961).

The tentative pharmacological identification of arginine-vasotocin as the naturally occurring water-balance principle was soon confirmed. Peptides with biological activities similar to those of arginine-vasotocin were isolated from pollack (HELLER and PICKERING, 1960) and chicken (CHAUVET et al., 1960) pituitaries.

Acid hydrolysis yielded the expected amino acids in both instances. Thus the first uniquely nonmammalian neurohypophysial principle had been identified. It had, however, been synthesized several years earlier by KATSOYANNIS and DU VIGNEAUD (1958) as part of their program relating specific molecular structures to the biological activities of neurohypophysial peptides.

CHAUVET et al. (1960) identified arginine-vasopressin as well as arginine-vasotocin in their chicken pituitary extracts. Other workers, however, have repeatedly failed to find any sign of vasopressin in avian neurohypophysial extracts (MUNSICK et al., 1960; HELLER and PICKERING, 1961; MUNSICK, 1964). Since CHAUVET et al. (1960) added equine neurophysin to their chicken pituitary extracts to facilitate

Table 3. *Avian neurohypophysial principles*

Species	Systems used[1] for separation	Evidence for identity of[1]: Arginine Vasopressin	Arginine vasotocin	Oxytocin	Ref.
O. Anseriformes:					
Duck	none	—	FB/RU	RU/ADH	1
(Anas platyrhyncos platyrhyncos)	PE	—	FB/RU	RU/VP	2
O. Galliformes:					
Domestic fowl	PC	—	FB/VP	RU/VP	3
Domestic fowl	PC	—	WB/RU	RU/VP	4
Domestic fowl	IRC	*Analysis*	*Analysis*	*Analysis*	5, 6
Domestic fowl	CMC	—	HO/VP	RU/VP	7
Domestic turkey	CMC	—	HO/VP	RU/VP	7
O. Columbiformes:					
Domestic pigeon	PC	—	VP/RU	RU/VP	4
Domestic pigeon	none	—	FB/RU	—	8
O. Psittaciformes:					
Parakeet *(Malopsittacus undulatus)*	none	—	FB/RU	—	1
O. Passeriformes:					
Zosterops pulpebrosa japonica . . .	none	—	FB/RU	—	8
White-crowned sparrow . . . . . *(Zonotrichia leucophrys gambelii)*	none	—	FB/RU	RU/VP	9

[1] Same abbreviations as in Table 2.

References: 1. HIRANO (1964); 2. HIRANO (1966); 3. MUNSICK et al. (1960); 4. HELLER and PICKERING (1961); 5. ACHER et al. (1960a); 6. CHAUVET et al. (1960); 7. MUNSICK (1964); 8. ISHII et al. (1962); 9. SAWYER and FARNER (unpublished data).

precipitation of the peptides it is possible that arginine-vasopressin could have been present as a contaminant in the preparation of neurophysin used. One cannot, however, dismiss the possibility that arginine-vasopressin is a natural principle in the pituitaries of some strains of chickens. ACHER et al. (1965a), however, now appear to agree that arginine-vasopressin only occurs in mammals despite the earlier report from this group that this peptide can be isolated from chicken pituitaries.

Chemical evidence for the presence of arginine-vasotocin in birds has only been obtained in the domestic fowl. Pharmacological evidence indicates a rather wide phyletic distribution among birds, although relatively few species have been examined (Table 3).

2. *Oxytocin*

Oxytocin was isolated from the neurohypophysis of domestic fowls and was shown to contain the appropriate amino acids (ACHER et al., 1960). The other birds that have been studied also appear to have a principle resembling oxytocin. This oxytocin-like principle from chickens (MUNSICK et al., 1960; HELLER and PICKERING, 1961), and pigeons (HELLER and PICKERING, 1961) has an R_F on paper chromatograms similar to that of oxytocin. In chicken and turkey extracts it appears to behave like oxytocin on CMC columns (MUNSICK, 1964). These criteria, however, are inadequate to distinguish oxytocin from many of its neutral analogues, as discussed above. The presence in birds of mesotocin (isoleucine^8-oxytocin), or other similar peptides, cannot be ruled out.

D. Reptilian Principles

1. Arginine-Vasotocin

Arginine-vasotocin has not been isolated and chemically identified from the neurohypophysis of any reptile. There is chromatographic and pharmacological evidence indicating its presence in all the species that have been examined (Table 4).

2. Oxytocin-like Principles

Oxytocic activity beyond that due to arginine-vasotocin is present in all reptilian pituitary extracts studied except one from the caiman (Table 4). This extract came from very young individuals (SAWYER et al., 1961b). The absence of a detectable oxytocin-like principle may be related to the immaturity of the specimens sampled.

Table 4. *Reptilian neurohypophysial principles*

Species	Systems used[1] for separation	Pharmacological or chemical criteria for identity of[1]:			Ref.
		Arginine vasotocin	Oxytocin-like principle	Mesotocin	
O. Chelonia:					
Green turtle *(Chelonia mydas)*	none	FB/RU	RU/VP	—	1
Tortoise *(Testudo graeca)*	PC	WB/RU	RU/VP	—	2
Turtle *(Clemmys japonica)*	PE	FB/RU	RU/VP	—	3
Slider *(Pseudemys scripta)*	none	FB/RU	RU/VP	—	4
O. Squamata:					
Iguana *(Iguana iguana)*	none	FB/RU	RU/VP	—	4
Grass snake *(Tropidonotus natrix)*	PC	WB/RU	RU/VP	—	2
Rattler *(Crotalus atrox)*	CMC	HO/VP	—	FD/RU	5
O. Crocodilia:					
Caiman *(Caiman crocodilus)*	none	FB/RU	none detected	—	1

[1] Same abbreviations as in Table 2.

References: 1. SAWYER et al. (1961b); 2. HELLER and PICKERING (1961); 3. HIRANO (1966); 4. SAWYER (unpublished data); 5. MUNSICK (1966).

The only evidence concerning the identity of the oxytocin-like principle from any reptile is that presented by MUNSICK (1966) for the rattlesnake. The pharmacological properties of the neutral oxytocin-like principle separated on CMC are definitely not those of oxytocin. It closely resembles mesotocin (isoleucine^8-oxytocin) in its pharmacological profile. The existence of this peptide in reptiles cannot be accepted as established until it has been isolated and chemically characterized.

Reptiles were ancestral to both birds and mammals. Their critical phylogenetic position would suggest that they deserve more detailed investigation, particularly with respect to their oxytocin-like principles.

E. Amphibian Principles

1. Arginine-Vasotocin

All amphibian species studied appear to possess a vasopressor principle with biological and chromatographic characteristics consistent with those of arginine-vasotocin (Table 5). ACHER et al. (1960b) isolated this principle from *Rana esculenta* pituitaries and found that it had the appropriate amino acid composition.

Table 5. *Amphibian neurohypophysial principles*

Species	Systems used[1] to separate	Evidence for identity of[1]: Arginine vasotocin	Oxytocin-like principle	Oxytocin	Mesotocin	Others	Ref.
O. Urodela:							
Necturus maculosus	PC	R_F	—	—	FD/RU	—	1
Triturus alpestris .	PC	VP/RU	R_F	—	—	—	1
O. Anura:							
Ranidae:							
Rana catesbiana .	none	FB/VP	RU/VP	—	—	—	2
R. catesbiana . . .	PE	FB/RU	RU/VP	—	—	—	3
R. temporaria. . .	PC	WB/VP	R_F	—	—	—	4
R. esculenta . . .	PC	—	—	—	FD/RU	—	1
R. esculenta . . .	IRC	*Analysis*	R_F	—	—	also arginine vasopressin	5
R. esculenta . . .	IRC	NF/VP	RU/VP	—	—	unknown natriferic principle	6
R. esculenta . . .	IRC	R_F	—	—	*Analysis*	—	7
R. esculenta . . .	IRC	FB/VP	R_F	—	—	—	8
R. pipiens	CMC	HO/VP	—	FD/RU	—	—	9
Bufonidae:							
Bufo americanus .	none	FB/RU	RU/VP	—	—	—	2
B. bufo	PC	WB/VP	—	—	FD/RU	—	4, 1
Pipidae:							
Xenopus laevis . .	PC	VP/RU	—	—	FD/RU	—	1
Xenopus laevis . .	IRC	VP/RU	R_F	—	—	—	8

[1] Same abbreviations as in Table 2.

References: 1. FOLLETT and HELLER (1964b); 2. SAWYER, MUNSICK, and VAN DYKE (1961b); 3. HIRANO (1966); 4. HELLER and PICKERING (1961); 5. ACHER et al. (1960b); 6. MOREL et al. (1961); 7. ACHER et al. (1964b); 8. ACHER et al. (1964a); 9. MUNSICK (1966).

They also found arginine-vasopressin in these extracts to which mammalian neurophysin had been added. It seems possible that the vasopressin had been inadvertently introduced as a contaminant of the neurophysin. Subsequent study of the same species by ACHER et al. (1964a) failed to reveal vasopressin. Neurophysin had not been used in the latter study. FOLLETT and HELLER (1964b) and MUNSICK (1966) have separated the active principles from *R. esculenta* and *R. pipiens* by paper and CMC column chromatography, respectively. No sign of arginine-vasopressin was detected in either instance.

2. Oxytocin and Mesotocin

FOLLETT and HELLER (1964b) separated "fast-moving" oxytocin-like fractions by paper chromatography of several amphibian neurohypophysial extracts. These fractions had pharmacological properties clearly differing from those of oxytocin.

They suggested that they might contain isoleucine^8-oxytocin. ACHER et al. (1964b) shortly thereafter identified this analogue by hydrolysis, amino acid analysis, and partial degradation of the oxytocin-like peptide from *R. esculenta* pituitaries. They named it "mesotocin." This was the second instance in which a peptide had been synthesized and studied pharmacologically (BERDE and KONZETT, 1960) before it had been recognized as a natural hormone. As in the case of arginine-vasotocin, the similarity of biological properties between synthetic isoleucine^8-oxytocin and natural pituitary principles had let to the first suggestions (SAWYER and VAN DYKE, 1963a; SAWYER, 1964; FOLLETT and HELLER, 1964b) that they might be identical.

FOLLETT and HELLER's (1964b) careful studies indicate that mesotocin is present in *R. esculenta*, *Bufo bufo*, *Xenopus laevis*, and *Necturus maculosus*. There is reason to believe, however, that oxytocin may also exist among amphibians. MUNSICK (1966) has presented strong evidence that the predominant neutral peptide in *R. pipiens* cannot be mesotocin. It resembles oxytocin closely. At present then we must admit the possibility that at least two neutral oxytocin-like principles occur among the amphibians and, more particularly, among members of the same genus or even among members of the same species.

3. The Natriferic Principle other than Arginine-Vasotocin

MOREL et al. (1961) reported that ion-exchange chromatography of a *R. esculenta* pituitary extract revealed the presence of two neutral principles. The leading edge of the neutral peak of oxytocic activity contained natriferic and rat uterus activities in ratios consistent with those of oxytocin or mesotocin. The trailing edge, however, contained about 15 times more natriferic and 90 times more frog bladder activities than it would if it were oxytocin. Mesotocin does not have such high relative activities on these assays. These activities could not be due to arginine-vasotocin since this section of the chromatogram contained very little vasopressor and frog or rat antidiuretic activities. This frog extract thus contained a previously unrecognized natriferic principle.

The only peptides known to have such high relative natriferic activities are analogues of oxytocin with deletions in the side chain (MOREL et al., 1965). Deglycine and deleucine oxytocins, for example, have little oxytocic or antidiuretic activities but do have natriferic activity greater than that of oxytocin or mesotocin (MOREL et al., 1965). It would be interesting if such a heptapeptide were present in the frog as a natriferic hormone. It would be an unexpected deviation from the generally assumed rule that active neurohypophysial hormones are octapeptides. A natriferic principle might serve as an independent humoral means for increasing salt uptake across the frog skin without causing antidiuresis, as would arginine-vasotocin. Such a neurohypophysial hormone could thus perform a useful adaptive function in amphibians.

Since a deletion of the C-terminal glycinamide of oxytocin can produce a natriferic peptide, however, we must be wary of accepting that the natriferic principle in frog extracts is a naturally occurring peptide. It is conceivable that enzymatic hydrolysis during collection or processing of the glands might have produced the natriferic principle from other peptides. FOLLETT and HELLER (1964b) were unable to detect excess natriferic activity in the oxytocic fraction obtained by paper chromatography of extracts from pituitaries of *R. esculenta* and *Xenopus laevis*. SAWYER (1960a, b) did not detect natriferic or frog bladder activities in *R. catesbiana* pituitary extracts in excess of that that could be attributed to arginine-vasotocin. The presence of a natural natriferic principle other than arginine-vasotocin in frog pituitary glands, therefore, must be considered uncertain until confirmatory evidence can be obtained.

F. Principles of Ray-finned (Actinopterygian) Fishes

1. Arginine-Vasotocin

The neurohypophysial principles from two species of gadid teleosts, *Gadus (Pollachius) virens* (the pollack or coalfish) and *Urophycis tenuis* (the Boston hake), have been more thoroughly studied than have principles of any other cold-blooded vertebrates. This is largely due to the availability of large amounts of material collected by Dr. GRACE E. PICKFORD and her co-workers from Yale University. This group gathered many kilograms of pollack and hake pituitaries over the course of several years. Lyophilized pituitary powders were then offered to interested investigators. Pollack pituitary powder from this source provided material for the first identification of arginine-vasotocin (HELLER and PICKERING, 1960, 1961) as a natural teleost neurohypophysial principle. Investigation of this powder also provided the first evidence for the presence of a unique teleost oxytocin-like principle (HELLER et al., 1961). Chemical identification (ACHER et al., 1962) of this principle and pharmacological confirmation of its identity (SAWYER and VAN DYKE, 1963b; FOLLETT and HELLER, 1964a) also resulted from studies on this powder. Pituitaries similarly collected from the Boston hake (*Urophycis tenuis*) by Dr. PICKFORD's group were used by RASMUSSEN and CRAIG (1961) for the isolation and identification of arginine-vasotocin. These authors erroniously identified the species from which the pituitary powder came as *Merluccius vulgaris*. The *Urophycis* powder was also used by ACHER et al. (1962) who reported that it came from *Merluccius merluccius*. These errors in identification are being pointed out here in an effort to prevent them from becoming irrevocably fixed in the scientific literature and again to emphasize the importance of the contribution made by the original collectors of this invaluable material.

Arginine-vasotocin has been chemically identified in pituitary extracts from carp, pollack, whiting-pout and Boston hake (Table 6). There is good pharmacological evidence for its presence in many other teleost, holostean and chondrostean species, including the primitive bichir *Polypterus*. There is little reason to doubt, therefore, that arginine-vasotocin is present in all actinopterygian fishes.

2. Oxytocin-like Principles

HELLER, PICKERING, MAETZ, and MOREL (1961) first recognized that the oxytocin-like principle in pollack pituitaries (SAWYER et al., 1961a; HELLER and PICKERING, 1961) clearly differed from oxytocin. It had relative activity on the rat uterus in the presence of magnesium (RU_{Mg}/RU) about four times that of oxytocin. It also had higher relative fowl vasodepressor activity and lower natriferic and water-balance activities than oxytocin. They called this new principle "ichthyotocin" (HELLER, 1963b). It was soon isolated and chemically identified as serine^4-isoleucine^8-oxytocin by ACHER et al. (1962) who named it "isotocin." GUTTMANN et al. (1962) synthesized this peptide. When directly compared, the pharmacological profiles of natural pollack isotocin and synthetic serine^4-isoleucine^8-oxytocin appeared identical (SAWYER and VAN DYKE, 1963b; FOLLETT and HELLER, 1964a). Thus it became clear that the pollack and related gadid teleosts, the Boston hake and the whiting-pout, possess a different oxytocin-like hormone than that found in mammals or birds.

Isotocin has been chemically identified in the carp (ACHER et al., 1965b) as well as in gadid teleosts (ACHER et al., 1962). Pharmacological studies on chromatographic fractions suggest that it is also present in many other teleosts and in three holostean species (TABLE 6). Although FOLLETT and HELLER (1964a) found an oxytocin-like principle in three species of sturgeon it was present in such small

Table 6. *Neurohypophysial principles in ray-finned fishes (Actinopterygians)*

Species	Systems used for separation[1]	Pharmacological or chemical criteria for identity of[1]: Arginine vasotocin	Oxytocin-like principle	Mesotocin	Isotocin	Ref.
Chondrostei:						
O. Polypterini:						
Bichir *(Polypterus senegalis)* . .	PC	FB/RU	—	RU_{Mg}/RU		1
P. senegalis	CMC	FB/RU	—	FD/RU	RU_{Mg}/RU	2
P. senegalis	none	NF/RU	—	—	—	3
O. Acipenseroidei:						
Paddlefish *(Polyodon spathula)* .	PC	NF/RU	none found	—	—	4
Sturgeon *(Acipenser guldenstadti)*	PC	VP/RU	R_F	—	—	4
Sturgeon *(A. persicus)*	PC	VP/RU	R_F	—	—	4
Sturgeon *(A. nudiventris)* . . .	PC	VP/RU	R_F	—	—	4
Holostei:						
Gar pike *(Lepisosteus [Lepidosteus] osseus)*	PC, CMC	FB/RU	—	—	RU_{Mg}/RU	5
Gar pike *(L. platystomus)* . . .	PC	VP/RU	—	—	RU_{Mg}/RU	4
Bowfin *(Amia calva)*	PC	VP/RU	—	—	RU_{Mg}/RU	4
Teleostei:						
O. Isospondyli:						
Trout *(Salmo [Trutta] trutta)*	none	NF/RU	—	—	—	6
Trout . . . . *(Salmo gairdneri = S. iridens)*	PC	WB/RU	R_F	—	—	7
O. Ostariophysi:						
Carp *(Cyprinus carpio)*.	PC, CMC	FB/RU	—	—	RU_{Mg}/RU	5
C. carpio	PC	NF/RU	—	—	RU_{Mg}/RU	4
C. carpio	IRC	*Analysis*	—	—	*Analysis*	8
O. Apodes:						
Eel *(Anguilla anguilla)*	PC	NF/RU	—	—	RU_{Mg}/RU	4
O. Mesichthyes:						
Killifish *(Fundulus heteroclitus)* .	PC	FB/RU	—	—	RU_{Mg}/RU	9
Pike *(Esox lucius)*.	PC	VP/RU	—	—	RU_{Mg}/RU	4
O. Acanthopterygii:						
Pollack *(Pollachius virens)* . . .	none	FB/RU	RU/VP	—	—	10
P. virens	IRC, PC	*Analysis*	R_F	—	—	7
P. virens	IRC	NF/RU	—	—	RU_{Mg}/RU	11
P. virens	IRC	R_F	—	—	*Analysis*	12
P. virens	CMC	FB/RU	—	—	RU_{Mg}/RU	13
Whiting-pout *(Gadus luscus)* . .	IRC	*Analysis*	R_F	—	—	14
G. luscus	IRC	R_F	—	—	*Analysis*	12
Boston hake *(Urophycis tenuis)*[2]	CCD	*Analysis*	—	—	—	15
U. tenuis[2]	IRC	NF/RU	R_F	—	*Analysis*	12
U. tenuis	CMC, PC	FB/RU	—	—	RU_{Mg}/RU	2
European hake . . . . *(Merluccius merluccius)*	IRC	NF/RU	—	—	—	16
Albacore *(Germo alalunga)* . . .	none	NF/RU	—	—	—	6
Mackerel *(Scomber scombrus)* . .	none	NF/RU	—	—	—	6
Blenny *(Blennius gattorugine)*. .	none	NF/RU	—	—	—	6

[1] Same abbreviations as in Table 2.

[2] Rasmussen and Craig (1961) and Acher et al. (1962) both reported analyses of hake pituitaries originally collected by Dr. G.E. Pickford of The Bingham Oceanographic Laboratory, Yale University. This material was from the Boston hake, *Urophycis tenuis*, not the European hake *Merluccius vulgaris* or *Merluccius merluccius* as reported by these authors.

References: 1. Sawyer (1964); 2. Sawyer (unpublished data); 3. Follett and Heller (1964b); 4. Follett and Heller (1964a); 5. Sawyer (1963c); 6. Maetz et al. (1959); 7. Heller and Pickering (1961); 8. Acher et al. (1965b); 9. Sawyer and Pickford (1963); 10. Sawyer et al. (1961a); 11. Heller et al. (1961); 12. Acher et al. (1962); 13. Sawyer and van Dyke (1963b); 14. Acher et al. (1961); 15. Rasmussen and Craig (1961); 16. Chauvet et al. (1961).

quantities that they could not determine whether it resembled isotocin, oxytocin or neither. The motility of this principle on paper chromatograms was similar to that of oxytocin, isotocin, and other "fast-moving" principles. FOLLETT and HELLER (1964a) could not detect any fast-moving oxytocic principle in pituitary extracts from a closely related chondrostean, the paddlefish *Polyodon*.

The most primitive living actinopterygian is the bichir *Polypterus*. This fish may be considered a primitive chondrostean (ROMER, 1945) or may be placed in a separate Subclass. It probably represents a separate line of descent from the paleoniscoids that were ancestral to all actinopterygians, and possesses many primitive characteristics. *Polypterus* pituitary extracts contain a fast-moving oxytocin-like fraction (SAWYER and VAN DYKE, 1963a; SAWYER, 1964). When isolated

Table 7. *Pharmacological characteristics of oxytocin-like principles separated from lungfish and bichir pituitaries and of synthetic oxytocin, mesotocin and isotocin*

Species	System used to separate[1]	RU_{Mg}/RU	FD/RU	GM/RU	FB/RU	ADH/RU	Ref.
Australian lungfish (*Neoceratodus forsteri*)	PC	1.19 ± 0.12	1.81 ± 0.06[2]	1.06 ± 0.06	—	—	1
African lungfish . . (*Protopterus aethiopicus*)	PC	1.00 ± 0.08	1.48 ± 0.13[2]	0.97 ± 0.16	—	—	1
S. Amer. lungfish (*Lepidosiren paradoxa*)	PC	1.0	1.1	—	—	—	2
Oxytocin	—	0.91 ± 0.03	0.98 ± 0.07	1.0	—	—	1
Mesotocin	—	1.30 ± 0.12	1.56 ± 0.08	—	—	—	1
Isotocin	—	2.9 ± 0.33	2.4 ± 0.16	2.5 ± 0.20	—	—	1
				ME/RU			
P. aethiopicus A	PC	0.91 ± 0.06	0.99 ± 0.07[3]	0.93 ± 0.15	2.1	0.004	3
P. aethiopicus A	CMC	0.95 ± 0.07	—	—	—	0.005	3
P. aethiopicus B	CMC	1.01 ± 0.05	1.46 ± 0.08[2]	—	—	—	4
P. aethiopicus C	CMC	1.19 ± 0.07[2]	1.57 ± 0.06[2]	—	3.0	—	4
P. aethiopicus D	CMC	1.30 ± 0.04[2]	1.84 ± 0.11[2]	—	4.9	—	4
Bichir (*Polypterus senegalis*) . . .	PC	1.33 ± 0.13[2]	—	—	—	< 0.008	3, 4
P. senegalis . . .	CMC	3.12 ± 0.15[2,3]	1.30 ± 0.14[2]	2.2 ± 0.11[2,3]	—	—	4
Oxytocin	—	1.00 ± 0.05	1.00	0.84	1.00	0.002	3, 4
Mesotocin	—	1.0—1.3	1.5	1.14 ± 0.11	3.7 ± 0.5	0.003	3, 4
Isotocin	—	2.8 ± 0.2	2.1	2.5 ± 0.3	0.04	< 0.0003	5

[1] Same abbreviations used in Table 2.

[2] Significantly different from corresponding ratio for oxytocin ($P < 0.05$).

[3] Significantly different from corresponding ratio for mesotocin ($P < 0.05$).

References: 1. FOLLET and HELLER (1964b); 2. PICKERING and MC WATTERS (1966); 3. SAWYER (1965a); 4. SAWYER (unpublished); 5. SAWYER and VAN DYKE (1963b).

by paper chromatography this fraction had a RU_{Mg}/RU ratio clearly differing from those of either oxytocin or isotocin (Table 7). This ratio was the same as that for isoleucine[8]-oxytocin, suggesting that this analogue might be a naturally occurring neurohypophysial principle (SAWYER and VAN DYKE, 1963a). Subsequent separation of the neutral peptide fraction on CMC, however, revealed a RU_{Mg}/RU ratio higher than that of isoleucine[8]-oxytocin (mesotocin). Relative fowl vasodepressor activity, however, was less than that of isotocin (Table 7). These preliminary studies suggest that the bichir pituitary may contain more than one active oxytocin-like principle. It is tempting to suggest that these are isotocin and mesotocin. This would be consistent with the pharmacological findings to date. Much work remains, however, to be done before the existence of either principle in this species can be considered established.

G. Lungfish Principles

1. Arginine-Vasotocin

Pituitaries from representative species of the three living genera of lungfishes (Dipnoi) contain activities suggesting the presence of arginine-vasotocin (FOLLETT and HELLER, 1964b). In the case of the African lungfish *Protopterus aethiopicus* this peptide has been thoroughly characterized and appears to have properties identical with those of arginine-vasotocin. It is reasonable to assume that all lungfishes have arginine-vasotocin, as do other bony fishes. The amounts of arginine-vasotocin present, compared to the total oxytocic activity of *Protopterus* pituitaries, are very small (FOLLETT and HELLER, 1964b; SAWYER, 1966). Pituitaries from South American lungfish (*Lepidosiren paradoxa*) contain relatively much more arginine-vasotocin (PICKERING and MC WATTERS, 1966). The meaning of this difference is not clear.

2. Oxytocin-like Principles

The Australian lungfish (*Neoceratodus forsteri*) appears to be the most primitive living dipnoan. The activities of the fast-moving fraction from paper chromatograms of extracts of its pituitary have a spectrum consistent with the assumption that mesotocin is the only peptide present (Table 7) (FOLLETT and HELLER, 1964b).

The activities found in the fast-moving fraction from paper chromatograms of pituitary extracts from the more specialized African lungfish *Protopterus aethiopicus* do not differ significantly from those of mesotocin as determined by FOLLETT and HELLER (1964b). These workers relied largely on the FD/RU ratio since it is the only clear difference they could demonstrate between oxytocin and mesotocin (Table 7). The low RU_{Mg}/RU ratio that they reported for this species might suggest, however, that all activities were not due to mesotocin. FOLLETT and HELLER (1964b) carefully point out that their results could reflect the presence of a new unknown neurohypophysial principle or to a mixture of one or more principles, one of which might be oxytocin.

SAWYER (1965a and unpublished) has examined extracts from four different collections of African lungfish of the same species (*Protopterus aethiopicus*). Extracts A, B, and C (Table 7) are from fish taken at the same season, but in different years, from the same fisheries (Lakes George and Edward, Uganda). When separated on paper or CMC columns the neutral fast-moving fraction from extract A appeared to have pharmacological properties clearly distinguishing it from mesotocin. The fowl depressor and rat uterus assays on which these ratios were based were done on the same preparations on which mesotocin as also assayed. There is no reason to suspect, therefore, that the differences between activity ratios for extract A and mesotocin (shown at the bottom of Table 7) could result merely from differing sensitivities of the assay preparations to this peptide. This was the basis for SAWYER's (1965a) conclusion that this *Protopterus* extract contained oxytocin and little or no mesotocin.

Extract B (Table 7) was collected at the same time as extract A but from female fish only. Its properties differ significantly from those of extract A. In having a high FD/RU ratio it resembles the *Protopterus* extract reported by FOLLETT and HELLER (1964b). Its pharmacological properties are consistent with those of mesotocin.

Extract C came from the same fisheries as did A and B but in a different year. Extract D came from Lake Victoria, where FOLLETT and HELLER (1964b) had obtained their fish. Both C and D also have properties entirely consistent with those of mesotocin.

The present situation, therefore, concerning the identity of the active oxytocin-like principle(s) in *Protopterus* remains confused. It is possible that individuals of this species may possess either oxytocin or mesotocin or both, as well as a possible unknown related peptide. The rather striking variations between pituitary extracts suggests that the relative quantities of these peptides may vary markedly, perhaps depending upon seasonal factors. There is another possibility that must be entertained, however. This is that artificial separation of active principles may have occurred prior to extraction. Loss of one or more neutral peptides might have occurred in some of these pituitaries. The methods of collection and preservation differed, at least in detail. Pituitaries of lots A and C were removed from heads severed several hours previously. These were not refrigerated. The fact that extracts A and C differ markedly suggests that autolysis is an unlikely cause for the differences. Pituitaries from lot B were obtained from freshly killed fish. The details concerning collection of lot D are not known. Pituitaries of lot A and B were kept in dry acetone for about one week and then dried in the sun. Pituitaries of lot C were kept in acetone for a similar length of time but were vacuum dried over phosphorus pentoxide. Pituitaries of lot D were stored and mailed in acetone and dried after a longer exposure to this solvent. In this respect their treatment resembled that of the pituitaries studied by FOLLETT and HELLER (1964b). Acetone containing water can dissolve oxytocin. Its effects upon mesotocin are not known. Watery acetone can also inactivate oxytocin (YAMASHIRO et al., 1965) reversibly. It is therefore conceivable that active peptides could have been lost prior to extraction of the pituitary powders. If the nature of the lost peptide varied among the collections this could explain variations between extracts.

The possibility that oxytocin occurs among lungfish has recently received support from studies of pituitaries from the South American lungfish *Lepidosiren paradoxa* by PICKERING and MC WATTERS (1966). The fast-moving principle isolated by paper chromatography resembles oxytocin more than mesotocin (Table 7).

Further study of more pituitaries by different methods are needed to help resolve the problem of exactly which oxytocin-like principles exist in lungfish pituitaries. At this point one can only conclude that *Neoceratodus* and some *Protopterus* extracts contain a principle clearly differing from oxytocin that could well be mesotocin. At least one *Protopterus* extract and one *Lepidosiren* extract contain activities consistent with the presence of oxytocin. Lungfish may, therefore, possess both oxytocin and mesotocin and, in this respect, resemble amphibians.

H. Cyclostome Principles

Arginine-Vasotocin

The cyclostomes occupy an important phyletic position as representative of the most primitive vertebrate group. Unfortunately their neurohypophysial principles have not been thoroughly characterized. HERRING (1913) could not demonstrate pharmacological activities similar to those of neurohypophyses from higher vertebrates in extracts from pituitaries of *Lampetra fluviatilis*, the river lamprey. He did detect weak vasopressor activity in pituitaries from the hagfish *Myxine*.

LANZING (1954) found weak oxytocic and frog water-balance activities in neurohypophyses from *Lampetra*, but he did not report quantitative estimates of either. SAWYER (1955) found considerable oxytocic, vasopressor and antidiuretic activities in forebrain extracts (including the neurohypophysis) from the marine lamprey *Petromyzon marinus*. SAWYER et al. (1961a) subsequently demonstrated vasopressor, antidiuretic, milk-ejection, hen oviduct and frog bladder activities in this species. These activities were present in proportions consistent with the assumption that arginine-vasotocin was the only active principle present. FOLLETT and HELLER (1964a) subjected *Lampetra* pituitary extracts to paper chromatography and only found evidence for a single principle with mobility and pharmacological characteristics resembling those of arginine-vasotocin. Their conclusion that the lamprey pituitary contained little or no active component other than arginine-vasotocin was supported by SAWYER's (1965d) failure to demonstrate any neutral oxytocin-like principle by ion-exchange chromatography of *Petromyzon* extracts. A basic peptide could be detected that resembled arginine-vasotocin in its frog bladder and vasopressor properties. The *Myxine* extract studied by FOLLETT and HELLER (1964a) was unfortunately so weakly active that chromatography could not be attempted. The extract did have natriferic activity consistent with the assumption that it also contained arginine-vasotocin. It thus seems possible that arginine-vasotocin is present in all cyclostomes. There is no evidence indicating the presence of any other active neurohypophysial principle. All cyclostome extracts studied to date have been very weakly active. It is quite possible that other active principles are present in quantities insufficient to be detected.

J. Chondrichthyan Principles

1. Properties of Crude Neurointermediate Lobe (NIL) Extracts

The elasmobranchs and holocephalians appear to have a wider variety of active neurohypophysial principles than do most other vertebrate groups. These peptides remain largely unknown, being characterized on the basis of their pharmacological and chromatographic properties, and are of an uncertain number. It would be impractical to attempt to discuss them individually. Instead I shall present the evidence that has been published concerning these principles and then try to interpret this in the simplest possible manner.

Several early investigators found weak pharmacological activities in elasmobranch neurointermediate (NIL) lobe extracts (HERRING, 1913; HELLER, 1941). PERKS, DODD, and DODD (1960) were the first to characterize such extracts from representative species by several assays. They found that these extracts contained rabbit milk-ejection, oxytocic, and rat antidiuretic activities in a ratio approximating 3:1:0.05 (Table 8). They suggested that the apparent constancy of this ratio among species indicated the presence of a single oxytocin analogue with unique biological properties. NIL extracts from many other species have properties consistent with this view (SAWYER et al., 1961a; PERKS and DODD, 1963a, b; PERKS, 1966). Very low antidiuretic and vasopressor activities of NIL extracts suggested that arginine-vasotocin could only be present in very small amounts, if at all. Crude extracts from *Squalus acanthias* were shown to have rather high FB/RU activity ratios (SAWYER et al., 1961a). The FB/RU ratio was lower and the FB/ADH ratio higher than those for arginine-vasotocin, however, suggesting that there was an oxytocin-like principle present that had relatively high frog bladder activity (SAWYER, 1961a).

NIL extracts from one species of skate *Raia ocellata* (PERKS and SAWYER, 1965) were found to differ strikingly from those of previously examined elasmobranchs (Table 8). On the other hand, extracts of NIL's from *Raia clavata*, *R. batis* and *R. naevis* had activities similar to those described for the majority of elasmobranch species (PERKS et al., 1960; PERKS and DODD, 1963a, b). *R. ocellata* extracts had

Table 8. *Pharmacological and chromatographic characteristics of extracts of chondrichthyan neurointermediate lobes*

Species	RU[1] mU/mg	RU_{Mg}/RU	ME/RU	ADH/RU	R_F of active spots on paper chromatograms[2] "Slow moving"	"Fast moving"	Ref.
Elasmobranchii. O. Selachii:							
Dogfish (*Scyliorinus caniculus*)	13	—	2.6	0.02	—	—	1
S. caniculus	—	—	—	—	0.35—0.45	0.5—0.6	2
S. caniculus	—	—	—	—	present	present	3
Dogfish (*Mustelus canis*)	1.1	2.0	—	<0.03	—	—	13
Lemon shark (*Negaprion brevirostris*)	0.7	—	—	—	—	—	4
N. brevirostris	—	—	—	—	0.35—0.45	0.5—0.8	3
Brown shark (*Eulania milberti*)	1.1	—	3.8	0.04	—	0.5—0.7	4
Blue shark (*Prionace glauca*)	0.78	2.1	—	<0.03	—	—	13
Bull shark (*Carcharinus leucas*)	0.5	—	4.2	0.07	—	0.5—0.7	4
Hammerhead shark (*Sphyrna mokarran*)	1.0	—	2.6	0.06	—	0.4—0.6	4
Dogfish (*Squalus acanthias*)	17	—	2.6	0.07	—	—	1
S. acanthias	33	1.7	1.7	0.03	—	—	5
S. acanthias	—	—	—	—	0.35—0.45	0.5—0.6	2
S. acanthias	20	1.6 ± 0.1	1.6	0.02	—	—	6
S. acanthias	46	2.6 ± 0.11	—	—	0.3—0.4	0.5—0.8	7
O. Batoidea:							
Thornback ray (*Raia clavata*)	15	—	3.5	0.03	—	—	1
R. clavata	—	—	—	—	0.04—0.36	0.45—0.74	8
R. clavata	4.5	10	—	—	—	—	9
Grey skate (*R. batis*)	7	—	4.5	0.07	—	—	1
R. batis	6.5	12	—	—	—	—	10
Cuckoo skate (*R. naevus*)	10	—	—	0.05	—	—	1
Bat ray (*R. lucuis*)	3	—	—	—	—	—	13
Skate (*Raia ocellata*)	19	—	10	0.06	—	—	11
Stingray (*Dasyatis sabina*)	59	—	3.4	0.004	—	0.6—0.8	4
Holocephali: O. Chimaerae:							
Ratfish (*Hydrolagus colliei*)	102	0.92 ± 0.02	0.98 ± 0.07	0.07	—	—	6
H. colliei	19	0.96 ± 0.04	—	—	—	—	12
Rabbitfish (*Chimaera monstrosa*)	—	—	—	—	present	present	3

[1] Abbreviations are the same as those used in preceding tables. — [2] Only data include from paper chromatograms run at room temperature, descending, on Whatman no. 1 or no. 3MM paper, with butanol:acetic acid:water = 4:1:5.

References: 1. PERKS et al. (1960), PERKS and DODD (1963b); 2. HELLER and PICKERING (1961); 3. HELLER and ROY (1965b); 4. PERKS (1966); 5. SAWYER et al. (1961a); 6. SAWYER (1965d); 7. SAWYER (unpublished); 8. HELLER and ROY (1965a); 9. ACHER et al. (1965c); 10. CHAUVET et al. (1965); 11. PERKS and SAWYER (1965); 12. SAWYER and FREER (unpublished); 13. PERKS, A.M. (pers. communication).

exceptionally high relative activity in rabbit milk-ejection assays (ME/RU = 10). This suggested the presence of a principle in *R. ocellata* differing from that found in other elasmobranchs.

2. Paper Chromatography of NIL Extracts

HELLER and PICKERING (1961) detected two areas of oxytocic activity on paper chromatograms of NIL extracts from *Squalus acanthias* and *Scyliorhinus caniculus*. They used descending chromatography developed with butanol:acetic acid:water = 4:1:5. The "fast-moving" area had the same R_F as oxytocin on this system. The "slow-moving" area had an R_F slightly greater than that of arginine-vasotocin. These authors did not further characterize these substances at that time.

PERKS (1966) has found "fast-moving" oxytocic activity in NIL extracts from several elasmobranchs using the same chromatographic method. He was unable to detect a slow-moving area on this system. Such principles could have been missed, however, if they were present in small amounts accounting for less than 10—30% of the total oxytocic activity.

SAWYER (unpublished) has found a slow-moving principle in *Squalus* extracts that resembles arginine-vasotocin (Table 9). It is present in small amounts, accounting for less than 2% of the total recovered oxytocic activity.

Table 9
Pharmacological characteristics of chondrichthyan principles separated by paper chromatography

Species	R_F[1]	R_{Mg}/RU[1]	GM/RU	FD/RU	ADH/RU	Ref.[1]
A. Fast-moving principles						
1. "EOP I"						
Squalus acanthias . .	0.5—0.8	2.5 ± 0.13	—	—	0.015	7
2. "E_2"						
Scyliorhinus caniculus.	"fast"	2.48 ± 0.06	—	—	—	3
Negaprion brevirostris .	0.5—0.8	2.58 ± 0.23	—	—	—	3
Raia clavata	0.45—0.74	2.07 ± 0.27	1.53 ± 0.09	2.4 ± 0.18	—	8
3. Others						
Chimaera monstrosa. .	"fast"	1.04 ± 0.07	—	—	—	3
B. *Slow-moving principles*						
1. Arginine-vasotocin-like						
Squalus acanthias . .	0.3—0.4	2.9 ± 0.15	—	—	2.1	7
2. "E_1"						
Scyliorhinus caniculus.	"slow"	6.28 ± 0.94	—	—	—	3
Raia clavata	0.04—0.45	6.14 ± 0.94	1.77 ± 0.30	7.2	—	8
3. Others						
Negaprion brevirostris	0.35—0.45	2.86	—	—	—	3
Chimaera monstrosa. .	"slow"	1.25 ± 0.12	—	—	—	8

[1] Footnotes and References the same as to Table 8.

HELLER and ROY (1965a, b) have succeeded in characterizing the slow-moving principles from several species. In *Raia clavata* and *Scyliorhinus caniculus* this principle has extraordinarily high relative activities when assayed on the rat uterus in the presence of magnesium and by fowl vasodepressor assays (Table 9). These activity ratios clearly distinguish it from the fast-moving principle and from arginine-vasotocin. HELLER and ROY (1965a) call this slow-moving principle "E_1". *Chimaera* and *Negaprion* have slow-moving principles clearly not E_1

(HELLER and ROY, 1965b). Fast-moving principles from most species appear similar, except for *Chimaera*. HELLER and ROY (1965a, b) call these "E_2." In *Chimaera* the fast-moving principle has a low RU_{Mg}/RU similar to those of oxytocin or mesotocin, and differing significantly from this ratio for E_2 (Table 9).

Paper chromatograms reveal, therefore, that there are several active principles among chondricthyes. These are: 1. slow-moving E_1 characterized by high RU_{Mg} and FD/RU ratios and little or no natriferic activity. 2. fast-moving E_2 with a RU_{Mg}/RU of about 2.5 and a lower FD/RU ratio than E_1. 3. a slow-moving principle resembling arginine-vasotocin. 4. a fast-moving principle resembling oxytocin or mesotocin.

3. Column Chromatography of NIL Extracts

PERKS and SAWYER (1965) used column chromatography of NIL extracts from *Raia ocellata* to isolate an oxytocin-like neutral principle. Only one peak of oxytocic activity was eluted from a CM-Sephadex column. It appeared in the position in which oxytocin is eluted from such columns. There was no evidence for the presence of a basic peptide resembling arginine-vasotocin.

The oxytocin-like peptide from *R. ocellata* appeared to be nearly pure. It contained 18 rat uterus (no Mg^{++}) units/mg. This principle had a unique pharmacological activity spectrum, differing from E_1 and E_2 in that the ME/RU ratio was about 7 (Table 10). It also had no detectable frog bladder activity. When

Table 10. *Pharmacological characteristics of chondrichthyan principles separated by ion exchange chromatography or paper electrophoresis*

Species	RU[1] U/mg	R_F	RU_{Mg}/RU	ME/RU	FB/RU	FD/RU	ADH/RU	Ref.[1]
A. "Oxytocin-like" (Neutral) peptides:								
1. "EOP I"								
Squalus acanthias	>30	—	1.8 ± 0.06	1.47 ± 0.05	3	1.4 ± 0.13	0.008	6
S. acanthias . .	>60	0.5–0.9	2.45 ± 0.13	—	4.2 ± 0.43	1.6 ± 0.11	0.005	7
2. "EOP II"								
Raia ocellata . .	~18	—	2.6 ± 0.2	6.9 ± 0.8	<0.45	—	0.04	11
3. Glumitocin								
Raia clavata. . .	8	—	10	—	—	—	—	9
Raia batis . . .	7.5	—	10	—	—	—	—	10
4. Oxytocin ?								
Hydrolagus colliei	—	—	0.89	—	1	—	0.003	6
H. colliei	—	—	1.05 ± 0.05	—	—	1.02 ± 0.06	0.008	12
B. Arginine-vasotocin-like (Basic) peptides:								
Squalus acanthias	—	0.4–0.5	2.85 ± 0.15	—	~250	—	1.8	7
Mustelus asterias	—	—	—	—	—	—	—	9
Raia clavata. . .	—	—	—	—	—	—	—	9
Raia batis. . . .	—	—	—	—	—	—	—	10
Hydrolagus colliei	—	—	—	—	~500	—	~1	6
H. colliei	—	—	3.09 ± 0.09	—	~1000	—	~3	7

[1] Footnotes and References the same as to Table 8.

hydrolyzed it yielded the amino acids of oxytocin except that the leucine residue was absent and was apparently replaced by serine. PERKS and SAWYER (1965) suggested that this might be serine^3-isoleucine^8-oxytocin. A sample of synthetic serine^3-isoleucine^8-oxytocin was subsequently found to have less than 1 unit/mg of activity on the rat uterus (SAWYER, unpublished). Unless the sample had lost activity before this assay this would indicate that the active *R. ocellata* principle could not be serine^3-isoleucine^8-oxytocin.

Sawyer (1965) separated the active principles from *Squalus* NIL extracts by CMC column chromatography. The neutral principle clearly differed from that obtained from. *R. ocellata*. It did resemble Heller and Roy's fast-moving principle E_2, having a similar RF on paper and a comparable activity profile. Sawyer called this elasmobranch oxytocin-like principle I (EOP I) to distinguish it from EOP II isolated from. *R. ocellata* NIL. The *Squalus* EOP I appears to have at least 60 rat uterus U/mg (Table 10).

Acher et al. (1965c) recently reported IRC-50 column chromatograms of extracts from *Mustelus asterias*, *Raia clavata* and *R. batis*. A peak of activity presumed due to arginine-vasotocin was detected in each case. The neutral peptide from *R. clavata* was subjected to hydrolysis and partial degradation. It appears to be serine^4-glutamine^8-oxytocin, which these authors named "glumitocin." Proof that this peptide accounts for the oxytocic activity of this chromatographic fraction must, of course, await studies on synthetic serine^4-glutamine^8-oxytocin. The amino acids of glumitocin have also been identified in a purified preparation of this peptide from *R. batis* (Chauvet et al., 1965).

Pharmacological evidence clearly indicates that glumitocin is neither EOP I nor EOP II. Glumitocin has a RU_{Mg}/RU ratio of 10 whereas EOP I and II have ratios about 2.5. It cannot explain the activities of Heller and Roy's (1965a, b) E_2 for the same reason. Glumitocin might well, however, be the slow-moving E_1 which has a RU_{Mg}/RU ratio above 6. The fact that E_1 and glumitocin have been found in the same species makes identity even more likely. The question remains as to why Acher et al. (1965c) and Chauvet et al. (1965) failed to find E_2 since it is clearly present in *R. clavata* (Heller and Roy, 1965a) and probably in *R. batis* (Perks, Dodd, and Dodd 1960).

The amino acid composition of the oxytocic fraction (EOP II) obtained from *R. ocellata* (Perks and Sawyer, 1965) is precisely that of glumitocin. Yet glumitocin could not provide the biological activities found in EOP II (Table 10). It has less than half the specific oxytocic activity of EOP II and a much higher RU_{Mg}/RU ratio. It appears possible that the fraction isolated by Perks and Sawyer (1965) contained two principles. Weakly active glumitocin may have constituted the bulk of the peptide present, explaining why its constituent amino acids appeared in nearly equimolar amounts in the hydrolysate. The activities ascribed to EOP II may have been for the most part those of a much more active peptide present in too low a concentration to contribute noticeably to the amino acid analysis.

Extracts of the holocephalian ratfish (*Hydrolagus colliei*) pituitary yield two active peaks when chromatographed on CMC or CM-Sephadex (Sawyer, 1965d; Sawyer and Freer, unpublished). The more neutral principle differs markedly from EOP I, EOP II, E_1, E_2 and glumitocin in having a RU_{Mg}/RU of about 1.0. It is thus indistinguishable from oxytocin. The basic peak contains much less activity and appears to be arginine-vasotocin.

4. *Interpretations*

The pituitaries of chondrichthyan fishes have thus yielded a variety of principles. Although one cannot draw firm conclusions based on assay data from different laboratories (see Section II-2) it still may be useful to introduce some simplifying assumptions. If one starts with the rule that principles may be identical unless there is clearly contrary evidence one may be able to reduce the chondrichthyan principles to the least number that could account for the reported activities.

There are many points of resemblance between EOP I and E_2. Both have similar activity spectra and chromatographic mobilities. There is little reason to doubt identity. This principle appears widely distributed, perhaps it occurs in all elasmobranch species except *R. ocellata* and the holocephalians (Table 11).

Table 11. *Summary suggesting the possible distribution of active NIL principles among those chondrichthyan species that have been studied, assuming the least number of active principles that could explain the biological properties of NIL extracts*

Species	Uncharacterized oxytocin-like	EOP I E_2	EOP II	E_1 glumitocin	Oxytocin	Arginine vasotocin
Elasmobranchs						
Selachians:						
Scyliorhinus	—	+	—	+	—	—
Mustelus	—	+	—	—	—	+
Negaprion	+	+	—	—	—	—
Eulania	—	+	—	—	—	—
Prionace	—	+	—	—	—	—
Carcharinus	—	+	—	—	—	—
Sphyrna	—	+	—	—	—	—
Squalus	—	+	—	—	—	+
Batoids:						
Raia clavata	—	+	—	*Analysis*	—	+
Raia batis	—	+	—	*Analysis*	—	+
Ravia naevus	—	+	—	—	—	—
Raia ocellata	—	—	+	*(?Analysis)*	—	—
Dasyatis	—	+	—	—	—	—
Holocephalians						
Chimaera	++	—	—	—	—	—
Hydrolagus	—	—	—	—	+	+

E_1 and glumitocin may be identical. The presence of E_1 in species as distantly related as *R. clavata* and *Scyliorhinus* suggests that this principle may also be of broad phyletic distribution.

EOP II has been detected in only one species. Arginine-vasotocin appears to be present in all groups although it has not been detected in all species.

Oxytocin could well be the neutral active fast-moving principle in the holocephalians.

We have thus, by avoiding postulation of more peptides than absolutely necessary, reduced chondrichthyan principles to arginine-vasotocin and four neutral peptides. Of the latter, one (glumitocin) is known and another may be oxytocin.

It may be possible to attempt a guess concerning the natures of the two unknown principles. EOP I has pharmacological characteristics suggesting that it has an intact oxytocin ring (Sawyer, 1965d). Vliegenthart and Versteeg (1965) suggest that glutamine^8-oxytocin would be a likely intermediate between previously identified principles and glumitocin. It is unfortunate that this analogue has not been synthesized. The characteristics of EOP II suggest that it contains a substitution within the oxytocin ring (Perks and Sawyer, 1965). It does not appear to be serine^4-oxytocin, or serine^4-isoleucine^8-oxytocin (Sawyer, 1965d), but it could be some other serine^4 analogue and thus related to isotocin and glumitocin. Further studies on this principle from *R. ocellata* may solve this interesting riddle.

IV. Phylogenetic Considerations

A. General

As information on the identities and distributions of active neurohypophysial principles has accumulated several investigators have tried to relate this to vertebrate phylogeny and thereby to describe the sequences by which these peptides may have evolved (SAWYER, 1961a, 1964, 1965b; ACHER, 1963; ACHER et al., 1964b, 1965a; FOLLETT and HELLER, 1964b; VLIEGENTHART and VERSTEEG, 1965). Unfortunately most such attempts have been made obsolete by discovery of new peptides and by more detailed studies of distributions. Hypothetical schemes of peptide phylogeny have, however, served a useful purpose in pointing out species that deserved attention and in suggesting possible structures for principles that had not been chemically identified. It is considered justifiable, therefore, to attempt again to relate present knowledge of peptide distribution to the probable phyletic relations among living vertebrates. We must bear in mind HELLER's (1963b) warning, however, that "so few Orders and Species within each vertebrate class have, as yet, been investigated that any statement on the distribution of the neurohypophysial hormones must at present be regarded as tentative."

To this warning we should add a few of our own. One is that we might expect that neurohypophysial peptides having important physiological functions are present in vertebrates but they have remained undetected because they do not affect our standard assay preparations. Such peptides could have served as intermediates in the evolution of the active principles that have been identified. It is also probable that peptides existed during evolution that are absent in living species. These also could have filled important gaps in the lines leading to the known principles. It is also quite possible that active peptides are present in many species but are stored in amounts too small to be readily detected and yet they could also be links in the evolution of the known active neurohypophysial principles.

B. Vasopressor Principles

Despite the limited number of species examined, and the other reservations expressed above, the evidence concerning the possible evolution of the active vasopressor-antidiuretic principles appears to lead toward some rather straightforward and simple hypotheses. This is because only three such principles have been discovered. Arginine-vasotocin appears to be present in almost all non-mammalian vertebrate groups. It is presumed present in the cyclostomes as well as the jawed vertebrates and can therefore be considered as the probable ancestor of all other active principles (SAWYER, 1961a; HELLER, 1963b; VLIEGENTHART and VERSTEEG, 1965), particularly since it is the only principle yet detected in cyclostome pituitaries.

The evolutionary stability of the arginine-vasotocin molecule appears remarkable (SAWYER, 1964). This suggests that arginine-vasotocin early acquired specific physiological functions that were dependent upon this exact molecular structure. Any mutation causing a change in amino acid composition would then be deleterious. This situation may not have prevented a mutation following gene doubling (VLIEGENTHART and VERSTEEG, 1965) from persisting as long as the gene for arginine vasotocin was also present. Mammals are the only group that appear to lack the genetic ability to manufacture arginine-vasotocin.

Defense of the hypothesis that a specific function could explain the evolutionary stability of arginine-vasotocin is impossible since there is little information suggesting what such a function might be among the fishes. If physiological responses of fishes to vasotocin are described it will be of great interest to see if they show narrow structural specificities which could help explain the persistence of this molecule throughout evolution of almost all nonmammalian vertebrates.

Among amphibians physiological responses to arginine-vasotocin do show a high degree of specificity for the exact structure of arginine-vasotocin (SAWYER, 1963b; MOREL et al., 1965). Substitution of phenylalanine^3 for isoleucine^3, or of lysine^8 for arginine^8 produces peptides that have much less antidiuretic, water-balance, and bladder permeability effects than does arginine-vasotocin. Amino acid changes elsewhere in the molecule have even more drastic effects on these activities. This suggests that mutations leading to substitution anywhere in the arginine-vasotocin molecule could be seriously deleterious if they occurred in amphibians.

A mutation did occur early in mammalian evolution which allowed the substitution of arginine-vasopressin for arginine-vasotocin. We can only guess at the relative effectiveness of these two antidiuretic peptides in the ancestors of living mammals. In rats or dogs, however, both arginine-vasopressin and arginine-vasotocin are highly potent antidiuretic agents. We might suppose that a mutation changing isoleucine^3 to phenylalanine^3 would not be clearly deleterious if the ancestral mammals showed a similar lack of discrimination between these two peptides.

Another mutation must have occurred early in the evolution of the Suina since many species possess lysine-vasopressin, either alone or in addition to arginine-vasopressin. In domestic swine these two vasopressin have essentially equal antidiuretic activity (MUNSICK et al., 1958). The change from arginine^8 to lysine^8 would not be clearly deleterious, therefore, if it occurred in pigs. In dogs, however, such a mutation would result in the substitution of an inferior antidiuretic hormone and would, all else being equal, probably not survive.

The reason that two vasopressins have peristed in some of the Suina is not clear. HELLER (1963b) has suggested that there might be some adaptive advantage to the heterozygous state, in having genes permitting the manufacture of both vasopressins. This is an interesting hypothesis which might explain a seemingly anomalous situation in which a mutation that does not appear clearly advantageous in itself has persisted in many species of Suina.

C. Oxytocin and Related Principles

The phylogenetic relationships among the neutral oxytocin-like principles appear to be much more complicated. Simple schemes that have been offered to explain the evolutionary changes among these molecules (SAWYER, 1961; ACHER, 1963) have become inadequate as the distribution of these principles becomes better known. The confusion concerning the exact natures and distributions of many of these peptides reflects the lack of simple and reliable means for pharmacological identification. It would appear to be foolish to attempt to outline their possible evolution at this time.

In past reviews (SAWYER, 1961, 1964, 1965b) we have tried to analyze phyletic distribution by the application of two assumptions. One is that no more mutations occurred than were absolutely necessary to account for the known peptides. The other was that if two species possess the same peptide it must have been present in a common ancestor. If, however, we try to apply these rules today we find ourselves having to postulate that there were several neutral oxytocin-like principles present in an ancestor common to all jawed vertebrates. For example, oxytocin may well be present in a holocephalian *Hydrolagus* as well as in birds and mammals. The dichotomy between lines leading to the holocephalians and elasmobranchs on one hand, and all other jawed vertebrates on the other, is generally believed to have occurred very early in fish evolution. This would date the first appearance of oxytocin, the leucine^{8} analogue of vasotocin, before the time of the divergence of the chondrichthyan line of descent from that leading to bony fishes.

Serine^{4} analogues (glumitocin and isotocin) occur among elasmobranchs and bony fishes. Applying the same assumptions, then, we would also have to conclude that the substitution of serine^{4} for glutamine^{4} must have occurred before the lines leading to chrondrichthyes and to bony fishes became distinct.

Isoleucine^{8} analogues (isotocin and mesotocin) appear among bony fishes and many tetrapods. This would not place the mutation leading to the substitution of isoleucine^{8} for arginine^{8} or leucine^{8} quite as far back in evolutionary history, since we do not have to assume that it occurred before the separation of the lines leading to chrondrichthyes and osteichthyes.

There are considerable areas in which the distributions of oxytocin and mesotocin appear to overlap. Both have been described as occurring in lungfish and amphibians, while mesotocin appears to be present among reptiles and oxytocin among birds. The common ancestor hypothesis would lead us to conclude that both these peptides were present very early in the evolutionary line leading to the lungfish and tetrapods. The persistence of one or the other of these principles or both, in any given species of lungfish or tetrapod seems to have occurred rather arbitrarily.

An alternative hypothesis is possible (Munsick, 1966). The natural active neutral peptides are quite uniform in their pharmacological properties. If one assumes that they have similar biological effects among the nonmammalian vertebrates, although their functions remain unknown, one could suggest that mutations involving the 4th and 8th positions have occurred rather frequently during evolution. If such mutations caused minimal changes in biological properties they might or might not survive. The presence, therefore, of serine^{4} or leucine^{8} moieties in peptides found among distantly related species might merely reflect parallel mutations that were not clearly deleterious to the species in which they occurred. Oxytocin and mesotocin, for example, are remarkably similar in their pharmacological properties when tested by assays done on amphibians, birds and mammals. It may make little difference, therefore, to most tetrapods whether their neutral neurohypophysial principle contains an isoleucine^{8} or a leucine^{8}.

Vliegenthart and Versteeg (1965) have attempted to interpret the phylogenetic distribution of neurohypophysial principles in terms of the genetic code. This requires several broad assumptions concerning the universality of the code and the degree to which the code shows systematic degeneracy. These authors then assume that each mutation occurred by the substitution of one base within a codon. Their application of these assumptions to an analysis of the probable course of evolution of neurohypophysial peptides has not, however, provided clearer insight. This is a promising approach, however, and may prove very useful as the details of the genetic code and the distribution of neurohypophysial peptides become better understood.

V. Conclusions

The pharmacological properties of neurohypophysial extracts indicate that at least nine active principles occur among the vertebrates. Seven have been chemically identified. These are all cyclic octapeptides that differ only in the identities of amino acids in three positions.

The biological properties of the three known neurohypophysial vasopressor peptides appear highly characteristic and pharmacological identifications can be quite reliable. The distribution of these principles can be easily reconciled with the course of vertebrate phylogeny. Arginine-vasotocin is most ubiquitous, occurring in all major vertebrate groups except mammals. In mammals it appears to be replaced by arginine-vasopressin and, among the Suina, by lysine-vasopressin. Each change, from arginine-vasotocin to arginine-vasopressin, and from arginine- to lysine-vasopressin, could result from a single mutation changing one amino acid moiety within a peptide.

The neutral neurohypophysial principles that resemble oxytocin are more difficult to isolate and characterize. Four have been chemically identified but there is pharmacological evidence for the existence of at least two more. It is impossible to relate current knowledge of their phyletic distributions to our usual concepts of vertebrate phylogeny. Some of these principles appear among distantly related species while closely related species often seem to secrete different oxytocin-like principles. Better methods for separating and characterizing these peptides must be developed and applied to neurohypophysial extracts from many more vertebrate species before their phyletic distributions can be meaningfully interpreted.

Acknowledgement

Previously unpublished work of the author reported in this article has been supported by research grants from the (U.S.) National Science Foundation (G-17660 and GB-4932X) and the National Institutes of Health (AM-01940), U.S. Public Health Service.

References

Acher, R.: The comparative chemistry of neurohypophysial hormones. Symp. Zool. Soc. London **9**, 83—91 (1963).

—, R. Beaupain, J. Chauvet, M.T. Chauvet, and D. Crepy: The neurohypophysial hormones of the amphibians: Comparison of the hormones of *Rana esculenta* and *Xenopus laevis*. Gen. comp. Endocr. **4**, 596—601 (1964a).

—, J. Chauvet, M.T. Chauvet, and D. Crepy: Les hormones neurohypophysaires des poissons. Isolement d'une vasotocine du tacaud (*Gadus luscus*). Biochim. biophys. Acta **51**, 419—420 (1961).

— — — — Isolement d'une nouvelle hormone neurohypophysaire, l'isotocine, présente chez les poissons osseux. Biochim. biophys. Acta **58**, 624—625 (1962).

— — — — Phylogénie des peptides neurohypophysaires: Isolement de la mesotocine ($Ileu_8$-ocytocine) de la grenouille, intermédiaire entre la Ser_4-$Ileu_8$-ocytocine des poissons osseux et l'ocytocine des mammifères. Biochim. biophys. Acta **90**, 613—615 (1964b).

— — — — Les hormones neurohypophysaires des vertébrés. Variations des structures au cours de l'evolution. Ann. Endocr. (Paris) **26**, 662—669 (1965a).

— — — — Caracterisation des hormones neurohypophysaires d'un poisson osseux d'eau douce, la carpe (*Cyprinus carpio*). Comparaison avec les hormones des poissons osseux marins. Comp. Biochem. Physiol. **14**, 245—254 (1965b).

— — — — Phylogénie des peptides neurohypophysaires: Isolement d'une nouvelle hormone, la glumitocine (Ser_4-gln_8-ocytocine) présente chez un poisson cartilagineax, la raie (*Raia clavata*). Biochim. biophys. Acta **107**, 393—396 (1965c).

— —, and M.-T. Lenci: L'ocytocine et la vasopressine du cheval. Bull. Soc. chim. biol. **40**, 2005—2018 (1958a).

— — — Purification et structure de l'ocytocine et de la vasopressine du mouton. C.R. Acad. Sci. (Paris) **1**, 1435—1438 (1959).

— — — Isolement de l'ocytocine du poulet. Biochim. biophys. Acta **38**, 344—345 (1960a).

— — —, F. Morel and J. Maetz: Présence d'une vasotocine dans la neurohypophyse de la grenouille (*Rana esculenta L*). Biochim. biophys. Acta **42**, 379—380 (1960b).

— —, and G. Olivry: Sur l'existence eventuelle d'une hormone unique neurohypophysaire. I. Relations entre l'ocytocine, la vasopressine et la proteine de van Dyke extraites de la neurohypophyse du boeuf. Biochim. biophys. Acta **22**, 421—427 (1956).

ACHER, R., A. LIGHT, and V. DU VIGNEAUD: Purification of oxytocin and vasopressin by way of a protein complex. J. Biol. Chem. **233**, 116—120 (1958b).

ADAMSONS, K., JR., S.L. ENGEL, H.B. VAN DYKE, B. SCHMIDT-NIELSEN, and K. SCHMIDT-NIELSEN: The distribution of oxytocin and vasopressin (antidiuretic hormone) in the neurohypophysis of the camel. Endocrinology **58**, 272—278 (1956).

BERDE, B., and H. KONZETT: Isoleucyl^8-oxytocin, ein biologisch hochwirksames Polypeptid. Med. exp. (Basel) **2**, 317—322 (1960).

CHAUVET, J., M.-T. CHAUVET, and R. ACHER: Les hormones neurohypophysaires des mammifères: Isolement et caractérisation de l'ocytocine et de la vasopressine de la baleine (*Balaenoptera physalus* L.). Bull. Soc. Chim. biol. **45**, 1369—1378 (1963).

— —, D. BEAUPAIN, and R. ACHER: Les hormones neurohypophysaires des raies: Comparaison des hormones du pocheteau blanc (*Raia batis*) et de la raie bouclée (*Raia clavata*). C.R. Acad. Sci. (Paris) **261**, 4234—4236 (1965).

—, M.-T. CHAUVET-LENCI, and R. ACHER: Quelques observations sur les hormones neurohypophysaires d'un poisson téléostéen, le merlu (*Merluccius merluccius L.*). C.R. Acad. Sci. (Paris) **252**, 2145 (1961).

—, M.-T. LENCI, and R. ACHER: Présence de deux vasopressines dans la neurohypophyse du poulet. Biochim. biophys. Acta. **38**, 571—573 (1960).

VAN DYKE, H.B., B.F. CHOW, R.O. GREEP, and A. ROTHEN: The isolation of a protein from the pars neuralis of the ox pituitary with constant oxytocic, pressor and diuresis-inhibiting effects. J. Pharmacol. exp. Ther. **74**, 190—209 (1941).

—, S.L. ENGEL, and K. ADAMSONS, jr.: Comparison of pharmacological effects of lysine and arginine vasopressins. Proc. Soc. exp. Biol. (N.Y.) **91**, 484—488 (1956).

FERGUSON, D.R.: Separation of mammalian neurohypophysial hormones by thin-layer chromatography. J. Endocr. **32**, 119—120 (1965).

—, and H. HELLER: Distribution of neurohypophysial hormones in mammals. J. Physiol. (Lond.) **180**, 846—863 (1965).

FOLLETT, B.K., and H. HELLER: The neurohypophysial hormones of bony fishes and cyclostomes. J. Physiol. (Lond.) **172**, 74—91 (1964a).

— — The neurohypophysial hormones of lungfishes and amphibians. J. Physiol. (Lond.) **172**, 92—106 (1964b).

GUTTMANN, S., B. BERDE, and E. STÜRMER: The synthesis and some pharmacological effects of serine^4-isoleucine^8-oxytocin, a probable neurohypophysial hormone. Experientia (Basel) **18**, 445 (1962).

HELLER, H.: Differentiation of an (amphibian) water balance principle from the antidiuretic principle of the posterior pituitary gland. J. Physiol. (Lond.) **100**, 124—141 (1941).

— Neurohypophysial hormones. In: Comparative Endocrinology, Vol. I, pp. 25—80. Ed. by U.S. VON EULER and H. HELLER. New York: Academic Press 1963a.

— Pharmacology and distribution of neurohypophysial hormones. Symp. Zool. Soc. Lond. **9**, 93—106 (1963b).

—, and K. LEDERIS: Paper chromatography of small amounts of vasopressins and oxytocins. Nature (Lond.) **182**, 1231—1232 (1958).

— — Posterior pituitary hormones of the hippopotamus. J. Physiol. (Lond.) **151**, 47—49 (abstract) (1960).

—, and B.T. PICKERING: Identification of a new neurohypophysial hormone. J. Physiol. (Lond.) **152**, 56—57 (abstract) (1960).

— — Neurohypophysial hormones of non-mammalian vertebrates. J. Physiol. (Lond.) **155**, 98—114 (1961).

— —, J. MAETZ, and F. MOREL: Pharmacological characterization of the oxytocic peptides in the pituitary of a marine teleost fish (*Pollachius virens*). Nature (Lond.) **191**, 670—671 (1961).

—, and B.P. ROY: Elasmobranch neurohypophysial hormones. J. Physiol. (Lond.) 50—51P (abstract) (1965a).

— — The neurohypophysial hormones of some elasmobranch species. Gen. comp. Endocr. **5**, 683—684 (abstract) (1965b).

HERRING, P.T.: A contribution to the comparative physiology of the pituitary body. Quart. J. exp. Physiol. **1**, 261—280 (1908).

— Further observations upon the comparative anatomy and physiology of the pituitary body. Quart. J. exp. Physiol. **6**, 73—108 (1913).

HIRANO, T.: Further studies on the neurohypophysial hormones in the avian median eminence. Endocr. jap. **11**, 87—95 (1964).

— Neurohypophysial hormones in the median eminence of the bullfrog, turtle and duck. Endocr. jap. **13**, 59—74 (1966).

ISHII, S., T. HIRANO, and H. KOBAYASHI: Neurohypophysial hormones in the avian median eminence and pars nervosa. Gen. comp. Endocr. **2**, 433—440 (1962).

Katsoyannis, P.G., and V. du Vigneaud: Arginine-vasotocin, a synthetic analogue of the posterior pituitary hormones containing the ring of oxytocin and the side chain of vasopressin. J. biol. Chem. **233**, 1352—1354 (1958).
Lanzing, W.J.R.: The occurrence of a water-balance-, a melanophore-expanding and an oxytocic principle in the pituitary gland of the river-lamprey (*Lampetra fluviatilis* L.). Acta endocr. (Kbh.) **16**, 277—284 (1954).
Light, A., and V. du Vigneaud: On the nature of oxytocin and vasopressin from human pituitary. Proc. Soc. exp. Biol. (N.Y.) **98** 692—696 (1958).
Maetz, J., F. Morel, and B. Lahlouh: Natriferin. A new hormonal principle in the neurohypophysis of certain vertebrates. Nature (Lond.) **184**, 1236—1237 (1959).
Morel, F., S. Jard, and F. Bastide: Correlations entre la structure des peptides neurohypophysaires et leur activité biologique sur la peau et le rein de grenouille. Ann. Endocr. (Paris) **26**, 643—654 (1965).
—, J. Maetz, R. Acher, J. Chauvet, and M.-T. Lenci: A "natriferic" principle other than arginine-vasotocin in the frog neurohypophysis. Nature (Lond.) **190**, 828 (1961).
Munsick, R.A.: Effect of magnesium ion on the response of the rat uterus to neurohypophysial hormones and analogues. Endocrinology **66**, 451—457 (1960).
— Neurohypophysial hormones of chickens and turkeys. Endocrinology **75**, 104—112 (1964).
— Chromatographic and pharmacological characterization of the neurohypophysial hormones of an amphibian and a reptile. Endocrinology **78**, 591—599 (1966).
—, and S.C. Jeronimus: Effects of diethylstilbestrol and magnesium on the rat oxytocic potencies of some neurohypophysial hormones and analogues. Endocrinology **76**, 90—96 (1965).
—, W.H. Sawyer, and H.B. van Dyke: The antidiuretic potency of arginine and lysine vasopressins in the pig with observations on porcine renal function. Endocrinology **63**, 688—693 (1958).
— — — Avian neurohypophysial hormones: Pharmacological properties and tentative identification. Endocrinology **66**, 860—871 (1960).
Oliver, G., and E.A. Schäfer: On the physiological action of extracts of pituitary body and certain other glandular organs. J. Physiol. (Lond.) **18**, 277—279 (1895).
Perks, A.M.: Pharmacological and chromatographic studies of the neurohypophysial activities of the pituitary of further elasmobranch species. Gen. comp. Endocr. **6**, 428—442 (1966).
—, and M.H.I. Dodd: The properties of the oxytocic, milk ejection and antidiuretic principle of the neurointermediate lobe of the elasmobranch pituitary. Gen. comp. Endocr. **3**, 194—195 (1963a).
— — Evidence for a neurohypophysial principle in the pituitary gland of certain elasmobranch species. Gen. comp. Endocr. **3**, 286—299 (1963b).
— —, and J.M. Dodd: A neurohypophysial principle in the elasmobranch pituitary. Nature (Lond.) **185**, 850—851 (1960).
—, and W.H. Sawyer: A new neurohypophysial principle in an elasmobranch *Raia ocellata*. Nature (Lond.) **205**, 154—156 (1965).
Pickering, B.T., and H. Heller: Chromatographic and biological characteristics of fish and frog neurohypophysial extracts. Nature (Lond.) **184**, 1463—1464 (1959).
—, and S. McWatters: Neurohypophysial hormones of the South American lungfish (*Lepidosiren paradoxa*). J. Endocr. **36**, 217—218 (1966).
Rasmussen, H., and L. Craig: The isolation of arginine vasotocin from fish pituitary glands. Endocrinology **68**, 1051—1055 (1961).
Romer, A.S.: Vertebrate Paleontology, Chicago: University of Chicago Press (1945).
Sawyer, W.H.: Oxytocic, antidiuretic and vasopressor activities in the neurohypophysis of the sea lamprey, *Petromyzon marinus*. Fed. Proc. **14**, 130 (abstract) (1955).
— The antidiuretic action of neurohypophysial hormones in Amphibia. In: The Neurohypophysis, pp. 171—179. Ed. by H. Heller. London: Butterworths (1957a).
— Increased renal reabsorption of osmotically free water by the toad (*Bufo marinus*) in response to neurohypophysial hormones. Amer. J. Physiol. **189**, 564—568 (1957b).
— Increased water permeability of the bullfrog (*Rana catesbiana*) bladder *in vitro* in response to synthetic oxytocin and arginine vasotocin and to neurohypophysial extracts from nonmammalian vertebrates. Endocrinology **66**, 112—120 (1960a).
— Evidence for the identity of natriferin, the frog water balance principle and arginine vasotocin. Nature (Lond.) **187**, 1030—1031 (1960b).
— Comparative pharmacology and physiology of the neurohypophysis. Recent Progr. Hormone Res. **17**, 437—465 (1961).
— Neurohypophysial secretions and their origin. In: Advances in Neuroendocrinology, pp. 68—89. Ed. by A.V. Nalbandov. Urbana: Univ. Illinois Press (1963a).
— Neurohypophysial peptides and water excretion in the vertebrates. In: Hormones and the Kidney, pp. 45—58. Ed. by P.C. Williams. London: Academic Press (1963b).

SAWYER, W.H.: Vertebrate neurohypophysial principles. Endocrinology **75**, 981—990 (1964).
— Evolution of neurohypophysial principles. Arch. Anat. Microscop. Morphol. Exp. 54, 295—312 (1965a).
— Neurohypophysial principles of vertebrates. In: The Pituitary, Vol. **3**, pp. 307—329. Ed. by G. HARRIS and B. DONOVAN. London: Butterworths (1965b).
— Biological assays for neurohypophysial principles in tissues and in blood. In: The pituitary, Vol. **3**, pp. 288—306. Ed. by G. HARRIS and B. DONOVAN. London: Butterworths (1965c).
— Active neurohypophysial principles from a cyclostome (*Petromyzon marinus*) and two cartilaginous fishes (*Squalus acanthias* and *Hydrolagus collei*). Gen. comp. Endocr. **5**, 427—439 (1965d).
— Diuretic and natriuretic responses of the lungfish (*Protopterus aethiopicus*) to arginine vasotocin. Amer. J. Physiol. **210**, 191—197 (1966).
—, and H.B. VAN DYKE: Principles resembling oxytocin in neurohypophysis of bony fishes. Fed. Proc. **22**, 386 (abstract) (1963a).
— — Isolation of the oxytocin-like pituitary principle of a teleost fish (*Pollachius virens*) and comparison of its properties with those of synthetic 4-serine, 8-isoleucine oxytocin. Endocrinology **73**, 394—396 (1963b).
—, R.A. MUNSICK, and H.B. VAN DYKE: Pharmacological evidence for the presence of arginine vasotocin and oxytocin in neurohypophysial extracts from cold-blooded vertebrates. Nature (Lond.) **184**, 1464—1465 (1959).
— — — Pharmacological characteristics of neurohypophysial hormones from a marsupial (*Didelphis virginiana*) and a monotreme (*Tachyglossus* [*Echidna*] *aculeatus*). Endocrinology **67**, 137—138 (1960).
— — — Pharmacological characteristics of the active principles of neurohypophysial extracts from several species of fishes. Endocrinology **68**, 215—225 (1961a).
— — — Evidence for the presence of arginine vasotocin (8-arginine oxytocin) and oxytocin in neurohypophysial extracts from amphibians and reptiles. Gen. comp. Endocr. **1**, 30—36 (1961b).
—, and G.E. PICKFORD: Neurohypophysial principles of *Fundulus heteroclitus:* Characteristics and seasonal changes. Gen. comp. Endocr. **3**, 439—445 (1963).
—, and R.M. SCHISGALL: Increased permeability of the frog bladder to water in response to dehydration and neurohypophysial extracts. Amer. J. Physiol. **187**, 312—314 (1956).
TAYLOR, S.P., jr.: Ion-exchange chromatography of oxytocin, arginine-vasopressin, and lysine-vasopressin. Proc. Soc. exp. Biol. (N.Y.) **85**, 226—228 (1954).
URANGA, J., and W.H. SAWYER: Renal responses of the bullfrog to oxytocin, arginine vasotocin and frog neurohypophysial extract. Amer. J. Physiol. **198**, 1287—1290 (1960).
DU VIGNEAUD, V.: Trail of sulfur research: from insulin to oxytocin. Science **123**, 967—974 (1956a).
— The isolation and proof of structure of the vasopressins and the synthesis of octapeptide amides with pressor-antidiuretic activity. Proc. 3rd Int. Congr. Biochem., Brussels, 1955, pp. 49—54. New York: Academic Press 1956b.
VLIEGENTHART, J.F.G.: The neurohypophyseal hormones of the finback whale (*Balaenoptera physalus* L.). Proc. kon. ned. Akad. Wet. **67**, 291—294 (1964).
—, and D.H.G. VERSTEEG: Some reflections on the evolution of the vertebrate neurohypophyseal hormones. Proc. Kon. ned. Akad. Wet. **68**, 131—140 (1965).
WARD, D.N., E.F. AALBORG, and R. GUILLEMIN: A simple method for preparation of highly purified vasopressin. Proc. Soc. exp. Biol. (N.Y.) **96**, 568—571 (1957).
— —, H.S. LIPSCOMB, and R. GUILLEMIN: Fractionation and analysis of monkey pituitary glands for posterior lobe hormones. Acta endocr. (Kbh.) **40**, 283—289 (1962).
YAMASHIRO, D.: Partition chromatography of oxytocin on "Sephadex." Nature (Lond.) **201**, 76—77 (1964).
—, H.L. AANING, and V. DU VIGNEAUD: Inactivation of oxytocin by acetone. Proc. nat. Acad. Sci. (Wash.) **54**, 166—171 (1965).
—, D. GILLESSEN, and V. DU VIGNEAUD: Simultaneous synthesis of 1-hemi-D-cystine-oxytocin and oxytocin and separation of the diastereoisomers by partition chromatography on Sephadex and by countercurrent distribution. J. Amer. chem. Soc. **88**, 1310—1313 (1966).

Antagonists of the Neurohypophysial Hormones

J. Rudinger and I. Krejčí

With 16 Figures

I. Introduction

Throughout the history of pharmacology the exploration of antagonism and the use of antagonists has played an important role both in the development of theoretical concepts and interpretations and in experimental practice. The use of antagonists to interfere with the physiological or pathological effects of endogenous mediators forms an important branch of rational drug therapy. The first synthesis of a peptide hormone — oxytocin — by du Vigneaud and his coworkers (1953) opened the way to structurally modified synthetic hormone analogues including, it was reasonable to hope, antagonists of the natural hormones. Moreover, synthesis made available unexceptionably homogeneous preparations of the individual hormones, thereby eliminated some of the uncertainties attaching to much of the earlier work with materials purified from natural sources, and in consequence stimulated extensive physiological and pharmacological studies including work on antagonism.

Antagonistic effects have been observed probably more frequently in studies with the neurohypophysial hormones than with any other peptides hormones and, in particular, an appreciable proportion of the synthetic analogues of oxytocin and vasopressin has shown inhibitor properties — in contrast with the present situation for instance in the gastrin or angiotensin field.

However, the multiplicity and complexity of the biological effects exerted by the neurohypophysial hormones offers possibilities for antagonism not only at the receptor level (competitive or non-competitive) but also at the tissue or organ level ("independent antagonism") or at the organismic level ("biological antagonism"); and on the other hand, much of the recorded information about antagonism in this field is descriptive rather than interpretative — sometimes, in fact, no more than a record of incidental observations. This situation must needs be reflected also in this review. It has not been possible to use a classification by mode of action of the antagonists and a classification by structure has therefore been used, though it is evident that even structurally related antagonists may — and in fact sometimes do — act by different mechanisms. The most detailed attention has been given to antagonists structurally resembling the agonist peptides, chiefly synthetic analogues of the neurohypophysial hormones but also the natural hormones themselves where they appear to inhibit each other's effects. Other antagonists are treated more briefly and selectively.

Where doses of the natural hormones are given in International Units or fractions thereof, these are understood to be oxytocic or avian depressor units for oxytocin and pressor units for the vasopressins and vasotocin. In presenting quantitative relations it has sometimes been expedient to restate doses and particularly dose ratios (recorded in the original papers in terms of pressor or oxytocic units) as weight or molar ratios; this has been done on the assumption that pure oxytocin has a potency of 500 uterotonic or avian depressor units per milligram, arginine-vasopressin at potency of 500 rat pressor units per milligram, and lysine-vasopressin 250 rat pressor units per milligram. The approximation involved is negligible compared with the variations in biological response. Where vasopressin preparations of unspecified composition were used they are referred to as "vasopressin" and assumed to contain mainly arginine-vasopressin.

II. Antagonism Between the Natural Hormones

The possibility of antagonism between the naturally occurring neurohypophysial peptides is a subject of particular interest. On the one hand, the structural similarities between the individual hormones are so extensive that all would be expected to interact in some degree with the same receptors, i.e. behave as analogues of each other; on the other hand, the structural differences could be sufficient to decrease, or abolish, the functional competence of one or other of the hormones at a particular receptor. Where both these possibilities are realised the conditions for antagonism exist. Physiologically a situation where two endogenous hormones have antagonistic effects is not unreasonable since it offers better possibilities for "fine" regulation than a system based on one hormone alone — provided, of course, that the two hormones can be released selectively by different stimuli.

A second possibility of antagonism arises from the wide range of target organs acted on by the neurohypophysial hormones. Thus action of one hormone on one particular organ can set in train a series of physiological events which counteracts the effect induced by the other hormone in another target organ. Such "biological" antagonism may account for some of the observed relations.

1. Renal responses

The clearest case of antagonism between two natural hormones is provided by the studies of Morel and Jard on water and sodium reabsorption in the frog kidney (Morel and Jard, 1963; Jard and Morel, 1961, 1963; Jard, 1966).

Table 1. *Effect of Neurohypophysial Peptides on Parameters of Kidney Performance in the Frog (R. esculenta)* (After Jard, 1966)

Peptide	Average dose (μg/100 g)	Effect on				
		C_{in}	C_{H_2O}/C_{in}	C_{Osm}/C_{in}	C_{Na}/C_{in}	C_K/C_{in}
Arginine-vasotocin .	0.035	↓	↓	—	↓	—
Lysine-vasotocin . .	0.052	↓	↓	—	↓	—
Oxytocin	0.52[1]	↓	—	—	—	—
Lysine-vasopressin .	0.89[1]	—	—	—	—	—
Mesotocin[2]	0.62	↑	↓	↑	↑	↑

[1] Maximum dose 4 μg. — [2] Qualitatively similar results were obtained with isotocin, deamino-oxytocin, Leu[3]-, Val[3]-, Phe[3]-, Gln[5]-, de-Pro[7]-, and de-Leu[8]-oxytocin and with Phe[2]-lysine-vasopressin (average doses 1.5—7.7 μg/100 g).

In these studies frogs (*Rana esculenta* L.) were prepared (Uranga and Sawyer, 1960) by catheterisation of the ureters and an iliac artery and kept hydrated by immersion in water. In this way urine and samples of blood could be collected, and inulin, peptides etc. injected or infused, under conditions which are thought to block secretion of endogenous neurohypophysial hormones. Injection of the hormone, arginine-vasotocin, or the synthetic analogue lysine-vasotocin in nanogram amounts caused antidiuresis, a decrease in glomerular filtration rate (GFR), and a decrease in the relative clearances of free water (C_{H_2O}/C_{in}) and of sodium (C_{Na}/C_{in}) with no significant change in the relative clearance of potassium and osmotic clearance (JARD and MOREL, 1963; JARD, 1966). Oxytocin in amounts up to 1000 times greater caused only a decrease in GFR, without changes in relative clearances of water or ions and lysine-vasopressin in similar doses had no effect whatever. Mesotocin (Ile^8-oxytocin), identified as the second endogenous neurohypophysial hormone of the frog (ACHER et al., 1964), caused diuresis with an increase in GFR and the changes in free water and ion clearances summarised in Table 1; these changes are thought to result from the change in GFR rather than a direct inhibition of tubular electrolyte reabsorption. Isotocin (ichthyotocin, Ser^4-Ile^8-oxytocin) and eight synthetic hormone analogues listed below Table 1 have effects similar to those of mesotocin in various degrees (JARD and MOREL, 1963; JARD, 1966).

When oxytocin was injected together with, or 5—10 min before, an active dose of arginine- or lysine-vasotocin the decrease in the relative clearance of free water and of sodium was largely or completely inhibited (Fig. 1). For oxytocin : vasotocin

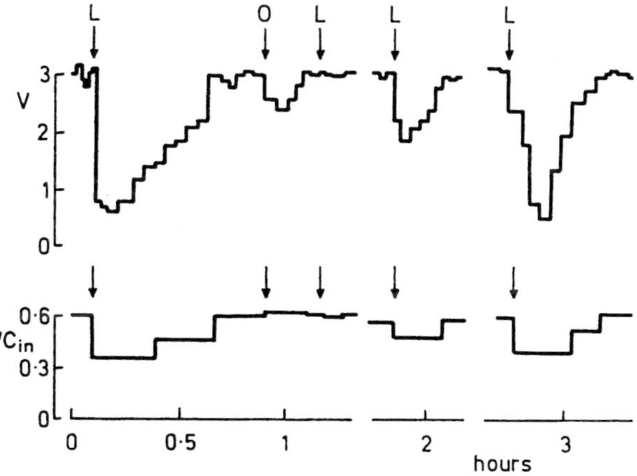

Fig. 1. Inhibition of the diuretic response of the frog kidney to lysine-vasotocin by oxytocin. Top: urine flow (ml/h/100 g), bottom: relative free water clearance; L lysine-vasotocin (5 ng), O oxytocin (550 ng). Note progressive fading of inhibition. From JARD (1966)

ratios between 7 and 40 the extent of inhibition was between 50 and 100% (see Table 2), with no regular dependence on the ratio of the two peptides over this range. The effect of oxytocin on the vasotocin-induced change in GFR was irregular. Lysine-vasopressin in analogous experiments had no effect on the responses to arginine- or lysine-vasotocin at ratios up to 70 or, in experiments with simultaneous infusion, up to 700:1 (MOREL and JARD, 1963; JARD, 1966).

Inhibition by oxytocin could be surmounted by increasing the dose of vasotocin. The dose dependence of the inhibition could be analysed by experiments in which oxytocin and lysine vasotocin were infused together in low dose ratios, between 1:1 and 10:1; the initial rate of infusion of vasotocin was chosen so as to elicit about 50% of the maximal response and kept constant while the amount of oxytocin was varied. A presentation of the results in double-reciprocal plots of dose ratio against percentage inhibition gave linear relations indicative of competitive inhibition. The ratio of affinity coefficients of oxytocin and lysine-vasotocin calculated from such experiments varied in different experiments but was of the order of 1 (JARD, 1966).

The action of the vasotocins on free water reabsorption was also inhibited by mesotocin and by six synthetic analogues of oxytocin* (Table 2) in ten- to hundred-fold excess; the effect on sodium excretion was not recorded because of the intrinsic natriuretic action of these peptides. On the other hand the natural hormone

Table 2. *Inhibition of the Responses of the Frog Kidney to the Vasotocins by Oxytocin and Related Peptides*[1] (From JARD, 1966)

Antagonist	Agonist[2]	Dose ratio antagonist: :agonist	Inhibition[3] (%) of effect on C_{H_2O}/C_{in}
Oxytocin	AVT	10—40	81 ± 17 (5)[4]
	LVT	7—36	88 ± 7 (18)[4]
Mesotocin	AVT	11—43	84 ± 7 (5)
	LVT	10—115	81 ± 14 (10)
Deamino-oxytocin . .	AVT	13—16	89 ± 12 (5)
	LVT	12—68	79 ± 24 (5)
Leu³-oxytocin	LVT	85	86 ± 20 (5)
Val³-oxytocin	AVT	43—103	80 ± 29 (5)
	LVT	13—143	99 ± 20 (8)
Gln⁵-oxytocin	LVT	25—100	79 ± 7 (7)
De-Leu⁸-oxytocin . . .	LVT	10—100	87 ± 24 (6)

[1] No significant inhibition was shown by the following peptides (highest antagonist:agonist ratios shown in parentheses): isotocin (104), Phe³- (17), and de-Pro⁷-oxytocin (100), lysine-vasopressin (700), Phe²-lysine-vasopressin (319). — [2] AVT is arginine-vasotocin, LVT lysine-vasotocin; the doses were 0.002—0.071 μg. — [3] Mean ± confidence interval for $P = 0.05$ (number of experiments). — [4] The decrease in C_{Na}/C_{in} due to AVT and LVT was inhibited to the extent of 87 ± 14 and 78 ± 11%, respectively.

isotocin and the synthetic analogues, Phe³-oxytocin, de-Pro⁷-oxytocin, and Phe²-Lys⁸-vasopressin in similar or greater excess had no effect on the response to the vasotocins (MOREL and JARD, 1963; JARD, 1966).

All these results are readily interpreted in terms of receptor theory (cf. ARIËNS, 1964). The reversibility of the inhibition and the quantitative dependence of the extent of inhibition on the relative concentrations of agonist and antagonist meet the criteria for competitive inhibition at a common set of receptors. The structural scope of agonism and antagonism suggests that attachment to the tubular receptors requires an oxytocin-like structure in the disulphide-bridged ("ring") sequence and in particular that an isoleucine or related aliphatic amino acid (leucine, valine) is required in sequence position 3; three peptides with phenylalanine in this position were inactive as either agonists or antagonists. The terminal amino group is not essential; the side-chain in position 4 appears to be of importance but that in position 5 is not critical. The structure of the carboxyl-terminal sequence ("side-chain") of the peptide has little effect on bonding to the receptor except that the

* Although they are not strictly within the scope of this section the effects of synthetic analogues are presented and discussed here to maintain the logical structure of the discussion.

omission of proline gives an inert peptide, perhaps because of the special conformational properties conferred by this residue (JARD, 1966).

For agonist properties, i.e. functionality of the complex formed from peptide and receptor, a basic amino acid in position 8 so far appears to be essential (MOREL and JARD, 1963; JARD, 1966). However, the structural differences in this position between the agonists and antagonists are not confined to the presence or absence of the basic group but also involve e.g. branching of the side-chain (Leu^8, Ile^8) or its absence (de-Leu^8) so that the conclusion about the role of basicity must be regarded as provisional, perhaps to be tested by the examination of additional analogues such as Nle^8-oxytocin.

A minute description of the molecular interactions involved in binding to the receptor and initiation of the response is obviously not yet possible, one reason being our ignorance of the conformational stereochemistry of these peptides and its sensitivity to particular changes in chemical structure (RUDINGER and JOŠT, 1964a); nevertheless the results of JARD and MOREL present as convincing a picture of antagonism at the receptor level as could be hoped for and lend strong support to the contention that the neurohypophysial peptides, like other, simpler biologically active compounds, initiate their effects by combining with and activating specific receptor sites, whatever the character of the processes resulting from this primary event and the nature of the ultimate response (RUDINGER and KREJČÍ, 1962).

It is instructive to note that the clear-cut conclusions emerging from the work discussed above were conditional upon an experimental approach in which the complex process of urine excretion was analysed into more fundamental parameters such as GFR and free water and ion clearances; the consideration merely of urine flow would obviously have given a more complicated and less informative picture.

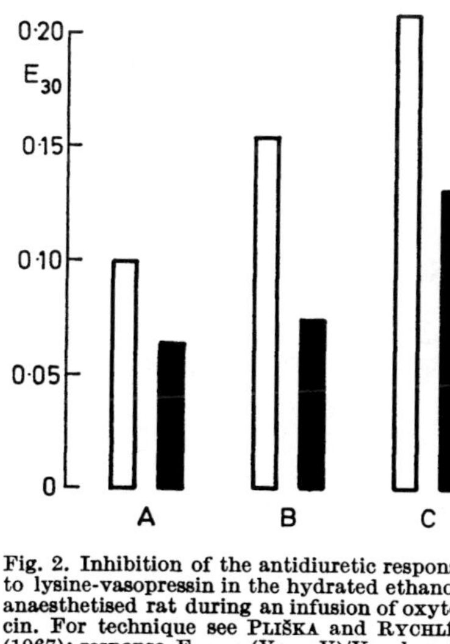

Fig. 2. Inhibition of the antidiuretic response to lysine-vasopressin in the hydrated ethanol-anaesthetised rat during an infusion of oxytocin. For technique see PLIŠKA and RYCHLÍK (1967); response $E_{30} = (V_0 — V)/V_0$ where V is the volume of urine excreted during 30 min following vasopressin injection and V_0 the volume excreted during a 30-min control period. Responses to 4.4 (A), 8.8 (B), and 17.6 μU (C) of lysine-vasopressin before (white columns) and during (black columns) infusion of oxytocin (100 μU/hr). PLIŠKA, unpublished results

The particular relations determined for *R. esculenta* may not necessarily be valid for other, even closely related species. In the bullfrog *R. catesbiana* and the toads *Bufo bufo* and *B. marinus* relatively high doses of oxytocin and the vasopressins have antidiuretic activity (cf. JØRGENSEN, 1950; SAWYER, 1960); in *B. bufo* oxytocin in equimolar amounts or tenfold excess inhibitis the antidiuretic response to nanogram doses of arginine-vasotocin though in microgram doses oxytocin itself has an antidiuretic effect (JØRGENSEN and LARSEN, 1962).

The antagonistic action of oxytocin on the antidiuretic response to vasopressin in rats was first reported by FRASER (1937). The existence of this antagonism has been repeatedly reaffirmed (FRASER, 1942; BRUNNER et al., 1956; SAWYER and VALTIN, 1965) and denied (VORHERR and FRIEDBERG, 1960; VORHERR, 1964). The use of hormone preparations obtained from pituitary extracts complicates the interpretation of the earlier work (see FRASER, 1942) but cannot account for the discrepancies; these appear to be due mainly to differences in the relative amounts used (Sawyer and Valtin, 1965). Antagonism was observed in conscious water-loaded rats at oxytocin: vasopressin ratios of 2—8:1 (Brunner et al., 1956) and in ethanol-anaesthetised rats at ratios of 40—50:1 (Sawyer and Valtin, 1965) though Vorherr (1964) failed to observe antagonism with ratios of 5:1 and 10:1 in the latter preparation; at higher ratios (800:1) oxytocin was inactive or potentiated the antidiuretic effect of vasopressin. It appears that in the hydrated rat the antagonistic relation is confined to a rather narrow range of oxytocin: vasopressin ratios. The maximal observed inhibition was about 35% (Sawyer and Valtin, 1965). These results have been confirmed (Pliška, unpublished results) in experiments in which the antidiuretic response to individual "challenge" doses of vasopressin was examined in hydrated, ethanol-anaesthetised rats during continuous infusions of oxytocin at various dose levels. Subthreshold infusion rates caused a significant though not dramatic decrease in the response to the challenge doses (Fig. 2).

It is by now generally accepted that oxytocin in low doses can have a diuretic effect; according to Brunner et al. (1956) this effect is more marked in thirsting, saline-loaded, or normal rats than in hydrated animals. However, oxytocin diuresis is unlikely to be caused by an inhibition of the antidiuretic response to endogenous vasopressin since it is also observed in hydrated, ethanol-anaesthetised rats (Berde and Cerletti, 1961; Kramár et al., 1966b) in which the release of endogenous neurohypophysial hormones, at least in response to osmotic stimuli (Eggleton, 1942; cf. Tata and Buzalkov, 1966) is thought to be blocked. Moreover, the relation of water and salt excretion during oxytocin diuresis shows that it is not due simply to a block in free-water reabsorption (Brunner et al., 1956; Kramár et al., 1966b) and finally, a diuretic response is also evoked by very low doses of vasopressin (Kramár et al., 1966a).

All these findings point to a biological antagonism rather than a competitive antagonism at the receptor level. The mechanism of oxytocin-induced diuresis and (by implication) of the oxytocin-vasopressin antagonism remains unclear. Although oxytocin can increase the GFR in hydrated rats it only does so at relatively high dose levels, well above the threshold for the *anti*diuretic action of oxytocin (Dicker and Heller, 1946; cf. Pliška and Rychlík, 1967). A primary action of oxytocin on renal medullary blood flow might be considered as the source of its diuretic effect.

The diuretic response to oxytocin in hydrated and non-hydrated rats is counteracted by vasopressin (Fraser, 1942; Brunner et al., 1956); thus the diuresis induced by oxytocin (125 mU) in thirsting rats was distinctly inhibited by vasopressin in a ratio of 1:1 (Brunner et al., 1956). Presumably this is merely another aspect of the same biological antagonism.

An inhibition by oxytocin of the antidiuretic response to vasopressin has also been observed in man (Frey et al., 1959); in hydrated subjects a two- to sixfold excess of oxytocin partly or completely blocked the effect of vasopressin (0.1 mU/kg) given 15 min later. No such antagonism was found in another series of experiments carried out under very similar conditions of water-loading, dosage etc. (Vorherr, 1964); the cause of this discrepancy remains unclear.

The interaction of oxytocin and vasopressin in their effect on the excretion of ions is complex though not generally antagonistic. However, Brooks and Pickford (1958) found that in dogs with diabetes insipidus infusion of vasopressin alone (0.067 mU/min/kg) reduced sodium excretion but the addition of oxytocin (0.13 mU/min/kg) counteracted this effect; the action of oxytocin could be due to changes in the GFR or renal plasma flow. Some evidence was also obtained that the effects of oxytocin on ion excretion may in part be of central origin. Following up suggestions of antagonism HOLEČEK and HORKÝ (1966) have treated some cases of oedema of premenstrual tension, thought to be due to salt retention caused by excess vasopressin, with oxytocin; an increase in sodium excretion was observed together with relief of subjective symptoms.

2. Vascular Responses

BROOKS and PICKFORD (1958) found that oxytocin (single doses up to 5 mU/kg, or infusions of 0.2 mU/min/kg) "markedly and for a long time" increased renal plasma flow in both hydrated and normal dogs; this effect was blocked by vasopressin at vasopressin:oxytocin ratios of 1:20 or 1:30. Extensive studies on the vascular effects of oxytocin and vasopressin in which these findings were followed up showed that in normal male or dioestrous female rats oxytocin (10—30 mU i.v., or 50 mU/ml topically) dilates the mesenteric blood vessels (without changing the systemic blood pressure) whereas vasopressin (0.05 to 0.5 mU) contracts them and increases the blood pressure (LLOYD, 1959a). In normal dogs, again, oxytocin dilates the blood vessels in the hind leg whereas vasopressin contracts them (LLOYD and PICKFORD, 1962)*. In this situation oxytocin and vasopressin would be expected to act antagonistically; and, indeed, the effect of oxytocin (200—600 mU, or 0.1 IU/min) in increasing blood flow in the human hand and forearm is inhibited by vasopressin at an oxytocin:vasopressin ratio of 20:1 (KITCHIN et al., 1958; PICKFORD, 1961).

3. Other Responses

The spontaneous uterine activity of intact, conscious puerperal rabbits is stimulated by oxytocin in the milliunit range; the simultaneous injection of lysine-vasopressin in tenfold excess (50 mU or more) inhibits this response after an initial brief phase of mainly tonic excitation (FUCHS, 1964). Both in this preparation and in the anaesthetised rabbit vasopressin also inhibits the spontaneous motility of the uterus, again after brief initial stimulation (CROSS, 1958; FUCHS, 1964).

Similarly, the tonic rise or rhythmic changes in the intramammary pressure of anaesthetised lactating rabbits caused by infusions of oxytocin (5—15 mU/min) are appreciably inhibited by the simultaneous infusion of vasopressin in equimolar concentration or fourfold excess; again there is an initial period of potentiation. After withdrawal of the vasopressin the original response is restored in 20—30 min. The responses to single doses of oxytocin (4 mU) are also inhibited when they are injected during an infusion of vasopressin (80 mU/min) (KULLANDER, 1963).

In both these cases it is unlikely that competitive antagonism is involved. It seems more probable that the vasopressin causes vasoconstriction and thereby decreases the amount of oxytocin supplied to the reactive tissue. The delayed onset and relatively long duration of the inhibition are compatible with such a vascular effect.

III. Synthetic Analogues as Antagonists

A. Analogues Modified in Sequence Position 1

The analogues modified in the amino-terminal hemicystine residue which show inhibitor properties appear to fall into three distinct groups: N^{α}-acetylated derivatives, analogues in which the carbon skeleton of the terminal hemicystine

* The critical experiments were carried out with purified oxytocin as well as a commercial preparation (BROOKS and PICKFORD, 1958) so that artifacts due to the presence of chlorobutanol in the latter (KATZ, 1964; SOMLYO et al., 1966) are excluded.

residue is modified, and derivatives in which the peptide chain of the hormone is extended at the amino end by additional amino-acid or peptide residues. These three groups differ in the particular biological preparations in which they are effective and in the characteristics of their inhibitor action and it therefore seems likely that they differ also in their mode of action.

1. N^{α}-Acetylated Derivatives

N^{α}-Acetyl-lysine-vasopressin (Ac-Cys¹-Lys⁸-vasopressin) (CASH and SMITH, 1963) shows no rat pressor or avian depressor activity in doses up to 100 μg and 600 μg, respectively, but in rather large excess (10^3:1 or 10^4:1) it markedly inhibits of the rat pressor and avian depressor responses to pituitary extracts given simultaneously or shortly afterwards. Similarly, N^{α}-acetyl-arginine-vasopressin (STUDER and CASH, 1963) has no pressor activity in doses up to 200 μg but inhibits the pressor response to arginine vasopressin in this dose range and acetyl-oxytocin (BOISSONNAS, PECHÈRE, and GUTTMANN, unpublished; see BOISSONNAS et al., 1961) inhibits the avian depressor action of oxytocin. The *in vitro* uterotonic and milk-ejection activities of acetyl-oxytocin and N^{α}-acetyl-lysine-vasopressin as well as the antidiuretic activity of the vasopressin derivative are low but apparently qualitatively normal. It therefore seems that the inhibitor properties of the N^{α}-acetylated analogues are confined to, or at any rate most prominent in, those assays involving changes in blood pressure. This fact has been related to possible differences between the receptors in vascular tissue and other target tissues (CASH and SMITH, 1963); in this connection studies on isolated blood vessels could be informative. It cannot be definitely excluded that the mechanism of inhibition by the acetyl derivatives is related to that considered for the hormonogen type analogues below.

The structural range of the inhibitor properties also remains to be defined. The N-methyl derivative, MeCys¹-oxytocin, and the acyl derivative, sarcosyl-oxytocin, show low but qualitatively normal activities in the avian depressor assay (BERÁNKOVÁ-KSANDROVÁ et al., 1966) and the inhibitor properties shown by the carbamylation product of oxytocin (BISSET et al., 1964) appear to be due to the N,O-dicarbamyl derivative rather than to the N-carbamyl derivative of oxytocin (SMYTH, 1965a, b; cf. p. 755). However, although N-carbamyl-oxytocin shows weak oxytocin-like activity on the rat uterus *in vitro* (SMYTH, 1965a, b) its behaviour in the avian depressor or rat pressor assays hase not yet been reported. In any case the preparation and study of other N^{α}-acylated derivatives of oxytocin and the vasopressins would be of some interest.

2. Analogues with a Modified Carbon Skeleton

Replacement of the hemicystine residue in position 1 of oxytocin by L-penicillamine or "deaminopenicillamine", i.e. β-mercaptoisovaleric acid (SCHULZ and DU VIGNEAUD, 1966a) leads to compounds which are the most potent specific antagonists of oxytocin so far known. Both are more effective inhibitors of the avian depressor activity of oxytocin than the acetyl derivatives discussed above but their most dramatic effect is on the uterotonic action of oxytocin which is markedly inhibited at molar ratios as low as 2.5:1. The contractions of the rat uterus *in situ* elicited by a continuous infusion of oxytocin are also suppressed by simultaneous infusion of either of the two analogues. 1-D-Penicillamine-oxytocin also inhibits the avian depressor and rat uterotonic action of oxytocin but is about ten times less effective in the latter assay system than the L- and deamino-derivatives. Preliminary results show that the inhibition is reversible, competitive, and specifically directed against the action of peptides related to the neurohypophysial hormones. The structural range of the inhibitor properties is defined to some extent by the finding that the diastereomeric 1-(β-mercaptobutyric acid)-oxytocins, formally related to the "deamino-penicillamine" analogue by omission of one or the other β-methyl group, no longer behave as antagonists but show fair oxytocin-like uterotonic and avian depressor activities (SCHULZ and DU VIGNEAUD, 1966b).

The feeble inhibitor properties shown by 1-hemi-homocystine-oxytocin in the avian depressor assay (JARVIS et al., 1961) are evidently unrelated; they appear to be lacking in the corresponding deamino derivative (JARVIS et al., 1965).

3. *Extended-Chain Analogues*

A series of analogues of oxytocin in which the terminal amino group is substituted with additional amino-acid residues (Gly, Leu, Phe, Pro) or short peptide chains (Gly-Gly, Leu-Leu, Leu-Gly-Gly) (DU VIGNEAUD et al., 1960; JOŠT et al., 1961, 1963b; KASAFÍREK et al., 1965) has been found to inhibit the action of oxytocin on the avian blood pressure (DU VIGNEAUD et al., 1960; BERÁNKOVÁ-KSANDROVÁ et al., 1966) and on the milk-ejection pressure in the lactating guinea pig (BISSET, 1962; BERÁNKOVÁ-KSANDROVÁ et al., 1966). The extent to which individual compounds of this group show oxytocin-like or inhibitor properties depends on the structure (i.e., the nature of the added amino-acid or peptide sequence), the biological preparation and the experimental conditions (dose sequence, route of administration).

Typically, after injection of such an analogue the blood pressure of the anaesthetised rooster decreases slowly and recovers slowly. There is marked tachyphylaxis, and the response to standard ("challenge") doses of oxytocin, given while the response to the analogue lasts and for some time after it has faded, is markedly decreased (Fig. 3a). With glycyl-glycyl-oxytocin and leucyl-glycyl-glycyl-oxytocin the onset of the response is sometimes rapid though recovery is again slow, and reactivity to subsequent doses of the analogue and to oxytocin is again decreased. Prolyl-oxytocin is exceptional in that doses up to 160 μg produce hardly any depressor effect but even 20 μg will inhibit the response to subsequent injections of oxytocin (BERÁNKOVÁ-KSANDROVÁ et al., 1966). DU VIGNEAUD et al. (1960) found that subthreshold doses of glycyl-oxytocin could also inhibit the avian depressor response to oxytocin; after higher doses of the analogue the inhibition lasted for 6 hours or more.

The action of this group of analogues on the mammary-gland pressure of the lactating guinea pig is described elsewhere in this volume by BISSET. Again, the most general response is a protracted increase in milk-ejection pressure followed by tachyphylaxis and inhibition of the response to oxytocin; sometimes the initial response is absent, particularly if the analogue is given in gradually increasing doses, and only the inhibitory action is observed. The type of response also depends on the route of administration (intravenous or close arterial injection).

No inhibition has been observed with isolated mammary gland strips, on the rat uterus *in vitro* or *in situ*, or in the rat pressor assay.

A clue to the probable mechanism by which this group of analogues inhibits the action of oxytocin is provided by their other properties which are those of "hormonogens", i.e. derivatives which in themselves are weakly active or inactive but are capable of releasing the active hormone by enzyme action, particularly *in vivo* (BERÁNKOVÁ-KSANDROVÁ et al., 1966). A causal relationship between their hormonogen character and inhibitor properties is suggested by the fact that the structural range of both these peculiarities is identical: Thus sarcosyl-oxytocin and D-leucyl-oxytocin, though formally similar in structure to the analogues discussed, would not be expected to be susceptible to activation by the common proteolytic enzymes and neither of these derivatives shows either protracted action* or inhibitor activity. To rationalise this parallelism it is simplest to assume that the "inhibitor" properties of these derivatives are due not to the analogues themselves but to the oxytocin released from them *in vivo*, i.e. that we are dealing not with true antagonism, but with oxytocin tachyphylaxis; both the mammary gland

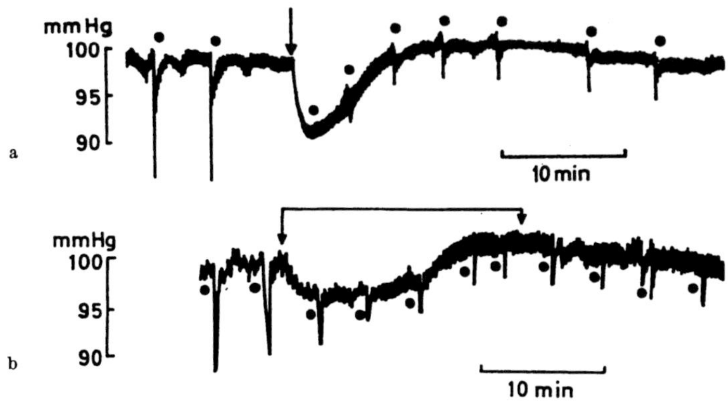

Fig. 3. Effect of phenylalanyl-oxytocin (a) and oxytocin infusion (b) on the avian blood pressure and its response to oxytocin. a) At arrow, (Phe-Cys)[1]-oxytocin (50 μg), at dots oxytocin (40 mU). b) Between arrows, infusion of oxytocin (20 mU/min), at dots single doses of oxytocin (20 mU). POLÁČEK and KREJČÍ, unpublished experiments; cf. BERÁNKOVÁ-KSANDROVÁ et al. (1966)

and the fowl preparation are known to be liable to tachyphylaxis. Differences in the rate of activation of individual hormonogens (depending also on the route of administration) would determine the rate at which the oxytocin level in the receptor tissue in built up, and this in turn would determine the balance between normal response and the development of tachyphylaxis.

This interpretation has been confirmed by experiments in which the "inhibitor" action of the hormonogens was closely mimicked by continuous infusions of oxytocin, both in the lactating guinea pig (see Fig. 7 on p. 530) and in the anaesthetised rooster (Fig. 3b). By varying the rate of infusion it was possible to imitate the situation where loss of sensitivity follows an initial response and (with subthreshold infusions) the case where "inhibition" alone is seen. It therefore seems beyond doubt that this particular class of oxytocin "antagonists" acts merely by creating conditions for the development of tachyphylaxis; though of course the molecular mechanism causing loss of responsiveness remains unclear.

It is conceivable that further structural variations in the hormonogen series may, by changing distribution properties and the susceptibility to particular enzymes, direct the tachyphylaxis-inducing effect of such analogues toward particular target tissues. The same principles might also serve to accentuate the inhibitor properties of certain other analogues of the neurohypophysial hormones.

B. Analogues Modified in Sequence Position 2

Variations in sequence position 2 have so far provided the richest crop of antagonists and partial agonists of the neurohypophysial hormones. In dealing with this group of analogues it will be convenient first do discuss the properties of its most extensively studied member in some detail, and then to illustrate the effect of further structural variations on these properties.

* The somewhat protracted antidiuretic action of D-leucyl-oxytocin in the rat is thought to be due to the presence of traces of the L-leucyl isomer (BERÁNKOVÁ-KSANDROVÁ et al., 1966).

1. *2-O-Methyltyrosine-oxytocin*

2-O-Methyltyrosine-oxytocin, referred to as methyloxytocin in the sequel, was early found to inhibit the pressor effect of arginine-vasopressin (LAW and DU VIGNEAUD, 1960) and the uterotonic action of oxytocin *in vitro* (JOŠT et al., 1961, 1963a; BERÁNKOVÁ et al., 1961). Later it was found to have abnormal properties, including inhibitor properties, in a number of other biological systems.

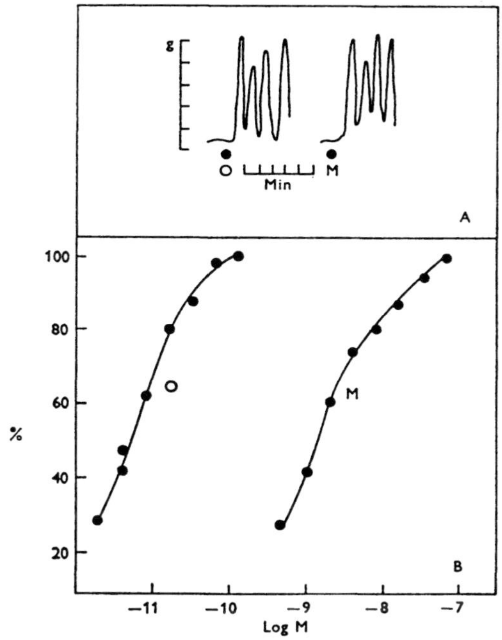

Fig. 4a

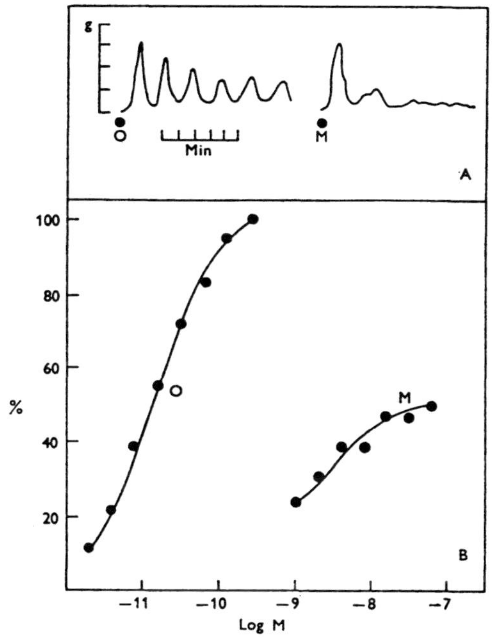

Fig. 4b

Fig. 4. Responses of isolated uteri from oestrogenised rats to oxytocin (O) and methyloxytocin (M). MUNSICK's (1960) medium without magnesium, calcium concentration 0.6 mM (a) or 0.3 mM (b), isometric recording, 30°. Top: time course of responses to oxytocin (1 mU/ml) and methyloxytocin (1 μg/ml), bottom: log dose–response curves recorded by cumulative dose procedure (doses in moles/5 ml). Examples of (a) full agonism, (b) "partial agonism". From KREJČÍ et al. (1966)

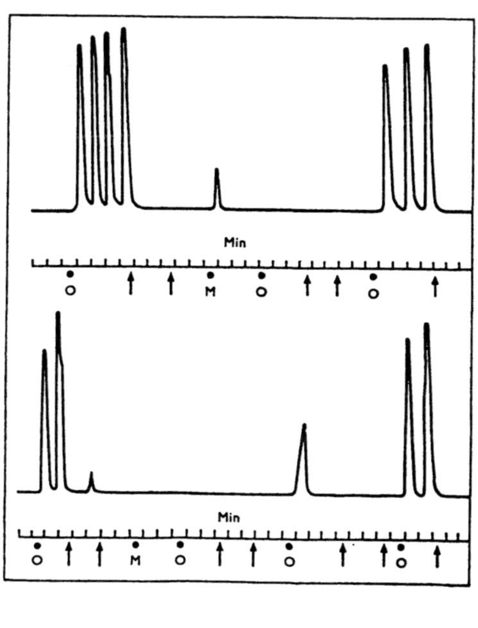

Fig. 5. Inhibition of the response of the isolated rat uterus to oxytocin by methyloxytocin. Top 30°, bottom 24°, other conditions and symbols as for Fig. 4b; arrows denote change of medium. From KREJČÍ et al. (1966)

a) *Action on the Uterus:* The apparently conflicting reports of *in vitro* uterotonic properties (LAW and DU VIGNEAUD, 1960) and inhibitor properties (BERÁNKOVÁ et al., 1961) for methyloxytocin were resolved when it was found that the type of response depends on the experimental conditions (RUDINGER and KREJČÍ, 1962; KREJČÍ et al., 1964, 1966, 1967b). Under some conditions, to be discussed below, the action of methyloxytocin on the rat uterus *in vitro* is qualitatively indistinguishable from that of oxytocin, the potency of the analogue being 1.0—1.5 IU/mg; the log dose–response curves for analogue and hormone are parallel and the maximal response at high doses is identical for both compounds (full agonism; Fig. 4a) though methyloxytocin does not cause contracture. In other experiments methyloxytocin still elicits rhythmic contractions of the uterus but their frequency is lower and their amplitude generally decreases rapidly with time; log dose–response curves for the analogue tend to have lower slopes and maxima, most markedly so when they are obtained by a cumulative dose procedure (RUDINGER and KREJČÍ, 1962). This type of behaviour (Fig. 4b) in many respects conforms to the definition of partial agonism. Finally, under suitable conditions methyloxytocin has no uterotonic effect, or at most causes a single contraction without

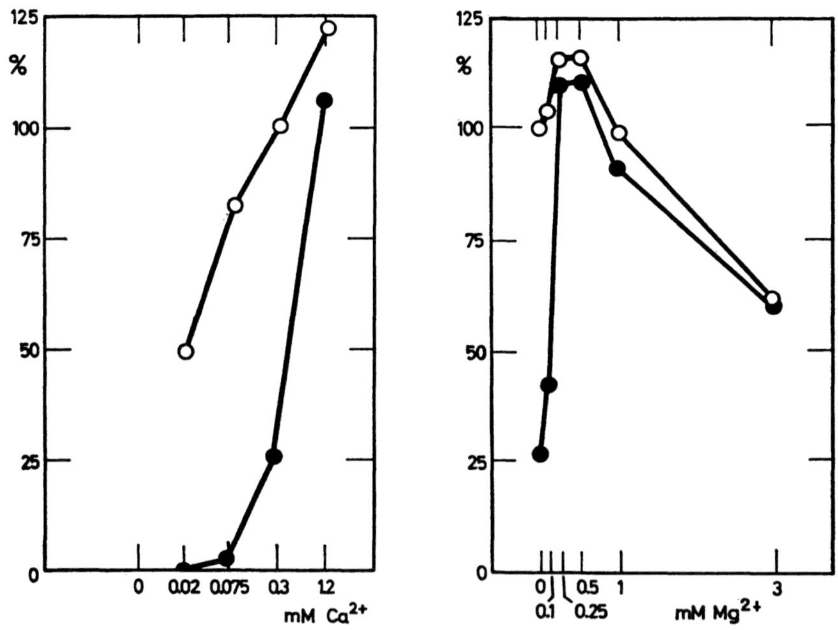

Fig. 6. Effect of the calcium and magnesium concentration on the response of the isolated rat uterus to oxytocin. Oestrogenised rats, HOLTON's (1948) medium, cumulative dose procedure; left: varying concentrations of calcium in the absence of magnesium, right: varying concentrations of magnesium in the presence of 0.3 mM calcium. The maximal response achieved at each ion concentration is expressed as a percentage of the maximal response to oxytocin in a medium containing 0.3 mM calcium and no magnesium. Each point is the mean of 3—8 experiments; ○ oxytocin, ● methyloxytocin. From KREJČÍ et al. (1967b)

regular dependence on dose, and the uterotonic action of oxytocin added to the organ bath is partly or wholly inhibited (Fig. 5); under these conditions, then, the analogue behaves as an antagonist of oxytocin.

It should be stressed that in all situations where spontaneous uterine activity is found, whatever the conditions, methyloxytocin, like oxytocin, stimulates this activity.

When oestrogen-dominated uteri (from rats in natural oestrus, or animals pretreated with oestrogen) are used, as is customary in the assay for uterotonic activity, the "anomalous" response to methyloxytocin (partial agonism or antagonism) is favoured by a decrease in the calcium concentration of the medium (from 0.6 mM in Holton's (1948) or Munsick's (1960) solution to 0.2—0.3 mM), the absence of magnesium, and low temperature (20—24°). The effect of the calcium concentration in altering the character of the response is illustrated in Fig. 4, the dependence of the maximal response to methyloxytocin and oxytocin in cumulative dose experiments on the concentration of calcium and magnesium is shown in Fig. 6 (Krejčí et al., 1964, 1967b). At very low calcium concentrations (0.05—0.1 mM) spontaneous activity appeared in some experiments which responded alike to oxytocin and methyloxytocin (Krejčí et al., 1966).

Progesterone-dominated rat uteri frequently show a tendency to irregular spontaneous contractions; again, these are stimulated by both oxytocin and methyloxytocin. In the absence of spontaneous activity, the type of response to methyloxytocin by such uteri shows little dependence on the calcium concentration.

On the relatively insensitive uterine strips taken from untreated rabbits methyloxytocin almost invariably acts as an antagonist of oxytocin. With the more sensitive preparations taken from rabbits pretrated with oestrogen contractile responses to methyloxytocin are also observed, and the tendency for the analogue to act as an agonist increases with the sensitivity of the muscle strip as indicated by the threshold active dose of oxytocin (Krejčí et al., 1967b).

When rat uterine strips are depolarised with increased potassium concentrations they respond to oxytocin by a single, slow, sustained contraction (Edman and Schild, 1962; Daniel et al., 1962). Under these conditions methyloxytocin may act either as an agonist or as an antagonist of oxytocin. In Krebs-Ringer media containing up to 100 mM K^+ both types of behaviour were observed, with no marked dependence on the calcium concentration; in K_2SO_4-Ringer solutions (Edman and Schild, 1962) the analogue behaved as an antagonist in all experiments (Krejčí et al., 1967b).

On the rat uterus *in situ* methyloxytocin exerts an oxytocin-like effect (Bisset, 1964; Krejčí et al., 1967b) with a potency of 20—50 IU/mg; an earlier report of inhibition (Beránková et al., 1961) could not be confirmed. Methyloxytocin also has a uterotonic effect qualitatively indistinguishable from that of oxytocin on the pregnant human uterus at term (Brotánek, Kazda, Hodr, Štembera, Rudinger, and Vondráček, unpublished results; cf. Hodr et al., 1964). In view of the ionic composition of serum and tissue fluids these results are not surprising.

The character of the antagonistic action of methyloxytocin was investigated using uterine strips from oestrogenised rats or from rabbits, in media with decreased calcium concentrations. When inhibition was observed it was found to be surmountable by increased doses of oxytocin, and reversible. The effect of the antagonist was greater when it was added to the organ bath 2—3 min before the oxytocin than when both peptides were added together but there was no further increase in the effect when the time interval was increased beyond 5 min. The inhibition was specifically directed against oxytocin and structurally related peptides (vasopressin, Val^3-oxytocin); methyloxytocin did not affect the response of the rat uterus to norepinephrine, acetylcholine, ergometrine, bradykinin, angiotensin, or Substance P (Rudinger and Krejčí, 1962; Bisset, 1962). In many experiments the inhibition met the criteria for competitive antagonism as expressed in the parallel displacement of log dose–response curves for oxytocin in the presence of the inhibitor (Fig. 7) or by the convergence in one point of the lines in the Lineweaver-Burk transformation of such curves (Rudinger and Krejčí,

1962; KREJČÍ et al., 1966, 1967b). However, the potency of the inhibitor was rather variable, sometimes even for repeated experiments on the same organ preparation; the molar ratio of methyloxytocin to oxytocin required to produce 50% inhibition of the response to a submaximal dose of the hormone varied from 12 to 125 in series of experiments with rat uteri and from 3 to 12 (occasionally up to 60) with rabbit uteri (KREJČÍ et al., 1967b). In another series of 35 experiments with rat uteri values of pA_2 between 9.80 and 9.95 were found (mean 9.85) (POLÁČEK and KREJČÍ, unpublished results). In a number of experiments with both rat and rabbit uterus the dose–response relations were more irregular and did not meet the requirements of competitive antagonism; however, this may be due not so much to a genuine variation in the character of the inhibition as to the experimental difficulties inherent in the use of the uterus preparation (the rhythmic nature of the contractions, importance of the propagated response, sensitivity to extrinsic factors etc.; KREJČÍ et al., 1967b).

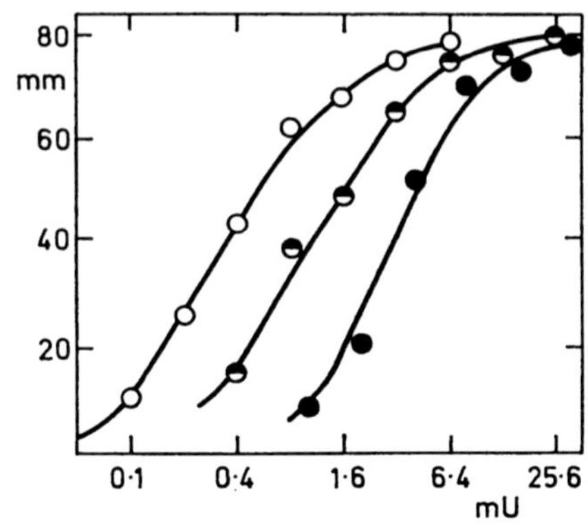

Fig. 7. Effect of methyloxytocin on the log dose–response relation for oxytocin on the isolated rat uterus. Rat in natural oestrus, Krebs-Ringer phosphate medium with 0.2 mM calcium, 30°, isometric recording, cumulative dose procedure. Concentration of methyloxytocin ○ nil, ◒ 0,2 μg/ml, ● 0.5 μg/ml. POLÁČEK and KREČÍ, unpublished experiment; cf. RUDINGER and KREJČÍ (1962), KREJČÍ et al. (1964, 1967b)

The most important variables affecting the character of the response to methyloxytocin appear to be the hormonal state of the uterus, the temperature, and the ion composition of the medium, in particular the calcium concentration. However, it should be stressed that the effect of calcium on the response of the uterus to methyloxytocin cannot be simply correlated with the interstitial concentration of this ion. An experiment which is particularly instructive in this respect (KREJČÍ et al., 1966) involves washing a rat uterine strip with calcium-free medium until the contractile response to both oxytocin and methyloxytocin disappears; if the calcium is now restored to the medium stepwise to concentrations of 0.1, 0.2, 0.4, and 0.8 mM with up to 1 hour allowed for equilibration at each step the response to oxytocin is restored at the lowest calcium concentrations but methyloxytocin still acts as an antagonist in the solution with 0.8 mM calcium, a concentration which invariably brings out the agonist properties of the analogue when a normal experimental protocol is followed. This result among others suggests that it is not the interstitial calcium concentration alone which governs the response to methyloxytocin but that a separate metabolic compartment of the ion, in slow equilibrium with the bulk of the solution, is involved in a critical way. The effect of the hormonal state of the uterus on the type of response to methyloxytocin and the difference in behaviour of the analogue in the two depolarising media (see above) may also be rationalised by considering the possible effects on membrane-bound calcium (see KREJČÍ et al., 1967b).

This conclusion links the somewhat complex behaviour of methyloxytocin to current ideas about the mode of action of oxytocin on the uterus (e.g. CSAPO, 1961; EDMAN and SCHILD, 1962; DANIEL et al., 1962) according to which the release of calcium from binding sites at or near the cell surface plays a crucial role in the initiation of uterine contraction by oxytocin.

On this basis the following model has been proposed for the action of methyloxytocin on the uterus (KREJČÍ et al., 1966, 1967b; RUDINGER, 1966): In relation to the oxytocin receptors of the uterus and the ("primary") process directly resulting from the peptide–receptor interaction, methyloxytocin is essentially a partial agonist. However, this primary process is linked to the final observed response of muscle contraction by a complex series of events. The excitation–contraction coupling may involve variable parameters affecting the magnitude of the final response which is elicited by a given intensity of the primary process. Under some conditions the maximal intensity of the primary process achieved on saturation of the receptors with the partial agonist, methyloxytocin, may be insufficient to lead to an observable final response whereas the higher intensity achieved by combination of the receptors with oxytocin will still initiate contraction; under such conditions the observed behaviour of methyloxytocin would be essentially that of a competitive antagonist. If, on the other hand, the maximal overt response is limited in such a way that it can be initiated by the degree of primary action of which even methyloxytocin is capable, and a further increase in the intensity of the primary process results in no further increase in the final response, then the observed behaviour of methyloxytocin will be that of a full agonist. Obviously, under intermediate conditions the behaviour of methyloxytocin even with respect to the observed response may be that of a partial agonist. If it is in addition assumed that at least one of the parameters regulating the relation between the primary

Table 3. *Action of 2-O-Alkyltyrosine Analogues of Oxytocin and Vasopressin on the Rat Pressor Response to the Natural Hormones*

Analogue[1])	Agonist[1,2]	Molar ratio antagonist: :agonist	Inhibition of response, %	Ref.
(OMe)Tyr²-OT	AVP	2000	50	3
	AVP	4000	100	3
	SPE	5000—10000	50	4
	OT	20—50	distinct	4
(OMe)Tyr²-LVP	SPE	160—320	25	4
	SPE	800—1600	30	4
(OEt)Tyr²-LVP	SPE	200—400	50	4
(Gly-Cys)¹-(OMe)Tyr²-LVP . .	SPE	5000—10000	20	4

[1] OT oxytocin, LVP lysine-vasopressin, AVP arginine-vasopressin, SPE standard posterior pituitary extract. — [2] Doses 2.5—10 mU of pressor activity. — [3] LAW and DU VIGNEAUD, 1960. — [4] KREJČÍ et al., 1967a.

process and the final response is closely related to the calcium concentration in a particular metabolic compartment ("membrane-bound" calcium) then a model of this kind accounts for many of the observed features of methyloxytocin action. Once more it appears (see p. 752) that the receptor theory, albeit in somewhat modified form, can be applied to relatively complex peptides as to simpler drugs.

It will be shown below that the inhibitor properties of methyloxytocin, or related anomalies in response, are patent in a wide range of biological preparations. This provides some experimental support for the speculation — attractive on the grounds of economy of hypothesis — that in a variety of target tissues the primary process resulting from interaction with the neurohypophysial hormones has certain common, fundamental features, however varied the character of the final observed response.

b) *Vascular Responses:* The inhibition by methyloxytocin of the pressor response to vasopressin was first reported by LAW and DU VIGNEAUD (1960) and studied in more detail by KREJČÍ et al. (1967a). The results in Table 3 show that the pressor action of the vasopressins in the rat preparation of DEKANSKI (1952) is distinctly inhibited by a 2000- to 5000-fold molar excess of methyloxytocin; the inhibitor is more effective against the pressor action of oxytocin in the same preparation. Methyloxytocin also inhibits the pressor response to the vasopressins in pithed rats and in anaesthetised cats but in rabbits the analogue often shows a slight pressor effect, with no distinct inhibition of the response to vasopressin (KREJČÍ et al., 1967a).

In the assay for avian depressor activity methyloxytocin has an oxytocin-like effect; however, it produces marked tachyphylaxis and a parallel loss of sensitivity to oxytocin (KREJČÍ and POLÁČEK, unpublished results).

The persistence of the inhibitor effect in these preparations suggest a relation more complicated than simple competitive antagonism and may reflect the complex nature of neurohypophysial hormone action on the vascular system. However, a direct peripheral interaction is suggested by the finding (PICKFORD, 1966)

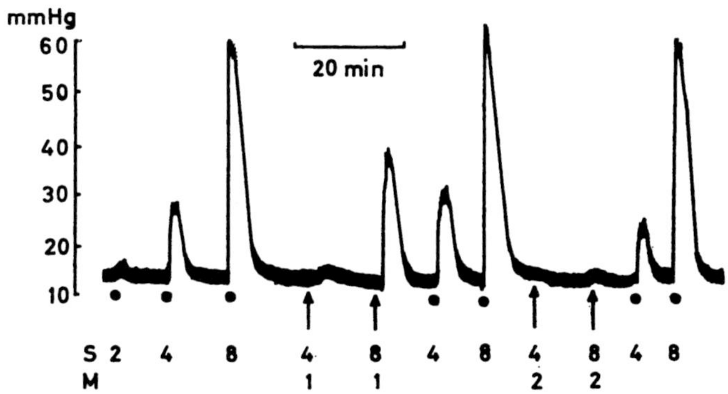

Fig. 8. Inhibition of the response of the isolated perfused rat tail artery to pituitary extract by methyloxytocin. Kymographic record of perfusion pressure for artery segment perfused with Tyrode solution (1 ml/min) containing 26 μM $CaNa_2$EDTA at 37°; pituitary extract (S, doses in mU) and methyloxytocin (M, doses in μg) were added to the organ bath (2.5 ml); the medium was changed when the contraction had passed its maximum. KUPKOVÁ, VÁVRA, and KREJČÍ, unpublished results

that methyloxytocin inhibits the effect of oxytocin on blood flow in the hind leg of the dog and in the rat (which may be vasodilator or vasoconstrictor according to conditions; LLOYD, 1959a, b; LLOYD and PICKFORD, 1961, 1962) regardless of the character of the original response. Furthermore, the direct effect of methyloxytocin at receptors in vascular tissue is confirmed by the observation that it inhibits the response of the perfused isolated rat tail artery to vasopressin (Fig. 8) and of the umbilical artery strip to oxytocin (KUPKOVÁ, VÁVRA, and KREJČÍ, unpublished results).

c) *Other Responses:* Methyloxytocin, like oxytocin, increases the milk-ejection pressure in the lactating guinea pig and contracts strips of guinea-pig or rat mammary gland tissue *in vitro* (BISSET, 1962, 1964). The rat mammary gland strip contracts more slowly in response to methyloxytocin than in response to oxytocin; the analogue causes distinct tachyphylaxis and loss of sensitivity to oxytocin (POLÁČEK et al., 1967).

Methyloxytocin increases the water permeability of the toad bladder, the maximal response being the same as that to oxytocin (RASMUSSEN et al., 1963). The analogue also increases sodium transport by the frog skin (NEMČEK et al., 1963; MOREL and BASTIDE, 1964); although in this preparation too the maximal effect is the same for methyloxytocin and for oxytocin, a decrease in the calcium concentration in the organ bath reduces the response to methyloxytocin more sharply than that to oxytocin so that the relative potency of the analogue decreases (JANÁČEK and KLEINZELLER, unpublished).

In the ethanol-anaesthetised water-loaded rat methyloxytocin has an antidiuretic effect (JOŠT et al., 1963a) and under the assay conditions used (PLIŠKA and RYCHLÍK, 1967) no inhibition of the response to oxytocin or vasopressin given subsequently has been noted. However, there is some evidence that large doses may cause tachyphylaxis in this preparation (VÁVRA, unpublished results).

The injection or infusion of oxytocin or lysine vasopressin into chloralosed cats causes an increase in blood pressure and in sodium excretion; similar changes are observed during carotid occlusion. Infusion of methyloxytocin abolishes the natriuretic (but not the pressor) effect of oxytocin and of leucyl-glycyl-glycyl-oxytocin (as well as the natriuretic response to carotid occlusion) and the pressor but not the natriuretic effect of lysine-vasopressin (CORT, 1964; CORT et al., 1966). The difference in the susceptibility of the natriuretic responses induced by oxytocin and by vasopressin to inhibition by methyloxytocin may be a matter of dosage.

2. Other Analogues of Oxytocin Modified in Position 2

In order to assess the importance of particular structural features for the inhibitor properties of methyloxytocin a series of additional oxytocin analogues was prepared in which the *p*-substituent in the aromatic side-chain was methyl, ethyl, ethoxyl (ZHUZE et al., 1964) and amino (RUDINGER, unpublished) (partial formulae in Fig. 9). Phe[2]-Oxytocin, with hydrogen as the "*p*-substituent" (BODANSZKY and DU VIGNEAUD, 1959a, b; JAQUENOUD and BOISSONNAS, 1959; JOŠT et al., 1963a) was also reinvestigated for purposes of comparison. Table 4 summarises the inhibitor properties of this series of analogues in three biological systems.

Table 4. *Summary of Inhibitor Properties shown by some Oxytocin Analogues Modified in Sequence Position 2* (After RUDINGER, 1965)

Amino acid in position 2	Inhibition of response: rat uterus in vitro[1]	avian depressor[2]	natriuretic (cat)[3]
(*p*-NH$_2$)Phe .	∸	—	—
Phe	∸	—	—
(*p*-Me)Phe .	∸/+	—	±
(*p*-Et)Phe . .	+	±	+
(O-Me)Tyr .	+	+	+
(O-Et)Tyr . .	+	+	+

[1] Under conditions favouring inhibition, cf. text; ∸ denotes partial agonism, + inhibition. See also Table 5. — [2] Pronounced tachyphylaxis and inhibition of response to oxytocin denoted by +. — [3] Inhibition of response to carotid occlusion or (in the case of methyloxytocin) infusion of oxytocin shown by +, natriuretic response by —; CORT et al., 1966.

Because of the complexity of the factors involved it had not proved possible to define the conditions which would guarantee a particular reactivity of rat uterine preparations toward methyloxytocin. A partial definition was achieved for the purpose of comparing the 2-substituted analogues by selecting organ preparations on which methyloxytocin acted as an antagonist of oxytocin in the media used (MUNSICK's (1960) or Krebs-Ringer phosphate without glucose, both with 0.2 mM calcium and no magnesium). Under these conditions Phe[2]-oxytocin and (*p*-NH$_2$)Phe[2]-oxytocin invariably acted as partial agonists of oxytocin, (O-Et)Tyr[2]-oxytocin as an antagonist, (*p*-Et)Phe[2]-oxytocin either as a partial agonist or antagonist; some quantitative relations are given in Table 5. In experiments with rabbit uterine strips of low sensitivity even Phe[2]-oxytocin occasionally behaved as a full antagonist of oxytocin; the *p*-amino derivative again acted as a partial agonist (POLÁČEK and KREJČÍ, unpublished results).

The results for the avian depressor assay in Table 4 refer to the occurrence of tachyphylaxis; in the case of (O-Et)Tyr²-oxytocin this becomes so marked that the potency of the analogue cannot be determined by the conventional assay pro-

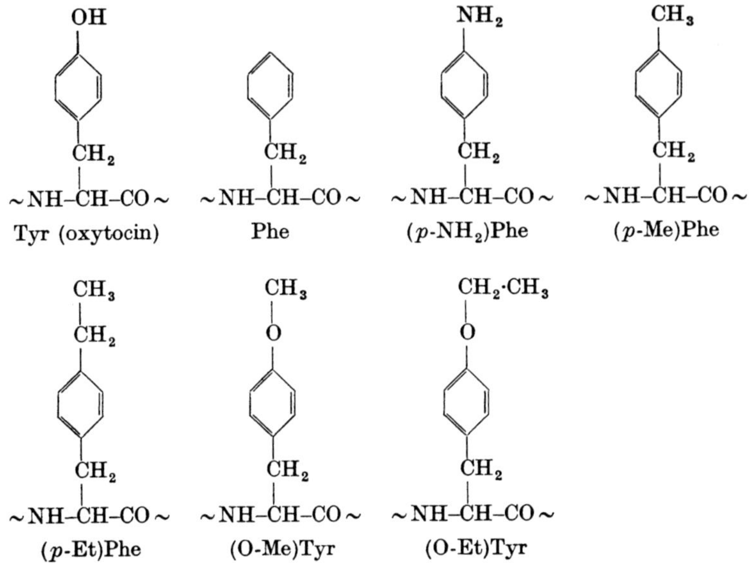

Fig. 9. Partial structures (amino-acid residue in sequence position 2) of some oxytocin analogues acting as partial agonists or antagonists

cedure (ZHUZE et al., 1964). (O-Et)Tyr²-oxytocin and (*p*-Et)Phe²-oxytocin inhibit the response of the isolated rat tail artery to vasopressin (KUPKOVÁ, VÁVRA, and KREJČÍ, unpublished results).

Table 5. *Inhibition of the Response of the Isolated Rat Uterus to Oxytocin and some Analogues Modified in Position 2* (KREJČÍ and POLÁČEK, unpublished results)[1 2]

Amino acid in position 2	Incidence of partial agonism	Incidence of antagonism	pA_2 ±S.E.
(p-NH_2)Phe	7/7	0/7	—
Phe	8/8	0/8	—
(p-Et)Phe	2/14	10/14	9.70 ± 0.06[3]
(O-Me)Tyr		35[2]	9.85 ± 0.03
(O-Et)Tyr	0/11	11/11	9.36 ± 0.13[4]

[1] Oestrous rats, Krebs-Ringer phosphate solution with 0.2 mM Ca, no Mg and no glucose, 30°, isometric recording. — [2] Only preparations on which methyloxytocin acted as antagonist were used. — [3] Not significantly different from pA_2 for methyloxytocin in parallel experiments. — [4] Significantly ($P < 0.05$) less than pA_2 for methyloxytocin in parallel experiments (9.81 ± 0.08).

The effects on the natriuresis induced by carotid occlusion in cats have been included in Table 4 because of their possible relation to the natriuresis caused by oxytocin; Phe²- and (p-NH_2)Phe²-oxytocin do, indeed, show an oxytocin-like natriuretic action in the chloralosed cat whereas (p-Et)Phe^2- and (O-Et)Tyr^2-oxytocin inhibit the natriuretic response to carotid occlusion and (p-Me)Phe^2-oxytocin is intermediate in properties, causing slight natriuresis followed by weak inhibition (CORT et al., 1966).

The response of the isolated rat mammary gland strip to (O-Et)Tyr^2-oxytocin develops still more slowly, and shows even more pronounced tachyphylaxis, than its response to the methyl derivative; in the case of (p-Et)Phe^2-oxytocin only the slowed response was noted (POLÁČEK et al., 1967).

In summary it appears that the inhibitor properties and related anomalies in this series of analogues increase in the order in which the compounds are listed in Table 4. Thus (O-Et)Tyr^2-oxytocin is apparently more effective an oxytocin antagonist than methyloxytocin in the sense that its inhibitor action is in evidence over a wider range of conditions though the pA_2 values in Table 5 indicate that it is somewhat less effective in terms of the molar concentration required to produce a given degree of inhibition. The structural feature of the p-substituent most important for the emergence of antagonism appears to be its bulk (the p-amino group being a possible exception, perhaps because of its similarity to the p-hydroxyl group of the hormone in size, polarity, and hydrogen-bonding ability). Partial agonism and antagonism may thus be associated both with loss of functionality at this site in the hormone molecule and with steric hindrance, suggesting that some process essential for activity but not for binding takes place in proximity to this site in the hormone-receptor complex (ZHUZE et al., 1964; RUDINGER, 1965; CORT et al., 1966).

Replacement of the aromatic side-chain in position 2 by an aliphatic residue, either non-functional (leucine; JOŠT et al., 1963a) or with functional substituents (α-amino-adipic acid or its δ-amide; MNDZHOYAN, JOŠT and RUDINGER, unpublished results) leads to analogues which once more behave as partial agonists or antagonists on the rat uterus *in vitro*; however, omission of the aromatic group in addition causes a considerable loss of affinity (KREJČÍ et al., 1964; POLÁČEK and KREJČÍ, unpublished results).

The diastereomer of oxytocin, D-Tyr^2-oxytocin, and its deamino analogue have fair avian depressor activity but low uterotonic activity and in addition they are reported to inhibit the oxytocic action of oxytocin (DRABAREK and DU VIGNEAUD, 1965); further pharmacological studies will show if the features of this antagonism permit these diastereomers to be classed with the group of analogues discussed above. No inhibitor properties are recorded for the oxytocin analogues with the tyrosine replaced by N-methyltyrosine (HUGUENIN and BOISSONNAS, 1961), serine (GUTTMANN and BOISSONNAS, 1960), or glycine (DRABAREK, 1964); the first of these in particular might merit reexamination.

The product obtained by reaction of oxytocin with cyanate (BISSET et al., 1963) behaved as an antagonist of oxytocin or vasopressin action on the rat uterus *in vitro*, the avian blood pressure, and the blood pressure of the rat (BISSET et al., 1964). Comparison of the properties of this product with those of N-acetyloxytocin and N-sarcosyloxytocin on the one hand and of the analogues modified in the tyrosine residue on the other suggested that an O-carbamyl derivative rather than a product substituted in the amino group alone might be responsible for the inhibitor action and SMYTH (1965a, b) has established that the inhibitor is, in fact, the N,O-dicarbamyloxytocin present together with the N-carbamyl derivative in the reaction mixture; N-carbamyloxytocin itself has weak oxytocin-like activity but apparently no inhibitor properties. The study of quantitative relations will presumably have to await the preparation of reasonably homogeneous specimens of N,O-dicarbamyloxytocin. An interesting property of dicarbamyloxytocin —

and one which is likely to complicate its pharmacological behaviour — is its sensitivity to hydrolysis. It is slowly converted to the N-carbamyl derivative in aqueous solution even under "physiological" conditions (pH 7.4, 37°) (SMYTH, 1965a).

Omission of the amino group from methyloxytocin, in deamino¹-(O-Me)Tyr²-oxytocin, seems to accentuate its inhibitor properties; according to preliminary results the analogue acts as an oxytocin antagonist even in media containing about 0.6 mM calcium but still has an oxytocin-like effect on the spontaneously contracting organ strip in Tyrode solution or on the rat uterus *in situ* (BERDE, unpublished results, cf. BERDE and SAAMELI, 1966; KREJČÍ and BISSET, unpublished results). A search for analogues with an increased range of inhibitor properties might therefore well be directed toward derivatives modified in positions 1 and 2 simultaneously.

3. *Analogues of Lysine-Vasopressin Modified in Position 2*

Inhibitor properties are also found in (O-Me)Tyr²-Lys⁸-vasopressin, referred to as methylvasopressin below (ŠORM, 1961; SIEDEL et al., 1963; ZAORAL et al., 1965) and the corresponding O-ethyl derivative (ZAORAL et al., 1965). Methylvasopressin retains fair pressor activity (50—100 IU/mg) in anaesthetised or decerebrated rabbits and cats, without any indication of antagonism, but in rats it shows low pressor activity (about 2 IU/mg) with marked tachyphylaxis and inhibition of the response to vasopressin (Fig. 10a) (VOGEL and HERGOTT, 1963; KREJČÍ et al., 1967a). In the rat preparation of DEKANSKI (1952) 1.6 μg methylvasopressin inhibited the response to vasopressin (2.5 and 5 mU) by about 25% (Table 3) but even with doses higher than 8 μg the degree of inhibition did not exceed about 30% (KREJČÍ et al., 1967a). In the anaesthetised rooster doses of about 65 and 130 μg had no effect on the blood pressure but inhibited the response to 0.1 mU of oxytocin by 20% in the first case and completely in the second (VOGEL and HERGOTT, 1963). On the isolated perfused rat tail artery methylvasopressin shows some constrictor activity but invariably inhibits the response to vasopressin. In most (but not all) experiments the analogue caused a parallel shift of the log dose–response curves for vasopressin, suggesting competitive inhibition (KUPKOVÁ, VÁVRA, and KREJČÍ, unpublished results).

The isolated rat uterus only in rare instances responds to high doses of methylvasopressin by slight contraction; however, the analogue inhibits the response to oxytocin even when the hormone is tested after the analogue has been washed out. In experiments in which the organ was exposed to about 0.25 and 25 μg/ml of the analogue for 3 min, rinsed for 3 min, and exposed to oxytocin (2.4 mU/ml) 4 min later the response to the hormone was inhibited by 20% and more than 90%, respectively. Reversal of the inhibition requires repeated or prolonged washing. The degree of inhibition depends on the time of exposure to the analogue (VOGEL and HERGOTT, 1963).

Although the action of methylvasopressin, like that of methyloxytocin, shows many features of competitive antagonism the slow reversal of the effects, not only in experiments *in vivo* but even on the isolated uterus or arterial segment, cannot as yet be accounted for. The similarity in the molecular size and structure of agonist and antagonist makes it unlikely that the two differ to any great extent in their diffusion coefficients.

In the O-ethyltyrosine analogue the agonist properties are further attenuated and the inhibitor properties more pronounced: in the rat, 100 μg of the analogue elicited a slight pressor reaction, or none at all, but completely blocked the response to 5 mU of vasopressin; a dose of 2 μg caused marked inhibition (Fig. 10b; Table 3). (O-Et)Tyr²-Lys⁸-vasopressin, unlike the O-methyl derivative, also inhibits the pressor response to vasopressin in anaesthetised or decerebrated cats though in these species the analogue still has appreciable pressor activity (KREJČÍ et al., 1967a). On the rat tail artery the ethyl derivative acts purely as a vasopressin antagonist.

In an attempt to combine the properties of (O-Me)Tyr²-Lys⁸-vasopressin with those of a hormonogen, the N^{α}-glycyl derivative has been synthesised (ZAORAL et al., 1963; ZAORAL and ŠORM, 1964, 1965). In dibenamine-treated rats the analogue generally causes a brief drop in the blood pressure or no change; only occasionally is there a slight protracted rise in the blood pressure. On the other hand, in pithed rats a protracted pressor response is obtained in more than half the experiments; the cause of this difference remains unclear. In dibenamine-treated rats the analogue inhibits the response to vasopressin (Table 3) (KREJČÍ et al., 1967a). The compound also inhibits the uterotonic action of oxytocin *in vitro*; with a 300-fold excess inhibition was complete (ZAORAL and ŠORM, 1965).

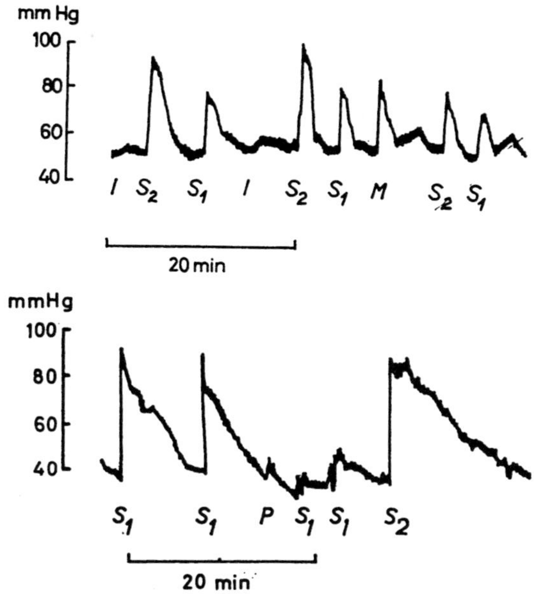

a

b

Fig. 10. Effect of (O-Me)Tyr²- and (O-Et)Tyr²-lysine-vasopressin on the blood pressure of the rat and its response to vasopressin. Rat preparation of DEKANSKI (1952); S_1, S_2 standard posterior pituitary extract (2.5 and 5.0 mU, respectively), M methylvasopressin (50 µg), P (O-Et)Tyr²-Lys⁸-vasopressin (25 µg). KREJČÍ, KUPKOVÁ, and VÁVRA, unpublished experiments; cf. KREJČÍ et al. (1967a)

It would have been predicted that under appropriate experimental conditions antagonism might be observed with Phe² derivatives of the vasopressin series. Although normal potency data are recorded for Phe²-Lys⁸-vasopressin (BOISSONNAS and GUTTMANN, 1960) it has been stated (BERDE et al., 1961) that in high doses the analogue showed some inhibitory action against oxytocin on the isolated rat uterus and, in some experiments, on the rabbit mammary gland. The slight pressor action in the anaesthetised rooster recorded for Phe²-Orn⁸-vasopressin and its 1-deamino derivative (HUGUENIN, 1966) might also indicate a potential for antagonism.

4. *Tyr²/³-Oxytocin*

An oxytocin analogue with a second tyrosine residue intercalated in the disulphide-bridged sequence of the molecule, Tyr²/³-oxytocin (Fig. 11a), was the earliest neurohypophysial hormone antagonist to be reported (GUTTMANN et al., 1957).

Cys–Tyr–**Tyr**–Ile–Glu(NH_2)–Asp(NH_2)–Cys–Pro–Leu–Gly–NH_2 (disulphide bridge Cys–Cys)

a

Cys–Tyr–**Ile**–Ile–Glu(NH_2)–Asp(NH_2)–Cys–Pro–Leu–Gly–NH_2 (disulphide bridge Cys–Cys)

b

Fig. 11. Structures of Tyr²/³-oxytocin (a) and Ile³/⁴-oxytocin (b)

The pure peptide has not been described; a solution of the reaction product obtained by removal of the protecting groups from the appropriate synthetic decapeptide intermediate and air oxidation, in analogy to the preparation of oxytocin, was used in the biological studies reported and the dosages refer to a solution containing the product from 1.25 mg of the protected material in 1 ml.

In the avian depressor assay the response to oxytocin (75 mU) was completely blocked by 0.3 or 0.4 ml of this solution given 15—30 sec before the hormone; when the time interval was extended to 2 min no inhibition was observed (Fig. 12). The action of oxytocin (0.16—0.4 mU/ml) on the isolated rat uterus was partly or completely inhibited by the solution of the analogue (0.8—3.2 μl per ml of medium) (Guttmann et al., 1957) and similar or somewhat higher concentrations inhibited the response of the spontaneously contracting rabbit uterine strip to oxytocin (1 mU/ml) added either after or before the analogue. In higher concentrations (10—20 μl per ml of medium) the analogue generally decreased the amplitude or frequency of the spontaneous contractions or both, and also the tone of the muscle strip. The peptide did not appreciably inhibit the response to methylergobasine on the same preparation and was without effect on the spontaneous activity of the rabbit uterus *in situ* or its response to oxytocin (Konzett, 1957).

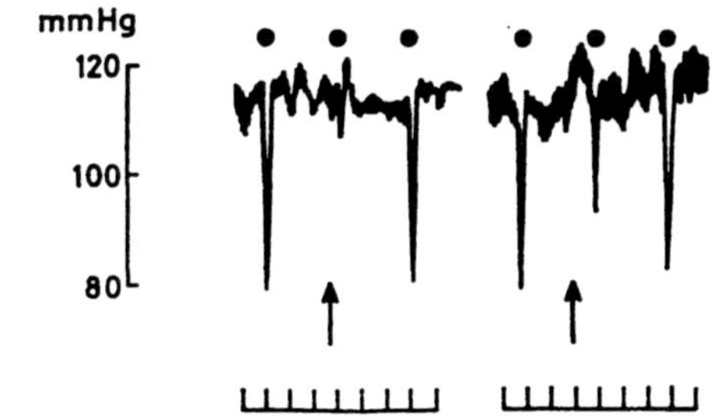

Fig. 12. Inhibition of the avian depressor response to pituitary extract by Tyr$^{2/3}$-oxytocin. At dots, 75 mU of standard; at arrows, 0.3 ml of antagonist solution (see text) given 15 sec (left) or 1 min (right) before the standard. Time markers 1 min. From Guttmann et al. (1957)

It is estimated that the analogue:oxytocin concentration ratios at which inhibition was observed were about 300—700:1 (Guttmann et al., 1957; Konzett, 1957).

A structurally related peptide with an isoleucine instead of a tyrosine residue in the same position (Fig. 11b), Ile$^{3/4}$-oxytocin, is reported to show no inhibitor properties (Berde et al., 1961). The protected decapeptide precursors of several additional analogues of the same general type have been synthetised (Beyerman et al., 1960a—d) but no information is available about the preparation or biological properties of the free peptides. However, the case of Ile$^{3/4}$-oxytocin shows (Berde et al., 1961) that the structural feature responsible for the inhibitor properties is not, as had been suggested (Ressler and Rachele, 1958), the increase in the size of the disulphide-bridged ring alone. Alternatively, Tyr$^{2/3}$-oxytocin can be regarded as an analogue modified in position 2 by replacement of tyrosine by tyrosyl-tyrosine. The rather general occurrence of inhibitor properties in analogues of this class lends colour to this suggestion. Tyr$^{2/3}$-oxytocin also resembles e.g. methyloxytocin in acting as an antagonist on the uterus *in vitro* but not *in situ* and in retaining milk-ejection activity (Guttmann et al., 1957); on the other hand, in the avian depressor assay Tyr$^{2/3}$-oxytocin has an inhibitory effect which rapidly fades whereas methyloxytocin on the contrary has depressor activity attended by a rather persistent loss of reactivity. In this context it would be interesting to know if the inhibitor properties of Tyr$^{2/3}$-oxytocin are affected by the calcium concentration.

C. Analogues modified in sequence positions 3, 4 and 5

The effect of some oxytocin analogues modified in positions 3, 4, and 5 on the tubular responses to the vasotocins in the frog kidney has already been noted

(p. 751; Morel and Jard, 1963; Jard, 1966). Replacement of the isoleucine in position 3 by valine or leucine affords active antagonists whereas its replacement by phenylalanine gives a product essentially inactive on the tubules. Substitution in position 4 of mesotocin (to give Ser^4-Ile^8-oxytocin or isotocin) leads to loss of antagonist properties whereas substitution in position 5 of oxytocin [Glu(NH_2)^5-oxytocin] does not; this finding is particularly interesting because it contrasts with the more usual situation in which biological activity is sensitive to changes in sequence position 5 but relatively insensitive to changes in position 4 (see du Vigneaud et al., 1964).

(γ-Glu-NH_2)^5-oxytocin (isoglutamine-oxytocin) (Ressler and du Vigneaud, 1957) has no detectable uterotonic, avian depressor, or rat pressor activity and inhibits the pressor response to arginine vasopressin in the rat (Ressler and Rachele, 1958). An analogue:hormone ratio of about 280—720:1 is required to decrease the response by 30—50%; at ratios above about 1500:1 the action of vasopressin is completely blocked. The time required to recover sensitivity increases markedly with the degree of inhibition. The structural features responsible for the antagonism are difficult to define. On the one hand, the shortening of the side-chain alone is unlikely to be responsible since the side-chain in this position can be omitted altogether (in Gly^4-oxytocin; Drabarek, 1964; Fosker and Law, 1965) without complete loss of activity or the appearance of inhibitor properties, and on the other hand merely increasing the ring does not create an antagonist: No inhibitor properties are reported for βAla^4-oxytocin (Manning and du Vigneaud, 1965), and although Tyr$^{2/3}$-oxytocin and Homocys^1-oxytocin act as inhibitors the closely related Ile$^{3/4}$-oxytocin and 1-(γ-mercaptobutyric acid)-oxytocin apparently do not. It is possible, of course, that closer scrutiny might yet reveal antagonism in some of these cases.

D. Analogues modified in sequence positions 7, 8 and 9

De-Pro^7-, de-Leu^8-, and de-Gly^9-oxytocin act as antagonists to oxytocin in the avian depressor assay and the latter two analogues also as antagonists of vasopressin in the rat pressor assay; the first two are effective at analogue:hormone mole ratios of 1000:1, the de-Gly^9-derivative appears ten times less effective (Jaquenoud and Boissonnas, 1962). The methylamide corresponding to de-Gly^9-oxytocin, 9-decarboxamido-oxytocin, also inhibits the response to the standard in the rat pressor assay (Branda and du Vigneaud, 1966), as does D-Leu^8-oxytocin (Schneider and du Vigneaud, 1962). A structural feature shared by all these analogues is the absence of the terminal carboxamide grouping from its proper position; more subtle ways of bringing about this situation should show whether this group is indeed essential for pressor action.

Two analogues have been described in which the glycine amide grouping of oxytocin is replaced by a hydrazinoacetamide residue (NH.Gly^9-oxytocin) and by a β-glycylhydrazinoacetamide grouping (Gly-NH.Gly^9-oxytocin; partial formulae in Fig. 13) (Niedrich et al., 1964). Both analogues induce contractions of the rat

Cys–Tyr–Ile–Glu(NH_2)–Asp(NH_2)–Cys–Pro–Leu–NH·NH·CH_2·CO·NH_2

NH-Gly^9-oxytocin

Cys–Tyr–Ile–Glu(NH_2)–Asp(NH_2)–Cys–Pro–Leu–NH·CH_2·CO–NH·NH·CH_2·CO·NH_2

Gly-NH-Gly^9-oxytocin

Fig. 13. Partial structural formulae for two oxytocin analogues with carboxyl-terminal hydrazinoacetic acid amide

uterus *in vitro* but if the responses to low concentrations (1 μg/ml) of either analogue are allowed to fade and the dose–response curve for oxytocin is then recorded by the cumulative dose procedure in the presence of the analogue it is found to be shifted to a higher concentration range as against the curve similarly recorded in the absence of the analogue, indicating antagonism by the analogues. Gly-NH.Gly^9-oxytocin appeared to be more effective both as an agonist and as an antagonist. It remains to be shown whether the antagonist properties of these analogues are due to the presence of the hydrazide grouping, substitution of the terminal amide nitrogen, or more complex structural requirements.

IV. Other Peptides; Amino Acids and Proteins

A. Amino-acids and simple peptides

Most of the common amino acids in low concentrations do not affect the response of the rat uterus to oxytocin (Ishida, 1961b; Aonuma et al., 1965; Khairallah et al., 1965). In concentrations above 4% the soluble common amino acids and also urea cause some inhibition of the uterine response to oxytocin, bradykinin, and serotonin; the response to angiotensin is sensitive even to low concentrations of amino acids and urea. The effect of high amino-acid concentrations is not readily reversed by washing (Khairallah et al., 1965).

Tyrosine ethyl ester (Ishida, 1961b), L-thyroxine, and 3,3′,5-triiodo-L-thyronine (Aonuma et al., 1965) inhibit the action of oxytocin on the rat uterus *in vitro*. The minimal concentration of thyroxine effective in antagonising the response to oxytocin (0.2 mU/ml) is given as 20 μg/ml for normal and 100 μg/ml for thyroidectomised rats; tyrosine ethyl ester is active in similar doses. Thyroxine, but not tyrosine ethyl ester, is also effective on the guinea-pig uterus. The response of the rat uterus to vasopressin, serotonin and "urinary oxytocic substance" is also inhibited (Aonuma et al., 1965).

Most simple peptides do not affect the uterotonic action of oxytocin; however, peptides of tyrosine and diiodotyrosine may act as inhibitors (Ishida and Hara, 1964; Aonuma et al., 1965; Ishida et al., 1966). Benzyloxycarbonyl-L-tyrosyl-L-tyrosine ethyl ester (Z-Tyr-Tyr-OEt) in 5.2 μM solution inhibited the response of the isolated rat uterus to oxytocin (0.2 mU/ml) by 50%. The peptide caused a parallel shift of the log dose-response curves for oxytocin proportional to the inhibitor concentration (pA_2 5.38). The response to acetylcholine and barium chloride was non-competitively inhibited at higher peptide concentrations. No inhibition was observed of the avian depressor response to oxytocin, or the pressor response to vasopressin in the rabbit or dog. The related derivatives, Z-Gly-Tyr-OEt, Z-Ala-Tyr-OEt, Z-Tyr-Tyr-OH (pA_2 3.64), and H-Tyr-Tyr-OEt (pA_2 3.96) (Ishida and Hara, 1964; Ishida et al., 1966) were less effective inhibitors of oxytocin, as was diiodotyrosylglycine which was active on the rat but not the rabbit uterus (Aonuma et al., 1965). Dibenzyloxycarbonyl-L-cystinyl-di-L-tyrosine diethyl ester, (Z-Cys-Tyr-OEt)$_2$, was a feeble inhibitor of the uterotonic response but 5 mg/kg caused a marked, persistent (more than 1 hour) inhibition of the avian depressor response to oxytocin and of the pressor response to vasopressin in dogs and rabbits (Ishida and Hara, 1964).

It has been suggested (Ishida and Hara, 1964; Ishida et al., 1966) that derivatives and peptides of tyrosine act as competitive antagonists of oxytocin by occupying the site on the specific uterine receptor which in the hormone–receptor complex accomodates the tyrosine side-chain of the hormone; the same mechanism is envisaged for inhibition by a number of other phenols (Ishida, 1961b; see p. 783) and this similarity is supported by the additive nature of the antagonism by

Z-Tyr-Tyr-OEt and oestradiol (ISHIDA et al., 1966). If the above interpretation is correct then, on general grounds, the effectiveness of an inhibitor would be expected to increase as its structural resemblance to the hormone becomes closer; this relation does not seem to be obeyed here, though examination of a wider range of structures appears desirable. The position of the cystinyl-tyrosine derivative is anomalous in that it inhibits vascular but not uterine responses, differing in this respect not only from the other tyrosine peptides but also from the disulphide-type inhibitors such as cystine diethyl ester.

The inhibitor properties of cysteine, cystine diethyl ester, and of glutathione and the corresponding disulphide are discussed together with those of other thiol and disulphide inhibitors on p. 774—778.

B. Biologically active peptides unrelated to the neurohypophysial hormones

The peptide kinins — bradykinin, kallidin, and angiotension — act on several tissues also susceptible to the neurohypophysial hormones (uterine and vascular smooth muscle, possibly also kidney tubules). However, there is a wealth of evidence that they do so at different receptors, including evidence from selective inhibition of responses to one or other of these peptides; thus methyloxytocin under suitable conditions (p. 760) inhibits the uterotonic action of oxytocin and vasopressin but not that of bradykinin or angiotensin (BISSET, 1962). Interaction between the various peptides would be expected chiefly at the higher levels of regulation.

Bradykinin (1 μg) markedly decreases the response of the rat uterus *in situ* to oxytocin (1 mU, i.e. 2 ng) given 5 min later, and abolishes the response when the interval is reduced to 2 min (BISSET et al., 1966). The rhythmic contractions of the rat uterus induced by infusion of oxytocin (8 mU/min) are unchanged in frequency or amplitude upon injection of bradykinin (2—4 μg) but there is a distinct decrease in uterine tone; similar effects are produced by eledoisin (2 μg) and by preparations of Substance P and "decontrin" (a pancreatic extract) while relaxin (20 μg) decreases the amplitude of the contractions (BIANCHINI, 1963).

No evidence for antagonism by bradykinin could be found on the rat uterus *in vitro*. The possibility that the inhibition *in vivo* is mediated by epinephrine has been considered but found to require release of an improbable amount of mediator (BISSET et al., 1966).

Although bradykinin (0.25—0.50 μg/ml) has no significant effect on the water permeability of the toad bladder or the short-circuit current through the toad skin (*B. marinus*) it inhibits the response of both tissues to vasopressin (1 mU/ml). The effect on the toad bladder was pronounced, that on the toad skin less marked but significant ($P = 0.05$) (FURTADO and MACHADO, 1966). The inhibitory effect on the water permeability response is only appreciable at molar ratios of bradykinin to vasopressin above about 20:1 (FURTADO, 1966). Bradykinin also inhibits the response of the toad bladder to oxytocin but not to theophylline; the inhibition shows features of competitive antagonism (FURTADO, personal communication).

C. Proteins

Proteins which inhibit the action of the neurohypophysial hormones may be either enzymes which inactivate the peptide by destroying the active molecule, or proteins capable of immobilising the hormone by binding.

The enzymic inactivation of the neurohypophysial hormones is discussed elsewhere in this volume; in this context it will suffice to illustrate the way in which such enzyme action can take on the appearance of antagonism. Injection of a preparation of human pregnancy serum oxytocinase into a hydrated ethanol-anaesthetised rat in which a constant submaximal level of urine flow was maintained by continuous infusion of oxytocin (Fig. 14) partly reversed the antidiuretic effect of the hormone, evidently by decreasing its steady-state concentration (PLIŠKA et al., 1967). The effect of the enzyme on the response to lysine-vasopressin in an analogous experiment was less marked.

The possibility has been considered that the inhibitory factor released from toad bladders (GOLDBERG et al., 1963; KARLIN, 1963; EDELMAN et al., 1964) is enzymic in character (KARLIN, 1963); an enzyme capable of inactivating vasopressin has in fact been extracted from toad bladders (CAMPBELL et al., 1965).

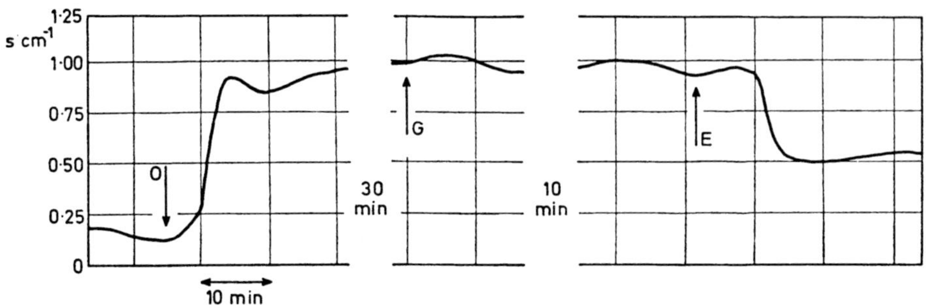

Fig. 14. Inhibition of the antidiuretic response to oxytocin by serum oxytocinase. Continuous recording of urine conductivity from water-loaded rat in ethanol narcosis (PLIŠKA and RYCHLÍK, 1967); at O, start of oxytocin infusion (0.5 mU/hr) continued to the end of the experiment; G—injection of γ-globulin (4 mg), E—injection of human pregnancy serum oxytocinase preparation (2.2 mg protein; 0.565 oxytocinase units). Cf. PLIŠKA et al. (1967)

However, because of the quantitative relations involved this explanation was rejected (KARLIN, 1963). The dialysable inhibitor obtained after heat-treatment of toad bladders (KARLIN and OVERWEG, 1965; OVERWEG, 1966) obviously cannot be an enzyme (p. 791).

In order to diminish the response to oxytocin or vasopressin by (non-destructive) binding, a protein must have a sufficient affinity and binding capacity for the peptide to decrease its concentration in the vicinity of the target tissue appreciably. This condition is likely to be met only where the protein–peptide binding is specific as a result of a high degree of complementarity, suggesting a functional adaptation. An obvious candidate would be neurophysin but no studies designed to translate hormone binding by this protein into inhibition have been reported, possibly because the conditions required for optimal binding (low pH, absence of calcium) are difficult to achieve in the standard assay systems.

A type of interaction more likely to be of interest from this point of view is that based on the antibody–antigen or antibody–hapten reaction. Recently, antibodies to oxytocin and vasopressin or their protein conjugates have been successfully produced (GILLILAND and PROUT, 1965; HOLLÄNDER et al., 1966; ROTH et al., 1966; PERMUTT et al., 1966; SCHÄKER, 1967; SCHÄKER and STERBA, personal communication) and it has been shown that such antibodies against an oxytocin-protein conjugate (HOLLÄNDER et al., 1966) or against oxytocin (SCHÄKER, 1967) may specifically inhibit biological responses to the hormone. For instance, the response of sensitive rat uterus preparations to threshold doses of oxytocin was blocked by suitable concentrations of rabbit antiserum added to the organ bath; higher concentrations of immune or normal serum themselves caused contractions (SCHÄKER, 1967). These results, together with those already obtained with antibodies against angiotensin conjugates (cf. GOODFRIEND et al., 1966) encourage the belief that under suitable conditions a useful degree of specific inhibition can be achieved. The question is of more than academic interest since it has been suggested that the resistance of certain cases of diabetes insipidus to vasopressin treatment may be of immune origin, and the serum of one such patient was shown to have a significantly increased binding capacity for lysine-vasopressin (ROTH et al., 1966).

The finding that antibodies discriminate between the different neurohypophysial hormones (ROTH et al., 1966; PERMUTT et al., 1966) whereas the neurohypophysial "carrier" proteins appear to bind both oxytocin and vasopressin about equally (e.g. BRESLOW and ABRASH, 1966) is instructive since it indicates that the regions of the peptide molecule involved in binding are different in the two instances.

V. Thiols, Disulphides and Thiol Reagents

A. Inactivation by thiols

The antidiuretic and *in vitro* uterotonic effects of neurohypophysial hormone preparations have long been known to be diminished by pretreatment with sulphydryl-containing compounds such as hydrogen sulphide (GULLAND and RANDALL, 1935; RESSLER, 1958), cysteine (VAN DYKE et al., 1942; AUDRAIN and CLAUSER, 1958; DICKER and GREENBAUM, 1958), thioglycollate (VAN DYKE et al., 1942; AMES et al., 1950; AMES and VAN DYKE, 1951; VOGT, 1953; RESSLER, 1958; BISSET, 1961; MARTIN and SCHILD, 1962a,b, 1964, 1965; BENTLEY, 1964), and glutathione (DICKER and GREENBAUM, 1958; BENTLEY, 1964). The effect of oxytocin or arginine vasopressin on water transport through the toad bladder is also antagonised by cysteine (RASMUSSEN et al., 1963; HANDLER and ORLOFF, 1964),

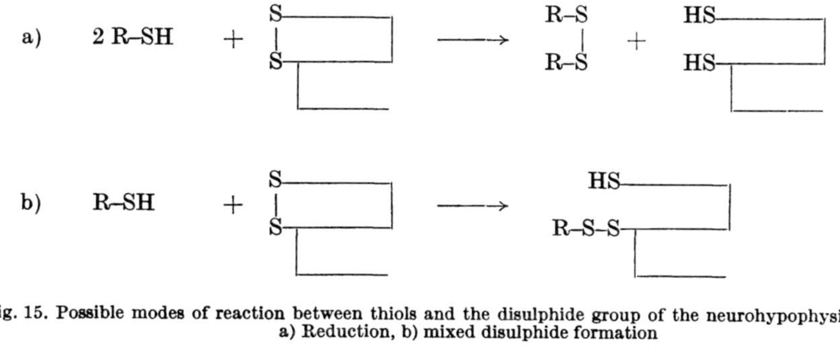

Fig. 15. Possible modes of reaction between thiols and the disulphide group of the neurohypophysial hormones. a) Reduction, b) mixed disulphide formation

thioglycollate (HANDLER and ORLOFF, 1964), and glutathione (BENTLEY, 1964) but the avian depressor or rat pressor response does not appear to be affected by such treatment (SEALOCK and DU VIGNEAUD, 1935; ACHER et al., 1956; DICKER and GREENBAUM, 1958; see, however, VOGT, 1953). It has generally been assumed, on good evidence, that thiols inactivate the hormones by reducing the disulphide bond (SEALOCK and DU VIGNEAUD, 1935) whose integrity is essential for biological activity (VAN DYKE et al., 1942) (Fig. 15a); this conclusion was supported by experiments in which the activity could be restored by oxidation (GULLAND and RANDALL, 1935; DICKER and GREENBAUM, 1958; AUDRAIN and CLAUSER, 1958). Ring-opening by disulphide exchange, with formation of a mixed disulphide between the reduced form of the hormone and the thiol (Fig. 15b) has been considered as an alternative mode of reaction (RESSLER, 1958; BISSET, 1961; RASMUSSEN et al., 1963). Those instances in which thiol pretreatment failed to reduce activity (SEALOCK and DU VIGNEAUD, 1935; ACHER et al., 1956; RESSLER,

1958; DICKER, 1960; BISSET, 1961; BENTLEY, 1964) have been explained by reoxidation of the hormone under the conditions of the incubation or the assay (AUDRAIN and CLAUSER, 1958; DICKER, 1964)* or by differences in equilibria, or reaction modes, with particular hormone–reagent combinations (RESSLER, 1958; BISSET, 1961).

The conditions under which inactivation takes place may be exemplified by the experiments of DICKER and GREENBAUM (1958) in which about 30% of the antidiuretic activity was destroyed when vasopressin (1.8 mU/ml) was incubated with cysteine (9 mM) or glutathione (0.18 mM) in Krebs-Ringer medium for 10 min, and of AUDRAIN and CLAUSER (1958) who recorded a 75% loss of uterotonic activity when oxytocin (25 mU/ml) was kept with 0.6 mM cysteine at pH 8 for 4 hours, both the pretreatment and the assay being done under anaerobic conditions. The inactivation by thioglycollate in particular has frequently served for the identification or selective assay of the hormones in biological material; a typical procedure (VOGT, 1953; BISSET, 1961) involves pretreatment of the material with 10 mM thioglycollate at pH 7—8 for 30—60 min. A recent kinetic study by MARTIN and SCHILD (1965) has shown that the rate of inactivation of oxytocin or lysine-vasopressin by excess thioglycollate is approximately exponential and that the pseudo-first-order rate constant is proportional to the concentration of thioglycollate. The times required for 90% inactivation at 20° and pH 7.4 at various thioglycollate concentrations (given in brackets) were about 57 min (5 mM), 35 min (10 mM), 20 min (20 mM), and 10 min (40 mM)**. Increasing the temperature from 20 to 30° approximately doubled the rate of inactivation. Incubation of oxytocin or lysine-vasopressin in 5 mM thioglycollate at 30° for 30 min caused 50% inactivation.

Recently MARTIN and SCHILD (1962a, b, 1964, 1965) have shown that in addition to inactivating oxytocin and vasopressin thioglycollic acid has a direct inhibitory effect on the response of the uterus to the hormones; similar conclusions have been reached about the effect of cysteine on the response of the toad bladder (HANDLER and ORLOFF, 1964) and of glutathione on both rat uterus and toad bladder (BENTLEY, 1964). These results do not, of course, invalidate the general conclusion that thiol compounds can inactivate peptides of this structural class by reaction at the disulphide bond but they do require a distinction to be made between the two modes of action wherever mechanistic inferences are to be drawn. Inactivation can be studied separately by chosing an experimental procedure in which the concentration conditions at the assay stage correspond to enough initial activity for reliable determination but reduce the amount of thiol below the known threshold for direct inhibition. MARTIN and SCHILD (1965) could deliberately establish such conditions on the basis of their kinetic results; a reexamination of the concentration ratios used in some of the earlier work on which current ideas of the inactivation are based (AUDRAIN and CLAUSER, 1958; RESSLER, 1958; BISSET, 1961)*** fortunately makes it almost certain that in these instances, too, the assays were uncomplicated by direct inhibition.

Thioglycollate given subcutaneously or intraperitoneally to rats has an antidiuretic effect which may complicate the results when inactivation with thioglycollate is followed by assay for antidiuretic activity after administration by

* The properties of carefully characterised S,S′-dihydro-oxytocin ("oxytoceine") and the corresponding deamino derivative in the avian depressor assay (lower potency but more protracted action) bear out this suggestion (YAMASHIRO, GILLESSEN, and DU VIGNEAUD, 1966).

** Estimated from the plots given in the paper of MARTIN and SCHILD (1965).

*** This applies to the model experiments of BISSET (1961) in which relatively high hormone: thiol ratios were used but not necessarily to the assays of biological materials.

these routes; however, no such effect is observed when thioglycollate is given intravenously, the more usual way of injecting samples for antidiuretic assay (AMES and VAN DYKE, 1951).

The inactivation of oxytocin, vasopressin and related peptides by thiols has been regarded as evidence that biological activity (at any rate on the uterus, kidney, and amphibian bladder) requires integrity of the disulphide bond (VAN DYKE et al., 1942; AUDRAIN and CLAUSER, 1958; DICKER and GREENBAUM, 1958; BISSET, 1961; RASMUSSEN et al., 1963) and this conclusion has in turn been used to support the hypothesis that the molecular event initiating the response involves reaction at the disulphide grouping of the peptide (RASMUSSEN et al., 1963). Since it has been shown that synthetic analogues isosteric with deamino-oxytocin but not containing a disulphide bond show qualitatively similar biological activities as the disulphide-containing prototype it is clear that disulphide *reactivity* is not a prerequisite for biological activity (RUDINGER and JOŠT, 1964b; SCHWARTZ et al., 1964; JOŠT and RUDINGER, 1967); on the other hand, there is also independent evidence that open-chain peptides with amino-acid sequences closely similar to those of active disulphide-bridged compounds have no appreciable hormone-like activity (SEALOCK and DU VIGNEAUD, 1935; TURNER et al., 1951; MUELLER et al., 1951; GORDON and DU VIGNEAUD, 1953; BERÁNKOVÁ and ŠORM, 1961; HUGUENIN and GUTTMANN, 1965) and it therefore appears that the disulphide bridge in the natural hormones is essential for maintaining the conformation and hence the topochemistry required for efficient interaction of the hormone molecule with the tissue receptors.

B. Inhibition by thiols

The direct inhibitory effect of thioglycollic acid on the response of the isolated rat uterus to oxytocin was studied under conditions under which inactivation of the hormone had been shown to be negligible and the results were confirmed using α-thioglycerol, an inhibitor which has only a slight inactivating effect when incubated with oxytocin (MARTIN and SCHILD, 1965).

Both thioglycollic acid and α-thioglycerol in concentrations up to 20 mM cause a parallel shift of the log dose–response curves for oxytocin; in 40 mM thioglycollic acid the slope of the curve is significantly decreased. The dose ratios (Table 6) increase somewhat more than in proportion to the concentration of the antagonist, indicating a departure from purely competitive antagonism. The responses to

Table 6. *Dose Ratios for the Response of the Isolated Rat Uterus to Oxytocin in the Presence of Thiols* (MARTIN and SCHILD, 1965)

Thiol	Thiol concentration 5 mM	10 mM	20 mM	40 mM
Thioglycollate (20°) . . .	—	7.0	26.0	—
Thioglycollate (30°) . . .	1.6	2.9	25.0	150.0
α-Thioglycerol (30°) . . .	—	4.8	16.3	—

acetylcholine and bradykinin are unaffected, or only slightly decreased (dose ratios 1.0—2.5) by both thiols in concentrations up to 20 mM showing that the antagonism is relatively specific for oxytocin and closely related peptides such as deamino-oxytocin and lysine-vasopressin. L-Cysteine, α- and β-mercaptopropionic acid, thiomalate, and α-mercaptoethanol also inhibit the response of the uterus to oxytocin, the dose ratios being 4—8 for 10 mM and 12—16 for 20 mM inhibitor; methyl thioglycollate (5 mM) is also active. In every case the dose ratios for bradykinin are less than half those for oxytocin. Thioethers (methionine, di-β-hydroxyethyl sulphide), a disulphide (dithioglycollic acid), and ethanethiol were found to be essentially inactive in similar of higher concentrations, a number of other compounds (dimercaprol, glycollate, cyanoacetate, ascorbic acid, sulphite) caused slight or marked but non-specific depression of the uterine response. It therefore appears that specific antagonism requires the presence of a thiol group together with a hydroxyl or carboxyl (or carbomethoxy) group in the molecule of the antagonist (MARTIN and SCHILD, 1964, 1965); the additional groups might be required to achieve the requisite distribution properties (RUDINGER, 1964).

The depolarised rat uterus responds to oxytocin (50 mU/ml) in the presence of 20 mM thioglycerol by a contraction followed by relatively rapid relaxation; the same organ preparation in the absence of thioglycerol responds to 5 mU/ml of oxytocin by a sustained contraction. The qualitative change in the response provides further evidence against a purely competitive antagonism. The contractile response of the rat or rabbit mammary gland strip to oxytocin (but not to acetylcholine) is inhibited by 15 or 20 mM thioglycollate; at the higher concentration the inhibition is sometimes insurmountable. Thioglycerol does not inhibit the response of the rat mammary gland strip in concentrations up to 100 mM. Injections of thioglycollate shown to produce a 40—60 mM concentration in the blood plasma inhibit the response of the uterus *in situ* to both oxytocin and angiotensin non-specifically (dose ratios 2—6) (MARTIN and SCHILD, 1965); by contrast, *pretreatment* of oxytocin with thioglycollate destroys its uterotonic activity *in vivo* (BISSET, 1961). No appreciable inhibition of the vasoconstrictor action of vasopressin in the perfused hind limb of the rat was observed when thioglycollate or thioglycerol (20 mM) was added to the perfusion fluid. It has been suggested that the difference between the effect of these thiols on the uterus and on vascular tissue might be due to a genuine difference in the receptors, but the difference in behaviour of the uterus *in vitro* and *in situ* remains unexplained (MARTIN and SCHILD, 1965).

Thioglycollate (10 mM) inhibits the permeability response of the toad bladder to oxytocin or vasopressin and to theophylline but not to adenosine 3′,5′-phosphate (cyclic AMP) (HANDLER and ORLOFF, 1964); these results will be discussed in connection with the effect of cysteine below.

BENTLEY (1964) has shown that 1—5 mM glutathione reduces the response of the isolated rat uterus to oxytocin; at the lower concentration of inhibitor, the response to acetylcholine is not affected. Double reciprocal plots of the dose–response relations for oxytocin in the presence of various concentrations of glutathione are suggestive of competitive antagonism. Control experiments confirmed that the decreased response was not due to inactivation of the hormone. Glutathione (2 mM) in the serosal, but not in the mucosal medium markedly decreased the water-permeability response of the toad bladder to oxytocin (10 mU/ml) given 25 min later (BENTLEY, 1964).

Cysteine added to the serosal medium also inhibits the effect of the neurohypophysial hormones and their analogues on the osmotic flow of water through the toad bladder (RASMUSSEN et al., 1963; HANDLER and ORLOFF, 1964). In 10 mM cysteine doses of oxytocin, lysine-vasopressin, Val^3-oxytocin, or deamino-oxytocin five times higher than those required to evoke a maximal response in control experiments failed to produce a change in permeability; 5 mM cysteine caused a parallel displacement of the log dose–response curves for lysine-vasopressin and

Cit[8]-oxytocin by about the same distance along the log dose axis. These results were interpreted in terms of inactivation of the hormones by disulphide exchange reactions with cysteine (Rasmussen et al., 1963). The observed effect of the inhibitor on the log dose–response relations is not inconsistent with this interpretation since, assuming the reaction to be first order with respect to the peptide and the rate to be independent of its detailed structure, this is the type of relation which would be expected. However, Handler and Orloff (1964) found that 1 mM cysteine inhibited the response not only to oxytocin (1—4 mU/ml) and vasopressin (0.5—1 mU/ml) but also to theophylline (10—20 mM) though not to cyclic AMP. Concentrations of cysteine as low as 0.1 mM were antagonistic to theophylline but even 10 mM cysteine had no effect on the nucleotide. D-Cysteine was equally effective. The results are thought to show that the inhibitory effect of cysteine (and thioglycollate) represents an action on the tissue and not on the drug in solution (Handler and Orloff, 1964). While this is undoubtedly correct for theophylline it does not necessarily follow for oxytocin and vasopressin since the cysteine or other thiol may well operate by two or even more distinct mechanisms. As a speculation, Handler and Orloff (1964) suggest that the thiols might act by inhibiting adenyl cyclase. Similar suggestions have been made with regard to other antagonists affecting the response to the hormones and theophylline but not to cyclic AMP (calcium, dichloroisoprenaline [DCI], hydrogen ions; Petersen and Edelman, 1964; Strauch and Langdon, 1964; Orloff and Handler, 1964) since, with this enzyme inactive, no increase in the concentration of the mediator (cyclic AMP) can be achieved either by stimulation of its production (hormone action) or by cumulation through a block on inactivation (theophylline effect). In the particular case of inhibition by thiols the objection may be raised that avian erythrocyte adenyl cyclase is activated (after aging), rather than inactivated, by thiols (Øye and Sutherland, 1966). In view of the multiplicity of thiol-sensitive molecules and processes in cells it seems not unlikely that in addition to any effect on the hormone several other modes of action may be involved, possibly including an action on the specific tissue receptors (Martin and Schild, 1962a, b, 1964, 1965; Bentley, 1964).

C. Disulphides

Somewhat surprisingly oxidised glutathione is a more effective inhibitor of the water permeability response to oxytocin than the reduced peptide, being active in concentrations as low as 0.5 mM; in higher concentrations (2 mM) it acts from the mucosal as well as the serosal side of the bladder. Oxidised glutathione also inhibits the response of the isolated rat uterus to oxytocin; as in the case of the thiol form, the inhibition appears competitive by the criterion of Lineweaver-Burk plots (Bentley, 1964). The antagonistic action of cystine diethyl ester (0.2—0.8 mM) on the uterotonic effect of oxytocin, which also appears competitive (pA_2 4.08; Ishida et al., 1966), may be related to the action of glutathione though the disulphide corresponding to thioglycollic acid, i. e. dithioglycollic acid, is inactive (Martin and Schild 1964, 1965) and dibenzyloxycarbonylcystinyl-bis-tyrosine diethyl ester (0.05 mg/ml) is only a weak oxytocin antagonist on the isolated rat uterus (Ishida and Hara, 1964; see p. 771).

To explain the inhibitor properties of thiols as well as disulphides Bentley (1964) suggests, in general terms, that both S-S groups and SH groups are involved in the uterus and bladder receptors. Studies with radioactively labelled disulphides might help to establish the mode and site of action of these compounds; as in the case of thiols, distribution properties could be important as well as the presence of disulphide bond.

D. Sulphydryl blocking reagents

Reagents known to react with sulphydryl groups to form covalent links (N-ethyl- or N-phenylmaleimide) or complex mercury mercaptides (methylmercuric bromide, *p*-hydroxymercuribenzoate, *p*-chloromercuribenzenesulphonate) inhibit the water permeability response of the toad bladder to the neurohypophysial hormones. The compounds act in 0.1—1 mM concentrations from both the serosal and mucosal sides of the bladder. The maleimides and methylmercuric bromide themselves also produce an increase in bladder permeability (RASMUSSEN et al., 1960). When N-methylmaleimide is added to the serosal medium after a permeability response to oxytocin or vasopressin has been established the bladder fails to return to the impermeable state after both agents have been washed out (RASMUSSEN et al., 1960; BENTLEY, 1964). Both N-ethylmaleimide and *p*-chloromercuribenzenesulphonate also inhibit the toad bladder response to theophylline and to cyclic AMP (ORLOFF and HANDLER, 1962).

Exposure of the isolated rat uterus to mercuric chloride (1 μg/ml) for 30 min sharply reduces the response to oxytocin; an analogous experiment with *p*-chloromercuribenzoate (10 μg/ml) is shown in Fig. 16. Both compounds also inhibit the barium-induced contractions of the uterus (ISHIDA et al., 1961). N-Ethylmaleimide reduces (0.1 mM) or abolishes (1 mM) the response of the rat uterus *in vitro* to oxytocin, and also to acetylcholine; when added during a contraction it prevents full relaxation of the muscle after removal of the stimulant (BENTLEY, 1964).

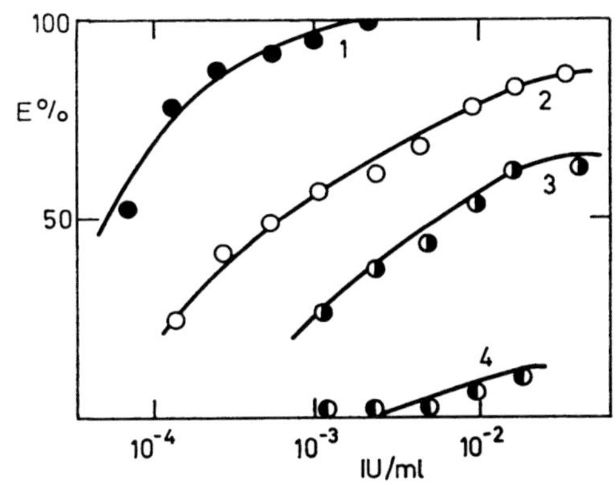

Fig. 16. Effect of *p*-chloromercuribenzoate (PCMB) on the response of the isolated rat uterus to oxytocin. Log dose–response curves for oxytocin: 1 control, 2 after treatment (30 min) with PCMB (10 μg/ml) in the presence of oxytocin (4.17 mU/ml), 3 after treatment with PCMB (30 min) followed by cysteine (100 μg/ml; 30 min), 4 after treatment with PCMB alone. From ISHIDA et al. (1961)

While the effects of N-ethylmaleimide are irreversible (RASMUSSEN et al., 1960; ORLOFF and HANDLER, 1962; BENTLEY, 1964) the action of methylmercuric bromide on the toad bladder can be partially reversed by washing (RASMUSSEN et al., 1960) or, more effectively, by treatment with cysteine (SCHWARTZ et al., 1960). Similarly, the sensitivity of the mercuribenzoate-treated uterus can in part be restored by exposing the muscle to cysteine (Fig. 16) (ISHIDA et al., 1961).

The original suggestion (RASMUSSEN et al., 1960) that compounds of this class act by blocking disulphide–sulphydryl interchange between the hormone and receptor is no longer tenable (see p. 776). The possibility remains that such inhibitors may react with sulphydryl groups on the receptor, among others; the finding that the presence of oxytocin during the pretreatment of the rat uterus with *p*-chloromercuribenzoate substantially reduces the degree of inhibition to subsequent doses of oxytocin (Fig. 16) suggests protection of the occupied oxytocin receptor against this reagent (ISHIDA et al., 1961) and hence a specific component in the inhibition. Maleimide and *p*-hydroxymercuribenzoate do inhibit the action of avian erythrocyte adenyl cyclase but only after the cells have been haemolysed (ØYE and SUTHERLAND, 1966). The ubiquity and functional importance of sulphydryl groups make it unlikely that a single mode of action is involved, and the low specificity of the inhibition (ORLOFF and HANDLER 1962; BENTLEY, 1964) could be a reflection of this. Effects on metabolism do not appear to be important since these only become evident after exposures much longer than those required for inhibition (RASMUSSEN et al., 1960; BENTLEY, 1964).

VI. Phenols

A. Catecholamines and compounds related to the adrenergic system

Epinephrine inhibits the milk-ejection response to oxytocin in a variety of mammalian species *in vivo* (ELY and PETERSEN, 1941; BRAUDE and MITCHELL, 1952; CROSS, 1953, 1955a, 1958; WHITTLESTONE, 1954; LINZELL, 1955; PICKFORD, 1960; BERDE and CERLETTI, 1960; KULLANDER, 1963; CHAN, 1965) and in the perfused mammary gland (PEETERS et al., 1952). This inhibition has been made responsible for the block in the milk-ejection reflex during stress (ELY and PETERSEN, 1941) which can also be simulated by nervous stimulation of the mammary gland or adrenal gland (CROSS, 1955a, b). In anaesthetised lactating rabbits epinephrine (0.2—5 μg) inhibits the intramammary pressure rise in response to oxytocin (10—50 mU) given 10—30 sec later (CROSS, 1953, 1955a, 1958; CHAN, 1965). The degree of inhibition is dose-dependent and the effect of epinephrine can be surmounted by increasing the dose of oxytocin (CHAN, 1965). Norepinephrine produces the same effect in doses 1.5—4 times higher (CROSS, 1955a, 1958; CHAN, 1965). Epinephrine also blocks the sustained response of the mammary gland to oxytocin infusion (CROSS, 1958; KULLANDER, 1963); an initial rapid biphasic effect is followed by a phase of inhibition developing and fading slowly (KULLANDER, 1963).

From the quantitative relations involved CROSS (1955b) has concluded that epinephrine inhibition cannot account for the emotional block in the milk-ejection reflex but that inhibition of oxytocin release must be a major factor in this block.

It has been widely accepted that epinephrine acts not directly on the alveolar tissue but through its vasoconstrictor effect, by limiting the access of oxytocin to this tissue (PEETERS et al., 1952; LINZELL, 1955; CROSS, 1955; KULLANDER, 1963), chiefly on the evidence that epinephrine does not inhibit the contraction of the alveoli induced by topically applied oxytocin in mice (LINZELL, 1955) or the response to local mechanical stimuli (LINZELL, 1955; CROSS, 1955a). However, CHAN (1965), using reserpinised rabbits, has shown that the vasodilator isoprenaline also inhibits the *in vivo* response of the mammary gland to oxytocin whereas the vasoconstrictor angiotensin does not, that α- and β-adrenergic blockade does not affect the inhibitory action of epinephrine while it abolishes the vascular effects, and finally that the contractile response of the isolated rabbit mammary gland strip to oxytocin is also inhibited by epinephrine, even though almost ten times higher ratios of epinephrine to oxytocin must be used. Isoprenaline was the most active inhibitor *in vivo*; phenylephrine was less active than norepinephrine, dextroamphetamine and ephedrine were essentially inactive.

It must be concluded that the inhibitory effect of epinephrine is not accounted for by its vascular effects but involves a direct action on mammary gland tissues. LINZELL's (1955) failure to observe antagonism in topical application to alveolar tissue remains to be explained; it could be due to species differences, the particular dose range chosen, or other experimental differences.

Epinephrine inhibits the spontaneous motility of the oestrogen-dominated rat and rabbit uterus *in situ*, after initial brief stimulation. It also inhibits the response to oxytocin of the spontaneously active rabbit uterus (CROSS, 1958; FUCHS, 1964) and of the quiescent rat uterus *in situ* (BISSET et al., 1966), in each case after initial stimulation. Higher molar ratios of epinephrine to oxytocin appear to be required for inhibition in the conscious, intact parturient rabbit (FUCHS, 1964) than in the spayed, oestrogenised rabbit anaesthetised with pentobarbital (CROSS, 1958). Norepinephrine is about half as active as epinephrine on the rabbit uterus *in situ* (CROSS, 1958).

The response of the isolated uterus to oxytocin is also inhibited by epinephrine (NISHIYAMA and CHUMA, 1955). In experiments with the rat uterus *in vitro*, epinephrine caused a parallel shift of the log dose–response curves for oxytocin; in the presence of 0.8 ng of the antagonist the oxytocin concentrations had to be roughly tripled to match the original response. However, the antagonism is clearly not at the receptor level since epinephrine inhibits the contractile responses to acetylcholine, serotonin, and urinary kinin in the same fashion, and to about the same degree, as those to oxytocin; it is concluded that epinephrine acts at an independent receptor in such a way as to counteract contractile stimuli, or by blocking a stage in excitation–contraction coupling common to all four agonists (JENSEN and SUND, 1960b). Attempts to block the inhibitory effect of epinephrine by DCI were inconclusive.

The concentrations of epinephrine, norepinephrine and several related compounds required to decrease or block the response of the oestrous rat uterus to oxytocin *in vitro* are shown in Table 7 (BERDE and SAAMELI, 1966). The same compounds also inhibit the spontaneous contractions of the rat uterus in Tyrode solution. Isoprenaline appears to be outstandingly effective; the concentrations reported to cause partial inhibition are of the same order, or smaller than, uterotonically active concentrations of oxytocin on a molar basis. Isoxsuprine also relaxes the uterine muscle of several species *in vitro* and *in situ* (LISH et al., 1960a); it inhibits the contractions of the isolated rat uterus induced by oxytocin more effectively than those due to serotonin, barium chloride, or acetylcholine, the concentration required for 50% inhibition of a submaximal response to oxytocin being 0.058 μg/ml (LISH et al., 1960b). In doses of 0.6 mg/kg isoxsuprine also reduces the response of the oestrous rabbit uterus and gravid dog uterus *in situ* to infusions of oxytocin (about 1.7 mU/min/kg) (LISH et al., 1960a).

Table 7. *Inhibition of the Response of the Rat Uterus in vitro to Oxytocin (100 to 200 μU/ml) by Epinephrine and Related Compounds* (BERDE, unpublished results; cf. BERDE and SAAMELI, 1966)[1]

Compound[2]	Effective concentration, μg/ml, for partial inhibition	total inhibition
Epinephrine	0.1—100	100
Norepinephrine	0.0001	0.001—1
Isoprenaline	10^{-13}—10^{-5}	10^{-4}—10^{-3}
Isoxsuprine	1	10
Pronethalol	0.01—10	100

[1] Oestrous rats, medium of Gaddum et al. (1949), 30°. — [2] The same compounds in similar dosages also inhibit the spontaneous motility of the uterus in Tyrode solution at 37°.

All these compounds are thought to act principally at β-adrenotropic receptors (although isoxsuprine appears to have a papaverine-like action as well); on the other hand, pronethalol (cf. Table 7) typically blocks such receptors.

On uterine strips taken from non-oestrous guinea pigs epinephrine (1—100 ng/ml) and norepinephrine (10—100 ng/ml) inhibit the contractile response to oxytocin and vasopressin as well as to acetylcholine; higher doses of norepinephrine have a biphasic effect. The inhibitory action is blocked by DCI, showing that it involves the β-adrenotropic receptors. Reserpine added to the organ bath inhibits the response to oxytocin and vasopressin but only on organ preparations taken from animals not pretreated with reserpine *in vivo*; this inhibition is thought to result from the release by reserpine of catecholamines from stores (CLEGG, 1963).

The interaction of the neurohypophysial hormones and catecholamines in the vascular system is complex and as yet unclear; a potentiating effect of the peptides on the response to catecholamines is most frequently observed (see e. g. BARTELSTONE and NASMYTH, 1965). However, in some situations the appearance of antagonism may result. It has been shown that the vasodilator action of oxytocin in rats can be converted to a vasoconstriction not only by oestrogen treatment but by sympathectomy and by ganglionic or peripheral sympathetic blockade (LLOYD and PICKFORD, 1962); the same is true for dogs, monkeys, and man. The vasodilator response can be restored in dogs and monkeys after lumbar sympathectomy by infusions of epinephrine (but not of norepinephrine); if now infusion rates below those capable of reversing the response are chosen, the vasoconstrictor response to oxytocin may be merely reduced, resulting in an apparent antagonism (HAIGH et al., 1965). The suggestion that "the fraction of adrenaline released by sympathetic nerves is . . . . . essential for the dilator effect of oxytocin" (HAIGH et al., 1965) is borne out by experiments in which the β-adrenotropic blocking agents DCI (WALASZEK et al., 1963) and pronethalol (POISNER, unpublished; see POISNER, 1964) were shown to inhibit the depressor response to oxytocin in the anaesthetised rooster. The response to oxytocin (7 mU/kg) was completely blocked by 10 mg/kg DCI, and the original response was not matched by four times the dose of oxytocin. DCI also blocks the response to isoprenaline but not to acetylcholine, ATP, or Substance P. The vasoconstriction caused by oxytocin in the isolated chicken wing preparation is diminished but not blocked by DCI (WALASZEK et al., 1963).

The neuropeptide–catecholamine relation is not confined to smooth muscle. The antidiuretic response to oxytocin (4 mU) in the hydrated, ethanol-anaesthetised rat was blocked by pronethalol (0.1 mg/kg) even when the drug itself had no effect on urine flow or blood pressure. In the conscious water-loaded rat pronethalol (2 mg/kg) significantly inhibited the antidiuretic effect of vasopressin (1 mU) given 30 min later but did not alter the diuretic response to oxytocin (30 mU) (POISNER, 1964). The possibility that the site of antagonism is vascular is considered, among others. However, inhibition of the response to vasopressin by a β-adrenotropic blocking agent, DCI, has been observed in yet another, simpler preparation — the toad bladder (STRAUCH and LANGDON, 1964). In molar ratios of about 10^5:1 and above DCI partly or completely blocked the increase in water permeability brought about by vasopressin (3—7.5 ng/ml). The analogous response to theophylline is also inhibited, the response to cyclic AMP apparently not; also when both theophylline and cyclic AMP are added inhibition by DCI is less pronounced than when stimulation is by theophylline alone.

Now the formation of cyclic AMP by pigeon erythrocytes, and by avian erythrocyte cell membranes, is stimulated by epinephrine (as well as by isoprenaline and norepinephrine) and this effect is inhibited by DCI (DAVOREN and SUTHERLAND, 1963; ØYE and SUTHERLAND, 1966). STRAUCH and LANGDON (1964) therefore argue that, since DCI inhibits adenyl cyclase (the enzyme which converts ATP to cyclic AMP), the inhibition by the same compound of the permeability response to vasopressin is consonant with the view (ORLOFF and HANDLER, 1962) that vasopressin acts on this tissue by stimulating the production of cyclic AMP. This argument is almost certainly oversimplified. Pressure-fragmented pigeon erythrocyte membranes retain cyclase activity but this is unaffected by catecholamines (ØYE and SUTHERLAND, 1966), suggesting that activation of the enzyme by epinephrine may be mediated rather than direct; there is no evidence that DCI inhibits adenyl cyclase, as distinct from preventing its activation by epinephrine;

and there seems to be no evidence for a role of epinephrine in maintaining normal responsiveness to vasopressin in the toad bladder. These objections in detail do not, however, invalidate the conclusion that the bladder provides yet another example of the recurrent interplay between the neurohypophysial hormones and catecholamines or related compounds, and that the interaction in this instance is at the cellular or subcellular rather than the organ level. The results also constitute suggestive, though not compelling, evidence for the involvement of the cyclic-AMP system in this interaction.

B. Other phenols

Phenol and its nitro derivatives inhibit the response of the isolated rat uterus to oxytocin, the effectiveness increasing in the order phenol (1.03), *o*-nitrophenol (1.0), *p*-nitrophenol (0.13), 2,4-dinitrophenol (0.107), picric acid (0.104) (the figures in brackets give the concentration, in mM, causing 50% inhibition of the response to 0.25 mU/ml of oxytocin). Tyramine and tyrosine ethyl ester appear somewhat less active than *p*-nitrophenol; oestradiol is effective in concentrations as low as 0.04 mM. The inhibition by *p*-nitrophenol, tyramine, and oestradiol shows the formal characteristics of competitive antagonism. *p*-Nitrophenol (25—50 μg/ml) also inhibits the contractile response to acetylcholine and barium chloride but in a non-competitive fashion. The inhibitor potency within the series of nitrophenols increases with increasing acidity and the phenolate anion is therefore thought to be the active form (Ishida, 1961b). The ethyl 2,4-, 2,5-, 3,4- and 3,5-dihydroxybenzoates (but not the free acids) in concentrations above 60—100 μg/ml also act as oxytocin antagonists on the rat uterus (Aonuma et al., 1965),

Ishida (1961b) regards the inhibition by phenols, including tyrosine derivatives and peptides (Ishida and Hara, 1964; Ishida et al., 1966) as true competitive antagonism at the receptor level (see p. 771); however, the inhibition of the response to other stimulants shows that other mechanisms must also operate.

VII. Steroids and Lipids

It is well known that endogenous and exogenous steroid hormones (oestrogens, progesterone) dramatically affect the reactivity of the uterus to oxytocin (e.g. Csapo, 1961) and also the responses of the vascular system to both oxytocin and vasopressin (Lloyd, 1959a, b; Lloyd and Pickford, 1961, 1962; Haigh et al., 1963, 1965).

When progesterone (10 μg/ml) is added to a rat uterine strip immersed in a medium containing oxytocin (50 μU/ml) the action potentials disappear in the course of 30 min, and the muscle is left refractory to the action of oxytocin (Marshall and Csapo, 1961). Exposure of a rat or guinea-pig uterus *in vitro* to progesterone (20 or 40 μg/ml) for 3 min depresses the mechanical response not only to oxytocin (0.4 mU/ml) but also to prostaglandin and electrical stimulation (Sullivan, 1966). However, oestradiol (1—10 μg/ml) is also reported to inhibit the response of the rat uterus to oxytocin *in vitro*; the effect has the appearance of competitive antagonism (Ishida, 1961b).

In spite of the probable physiological significance of the interrelations between steroid and neurohypophysial peptide hormones relatively little is known about their molecular basis. It has been suggested (Woolley, 1964) that oestrogens might participate in the structure of the specific uterine receptor for oxytocin; however, this could at most be one of several mechanisms involved since the steroids affect numerous other properties of the uterus, including its gross morphology, electrical activity, and reactivity to other drugs. Progesterone is thought to act primarily on the electrical properties of the myometrial cell membranes (MARSHALL and CSAPO, 1961); the inhibition by oestradiol is regarded as analogous to that by other phenols (ISHIDA, 1961b; see p. 783). The action of oestrogens in reversing the vascular reaction to oxytocin may be exerted by way of the neural mediator systems (HAIGH et al., 1965). Steroids of all hormonal types, as the water-soluble sulphates, inhibit the action of oxytocin on the uterus (HEMPEL and NEUMANN, 1965).

The neurohypophysial hormones and mineralocorticoids share common target organs in the kidney and amphibian bladder; however, their respective effects on salt and water excretion represent the operation of largely independent regulating systems. Even in the toad bladder preparation the vasopressin-induced change in short-circuit current is independent of pretreatment with aldosterone *in vitro* and *in vivo* (CRABBÉ and DE WEER, 1965), a relation suggesting different sites of action.

The interaction of oxytocin and lysine-vasopressin with prostaglandins on the uterus has been studied (ELIASSON, 1966) but no clear-cut antagonism has been observed. On the other hand, the water permeability response of the toad bladder to vasopressin (1 mU/ml, i.e. about 2 nM) was significantly inhibited by a purified prostaglandin, PGE_1, in concentrations as low as 1.7 and 0.17 nM. PGE_1 also inhibited the response to theophylline (10 mM) but not to cyclic AMP; ricinoleic acid had no effect. It is thought possible that PGE may serve as a physiological regulator of the antidiuretic response to vasopressin (ORLOFF et al., 1965).

VIII. Hydrogen and Metal Ions

Although it is hardly customary to include the pH dependence of a response under the heading of antagonism, in the cases to be discussed below the relation appears to be sufficiently clear, and informative, to justify such an inclusion. The physiological role of the neurohypophysial hormones in regulating ion movements lends particular interest to any antagonistic action of the common ions on these hormones; such action may in addition be of some practical importance since it is suspected that certain nephropathies involving refractoriness to antidiuretic hormone may result from ion imbalances such as hypercalcaemia or hypokalaemia (see e.g. HAYS and LEAF, 1961; BUCHBORN, 1965; FINN et al., 1966).

A. Hydrogen ions

The action of vasopressin in increasing the osmotic flow of water through the toad bladder is almost completely inhibited by acidification of the serosal medium from the usual pH of 8.4 to 6.5 (BENTLEY, 1958; SCHWARTZ et al., 1960). Detailed analyses of the pH dependence of this response by two groups of authors using somewhat different experimental produres and mathematical treatment but essentially the same premises (RASMUSSEN et al., 1963; GULYASSY and EDELMAN, 1965) gave consonant results. The inhibition was reversible between pH 8.4 and 6.7, surmountable by increased concentrations of the hormone, and over the pH range from 8.4 to 7.0 it showed the characteristics of a competitive antagonism; at lower pH values the maximal response was decreased as well as the response to a given concentration of peptide. The dissociable group responsible for the pH dependence between pH 8.4 and 7.0 was found to have a pK_a of about 8; the values for this constant reported in the two papers, and for different peptides — arginine-vasopressin, oxytocin, and deamino-oxytocin — do not appear to differ significantly. The result for deamino-oxytocin clearly shows that the ionising group is associated with the target tissue. Since the action of cyclic

AMP has a pH optimum of 7.0 it is unlikely that the step determining the pH dependence of hormone action is subsequent to formation of the mediator (GULYASSY and EDELMAN, 1965) — provided the pH dependence for exogenous cyclic AMP is not composite in character. Partially purified preparations of adenyl cyclase show a broad pH optimum between pH 7.2 and 8.2 (SUTHERLAND et al., 1962) which also by itself cannot account for the observed pH dependence of the hormone effect in this range, although the low activity of the enzyme at pH 6.5 may be related to the sharply decreased effect of both vasopressin and theophylline at this pH (ORLOFF and HANDLER, 1962, 1964). The simplest assumption is that the dissociable group is located on the receptor itself; from its pK_a, this group might be a sulphydryl (RASMUSSEN et al., 1963) but also a peptide α-amino group or substituted imidazole (GULYASSY and EDELMAN, 1965) — in either case the result carries the suggestion that the functional receptor is chemically a protein, or closely associated with a protein.

Acidification of the serosal medium to pH 6.7 also decreases the rate of uptake of radioactivity by the toad bladder exposed to tritiated oxytocin; however, since this uptake continues even after the response has reached its peak the precise significance of this result remains doubtful, though it is thought to point to an intracellular locus of vasopressin action; the second dissociable group whose presence has been inferred, with a pK_a of about 7, may then act by impairing peptide transport into the cell (GULYASSY and EDELMAN, 1965). Alternatively it may be associated with the adenyl cyclase system (see above).

The transport of sodium (but not of water, urea, potassium or chloride) through the toad bladder is increased when the mucosal medium is acidified to pH 5.5. Addition of vasopressin to the serosal solution causes a further increase in the short-circuit current (LEAF et al., 1964). Whereas acidification of the serosal medium increases the intracellular hydrogen ion concentration, acidification of the mucosal solution does not (LEAF et al., 1964; GULYASSY, 1965), nor does it alter the serosal pH, so that the site of action of the hormone remains unaffected. The stimulation of sodium transport from the acidified mucosal medium may be due to increased sodium permeation into the cells through the mucosal barrier (LEAF et al., 1964).

Lysine-vasopressin in rather high concentrations (100 mU/ml) inhibits the efflux of sodium from the single muscle fibres of the crab, *Maia squinado*, at pH 8.4; the effect is abolished if the pH is decreased below 7.4. This pH dependence is discussed in terms of possible changes in the inward diffusion of the hormone and competition between hormone and hydrogen ions for a site on the postulated intracellular receptor (BITTAR, 1966). The examination of uncharged analogues should, as in the case of the toad bladder, afford evidence on the first possibility.

The sensitivity to oxytocin of the isolated human myometrium, as well as its spontaneous activity, is decreased as the pH is lowered from 7.7 to 7.1 (MARKS, 1961). For the isolated rat uterus it has been shown that a change in the pH of the medium from 7.3 to 7.0 and 6.6 causes a parallel displacement of the log dose–response curves for oxytocin along the concentration axis by an amount proportional to the hydrogen ion concentration; this apparent competitive inhibition by hydrogen ion has been ascribed to a decrease in the concentration of the anionic (phenolate) species which is thought to be the active form of the hormone (ISHIDA, 1961a). The relatively high uterotonic activity of several oxytocin analogues lacking the ionisable phenolic group, such as Phe^2-oxytocin (BODANSZKY and DU VIGNEAUD, 1959a, b; JAQUENOUD and BOISSONNAS, 1959) and (p-Me)Phe^2-oxytocin (ZHUZE et al., 1964) makes it unlikely that this explanation is correct.

B. Calcium

When the calcium concentration of the Ringer medium in contact with the serosal surface of the toad bladder is raised from 2.7 mM to 8—10 mM the increase in water permeability which is the normal response to pituitrin or vasopressin is significantly inhibited; no such inhibition is observed when the calcium concentration is raised in the mucosal medium (BENTLEY, 1959, PETERSEN and EDELMAN, 1964). The response to 1 mU/ml of vasopressin was lowered by 60—65% in 10 mM calcium (serosal), but the response to 66 mU/ml was not significantly inhibited, showing that the inhibition is surmountable. Under the same conditions the effect of vasopressin (1 mU/ml) on the permeability to urea was inhibited by 40—45% (PETERSEN and EDELMAN, 1964). Independent evidence of the same effect has been obtained by a completely different experimental approach using kidney slices from the newt, *Necturus maculosus* (WHITTEMBURY et al., 1960). Administration of vasopressin (10 IU) to the animal $2^1/_2$—$3^1/_2$ hours before removal of the kidney increases the equivalent pore radius as measured *in vitro* by the iso-osmotic concentrations of a graded series of probing molecules; but the increase in the iso-osmotic concentration of glycerol and erythritol normally resulting from vasopressin pretreatment is partly or completely inhibited when the calcium concentration in the medium is increased from 1 mM to 5 mM and 10 mM, respectively (WHITTEMBURY et al., 1960).

By contrast, increased calcium does not affect the action of vasopressin on sodium transport through the toad bladder (BENTLEY, 1960; PETERSEN and EDELMAN, 1964). In the frog skin (*Rana temporaria*) the short-circuit current is decreased when the calcium concentration in the serosal medium is raised so that, in appropriately arranged experiments, calcium appears to reverse the action of vasopressin; however, quantitative analysis of this interrelation shows that calcium and vasopressin act on sodium transport at separate sites and, moreover, that these sites are in parallel on independent pathways of sodium transport rather than consecutive on a single pathway (HERRERA and CURRAN, 1963).

The difference between the calcium effect on vasopressin-stimulated movement of water and small uncharged solutes on the one hand and of sodium ions on the other must be accomodated within any model of neurohypophysial hormone action on the amphibian membranes. If such a model assumes that the effects of the hormones on the osmotic flow of water and uncharged solutes, and on the transport of sodium, are initiated by interaction with a single set of receptors, with the pathways leading to the separate observed effects diverging at some later point, then the stage at which calcium affects the water permeability response must be located after the point of divergence. If, on the other hand, the two responses are assumed to be initiated by interaction of the hormone with two distinct sets of receptors, then calcium might affect the one but not the other at any stage, including the primary event of hormone–receptor interaction. PETERSEN and EDELMAN (1964) have found that the action of cyclic AMP on the water permeability of the toad bladder, unlike that of vasopressin, is unaffected by calcium; accepting the strong evidence which indicates that the effects of neurohypophysial hormones on the toad bladder are mediated by cyclic AMP they conclude that this result is incompatible with the existence of a single set of receptors. They propose a model in which vasopressin acts on the toad bladder to generate cyclic AMP at two different loci, one at the mucosal and one at the serosal border of the epithelial cells; at the first of these the ultimate effect is a change in the permeability to water and urea (and possibly also sodium), at the second activation of the mechanism of active transport of sodium (the "sodium pump"). Calcium competes with vasopressin at the first of these sites only.

However, most of the evidence goes to show that vasopressin does not activate the "sodium pump" as such but increases permeation of sodium from the mucosal medium into the epithelial cells and thereby increases the amount available to the "pump;" the site of this action, as of the action on water permeability, is thought to be at the urinary border of the mucosal cells (LEAF, 1960; FRAZIER et al., 1962; HERRERA and CURRAN, 1963; CURRAN et al., 1963; LICHTENSTEIN and LEAF, 1965; CRABBÉ and DE WEER, 1965; CIVAN et al., 1966). In the double series barrier model of permeability regulation (ANDERSEN and USSING, 1957) it is the outer, dense diffusion barrier which is thought to limit the entry into the cell of sodium as well as small solutes whereas the inner, porous barrier is decisive for the osmotic flow of water (ANDERSEN and USSING, 1957; LEAF and HAYS, 1962; HAYS and LEAF, 1962a, b; LICHTENSTEIN and LEAF, 1965). It is conceivable that these sites are sufficiently distinct topographically to permit localised generation and action of cyclic AMP as envisaged in the model of PETERSEN and EDELMAN (1964). On the other hand, if it is conceded that cyclic AMP added to the serosal medium is not fully equivalent to the endogenous nucleotide a single-receptor model could yet be proposed in which calcium prevents access of endogenous (but not exogenous) nucleotide to one but not the other class of sites.

The evidence from calcium inhibition suggests that the site of action of vasopressin on urea transport, as on the osmotic flow of water through the toad bladder, is the porous barrier; on the other hand, amphotericin B inhibits the vasopressin effect on the permeability to urea and sodium but not to water, apparently implicating the outer diffusion barrier as the main hindrance to the movement of urea (LICHTENSTEIN and LEAF, 1965; see p. 791). If, in fact, both barriers can appreciably affect the permeation of urea this conflict of evidence may arise from the different experimental conditions used in the two sets of inhibitor studies, particularly perhaps the lower osmotic gradient in the work with amphotericin B (LICHTENSTEIN and LEAF, 1965).

C. Other cations

The water permeability response of the toad bladder to pituitrin is inhibited when the potassium concentration in the serosal medium is changed in either direction from the normal value of 3.35 mM. An increase to 5 mM inhibited the response to 1 mU/ml of pituitrin by about 26%, an increase to 10 mM by about 80%; reversal of the effect required rather prolonged exposure to normal Ringer solution (BENTLEY, 1959).

Exposure of the inner surface of the frog skin to increased concentrations of potassium chloride (but not potassium sulphate) inhibits the sodium transport response to vasopressin. The effect is associated with swelling of the epithelial cells and is thought to result from the stretching of the cell membranes, possibly because this mimics the action of vasopressin, or because it opens alternative pathways for sodium permeation which make the vasopressin-stimulated entry negligible (USSING et al., 1965).

Magnesium in concentrations up to about 0.3 mM is well known to potentiate the response of the uterus to the neurohypophysial hormones and their analogues; however, higher concentrations inhibit the response (VAN DYKE and HASTINGS, 1928; KREJČÍ et al., 1964), possibly as a result of the general depressant action of this ion (SCHILD, 1964).

The effect of pituitrin on the water permeability of the toad bladder is also inhibited by the addition of magnesium to the serosal medium; the decrease in response to 1 mU/ml pituitrin is about 18% in 1 mM and 48% in 3 mM magnesium. A similar effect is shown by barium, strontium, and manganese (BENTLEY, 1959).

IX. Other Antagonists

At this point, an attempt to classify the remaining miscellaneous cases of antagonism according to the chemical structure of the antagonists would be merely formal, and biochemical or pharmacological categories will therefore be used.

A. Metabolic inhibitors

The action of the neurohypophysial hormones on the osmotic flow of water and on sodium transport through the toad bladder is decreased or blocked by a number of metabolic inhibitors (BENTLEY, 1958; RASMUSSEN et al., 1960; HANDLER et al., 1966). Iodoacetate (0.5 mM), malonate (7 mM), cyanide (1 mM), and 2,4-dinitrophenol (0.1 mM) added to the serosal medium each decreased the water permeability response to pituitary extract (1 mU/ml) by 20—40% (BENTLEY, (1958); azide (1 mM) was also effective but fluoroacetate was not. Iodoacetate, dinitrophenol, azide, and fluoroacetate all decrease the short-circuit current through the toad bladder and in addition inhibit its response to vasopressin. Inhibition of the water permeability response to vasopressin by iodoacetate and dinitrophenol persists in sodium-free (choline-Ringer) media (HANDLER et al., 1966).

The active transport of sodium is well known to require metabolic energy and the lessened sensitivity to hormone stimulation of a process itself subject to inhibition is perhaps not surprising. It is more difficult to see why the mechanism by which the neurohypophysial hormones induce changes in the osmotic flow of water should be dependent, at least in part, on oxidative metabolism (BENTLEY, 1958); perhaps this dependence is indirect, involving such factors as potassium depletion (HANDLER et al., 1966).

Exposure of rat uterine strips to 2,4-dinitrophenol (1 mM) for 40 min decreased their electrical activity and inhibited both spotaneous activity and the response to oxytocin or electrical stimulation; the effects were greater for progesterone-dominated than for oestrogen-dominated muscles. Iodoacetate (0.2 mM) abolished the contractile response to oxytocin and electrical stimulation without altering the membrane potential. The effects of dinitrophenol but not of iodoacetate could be reversed by washing. The inhibition of the response to oxytocin by both compounds may be associated with their action on the cell membrane: depolarisation in the first case and stabilisation in the second (MARSHALL and MILLER, 1964). Other authors (ISHIDA, 1961b; AONUMA et al., 1965) habe interpreted the antagonistic effects of dinitrophenol and thyroxine in terms of their chemical properties as phenols rather than their biochemical effects (p. 783).

B. Some natural and synthetic drugs

Histamine inhibits the action of the neurohypophysial hormones (NISHIYAMA and CHUMA, 1955; JENSEN and SUND, 1960a) as well as other agents on the isolated uterus. In about 10 μM solution it causes a parallel displacement of the log dose–response curves for oxytocin, acetylcholine, serotonin, and urinary kinin to about the same extent. As in the case of epinephrine (JENSEN and SUND, 1960b; p. 781) the unspecific inhibition presumably affects some stage in the excitation–contraction coupling subsequent to the specific receptor interactions (JENSEN and SUND, 1960a).

Papaverine (1—10 μg/ml) inhibits the response of the isolated rat uterus to oxytocin in the normal dose range (LISH et al., 1960a; TAKAGI et al., 1961; BERDE and SAAMELI, 1966). The inhibition is non-competitive in character (TAKAGI et al., 1961) and non-specific since spontaneous activity and responses to acetylcholine, barium chloride and serotonin are also affected (LISH et al., 1960a, b; TAKAGI et al., 1961; BERDE and SAAMELI, 1966). Papaverine (10 mg/kg) also inhibits the contractions of the oestrogenised rat uterus *in situ* evoked by oxytocin infusion (100 mU/h/kg) (LISH et al., 1960b). Diphenhydramine is about as effective as papaverine on the rat uterus *in vitro* (TAKAGI et al., 1961), pethidine and tolazoline somewhat less (BERDE and SAAMELI, 1966).

The contractile response of the guinea-pig proximal colon to vasopressin (0.8 mU/ml) is markedly inhibited by hexamethonium (10 μg/ml) and pentolinium (1 μg/ml) but only slightly by atropine (1 μg/ml); the response to acetylcholine or histamine is unaffected, or slightly potentiated, by hexamethonium. The inhibition byganglionic blocking agents indicates the participation of nervous elements in the response of this preparation to vasopressin (BOTTING, 1965).

Diphenhydramine, orphenandrine, tripelennamine, and chlorpheniramine (about 10 mg/kg) as well as atropine and propantheline bromide (1 mg/kg) reduce the inhibitory effect of oxytocin, vasopressin, and bradykinin on the spontaneous intestinal motility of the anaesthetised dog*. The effect correlates neither with the antihistaminic nor with the anticholinergic properties within this series of drugs and its basis remains unclear (LEVY, 1963).

A number of antihistamine and related drugs (Table 8) inhibit the water permeability response of the frog (*R. temporaria*) bladder to pituitary extract. The relation between log concentration and percentage inhibition for tiphenamil is sigmoid over the concentration range 10^{-6}—10^{-3}M (NATOCHIN and MAGAZANIK, 1964). The investigation of these compounds was based on the hypothesis (GINETZINSKY, 1958) that the effects of the neurohypophysial hormones on water permeability are due to the release of hyaluronidase which depolymerises the interstitial hyaluronic acid, on the observation (GINETSINSKII and VASIL'EVA, 1963) that some hyaluronidase inhibitors are diuretic in dogs, and on the finding (ŠMAHEL, 1960) that certain antihistamine agents inhibit hyaluronidase *in vivo*. However, the relative inhibitor potency of the compounds in Table 8 shows no clear relation to antihistamine activity, or to chemical structure except that the quaternary methyl methosulphates of several active drugs are ineffective as inhibitors, indicating an intracellular locus of action (NATOCHIN and MAGAZANIK, 1964).

Chlorobutanol (1,1,1-trichloro-2-methyl-2-propanol), an anaesthetic commonly added to commercial preparations of oxytocin and vasopressin, has a vasodilator effect in cats (KATZ, 1964) and relaxes canine artery strips (SOMLYO et al., 1966). The concentrations present in oxytocin preparations (1 mg chlorobutanol with 2 IU oxytocin) are such that they may partly or wholly reverse the vasoconstrictor action as shown by oxytocin without the additive in parallel experiments (KATZ, 1964, SOMLYO et al., 1966). The danger that the use of such commercial preparations, without proper controls, may lead to spurious results is obvious but nevertheless requires continued emphasis.

Phenacetin (0.5 mg/ml) in the serosal medium significantly inhibits the water permeability response of the toad bladder to vasopressin (5 mU/ml); sodium acetylsalicylate has no such effect. This finding suggests (on the assumption that the toad bladder is a valid model for the human kidney tubule) that phenacetin

* It has since been reported that only commercial preparations of oxytocin and vasopressin containing chlorobutanol, as well as chlorobutanol itself, inhibit the motility of rabbit and guinea-pig ileum (BOTTING and MANLEY, 1867) though preservative-free arginine-vasopressin does relax rabbit lower colon muscle (WOO and SOMLYO, 1967). It is possible that the antagonism observed by LEVY (1963) is directed not against an effect of the neurohypophysial hormones but against the action of chlorobutanol (BOTTING and MANLEY, 1967).

is responsible for the vasopressin-resistant hyposthenuria resulting from the abuse of analgesics (NUSYNOWITZ et al., 1966).

Acetazolamide (80 mg/kg) inhibits the response of conscious water-load rats to lysine-vasopressin (5 mU/kg i. p.). This effect of acetazoalamide is ascribed to its ability to inhibit carbonic anhydrase and interpreted as evidence that the action of vasopressin on the tubular resorption of water involves activation of carbonic anhydrase by the hormone (TABORSKY, 1966; cf. KASHIWAGA, 1959). In high concentrations (1 mg/ml) acetazolamide inhibits the water permeability response of the toad bladder to pituitary extract (1 mU) (BENTLEY, 1958).

The diuresis induced by furosemide and ethacrynic acid in human subjects does not respond to vasopressin, a situation which "formally . . . corresponds to a partial tubular refractoriness to ADH" (BUCHBORN, 1965). Furosemide and acetazolamide have been shown to abolish the sodium and urea concentration

Table 8. *Inhibition of the Water-permeability Response of the Frog (R. temporaria) Bladder to Pituitrin by Some Drugs* (After NATOCHIN and MAGAZANIK, 1964)

No.	Drug[1]	Chemical character[2]	Inhibition[3] %
1	Promazine	A	100
2	Chlorpromazine	A	100
3	Tiphenamil	B	97
4	Diethazine	A	94
5	Meflophenhydramine	C	92
6	Cyclizine	D	90
7	Chloracyzine	A	87
8	Diphenhydramine	C	86
9	Caramiphen	B	84
10	Diphazine	A	84
11	Moxastine	C	84
12	N-(N'-Diethylaminoethylalanyl)phenothiazine	A	82
13	Antazoline	E	77
14	Arpenal	B	74
15	Perastine	C	73
16	Mebhydroline	F	60

[1] The benzilic acid esters of dimethylaminoethanol (benactyzine, 17), diethylaminoethanol (benzazine, 18) and 3-dimethylamino-2-methylbutanol were marginally active; the methyl methosulphates of 1, 3, 9, 10, 14, 17, and 18 were inactive. — [2] A Phenothiazine derivatives, B diphenylacetic or related basic esters, C benzhydryl basic ethers, D benzhydrylamine, E imidazoline, F carboline. — [3] Percentage inhibition of response to pituitrin (1 mU/ml) by drug (1 mM) in serosal medium.

gradients in the rat kidney (HELLER et al., 1965) and the absence of an antidiuretic response to vasopressin after treatment with these diuretics is presumably due largely to the elimination of the countercurrent concentrating system, though BUCHBORN (1965) concludes that furosemide and ethacrynic acid in addition decrease the water permeability of the collecting tubules. The water-permeability response of the toad bladder to arginine-vasopressin (5 or 10 mU/ml) is unaffected by furosemide (76 μM) in the serosal medium but the action of the hormone, and also of coffeine and of cyclic AMP, on the short-circuit current is reduced or blocked. A certain structural resemblance suggests that furosemide might act as a competitive antagonist of the cyclic nucleotide (FERGUSON, 1966).

The diuretic action of cyclophosphamide and its metabolite, β,β'-dichlorodiethylamine ("nor-nitrogen mustard") in rats and dogs has been traced to inhibition of the response to endogenous vasopressin; both compounds (100 and

50 mg/kg, respectively) also decrease the response to exogenous vasopressin. The antagonism appears to be peripheral but in view of the varied reactivity of these alkylating agents the molecular site of action remains uncertain*. The diuretic effects of other alkylating agents reported in the literature could be due to the same cause (ZEDECK et al., 1966).

The polyene antibiotics amphotericin B and nystatin added to the mucosal medium (2—13 μg/ml) increase the short-circuit current through the toad bladder and decrease or abolish its response to vasopressin (50 mU/ml) without affecting the water-permeability response to the hormone. The antibiotics are thought to "open" the mucosal diffusion barrier to sodium, urea and other small molecules, possibly as a result of their ability to form complexes with steroids (LICHTENSTEIN and LEAF, 1965); the effect in some respects resembles that of calcium and is discussed in this context on p. 787).

Prolonged (90 min) exposure of the toad bladder to ouabain (0.1 mM) inhibits the water permeability response to vasopressin, probably as a result of potassium depletion (FINN et al., 1966).

C. Inhibitors of unknown structure

Commercial "cholera filtrates" briefly stimulate and then depress sodium transport through the frog (*R. temporaria*) skin and inhibit its response to vasopressin; the material is more active in contact with the mucosal than with the serosal surface. The effect on sodium transport may by related to pathological mechanisms (LYNG, 1964).

On prolonged exposure of toad bladders to the neurohypophysial hormones the permeability gradually decreases (GOLDBERG et al., 1963; KARLIN, 1963; EDELMAN et al., 1964). When such bladders are transferred to fresh medium their reactivity to the hormones remains low, pointing to an intrinsic factor; but the original medium also inhibits the response of fresh bladders, indicating the existence in addition of a soluble inhibitor (GOLDBERG et al., 1963). The inhibitor extracted from homogenised toad bladders (KARLIN and OVERWEG, 1965; OVERWEG, 1966) is non-dialysable but after heating (100°, 10 min) it passes into the dialysate. Such preparations inhibit the water-permeability response of toad bladders to oxytocin, arginine-vasotocin, and theophylline but not to cyclic AMP, and also the contractile response of the isolated rat uterus to oxytocin and (less effectively) to acetylcholine and serotin. Concentrations corresponding to the extract of 2 bladders in 1000 ml still have appreaciable activity. The inhibitor is inactivated by heating with strong acid and alkali but not by incubation with trypsin, chymotrypsin, pepsin, and pronase; its chemical nature remains unclear (OVERWEG, 1966).

X. Conclusions

Studies of antagonism have already contributed toward a definition of the specificities of the neurohypophysial hormones on the one hand and toward a knowledge of interrelations between various systems of humoral and nervous regulation on the other. They have yielded information about the cellular sites of action of the hormones in some instances but as yet done little to elucidate the molecular nature of the primary event in hormone action, or the identity of the receptor. On the whole more questions have so far been raised than answered.

* Ethylene imine, which inhibits the antidiuretic response of dogs with experimental diabetes insipidus to vasopressin (GOLDBLATT, KAUKER, HARE, and HARE, 1966) is a related alkylating agent. It is thought to act primarily on the vasopressin-sensitive urea transport in the kidney (GOLDBLATT et al., 1966).

It seems likely that future work on this topic will be concerned, among other problems, with the design of more effective specific inhibitors of potential practical interest and the definition of molecular features required for activity as against binding to the specific receptors; attempts to identify the receptors, perhaps with the aid of inhibitors irreversibly bound at the site of action; and the more precise definition of the interrelations with other humoral systems at both the physiological and the biochemical level. A close coordination between the chemical, biochemical, pharmacological, and physiological approaches to these problems is likely to prove particularly effective.

Acknowledgements

The authors are obliged to the following for permission to use Figures previously published: To Dr. S. Jard and Masson et Cie, Paris (Fig. 1), to the Cambridge University Press (Fig. 4 and 5), to the Editors and Publishers of the British Journal of Pharmacology and Chemotherapy, B.M.A. House, Tavistock Square, London (Fig. 6), to Dr. B. Berde (Fig. 12), and to Prof. Y. Ishida and the Pharmaceutical Society of Japan (Fig. 16).

References

Acher, R., J. Chauvet, M.T. Chauvet, and D. Crepy: Phylogénie des peptides neurohypophysaires: Isolement de la mesotocine (Ileu$_8$-ocytocine) de la grenouille, intermédiaire entre la Ser$_4$-Ileu$_8$-ocytocine des poissons osseux et l'ocytocine des mammifères. Biochim. biophys. Acta (Amst.) **90**, 613—615 (1964).

— —, and G. Olivry: Sur l'existence éventuelle d'une hormone unique neurohypophysaire. I. Relations entre l'ocytocine, la vasopressine et la protéine de van Dyke extraites de la neurohypophyse du boeuf. Biochim. biophys. Acta (Amst.) **22**, 421—427 (1956).

Ames, R.G., and H.B. van Dyke: Thioglycollate inactivation of posterior pituitary antidiuretic principle as determined in the rat. Proc. Soc. exp. Biol. (N.Y.) **76**, 576—578 (1951).

—, D.H. Moore, and H.B. van Dyke: The excretion of posterior pituitary antidiuretic hormone in the urine and its detection in the blood. Endocrinology **46**, 215—227 (1950).

Andersen, B., and H.H. Ussing: Solvent drag on non-electrolytes during osmotic flow through isolated toad skin and its response to antidiuretic hormone. Acta physiol. scand. **39**, 228—239 (1957).

Aonuma, S., T. Mimura, M. Okui, J. Mori, and K. Sasahara: Studies on posterior pituitary hormones. VI. The effects of thyroidhormone related compounds upon the uterine inhibitory responses to posterior pituitary hormones. Yakugaku Zasshi **85**, 703—709 (1965) [in Japanese].

Ariëns, E.J.: Molecular Pharmacology, Vol. 1. New York: Academic Press 1964.

Audrain, L., and H. Clauser: Relation entre l'activité physiologique de l'ocytocine et l'état de son pont disulfure. Biochim. biophys. Acta (Amst.) **30**, 191—192 (1958).

Bartelstone, H.J., and P.A. Nasmyth: Vasopressin potentiation of catecholamine actions in dog, rat, cat, and rat aortic strip. Amer. J. Physiol. **208**, 754—762 (1965).

Bentley, P.J.: The effects of neurohypophysial extracts on water transfer across the wall of the isolated urinary bladder of the toad Bufo marinus. J. Endocr. **17**, 201—209 (1958).

— The effects of ionic changes on water transfer across the isolated urinary bladder of the toad Bufo marinus. J. Endocr. **18**, 327—333 (1959).

— The effects of vasopressin on the short-circuit current across the wall of the isolated bladder of the toad, Bufo marinus. J. Endocr. **21**, 161—170 (1960).

— The effects of N-ethylmaleimide and glutathione on the isolated rat uterus and frog bladder with special reference to the action of oxytocin. J. Endocr. **30**, 103—113 (1964).

Beránková, Z., I. Rychlík, K. Jošt, J. Rudinger, and F. Šorm: Inhibition of the uterus-contracting effect of oxytocin by O-methyloxytocin. Collection Czech. chem. Commun. **26**, 2673—2675 (1961).

—, and F. Šorm: Enzymic inactivation of oxytocin. III. Desthiooxytocin and S,S′-dibenzyldihydrooxytocin as oxytocinase inhibitors and substrates. Collection Czech. chem. Commun. **26**, 2557—2761 (1961).

Beránková-Ksandrová, Z., G.W. Bisset, K. Jošt, I. Krejčí, V. Pliška, J. Rudinger, I. Rychlík, and F. Šorm: Synthetic analogues of oxytocin acting as hormonogens. Brit. J. Pharmacol. **26**, 615—632 (1966).

BERDE, B., and A. CERLETTI: Über die Wirkung pharmakologischer Oxytocindosen auf die Milchdrüse. Acta endocr. (Kbh) **34**, 543—557 (1960).

— — Über die antidiuretische Wirkung von synthetischem Lysin-Vasopressin. Helv. physiol. pharmacol. Acta **19**, 135—150 (1961).

— —, and H. KONZETT: The biological activity of a series of peptides related to oxytocin. In: Oxytocin, pp. 247—264. Ed. by R. CALDEYRO-BARCIA and H. HELLER. Proc. Int. Symp., Montevideo 1959. Oxford: Pergamon Press 1961.

—, and K. SAAMELI: Evaluation of substances acting on the uterus. In: Methods in Drug Evaluation, pp. 481—514. Ed. by P. MANTEGAZZA and F. PICCININI. Proc. Int. Symp., Milano 1965. Amsterdam: North-Holland 1966.

BEYERMAN, H.C., and J.S. BONTEKOE: Synthesis of a tyrosine "homologue" of lysine-vasotocin. Rec. Trav. chim. Pays-Bas **79**, 1044—1049 (1960a).

— — Synthesis of an analogue of lysine-vasopressin, with the phenylalanine "replaced" by two consecutive tyrosyl radicals. Rec. Trav. chim. Pays-Bas **79**, 1165—1173 (1960b).

— —, and A.C. KOCH: Synthesis of a tyrosine "homologue" of lysine-vasopressin. Rec. Trav. chim. Pays-Bas **79**, 1034—1038 (1960c).

— — — Synthesis of a tyrosine "homologue" of oxypressin. Rec. Trav. chim. Pays-Bas **79**, 1039—1043 (1960d).

BIANCHINI, P.: Attività di alcuni polipeptidi sull'utero in situ di ratta. Farmaco Ed. sci. **18**, 773—779 (1963).

BISSET, G.W.: The assay of oxytocin and vasopressin in blood and the mechanism of inactivation of these hormones by sodium thioglycollate. In: Oxytocin, pp. 380—398. Ed. by R. CALDEYRO-BARCIA and H. HELLER. Proc. Int. Symp., Montevideo 1959. Oxford: Pergamon Press 1961.

— Synthetic analogues of oxytocin acting as antagonists. J. Physiol. (Lond.) **165**, 69—71P (1962).

— The effect on milk-ejecting activity of modifying two functional groups in oxytocin. In: Oxytocin, Vasopressin and their Structural Analogues, pp. 21—29. Ed. by J. RUDINGER. Proc. 2nd Int. Pharmacol. Meeting, Prague 1963, Vol. 10. Oxford: Pergamon Press 1964.

—, J. HALDAR and J.E. LEWIN: Actions of oxytocin and other biologically active peptides on the rat uterus. In: Endogenous Substances affecting the Myometrium, pp. 185—197. Ed. by V.R. PICKLES and R.J. FITZPATRICK. Mem. Soc. Endocrinol. No. 14. London: Cambridge University Press 1966.

—, A.M. POISNER and D.G. SMYTH: Carbamylation of oxytocin and arginine-vasopressin. Nature (Lond.) **199**, 69—70 (1963).

— — — 1-N-Carbamyl-oxytocin — a new analogue with inhibitory properties toward oxytocin and vasopressin. J. Physiol. (Lond.) **170**, 12—13P (1964).

BITTAR, E.E.: On the natriferic action of 8-lysine vasopressin. Biochem. biophys. Res. Commun. **23**, 96—101 (1966).

BODANSZKY, M., and V. DU VIGNEAUD: Synthesis of a biologically active analog of oxytocin, with phenylalanine replacing tyrosine. J. Amer. chem. Soc. **81**, 1258—1259 (1959a).

— — Synthesis of a biologically active analog of oxytocin, with phenylalanine replacing tyrosine. J. Amer. chem. Soc. **81**, 6072—6075 (1959b).

BOISSONNAS, R.A., and S. GUTTMANN: Synthese d'analogues de l'ocytocine et de la lysine-vasopressine contenant de la phénylalanine ou de la tyrosine en positions 2 et 3. Helv. chim. Acta **43**, 190—200 (1960).

— — B. BERDE and H. KONZETT: Relationships between chemical structure and the biological properties of posterior pituitary hormones and their synthetic analogues. Experientia (Basel) **17**, 377—390 (1961).

BOTTING, J.H.: An isolated preparation with a selective sensitivity to vasopressin. Brit. J. Pharmacol. **24**, 156—162 (1965).

— and D.G. MANLEY: The action of commercial preparations of oxytocin and vasopressin on the smooth muscle of the gut. J. Pharm. Pharmacol. **19**, 66 (1967).

BRANDA, L.A., and V. DU VIGNEAUD: Synthesis and pharmacological properties of 9-decarboxamido-oxytocin. J. med. Chem. **9**, 169—172 (1966).

BRAUDE, R., and K.G. MITCHELL: Observations on the relationship between oxytocin and adrenaline in milk ejection in the sow. J. Endocr. **8**, 238—241 (1952).

BRESLOW, E., and L. ABRASH: The binding of oxytocin and oxytocin analogues by purified bovine neurophysins. Proc. nat. Acad. Sci. (Wash.) **56**, 640—646 (1966).

BROOKS, F.P., and M. PICKFORD: The effect of posterior pituitary hormones on the excretion of electrolytes in dogs. J. Physiol. (Lond.) **142**, 468—493 (1958).

BRUNNER, H., G. KUSCHINSKY and G. PETERS: Der Einfluß von Oxytocin auf die renale Wasser- und Salzausscheidung der Ratte. Arch. exp. Pathol. Pharmakol. **228**, 457—473 (1956).

Buchborn, E.: Nephrogener Diabetes insipidus und symptomatische ADH-Refraktärität. In: Normale und pathologische Funktionen des Nierentubulus, pp. 247—264. Ed. by K.J. Ullrich und K. Hierholzer. Bern und Stuttgart: Hans Huber 1965.

Campbell, B.J., B. Thysen and F.S. Chu: Peptidase catalysed hydrolysis of antidiuretic hormone in toad bladder. Life Sci. **4**, 2129—2140 (1965).

Cash, W.D., and B.L. Smith: Synthesis and biological properties of 1-acetyl-8-lysine-vasopressin. J. biol. Chem. **238**, 994—997 (1963).

Chan, W.Y.: Mechanism of epinephrine inhibition of the milk ejecting response to oxytocin. J. Pharmacol. exp. Ther. **147**, 48—53 (1965).

Civan, M.M., O. Kedem and A. Leaf: Effect of vasopressin on toad bladder under conditions of zero net sodium transport. Amer. J. Physiol. **211**, 569—575 (1966).

Clegg, P.C.: The effect of adrenergic blocking agents on the guinea-pig uterus in vitro, and a study of the histology of the intrinsic myometrial nerves. J. Physiol. (Lond.) **169**, 73—90 (1963).

Cort, J.H.: Discussion. In: Oxytocin, Vasopressin and their Structural Analogues, pp. 72—74. Ed. by J. Rudinger. Proc. 2nd Int. Pharmacol. Meeting, Prague 1963, Vol. 10. Oxford: Pergamon Press 1964.

—, J. Rudinger, B. Lichardus and I. Hagemann: Effects of oxytocin antagonists on the saluresis accompanying carotid occlusion. Amer. J. Physiol. **210**, 162—168 (1966).

Crabbé, J., and P. de Weer: Action of aldosterone and vasopressin on the active transport of sodium by the isolated toad bladder. J. Physiol. (Lond.) **180**, 560—568 (1965).

Cross, B.A.: Sympathetico-adrenal inhibition of the neurohypophysial milk-ejection mechanism. J. Endocr. **9**, 7—18 (1953).

— The hypothalamus and the mechanism of sympathetico-adrenal inhibition of milk ejection. J. Endocr. **12**, 15—28 (1955a).

— Neurohormonal mechanisms in emotional inhibition of milk ejection. J. Endocr. **12**, 29—37 (1955b).

— The motility and reactivity of the oestrogenized rabbit uterus in vivo; with comparative observations on milk ejection. J. Endocr. **16**, 237—260 (1958).

Csapo, A.: The effect of oxytocic substances on the excitability of the uterus. In: Oxytocin, Proc. Int. Symp., Montevideo 1959, pp. 100—121. Ed. by Caldeyro-Barcia and H. Heller. Oxford: Pergamon Press 1961.

Curran, P.F., F.C. Herrera and W.J. Flanigan: The effect of Ca and antidiuretic hormone on Na transport across frog skin. II. Sites and mechanisms of action. J. gen. Physiol. **46**, 1011—1027 (1963).

Daniel, E.E., H. Sehdev and K. Robinson: Mechanisms for activation of smooth muscle. Physiol. Rev. **42**, Suppl. 5, 228—260 (1962).

Davoren, P.R., and E.W. Sutherland: The effect of L-epinephrine and other agents on the synthesis and release of adenosine 3′,5′-phosphate by whole pigeon erythrocytes. J. biol. Chem. **238**, 3009—3015 (1963).

Dekanski, J.: The quantitative assay of vasopressin. Brit. J. Pharmacol. **7**, 567—572 (1952).

Dicker, S.E.: The inactivation of vasopressin and of oxytocin, *in vitro*. In: Polypeptides which affect Smooth Muscles and Blood Vessels, pp. 79—82. Ed. by M. Schachter. Oxford: Pergamon Press 1960.

— The mechanism of action of oxytocin and vasopressin and their analogues on the kidney of mammals. In: Oxytocin, Vasopressin and their Structural Analogues, pp. 57—71. Ed. by J. Rudinger. Proc. 2nd Int. Pharmacol. Meeting, Prague 1963, Vol. 10. Oxford: Pergamon Press 1964.

—, and A.L. Greenbaum: The destruction of the antidiuretic activity of vasopressin by —SH active compounds. J. Physiol. (Lond.) **141**, 107—116 (1958).

—, and H. Heller: The renal action of posterior pituitary extract and its fractions as analysed by clearance experiments on rats. J. Physiol. (Lond.) **104**, 353—360 (1946).

Drabarek, S.: Analogs of oxytocin containing glycine in place of tyrosine, isoleucine, or glutamine. J. Amer. chem. Soc. **86**, 4477—4481 (1964).

—, and V. du Vigneaud: 2-D-Tyrosine-oxytocin and 2-D-tyrosine-deamino-oxytocin, diastereomers of oxytocin and deamino-oxytocin. J. Amer. chem. Soc. **87**, 3974—3978 (1965).

van Dyke, H.B., B.F. Chow, R.O. Greep, and A. Rothen: The isolation of a protein from the *pars neuralis* of the ox pituitary with constant oxytocic, pressor and diuresis-inhibiting activities. J. Pharmacol. exp. Ther. **74**, 190—209 (1942).

—, and A.B. Hastings: The response of smooth muscle in different ionic environments. Amer. J. Physiol. **83**, 563—570 (1928).

Edelman, I.S., M.J. Petersen and P.F. Gulyassy: Kinetic analysis of the antidiuretic action of vasopressin and adenosine-3′,5′-monophosphate. J. clin. Invest. **43**, 2185—2194 (1964).

Edman, K.A.P., and H.O. Schild: The need for calcium in the contractile responses induced by acetylcholine and potassium in the rat uterus. J. Physiol. (Lond.) **161**, 424—441 (1962).

Eggleton, M.G.: The diuretic action of alcohol in man. J. Physiol. (Lond.) **101**, 172—191 (1942).

Eliasson, R.: Effect of posterior pituitary hormones on the myometrial response to prostaglandin. Acta physiol. scand. **66**, 249—250 (1966).

Ely, F., and W.E. Petersen: Factors involved in the ejection of milk. J. Dairy Sci. **24**, 211—223 (1941).

Ferguson, D.R.: Effect of Frusemide on sodium and water transport by the isolated toad bladder. Brit. J. Pharmacol. **27**, 528—531 (1966).

Finn, A.L., J.S. Handler and J. Orloff: Relation between toad bladder potassium content and permeability response to vasopressin. Amer. J. Physiol. **210**, 1279—1284 (1966).

Fosker, A.P., and H.D. Law: Oxytocin and 4-glycine oxytocin. J. chem. Soc. 4922—4929 (1965).

Fraser, A.M.: The diuretic action of the oxytocic hormone of the pituitary gland and its effect on the assay of pituitary extracts. J. Pharmacol. exp. Ther. **60**, 89—95 (1937).

— Pituitary oxytocic hormone and urine secretion. J. Physiol. (Lond.) **101**, 236—251 (1942).

Frazier, H.S., E.F. Dempsey and A. Leaf: Movement of sodium across the mucosal surface of the isolated toad bladder and its modification by vasopressin. J. gen. Physiol. **45**, 529—543 (1962).

Frey, J., L. Kerp u. W. Reichardt: Zum Vasopressin-Oxytocin-Antagonismus beim Menschen. Klin. Wschr. **37**, 325—329 (1959).

Fuchs, A.-R.: Effect of adrenaline and vasopressin on the uterine response to oxytocin in conscious rabbits. Acta endocr. (Kbh.) **45**, 272—280 (1964).

Furtado, M.R.: The antagonistic action of bradykinin upon the effect of pitressin on the permeability to water of the toad bladder. Abstr. 3rd Int. Pharmacol. Congr., São Paulo, No. 451, 1966.

Furtado, M.R.F., and M.M. Machado: Effects of bradykinin on the movement of water and sodium in some isolated living membranes. Acta physiol. lat.-amer. **16**, 63—65 (1966).

Gaddum, J.H., W.S. Peart and M. Vogt: The estimation of adrenaline and allied substances in blood. J. Physiol. (Lond.) **108**, 467—481 (1949).

Gilliland, P.F., and T.E. Prout: Immunologic studies of octapeptides. II. Production and detection of antibodies to oxytocin. Metabolism **14**, 918—923 (1965).

Ginetsinskii, A.G., and V.F. Vasil'eva: Effect of hyaluronidase and its inhibitors on renal function. Fiziol. Zh. (Mosk.) **49**, 519—524 (1963) [in Russian].

Ginetzinsky, A.G.: Role of hyaluronidase in the re-absorption of water in renal tubules: the mechanism of action of the antidiuretic hormone. Nature (Lond.) **182**, 1218—1219 (1958).

Goldberg, D.C., M.A. Schoessler, and I.L. Schwartz: Intrinsic and extrinsic inhibition of the reactivity of the toad bladder to vasopressin. Physiologist **6**, 188 (1963).

Goldblatt, E.L., M.L. Kauker, R.S. Hare, and K. Hare: Effect of ethyleneimine on renal action of vasopressin. Proc. Soc. exp. Biol. (N.Y.) **123**, 845—847 (1966).

Goodfriend, T., G. Fasman, D. Kemp, and L. Levine: Immunochemical studies on angiotensin. Immunochemistry **3**, 223—231 (1966).

Gordon, S., and V. du Vigneaud: Preparation of S,S′-dibenzyloxytocin and its reconversion to oxytocin. Proc. Soc. exp. Biol. (N.Y.) **84**, 723—725 (1953).

Gulland, J.M., and S.S. Randall: The oxytocic hormone of the posterior lobe of the pituitary gland. V. Recognition as an oxidation-reduction system. Biochem. J. **29**, 378—390 (1935).

Gulyassy, P.F.: Intracellular H^+ concentration of the isolated urinary bladder of the toad. Nature (Lond.) **206**, 511—512 (1965).

—, and I.S. Edelman: Hydrogen-ion dependence of the antidiuretic action of vasopressin, oxytocin and deaminooxytocin. Biochim. biophys. Acta (Amst.) **102**, 185—197 (1965).

Guttmann, S., and R.A. Boissonnas: Synthèse de dix analogues de l'oxytocine et de la lysine-vasopressine, contenant de la sérine, de l'histidine ou du tryptophane en position 2 our 3. Helv. chim. Acta **43**, 200—216 (1960).

—, P.-A. Jaquenoud, R.A. Boissonnas, H. Konzett, and B. Berde: Ein Nonapeptid mit Oxytocin hemmenden Eigenschaften. Naturwissenschaften **44**, 632—633 (1957).

Haigh, A.L., A.H. Kitchin, and M. Pickford: The effect of oxytocin on hand blood flow in man following the administration of an oestrogen and isoprenaline. J. Physiol. (Lond.) **169**, 161—166 (1963).

—, S. Lloyd, and M. Pickford: A relationship between adrenaline and the mode of action of oxytocin and oestrogen on vascular smooth muscle. J. Physiol. (Lond.) **178**, 563—576 (1965).

HANDLER, J.S., and J. ORLOFF: Cysteine effect on toad bladder response to vasopressin, cyclic AMP, and theophylline. Amer. J. Physiol. **206**, 505—509 (1964).
—, M. PETERSEN, and J. ORLOFF: Effect of metabolic inhibitors on the response of the toad bladder to vasopressin. Amer. J. Physiol. **211**, 1175—1180 (1966).
HAYS, R.M., and A. LEAF: The problem of clinical vasopressin resistance: *in vitro* studies. Ann. intern. Med. **54**, 700—709 (1961).
— — Studies on the movement of water through the isolated toad bladder and its modification by vasopressin. J. gen. Physiol. **45**, 905—919 (1962a).
— — The state of water in the isolated toad bladder in the presence and absence of vasopressin. J. gen. Physiol. **45**, 933—948 (1962b).
HELLER, J., V. ŠKRHOVÁ, and J. VOSTÁL: The effect of various diuretic agents on renal electrolyte and urea concentration gradients in rats. Experientia (Basel) **21**, 454—455 (1965).
HEMPEL, R., and F. NEUMANN: Hemmung der Uteruswirkung von Oxytocin durch wasserlösliche Steroide. Acta endocr. (Kbh.) **48**, 656—663 (1965).
HERRERA, F.C., and P.F. CURRAN: The effect of Ca and antidiuretic hormone on Na transport across frog skin. I. Examination of interrelationships between Ca and hormone. J. gen. Physiol. **46**, 999—1010 (1963).
HODR, J., Z.K. ŠTEMBERA, V. ŠABATA, S. Kazda, V. BROTÁNEK, and J. RUDINGER: Effect of O-methyl-tyrosyl^2-oxytocin on carbohydrate and lipid metabolism in women during labour. In: Oxytocin and its Analogues, pp. 109—112. Ed. by R. KLIMEK and W. KRÓL. Kraków: Polish Endocrinological Society 1964.
HOLEČEK, V., and K. HORKÝ: Natriuretic effect of oxytocin in premenstrual tension. Čas. Lék. čes. **105**, 924—926 (1966) [in Czech].
HOLLÄNDER, L.P., J. FRANZ, and B. BERDE: An attempt to produce antibodies to oxytocin and vasopressin. Experientia (Basel) **22**, 325—328 (1966).
HOLTON, P.: A modification of the method of Dale and Laidlaw for standardization of posterior pituitary extract. Brit. J. Pharmacol. **3**, 328—334 (1948).
HUGUENIN, R.L.: Synthèse de la désamino^1-Orn^8-vasopressine, de la désamino^1-Phe^2-Orn^8-vasopressine, de la désamino^1-Ile^3-Orn^8-vasopressine (= désamino^1-Orn^8-oxytocine) et de la désamino^1-Phe^2-Ile^3-Orn^8-vasopressine (= désamino^1-Phe^2-Orn^8-oxytocine). Helv. chim. Acta **49**, 711—725 (1966).
—, and R.A. BOISSONNAS: Synthese de la (N-méthyl-Tyr)^2-oxytocine. Helv. chim. Acta **44**, 213—231 (1961).
—, and S. GUTTMANN: Synthese de l'Ala^1-Ala^6-Arg^8-vasopressine et de l'Ala^1-Ala^6-Lys^8-vasopressine, ainsi que de la (désamino-Ala)^1-Ala^6-Arg^8-vasopressine et de la (désamino-Ala^1)-Ala^6-Lys^8-vasopressine. Helv. chim. Acta **48**, 1885—1898 (1965).
ISHIDA, Y.: Studies of drug receptors on the plain muscle. III. Effect of hydrogen ion concentration upon ACh-, Ba-, and oxytocin-receptors of isolated rat uterus. Yakugaku Zasshi **81**, 1717—1721 (1961a) [in Japanese]. (In English: Ann. Rept. Fac. Pharm. Sci. Tokushima Univ. **11**, 45—51 (1962)).
— Studies of drug receptors on the plain muscle. IV. On the antagonistic action of phenolic compounds to oxytocin on isolated rat uterus. Yakugaku Zasshi **81**, 1722—1726 (1961b) [in Japanese]. (In English: Ann. Rept. Fac. Pharm. Sci. Tokushima Univ. **11**, 52—58 (1962)).
—, and K. HARA: Studies on inhibitory actions of synthetic peptides on the effects of oxytocin and vasopressin. Chem. pharm. Bull. **12**, 872—877 (1964).
—, H. MORITOKI, and K. HARA: Studies of drug receptors on the plain muscle. II. Influence of heavy metal ions on the oxytocin- and barium-receptor of isolated rat uterus. Yakugaku Zasshi **81**, 1713—1717 (1961) [in Japanese]. (In English: Ann. Rept. Fac. Pharm. Sci. Tokushima Univ. **11**, 38—44 (1962)).
— —, and M. ONISHI: Two kinds of oxytocin antagonists on the isolated rat uterus. Chem. pharm. Bull. **14**, 748—752 (1966).
JAQUENOUD, P.-A., and R.A. BOISSONNAS: Synthèse de la Phe^2-oxytocine. Helv. chim. Acta **42**, 788—793 (1959).
— — Synthèse de la Dé-Pro^7-oxytocine, de la Dé-Leu^8-oxytocine et de la Dé-Gly^9-oxytocine. Helv. chim. Acta **45**, 1462—1472 (1962).
JARD, S.: Étude des effecs de la vasotocine sur l'excrétion de l'eau et des électrolytes par le rein de la grenouille *Rana esculenta* L: Analyse à l'aide d'analogues artificiels de l'hormone naturelle des caractères structuraux requis pour son activité biologique. J. Physiol. (Paris) **58**, Suppl. 15 (1966).
—, and F. MOREL: Inhibition compétitive de l'action antidiurétique de la lysine-vasotocine par l'ocytocine chez *Rana esculenta*. Compt. rend. **252**, 339—341 (1961).
— — Actions of vasotocin and some of its analogues on salt and water excretion by the frog. Amer. J. Physiol. **204**, 222—226 (1963).

Jarvis, D., M. Bodanszky, and V. du Vigneaud: The synthesis of 1-(hemi-homocystine)-oxytocin and a study of some of its pharmacological properties. J. Amer. chem. Soc. **83**, 4780—4784 (1961).

—, B.M. Ferrier, and V. du Vigneaud: The effect of increasing the size of the ring present in deamino-oxytocin by one methylene group on its biological properties. J. biol. Chem. **240**, 3553—3557 (1965).

Jensen, K.B., and R.B. Sund: The inhibitory action of histamine on the isolated rat uterus. Acta pharmacol. (Kbh.) **17**, 161—172 (1960a).

— — The inhibitory action of adrenaline on the isolated rat uterus. Acta pharmacol. (Kbh.) **17**, 173—181 (1960b).

Jørgensen, C.B.: The amphibian water economy, with special regard to the effect of hypophyseal extracts. Acta physiol. scand. **22**, Suppl. 78 (1950).

—, and L.O. Larsen: Inhibition by oxytocin of vasotocin-induced activities in toads. Proc. Soc. exp. Biol. (N.Y.) **110**, 293—294 (1962).

Jošt, K., and J. Rudinger: Amino acids and peptides. LXIX. Synthesis of two biologically active analogues of deamino-oxytocin not containing a disulphide bond. Collection Czech. chem. Commun. **32**, 1229—1241 (1967).

— —, and F. Šorm: Amino-acids and peptides. XXXV. Analogues of oxytocin modified in positions 1 and 2 of the peptide chain: protected intermediates. Collection Czech. chem. Commun. **26**, 2496—2510 (1961).

— — — Amino acids and peptides. XXXVIII. Structural analogues of oxytocin modified in position 2 of the peptide chain: preparation and some chemical and biological properties. Collection Czech. chem. Commun. **28**, 1706—1714 (1963a).

— — — Amino acids and peptides. XXXIX. Analogues of oxytocin exerting protracted biological effects. Collection Czech. chem. Commun. **28**, 2021—2030 (1963b).

Karlin, A.: The *in vitro* release by the toad bladder of an inhibitor of oxytocin. Biochem. biophys. Res. Commun. **11**, 44—49 (1963).

—, and N.I.A. Overweg: An inhibitor of oxytocin from the urinary bladder of the toad, *Bufo marinus*. Nature (Lond.) **207**, 1401—1402 (1965).

Kasafírek, E., K. Jošt, J. Rudinger, and F. Šorm: Amino acids and peptides. LIV. Synthesis of further extended-chain analogues of oxytocin. Collection Czech. Chem. Commun. **30**, 2600—2608 (1965).

Kashiwagi, T.: Mechanism of the antidiuretic effect of vasopressin. Nature (Lond.) **184**, 991 (1959).

Katz, R.L.: Antiarrhythmic and cardiovascular effects of synthetic oxytocin. Anesthesiology **25**, 653—661 (1964).

Khairallah, P. A., R.R. Smeby, I.H. Page, and F.M. Bumpus: Effect of urea and amino acids on angiotensin interaction with smooth muscle. Biochim. biophys. Acta (Amst.) **104**, 85—91 (1965).

Kitchin, A.H., S. Lloyd, and M. Pickford: Some actions of oxytocin on the cardiovascular system in man. Clin. Sci. **18**, 399—408 (1958).

Konzett, H.: Zur Uteruswirkung eines oxytocinhomologen Polypeptids. Helv. physiol. pharmacol. Acta **15**, 419—425 (1957).

Kramár, J., E.H. Grinnell, and W.M. Duff: Observations on the diuretic activity of antidiuretic hormone. Amer. J. med. Sci. **252**, 53—61 (1966a).

— — — Studies on the renal activity of oxytocin. Amer. J. med. Sci. **252**, 331—339 (1966b).

Krejčí, I., B. Kupková, and I. Vávra: The effect of some 2-O-alkyltyrosine analogues of oxytocin and lysine vasopressin on the blood pressure of the rat, rabbit, and cat. Brit. J. Pharmacol. **30**, 497—505 (1967a).

—, I. Poláček, B. Kupková, and J. Rudinger: Dose-response analysis of the action of some oxytocin analogues on the isolated uterus: the effect of ions. In: Oxytocin, Vasopressin and their Structural Analogues, pp. 117—122. Ed. by J. Rudinger. Proc. 2nd Int. Pharmacol. Meeting, Prague 1963, Vol. 10. Oxford: Pergamon Press 1964.

— —, and J. Rudinger: The effect of an oxytocin analogue on the uterus and its dependence on the functional state of the myometrium. In: Endogenous Substances affecting the Myometrium, pp. 171—182. Ed. by V.R. Pickles and R.J. Fitzpatrick. Mem. Soc. Endocrinol. No. 14. London: Cambridge University Press 1966.

— — — The action of 2-O-methyltyrosine-oxytocin on the rat and rabbit uterus: effect of some experimental conditions on the change from agonism to antagonism. Brit. J. Pharmacol. **30**, 506—517 (1967b).

Kullander, S.: Studies on the hormonal control of the milkejection activity in lactating rabbits. Acta endocr. (Kbh.) **44**, 313—324 (1963).

Law, H.B., and V. du Vigneaud: Synthesis of 2-p-methoxyphenylalanine oxytocin (O-methyl-oxytocin) and some observations on its pharmacological behaviour. J. Amer. chem. Soc. **82**, 4579—4581 (1960).

Leaf, A.: Some actions of neurohypophyseal hormones on a living membrane. J. gen. Physiol. **43**, 175—189 (1960).
—, and R.M. Hays: Permeability of the isolated toad bladder to solutes and its modification by vasopressin. J. gen. Physiol. **45**, 921—932 (1962).
—, A. Keller, and E.F. Dempsey: Stimulation of sodium transport in the toad bladder by acidification of mucosal medium. Amer. J. Physiol. **207**, 547—552 (1964).
Levy, B.: The intestinal inhibitory response to oxytocin, vasopressin and bradykinin. J. Pharmacol. exp. Ther. **140**, 356—366 (1963).
Lichtenstein, N.S., and A. Leaf: Effect of amphotericin B on the permeability of the toad bladder. J. clin. Invest. **44**, 1328—1342 (1965).
Linzell, J.L.: Some observations on the contractile tissue of the mammary gland. J. Physiol. (Lond.) **130**, 257—267 (1955).
Lish, P.M., K.W. Dungan, and E.L. Peters: A survey of the effects of isoxsuprine on non-vascular smooth muscle. J. Pharmacol. exp. Ther. **129**, 191—199 (1960a).
—, I.W. Hillyard, and K.W. Dungan: The uterine relaxant properties of isoxsuprine. J. Pharmacol. exp. Ther. 129, 438—444 (1960b).
Lloyd, S.: The vascular responses of the rat during the reproductive cycle. J. Physiol. (Lond.) **148**, 625—632 (1959a).
— Changes in the vascular responses of the rat during pregnancy. J. Physiol. (Lond.) **149**, 586—592 (1959b).
—, and M. Pickford: The action of posterior pituitary hormones and oestrogens on the vascular system of the rat. J. Physiol. (Lond.) **155**, 161—174 (1961).
— — The effect of oestrogens and sympathetic denervation on the response to oxytocin of the blood vessels in the hind limb of the dog. J. Physiol. (Lond.) **163**, 362—371 (1962).
Lyng, J. Cholera filtrate and vasopressin. Antagonistic effect on the isolated frog skin. Acta path. microbiol. scand. **62**, 349—355 (1964).
Manning, M., and V. du Vigneaud: 4-β-Alanine-oxytocin: an oxytocin analog containing a twenty-one-membered disulfide ring. Biochemistry **4**, 1884—1888 (1965).
Marks, R.F.: The dependence of uterine muscular contraction on pH, with reference to prolonged labour. J. Obstet. Gynaec. Brit. Cwlth. **68**, 584—591 (1961).
Marshall, J.M., and A. Csapo: Hormonal and ionic influences on the membrane activity of uterine smooth muscle cells. Endocrinology **68**, 1026—1035 (1961).
—, and M.D. Miller: Effects of metabolic inhibitors on the rat uterus and on its response to oxytocin. Amer. J. Physiol. **206**, 437—442 (1964).
Martin, P.J., and H.O. Schild: Pharmacological antagonism of oxytocin and vasopressin by thiol compounds. J. Physiol. (Lond.) **163**, 51—52P (1962a).
— — Effect of thiols on oxytocin and vasopressin receptors. Nature (Lond.) **196**, 382—383 (1962b).
— — Pharmacological antagonism between SH compounds and S-S polypeptides. In: Oxytocin, Vasopressin, and their Structural Analogues, pp. 109—115. Ed. by J. Rudinger. Proc. 2nd Int. Pharmacol. Meeting, Prague 1963, Vol. 10. Oxford: Pergamon Press 1964.
— — The antagonism of disulphide polypeptides by thiols. Brit. J. Pharmacol. **25**, 418—431 (1965).
Morel, F., and F. Bastide: Relationship between the structure of several analogues of oxytocin and their "natriferic" activity *in vitro*. In: Oxytocin, Vasopressin and their Structural Analogues, pp. 47—55. Ed. by J. Rudinger. Proc. 2nd Int. Pharmacol. Meeting, Prague 1963, Vol. 10. Oxford: Pergamon Press 1964.
—, and S. Jard: Inhibition of frog *(Rana esculenta)* antidiuretic action of vasotocin by some analogues. Amer. J. Physiol. **204**, 227—232 (1963).
Mueller, J.M., J.G. Pierce, H. Davoll, and V. du Vigneaud: The oxidation of oxytocin with performic acid. J. biol. Chem. **191**, 309—313 (1951).
Munsick, R.A.: Effect of magnesium ion on the response of the rat uterus to neurohypophysial hormones and analogues. Endocrinology **66**, 451—457 (1960).
Natochin, Yu. V., and L.G. Magazanik: Search for pharmacological agents capable of inhibiting the effect of the antidiuretic hormone. Byul. eksp. Biol. Med. No. 1, 58—62 (1964) [in Russian].
Nemček, O., A. Kleinzeller, and J. Rudinger: Effect of some synthetic analogues of oxytocin on the active transport of sodium through the frog skin. Biochem. Pharmacol. **12**, Suppl., 227 (1963).
Niedrich, H., B. Wiegershausen, and E. Göres: Synthesis and activity of oxytocin analogues with carboxyl-terminal hydrazinoacetic acid. In: Oxytocin, Vasopressin and their Structural Analogues, pp. 173—176. Ed. by J. Rudinger. Proc. 2nd Int. Pharmacol. Meeting, Prague 1963, Vol. 10. Oxford: Pergamon Press 1964.

NISHIYAMA, Y., and S. CHUMA: Pharmacological studies on the uterine movement of albino rat *in vitro* and *in vivo*. Osaka Cy med. J. **2**, 1—6 (1955).
NUSYNOWITZ, M.L., L.C. WEGIENKA, B.F. BOWER, P.H. FORSHAM, and J.H. HALE: Effect on vasopressin action of analgesic drugs *in vitro*. Am. J. med. Sci. **252**, 424—428 (1966).
ØYE, I., and E.W. SUTHERLAND: The effect of epinephrine and other agents on adenyl cyclase in the cell membrane of avian erythrocytes. Biochim. biophys. Acta (Amst.) **127**, 347—354 (1966).
ORLOFF, J., and J.S. HANDLER (with the technical assistance of A.S. PRESTON): The similarity of effects of vasopressin, adenosine-3′,5′-phosphate (cyclic AMP) and theophylline on the toad bladder. J. clin. Invest. **41**, 702—709 (1962).
— — The role of adenosine 3′,5′-monophosphate (cyclic AMP) in the action of neurohypophyseal hormones. In: Oxytocin, Vasopressin and their Structural Analogues, pp. 133—139. Ed. by J. RUDINGER. Proc. 2nd Int. Pharmacol. Meeting, Prague 1963, Vol. 10. Oxford: Pergamon Press 1964.
— —, and S. BERGSTROM: Effect of prostaglandin (PGE_1) on the permeability response of toad bladder to vasopressin, theophylline and adenosine 3′,5′-monophosphate. Nature (Lond.) **205**, 397—398 (1965).
OVERWEG, N.I.A.: Inhibition of toad bladder and rat uterus responses to oxytocin and other agents by toad bladder extracts. J. Pharmacol. exp. Ther. **153**, 314—320 (1966).
PEETERS, G., G. SIERENS, and M. SILVER: Expulsion of milk in the isolated perfused udder of the cow. Arch. int. Pharmacodyn. **88**, 413—424 (1952).
PERMUTT, M.A., C.W. PARKER, and R.D. UTIGER: Immunochemical studies with lysine vasopressin. Endocrinology **78**, 809—814 (1966).
PETERSEN, M.J., and I.S. EDELMAN: Calcium inhibition of the action of vasopressin on the urinary bladder of the toad. J. clin. Invest. **43**, 583—594 (1964).
PICKFORD, M.: Factors affecting milk release in the dog and the quantity of oxytocin liberated during suckling, J. Physiol. (Lond.) **152**, 515—526 (1960).
— Some extra-uterine actions of oxytocin. In: Oxytocin, pp. 68—79. Ed. by R. CALDEYRO-BARCIA, and H. HELLER. Proc. Int. Symp., Montevideo 1959. Oxford: Pergamon Press 1961.
— Comment. In: Endogenous Substances affecting the Myometrium, p. 183. Ed. by V.R. PICKLES and R.J. FITZPATRICK. Mem. Soc. Endocrinol. No. 14. London: Cambridge University Press 1966.
PLIŠKA, V., T. BARTH, and I. RYCHLÍK: Effect of human serum oxytocinase on the antidiuretic action of lysine vasopressin and oxytocin in the rat. Experientia (Basel), **24**, 196—197 (1967).
—, and I. RYCHLÍK: Determination of antidiuretic activity in the rat for structural analogues of the neurohypophysial hormones. Acta endocr. (Kbh.) **54**, 129—140 (1967).
POISNER, A.M.: Interaction of oxytocin and vasopressin with β-adrenergic receptors in the kidney. Nature (Lond.) **201**, 199—200 (1964).
POLÁČEK, I., I. KREJČÍ, and J. RUDINGER: The action of oxytocin and synthetic analogues on the isolated mammary-gland myoepithelium of the lactating rat; effect of some ions. J. Endocr. **38**, 13—24 (1967).
RASMUSSEN, H., I.L. SCHWARTZ, M.A. SCHOESSLER, and G. HOCHSTER: Studies on the mechanism of action of vasopressin. Proc. nat. Acad. Sci. (Wash.). **46**, 1278—1287 (1960).
— —, R. YOUNG, and J. MARC-AURELE: Structural requirements for the action of neurohypophyseal hormones upon the isolated amphibian urinary bladder. J. gen. Physiol. **46**, 1171—1189 (1963).
RESSLER, C.: Inactivations of oxytocin suggesting peptide denaturation. Science **128**, 1281—1282 (1958).
—, and J.R. RACHELE: Further properties of isoglutamine-oxytocin; inhibition of pressor activity of vasopressin. Proc. Soc. exp. Biol. (N.Y.) **98**, 170—174 (1958).
—, and V. DU VIGNEAUD: The isoglutamine isomer of oxytocin: its synthesis and comparison with oxytocin. J. Amer. chem. Soc. **79**, 4511—4515 (1957).
ROTH, J., S.M. GLICK, L.A. KLEIN, and M.J. PETERSEN: Specific antibody to vasopressin in man. J. clin. Endocr. **26**, 671—675 (1966).
RUDINGER, J.: Discussion. In: Oxytocin, Vasopressin and their Structural Analogues, p. 116. Ed. by J. RUDINGER. Proc. 2nd Int. Pharmacol. Meeting, Prague 1963, Vol. 10. Oxford: Pergamon Press 1964.
— Synthetic analogues of oxytocin with inhibitor activity or protracted action. Proc. 2nd Int. Congr. Endocrinol., London 1964, 1202—1206. Amsterdam: Excerpta med. (Amst.) 1965.
— Comment. In: Endogenous Substances affecting the Myometrium, pp. 183—184. Ed. by V.R. PICKLES and R.J. FITZPATRICK. Mem. Soc. Endocrinol. No. 14. London: Cambridge University Press 1966.

Rudinger, J., and K. Jošt: Synthetic analogues of oxytocin and vasopressin: structural relations. In: Oxytocin, Vasopressin and their Structural Analogues, pp. 3—19. Ed. by J. Rudinger. Proc. 2nd Int. Pharmacol. Meeting, Prague 1963, Vol. 10. Oxford: Pergamon Press 1964a.
— — A biologically active analogue of oxytocin not containing a disulphide group. Experientia (Basel) **20**, 570—571 (1964b).
—, and I. Krejčí: Dose-response relations for some synthetic analogues of oxytocin, and the mode of action of oxytocin on the isolated uterus. Experientia (Basel) **18**, 585—588 (1962).
Sawyer, W. H.: Increased water permeability of the bull frog *(Rana catesbiana)* bladder *in vitro* in response to synthetic oxytocin and arginine vasotocin and to neurohypophysial extracts from nonmammalian vertebrates. Endocrinology **66**, 112—120 (1960).
—, and H. Valtin: Inhibition of vasopressin antidiuresis by extracts of pituitaries from rats with hereditary hypothalamic diabetes insipidus and by oxytocin. Endocrinology **76**, 999—1001 (1965).
Schäker, W.: Disertation, Karl-Marx-Universität, Leipzig 1967.
Schild, H. O.: Discussion. In: Oxytocin, Vasopressin and their Structural Analogues, p. 123. Proc. 2nd Int. Pharmacol. Meeting, Prague 1963, Vol. 10. Oxford: Pergamon Press 1964.
Schneider, C. H., and V. du Vigneaud: Synthesis of D-leucine-oxytocin, a biologically active diastereoisomer of oxytocin, and demonstration of its separability from oxytocin upon countercurrent distribution. J. Amer. chem. Soc. **84**, 3005—3008 (1962).
Schulz, H., and V. du Vigneaud: Synthesis of 1-L-penicillamine-oxytocin, 1-D-penicillamine-oxytocin, and 1-deaminopenicillamine-oxytocin, potent inhibitors of the oxytocic response to oxytocin. J. med. Chem. **9**, 647—650 (1966a).
— — The effect of replacing one of the hydrogens of the β-carbon of the β-mercaptopropionic acid residue in deamino-oxytocin by a methyl group on its oxytocic and avian vasodepressor activity. J. Amer. chem. Soc. **88**, 5015—5018 (1966b).
Schwartz, I. L., H. Rasmussen, and J. Rudinger: Activity of neurohypophysial hormone analogues lacking a disulfide bridge. Proc. nat. Acad. Sci. (Wash.) **52**, 1044—1045 (1964).
— —, M. A. Schoessler, and C. T. O. Fong: Relation of chemical attachment to physiological action of vasopressin. Proc. nat. Acad. Sci. (Wash.) **46**, 1288—1298 (1960).
Sealock, R. R., and V. du Vigneaud: Studies on the reduction of Pitressin and Pitocin with cysteine. J. Pharmacol. exp. Ther. **54**, 433—447 (1935).
Siedel, W., K. Sturm, and R. Geiger: Synthese eines vasopressorisch wirkenden Peptids: [O-Methyl-tyrosin]^2-Lysin^8-Vasopressin (OMTLV). Chem. Ber. **96**, 1436—1440 (1963).
Šmahel, O.: The relation of hyaluronidase, histamine and antihistamine substances. Acta allerg. (Kbh.) **15**, Suppl. 7, 497—499 (1960).
Smyth, D. G.: Proteins and Peptides. Ann. Rep. Progr. Chem. for 1964, 59, 507—525 (1965a).
— Reactions of cyanate with amino and hydroxyl groups; application to oxytocin. Acta chim. Acad. Sci. Hung. **44**, 197—204 (1965b).
Somlyo, A. V., C.-Y. Woo, and A. P. Somlyo: Effect of magnesium on posterior pituitary hormone action on vascular smooth muscle. Amer. J. Physiol. **210**, 705—714 (1966).
Šorm, F.: Proteins: Structure and function. Plenary Lecture, 5th Int. Congr. Biochem., Moscow. Prague: Czechoslovak Academy of Science 1961.
Strauch, B. S., and R. G. Langdon: The role of adenosine 3′,5′-phosphate in the action of vasopressin on water permeability of toad bladders. Biochem. biophys. Res. Commun. **16**, 27—33 (1964).
Studer, R. O., and W. D. Cash: Synthesis of 1-acetyl-8-arginine vasopressin and a study of its effects in the rat pressor assay. J. biol. Chem. **238**, 657—659 (1963).
Sullivan, T. J.: Response of the mammalian uterus to prostaglandins under differing hormonal conditions. Brit. J. Pharmacol. **26**, 678—685 (1966).
Sutherland, E. W., T. W. Rall, and T. Menon: Adenyl cyclase. I. Distribution, preparation and properties. J. biol. Chem. **237**, 1220—1227 (1962).
Taborsky, J.: Über die Hemmung der antidiuretischen Wirkung von Vasopressin und Nikotin mittels Acetazolamid bei Wasserbelasteten Ratten. Med. Pharmacol. Exp. **15**, 427—431 (1966).
Takagi, K., Y. Ishida, H. Moritoki, and K. Hara: Studies of drug receptors on the plain muscle. I. Antagonistic action on the activities of acetylcholine, barium chloride, and oxytocin on the isolated rat uterus. Yakugaku Zasshi **81**, 1708—1712 (1961) [in Japanese]. (In English: Ann. Rept. Fac. Pharm. Sci. Tokushima Univ. **11**, 31—37 (1962)).
Tata, P. S., and R. Buzalkov: Vasopressin studies in the rat. III. Inability of ethanol anesthesia to prevent ADH secretion due to pain and hemorrhage. Arch. ges. Physiol. **290**, 294 to 297 (1966).
Turner, R. A., J. G. Pierce, and V. du Vigneaud: The desulfurization of oxytocin. J. biol. Chem. **193**, 359—361 (1951).
Uranga, J., and W. H. Sawyer: Renal responses of the bullfrog to oxytocin, arginine-vasotocin and frog neurohypophysial extracts. Amer. J. Physiol. **198**, 1287—1290 (1960).

USSING, H.H., T.U.L. BIBER, and N.S. BRICKER: Exposure of the isolated frog skin to high potassium concentrations at the internal surface. II. Changes in epithelial cell volume, resistance, and response to antidiuretic hormone. J. gen. Physiol. **48**, 425—433 (1965).

DU VIGNEAUD, V., G.S. DENNING, S. DRABAREK, and W.Y. CHAN: The synthesis and pharmacological study of 4-decarboxamido-oxytocin (4-α-aminobutyric acid-oxytocin) and 5-decarboxamido-oxytocin (5-alanine-oxytocin). J. biol. Chem. **239**, 472—478 (1964).

—, P.S. FITT, M. BODANSZKY, and M. O'CONNELL: Synthesis and some pharmacological properties of a peptide derivative of oxytocin: glycyloxytocin. Proc. Soc. exp. Biol. (N.Y.) **104**, 653—656 (1960).

—, C. RESSLER, J.M. SWAN, C.W. ROBERTS, P.G. KATSOYANNIS, and S. GORDON: The synthesis of an octapeptide amide with the hormonal activity of oxytocin. J. Amer. chem. Soc. **75**, 4879—4880 (1953).

VOGEL, G., u. J. HERGOTT: Pharmakologische Untersuchungen über O-Methyl-tyrosin^2-lysin^8-Vasopressin. Arzneimittel-Forsch. **13**, 415—421 (1963).

VOGT, M.: Vasopressor, antidiuretic and oxytocic activities of extracts of the dog's hypothalamus. Brit. J. Pharmacol. **8**, 193—196 (1953).

VORHERR, H.: Zur Frage des Oxytocin-Vasopressin-Antagonismus bei Mensch und Tier. Klin. Wschr. **42**, 198—201 (1964).

—, and V. FRIEDBERG: Über die Wirkung von synthetischem Oxytocin auf die Wasserdiurese der Ratte. Z. ges. exp. Med. **133**, 602—608 (1960).

WALASZEK, E.J., C.G. HUGGINS, and C.M. SMITH: Drugs that modify actions of pharmacologically active polypeptides. Ann. N.Y. Acad. Sci. **104**, 281—289 (1963).

WHITTEMBURY, G., N. SUGINO, and A.K. SOLOMON: Effect of anti-diuretic hormone and calcium on the equivalent pore radius of kidney slices from Necturus. Nature (Lond.) **187**, 699—701 (1960).

WHITTLESTONE, W.G.: The effect of adrenaline on the milk-ejection response of the sow. J. Endocr. **10**, 167—172 (1954).

WOO, C.-Y., and A.P. SOMLYO: Interaction of magnesium with vasopressin in intestinal smooth muscle. J. Pharmacol. exp. Ther. **155**, 357—366 (1967).

WOOLLEY, D.W.: Discussion, In: Oxytocin, Vasopressin and their Structural Analogues, p. 35. Ed. by J. RUDINGER. Proc. 2nd Int. Pharmacol. Meeting, Prague 1963, Vol. 10. Oxford: Pergamon Press 1964.

YAMASHIRO, D., D. GILLESSEN, and V. DU VIGNEAUD: Oxytoceine and deamino-oxytoceine. Biochemistry **5**, 3711—3720 (1966).

ZAORAL, M., E. KASAFÍREK, J. RUDINGER, and F. ŠORM: Amino Acids and peptides. LI. Synthesis of 2-O-methyltyrosine- and 2-O-ethyltyrosine-lysine-vasopressin. Collection Czech. chem. Commun. **30**, 1869—1873 (1965).

—, V. PLIŠKA, K. ŘEŽÁBEK, and F. ŠORM: Synthesis of two lysine-vasopressin analogues with protracted hormonal activity. Collection Czech. chem. Commun. **28**, 747—749 (1963).

—, and F. ŠORM: Preparation and biological activity of some new lysine vasopressin analogues. In: Oxytocin, Vasopressin and their Structural Analogues, pp. 167—171. Ed. by J. RUDINGER. Proc. 2nd Int. Pharmacol. Meeting, Prague 1963, Vol. 10. Oxford: Pergamon Press 1964.

— — Synthesis of Gly-Cys^1-lysine-vasopressin and Gly-Cys^1-Tyr(Me)^2-lysine-vasopressin. Collection Czech. chem. Commun. **30**, 2812—2816 (1965).

ZEDECK, M.S., L.B. MELLETT, and E.J. CAFRUNY: The diuretic effects of cyclophosphamide and nor-nitrogen mustard: Relationship to antidiuretic hormone. J. Pharmacol. exp. Therap. **153**, 550—561 (1966).

ZHUZE, A.L., K. JOŠT, E. KASAFÍREK, and J. RUDINGER: Amino Acids and Peptides. XLV. Analogues of oxytocin with O-ethyltyrosine, p-methylphenylalanine, and p-ethylphenylalanine replacing tyrosine. Collection Czech. chem. Commun. **29**, 2648—2662 (1964).

Basic Pharmacological Properties of Synthetic Analogues and Homologues of the Neurohypophysial Hormones

B. BERDE and R. A. BOISSONNAS

With 2 Figures

During the last decade, nearly 200 analogues and homologues of the neurohypophysial hormones have been synthesised in various laboratories, and the biological activities of these synthetic peptides structurally related to the neurohypophysial hormones have been more or less extensively investigated. The principal aim of all this work was to try to establish relationships between the chemical structure and the biological activities of these hormones.

Furthermore, attempts were made to produce analogues or homologues which (a) are more potent than the hormones occurring in nature, (b) exhibit one of the inherent and therapeutically useful pharmacological qualities of these hormones more selectively than the molecules built up by nature or (c) antagonise some effects of oxytocin or the vasopressins. The first two aims were pursued with considerable success (see e.g. De-Amino^1-oxytocin [CHAN and DU VIGNEAUD, 1962], De-Amino^1-Arg^8-vasopressin [HUGUENIN et al., 1965], De-Amino^1-Phe^2-Arg^8-vasopressin [STÜRMER et al., 1965], Orn^8-vasopressin and Phe^2-Orn^8-oxytocin [BERDE et al., 1964], etc.). The question of antagonism is more complex, and a separate chapter in this volume (RUDINGER and KREJČÍ) goes into this topic in detail.

The availability of synthetic analogues of the neurohypophysial hormones also afforded greater scope for studying the influence of enzymes on these compounds (e.g. GOLUBOW and DU VIGNEAUD, 1963; GOLUBOW et al., 1963), thereby contributing to a better understanding of their metabolism.

Last but not least the quantitatively well-defined biological activities and physico-chemical properties of these synthetic peptides played a considerable rôle:

a) in the discovery and identification of hitherto unknown neurohypophysial hormones (e.g. arginine-vasotocin [CHAUVET et al., 1960; KATSOYANNIS and DU VIGNEAUD, 1959; PICKERING and HELLER, 1959; SAWYER et al., 1959], ichthyotocin or isotocin [ACHER et al., 1962; FOLLETT and HELLER, 1964a; GUTTMANN et al., 1962; SAWYER and VAN DYKE, 1963a, 1963b], mesotocin [BERDE and KONZETT, 1960; FOLLETT and HELLER, 1963, 1964b; SAWYER, 1964; SAWYER and VAN DYKE, 1963a, b]).

b) in attempts to identify ectopically produced pathological hormone(s) (BERDE, 1965; DE SOUSA et al., 1965).

I. Methodical Remarks

The aim of the present chapter is to discuss possible relationships between the chemical structure and the biological activities of synthetic analogues and homologues of the neurohypophysial hormones. For this purpose, only those activities can be considered which have been established with a reasonable degree of accuracy for all the compounds in question or at least for the majority of them. In Tables 2—24, therefore, only five activities are considered, namely three "oxytocin-like properties": uterotonic, avian depressor and milk-ejecting potencies, and two "vasopressin-like properties": pressor and antidiuretic effects. In spite of this narrowing of the field, some limitations still remain and call for a few brief remarks.

There are well-established ("classical") pharmacological methods for measuring the five above-mentioned activities and the experimental procedures employed in different laboratories are substantially similar. However, such small technical variations as there are from one laboratory to another may lead to differences in results and may have affected our deductions.

Uterotonic activity is generally measured on the non-pregnant rat uterus *in vitro*, along the lines described by HOLTON (1948). The results obtained may, however, show considerable variation depending on the hormonal state of the animal used (CHAN et al., 1963) and on the ionic composition of the physiological

Table 1. *The composition — in grammes per litre — of some organ bath solutions used for in vitro uterus preparations (from* BERDE *and* SAAMELI *1966)*

Authors / Ingredients	GADDUM et al. (1949)	BEAU-VILLAIN (1943)	GARCIA DE JALON et al. (1945)	British Pharmacopoeia (1963)	SUND (1963)	MUNSICK I (1960)	MUNSICK II (1960)	TYRODE (1910)
NaCl	9.00	9.000	9.000	9.0000	9.000	6.6230	6.6230	8.00
KCl	0.42	0.420	0.420	0.4200	0.420	0.4540	0.4540	0.20
$CaCl_2$	0.06	0.060	0.012	0.1200	0.060	0.0555	0.0555	0.20
$MgCl_2$ . . .	—	0.005	0.005	0.0025	0.096	—	0.0476	0.10
$NaHCO_3$ . .	0.50	0.500	0.500	0.5000	0.500	2.5590	2.5590	1.00
NaH_2PO_4 . .	—	—	—	—	—	0.0244	0.0244	0.05
Na_2HPO_4 . .	—	—	—	—	—	0.1130	0.1130	—
Glucose . . .	0.50	0.500	0.500	0.2500	0.500	0.500	0.500	1.00

solution — particularly its magnesium content (MUNSICK, 1960). In most laboratories, therefore, the assays are performed on rats in artificially induced oestrus, and as a rule a magnesium-free physiological solution (GADDUM et al., 1949; MUNSICK, 1960, see Table 1) is used. The organ bath temperature (maintained at 30 or 32 °C in many laboratories) may also influence the results.

The determination of avian depressor activity is based on the method of COON (1939). Differences in experimental design (THOMPSON, 1944; *British Pharmacopoeia*, 1963; *United States Pharmacopeia*, 1965) may give rise to some discrepancies.

For the assessment of milk-ejecting activity an *in situ* lactating rabbit preparation is widely used, the substances being injected intravenously (CROSS and HARRIS, 1951/52; VAN DYKE et al., 1955; BERDE and CERLETTI, 1960). Most data were obtained under these experimental conditions. In later years an *in situ* guinea-pig preparation has been used in some laboratories (TINDAL and YOKOYAMA, 1962), the substances being applied intra-arterially. In Tables 2—24 milk-ejecting activities are collected under the heading "Rabbit mammary gland," and where a value was obtained in the guinea-pig this is stated. It is clear that species differences and different routes of administration make a comparative evaluation of these data hazardous.

Pressor activity is generally measured on anaesthetised rats pretreated with an adrenergic blocking agent, as suggested by DEKANSKI (1952) and adopted by the Pharmacopoeias (*British Pharmacopoeia*, 1963; *United States Pharmacopeia*, 1965).

The values for antidiuretic activity are those obtained in rats loaded with water and treated with alcohol, according to an original suggestion by JEFFERS et al. (1942). In different laboratories, variations of this method are used (see e.g. DICKER, 1953; BOURA and DICKER, 1953; THORN, 1957; DETTELBACH, 1958; SAWYER, 1958; BERDE and CERLETTI, 1961) which may be a source of some discrepancies in the results.

A further limit to the validity of the values in Tables 2—24 is that the activities of the synthetic analogues and homologues have to be established by comparing them with some standard, such as the 3rd International Standard for Oxytocic, Vasopressor and Antidiuretic Substances (BANGHAM and MUSSET, 1958) or the United States Pharmacopeia Posterior Pituitary Reference Standard (*United States Pharmacopeia*, 1965) both containing oxytocin and arginine-vasopressin. This means that the activity of the analogues and homologues is quantitatively compared with that of chemically different substances. If the dose-response lines happen to be parallel —or do not significantly diverge — the results are of course more precise than if the slopes of the dose-response lines differ widely. However, it is exceptional for the potencies of two neurohypophysial compounds to be compared over a very wide section of the possible dose-response line (e.g. smallest dose: highest dose = 1:36 and 6 different doses per compound) (BERDE and CERLETTI, 1961). Even six-point assays, i. e. three doses of each compound, are rather infrequently used, the four-point assay (SCHILD, 1942) being more popular, i. e. two doses per substance. With certain well established experimental designs (e. g. that of THOMPSON, 1944) or with comparisons based on three-point matching assays and probit evaluation (e. g. BERDE and SAAMELI, 1959), it is impossible to judge whether or not the dose-response curves are parallel.

In spite of all these limitations, the five methods widely used to quantify the "basic pharmacological properties" of analogues and homologues of neurohypophysial peptides yield remarkably constant values: Many synthetic analogues produced in our laboratories and tested against the 3rd International Standard for Oxytocic, Vasopressor and Antidiuretic Substances were also assayed by Dr. WILBUR SAWYER (Department of Pharmacology, Columbia University, New York) and no major discrepancies were encountered (see e. g. SAWYER, 1961; SAWYER, 1965), although he used the United States Pharmacopeia Posterior Pituitary Reference Standard and the techniques used in New York and in Basle differ in some details. Only in exceptional cases is marked divergence of the dose-response curve responsible for an appreciable discrepancy between the quantitative data from different laboratories for a given synthetic analogue (e. g. PLIŠKA and KREJČÍ, 1966).

II. Tabulated Data

In order to facilitate a systematic study of the changes in pharmacological activities brought about by limited modifications of the structure of the natural hormones, a series of Tables have been drawn up. The Tables include only chemically pure peptides, which have been demonstrated, by appropriate analytical tests, to be homogeneous.

In addition to the name, the abbreviated chemical formula* and the molecular weight of the compounds presented for comparison, the detailed chemical structure of the grouping by which the compounds of a given Table differ among themselves, is also indicated in most cases. The quantitative data obtained in the above-mentioned pharmacological assays are given in International Units (IU) per micromole (not per milligramme!), in order to allow a direct comparison of the activities on a *molecular* basis. The relation between IU per micromole and IU per milligramme is as follows: IU per micromole = IU per milligramme × molecular weight/1000. When available, the standard deviations of the values are also indicated. "Anti" means that the compound in question shows some antagonism to oxytocin or vasopressin in that particular test. In the extreme right-hand column of the Tables, references to papers on the chemistry and the pharmacology of the synthetic analogues in question are cited.

The neurohypophysial hormones which have so far been found in nature are listed in Table 2. These hormones differ among themselves in having different amino acids in positions 3, 4 or 8, but the general pattern of their structure is the same. They can all be considered to be variants of oxytocin (Fig. 1) or of vasopressin (Fig. 2), which are the two natural hormones on which the nomenclature of these peptides is based.

Examination of the biological properties of these natural hormones shows that vasotocin, which has a structure intermediate between that of oxytocin and of vasopressin, also exhibits biological properties, which are intermediate between those of these two hormones.

Let us first examine the effect of single modifications in positions 2, 3, 4, 5, 8 and 9 of oxytocin and vasopressin, i. e. modifications which do not directly affect the two half cystine residues which close the ring in positions 1 and 6 (Tables 2—13).

The modifications which have hitherto been effected at position 2 of oxytocin are summarized in Table 3. Suppression of the phenolic group in oxytocin, i. e. the replacement of tyrosine by phenylalanine (Phe^2-oxytocin) lowers the different activities in varying degree. The fact that quite appreciable oxytocin-like effects are still present demonstrates that the hydroxyl group is not vital for oxytocic activity. Replacement of the hydroxyl group by a methyl group ([p-Me] Phe^2-oxytocin) or an ethyl group ([p-Et] Phe^2-oxytocin) is also compatible with an appreciable degree of activity. Methylation and still more ethylation of the hydroxyl group ([O-Me] Tyr^2-oxytocin) and ([O-Et] Tyr^2-oxytocin) diminishes the activities still further. It therefore appears that the hydroxyl group favours the biological effects but can be eliminated or replaced by a small group without greatly affecting the activities. Its replacement by a more bulky group has a

* In accordance with the recommendations of IUPAC (Information Bulletin No. 25, February 1966), the following abbreviations are used for amino acids:

Abu	= L-α-aminobutyric acid	Leu	= L-leucine
Ala	= L-alanine	Lys	= L-lysine
β-Ala	= β-alanine	Met	= L-methionine
Arg	= L-arginine	Nle	= L-norleucine
Asn	= L-asparagine	Nva	= L-norvaline
Asp	= L-aspartic acid	Orn	= L-ornithine
Cys	= L-cysteine (or L-half cystine)	Pro	= L-proline
Dbu	= L-α, γ-diamino-butyric acid	Sar	= sarcosine
Gln	= L-glutamine	Ser	= L-serine
Glu	= L-glutamic acid	Thr	= L-threonine
Gly	= glycine	Trp	= L-tryptophan
His	= L-histidine	Tyr	= L-tyrosine
Ile	= L-isoleucine	Val	= L-valine
aIle	= L-allo-isoleucine		

Table 2. *Neurohypophysial*

Name, abbreviated chemical formula and molecular weight	Structure of amino acid in position 3	Structure of amino acid in position 4
Cys–Tyr–*Ile*–*Gln*–Asn–Cys–Pro–*Leu*–Gly–NH_2 (Cys–Cys bridge) Oxytocin 1007.2	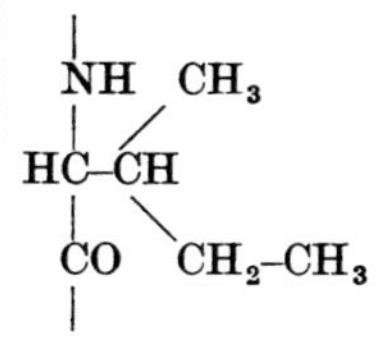	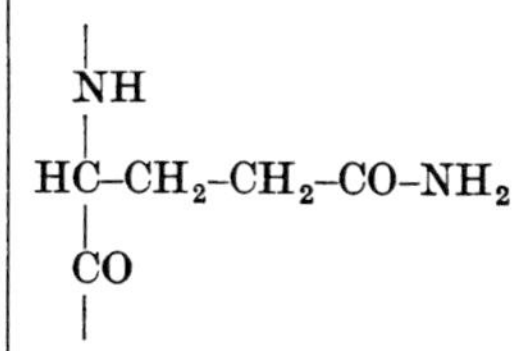
Cys–Tyr–*Phe*–*Gln*–Asn–Cys–Pro–*Lys*–Gly–NH_2 (Cys–Cys bridge) Lysine-vasopressin = Lys[8]-vasopressin 1056.2	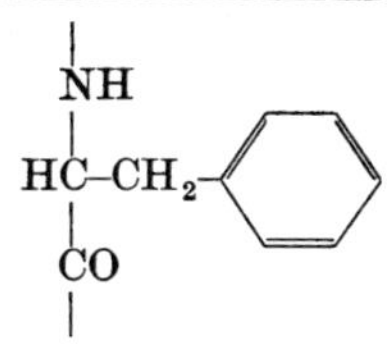	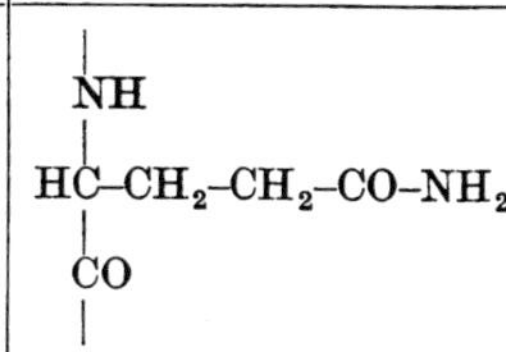
Cys–Tyr–*Phe*–*Gln*–Asn–Cys–Pro–*Arg*–Gly–NH_2 (Cys–Cys bridge) Vasopressin = Arginine-vasopressin 1084.2	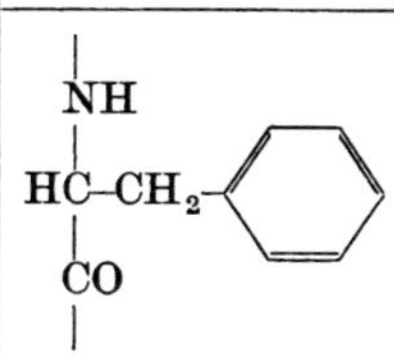	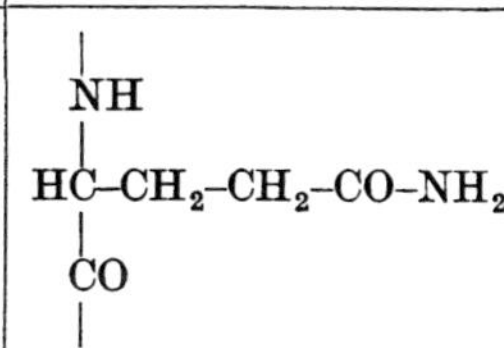
Cys–Tyr–*Ile*–*Gln*–Asn–Cys–Pro–*Arg*–Gly–NH_2 (Cys–Cys bridge) Vasotocin = Arginine-vasotocin = Ile[3]-vasopressin = Arg[8]-oxytocin 1050.2	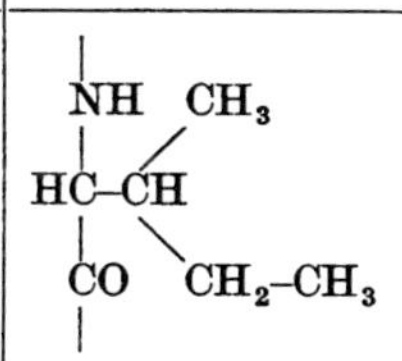	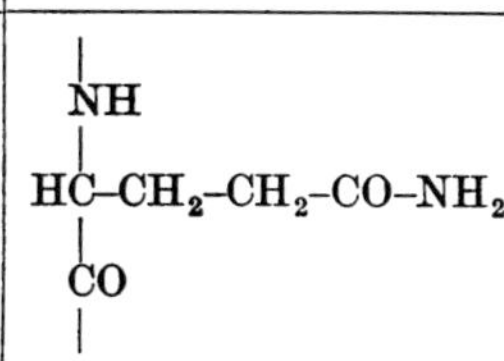
Cys–Tyr–*Ile*–*Gln*–Asn–Cys–Pro–*Ile*–Gly–NH_2 (Cys–Cys bridge) Mesotocin = Ile[8]-oxytocin 1007.2	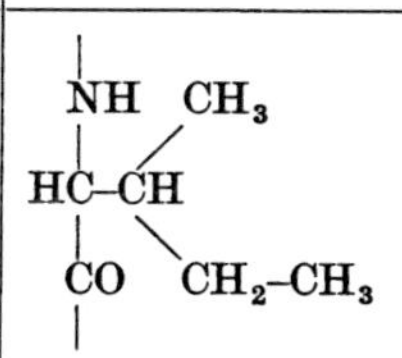	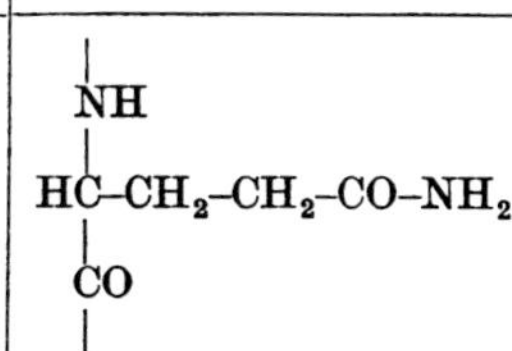
Cys–Tyr–*Ile*–*Ser*–Asn–Cys–Pro–*Ile*–Gly–NH_2 (Cys–Cys bridge) Isotocin = Ichthyotocin = Ser[4]-Ile[8]-oxytocin 966.2	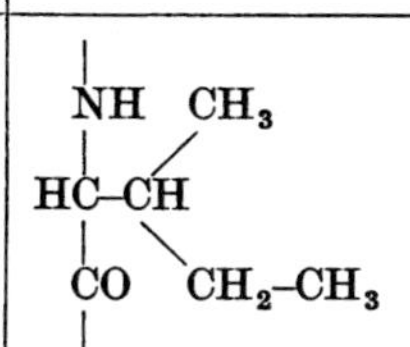	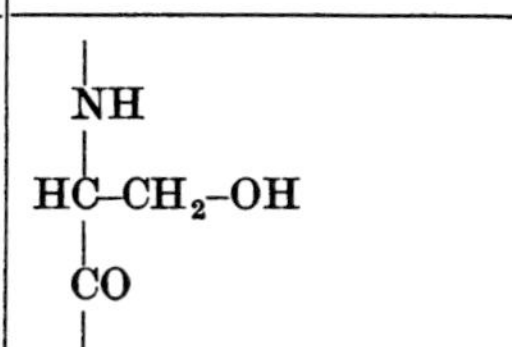
Cys–Tyr–*Ile*–*Ser*–Asn–Cys–Pro–*Gln*–Gly–NH_2 (Cys–Cys bridge) Glumitocin = Ser[4]-Glu[8]-oxytocin 981.1	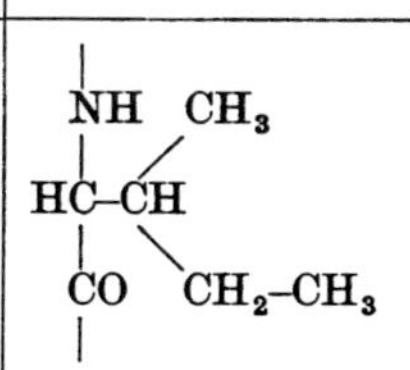	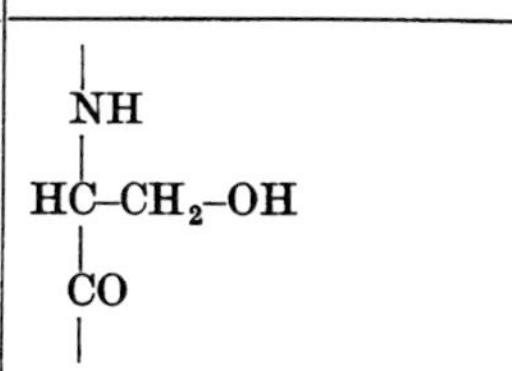

hormones occurring in nature

Structure of amino acid in position 8	Oxytocin-like activities in International Units per micromole			Vasopressin-like activities in International Units per micromole		Occurs in:
	Rat uterus	Chicken blood pressure	Rabbit mammary gland	Rat blood pressure	Rat antidiuresis	
$-NH-HC(CO-)-CH_2-CH(CH_3)_2$	450 ± 30	450 ± 30	450 ± 30	5 ± 1	5 ± 1	Many vertebrates
$-NH-HC(CO-)-CH_2-CH_2-CH_2-CH_2-NH_2$	5 ± 0.5	42 ± 5	63 ± 10	285 ± 21	~260	Pig, hippopotamus, peccary
$-NH-HC(CO-)-CH_2-CH_2-CH_2-NH-C(=NH)-NH_2$	17 ± 4	62 ± 6	69 ± 9	412 ± 41	465 ± 45	Most mammals
$-NH-HC(CO-)-CH_2-CH_2-CH_2-NH-C(=NH)-NH_2$	120 ± 16	300 ± 42	~220	255 ± 16	260 ± 37	Some non-mammalian vertebrates
$-NH-HC(CO-)-CH(CH_3)-CH_2-CH_3$	291 ± 21	502 ± 37	330 ± 21	6.3 ± 0.8	1.1 ± 0.1	Some amphibians and lung fishes
$-NH-HC(CO-)-CH(CH_3)-CH_2-CH_3$	145 ± 12	310 ± 15	290 ± 15	0.06 ± 0.01	0.18 ± 0.03	Some teleost fishes
$-NH-HC(CO-)-CH_2-CH_2-CO-NH_2$	~8	—	—	—	—	Some cartilaginous fishes

Fig. 1. *Developped chemical formula of oxytocin*

Position number	Chemical structure	Amino acid residue	
1	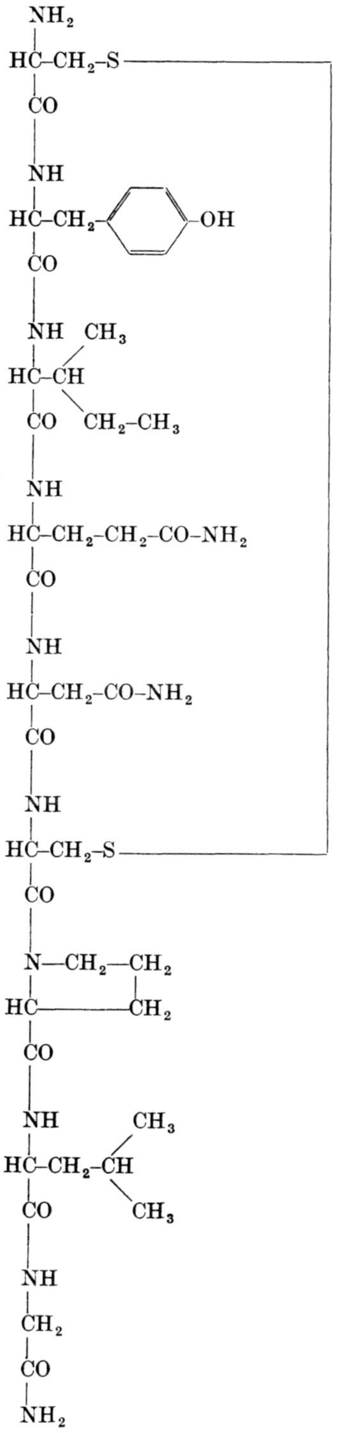	L-halfcystine	(Cys)
2		L-tyrosine	(Tyr)
3		L-isoleucine	(Ile)
4		L-glutamine	(Gln)
5		L-asparagine	(Asn)
6		L-halfcystine	(Cys)
7		L-proline	(Pro)
8		L-leucine	(Leu)
9		glycine	(Gly)

Fig. 2. *Developped chemical formula of vasopressin*

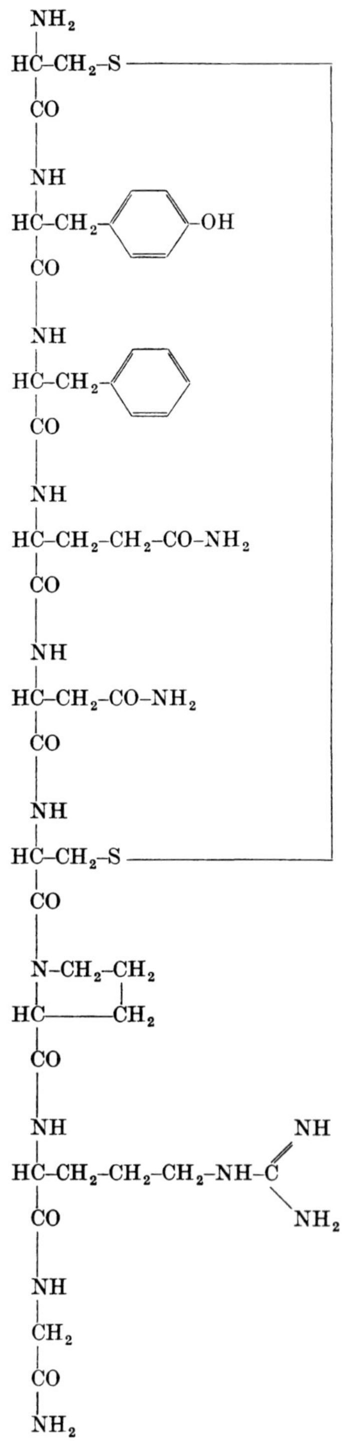

Position number	Chemical structure	Amino acid residue	
1		L-halfcystine	(Cys)
2		L-tyrosine	(Tyr)
3		L-phenylalanine	(Phe)
4		L-glutamine	(Gln)
5		L-asparagine	(Asn)
6		L-halfcystine	(Cys)
7		L-proline	(Pro)
8		L-arginine	(Arg)
9		glycine	(Gly)

Table 3. *Variations in position 2*

Name, abbreviated chemical formula and molecular weight		Structure of amino acid in position 2
Cys–*Tyr–Ile*–Gln–Asn–Cys–Pro–Ile–Gly–NH_2 Oxytocin	1007.2	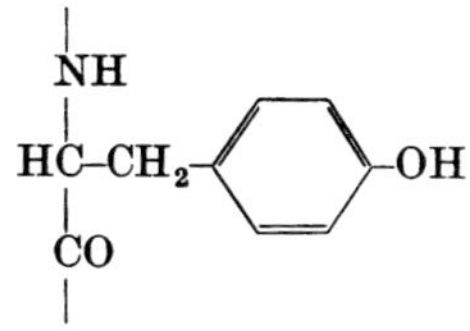
Cys–*Phe–Ile*–Gln–Asn–Cys–Pro–Leu–Gly–NH_2 Phe[2]-oxytocin	991.2	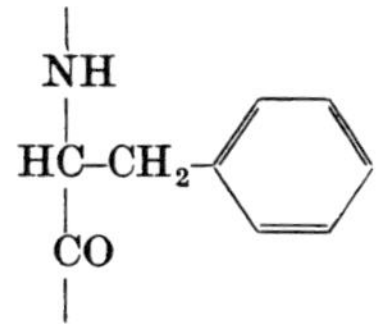
Cys–*(p-Me)Phe–Ile*–Gln–Asn–Cys–Pro–Leu–Gly–NH_2 (p-Me)Phe[2]-oxytocin	1005.2	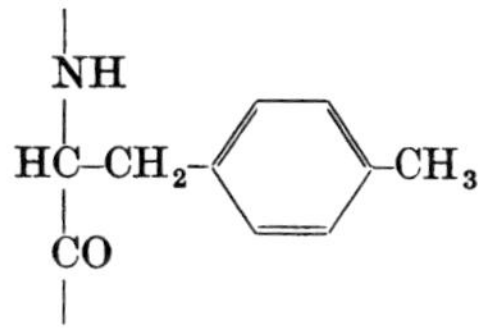
Cys–*(p-Et)Phe–Ile*–Gln–Asn–Cys–Pro–Leu–Gly–NH_2 (p-Et)Phe[2]-oxytocin	1019.2	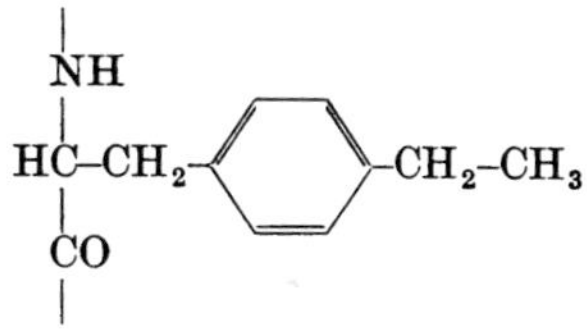
Cys–*(O-Me)Tyr–Ile*–Gln–Asn–Cys–Pro–Leu–Gly–NH_2 (O-Me)Tyr[2]-oxytocin	1021.2	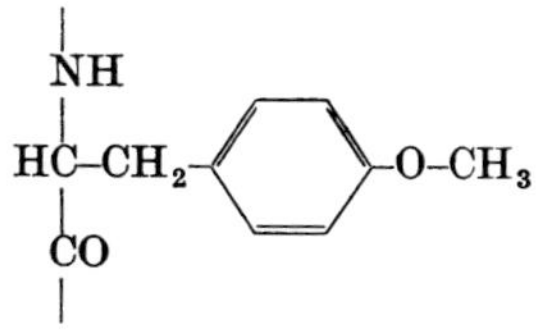
Cys–*(O-Et)Tyr–Ile*–Gln–Asn–Cys–Pro–Leu–Gly–NH_2 (O-Et)Tyr[2]-oxytocin	1035.1	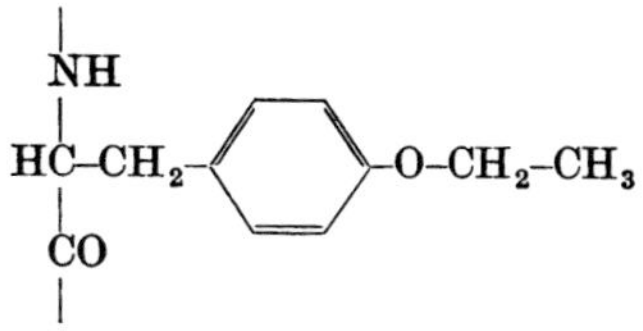
Cys–*D–Tyr–Ile*–Gln–Asn–Cys–Pro–Leu–Gly–NH_2 D-Tyr[2]-oxytocin	1007.2	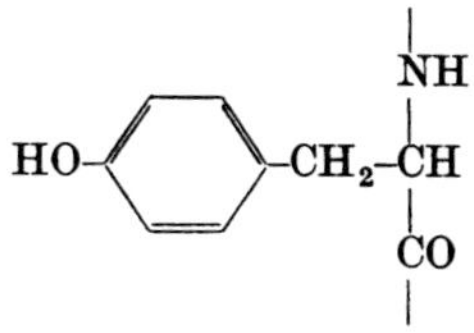

of oxytocin and oxypressin

Structure of amino acid in position 3	Oxytocin-like activities in International Units per micromole			Vasopressin-like activities in International Units per micromole		References S = synthesis P = pharmacology 1 = also contains pharmacological data
	Rat uterus (isolated)	Chicken blood pressure	Rabbit mammary gland	Rat blood pressure	Rat anti-diuresis	
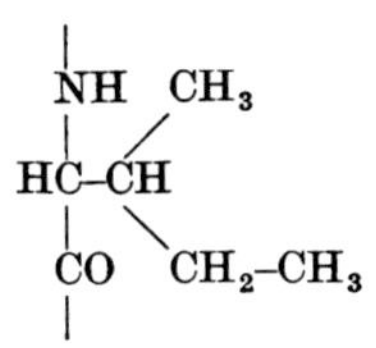	450 ± 30	450 ± 30	450 ± 30	5 ± 1	5 ± 1	Occurs in nature
as above	32 ± 2	63 ± 9	140 ± 21	~0.4	~0.5	S: JAQUENOUD, BOISSONNAS (1959)[1] BODANSZKY, DU VIGNEAUD (1959)[1] ZHUZE et al. (1964)[1] P: KONZETT, BERDE (1959)
as above	~19 or Anti	~58	~240	Anti	1.5	S: ZHUZE et al. (1964)[1]
as above	~6.5 or Anti	~46	~60	Anti	1.1	S: ZHUZE et al. (1964)[1]
as above	~2.0 or Anti	~8	~30	Anti (1.000:1)	~0.01	S: LAW, DU VIGNEAUD (1960)[1] BERANKOVA et al. (1961)[1] JOŠT et al. (1963a)[1] ZHUZE et al. (1964)[1]
as above	0.15	~0.1	~6	Anti	~0.005	S: ZHUZE et al. (1964)[1]
as above	6.6 ± 1	34 ± 3	34 ± 9	~0.02	~0.02	S: DRABAREK, DU VIGNEAUD (1965)[1]

Continuation Table 3.

Name, abbreviated chemical formula and molecular weight		Structure of amino acid in position 2
Cys–*(N-Me)Tyr–Ile*–Gln–Asn–Cys–Pro–Leu–Gly–NH_2 (N-Me)Tyr²-oxytocin	1021.1	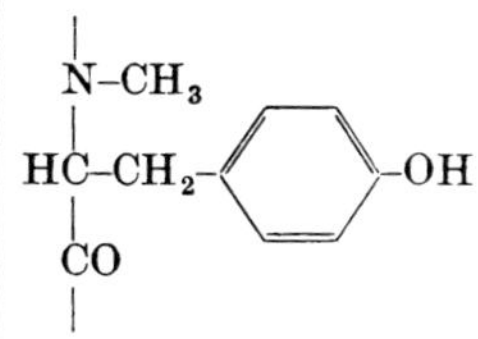
Cys–*Leu–Ile*–Gln–Asn–Cys–Pro–Leu–Gly–NH_2 Leu²-oxytocin	957.2	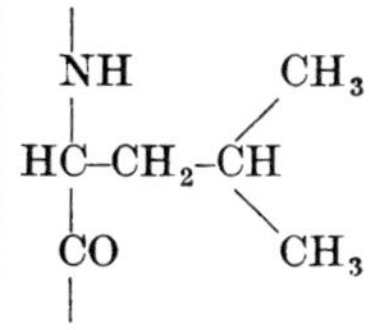
Cys–*Ser–Ile*–Gln–Asn–Cys–Pro–Leu–Gly–NH_2 Ser²-oxytocin	931.1	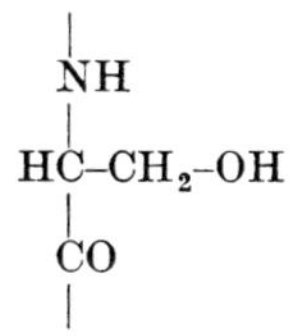
Cys–*Gly–Ile*–Gln–Asn–Cys–Pro–Leu–Gly–NH_2 Gly²-oxytocin	901.1	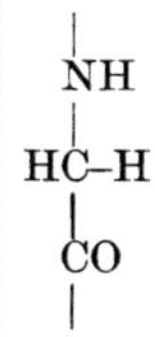
Cys–*Tyr–Phe*–Gln–Asn–Cys–Pro–Leu–Gly–NH_2 Oxypressin = Phe³-oxytocin	1075.3	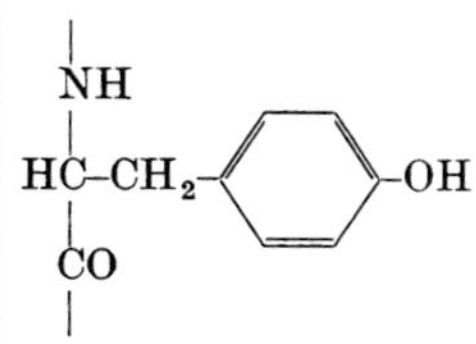
Cys–*His–Phe*–Gln–Asn–Cys–Pro–Leu–Gly–NH_2 Phe²-oxypressin = Phe²-Phe³-oxytocin	1059.3	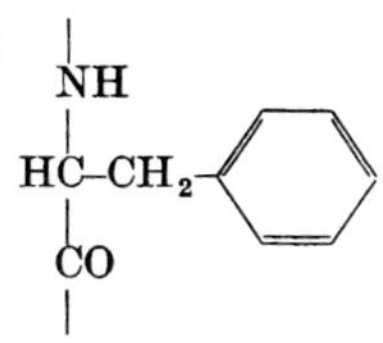
Cys–*His–Phe*–Gln–Asn–Cys–Pro–Leu–Gly–NH_2 His²-oxypressin = His²-Phe³-oxytocin	981.1	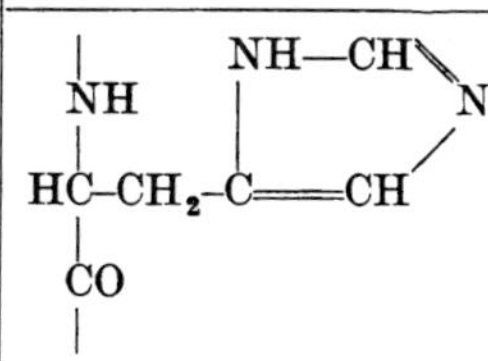

Structure of amino acid in position 3	Oxytocin-like activities in International Units per micromole			Vasopressin-like activities in International Units per micromole		References S = synthesis P = pharmacology 1 = also contains pharmacological data
	Rat uterus (isolated)	Chicken blood pressure	Rabbit mammary gland	Rat blood pressure	Rat antidiuresis	
as above	1.2 ± 0.4	0.32 ± 0.05	3.1 ± 0.7	—	<0.01	S: Huguenin, Boissonnas (1961)[1] P: Berde et al. (1960)
as above	~0.44	~1.2	~1.7	—	~0.02	S: Jošt et al. (1963a)
as above	<0.01	<0.01	<0.01	<0.01	<0.01	S: Guttmann, Boissonnas (1960)[1] P: Berde et al. (1961a)
as above	<0.01	<0.01	—	<0.01	—	S: Drabarek (1964)[1]
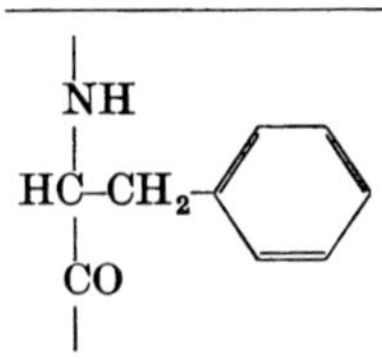	~20	~30	~65	~3	~30	S: Boissonnas et al. (1956) Katsoyannis (1957)[1] P: Berde et al. (1957)
as above	3.5 ± 0.3	5.7 ± 0.9	26 ± 9	~0.9	6.0 ± 0.6	S: Boissonnas, Guttmann (1960)[1] P: Berde et al. (1961a)
as above	<0.1	<0.1	—	<0.1	—	S: Guttmann, Boissonnas (1960)[1] P: Berde et al. (1961a)

Table 4. *Variations in position 2 of vasotocin*

Name, abbreviated chemical formula and molecular weight		Structure of amino acid in position 2
Cys–*Tyr*–Ile–Gln–Asn–Cys–Pro–*Arg*–Gly–NH_2 (Cys¹–Cys⁶ bridged) Vasotocin = arginine-vasotocin = Arg[8]-oxytocin	1050.2	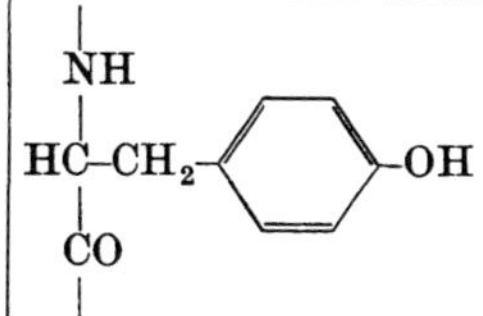
Cys–*Phe*–Ile–Gln–Asn–Cys–Pro–*Arg*–Gly–NH_2 (Cys¹–Cys⁶ bridged) Phe[2]-vasotocin = Phe[2]-Arg[8]-oxytocin	1034.2	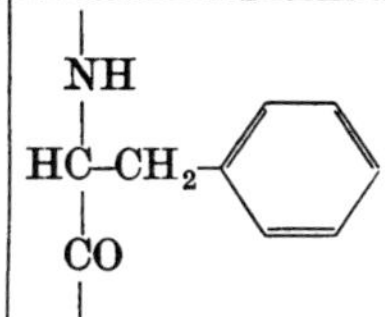
Cys–*Tyr*–Ile–Gln–Asn–Cys–Pro–*Lys*–Gly–NH_2 (Cys¹–Cys⁶ bridged) Lysine-vasotocine = Lys[8]-oxytocin	1022.2	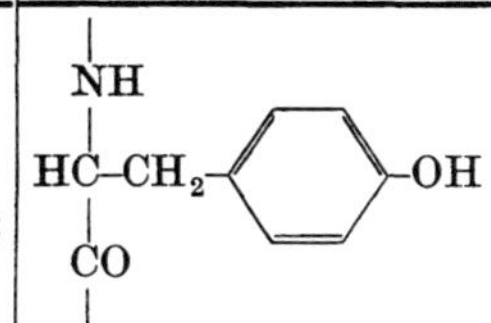
Cys–*Phe*–Ile–Gln–Asn–Cys–Pro–*Lys*–Gly–NH_2 (Cys¹–Cys⁶ bridged) Phe[2]-lysine-vasotocin = Phe[2]-Lys[8]-oxytocin	1006.2	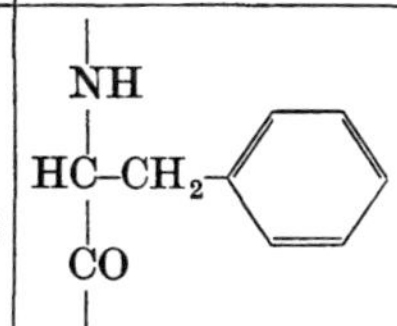
Cys–*Ser*–Ile–Gln–Asn–Cys–Pro–*Lys*–Gly–NH_2 (Cys¹–Cys⁶ bridged) Ser[2]-lysine-vasotocin = Ser[2]-Lys[8]-oxytocin	945.1	NH HC–CH_2–OH CO
Cys–*Tyr*–Ile–Gln–Asn–Cys–Pro–*Orn*–Gly–NH_2 (Cys¹–Cys⁶ bridged) Ornithine-vasotocin = Orn[8]-oxytocin	1008.2	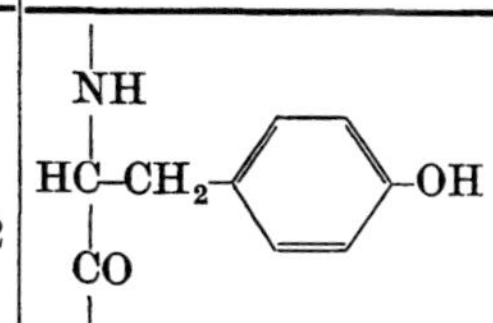
Cys–*Phe*–Ile–Gln–Asn–Cys–Pro–*Orn*–Gly–NH_2 (Cys¹–Cys⁶ bridged) Phe[2]-Orn[8]-vasotocin = Phe[2]-Orn[8]-oxytocin	992.2	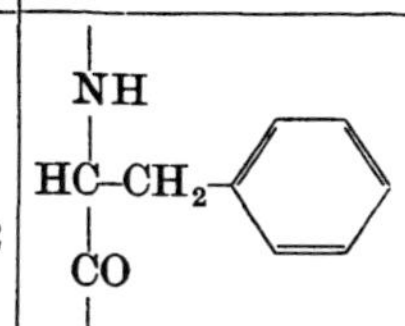

References S = synthesis P = pharmacology [1] also contains pharmacological data

1 = Occurs in nature. 2 = S: Huguenin, Boissonnas (1962)[1]; P: Berde, Stürmer (1962). 3 = S: Boissonnas, Huguenin (1960)[1], Kimbrough, du Vigneaud (1961)[1], Huguenin, Boissonnas (1962)[1];

(arginine-vasotocin), lysine-vasotocin and ornithine-vasotocin.

Structure of amino acid in position 8	Oxytocin-like activities in International Units per micromole			Vasopressin-like activities in International Units per micromole		Ref.
	Rat uterus (isolated)	Chicken blood pressure	Rabbit mammary gland	Rat blood pressure	Rat antidiuresis	
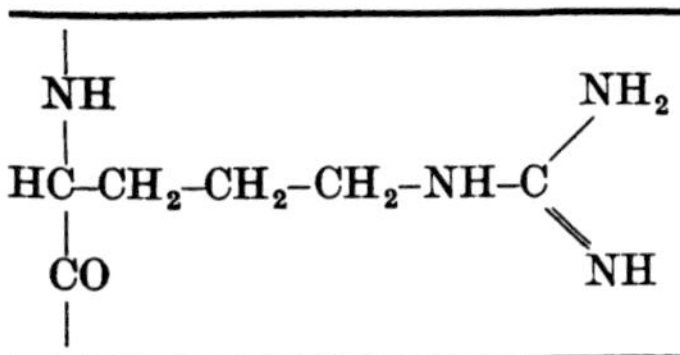	120 ± 16	300 ± 42	~220	255 ± 16	260 ± 37	1
as above	2 ± 0.4	~10	~10	130 ± 15	113 ± 13	2
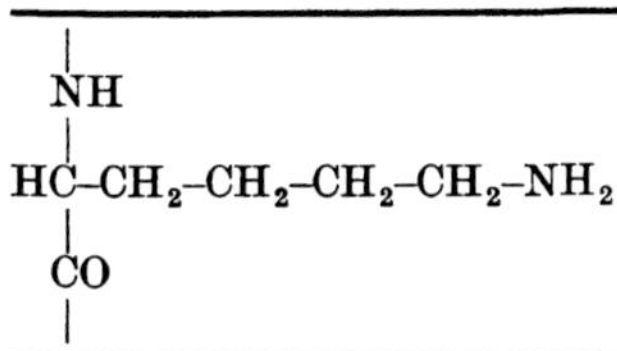	80 ± 10	215 ± 3	185 ± 25	133 ± 13	25 ± 3	3
as above	1.0 ± 0.1	~8	12 ± 3	32 ± 6	1.0 ± 0.1	4
as above	<0.01	<0.01	<0.01	~0.1	~0.06	5
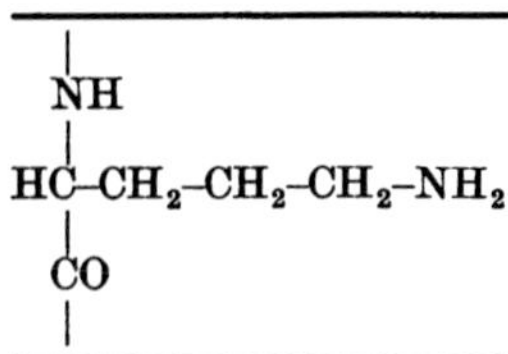	42 ± 5	90 ± 3	95 ± 6	104 ± 10	2.5 ± 0.3	6
as above	~1	~3	7 ± 2	123 ± 10	0.55 ± 0.08	7

P: BERDE et al. (1961a), BERDE, STÜRMER (1962). 4 = S: JAQUENOUD, BOISSONNAS (1960)[1], BOISSONNAS et al. (1961)[1]; P: BERDE et al. (1960). 5 = S: GUTTMANN, BOISSONNAS (1960)[1]; P: BERDE et al. (1961a). 6 = S: HUGUENIN, BOISSONNAS (1963)[1]; P: BERDE et al. (1964). 7 = S: HUGUENIN (1964)[1]; P: BERDE et al. (1964).

Table 5. *Variations in position 2 of vasopressin (arginine-vasopressin),*

Name, abbreviated chemical formula and molecular weight		Structure of amino acid in position 2
Cys–*Tyr*–Phe–Gln–Asn–Cys–Pro–*Arg*–Gly–NH_2 Vasopressin = Arginine-vasopressin	1084.2	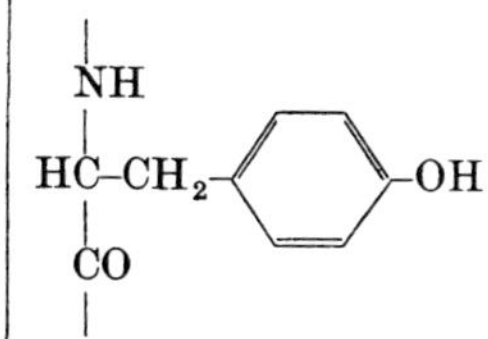
Cys–*Phe*–Phe–Gln–Asn–Cys–Pro–*Arg*–Gly–NH_2 Phe^2-vasopressin	1068.2	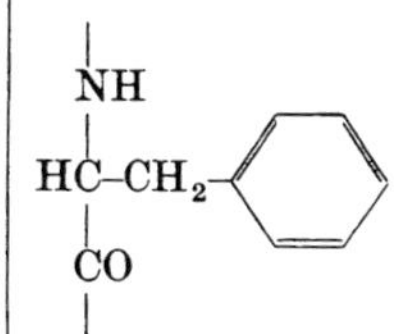
Cys–*Tyr*–Phe–Gln–Asn–Cys–Pro–*Lys*–Gly–NH_2 Lysine-vasopressin = Lys^8-vasopressin	1056.2	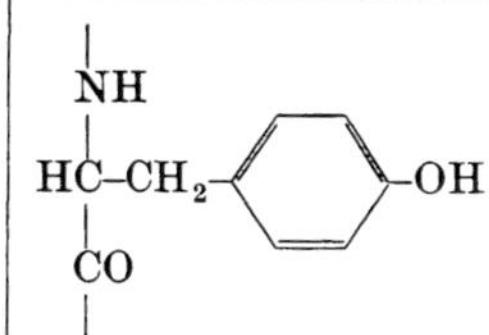
Cys–Phe–*Phe*–Gln–Asn–Cys–Pro–*Lys*–Gly–NH_2 Phe^2-lysine-vasopressin	1040.2	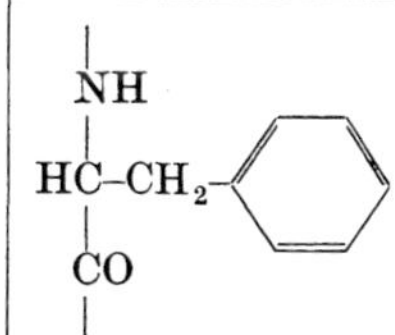
Cys–*(O-Me)Tyr*–Phe–Gln–Asn–Cys–Pro–*Lys*–Gly–NH_2 (O-Me)Tyr^2-lysine-vasopressin	1070.3	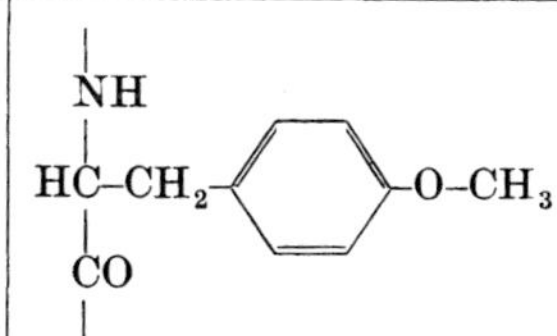
Cys–*(O-Et)Tyr*–Phe–Gln–Asn–Cys–Pro–*Lys*–Gly–NH_2 (O-Et)Tyr^2-lysine-vasopressin	1084.3	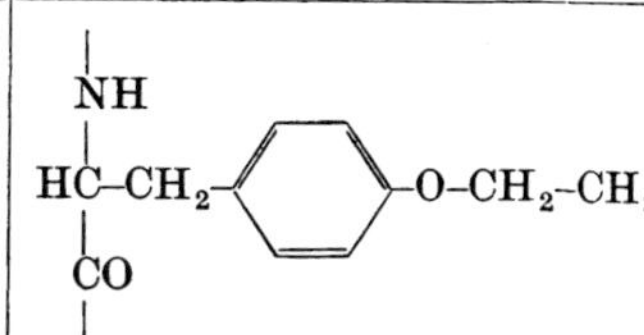

References S = synthesis P = pharmacology [1] = also contains pharmacological data

1 = Occurs in nature. 2 = S: HUGUENIN, BOISSONNAS (1962)[1]; P: BERDE, STÜRMER (1962). 3 = Occurs in nature. 4 = S: BOISSONNAS, GUTTMANN (1960)[1]; MEIENHOFER, DU VIGNEAUD (1960)[1];

lysine-vasopressin and ornithine-vasopressin

Structure of amino acid in position 8	Oxytocin-like activities in International Units per micromole			Vasopressin-like activities in International Units per micromole		Ref.
	Rat uterus (isolated)	Chicken blood pressure	Rabbit mammary gland	Rat blood pressure	Rat antidiuresis	
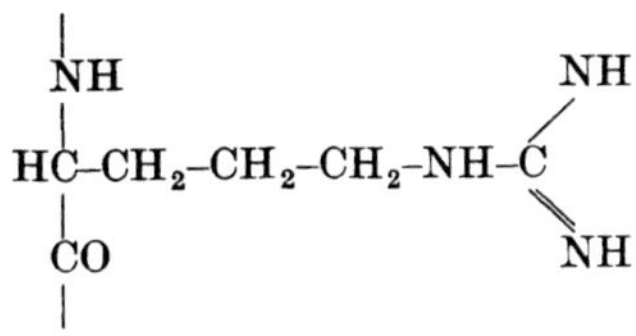	17 ± 4	65 ± 6	70 ± 9	435 ± 45	435 ± 45	1
as above	~0.2	<1	3 ± 0.4	130 ± 13	~375	2
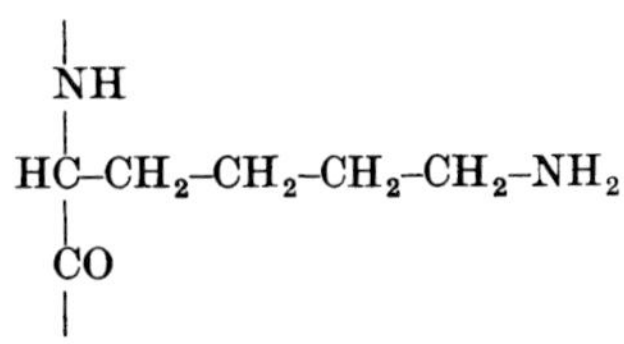	5 ± 0.5	42 ± 5	63 ± 10	285 ± 21	~260	3
as above	0.3	~0.15	~2.5	57 ± 7	21 ± 2	4
as above	Anti	Anti	—	2.4 ± 0.7	79 ± 11	5
as above	Anti	—	—	Anti	~5	6

P: Berde et al. (1961a, b). 5 = S: Siedel et al. (1963); Zaoral et al. (1965)[1]; P: Vogel, Hergott (1963). 6 = S: Zaoral et al. (1965)[1]. 7 = S: Guttmann, Boissonnas (1960)[1]; P: Berde et al. (1961a). 8 = S: Huguenin, Boissonnas (1963)[1]; P: Berde et al. (1964). 9 = S: Huguenin (1964)[1]; P: Berde et al. (1964).

Continuation Table 5.

Name, abbreviated chemical formula and molecular weight		Structure of amino acid in position 2
Cys–*His*–Phe–Gln–Asn–Cys–Pro–*Lys*–Gly–NH_2 His²-lysine-vasopressin	1030.2	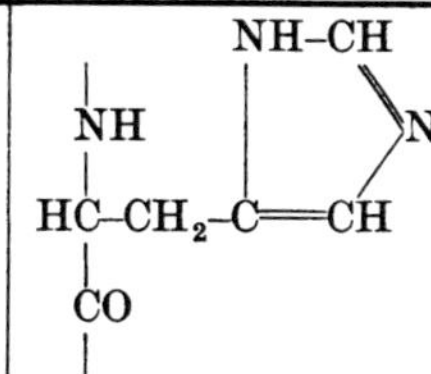
Cys–*Tyr*–Phe–Gln–Asn–Cys–Pro–*Orn*–Gly–NH_2 Ornithine-vasopressin	1042.2	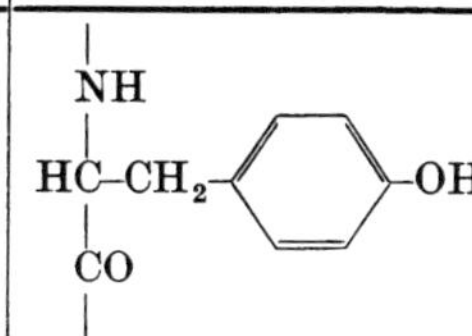
Cys–*Phe*–Phe–Gln–Asn–Cys–Pro–*Orn*–Gly–NH_2 Phe²-Orn⁸-vasopressin	1024.2	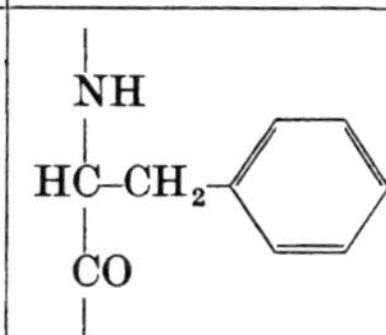

References S = synthesis P = pharmacology [1] = also contains pharmacological data

1 = Occurs in nature. 2 = S: Huguenin, Boissannas (1962)[1]; P: Berde, Stürmer (1962). 3 = Occurs in natura. 4 = S: Boissannas, Guttmann (1960)[1]; Meienhofer, du Vigneaud (1960)[1];

deleterious result. One is tempted to conclude that steric factors play a decisive role in this region of the molecule, but the relatively high level of activity still exhibited by the analogue having a D-tyrosine residue instead of a L-tyrosine residue (D-Tyr²-oxytocin) calls for a more cautious interpretation.

The presence of a methyl group on the nitrogen atom of the tyrosine residue ([N-Me] Tyr²-oxytocin) is seemingly a small modification, but a study of a molecular model shows that it limits the degrees of freedom of the peptide chain, this explaining its deleterious effect on biological activity.

Replacement of the aromatic group by an aliphatic group (Leu²-oxytocin) also greatly decreases the activities. The introduction of a hydroxyl group (Ser²-oxytocin) or total suppression of the side group (Gly²-oxytocin) abolishes them completely.

When the hydroxyl group of oxypressin is eliminated (Phe²-Phe³-oxytocin), the effect is the same as in the case of oxytocin.

It is interesting to note that, when oxytocin-like activities are reduced by modifications in position 2, uterotonic activity is always more greatly affected than milk-ejecting activity. The effect on avian depressor activity generally falls somewhere in-between.

Stucture of amino acid in position 8	Oxytocin-like activities in International Units per micromole			Vasopressin-like activities in International Units per micromole		Ref.
	Rat uterus (isolated)	Chicken blood pressure	Rabbit mammary gland	Rat blood pressure	Rat antidiuresis	
ıs above	<0.01	<0.01	<0.01	<0.01	—	7
NH HC–CH_2–CH_2–CH_2–NH_2 CO	10 ± 2	22 ± 1	~50	375 ± 27	92 ± 18	8
ıs above	~0.5	<0.01	~3	157 ± 11	16 ± 2	9

?: Berde et al. (1961 a, b). 5 = S: Siedel et al. (1963), Zaoral et al. (1965)[1]; P: Vogel, Hergott 1963). 6 = S: Zaoral et al. (1965)[1]. 7 = S: Guttmann, Boissannas (1960)[1]; P: Berde et al. (1961 a). 3 = S: Huguenin, Boissannas (1963)[1]; P: Berde et al. (1964). 9 = S: Huguenin (1964); P: Berde ›t al. (1964).

Variations in position 2 of the vasotocins (Table 4) mainly relate to the suppression of the phenolic group. The effects on the oxytocin-like activities are the same as in the oxytocin series.

In all these compounds, with the exception of arginine-vasotocin, antidiuretic activity is more strongly affected than pressor activity. As a result, the selectivity of the vasoconstrictor effect is enhanced.

In the vasopressin series (Table 5) suppression of the phenolic group also causes a greater decrease of antidiuretic than of pressor activity, with the notable exception again of the arginine-containing representative, in which the reverse effect occurs. Methylation of the phenolic group of lysine-vasopressin also favours the antidiuretic property of the hormone, whereas ethylation sharply decreases all activities, as in the case of oxytocin.

Modifications in position 3 of oxytocin (Table 6) are especially interesting, for the isoleucine residue, which is present in this position, bears two asymmetric carbon atoms. Inversion at the second centre of asymmetry yields allo-isoleucine^3-oxytocin, which is considerably less active than oxytocin (the latter contains isoleucine in the threo form). The low activity of Leu^3-oxytocin by comparison with Val^3-oxytocin shows that the tertiary carbon must be kept close to the

Table 6. *Variations in*

Name, abbreviated chemical formula and molecular weight		Structure of amino acid in position 3
Cys–Tyr–*Ile*–Gln–Asn–Cys–Pro–Leu–Gly–NH_2 Oxytocin	1007.2	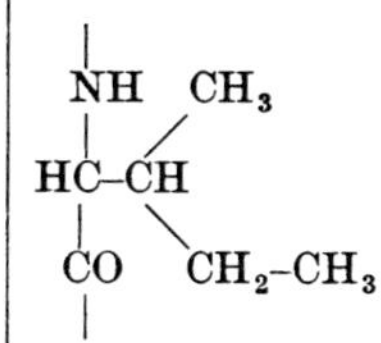
Cys–Tyr–*aIle*–Gln–Asn–Cys–Pro–Leu–Gly–NH_2 aIle³-oxytocin = alloisoleucine³-oxytocin	1007.2	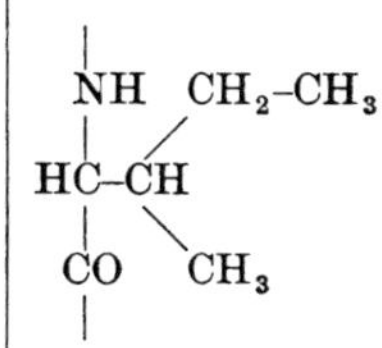
Cys–Tyr–*Val*–Gln–Asn–Cys–Pro–Leu–Gly–NH_2 Val³-oxytocin	993.2	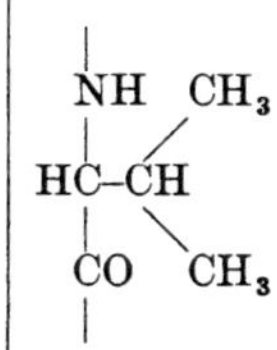
Cys–Tyr–*Leu*–Gln–Asn–Cys–Pro–Leu–Gly–NH_2 Leu³-oxytocin	1007.2	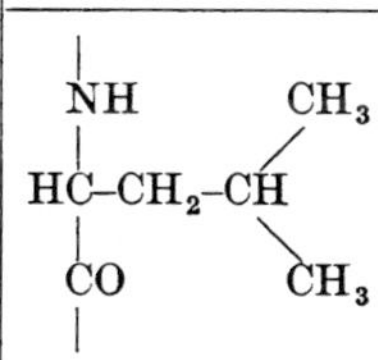
Cys–Tyr–*Nva*–Gln–Asn–Cys–Pro–Leu–Gly–NH_2 Nva³-oxytocin	993.2	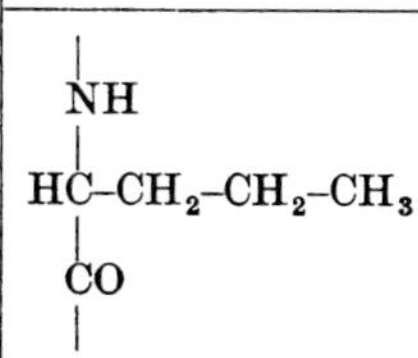
Cys–Tyr–*Nle*–Gln–Asn–Cys–Pro–Leu–Gly–NH_2 Nle³-oxytocin	1007.2	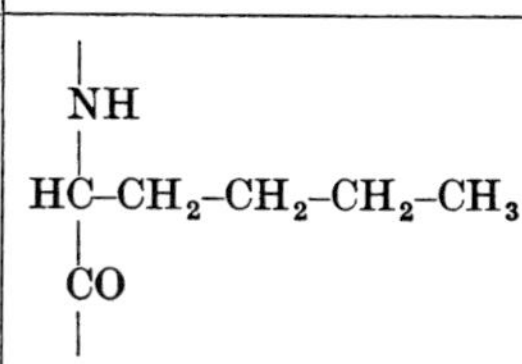
Cys–Tyr–*(O-Me)Thr*–Gln–Asn–Cys–Pro–Leu–Gly–NH_2 (O-Me)Thr³-oxytocin	1009.2	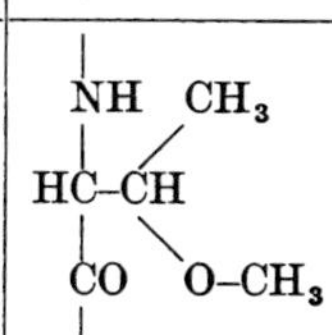

position 3 of oxytocin

Oxytocin-like activities in International Units per micromole			Vasopressin-like activities in International Units per micromole		References S = synthesis P = pharmacology [1] = also contains pharmacological data
Rat uterus (isolated)	Chicken blood pressure	Rabbit mammary gland	Rat blood pressure	Rat antidiuresis	
450 ± 30	450 ± 30	450 ± 30	5 ± 1	5 ± 1	Occurs in nature
~25	~20	~125 (guinea pig)	~0.2	~0.05	S: NESVADBA et al. (1963)[1]
59 ± 8	58 ± 4	206 ± 14 (guinea pig 67)	~0.1	~0.8	S: BOISSONNAS et al. (1956) RUDINGER et al. (1956) NESVADBA et al. (1963)[1] P: BERDE et al. (1957, 1961a)
~4	~9	~35 (guinea pig)	~0.03	~1	S: BOISSONNAS et al. (1956) NESVADBA et al. (1963)[1] P: BERDE et al. (1957)
~7	~12	~85 (guinea pig)	~0.1	~5	S: NESVADBA et al. (1963)[1]
~10	~20	~25 (guinea pig)	~0.2	~0.5	S: NESVADBA et al. (1963)[1]
~35	~20	~65 (guinea pig)	~0.07	~0.16	S: CHIMIAK and RUDINGER (1965)[1]

Continuation Table 6.

Name, abbreviated chemical formula and molecular weight		Structure of amino acid in position 3
Cys–Tyr–*Gly*–Gln–Asn–Cys–Pro–Leu–Gly–NH_2 Gly³-oxytocin	951.1	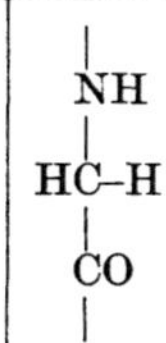
Cys–Tyr–*Phe*–Gln–Asn–Cys–Pro–Leu–Gly–NH_2 Phe³-oxytocin = oxypressin	1075.3	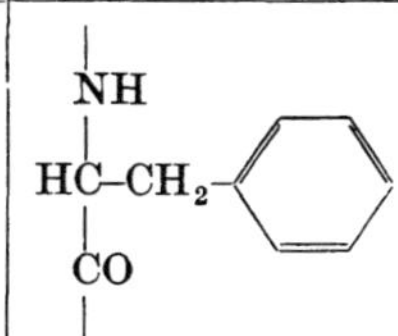
Cys–Tyr–*Tyr*–Gln–Asn–Cys–Pro–Leu–Gly–NH_2 Tyr³-oxytocin	1057.2	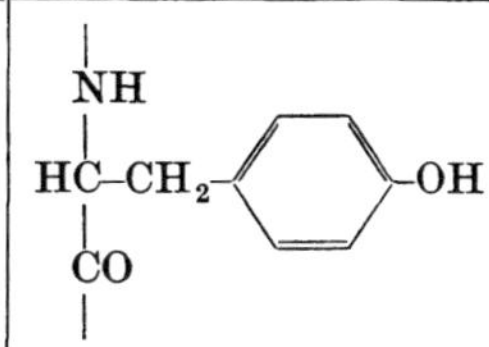
Cys–Tyr–*Trp*–Gln–Asn–Cys–Pro–Leu–Gly–NH_2 Trp³-oxytocin	1081.2	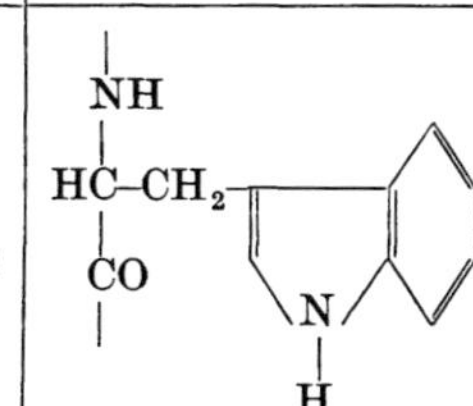

peptide chain. It is interesting that (O-Me) Thr³-oxytocin, in which a methylene group has been replaced by an oxygen atom and which is isosteric with oxytocin, still has a fair level of activity.

Here again, complete suppression of the side group (Gly³-oxytocin) completely abolishes all activity.

Introduction of a phenylalanine residue in position 3 of oxytocin (Phe³-oxytocin or oxypressin) gives an analogue which is a structural intermediate between oxytocin and vasopressin and is thus the counterpart of vasotocin. Like the latter, oxypressin also exhibits biological properties both of oxytocin and vasopressin, but at an appreciable lower level. It is interesting to note that the pressor activity of this compound is ten times lower than its antidiuretic activity.

From the fact that in all cases investigated, tyrosine in position 2 can be replaced by phenylalanine without drastically affecting the biological activities, one is tempted to infer that the reverse must also be true and that phenylalanine in position 3 should be replaceable by tyrosine. The very low activity of Tyr³-oxytocin proves this inference to be fallacious.

Oxytocin-like activities in International Units per micromole			Vasopressin-like activities in International Units per micromole		References S = synthesis P = pharmacology [1] = also contains pharmacological data
Rat uterus (isolated)	Chicken blood pressure	Rabbit mammary gland	Rat blood pressure	Rat antidiuresis	
<0.01	<0.01	—	<0.01	—	S: DRABAREK (1964)[1]
~20	~30	~65	~3	~30	S: BOISSONNAS et al. (1956) KATSOYANNIS (1957)[1] P: BERDE et al. (1957)
0.10 ± 0.03	~0.03	1.5 ± 0.3	~0.01	~0.01	S: BOISSONNAS, GUTTMANN (1960)[1] P: BERDE et al. (1961a)
0.04 ± 0.01	~0.1	0.10 ± 0.06	<0.01	<0.01	S: GUTTMANN, BOISSONNAS (1960)[1] P: BERDE et al. (1961a)

From Table 7 it is evident that in the vasopressin series too, replacement of phenylalanine in position 3 by tyrosine abolishes all activity. Introduction of an isoleucine residue in position 3 (Ile^{3}-Lys^{8}-vasopressin = lysine-vasotocin) yields a compound which differs from natural vasotocin (arginine-vasotocin) only in having a lysine residue instead of an arginine residue in position 8. The spectrum of activities of this analogue is the same as that of vasotocin with the exception of the antidiuretic effect which is considerably lower.

Introduction of a serine residue in position 3 of lysine-vasopressin has the same effect as the introduction of the same residue in position 2 of oxytocin or lysine-vasotocin, i. e. all activities are abolished. This is surprising, for we have seen that the natural hormones, isotocin and glumitocin, contain a serine residue in position 4 and we shall see below that Ser^{4}-oxytocin and Ser^{4}-Lys^{8}-vasopressin are active analogues.

Many modifications have been effected recently in position 4 of oxytocin (Table 8). Hydrolysis of the lateral amide group (Glu^{4}-oxytocin) sharply decreases the activities. As this amide group is particularly susceptible to hydrolysis in

Table 7. *Variations in*

Name, abbreviated chemical formula and molecular weight		Structure of amino acid in position 3
Cys–Tyr–*Phe*–Gln–Asn–Cys–Pro–Lys–Gly–NH_2 Lysine-vasopressin	1056.2	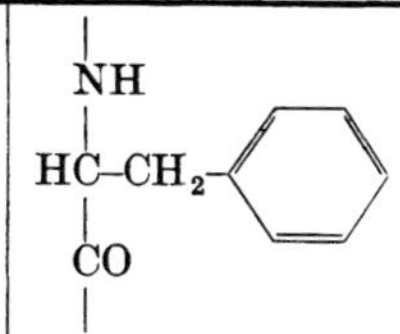
Cys–Tyr–*Tyr*–Gln–Asn–Cys–Pro–Lys–Gly–NH_2 Tyr[3]-Lys[8]-vasopressin	1072.2	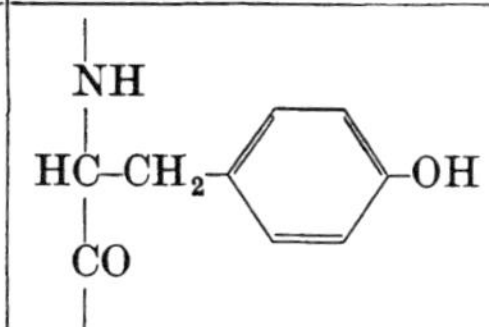
Cys–Tyr–*Ile*–Gln–Asn–Cys–Pro–Lys–Gly–NH_2 Ile[3]-Lys[8]-vasopressin = Lysine-vasotocin	1022.2	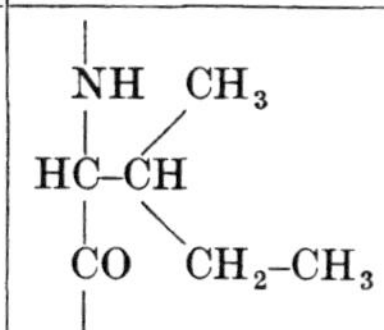
Cys–Tyr–*Ser*–Gln–Asn–Cys–Pro–Lys–Gly–NH_2 Ser[3]-Lys[8]-vasopressin	996.1	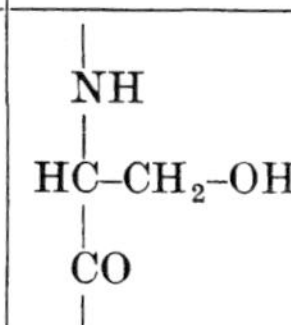
Cys–Tyr–*Trp*–Gln–Asn–Cys–Pro–Lys–Gly–NH_2 Trp[3]-Lys[8]-vasopressin	1096.2	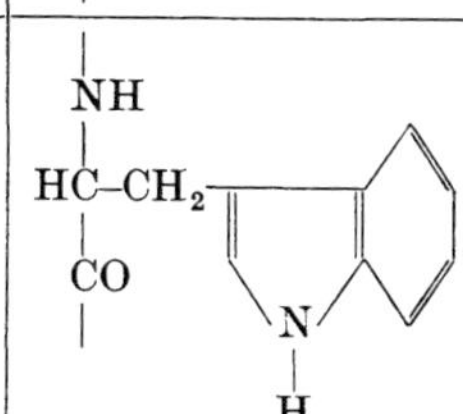

oxytocin, it is likely that the limited stability of the hormone under strongly acid or basic conditions is due to the conversion of oxytocin to Glu[4]-oxytocin. In view of the relatively high activity of Asn[4]-oxytocin, from which a methylene group has been omitted but in which the amide group is still present, it would be wrong to conclude that this amide group is necessary for activity: Abu[4]-oxytocin, in which the carboxamide group has been suppressed, is fairly active, as also is Val[4]-oxytocin, Ala[4]-oxytocin and Ser[4]-oxytocin. The high activity of the latter compound is remarkable, for introduction of a serine in the adjoining positions is always associated with loss of activity. Even Gly[4]-oxytocin still has some activity, whereas introduction of a glycine residue, i. e. suppression of the side group, in the other positions always abolishes activity.

position 3 of lysine-vasopressin

Oxytocin-like activities in International Units per micromole			Vasopressin-like activities in International Units per micromole		References S = synthesis P = pharmacology [1] = also contains pharmacological data
Rat uterus (isolated)	Chicken blood pressure	Rabbit mammary gland	Rat blood pressure	Rat antidiuresis	
5 ± 0.5	42 ± 5	63 ± 10	285 ± 21	~ 260	Occurs in nature
~ 0.01	~ 0.1	~ 0.2	1.6 ± 0.2	0.18 ± 0.08	S: Boissonnas, Guttmann (1960)[1] P: Berde et al. (1961 a)
80 ± 10	215 ± 3	185 ± 25	133 ± 13	25 ± 3	S: Boissonnas, Huguenin (1960)[1] Kimbrough, du Vigneaud (1961)[1] Huguenin, Boissonnas (1962)[1] P: Berde et al. (1961 a) Berde, Stürmer (1962)
<0.01	<0.01	~ 0.04	<0.01	~ 0.02	S: Guttmann, Boissonnas (1960)[1] P: Berde et al. (1961 b)
<0.01	~ 0.08	<0.01	~ 0.07	—	S: Guttmann, Boissonnas (1960)[1] P: Berde et al. (1961 a)

We have seen that position 2 of oxytocin is very sensitive to modification, but that inversion of the amino acid occupying that position yields a compound which is still appreciably active. It is therefore surprising, that in position 4 of oxytocin, which is rather insensitive to modification, inversion of the amino acid occupying this position inactivates the molecule.

No modifications have so far been effected in position 4 of vasotocin and vasopressin. Modifications in position 4 of lysine-vasopressin are listed in Table 9. The same conclusions can be drawn as in the case of oxytocin. The low pressor activity of Ser^4-Lys^8-vasopressin in comparison with its appreciable antidiuretic effect confers an interesting selectivity upon this analogue.

Table 8. *Variations in*

Name, abbreviated chemical formula and molecular weight		Structure of amino acid in position 4
Cys–Tyr–Ile–*Gln*–Asn–Cys–Pro–Leu–Gly–NH_2 Oxytocin	1007.19	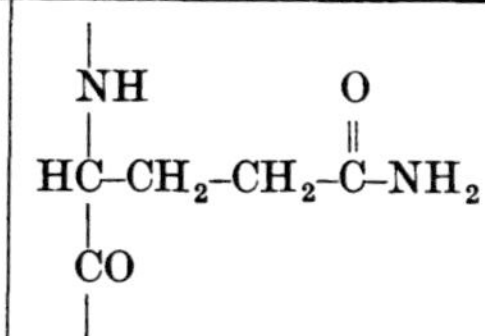
Cys–Tyr–Ile–*Glu*–Asn–Cys–Pro–Leu–Gly–NH_2 Glu[4]-oxytocin	1008.2	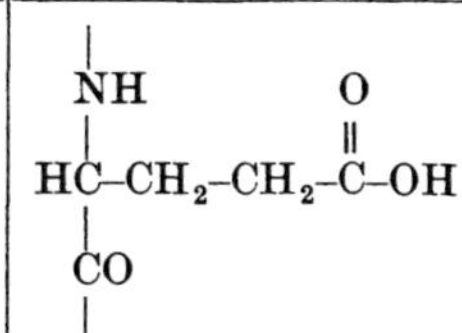
Cys–Tyr–Ile–*Asn*–Asn–Cys–Pro–Leu–Gly–NH_2 Asn[4]-oxytocin	993.2	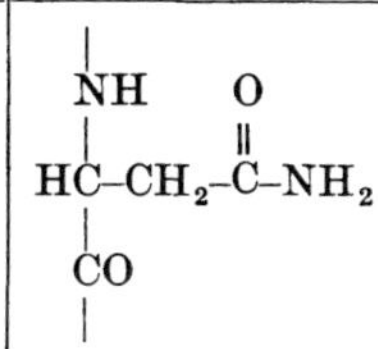
Cys–Tyr–Ile–*Abu*–Asn–Cys–Pro–Leu–Gly–NH_2 Abu[4]-oxytocin	964.2	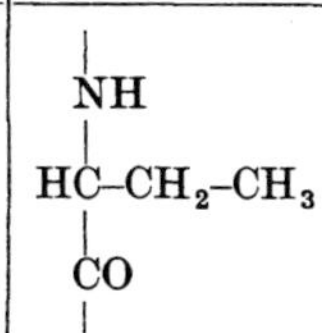
Cys–Tyr–Ile–*Val*–Asn–Cys–Pro–Leu–Gly–NH_2 Val[4]-oxytocin	978.2	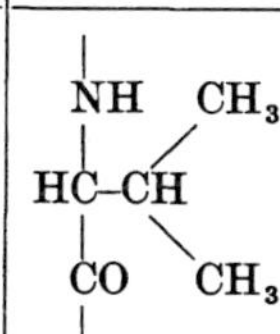
Cys–Tyr–Ile–*Ala*–Asn–Cys–Pro–Leu–Gly–NH_2 Ala[4]-oxytocin	950.2	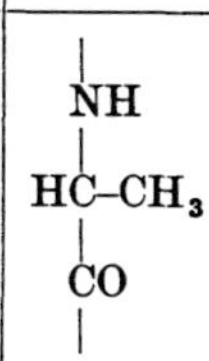
Cys–Tyr–Ile–*Ser*–Asn–Cys–Pro–Leu–Gly–NH_2 Ser[4]-oxytocin	966.2	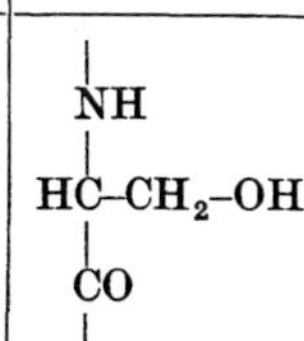

position 4 of oxytocin

Oxytocin-like activities in International Units per micromole			Vasopressin-like activities in International Units per micromole		References S = synthesis P = pharmacology [1] = also contains pharmacological data
Rat uterus (isolated)	Chicken blood pressure	Rabbit mammary gland	Rat blood pressure	Rat antidiuresis	
450 ± 30	450 ± 30	450 ± 30	5 ± 1	5 ± 1	Occurs in nature
~1.5	~0.5	~11	<0.01	<0.01	S: PHOTAKI, DU VIGNEAUD (1965)[1]
107 ± 29	201 ± 12	298 ± 128	0.13 ± 0.03	0.044 ± 0.005	S: JAQUENOUD, BOISSONNAS (1962a)[1] P: BERDE, STÜRMER (1962)
70 ± 2	104 ± 5	217 ± 7	~0.1	~0.25	S: DU VIGNEAUD et al (1963; 1964)[1]
~135	~230	—	<0.01	—	S: DU VIGNEAUD et al. (1966)[1]
34 ± 6	62 ± 3	228 ± 55	<0.01	<0.01	S: GUTTMANN, BOISSONNAS (1963)[1] P: BERDE, STÜRMER (1962)
190 ± 30	220 ± 20	245 ± 45	<0.1	0.06 ± 0.01	S: GUTTMANN, BOISSONNAS (1963)[1] P: BERDE, STÜRMER (1962)

Continuation Table 8.

Name, abbreviated chemical formula and molecular weight		Structure of amino acid in position 4
Cys–Tyr–Ile–*Gly*–Asn–Cys–Pro–Leu–Gly–NH_2 (disulfide bridge Cys–Cys) Gly[4]-oxytocin	936.2	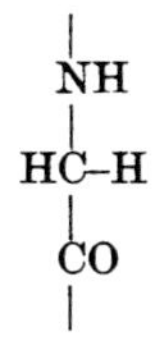
Cys–Tyr–Ile–*D–Gln*–Asn–Cys–Pro–Leu–Gly–NH_2 (disulfide bridge Cys–Cys) D-Gln[4]-oxytocin	1007.2	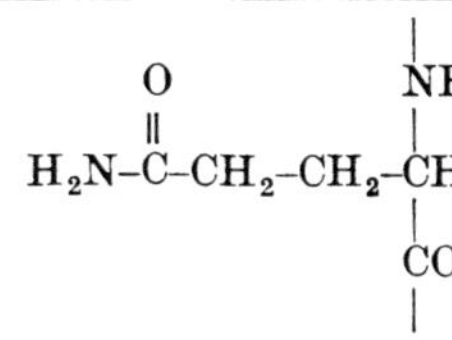

Table 9. *Variations in position 4*

Name, abbreviated chemical formula and molecular weight		Structure of amino acid in position 4
Cys–Tyr–Phe–*Gln*–Asn–Cys–Pro–Lys–Gly–NH_2 (disulfide bridge Cys–Cys) Lysine-vasopressin	1056.2	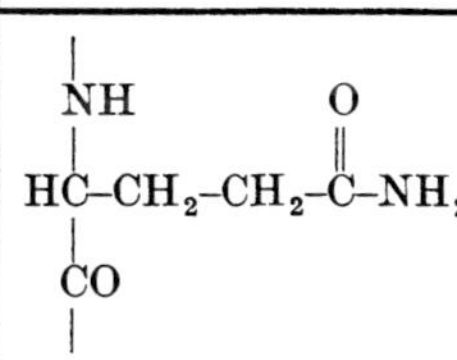
Cys–Tyr–Phe–*Asn*–Asn–Cys–Pro–Lys–Gly–NH_2 (disulfide bridge Cys–Cys) Asn[4]-Lys[8]-vasopressin	1042.2	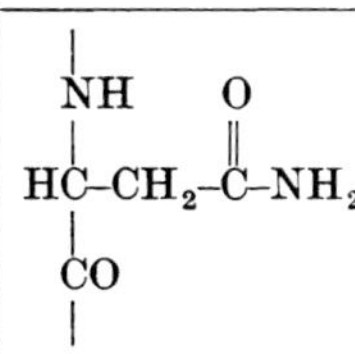
Cys–Tyr–Phe–*Ala*–Asn–Cys–Pro–Lys–Gly–NH_2 (disulfide bridge Cys–Cys) Ala[4]-Lys[8]-vasopressin	1001.2	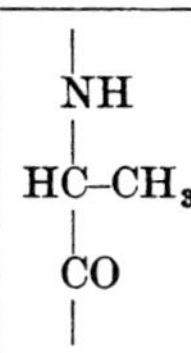
Cys–Tyr–Phe–*Ser*–Asn–Cys–Pro–Lys–Gly–NH_2 (disulfide bridge Cys–Cys) Ser[4]-Lys[8]-vasopressin	1017.2	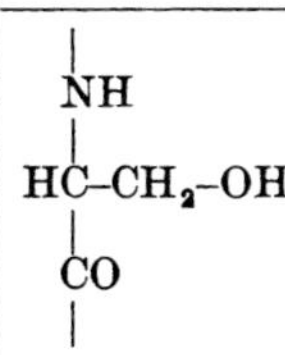

Oxytocin-like activities in International Units per micromole			Vasopressin-like activities in International Units per micromole		References S = synthesis P = pharmacology [1] = also contains pharmacological data
Rat uterus (isolated)	Chicken blood pressure	Rabbit mammary gland	Rat blood pressure	Rat antidiuresis	
2.8 ± 0.1	5.5 ± 0.2	17 ± 1	< 0.002	< 0.005	S: DRABAREK (1964)[1] FOSKER, LAW (1965)[1]
~0.1	~1.0	—	—	—	S: DUTTA, ANAND (1965) P: DUTTA, ANAND (1966)

f lysine-vasopressin

Oxytocin-like activities in International Units per micromole			Vasopressin-like activities in International Units per micromole		References S = synthesis P = pharmacology [1] = also contains pharmacological data
Rat uterus (isolated)	Chicken blood pressure	Rabbit mammary gland	Rat blood pressure	Rat antidiuresis	
5 ± 0.5	42 ± 5	63 ± 10	285 ± 21	~260	Occurs in nature
3 ± 0.4	23 ± 1	19 ± 3	56 ± 12	25 ± 3	S: BOISSONNAS et al. (1963)[1] P: BERDE, STÜRMER (1962)
0.5 ± 0.05	2.2 ± 0.1	~2	1.6 ± 0.3	30 ± 0.3	S: BOISSONNAS et al. (1963)[1] P: BERDE, STÜRMER (1962)
0.9 ± 0.2	10 ± 0.7	7 ± 4	3.3 ± 0.5	70 ± 11	S: BOISSONNAS et al. (1963)[1] P: BERDE, STÜRMER (1962)

Table 10. *Variations in position 5*

Name, abbreviated chemical formula and molecular weight		Structure of amino acid in position 5
Cys–Tyr–Ile–Gln–*Asn*–Cys–Pro–Leu–Gly–NH_2 Oxytocin	1007.2	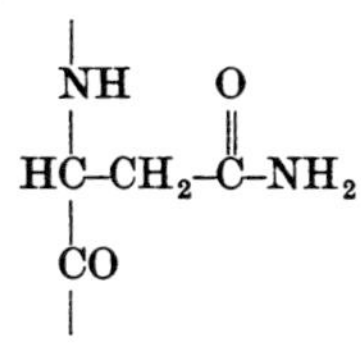
Cys–Tyr–Ile–Gln–*Gln*–Cys–Pro–Leu–Gly–NH_2 Gln[5]-oxytocin	1021.2	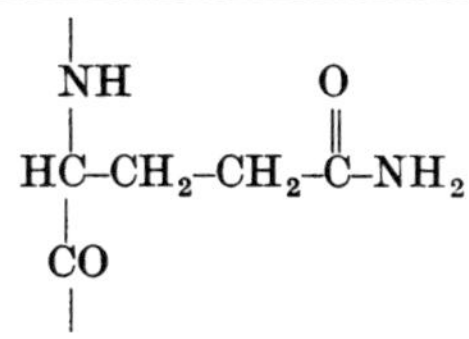
Cys–Tyr–Ile–Gln–*Ala*–Cys–Pro–Leu–Gly–NH_2 Ala[5]-oxytocin	950.2	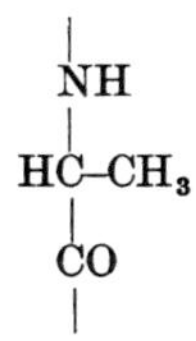
Cys–Tyr–Ile–Gln–*Ser*–Cys–Pro–Leu–Gly–NH_2 Ser[5]-oxytocin	966.2	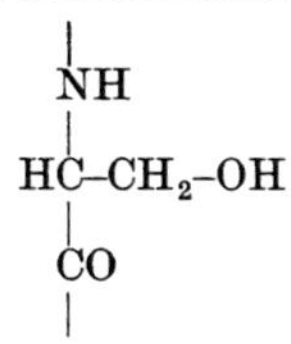
Cys–Tyr–Ile–Gln–*D–Asn*–Cys–Pro–Leu–Gly–NH_2 D-Asn[5]-oxytocin	1007.2	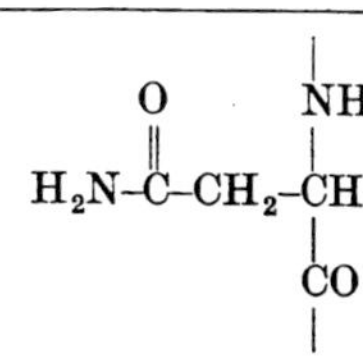
Cys–Tyr–Phe–Gln–*Asn*–Cys–Pro–Lys–Gly–NH_2 Lysine-vasopressin	1056.2	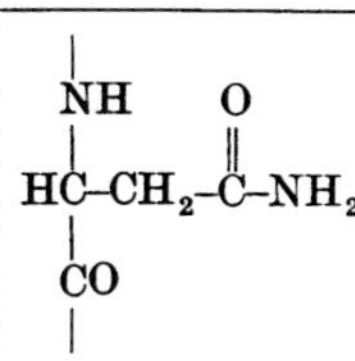
Cys–Tyr–Phe–Gln–*Ser*–Cys–Pro–Lys–Gly–NH_2 Ser[5]-Lys[8]-vasopressin	1017.2	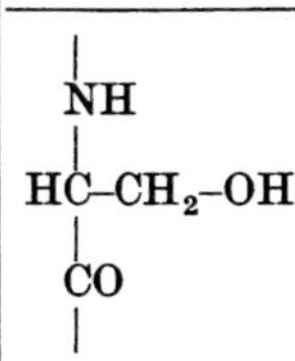

of oxytocin and lysine-vasopressin

Oxytocin-like activities in International Units per micromole			Vasopressin-like activities in International Units per micromole		References S = synthesis P = pharmacology [1] = also contains pharmacological data
Rat uterus (isolated)	Chicken blood pressure	Rabbit mammary gland	Rat blood pressure	Rat antidiuresis	
450 ± 30	450 ± 30	450 ± 30	5 ± 1	5 ± 1	Occurs in nature
1 ± 0.2	0.8 ± 0.03	7.3 ± 1.1	< 0.01	—	S: JAQUENOUD, BOISSONNAS (1962a)[1] P: BERDE, STÜRMER (1962)
0.03 or less	0.03 or less	< 0.05	< 0.01	< 0.01	S: GUTTMANN, BOISSONNAS (1963)[1] DU VIGNEAUD et al. (1963; 1964)
0.7 ± 0.2	0.20 ± 0.01	4.1 ± 0.8	< 0.1	< 0.01	S: GUTTMANN, BOISSONNAS (1963)[1] P: BERDE, STÜRMER (1962)
~0.2	~0.36	—	—	—	S: DUTTA et al. (1966)[1]
5 ± 0.5	42 ± 5	63 ± 10	285 ± 21	~260	Occurs in nature
< 0.05	< 0.1	0.06 ± 0.01	< 0.1	0.04 ± 0.01	S: BOISSONNAS et al. (1963)[1] P: BERDE, STÜRMER (1962)

Table 11. *Variations in*

Name, abbreviated chemical formula and molecular weight		Structure of amino acid in position 8
Cys–Tyr–Ile–Gln–Asn–Cys–Pro–*Leu*–Gly–NH_2 (Cys¹–Cys⁶ bridged) Oxytocin	1007.2	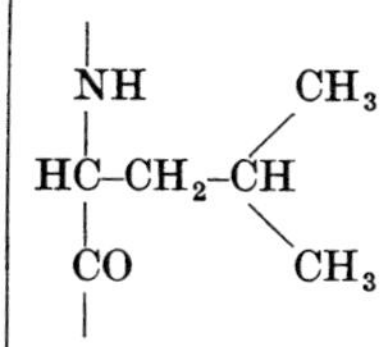
Cys–Tyr–Ile–Gln–Asn–Cys–Pro–*Ile*–Gly–NH_2 (Cys¹–Cys⁶ bridged) Ile^8-oxytocin = mesotocin	1007.2	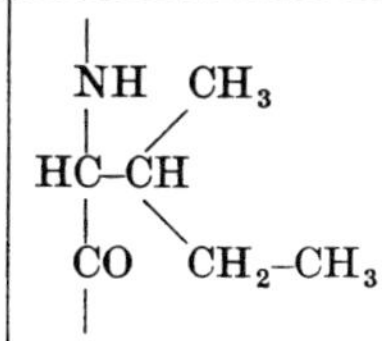
Cys–Tyr–Ile–Gln–Asn–Cys–Pro–*Val*–Gly–NH_2 (Cys¹–Cys⁶ bridged) Val^8-oxytocin	993.2	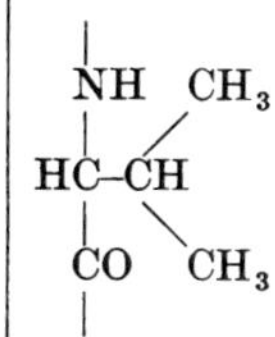
Cys–Tyr–Ile–Gln–Asn–Cys–Pro–*Abu*–Gly–NH_2 (Cys¹–Cys⁶ bridged) Abu^8-oxytocin	979.2	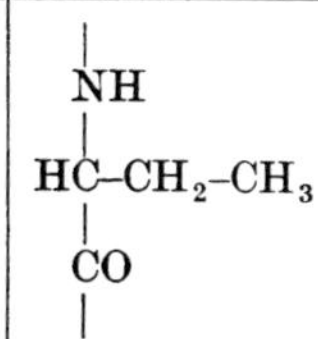
Cys–Tyr–Ile–Gln–Asn–Cys–Pro–*Ala*–Gly–NH_2 (Cys¹–Cys⁶ bridged) Ala^8-oxytocin	965.1	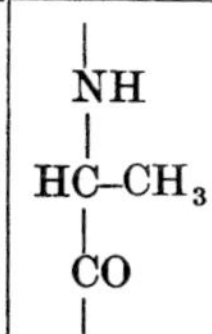
Cys–Tyr–Ile–Gln–Asn–Cys–Pro–*Gly*–Gly–NH_2 (Cys¹–Cys⁶ bridged) Gly^8-oxytocin	951.1	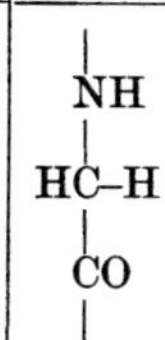
Cys–Tyr–Ile–Gln–Asn–Cys–Pro–*D–Leu*–Gly–NH_2 (Cys¹–Cys⁶ bridged) D-Leu^8-oxytocin	1007.2	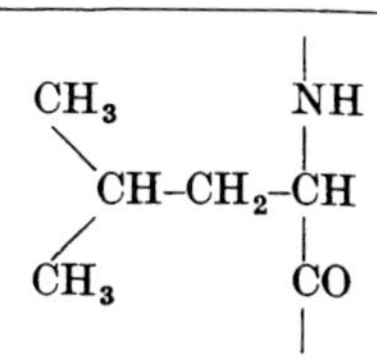

position 8 of oxytocin

Oxytocin-like activities in International Units per micromole			Vasopressin-like activities in International Units per micromole		References S = synthesis P = pharmacology [1] = also contains pharmacological data
Rat uterus (isolated)	Chicken blood pressure	Rabbit mammary gland	Rat blood pressure	Rat antidiuresis	
450 ± 30	450 ± 30	450 ± 30	5 ± 1	5 ± 1	Occurs in nature
291 ± 21	502 ± 37	330 ± 21	6.3 ± 0.8	1.1 ± 0.1	S: JAQUENOUD, BOISSONNAS (1961)[1] P: BERDE, KONZETT (1960)
199 ± 15	278 ± 17	308 ± 20	9 ± 1	0.8 ± 0.1	S: JAQUENOUD, BOISSONNAS (1961)[1] P: BERDE et al. (1960)
—	430 ± 31	—	32 ± 2	—	S: JAQUENOUD (1965)[1] P: BERDE, STÜRMER (1965)
136 ± 17	130 ± 13	201 ± 8	11.2 ± 0.6	0.08 ± 0.01	S: JAQUENOUD (1965)[1] P: BERDE, STÜRMER (1964)
15 ± 1.4	7 ± 1.4	44 ± 7	0.6 ± 0.1	0.15 ± 0.03	S: JAQUENOUD (1965)[1] P: BERDE, STÜRMER (1965)
~20	~20	~50	<0.01	~0.01	S: SCHNEIDER, DU VIGNEAUD (1962)[1]

Table 12. *Variations in*

Name, abbreviated chemical formula and molecular weight		Structure of amino acid in position 8
Cys–Tyr–Ile–Gln–Asn–Cys–Pro–*Arg*–Gly–NH_2 Vasotocin = Arginine-vasotocin = Arg^8-oxytocin	1050.2	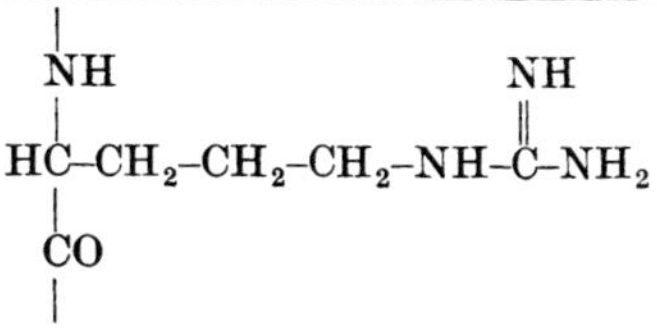
Cys–Tyr–Ile–Gln–Asn–Cys–Pro–*Lys*–Gly–NH_2 Lysine-vasotocin = Lys^8-oxytocin	1022.2	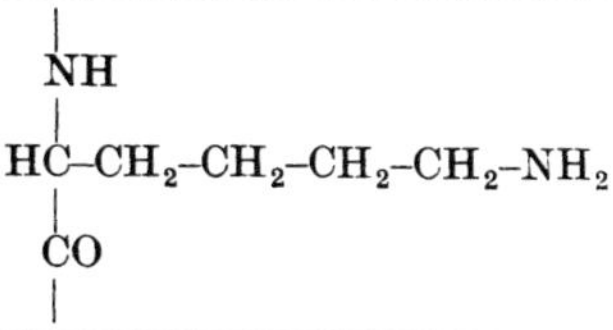
Cys–Tyr–Ile–Gln–Asn–Cys–Pro–*Orn*–Gly–NH_2 Ornithine-vasotocin = Orn^8-oxytocin	1008.2	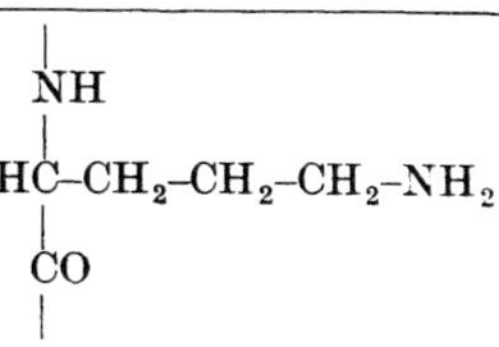
Cys–Tyr–Ile–Gln–Asn–Cys–Pro–*Cit*–Gly–NH_2 Citrulline-vasotocin = Cit^8-oxytocin	1051.2	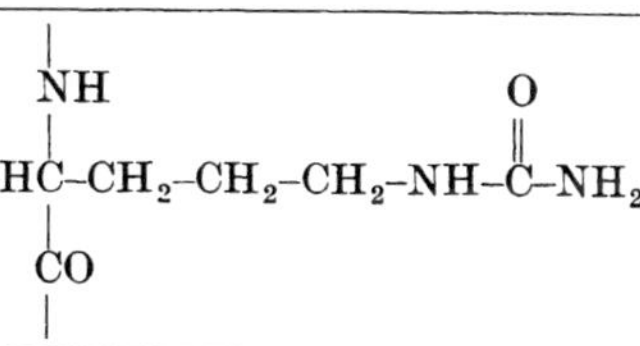
Cys–Tyr–Ile–Gln–Asn–Cys–Pro–*(For)Lys*–Gly–NH_2 (N^{ε}-For-Lys)^8-oxytocin	1050.2	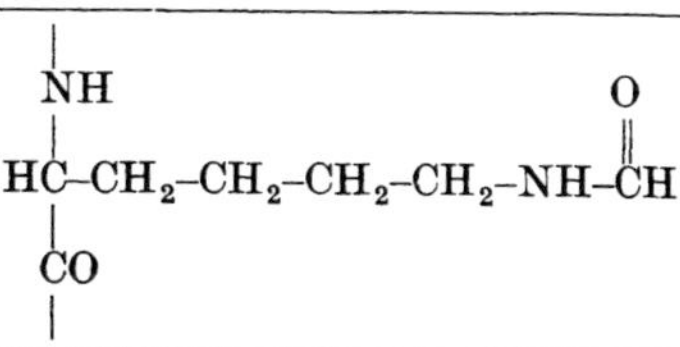

All variations so far in position 5 of oxytocin and lysine-vasopressin (Table 10) have yielded compounds with low or negligible activity. It seems therefore that position 5 does not tolerate modification, although the neighbouring position 4 has proved surprisingly tolerant.

The effect of modifying the neurohypophysial hormones at position 8 (i. e. outside the disulphide ring) is of particular interest, for the natural hormones also differ among themselves in this position.

In the oxytocin series (Table 11) replacement of the leucine residue by the isomeric isoleucine residue has only a slight influence on biological activity. The replacement of leucine by valine (Val^8-oxytocin) is identical to the shortening by one methylene group of the distance between the peptide chain and the isopropyl side group. This analogue is less active than Abu^8-oxytocin, which possesses one methyl group less, this implying that steric hindrance at the α-carbon atom of the

osition 8 of vasotocin

Oxytocin-like activities in International Units per micromole			Vasopressin-like activities in International Units per micromole		References
Rat uterus (isolated)	Chicken blood pressure	Rabbit mammary gland	Rat blood pressure	Rat antidiuresis	S = synthesis P = pharmacology 1 = also contains pharmacological data
120 ± 16	300 ± 42	~220	255 ± 16	260 ± 37	Occurs in nature
80 ± 10	215 ± 3	185 ± 25	133 ± 13	25 ± 3	S: BOISSONNAS, HUGUENIN (1960)[1] KIMBROUGH, DU VIGNEAUD (1961)[1] HUGUENIN, BOISSONNAS (1962)[1] P: BERDE et al. (1961a) BERDE, STÜRMER (1962)
42 ± 5	90 ± 3	95 ± 6	104 ± 10	2.5 ± 0.3	S: HUGUENIN, BOISSONNAS (1963)[1] P: BERDE et al. (1964)
~525	~260	—	~7	—	S: BODANSZKY et al. (1962a, b)[1]
155 ± 13	210 ± 4	230 ± 12	17 ± 1	0.3 ± 0.03	S: HUGUENIN (1965) P: BERDE, BOISSONNAS (1966)

amino acid residue in position 8 is unfavourable to activity. Further shortening of the side chain, as in Ala^{8}-oxytocin, causes an additional slight loss of activity, whereas complete elimination of the side chain, as in Gly^{8}-oxytocin, brings about sharp decrease in activity. It is surprising that an analogue containing D-leucine instead of L-leucine (D-Leu^{8}-oxytocin) possesses appreciable biological activities.

By replacing leucine in oxytocin by the basic amino acid arginine, Arg^{8}-oxytocin or vasotocin is obtained. This compound was discovered in some non-mammalian vertebrates, and its biological properties were discussed above. On replacing arginine by lysine, Lys^{8}-oxytocin or lysine-vasotocin (Table 12) is obtained. This has the same profile of activities as vasotocin itself, as far as its oxytocic and pressor properties are concerned, but it has much lower antidiuretic activity. When arginine is replaced by ornithine (Orn^{8}-oxytocin), this tendency is still further enhanced, and the antidiuretic activity amounts to only 1/40 of the

Table 13. *Variations in*

Name, abbreviated chemical formula and molecular weight		Structure of amino acid in position 8
Cys–Tyr–Phe–Gln–Asn–Cys–Pro–*Arg*–Gly–NH_2 Vasopressin = Arginine-vasopressin = Arg[8]-vasopressin	1084.2	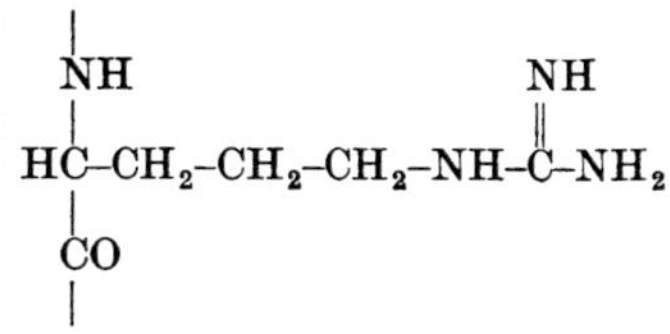
Cys–Tyr–Phe–Gln–Asn–Cys–Pro–*Lys*–Gly–NH_2 Lysine-vasopressin = Lys[8]-vasopressin	1056.2	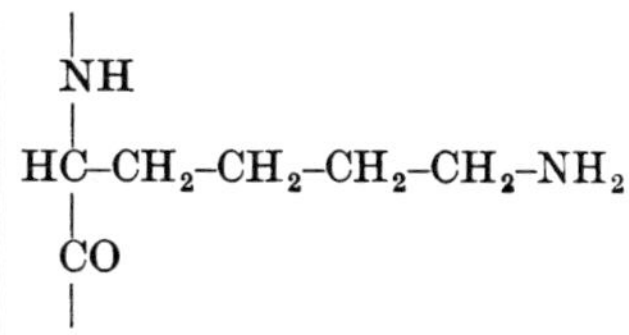
Cys–Tyr–Phe–Gln–Asn–Cys–Pro–*Orn*–Gly–NH_2 Orn[8]-vasopressin	1042.2	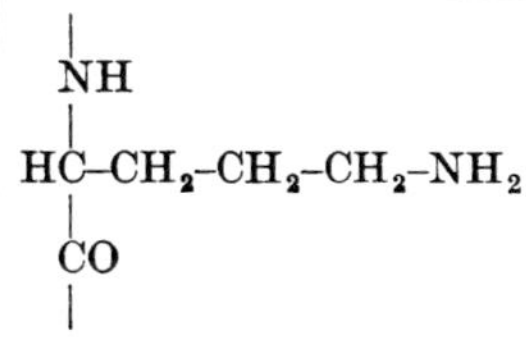
Cys–Tyr–Phe–Gln–Asn–Cys–Pro–*Dbu*–Gly–NH_2 Dbu[8]-vasopressin	1028.2	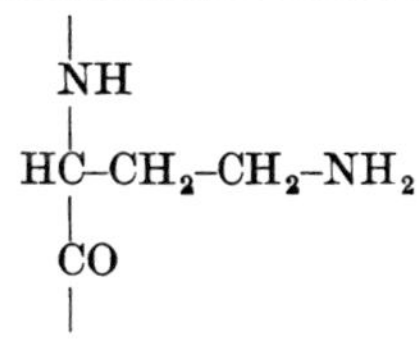
Cys–Tyr–Phe–Gln–Asn–Cys–Pro–*Tly*–Gly–NH_2 Thialysine[8]-vasopressin	1074.3	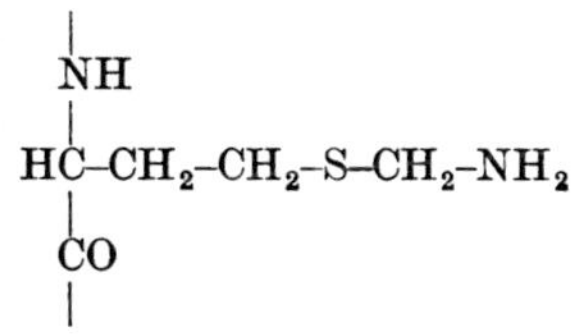
Cys–Tyr–Phe–Gln–Asn–Cys–Pro–*His*–Gly–NH_2 His[8]-vasopressin	1062.2	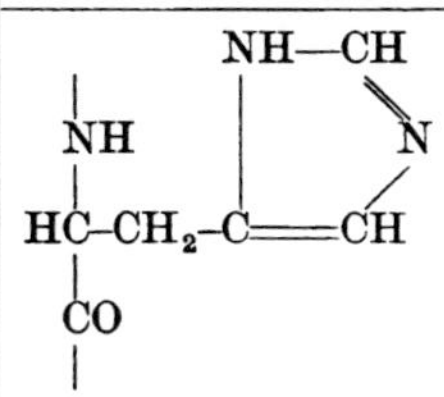
Cys–Tyr–Phe–Gln–Asn–Cys–Pro–*Cit*–Gly–NH_2 Cit[8]-vasopressin = citrulline[8]-vasopressin	1085.3	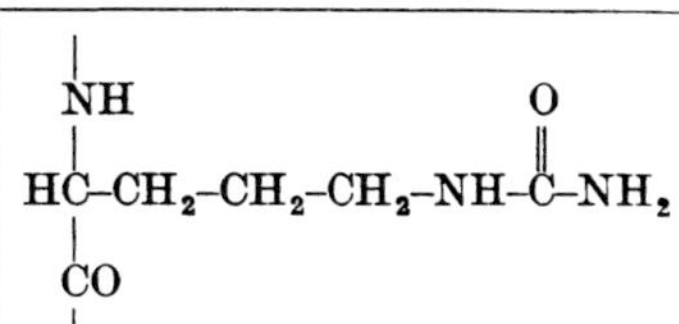

position 8 of vasopressin

Oxytocin-like activities in International Units per micromole			Vasopressin-like activities in International Units per micromole		References S = synthesis P = pharmacology 1 = also contains pharmacological data
Rat uterus (isolated)	Chicken blood pressure	Rabbit mammary gland	Rat blood pressure	Rat antidiuresis	
17 ± 4	65 ± 6	70 ± 9	435 ± 45	435 ± 45	Occurs in nature
5 ± 0.5	42 ± 5	63 ± 10	285 ± 21	~260	Occurs in nature
10 ± 2	22 ± 0.7	~50	375 ± 27	92 ± 18	S: Huguenin, Boissonnas (1963)[1] P: Berde et al. (1964)
~3.5	—	—	~149	120 ± 30	S: Zaoral, Šorm (1966a)[1]
~5	—	—	55 ± 5	400 ± 50	S: Hermann, Zaoral (1965)
~1.5	~4.6	~15	~1.5	—	S: Katsoyannis, du Vigneaud (1958)[1]
~3	—	78 ± 5	~43	~16 (dog)	S: Bodanszky et al. (1962a, b)[1]

Continuation Table 13.

Name, abbreviated chemical formula and molecular weight	Structure of amino acid in position 8
Cys–Tyr–Phe–Gln–Asn–Cys–Pro–*(For)Lys*–Gly–NH_2 (Nε-For-Lys)^8-vasopressin 1084.3	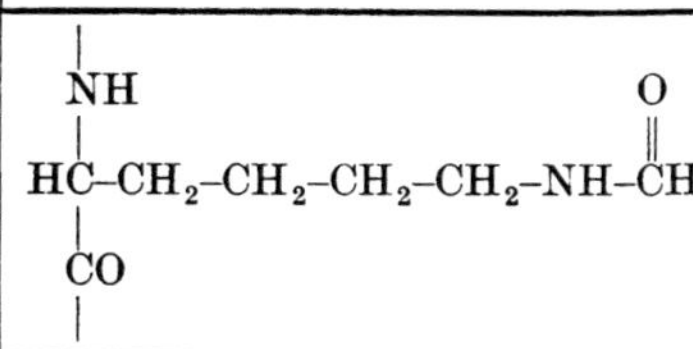
Cys–Tyr–Phe–Gln–Asn–Cys–Pro–*Leu*–Gly–NH_2 Leu^8-vasopressin = Phe^3-oxytocin = Oxypressin 1075.3	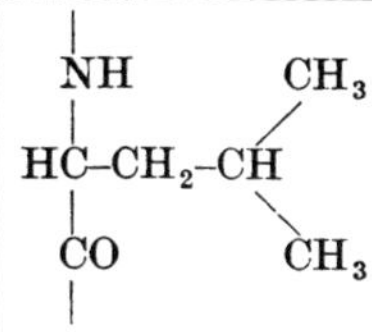
Cys–Tyr–Phe–Gln–Asn–Cys–Pro–*D–Arg*–Gly–NH_2 D-Arg^8-vasopressin 1084.2	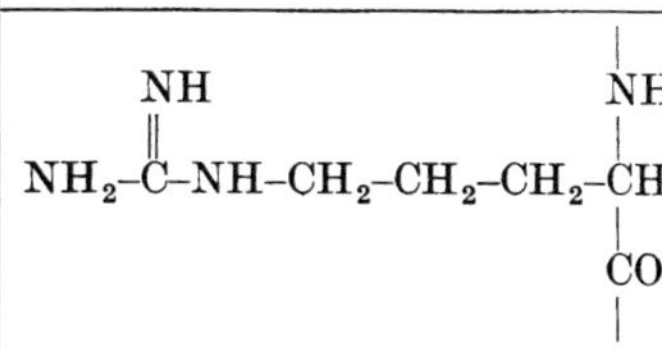
Cys–Tyr–Phe–Gln–Asn–Cys–Pro–*D–Lys*–Gly–NH_2 D-Lys^8-vasopressin 1056.2	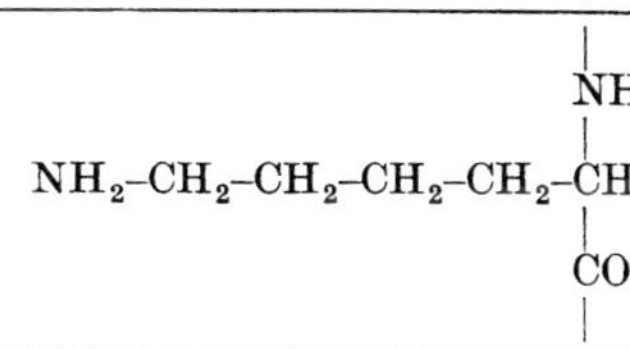
Cys–Tyr–Phe–Gln–Asn–Cys–Pro–*D–Dbu*–Gly–NH_2 D-Dbu^8-vasopressin 1028.1	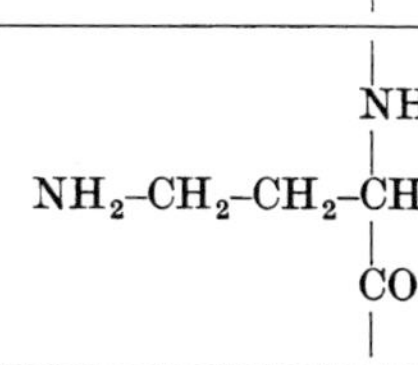

vasopressor activity. On replacing the basic amino acid arginine in vasotocin by its neutral structural analogue citrulline (Cit^8-oxytocin), the activity on the rat uterus is, as might be expected, raised and, in fact, it equals that of oxytocin itself. Masking the basic group of lysine in lysine-vasotocin by a formyl group ([Nε-For-Lys]^8-oxytocin) has little influence on the oxytocin-like activities, but depresses the vasopressin-like properties.

Examples of variations in position 8 of the vasopressins (Table 13) are found in nature: lysine-vasopressin occurs in the pig, the hippopotamus and the peccary, while vasopressin is found in all other mammalian vertebrates investigated so far. Vasopressin is somewhat more potent than lysine-vasopressin in every respect. Orn^8-vasopressin, although a strong pressor agent, differs from the natural vasopressins in possessing a relatively low antidiuretic activity.

Oxytocin-like activities in International Units per micromole			Vasopressin-like activities in International Units per micromole		References S = synthesis P = pharmacology [1] = also contains pharmacological data
Rat uterus (isolated)	Chicken blood pressure	Rabit mammary gland	Rat blood pressure	Rat antidiuresis	
14 ± 2	45 ± 1	~80	35 ± 2	11 ± 1	S: Boissonnas et al. (1963)[1] P: Berde, Stürmer (1962)
~20	~30	~65	~3	~30	S: Boissonnas et al. (1956) Katsoyannis (1957)[1] P: Berde et al. (1957)
—	—	—	~4.1	~114	S: Zaoral et al. (1966)[1]
—	—	—	~1	~20	S: Zaoral et al. (1966)[1]
~0.1	—	—	~3.6	120 ± 40	S: Zaoral, Šorm (1966b)[1]

By contrast, the next lower homologue, Dbu^8-vasopressin, is as strongly antidiuretic as pressor. In the case of thialysine^8-vasopressin, the antidiuretic activity is almost four times higher than the vasopressor activity. These results exemplify how relatively small changes can have opposite effects on the vasopressor/antidiuretic ratio, thus affording a means of producing closely related substances with different selectivities.

Introduction of the slightly basic histidine residue in position 8 yields an analogue with a surprisingly low level of activity.

Replacement of arginine by its neutral analogue, citrulline, lowers the vasopressin-like activities. The same effect is obtained when the basic lateral amino group of lysine is masked by a formyl group.

Table 14. *Interchange*

<table>
<tr><th>Name, abbreviated chemical formula and molecular weight</th><th></th><th>Structures of permuted amino acids</th><th></th></tr>
<tr><td>Cys–Tyr–Ile–Gln–Asn–Cys–Pro–Leu–Gly–NH$_2$
Oxytocin</td><td>1007.2</td><td>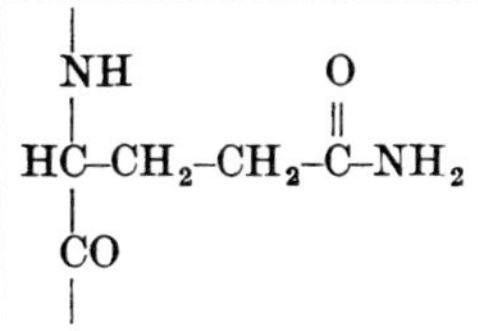</td><td>Gln</td></tr>
<tr><td>Cys–Tyr–Ile–Asn–Gln–Cys–Pro–Leu–Gly–NH$_2$
Asn[4]-Gln[5]-oxytocin</td><td>1007.2</td><td>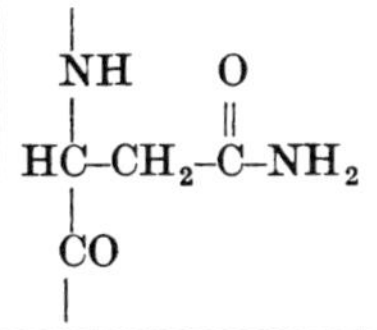</td><td>Asn</td></tr>
<tr><td>Cys–Tyr–Phe–Gln–Asn–Cys–Pro–Leu–Gly–NH$_2$
Phe[3]-oxytocin = oxypressin</td><td>1075.3</td><td>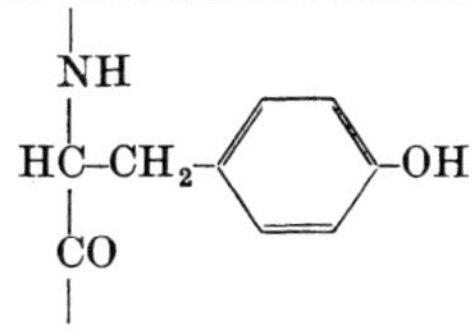</td><td>Tyr</td></tr>
<tr><td>Cys–Phe–Tyr–Gln–Asn–Cys–Pro–Leu–Gly–NH$_2$
Phe[2]-Tyr[3]-oxytocin</td><td>1075.3</td><td>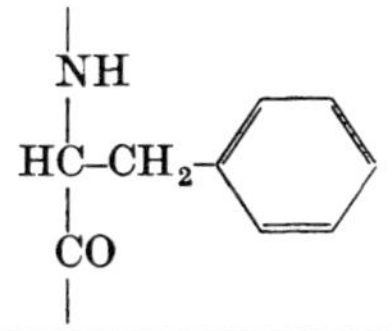</td><td>Phe</td></tr>
<tr><td>Cys–Tyr–Phe–Gln–Asn–Cys–Pro–Lys–Gly–NH$_2$
Lysine-vasopressin</td><td>1056.2</td><td>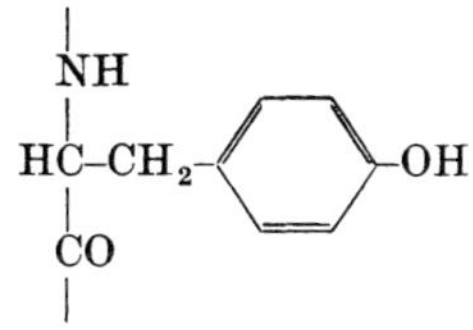</td><td>Tyr</td></tr>
<tr><td>Cys–Phe–Tyr–Gln–Asn–Cys–Pro–Lys–Gly–NH$_2$
Phe[2]-Tyr[3]-Lys[8]-vasopressin</td><td>1056.2</td><td>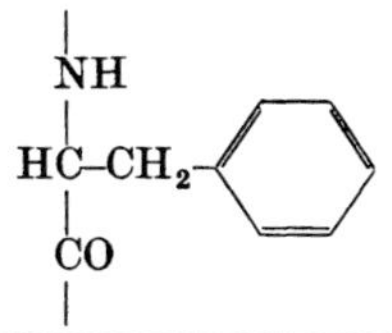</td><td>Phe</td></tr>
</table>

Introduction of leucine in the same position yields oxypressin (Phe[3]-oxytocin = Leu[8]-vasopressin), a compound discussed above, which has properties intermediate between those of oxytocin and the vasopressins. It is interesting that in this case the pressor effect is ten times lower than the antidiuretic effect, whereas the two preceding compounds were more strongly pressor than antidiuretic.

Introduction of D-amino acids in position 8 yields compounds with low pressor activity, but with quite unexpectedly high antidiuretic activity. It there-

between two positions

Oxytocin-like activities in International Units per micromole			Vasopressin-like activities in International Units per micromole		References S = synthesis P = pharmacology 1 = also contains pharmacological data
Rat uterus (isolated)	Chicken blood pressure	Rabbit mammary gland	Rat blood pressure	Rat antidiuresis	
450 ± 30	450 ± 30	450 ± 30	5 ± 1	5 ± 1	Occurs in nature
0.4 ± 0.08	0.3 ± 0.01	—	<0.01	—	S: JAQUENOUD, BOISSONNAS (1962a)[1] P: BERDE, STÜRMER (1962)
~20	~30	~65	~3	~30	S: BOISSONNAS et al. (1956) KATSOYANNIS (1957)[1] P: BERDE et al. (1957)
<0.01	<0.01	—	<0.01	~0.001	S: BOISSONNAS, GUTTMANN (1960)[1] P: BERDE et al. (1960)
5 ± 0.5	42 ± 5	63 ± 10	285 ± 21	~260	Occurs in nature
<0.01	<0.01	—	0.14 ± 0.01	0.013 ± 0.002	S: BOISSONNAS, GUTTMANN (1960)[1] P: BERDE et al. (1960)

fore seems that the structural requirements for the amino acid in position 8 are more limiting at the vasopressor receptor site than at the antidiuretic site.

Interchanging two amino acids in neurohypophysial hormones has been effected in a few instances (Table 14). Although these interchanges involved amino acids closely related structurally and occupying adjoining positions, they invariably led to complete inactivation. This may appear surprising for these interchanges have practically no influence on physial properties.

Table 15. *Introduction of D-amino*

Name, abbreviated chemical formula and molecular weight		Rat uterus (isolated)
D-Cys–Tyr–Ile–Gln–Asn–Cys–Pro–Leu–Gly–NH_2 D-Cys[1]-oxytocin	1007.2	1.9 ± 0.1
Cys–*D–Tyr*–Ile–Gln–Asn–Cys–Pro–Leu–Gly–NH_2 D-Tyr[2]-oxytocin	1007.2	6.6 ± 1
Cys–Tyr–Ile–*D–Gln*–Asn–Cys–Pro–Leu–Gly–NH_2 D-Gln[4]-oxytocin	1007.2	~ 0.1
Cys–Tyr–Ile–Gln–*D–Asn*–Cys–Pro–Leu–Gly–NH_2 D-Asn[5]-oxytocin	1007.2	~ 0.2
Cys–Tyr–Ile–*D–Gln–D–Asn*–Cys–Pro–Leu–Gly–NH_2 D-Gln[4]-D-Asn[5]-oxytocin	1007.2	<0.01
Cys–Tyr–Ile–Gln–Asn–*D–Cys*–Pro–Leu–Gly–NH_2 D-Cys[6]-oxytocin	1007.2	~ 0.62
Cys–Tyr–Ile–Gln–Asn–Cys–Pro–*D–Leu*–Gly–NH_2 D-Leu[8]-oxytocin	1007.2	~ 20
D–Cys–D–Tyr–D–Ile–D–Gln–D–Asn–D–Cys–D–Pro–D–Leu–Gly–NH_2 All-D-oxytocin	1007.2	<0.01

Table 16. *Removal of the N-terminal amino*

Name, abbreviated chemical formula and molecular weight		
S–$(CH_2)_2$–CO–Tyr–Ile–Gln–Asn–Cys–Pro–Leu–Gly–NH_2 De-Amino[1]-oxytocin	992.2	Biological properties of the amino homologue, oxytocin, are given in table 2
S–$(CH_2)_2$–CO–Phe–Ile–Gln–Asn–Cys–Pro–Leu–Gly–NH_2 De-Amino[1]-Phe[2]-oxytocin	976.2	Biological properties of the amino homologue, Phe[2]-oxytocin, are given in table 3

acids in oxytocin

Oxytocin-like activities in International Units per micromole		Vasopressin-like activities in International Units per micromole		References S = synthesis P = pharmacology 1 = also contains pharmacological data
Chicken blood pressure	Rabbit mammary gland	Rat blood pressure	Rat antidiuresis	
~0.2	6.2 ± 0.2	<0.01	~0.02	S: JOŠT et al. (1963b)[1] HOPE et al. (1963)[1] YAMASHIRO et al. (1966)[1]
34 ± 3	34 ± 9	~0.02	~0.02	S: DRABAREK, DU VIGNEAUD (1965)[1]
~1.0	—	—	—	S: DUTTA, ANAND (1965) P: DUTTA et al. (1966)
~0.36	—	—	—	S: DUTTA et al. (1966)[1]
<0.01	—	—	—	S: DUTTA et al. (1966)[1]
<0.01	<0.002	<0.002 (Anti)	(0.002)	S: MANNING, DU VIGNEAUD (1965b)[1]
~20	~50	<0.01	<0.01	S: SCHNEIDER, DU VIGNEAUD (1962)[1]
<0.01	—	—	—	S: FLOURET, DU VIGNEAUD (1965)

group of oxytocin and its analogues

Oxytocin-like activities in International Units per micromole			Vasopressin-like activities in International Units per micromole		References S = synthesis P = pharmacology 1 = also contains pharmacological data
Rat uterus (isolated)	Chicken blood pressure	Rabbit mammary gland	Rat blood pressure	Rat antidiuresis	
795 ± 36	965 ± 24	536 ± 13	1.43 ± 0.1	~19	S: DU VIGNEAUD et al. (1960b)[1] HOPE et al. (1962)[1] P: CHAN, DU VIGNEAUD (1962) FERRIER et al. (1965)
~25	60 ± 2	—	~0.04	~0.35	S: HOPE, DU VIGNEAUD (1962)[1] HOPE (1962)[1]

Continuation Table 16.

Name, abbreviated chemical formula and molecular weight		
S–$(CH_2)_2$–CO–(O-Me)Tyr–Ile–Gln–Asn–Cys–Pro–Leu–Gly–NH_2 De-Amino^{1}-(O-Me)Tyr^{2}-oxytocin	1006.2	Biological properties of the amino homologue, (O-Me)Tyr^{2}-oxytocin, are given in table 3
S–$(CH_2)_2$–D–Tyr–Ile–Gln–Asn–Cys–Pro–Leu–Gly–NH_2 De-Amino^{1}-D-Tyr^{2}-oxytocin	992.2	Biological properties of the amino homologue, D-Tyr^{2}-oxytocin, are given in table 3
S–$(CH_2)_2$–CO–Tyr–Ile–Val–Asn–Cys–Pro–Leu–Gly–NH_2 De-Amino^{1}-Val^{4}-oxytocin	963.2	Biological properties of the amino homologue, Val^{4}-oxytocin, are given in table 8
S–$(CH_2)_2$–CO–Tyr–Ile–Abu–Asn–Cys–Pro–Leu–Gly–NH_2 De-Amino^{1}-Abu^{4}-oxytocin	949.2	Biological properties of the amino homologue, Abu^{4}-oxytocin, are given in table 8
S–$(CH_2)_2$–CO–Tyr–Ile–Gln–Asn–Selenocys–Pro–Leu–Gly–NH_2 De-Amino^{1}-hemiselenocystine^{6}-oxytocin	1039.2	Biological properties of the amino homologue, hemiselenocystine^{6}-oxytocin, are given in table 21

Table 17. *Removal of the N-terminal amino group*

Name, abbreviated chemical formula and molecular weight		
S–$(CH_2)_2$–CO–Tyr–Phe–Gln–Asn–Cys–Pro–Arg–Gly–NH_2 De-Amino^{1}-vasopressin	1069.3	Biological properties of the amino homologue, vasopressin, are given in Table 2
S–$(CH_2)_2$–CO–Phe–Phe–Gln–Asn–Cys–Pro–Arg–Gly–NH_2 De-Amino^{1}-Phe^{2}-vasopressin	1053.3	Biological properties of the amino homologue, Phe^{2}-vasopressin, are given in table 5
S–$(CH_2)_2$–CO–Tyr–Phe–Gln–Asn–Cys–Pro–Lys–Gly–NH_2 De-Amino^{1}-Lys^{8}-vasopressin	1041.3	Biological properties of the amino homologue, lysine-vasopressin, are given in table 2
S–$(CH_2)_2$–CO–Tyr–Phe–Gln–Asn–Cys–Pro–Orn–Gly–NH_2 De-Amino^{1}-Orn^{8}-vasopressin	1027.3	Biological properties of the amino homologue, Orn^{8}-vasopressin, are given in table 5

Oxytocin-like activities in International Units per micromole			Vasopressin-like activities in International Units per micromole		References S = synthesis P = pharmacology [1] = also contains pharmacological data
Rat uterus (Isolated)	Chicken blood pressure	Rabbit mammary gland	Rat blood pressure	Rat antidiuresis	
Oxytocic (Anti 20:1)	Pressor (Anti 6:1)	~4	Depressor (Anti)	~0.13	S: HUGUENIN (1965) P: BERDE, SAAMELI (1966) BERDE, STÜRMER (1965)
~1	30 ± 1	16 ± 1	~0.04	~0.07	S: DRABAREK, DU VIGNEAUD (1965)[1]
~350	~800	~350	<0.01	~5	S: DU VIGNEAUD et al. (1966)[1]
88 ± 2	183 ± 9	253 ± 2	<0.05	<0.2	S: BRANDA et al. (1966)[1]
~520	~650	~415	~1	—	S: WALTER, DU VIGNEAUD (1965)[1]

of vasopressin and vasotocin, and of their analogues

Oxytocin-like activities in International Units per micromole			Vasopressin-like activities in International Units per micromole		References S = synthesis P = pharmacology [1] = also contains pharmacological data
Rat uterus (isolated)	Chicken blood pressure	Rabbit mammary gland	Rat blood pressure	Rat antidiuresis	
29 ± 4	160 ± 4	85 ± 30	395 ± 20	1400 ± 200	S: HUGUENIN, BOISSONNAS (1966)[1] P: HUGUENIN et al. (1965)
0.32 ± 0.09	<1	~4.0	31 ± 7	850 ± 180	S: HUGUENIN, BOISSONNAS (1966)[1] P: STÜRMER et al. (1965)
12 ± 0.5	63 ± 2	33 ± 2	131 ± 2	313 ± 11	S: KIMBROUGH et al. (1963)[1]
16 ± 2	44 ± 9	44 ± 7	365 ± 31	208 ± 24	S: HUGUENIN (1966)[1] P: BERDE, STÜRMER (1965)

Continuation Table 17.

Name, abbreviated chemical formula and molecular weight	
S–$(CH_2)_2$–CO–Phe–Phe–Gln–Asn–Cys–Pro–Orn–Gly–NH_2 De-Amino[1]-Phe[2]-Orn[8]-vasopressin 1011.3	Biological properties of the amino homologue, Phe[2]-Orn[8]-vasopressin, are given in table 5
S–$(CH_2)_2$–CO–Tyr–Ile–Gln–Asn–Cys–Pro–Orn–Gly–NH_2 De-Amino[1]-Orn[8]-vasotocin 1008.2	Biological properties of the amino homologue, Orn[8]-vasotocin, are given in table 4
S–$(CH_2)_2$–CO–Phe–Ile–Gln–Asn–Cys–Pro–Orn–Gly–NH_2 De-Amino[1]-Phe[2]-Orn[8]-vasotocin 993.2	Biological properties of the amino homologue, Phe[2]-Orn[8]-vasotocin, are given in table 4

Table 18. *Substitution of the N-terminal*

Name, abbreviated chemical formula and molecular weight	Structure of the N-terminal extremity
MeCys–Tyr–Ile–Gln–Asn–Cys–Pro–Leu–Gly–NH_2 (N-Me)Cys[1]-oxytocin 1021.2	CH_3–NH HC–CH_2–S– CO
Ac–Cys–Tyr–Ile–Gln–Asn–Cys–Pro–Leu–Gly–NH_2 N-Acetyl-oxytocin 1049.2	CH_3–CO–NH HC–CH_2–S– CO
Gly–Cys–Tyr–Ile–Gln–Asn–Cys–Pro–Leu–Gly–NH_2 N-Glycyl-oxytocin = (Gly-Cys)[1]-oxytocin 1064.2	NH_2–CH_2–CO–NH HC–CH_2–S– CO
MeGly–Cys–Tyr–Ile–Gln–Asn–Cys–Pro–Leu–Gly–NH_2 N-Sarcosyl-oxytocin = (MeGly-Cys)[1]-oxytocin 1021.2	CH_3–NH–CH_2–CO–NH HC–CH_2–S– CO

Oxytocin-like activities in International Units per micromole			Vasopressin-like activities in International Units per micromole		References S = synthesis P = pharmacology 1 = also contains pharmacological data
Rat uterus (isolated)	Chicken blood pressure	Rabbit mammary gland	Rat blood pressure	Rat antidiuresis	
<1	slightly pressoric	2.6 ±0.3	45 ±2	13 ±2.5	S: HUGUENIN (1966)[1] P: BERDE, STÜRMER (1965)
~80	400 ±30	~300	270 ±12	~70	S: HUGUENIN (1966)[1] P: BERDE, STÜRMER (1965)
<2	18 ±2	~10	100 ±11	~4	S: HUGUENIN (1966)[1] P: BERDE, STÜRMER (1965)

amino group of oxytocin

Oxytocin-like activities in International Units per micromole			Vasopressin-like activities in International Units per micromole		References S = synthesis P = pharmacology 1 = also contains pharmacological data
Rat uterus (isolated)	Chicken blood pressure	Rabbit mammary gland	Rat blood pressure	Rat antidiuresis	
~0.25	~0.025	~1 (guinea pig)	<0.01	~0.004	S: JOŠT et al. (1963b)[1] P: BERANKOVA et al. (1966)
1.7 ±0.2	Anti (5.000:1)	2.1 ±0.2	—	—	S: BOISSONNAS et al. (1959) P: BERDE et al. (1960)
~0.33	~0.7 Anti (20:1)	Anti (guinea pig)	~0.05	~0.11	S: DU VIGNEAUD et al. (1960a)[1] JOŠT et al. (1963b)[1] P: BERANKOVA et al. (1966)
~2.3	~0.85	~1.3 (guinea pig)	—	~0.027	S: JOŠT et al. (1963b)[1] P: BERANKOVA et al. (1966)

Continuation Table 18.

Name, abbreviated chemical formula and molecular weight	Structure of the N-terminal extremity
Leu–Cys–Tyr–Ile–Gln–Asn–Cys–Pro–Leu–Gly–NH_2 N-Leucyl-oxytocin = (Leu-Cys)[1]-oxytocin 1120.4	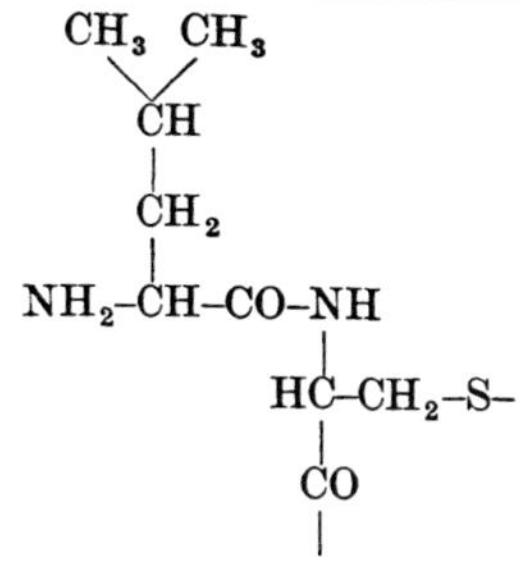
His–Ser–Cys–Tyr–Ile–Gln–Asn–Cys–Pro–Leu–Gly–NH_2 N-(Histidyl-Seryl)-oxytocin = (His-Ser-Cys)[1]-oxytocin 1231.4	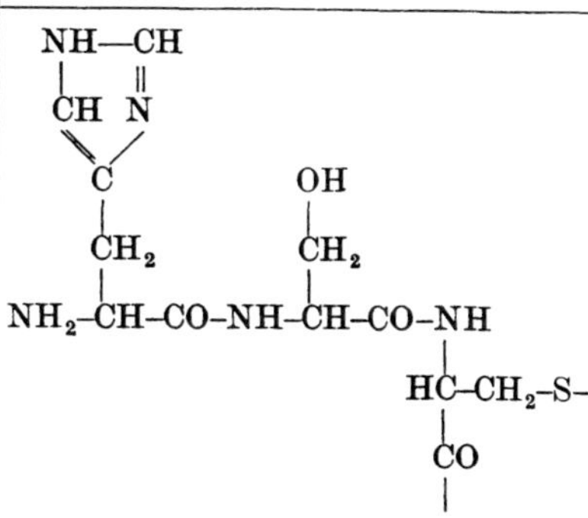
Ser–His–Cys–Tyr–Ile–Gln–Asn–Cys–Pro–Leu–Gly–NH_2 N-(Seryl-Histidyl)-oxytocin = (Ser-His-Cys)[1]-oxytocin 1231.4	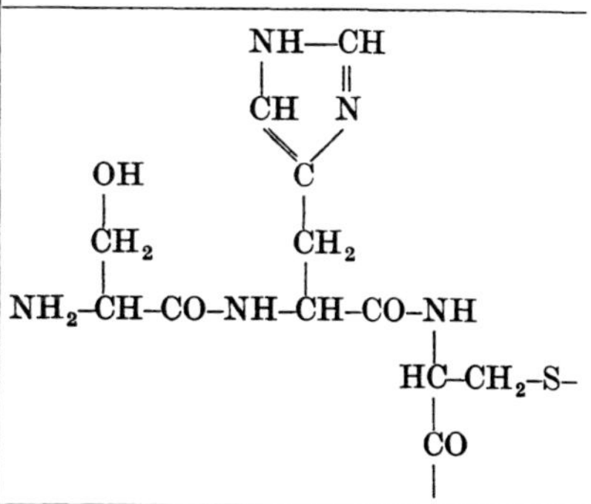

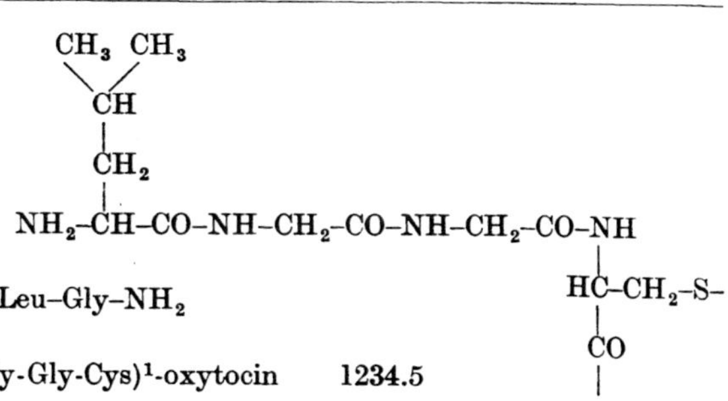

Leu–Gly–Gly–Cys–Tyr–Ile–Gln–Asn–Cys–Pro–Leu–Gly–NH_2

N-(Leucyl-Glycyl-Glycyl)-oxytocin = (Leu-Gly-Gly-Cys)[1]-oxytocin 1234.5

Oxytocin-like activities in International Units per micromole			Vasopressin-like activities in International Units per micromole		References S = synthesis P = pharmacology [1] = also contains pharmacological data
Rat uterus (isolated)	Chicken blood pressure	Rabbit mammary gland	Rat blood pressure	Rat antidiuresis	
~23	~3	Anti (guinea pig)	—	~0.27	S: Jošt et al. (1963b)[1] P: Berankova et al. (1966)
19.2 ± 1.5	19.1 ± 1.0	15.5 ± 0.7	0.33 ± 0.03	—	S: Guttmann, Boissonnas (1961)[1] P: Doepfner et al. (1963)
3.7 ± 0.5	3.1 ± 0.1	3.1 ± 0.5	0.05 ± 0.02	—	S: Guttmann, Boissonnas (1961)[1] P: Doepfner et al. (1963)
~0.2	—	Anti (guinea pig)	—	~0.034	S: Jošt et al. (1963b)[1] P: Berankova et al. (1966)

Table 19. *Substitution of the N-terminal*

Name, abbreviated chemical formula and molecular weight	Structure of the N-terminal extremity
Ac–Cys–Tyr–Phe–Gln–Asn–Cys–Pro–Arg–Gly–NH_2 N^a-Acetyl-vasopressin 1126.2	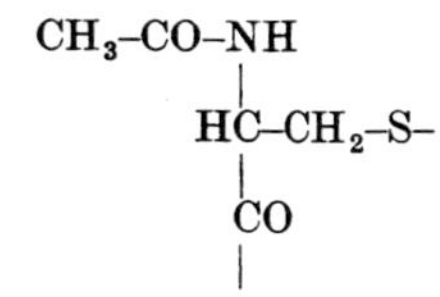
Ac–Cys–Tyr–Phe–Gln–Asn–Cys–Pro–Lys–Gly–NH_2 N^a-Acetyl-Lys^8-vasopressin 1098.2	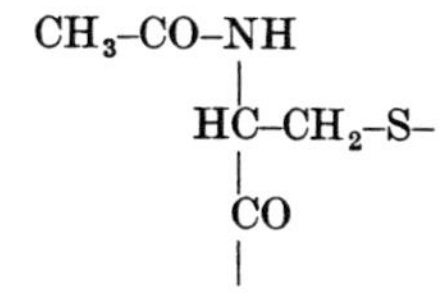
Gly–Cys–Tyr–Phe–Gln–Asn–Cys–Pro–Lys–Gly–NH_2 N^a-(Gly-Cys)^1-Lys^8-vasopressin 1113.3	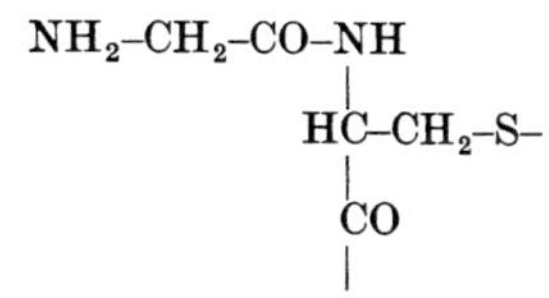
His–Ser–Cys–Tyr–Phe–Gln–Asn–Cys–Pro–Lys–Gly–NH_2 N^a-Histidyl-seryl-Lys^8-vasopressin = (His-Ser-Cys)^1-Lys^8-vasopressin 1280.4	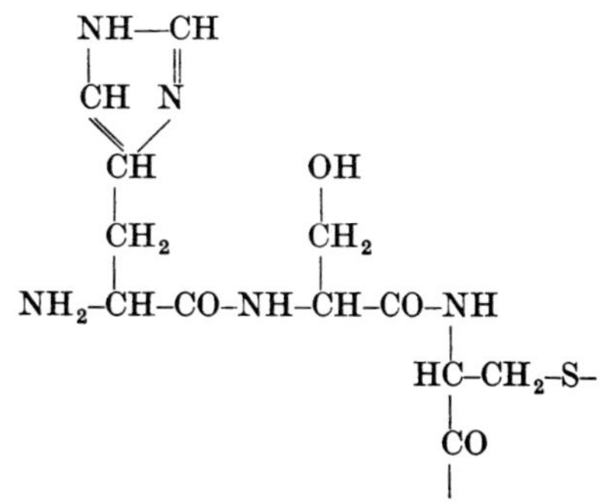
His–Ser–Cys–Tyr–Phe–Gln–Asn–Cys–Pro–Arg–Gly–NH_2 N-Histidyl-seryl-vasopressin = (His-Ser-Cys)^1-vasopressin 1308.4	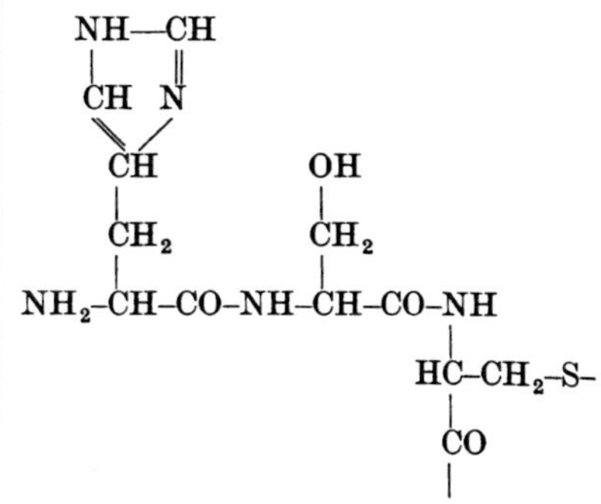

amino group of the vasopressins

Oxytocin-like activities in International Units per micromole			Vasopressin-like activities in International Units per micromole		References S = synthesis P = pharmacology 1 = also contains pharmacological data
Rat uterus (isolated)	Chicken blood pressure	Rabbit mammary gland	Rat blood pressure	Rat antidiuresis	
—	—	—	Anti	—	S: STUDER, CASH (1963)[1]
<0.03	Anti	~0.1	Anti	~0.001	S: CASH, SMITH (1963)[1]
—	—	—	~15	15—50	S: ZAORAL, ŠORM (1965)[1]
0.18 ± 0.05	~0.4	~0.9	14.1 ± 1.7	7.8 ± 1.0	S: GUTTMANN, BOISSONNAS (1961, 1962)[1] P: DOEPFNER et al. (1963)
<0.01	—	—	13 ± 2	11.1 ± 2.0	S: GUTTMANN, BOISSONNAS (1961) P: DOEPFNER et al. (1963)

Continuation Table 19.

Name, abbreviated chemical formula and molecular weight		Structure of the N-terminal extremity
Ser–His–Cys–Tyr–Phe–Gln–Asn–Cys–Pro–Lys–Gly–NH_2 N^{α}-Seryl-histidyl-Lys^8-vasopressin = (Ser-His-Cys)^1-Lys^8-vasopressin	1280.4	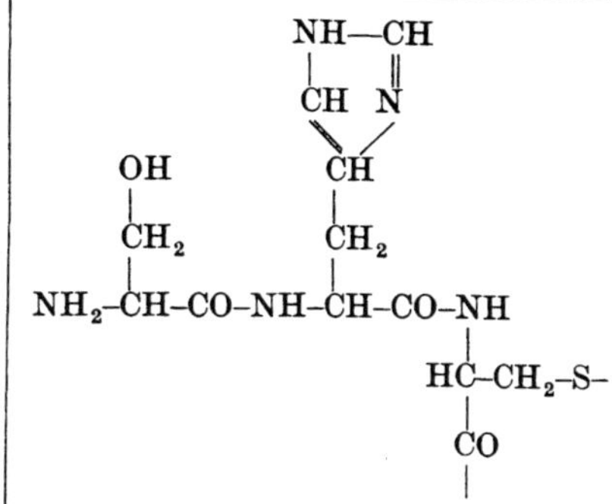
Ac–Ser–Tyr–Ser–Cys–Tyr–Phe–Gln–Asn–Cys–Pro–Lys–Gly–NH_2 (Ac-Ser-Tyr-Ser-Cys)^1-Lys^8-vasopressin	1435.6	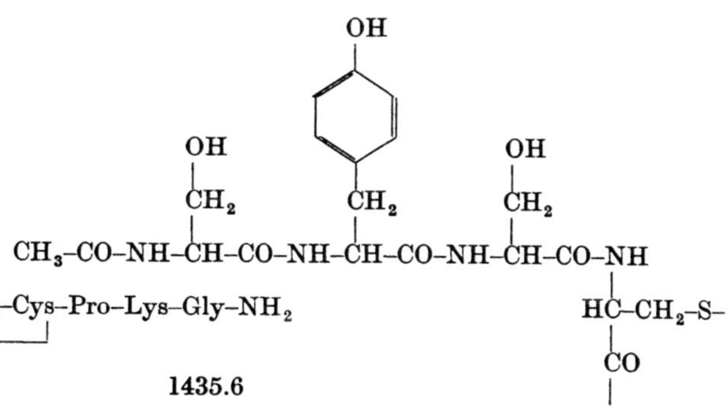

Table 20. *Methylation*

Name, abbreviated chemical formula and molecular weight		Structure of the methylated amino acid
Cys–*MeTyr*–Ile–Gln–Asn–Cys–Pro–Leu–Gly–NH_2 (N-Me)Tyr^2-oxytocin	1021.2	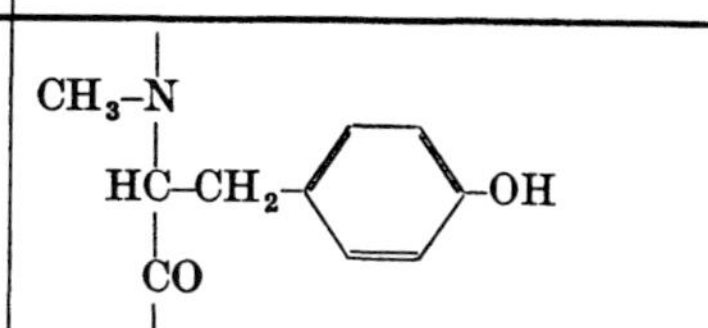
Cys–Tyr–Ile–Gln–Asn–Cys–Pro–Leu–*MeGly*–NH_2 (N–Me)Gly^9-oxytocin = Sar^9-oxytocin	1021.2	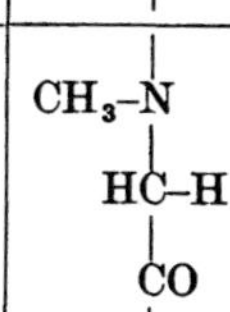

Oxytocin-like activities in International Units per micromole			Vasopressin-like activities in International Units per micromole		References S = synthesis P = pharmacology [1] = also contains pharmacological data
Rat uterus (isolated)	Chicken blood pressure	Rabbit mammary gland	Rat blood pressure	Rat antidiuresis	
~1.0	~0.4	~0.8	2.6 ± 0.4	—	S: GUTTMANN, BOISSONNAS (1961, 1962)[1] P: DOEPFNER et al. (1963)
<0.05	—	—	0.06 ± 0.01	—	S: GUTTMANN, BOISSONNAS (1961) P: DOEPFNER et al. (1963)

of a peptide amide group

Oxytocin-like activities in International Units per micromole			Vasopressin-like activities in International Units per micromole		References S = synthesis P = pharmacology [1] = also contains pharmacological data
Rat uterus (isolated)	Chicken blood pressure	Rabbit mammary gland	Rat blood pressure	Rat antidiuresis	
1.2 ± 0.4	0.32 ± 0.05	3.1 ± 0.7	—	<0.01	S: HUGUENIN, BOISSONNAS (1961)[1]; JOŠT et al. (1961)[1] P: BERDE et al. (1960)
~36	~9	~55	~0.01	~0.1	S: CASH et al. (1962)[1]

Continuation Table 20.

Name, abbreviated chemical formula and molecular weight		Structure of the methylated amino acid
Cys–Tyr–Phe–Gln–Asn–Cys–Pro–Lys–*MeGly*–NH_2 (N–Me)Gly[9]-Lys[8]-vasopressin = Sar[9]-Lys[8]-vasopressin	1070.2	CH_3–N HC–H CO

Table 21. *Replacement of sulphur by*

Name, abbreviated chemical formula and molecular weight		Structure of residue in position 1
$(CH_2)_3$–CO–Tyr–Ile–Gln–Asn–Cys–Pro–Leu–Gly–NH_2 Methylene[1]-De-Thio[1]-oxytocin	989.2	H HC–CH_2–CH_2– CO
Cys–Tyr–Ile–Gln–Asn–Selenocys–Pro–Leu–Gly–NH_2 Seleno[6]-De-Thio[6]-oxytocin = Hemiselenocystine[6]-oxytocin	1054.2	NH_2 HC–CH_2–S– CO
S–$(CH_2)_2$–CO–Tyr–Ile–Gln–Asn–Selenocys–Pro–Leu–Gly–NH_2 De-Amino[1]-Seleno[6]-De-Thio[6]-oxytocin = De-Amino[1]-Hemiselenocystine[6]-oxytocin	1039.2	H HC–CH_2–S– CO
Se–$(CH_2)_2$–CO–Tyr–Ile–Gln–Asn–Selenocys–Pro–Leu–Gly–NH_2 De-Amino[1]-Seleno[1,6]-De-Thio[1,6]-oxytocin	1086.2	H HC–CH_2–Se– CO
S–CH_2–CO–Tyr–Ile–Gln–Asn–Homocys–Pro–Leu–Gly–NH_2 Mercaptoacetic[1]-Hemihomocystine[6]-oxytocin	992.2	H HC–S– CO

Oxytocin-like activities in International Units per micromole			Vasopressin-like activities in International Units per micromole		References S = synthesis P = pharmacology [1] = also contains pharmacological data
Rat uterus (isolated)	Chicken blood pressure	Rabbit mammary gland	Rat blood pressure	Rat antidiuresis	
—	<0.01	—	~0.5	—	S: MEIENHOFER, DU VIGNEAUD (1961)[1]

selenium or a methylene group in oxytocin

Structure of residue in position 6	Oxytocin-like activities in International Units per micromole			Vasopressin-like activities in International Units per micromole		References S = synthesis P = pharmacology [1] = also contains pharmacological data
	Rat uterus (isolated)	Chicken blood pressure	Rabbit mammary gland	Rat blood pressure	Rat antidiuresis	
| NH | HC–CH_2–S– | CO |	~60	~25	—	—	~1	S: RUDINGER, JOŠT (1964)[1]
| NH | HC–CH_2–Se– | CO |	~440	~420	~420	~4	—	S: WALTER, DU VIGNEAUD (1965)[1]
| H | HC–CH_2–Se– | CO |	~520	~650	~415	~1	—	S: WALTER, DU VIGNEAUD (1965)[1]
| NH | HC–CH_2–Se– | CO |	~565	~920	—	—	—	S: WALTER, DU VIGNEAUD (1966)[1]
| NH | HC–CH_2–CH_2–S– | CO |	~16	<0.01	—	—	—	S: JARVIS, DU VIGNEAUD (1964)[1]

Table 22. *Linear*

Name, abbreviated chemical formula and molecular weight		Structure of amino acid in position 1
Ala–Tyr–Ile–Gln–Asn–*Ala*–Pro–Leu–Gly–NH_2 Ala[1]-Ala[6]-oxytocin	945.1	NH_2 | $HC–CH_3$ | CO |
Ala–Tyr–Phe–Gln–Asn–*Ala*–Pro–Arg–Gly–NH_2 Ala[1]-Ala[6]-vasopressin	1022.1	NH_2 | $HC–CH_3$ | CO |
Ala–Tyr–Phe–Gln–Asn–*Ala*–Pro–Lys–Gly–NH_2 Ala[1]-Ala[6]-Lysine-vasopressin	994.1	NH_2 | $HC–CH_3$ | CO |
CH_3–CH_2–*CO*–Tyr–Phe–Gln–Asn–*Ala*–Pro–Arg–Gly–NH_2 Propionyl[1]-Ala[6]-vasopressin	1007.1	H | $HC–CH_3$ | CO |
CH_3–CH_2–*CO*–Tyr–Phe–Gln–Asn–*Ala*–Pro–Lys–Gly–NH_2 Propionyl[1]-Ala[6]-Lysine-vasopressin	979.1	H | $HC–CH_3$ | CO |

Replacement of L-amino-acids by D-amino acids in oxytocin are summarized in Table 15. It is interesting that inversion of the amino acids occupying the positions 1, 2 or 8 is still compatible with some activity, whereas in positions 4, 5 and 6 it brings about complete inactivation.

Suppression of the N-terminal amino group in oxytocin and its analogues (Table 16) only slightly alters the activity of the moderately active analogues, but quite significantly enhances the effect of the active compounds. This shows that the terminal amino group is not indispensable for the biological action and, in addition, that its removal probably extends the half life of these compounds by making them less susceptible to aminopeptidases (GOLUBOW and DU VIGNEAUD, 1963; GOLUBOW et al., 1963). All the oxytocin-like activities of De-Amino[1]

dethio analogues

Structure of amino acid in position 6	Oxytocin-like activities in International Units per micromole			Vasopressin-like activities in International Units per micromole		References S = synthesis P = pharmacology ¹ = also contains pharmacological data
	Rat uterus (isolated)	Chicken blood pressure	Rabbit mammary gland	Rat blood pressure	Rat antidiuresis	
NH HC–CH_3 CO	<0.01	<0.01	—	—	—	S: Jošt et al. (1964)[1]
NH HC–CH_3 CO	<0.2	<0.1	—	~0.025	0.08 ± 0.02	S: Huguenin, Guttmann (1965)[1] P: Berde, Stürmer (1965)
NH HC–CH_3 CO	<0.2	<0.1	—	~0.012	0.05 ± 0.01	S: Huguenin, Guttmann (1965)[1] P: Berde, Stürmer (1965)
NH HC–CH_3 CO	<0.2	<0.1	—	~0.041	0.20 ± 0.03	S: Huguenin, Guttmann (1965)[1] P: Berde, Stürmer (1965)
NH HC–CH_3 CO	<0.2	<0.1	—	~0.008	0.05 ± 0.01	S: Huguenin, Guttmann (1965)[1] P: Berde, Stürmer (1965)

oxytocin are significantly higher than those of oxytocin itself; thus it is an analogue which is more active than the natural hormone.

On the isolated rat uterus, De-Amino[1]-(O-Me)Tyr[2]-oxytocin shows an ambivalent effect, depending on the experimental conditions (Berde and Saameli, 1966). The effects on chicken and rat blood pressure are the reverse of those of oxytocin. On the chicken blood pressure, there is some antagonism to oxytocin, on the rat blood pressure some antagonism to vasopressin. In spite of these marked differences to oxytocin, this compound still exhibits milk-ejecting activity.

In the vasopressin and vasotocin series (Table 17) oxytocin-like activities are also generally enhanced by the suppression of the amino group. In most instances pressor activities are somewhat decreased, but antidiuretic activities increased.

Table 23. *Enlargement*

Name, abbreviated chemical formula and molecular weight		Structure of the residue different from the one in oxytocin
Homocys–Tyr–Ile–Gln–Asn–Cys–Pro–Leu–Gly–NH_2 Hemihomocystine[1]-oxytocin	1021.1	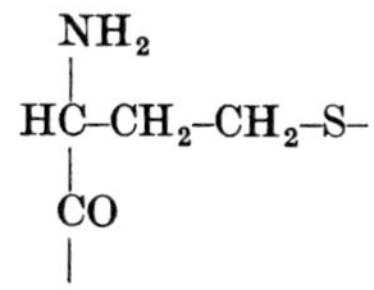
S–$(CH_2)_3$–*CO*–Tyr–Ile–Gln–Asn–Cys–Pro–Leu–Gly–NH_2 De-Amino-Hemihomocystine[1]-oxytocin = γ Mercaptobutyric[1]-oxytocin	1006.2	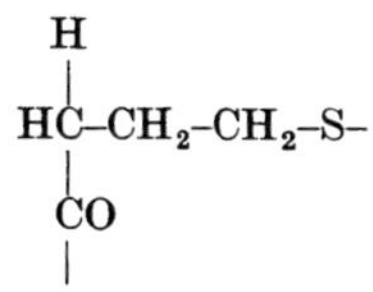
Cys–Tyr–Ile–*βAla*–Asn–Cys–Pro–Leu–Gly–NH_2 (βAla)[4]-oxytocin	950.2	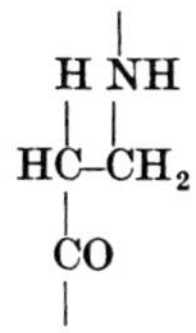
Cys–Pro–Leu–Gly–NH_2 Cys–Tyr–Ile–Gln–*Asp–NH*$_2$ Isoasparagine[5]-oxytocin	1007.2	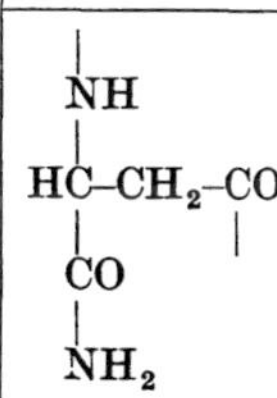
Asn–Cys–Pro–Leu–Gly–NH_2 Cys–Tyr–Ile–*Gln–NH*$_2$ Isoglutamine[4]-oxytocin	1007.2	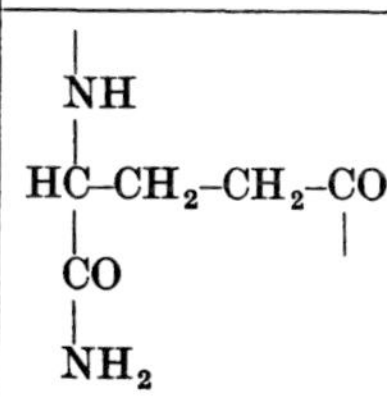
Cys–Tyr–*Tyr*–Ile–Gln–Asn–Cys–Pro–Leu–Gly–NH_2 Homo-Tyr[2]/[3]-oxytocin	1170.4	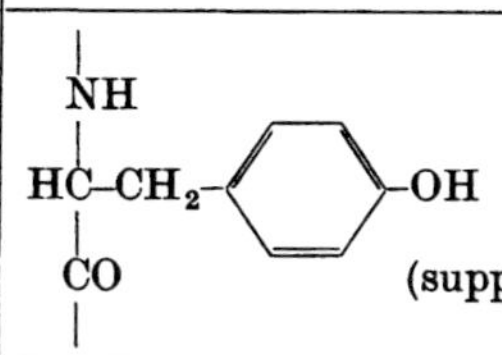 (supplementary)
Cys–Tyr–Ile–*Ile*–Gln–Asn–Cys–Pro–Leu–Gly–NH_2 Homo-Ile[3]/[4]-oxytocin	1120.4	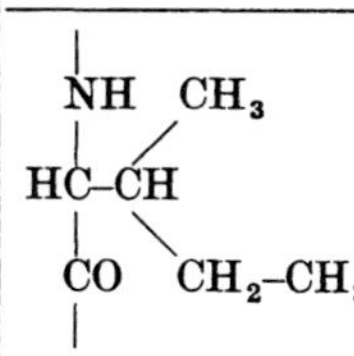 (supplementary)

of the disulphide ring

Number of atoms in the ring (oxytocin: 20)	Oxytocin-like activities in International Units per micromole			Vasopressin-like activities in International Units per micromole		References S = synthesis P = pharmacology [1] = also contains pharmacological data
	Rat uterus (isolated)	Chicken blood pressure	Rabbit mammary giand	Rat blood pressure	Rat antidiuresis	
21	~0.75	<0.01	—	<0.01	—	S: JARVIS et al. (1961)[1]
21	~3	<0.01	—	—	—	S: JARVIS et al. (1965)[1]
21	~0.12	~0.4	~0.5	~0.03	<0.01	S: MANNING, DU VIGNEAUD (1965a)[1]
21	<0.01	<0.05	—	<0.01	—	S: LUTZ et al. (1959)[1]
22	<0.01	<0.05	—	Anti (500:1)	—	S: RESSLER, DU VIGNEAUD (1957)[1] RESSLER, RACHELE (1958)
23	Anti (500:1)	Anti (500:1)	~0.5	—	—	S: GUTTMANN et al. (1957)[1]
23	~0.1	~0.05	~0.2	—	<0.01	S: JAQUENOUD et al. (1958) BOISSONNAS et al. (1961)[1] P: KONZETT, BERDE (1958)

Table 24. *Shortening of*

Name, abbreviated chemical formula and molecular weight		Structure of the lateral peptide chain
Cys–Tyr–Ile–Gln–Asn–Cys–*Pro–Leu–Gly–*NH_2 Oxytocin	1007.2	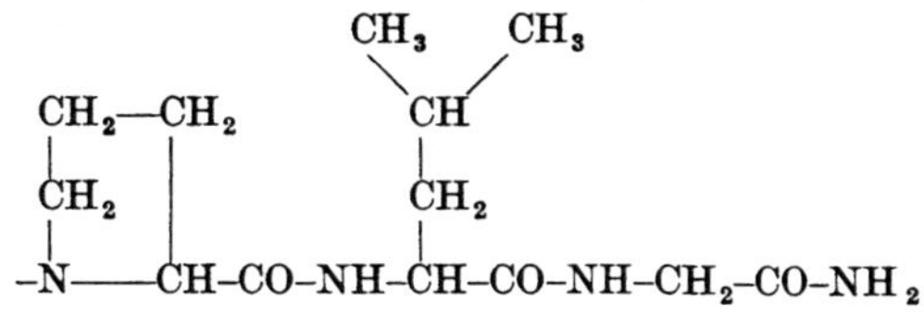
Cys–Tyr–Ile–Gln–Asn–Cys–*Pro–Leu–Gly–OH* (Gly–OH)^{9}-oxytocin = Deamido^{9}-oxytocin	1008.2	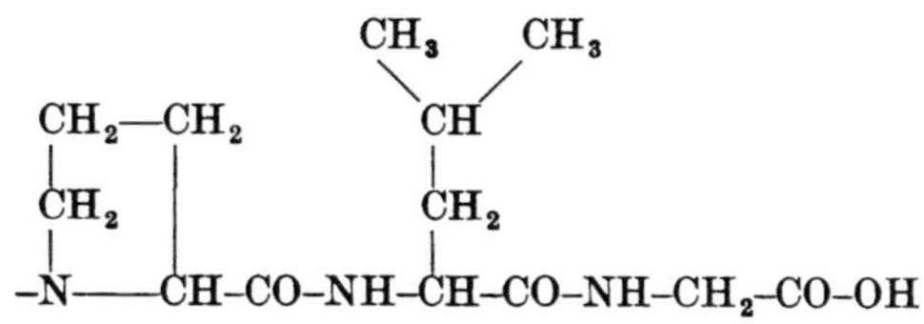
Cys–Tyr–Ile–Gln–Asn–Cys–*Pro–Leu–*$NH{-}CH_3$ De-Carboxamido^{9}-oxytocin	964.1	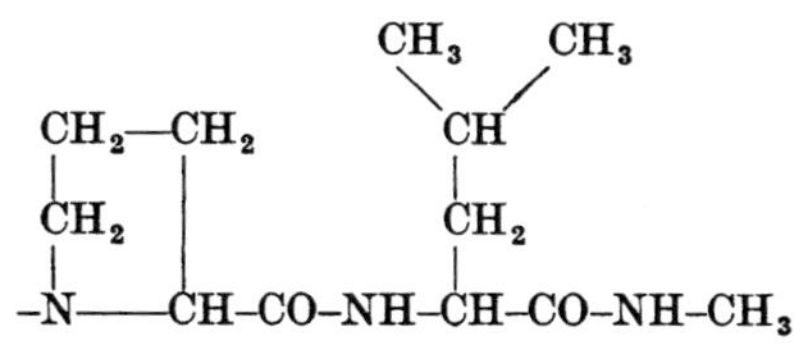
Cys–Tyr–Ile–Gln–Asn–Cys–*Pro–Leu–*NH_2 De-Gly^{9}-oxytocin	950.1	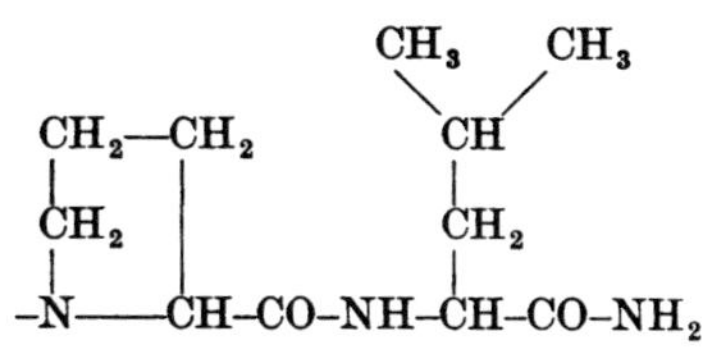
Cys–Tyr–Ile–Gln–Asn–Cys–*Pro–Gly–*NH_2 De-Leu^{8}-oxytocin	894.0	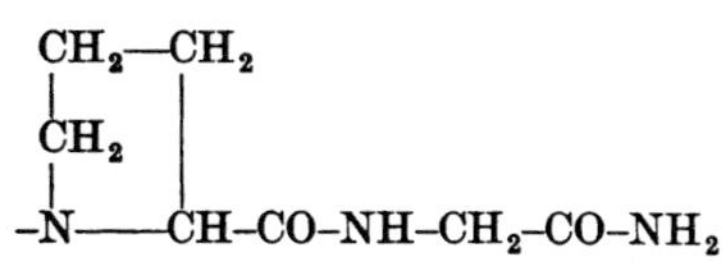
Cys–Tyr–Ile–Gln–Asn–Cys–*Leu–Gly–*NH_2 De-Pro^{7}-oxytocin	910.1	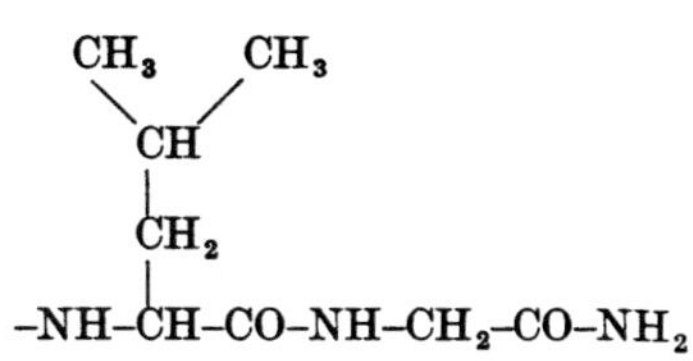
Cys–Tyr–Ile–Gln–Asn–Cys–NH_2 De-(Pro-Leu-Gly)^{9}-oxytocin	739.9	$-NH_2$

the lateral peptide chain

Oxytocin-like activities in International Units per micromole			Vasopressin-like activities in International Units per micromole		References S = synthesis P = pharmacology [1] = also contains pharmacological data
Rat uterus (isolated)	Chicken blood pressure	Rabbit mammary gland	Rat blood pressure	Rat antidiuresis	
450 ± 30	450 ± 30	450 ± 30	5 ± 1	5 ± 1	Occurs in nature
1.3	~0.2	1.2	~0.02	<0.01	S: FERRIER, DU VIGNEAUD (1966)[1]
7.2 ± 0.2	<0.02	3.8 ± 0.1	<0.01	~0.2	S: BRANDA, DU VIGNEAUD (1966)[1]
4.0 ± 0.7	Anti (10′000:1)	~3	Anti (10′000:1)	~0.02	S: JAQUENOUD, BOISSONNAS (1962b)[1] P: BERDE, STÜRMER (1962)
4.0 ± 1	Anti (1′000:1)	~3	Anti (1′000:1)	0.07 ± 0.01	S: JAQUENOUD, BOISSONNAS (1962b)[1] P: BERDE, STÜRMER (1962)
3.5 ± 0.8	Anti (1′000:1)	1.5 ± 0.2	~0.01	~0.01	S: JAQUENOUD, BOISSONNAS (1962b)[1] P: BERDE, STÜRMER (1962)
~2.4	<0.02	~0.8	<0.01	—	S: RESSLER (1956)[1]

The antidiuretic activity of De-Amino[1]-arginine-vasopressin — three times higher than that of the natural parent hormone — is quite remarkable. Also De-Amino[1]-Phe[2]-Arg[8]-vasopressin is a more potent antidiuretic compound than vasopressin itself. Due to its relatively low pressor activity, this analogue is the most potent selective antidiuretic compound known up to now.

Substitution of the terminal amino group of oxytocin (Table 18) sharply decreases all activities. It is not impossible that the low activity exhibited by the oxytocin derivatives with an amino acid or a short peptide residue at the amino end is not intrinsic but due to their partial transformation to oxytocin itself under the action of aminopeptidases. These derivatives have therefore been called "oxytocinogens" (BERÁNKOVÁ et al., 1966). Similarly, after addition of an amino acid or a short peptide residue to vasopressin and lysine-vasopressin (Table 19) noteworthy pressor and antidiuretic activities are retained, but when an acetyl group or an acetyl peptide, which cannot be split by aminopeptidases, is added to the amino end, inactivation occurs.

The effect of methylating a peptide linkage is shown in Table 20. The low activity of (N-Me)Tyr[2]-oxytocin has already been mentioned above. It is noteworthy that methylation of the nitrogen of the glycine residue in position 9 of oxytocin yields a compound with still appreciable oxytocin-like activities, whereas, when the same modification is performed on lysine-vasopressin, the pressor effect is lost.

The effect of replacing sulphur by selenium or a methylene group in oxytocin are summarized in Table 21. Introduction of a methylene group for a sulphur atom does not abolish the oxytocin-like activities, this showing that a disulphide bridge is not indispensable for the biological effect. As the thioether linkage resulting from this modification cannot reversibly generate a thiol group, this also proves that oxytocin need not be bound by a sulphur bridge to its receptor site in order to exhibit its biological action. Quite surprisingly, replacement of one of the sulphur atoms in oxytocin by selenium yields a very active analogue. Indeed, replacement of the two sulphur atoms by selenium increases the activity above that of oxytocin. It is interesting that displacement of the disulphide bridge by one methyl group is still compatible with a biological effect.

On the other hand, all modifications which eliminate the two sulphur atoms with concomitant opening of the ring (Table 22) or which lead to enlargement of the ring (Table 23) cause almost complete inactivation.

Analogues of oxytocin, from which part of the peptide chain outside the ring has been omitted, are listed in Table 24. It is noteworthy that none of these six compounds appreciably lowers chicken blood pressure. In fact, three of them slightly inhibit the response to a subsequent dose of oxytocin. Shortening of the side chain does not have such a drastic effect on the two other oxytocin-like activities, which are still present at a low but measurable level.

III. Activities in the Human

Comparatively little is known about the activities of synthetic analogues and homologues of the neurohypophysial hormones in man. In a systematic study (SAAMELI, 1964) the oxytocic activity of 5 analogues of oxytocin was compared with that of oxytocin on the postpartum uterus using an external strain-gauge tocodynamometer soon after uncomplicated vaginal delivery. The results are given in the last column of Table 25, which also lists the activities of these compounds in four tests which are frequently used to define the oxytocin-like activities of this type of compounds in animals. It will be seen that all those peptides which were found in animals to show a high oxytocin-like activity were also found to be potent oxytocics on the postpartum human uterus *in situ*. On the other hand, none of the four experimental procedures in animals listed can predict the activity in the human exactly. This, of course, is not surprising. The chicken blood pressure

Table 25. *Oxytocin-like activities of neurohypophysial peptides in conventional bioassay procedures and on the human uterus in vivo (from* SAAMELI *1964; slightly modified)*

Values are means and standard errors. Figures in italics indicate nearest corresponding values for each peptide

Neurohypophysial peptides	Oxytocin-like activities (I.U. per micromole) on				
	Rat uterus (isolated)	Chicken blood pressure	Rabbit mammary gland	Cat uterus (in situ)	Human uterus (in situ)
Oxytocin	450 ± 30	450 ± 30	450 ± 30	450 ± 30	450 ± 30
De-Amino¹-oxytocin	357 ± 55	705 ± 60	436 ± 45	*895* ± 130	*1020* ± 300
Val³-oxytocin	59 ± 8	58 ± 4	206 ± 14	*225* ± 17	*275* ± 65
Asn⁴-oxytocin	*107* ± 29	201 ± 12	298 ± 128	333 ± 75	*149* ± 40
Ser⁴-Ile⁸-oxytocin	145 ± 12	*310* ± 15	290 ± 15	242 ± 40	*324* ± 95
Ile⁸-oxytocin	291 ± 21	502 ± 37	*330* ± 21	567 ± 74	*367* ± 70

method favoured by the Pharmacopoeias for the standardisation of oxytocin is certainly not the best guide. The cat uterus *in situ* has perhaps the highest predictive value, but the series is too small to allow any final judgement to be made.

The activity on the human uterus of De-Amino¹-oxytocin was also measured by other investigators (EMBREY, 1965; MASSI et al., 1965), and they confirmed the high activity of this analogue on the human uterus *in situ*. Clinical trials — mainly concerning the induction of labour — have also been successfully carried out with De-Amino¹oxytocin (JANSSON, 1966).

Pressor and antidiuretic activities in man have been determined in quantitative terms only for one of the synthetic analogues of vasopressin, namely Phe²-Lys⁸-vasopressin (Octapressin®), this being the sole analogue that has been investigated with sufficient thoroughness to make this possible. The pressor activity of this analogue, by the intravenous route, is about five times higher in man than in the rat, and its antidiuretic activity in man is thirteen to fourteen times weaker than that of lysine-vasopressin in man, i. e. similar to that in the rat (GUHL, 1961). From these findings it may be calculated that in man Phe²-Lys⁸-vasopressin has a potency of about 270 pressor units per mg and about 20 antidiuretic units per mg (281 and 21 per micromole respectively). This compound is finding wide use clinically for its vasoconstrictor activity (e. g. AGUET, 1964; BOSOMWORTH, 1964; BURGHARDT, 1963; CRAWFORD, 1965; FISHER et al., 1965; GREEN and BLUMBERG, 1965; HAEMMERLI, 1965; HERSHEY and ALTURA, 1966; HOCHULI, 1962; KLINGENSTRÖM et al., 1966a; MISSURA and WEDER, 1962; RAWSTRON, 1964; TSAKIRIS et al., 1964).

Two other vasopressin-analogues with highly selective vasoconstrictor activities, namely ornithine⁸-vasopressin and Phe²-Orn⁸-oxytocin have been tested in man, and attention has been drawn to their potent local vasoconstrictor activity — particularly to that of Orn⁸-vasopressin (KLINGENSTRÖM et al., 1966b). However, from the data at present available it is not possible to calculate their activity in the human in terms of units per mg.

References

Acher, R., J. Chauvet, M. T. Chauvet, et D. Crepy: Isolement d'une nouvelle hormone neurohypophysaire, l'isotocine, présente chez les poissons osseux. Biochim. biophys. Acta (Amst.) **58**, 624 (1962).

Aguet, F.: Les hémoptysies et leurs traitements. Schweiz. med. Wschr. **94**, 628 (1964).

Bangham, D. R., and M. V. Mussett: Third International Standard for Posterior Pituitary. Bull. Org. mond. Santé **19**, 325 (1958).

Beauvillain, A.: Titrage des préparations posthypophysaires par leur seuil d'action sur l'utérus isolé de rat adulte. C. R. Soc. Biol. (Paris) **137**, 284 (1943).

Beránková, Z., I. Rychlík, K. Jošt, J. Rudinger, and F. Šorm: Inhibition of the uterus-contracting effect of oxytocin by O-methyloxytocin. Coll. Czechoslov. Chem. Commun. **26**, 2673 (1961).

Beránková-Ksandrová, Z., G. W. Bisset, K. Jošt, I. Krejčí, V. Pliška, J. Rudinger, I. Rychlík, and F. Šorm: Synthetic analogues of oxytocin acting as hormonogens. Brit. J. Pharmacol. **26**, 615 (1966).

Berde, B.: Les analogues synthétiques des hormones neurohypophysaires sont-ils une clef de l'étude des troubles de l'hormonogénèse de ce systeme? In: Les Troubles Congénitaux de l'Hormonogénèse, p. 33. Paris: Masson 1965.

—, and R. A. Boissonnas: Synthetic analogues and homologues of the posterior pituitary hormones. In: The pituitary gland, p. 624. Ed. by G. W. Harris and B. T. Donovan. London: Butterworths 1966.

— —, R. Huguenin, and E. Stürmer: Vasopressin analogues with selective pressor activity. Experientia (Basel) **20**, 42 (1964).

—, u. A. Cerletti: Über die Wirkung pharmakologischer Oxytocindosen auf die Milchdrüse. Acta endocr. **34**, 543 (1960).

— — Über die antidiuretische Wirkung von synthetischem Lysin-Vasopressin. Helv. physiol. pharmacol. Acta **19**, 135 (1961).

— —, and H. Konzett: The biological activity of a series of peptides related to oxytocin. In: Oxytocin, p. 247. Ed. by R. Caldeyro-Barcia and H. Heller. Oxford: Pergamon Press 1961a.

—, W. Doepfner, and H. Konzett: Some pharmacological actions of four synthetic analogues of oxytocin. Brit. J. Pharmacol. **12**, 209 (1957).

—, and H. Konzett: Isoleucyl[8]-Oxytocin, ein biologisch hochwirksames Polypeptid. Med. Exp. **2**, 317 (1960).

— —, and E. Stürmer: Personal communication (1960).

—, and K. Saameli: The action of the synthetic polypeptide valyl-oxytocin on the human uterus *in vitro* and *in vivo*. Acta endocr. (Kbh.) **32**, 391 (1959).

— — Evaluation of substances acting on the uterus. In: Methods in drug evaluation, p. 481. Ed. by P. Mantegazza and F. Piccinini. Amsterdam: North-Holland Publ. Co. 1966.

—, and E. Stürmer: Personal communication (1962, 1964, 1965).

—, H. Weidmann, and A. Cerletti: Über Phenylalanin[2] Lysin-Vasopressin. Helv. physiol. pharmacol. Acta **19**, 285 (1961b).

Bodanszky, M., and C. A. Birkhimer: 8-L-citrulline vasopressin and 8-L-citrulline oxytocin. J. Amer. chem. Soc. **84**, 4943 (1962a).

—, M. A. Ondetti, B. Rubin, J. J. Piala, J. Fried, J. T. Sheehan, and C. A. Birkhimer: Biologically active citrulline peptides. Nature (Lond.) **194**, 485 (1962b).

—, and V. du Vigneaud: Synthesis of a biologically active analog of oxytocin, with phenylalanine replacing tyrosine. J. Amer. chem. Soc. **81**, 1258 (1959).

Boissonnas, R. A., and St. Guttmann: Synthèse d'analogues de l'oxytocine et de la lysine-vasopressine contenant de la phénylalanine ou de la tyrosine en positions 2 et 3. Helv. chim. Acta **43**, 190 (1960).

— —, B. Berde, and H. Konzett: Relationships between the chemical structures and the biological properties of the posterior pituitary hormones and their synthetic analogues. Experientia (Basel) **17**, 377 (1961).

— —, R. L. Huguenin, P.-A. Jaquenoud, and Ed. Sandrin: Synthèse de nouveaux analogues de la lysine-vasopressine (Asp[NH_2][4]-lysine-vasopressine, Ala[4]-lysine-vasopressine, Ser[4]-lysine-vasopressine, Ser[5]-lysine-vasopressine, Val[7]-lysine-vasopressine et [Nε-For-Lys][8]-vasopressine). Helv. chim. Acta **46**, 2347 (1963).

— —, P.-A. Jaquenoud, and J.-P. Waller: Synthèse d'analogues structuraux de l'ocytocine. Helv. chim. Acta **39**, 1421 (1956).

BOISSONNAS, R. A., and R. L. HUGUENIN: Synthèse de la Lys[8]-oxytocine (lysine-vasotocine) et nouvelle synthèse de la lysine-vasopressine. Helv. chim. Acta **43**, 182 (1960).

—, J.-F. PECHÈRE, and ST. GUTTMANN: Personal communication (1959).

BOSOMWORTH, P. P.: Anesthetic implications of phenylalanine[2]-lysine[8]-vasopressin. J. New Drugs **4**, 221 (1964).

BOURA, A., and S. E. DICKER: An apparatus for the maintenance of a constant water load and the recording of urine flow in rats. J. Physiol. (Lond.) **122**, 144 (1953).

BRANDA, L. A., S. DRABAREK, and V. DU VIGNEAUD: The synthesis and pharmacological properties of deamino-4-decarboxamido-oxytocin (1-β-mercaptopropionic acid-4-α-aminobutyric acid-oxytocin). J. Biol. Chem. **241**, 2572 (1966).

—, and V. DU VIGNEAUD: Synthesis and pharmacological properties of 9-decarboxamido-oxytocin. J. Med. Chem. **9**, 169 (1966).

British Pharmacopoeia: The Pharmaceutical Press. London: 1963.

BURGHARDT, E: Zur Operationstechnik der diagnostischen Konisation. Geburtsh. u. Frauenheilk. **23**, 548 (1963).

CASH, W. D., L. M. MAHAFFEY, A. S. BUCK, D. E. NETTLETON jr., C. ROMAS, and V. DU VIGNEAUD: Synthesis and biological properties of 9-sarcosine oxytocin. J. Med. Pharm. Chem. **5**, 413 (1962).

—, and B. L. SMITH: Synthesis and biological properties of 1-Acetyl-8-lysine-vasopressin. J. Biol. Chem. **238**, 994 (1963).

CHAN, W. Y., M. O'CONNELL, and S. R. POMEROY: Effects of the estrous cycle on the sensitivity of rat uterus to oxytocin and desamino-oxytocin. Endocrinology **72**, 279 (1963).

—, and V. DU VIGNEAUD: Comparison of the pharmacologic properties of oxytocin and its highly potent analogue, desamino-oxytocin. Endocrinology **71**, 977 (1962).

CHAUVET, J., M.-T. LENCI, and R. ACHER: Présence de deux vasopressines dans la neurohypophyse du poulet. Biochim. biophys. Acta **38**, 571 (1960).

CHIMIAK, A., and J. RUDINGER: Amino acids and peptides. LIII. Synthesis and some biological properties of 3-O-methylthreonine-oxytocin. Collection Czech. Chem. Commun. **30**, 2592 (1965); and personal communication.

COON, J. M.: A new method for the assay of posterior pituitary extracts. Arch. int. pharmacodyn. **62**, 79 (1939).

CRAWFORD, R. A. D.: Preliminary trial of a new haemostatic, Octapressin-Sandoz. Brit. J. Ophthal. **49**, 49 (1965).

CROSS, B. A., and G. W. HARRIS: The role of the neurohypophysis in the milk-ejection reflex. J. Endocr. **8**, 148 (1951/52).

DEKANSKI, J.: The quantitative assay of vasopressin. Brit. J. Pharmacol. **7**, 567 (1952).

DETTELBACH, H. R.: A method for assaying small amounts of antidiuretic substances with notes on some properties of vasopressin. Amer. J. Physiol. **192**, 379 (1958).

DICKER, S. E.: A method for the assay of very small amounts of antidiuretic activity with a note on the antidiuretic titre of rats' blood. J. Physiol. (Lond.) **122**, 149 (1953).

DOEPFNER, W., E. STÜRMER, and B. BERDE: On the corticotrophin-releasing activity of synthetic neurohypophysial hormones and some related peptides. Endocrinology **72**, 897 (1963).

DRABAREK, S.: Analogues of oxytocin containing glycine in place of tyrosine, isoleucine, or glutamine. J. Amer. chem. Soc. **86**, 4477 (1964).

—, and V. DU VIGNEAUD: 2-D-Tyrosine-oxytocin and 2-D-Tyrosine-deamino-oxytocin, diastereoisomers of oxytocin and deamino-oxytocin. J. Amer. chem. Soc. **87**, 3974 (1965).

DUTTA, A. S., and N. ANAND: Synthesis of 9-β-alanine-oxytocin and 4-D-glutamine-oxytocin. Indian J. Chem. **3**, 232 (1965).

— —, and K. KAR: Synthesis and pharmacological activity of 4-D-glutamine-oxytocin, 5-D-asparagine-oxytocin and 4-D-glutamine-5-D-asparagine-oxytocin. J. Med. Chem. **9**, 497 (1966).

DYKE, H. B. VAN, K. ADAMSONS jr., and S. L. ENGEL: Aspects of the biochemistry and physiology of the neurohypophyseal hormones. Recent Progr. Hormone Res. **11**, 1 (1955).

EMBREY, M. P.: The action of desamino-oxytocin on the human pregnant uterus. J. Endocr. **31**, 185 (1965).

FERRIER, B. M., D. JARVIS, and V. DU VIGNEAUD: Deamino-oxytocin, its isolation by partition chromatography on Sephadex and crystallization from water, and its biological activities. J. biol. Chem. **240**, 4264 (1965).

Ferrier, B. M., and V. du Vigneaud: 9-Deamidooxytocin, an analog of the hormone containing a glycine residue in place of the glycinamide residue. J. Med. Chem. **9**, 55 (1966).

Fisher, S. J., J. Gehrig, and H. Green: Non-catechol amine vasopressor (PLV-2) for use as adjunct to local anesthesia. J. Amer. dent. Ass. **70**, 1189 (1965).

Flouret, G., and V. du Vigneaud: The synthesis of D-oxytocin, the enantiomer of the posterior pituitary hormone, oxytocin. J. Amer. chem. Soc. **87**, 3775 (1965).

Follett, B. K., and H. Heller: Pharmacological characteristics of neurohypophysial hormones in lungfish and amphibians. Nature (Lond.) **199**, 611 (1963).

— — The neurohypophysial hormones of bony fishes and cyclostomes. J. Physiol. (Lond.) **172**, 74 (1964a).

— — The neurohypophysial hormones of lungfishes and amphibians. J. Physiol. (Lond.) **172**, 92 (1964b).

Fosker, A. P., and H. D. Law: Oxytocin and 4-glycine-oxytocin. J. chem. Soc. **1965**, 4922.

Gaddum, J. H., W. S. Peart, and M. Vogt: The estimation of adrenaline and allied substances in blood. J. Physiol. (Lond.) **108**, 467 (1949).

Garcia de Jalon, P., J. Bayo Bayo, y M. Garcia de Jalon: Sensible y nuevo método de valoracion de adrenalina en utero aislado de rata (A sensitive and new method for the bioassay of adrenaline on the isolated rat uterus). Farmacoterap. act. **2**, 313 (1945) [in Spanish].

Golubow, J., W. Y. Chan, and V. du Vigneaud: Effect of human pregnancy serum on avian depressor activities of oxytocin and desamino-oxytocin. Proc. Soc. exp. Biol. (N.Y.) **113**, 113 (1963).

—, and V. du Vigneaud: Comparison of susceptibility of oxytocin and desamino-oxytocin to inactivation by leucine aminopeptidase and α-chymotrypsin. Proc. Soc. exp. Biol. (N.Y.) **112**, 218 (1963).

Green, H. D., and J. B. Blumberg: The use of a synthetic analogue of posthypophysial vasopressin (PLV-2) for local hemostasis. Surgery **58**, 524 (1965).

Guhl, U.: Die antidiuretische und pressorische Wirksamkeit von Arginin^8-Vasopressin, Lysin^8-Vasopressin und Phenylalanin^2-lysin^8-Vasopressin beim Menschen. Schweiz. med. Wschr. **91**, 798 (1961).

Guttmann, St., B. Berde, and E. Stürmer: The synthesis and some pharmacological effects of serine^4-isoleucine^8-oxytocin, a probable neurohypophysial hormone. Experientia (Basel) **18**, 445 (1962).

—, and R. A. Boissonnas: Synthèse de dix analogues de l'oxytocine et de la lysine-vasopressine, contenant de la sérine, de l'histidine ou du tryptophane en position 2 ou 3. Helv. chim. Acta **43**, 200 (1960).

— — Synthèse de nouveaux analogues de l'oxytocine et de la vasopressine. Chimia (Zürich) **15**, 575 (1961).

— — Synthèse d'homologues de la lysine-vasopressine et de l'oxytocine contenant une séquence His-Sér ou Sér-His en position N-terminale. Helv. chim. Acta **45**, 2517 (1962).

— — Synthèse de la Sér^4-oxytocine, de l'Ala^4-oxytocine, de la Sér^5-oxytocine et de l'Ala^5-oxytocine. Helv. chim. Acta **46**, 1626 (1963).

—, P.-A. Jaquenoud, R. A. Boissonnas, H. Konzett, and B. Berde: Ein Nonapeptid mit Oxytocin hemmenden Eigenschaften. Naturwissenschaften **44**, 632 (1957).

Haemmerli, U. P.: Die Therapie der Ösophagusvarizenblutung. Dtsch. med. Wschr. **90**, 311 (1965).

Hermann, P., u. M. Zaoral: Aminosäuren und Peptide. LVI. Synthese von Thialysin^8-Vasopressin. Collection Czech. Chem. Commun. **30**, 2817 (1965).

Hershey, S. G., u. B. M. Altura: Behandlung des Schocks durch Beeinflussung der peripheren Zirkulation mit vasoaktiven Wirkstoffen. Eine mikrozirkulatorische Basis für die Therapie. Schweiz. med. Wschr. **96**, 1467 und 1516 (1966).

Hochuli, E.: Klinische Erfahrungen mit der lokalen Anwendung von Octapressin in der Gynäkologie und Geburtshilfe. Schweiz. med. Wschr. **92**, 654 (1962).

Holton, P.: A modification of the method of Dale and Laidlaw for standardization of posterior pituitary extract. Brit. J. Pharmacol. **3**, 328 (1948).

Hope, D. B.: The biological activity of analogues of oxytocin lacking basic and acidic groups. Brit. Pharmacol. Soc. Meeting, Oxford 1962.

—, V. V. S. Murti, and V. du Vigneaud: A highly potent analogue of oxytocin, desamino-oxytocin. J. biol. Chem. **237**, 1563 (1962).

— — — Synthesis of 1-hemi-D-cystine-oxytocin. J. Amer. chem. Soc. **85**, 3686 (1963).

—, and V. du Vigneaud: Synthesis of desamino-desoxy-oxytocin, a biologically active analogue of oxytocin. J. biol. Chem. **237**, 3146 (1962).

HUGUENIN, R.L.: Synthèse de la Phe[2]-Orn[8]-vasopressine et de la Phe[2]-Orn[8]-oxytocine, deux analogues de la vasopressine doués d'une activité pressorique sélective. Helv. chim. Acta **47**, 1934 (1964).

— Personal communication (1965).

— Synthèse de la désamino[1]-Orn[8]-vasopressine, de la désamino[1]-Phé[2]-Orn[8]-vasopressine, de la désamino[1]-Ile[3]-Orn[8]-vasopressine (= désamino[1]-Orn[8]-oxytocine) et de la désamino[1]-Phé[2]-Ile[3]-Orn[8]-vasopressine (= désamino[1]-Phé[2]-Orn[8]-oxytocine). Helv. chim. Acta **49**, 711 (1966).

—, and R.A. BOISSONNAS: Synthèse de la (N-méthyl-Tyr)[2]-oxytocine. Helv. chim. Acta **44**, 213 (1961).

— — Synthèses de la Phé[2]-arginine-vasopressine et de la Phé[2]-arginine-vasotocine et nouvelles synthèses de l'arginine-vasopressine et de l'arginine-vasotocine. Helv. chim. Acta **45**, 1629 (1962).

— — Synthèse de l'Orn[8]-vasopressine et de l'Orn[8]-oxytocine. Helv. chim. Acta **46**, 1669 (1963).

— — Synthèse de la désamino[1]-Arg[8]-vasopressine et de la désamino[1]-Phé[2]-Arg[8]-vasopressine, deux analogues possédant une activité antidiurétique plus élevée et plus sélective que celle des vasopressines naturelles. Helv. chim. Acta **49**, 695 (1966).

—, and ST. GUTTMANN: Synthèse de l'Ala[1]-Ala[6]-Arg[8]-vasopressine et de l'Ala[1]-Ala[6]-Lys[8]-vasopressine, ainsi que de la (désamino-Ala)[1]-Ala[6]-Arg[8]-vasopressine et de la (désamino-Ala)[1]-Ala[6]-Lys[8]-vasopressine. Helv. chim. Acta **48**, 1885 (1965).

—, E. STÜRMER, R.A. BOISSONNAS, and B. BERDE: Desamino-arginine-vasopressin, an analogue of arginine-vasopressin with high antidiuretic activity. Experientia (Basel) **21**, 68 (1965).

JANSSON, I.: Effect of desamino-oxytocin on the human pregnant uterus at term. Acta obstet. gynec. scand. **45**, 29 (1966).

JAQUENOUD, P.-A.: Synthèse de la Gly[8]-oxytocine, de l'Ala[8]-oxytocine et de la But[8]-oxytocine. Helv. chim. Acta **48**, 1899 (1965).

—, and R.A. BOISSONNAS: Synthèse de la Phé[2]-oxytocine. Helv. chim. Acta **42**, 788 (1959).

— — Personal communication (1960).

— — Synthèse de la Ileu[8]-oxytocine et de la Val[8]-oxytocine, deux analogues de l'oxytocine modifiés dans la chaîne latérale. Helv. chim. Acta **44**, 113 (1961).

— — Synthèse de l'Asp(NH_2)[4]-oxytocine, de la Glu(NH_2)[5]-oxytocine et de l'Asp(NH_2)[4]-Glu(NH_2)[5]-oxytocine. Helv. chim. Acta **45**, 1601 (1962a).

— — Synthèse de la Dé-Pro[7]-oxytocine, de la Dé-Leu[8]-oxytocine et de la Dé-Gly[9]-oxytocine. Helv. chim. Acta **45**, 1462 (1962b).

—, ST. GUTTMANN, and R.A. BOISSONNAS: Personal communication (1958).

JARVIS, D., M. BODANSZKY, and V. DU VIGNEAUD: The synthesis of 1-(Hemi-homocystine)-oxytocin and a study of some of its pharmacological properties. J. Amer. chem. Soc. **83**, 4780 (1961).

—, B.M. FERRIER, and V. DU VIGNEAUD: The effect of increasing the size of the ring present in deamino-oxytocin by one methylene group on its biological properties. J. biol. Chem. **240**, 3553 (1965).

—, and V. DU VIGNEAUD: Crystalline deamino-oxytocin. Science **143**, 545 (1964).

JEFFERS, W.A., M.M. LIVEZEY, and J.H. AUSTIN: A method for demonstrating an antidiuretic action of minute amounts of pitressin: statistical analysis of results. Proc. Soc. exp. Biol. (N.Y.) **50**, 184 (1942).

JOŠT, K., V.G. DEBABOV, H. NESVADBA, and J. RUDINGER: Amino acids and peptides. XLII. A synthesis of dethiooxytocin and other acyclic peptides related to oxytocin. Collection Czech. Chem. Commun. **29**, 419 (1964).

—, J. RUDINGER, and F. ŠORM: Analogues of oxytocin modified in positions 1 and 2 of the peptide chain: protected intermediates. Collection Czech. Chem. Commun. **26**, 2496 (1961).

— — — Structural analogues of oxytocin modified in position 2 of the peptide chain: preparation and some chemical and biological properties. Collection Czech. Chem. Commun. **28**, 1706 (1963a).

— — — Analogues of oxytocin exerting protracted biological effects. Collection Czech. Chem. Commun. **28**, 2021 (1963b).

KATSOYANNIS, P.G.: Oxypressin, a synthetic octapeptide amide with hormonal properties. J. Amer. chem. Soc. **79**, 109 (1957).

—, and V. DU VIGNEAUD: The synthesis of the histidine analog of the vasopressins. Arch. Biochem. **78**, 555 (1958).

— — Arginine-vasotocin. Nature (Lond.) **184**, 1465 (1959).

Kimbrough, R. D. jr., W. D. Cash, L. A. Branda, W. Y. Chan, and V. du Vigneaud: Synthesis and biological properties of 1-desamino-8-lysine-vasopressin. J. biol. Chem. **238**, 1411 (1963).

—, and V. du Vigneaud: Lysine-vasotocin, a synthetic analogue of the posterior pituitary hormones containing the ring of oxytocin and the side chain of lysine-vasopressin. J. biol. Chem. **236**, 778 (1961).

Klingenström, P., B. Nylén, and L. Westermark: A clinical comparison between adrenaline and Octapressin as vasoconstrictors in local anaesthesia. Acta anaesth. scand. **11**, 35 (1967).

— — — Synthetic pituitary posterior-lobe hormones as vasoconstrictors in local anaesthesia. 2nd European Congress of Anaesthesiology, Copenhagen, 8—13 August, 1966.

Konzett, H., and B. Berde: Personal communication (1958).

— — The biological activity of a new analogue of oxytocin in which the tyrosyl group is replaced by phenylalanyl. Brit. J. Pharmacol. **14**, 133 (1959).

Law, H. D., and V. du Vigneaud: Synthesis of 2-p-methoxy-phenylalanine oxytocin (O-methyl-oxytocin) and some observations on its pharmacological behavior. J. Amer. chem. Soc. **82**, 4579 (1960).

Lutz, W. B., C. Ressler, D. E. Nettleton jr., and V. du Vigneaud: Isoasparagine-oxytocin: the isoasparagine isomer of oxytocin. J. Amer. chem. Soc. **81**, 167 (1959).

Manning, M., and V. du Vigneaud: 4-β-alanine-oxytocin: an oxytocin analog containing a twenty-one-membered disulfide ring. Biochemistry **4**, 1884 (1965a).

— — 6-hemi-D-cystine-oxytocin, a diastereoisomer of the posterior pituitary hormone oxytocin. J. Amer. chem. Soc. **87**, 3978 (1965b).

Massi, G. B., J. J. Poseiro, R. Caldeyro-Barcia, and V. du Vigneaud: Effetti della desamino-ossitocina sulla contrattilità dell'utero umano a termine di gravidanza. Riv. Ostet. Ginec. **20**, 77 (1965).

Meienhofer, J., and V. du Vigneaud: Synthesis of a biologically active analog of lysine-vasopressin, with phenylalanine replacing tyrosine: 2-phenylalanine lysine-vasopressin. J. Amer. chem. Soc. **82**, 6336 (1960).

— — Synthesis of a lysine-vasopressin derivative with a methyl substituent on the imino nitrogen of the peptide bond between lysine and glycinamide (9-sarcosine lysine-vasopressin). J. Amer. chem. Soc. **83**, 142 (1961).

Missura, T., u. A. Weder: Vergleichende Untersuchungen über das Verhalten des Kreislaufes bei der Tonsillektomie in LA mit vasokonstriktorischem Zusatz von Adrenalin bzw. PLV 2. Pract. oto-rhino-laryng. (Basel) **24**, 249 (1962).

Munsick, R. A.: Effect of magnesium ion on the response of the rat uterus to neurohypophysial hormones and analogues. Endocrinology **66**, 451 (1960).

Nesvadba, H., J. Honzl, and J. Rudinger: Some structural analogues of oxytocin modified in position 3 of the peptide chain: synthesis and some chemical and biological properties. Collection Czech. Chem. Commun. **28**, 1691 (1963).

Photaki, I., and V. du Vigneaud: 4-deamido-oxytocin, an analog of the hormone containing glutamic acid in place of glutamine. J. Amer. chem. Soc. **87**, 908 (1965).

Pickering, B. T., and H. Heller: Chromatographic and biological characteristics of fish and frog neurohypophysial extracts. Nature (Lond.) **184**, 1463 (1959).

Pliška, V., and I. Krejčí: The dose-response relation of the antidiuretic and vasopressor activities of 4-asparagine-8-lysine-vasopressin. Arch. int. Pharmacodyn. **161**, 289 (1966).

Rawstron, R. E.: A trial of phenyl-lysine-vasopressin (Octapressin) as a haemostatic agent. N. Z. med. J. **63**, 297 (1964).

Ressler, Ch.: The cyclic disulfide ring of oxytocin. Proc. Soc. exp. Biol. (N.Y.) **92**, 725 (1956).

—, and J. R. Rachele: Further properties of isoglutamine-oxytocin; inhibition of pressor activity of vasopressin. Proc. Soc. exper. Biol. (N.Y.) **98**, 170 (1958).

—, and V. du Vigneaud: The isoglutamine isomer of oxytocin: its synthesis and comparison with oxytocin. J. Amer. chem. Soc. **79**, 4511 (1957).

Rudinger, J., J. Honzl and M. Zaoral: Syntheses in the oxytocin field. IV. Two analogues. Collection Czech. Chem. Commun. **21**, 770 (1956).

—, and K. Jošt: A biologically active analogue of oxytocin not containing a disulfide group. Experientia (Basel) **20**, 570 (1964).

Saameli, K.: Quantitative comparison between oxytocin and four related neurohypophysial peptides on the human uterus in situ. Brit. J. Pharmacol. **23**, 176 (1964).

SAWYER, W.H.: Differences in the antidiuretic responses of rats to the intravenous administration of lysine and arginine vasopressins. Endocrinology **63**, 694 (1958).

— Neurohypophysial hormones. Pharmacol. Rev. **13**, 225 (1961).

— Vertebrate neurohypophysial principles. Endocrinology **73**, 981 (1964).

— Active neurohypophysial principles from a cyclostome (Petromyzon marinus) and two cartilaginous fishes (Squalus acanthias and Hydrolagus collei). Gen. comp. Endocr. **5**, 427 (1965).

—, and H.B. VAN DYKE: Isolation of the oxytocin-like pituitary principle of a teleost fish (Pollachius virens) and comparison of its properties with those of synthetic 4-serine, 8-isoleucine oxytocin. Endocrinology **73**, 394 (1963a).

— — Principles resembling oxytocin in neurohypophyses of fishes. Fed. Proc. **22**, 386 (1963b).

—, R.A. MUNSICK, and H.B. VAN DYKE: Pharmacological evidence for the presence of arginine vasotocin and oxytocin in neurohypophysial extracts from cold-blooded vertebrates. Nature (Lond.) **184**, 1464 (1959).

SCHILD, H.O.: A method of conducting a biological assay on a preparation giving repeated graded responses illustrated by the estimation of histamine. J. Physiol. (Lond.) **101**, 115 (1942).

SCHNEIDER, C.H., and V. DU VIGNEAUD: Synthesis of D-leucine-oxytocin, a biologically active diastereoisomer of oxytocin, and demonstration of its separability from oxytocin upon countercurrent distribution. J. Amer. chem. Soc. **84**, 3005 (1962).

SIEDEL, W., K. STURM u. R. GEIGER: Synthese eines vasopressorisch wirkenden Peptids: [O-Methyl-tyrosin]^2-Lysin^8-Vasopressin (OMTLV). Chem. Ber. **96**, 1436 (1963).

SOUSA, R.C. DE, J. DELAERE, and B. BERDE: Inappropriate secretion of vasopressin. Lancet **1965/I**, 436.

SUND, R.B.: A sensitive method for estimation of ergometrine, based upon serotonin antagonism on isolated rat uterus. Acta pharmacol. (Kbh). **20**, 233 (1963).

STUDER, R.O., and W.D. CASH: Synthesis of 1-acetyl-8-arginine-vasopressin and a study of its effects in the rat pressor assay. J. biol. Chem. **238**, 657 (1963).

STÜRMER, E., R.L. HUGUENIN, R.A. BOISSONNAS, and B. BERDE: Deamino^1-phenylalanine^2-arginine^8-vasopressin: a peptide with highly selective antidiuretic activity. Experientia (Basel) **21**, 583 (1965).

THOMPSON, R.E.: Biological assay of posterior pituitary. J. Pharmacol. exp. Ther. **80**, 373 (1944).

THORN, N.A.: A densimetric method for assay of small amounts of antidiuretic hormone. J. exp. Med. **105**, 585 (1957).

TINDAL, J.S., and A. YOKOYAMA: Assay of oxytocin by the milk-ejection response in the anesthetized lactating guinea-pig. Endocrinology **71**, 196 (1962).

TSAKIRIS, A., U. P. HAEMMERLI, and A. BÜHLMANN: Reduction of portal venous pressure in cirrhotic patients with bleeding from oesophageal varices, by administration of a vasopressin derivative, phenylalanine^2-lysine^8-vasopressin. Amer. J. Med. **36**, 825 (1964).

TYRODE, M.V.: The mode of action of some purgative salts. Arch. int. Pharmacodyn. **20**, 205 (1910).

United States Pharmacopeia, 17th Rev. Easton, Pa: Mack Printing Co. 1965.

VIGNEAUD, V. DU, G.S. DENNING, S. DRABAREK, and W.Y. CHAN: The effect of replacement of the carboxamide group by hydrogen in the glutamine or asparagine residue of oxytocin on its biological activity. J. biol. Chem. **238**, PC 1560 (1963).

— — — — The synthesis and pharmacological study of 4-decarboxamido-oxytocin (4-α-aminobutyric acid-oxytocin) and 5-decarboxamido-oxytocin (5-alanine-oxytocin). J. biol. Chem. **239**, 472 (1964).

—, P.S. FITT, M. BODANSZKY, and M. O'CONNELL: Synthesis and some pharmacological properties of a peptide derivative of oxytocin: glycyloxytocin. Proc. Soc. exp. Biol. (N.Y.) **104**, 653 (1960a).

—, G. FLOURET, and R. WALTER: Synthesis and some biological properties of 4-valine-oxytocin and 1-deamino-4-valine-oxytocin. J. biol. Chem. **241**, 2093 (1966).

—, G. WINESTOCK, V.V.S. MURTI, D.B. HOPE, and R.D. KIMBROUGH jr.: Synthesis of 1-β-mercaptopropionic acid oxytocin (desamino-oxytocin), a highly potent analogue of oxytocin. J. biol. Chem. **235**, PC 64 (1960b).

VOGEL, G., u. J. HERGOTT: Pharmakologische Untersuchungen über O-Methyl-tyrosin^2-lysin^8-Vasopressin. Arzneimittel-Forsch. **13**, 415 (1963).

Walter, R., and V. du Vigneaud: 6-hemi-L-selenocystine-oxytocin and 1-deamino-6-hemi-L-selenocystine-oxytocin, highly potent isologs of oxytocin and 1-deamino-oxytocin. J. Amer. chem. Soc. **87**, 4192 (1965).

— — 1-deamino-1,6-L-selenocystine-oxytocin, a highly potent isolog of 1-deamino-oxytocin. J. Amer. chem. Soc. **88**, 1331 (1966).

Yamashiro, D., D. Gillessen, and V. du Vigneaud: Simultaneous synthesis of 1-hemi-D-cystine-oxytocin and oxytocin and separation of the diastereoisomers by partition chromatography on Sephadex and by countercurrent distribution. J. Amer. chem. Soc. **88**, 1310 (1966).

Zaoral, M., E. Kasafírek, J. Rudinger, and F. Šorm: Amino acids and peptides. LI. Synthesis of 2-O-methyltyrosine- and 2-O-ethyltyrosine-lysine-vasopressin. Collection Czech. Chem. Commun. **30**, 1869 (1965).

—, J. Kolc, and F. Šorm: Synthesis of D-Arg^8- and D-Lys^8-vasopressin. Collection Czech. Chem. Commun. **31**, 382 (1966).

—, and F. Šorm: Amino acids and peptides. LV. Synthesis of Gly-Cys^1-lysine-vasopressin and Gly-Cys^1-Tyr(Me)^2-lysine-vasopressin. Collection Czech. Chem. Commun. **30**, 2812 (1965).

— — Amino acids and peptides. LIX. Synthesis and some biological properties of L-Dab^8-vasopressin. Collection Czech. Chem. Commun. **31**, 90 (1966a).

— — Amino acids and peptides. LX. Synthesis of D-Dab^8-vasopressin. Collection Czech. Chem. Commun. **31**, 310 (1966b).

Zhuze, A. L., K. Jošt, E. Kasafírek, and J. Rudinger: Amino acids and peptides. XLV. Analogues of oxytocin with O-ethyltyrosine, p-methylphenylalanine and p-ethylphenylalanine replacing tyrosine. Collection Czech. Chem. Commun. **29**, 2648 (1964).

Author Index

Page numbers in *italics* refer to the references

Subject Index

Joh. Roth sel. Ww., Graphische Kunstanstalt, München

FSC
www.fsc.org
MIX
Papier | Fördert
gute Waldnutzung
FSC® C083411

Kolibri 360 GmbH
Ferdinand-Jühlke-Straße 7
99095 Erfurt, Deutschland
produktsicherheit@kolibri360.de